REHABILITATION OF THE ADULT AND CHILD

WITH TRAUMATIC BRAIN INJURY

Third Edition

REHABILITATION OF THE ADULT AND CHILD WITH TRAUMATIC BRAIN INJURY

Third Edition

Mitchell Rosenthal, Ph.D.
Professor and Associate Chair
Department of Physical Medicine and
    Rehabilitation
Adjunct Professor of Psychology
Wayne State University
Administrator, Research and Education
Rehabilitation Institute of Michigan
Detroit, Michigan

Ernest R. Griffith, M.D.
Private Practice, Physical Medicine and
    Rehabilitation
Associate Medical Director
HealthSouth Meridian Point
    Rehabilitation Hospital
Medical Director, Outpatient
    Rehabilitation
Sun Grove Village Care Center
Scottsdale, Arizona

Jeffrey S. Kreutzer, Ph.D., A.B.P.P.
Professor and Director, Rehabilitation
    Psychology and Neuropsychology
Department of Physical Medicine and
    Rehabilitation
Medical College of Virginia
Virginia Commonwealth University
Richmond, Virginia

**Brian Pentland, M.B.Ch.B.,
    F.R.C.P., F.R.C.S.L.T**
Head of Unit
Scottish Brain Injury Rehabilitation
    Service
Astley Ainslie Hospital
Edinburgh Healthcare
Edinburgh, Scotland, United Kingdom

F. A. Davis Company
1915 Arch Street
Philadelphia, PA 19103

Printed in the United States of America

Last digit indicates print number: 10 9 8 7 6 5 4 3 2 1

Acquisitions Editor: Jean-François Vilain
Developmental Editor: Marianne Fithian
Production Editor: Samuel A. Rondinelli
Designer: Bill Donnelly
Cover Designer: Louis Forgione

As new scientific information becomes available through basic and clinical research, recommended treatments and drug therapies undergo changes. The author(s) and publisher have done everything possible to make this book accurate, up to date, and in accord with accepted standards at the time of publication. The authors, editors, and publisher are not responsible for errors or omissions or for consequences from application of the book, and make no warranty, expressed or implied, in regard to the contents of the book. Any practice described in this book should be applied by the reader in accordance with professional standards of care used in regard to the unique circumstances that may apply in each situation. The reader is advised always to check product information (package inserts) for changes and new information regarding dose and contraindications before administering any drug. Caution is especially urged when using new or infrequently ordered drugs.

Library of Congress Cataloging in Publication Data

Rehabilitation of the adult and child with traumatic brain injury /
    [edited by] Mitchell Rosenthal ... [et al.] — 3rd ed.
        p.   cm.
    Includes bibliographical references and index.
    ISBN 0-8036-0391-6
    1. Brain—Wounds and injuries—Patients—Rehabilitation. 2. Brain-
damaged children—Rehabilitation.   I. Rosenthal, Mitchell, 1949–.
    [DNLM: 1. Brain Injuries—rehabilitation.   WL 354 R34534   1998]
RD594.R44   1998
617.5' 1044—dc21
DNLM/DLC
for Library of Congress   98-37319
                                                                                                        CIP

*To the memory of Sheldon Berrol, M.D., and J. Douglas Miller, M.D., Ph.D.,
both pioneers in the art and science of brain injury rehabilitation,
whose contributions have been immeasurable.*

PREFACE TO THE THIRD EDITION

It has been almost a decade since the publication of the second edition of this textbook. During that time substantial changes have occurred in health care delivery, not only in the United States, but throughout the world. Scientific advances have occurred at levels of brain injury investigation ranging from basic science to outcome measurement. Funding sources have pressured service providers to demonstrate the reliability, validity, functional significance, and cost-effectiveness of medical and rehabilitative interventions. In some cases, consumers as well as legislative and other regulatory groups have questioned the value and ethics of brain injury service delivery practices. The eras of "enlightenment" and "proliferation," which characterized brain injury rehabilitation in the 1970s and 1980s, have yielded to the more skeptical periods of "accountability" and "consolidation." Yet we remain hopeful that the dawn of a new millenium will usher in a period of "renaissance," fueled by a greater understanding of the mechanisms underlying neurologic recovery and a more sophisticated use of technology and rehabilitation therapy that will enhance quality of life for persons with traumatic brain injury and their families.

What is different about his edition? The organization and chapter headings are quite similar, but much of the content is new. In a response to suggestions from reviewers, we decided to add chapters and sections that cover some specialty areas of increased importance: the low-level patient, the older adult with brain injury, life care planning, advances in neuroradiology, functional assessment, behavioral and personality assessment, psychotherapy, psychopharmacology, and ethical issues. We hope the result is an even more comprehensive book that will serve as a premier reference book in the field of traumatic brain injury. While retaining many of the authors from the previous edition, we have added over sixty new authors to the "mixture"; they provide some fresh insights and perspectives. As in the past, the authorship is quite multidisciplinary, though admittedly not all disciplines within rehabilitation are represented within the list of contributors.

As with our previous editions, our intent is to present a reasonably up-to-date discussion of issues that are of greatest relevance to the practitioner, whether student, novice, or expert. We have attempted to include updated research findings, so that suggestions for clinical practice are well grounded in science. We recognize that, as a medical science, rehabilitation—specifically brain injury rehabilitation—does not have a history of randomized clinical trials or a similar gold standard for judging the efficacy of the treatments commonly used in the field. We acknowledge that some of the methodologies described in this textbook have yet to demonstrate their ultimate value in scientific terms. Thus, brain injury rehabilitation remains part "art," though more grounded in science than a decade ago. It is also important to appreciate the scope of the audience who have found this textbook to be a useful reference—from experienced clinicians and researchers, to survivors of brain injury and their family members. We have taken great pleasure in the wide reach of this book and are especially pleased that it has proven beneficial for consumers as well as professionals.

Some would argue that subsequent editions of a textbook are easier to produce than the initial endeavor. Though memory fades somewhat after twenty years, it does seem that the third edition has been more challenging than the earlier ones. First, our distinguished co-editor, J. Douglas Miller, M.D., Ph.D., died an untimely death in 1995. Fortunately, his colleague, Brian Pentland, M.D., a well-recognized neurologist from the same department at the University of Edinburgh, was willing and able to pick up the gauntlet and assist in the process. Second, another of our co-editors, Michael Bond, M.D., Ph.D., had become more engaged in higher administrative challenges at the University of Glasgow (becoming "Sir Michael Bond" in the process), and was unable to continue for the third edition. Luckily, an esteemed colleague and in-

vii

ternationally regarded brain injury researcher and practitioner, Jeffrey Kreutzer, Ph.D., from the Medical College of Virginia, was recruited to complete the editorial team. Finally, I was most pleased that Dr. Griffith, who himself was largely responsible for the previous edition, was willing to endure the trials and tribulations of working on yet another edition of this textbook. We are also most grateful for the continued support and guidance of Jean-François Villain at F.A. Davis who, along with his colleagues at F.A. Davis Company, have been instrumental in the production of the third edition.

I would also like to express thanks to my chairman, Bruce M. Gans, M.D., who has been appreciative and supportive of my scholarly endeavors throughout my career. Finally, thanks to my wife Peggy, daughter Michelle, and son David, who have been a continuing source of love, strength, and support.

Mitchell Rosenthal

PREFACE TO THE SECOND EDITION

Why publish a second edition of our textbook on rehabilitation of the head-injured adult? And why expand the scope of the book to include pediatric aspects? Dr. Rosenthal's preface to the first edition merits rereading as an introduction to the answers to these questions. Our first book was a response to a long-identified need for a current state-of-the-art text on the subject. The awakening of a professional and public consciousness to the presence of a "silent epidemic" has become a dramatic reality in the 6 years since our first publication. That former silent epidemic is now an audible, visible, and palpable epidemic. A number of textbooks relating to rehabilitation of the head-injured patient have appeared, with notable emphasis on psychosocial aspects. Two books on pediatric head trauma have been published. However, no single work encompassing the spectrum of disabilities resulting from brain injury in adults and children has been assembled—until now.

Meanwhile a worldwide quest continues for enhanced knowledge and skills of rehabilitation and related professionals in this discipline. The genesis of an international head trauma society, the appearance of two scientific journals devoted exclusively to brain injury, continuing productivity of educational seminars throughout the United States and in other countries attest the mounting attention that is accorded the topic. Specialization of brain injury rehabilitation is expanding with the development of national systems of care, and increasing numbers of head trauma units within hospitals, rehabilitation centers, and other facilities. Other forms of rehabilitation programs proliferate, ranging from those within intensive care units to community-based educational, vocational, behavioral, residential, and respite programs. Training fellowships for physicians and other rehabilitation professionals are increasingly available.

The National Head Injury Foundation (NHIF) has become a potent and articulate voice in patient and family advocacy, dissemination of information, and reformation of legislative and public policy.[1] The National Institute of Disability and Rehabilitation Research (formerly NIHR) has designated head injury as a priority area of research. A federal interagency agreement has been concluded in order to promote coordinated research and training. Standards of care for rehabilitation of traumatic brain-injured patients have been adopted by the Commission on the Accreditation of Rehabilitation Facilities (CARF). A Special Education Task Force has produced a manual for educators. In addition, NHIF has promulgated the development of revised disability criteria by the Social Security Disability Insurance Administration, thereby allowing more equitable assessment of brain injury clients. The Foundation has provided evidence to third-party payers of the urgency of funding post-acute rehabilitation services.

The Head Injury Task Force has assumed an influential and productive role as a national organization of concerned educational, research, and care provider professionals. The standards of care for head injury adopted by CARF were generated by this body. It has developed close liaisons with NHIF, the American Congress of Rehabilitation Medicine, and other organizations concerned with head injury. The Task Force has focused on such subjects as innovations in service delivery, coordination of educational and research activities, and dissemination of information and resources among professionals. The Head Injury Special Interest Group of the American Academy of Physical Medicine and Rehabilitation is an organization of concerned physiatrists. This body has produced major academic courses at the Academy annual scientific meetings. It is currently addressing academic issues including standards of training and education in head injury for residents and fellows, and research priorities.

Here, then, are some instances of the accelerating interest and activity engendered by this provocative field. The spirit of inquiry, of exchange of information, of advancing expertise proceeds unabatedly; what has been more art is evolving into an applied science, with many questions yet to be answered.

How will this book compare and contrast with its predecessor? In response to constructive criticisms of the first edition, we have attempted to rectify omissions, upgrade information, and delete material that seemed unessential. Hence, several chapters have been omitted, a number added, surviving chapters extensively rewritten, and a section on pediatric head injury appended. Our authors include many who contributed to the first edition and a host of new contributors, experienced and knowledgeable in the discipline. We have sought to retain the essence of the first book: a resource of practical information to aid clinicians and students who work with the brain injured in all of the health care and related professions.

The original editorial team remains intact. My colleagues, Drs. Rosenthal, Bond, and Miller, have adhered to the core of our mission: to provide a book of quality and practicality that will compare favorably with the original. The expansive presence of the Atlantic Ocean notwithstanding, we have communicated closely and harmoniously throughout the preparation. I salute each of these scholars and friends for his estimable work as author and editor. My grateful appreciation extends to each of the contributing authors for his or her thoughtful, enthusiastic participation. Once again, we have enjoyed a fully supportive relationship with F.A. Davis Company, particularly with Jean-François Vilain, Senior Editor. To Brenda Thomas, my secretary: profound thanks for your devoted efforts. To my wife, Anna, and children, Ann, Jean Ellen, Drew, and Wesley: Bless you for your steadfast love and support. And to you, the reader, our ultimate gratitude: for the study and application of the contents of this book for the benefit of your patients and their families.

Ernest R. Griffith

Reference

1. Rosenthal, M, and Berrol, S: From the editors. J Head Trauma Rehabil 2(1):viii, 1987.

PREFACE TO THE FIRST EDITION

For the victim, family member, and health-care professional, head injury has always been something of a "puzzle." The event creating the injury occurs suddenly without warning. From that instant, the course of medical and rehabilitative management proceeds, but ultimately may not resolve the nagging questions posed by family members: "Will he ever be the same person again?" "What kind of life can he have now that he is brain-damaged?" Head injury often strikes persons within the prime of their lives—aged 16 to 35 years. Often, these victims are, at the time of injury, in the midst of carving out social, vocational, and economic patterns that typically last a lifetime. Yet, in the case of severe head injury, all of this has changed—often permanently. Within the past few decades, the advances in neurosurgical diagnostic and management techniques have enabled many persons to survive the immediate consequences of the injury. However, this newly head-injured person and the family are then faced with the difficulties inherent in continued survival and the challenge of regaining a measure of productivity and happiness.

Those professionals concerned with rehabilitation have only recently truly awakened to the plight of head-injured persons. That is not to say that head-injured persons have not received rehabilitative services for the past 30 years. Instead, I would suggest that the impression of "irreversibility of damage to brain tissue" has led many to behave as if rehabilitation efforts were rarely successful in restoring the person to a meaningful, productive existence. The public has also been frightened by head injury, perhaps because of its close association with the concept of brain damage, which has often incorrectly been equated with "mentally retarded," "emotionally disturbed," "physically crippled," and the like. Though the process of neural reconstitution and recovery from head injury is still not fully understood, those practicing within the medical and allied health community appear to be more hopeful about the future prospects of head-injured patients.

The "puzzle" of head injury is partly attributable to the extraordinary array of physical and mental sequelae of the injury, and the lack of adequate, scientifically based methods of treating these deficits in a systematic, effective manner. The fact that no two head injuries result in the exact same sequelae precludes broad generalizations for rehabilitation management and necessitates individualized treatment programs. In the not-so-distant past, many well-meaning practitioners equated head injury with stroke and dealt with these two populations in a similar manner. However, the research and clinical experiences gained in the past decade have highlighted the important differences in the initial neurologic insult and eventual residual deficits. One such finding—namely, that head injury usually results in diffuse brain damage, while stroke often is focal and unilateral in its locus—has helped to explain the greater variety of physical and mental deficits following head injury. For example, a stroke patient with a right brain insult may experience motor paralysis on the left side, spatial disorientation, dysarthria, and emotional liability. In contrast, a closed head injury impacting on the right hemisphere may cause a "contre-coup effect, which may result in diffuse damage. The manifestations of this injury could include bilateral motor weakness, subtle language deficits, post-traumatic amnesia, motor slowing, impaired perception, emotional blunting, altered sensation, and so forth. In addition, the head-injured victim often sustains associated injuries, which may include leg fractures, spinal cord injury, and facial lacerations.

The sum total of head injury may often be the temporary or permanent displacement of the victim and family. The victim may struggle for many years to accept and understand what has really happened. Life can become a series of frustrations and obstacles that often lead to exasperating failures. Head-injured persons return to the community to find that previous friendships and rewarding activities have been greatly restricted. After the euphoria accompanying discharge from the hospital subsides, relationships with spouse, family members, and significant others become strained. Economic hardship becomes a new reality. Some head-injured persons describe their houses as "feeling like a prison." A fight for emotional, social, and economic independence is likely to be a long, painful one.

The initial impetus for the writing of this text comes from our collective involvement in the Annual Post-Graduate Course on the Rehabilitation of the Brain Injured Adult, sponsored by the Medical College of Virginia. When initiated in 1977, no other annual course on head injury was ongoing in the United States. The first program was planned with the hope that 50 to 100 rehabilitation professionals would attend. More than 250 applications were received for that course. By 1981, at least 10 major hospitals and initiated annual courses in head injury, involving more than 2000 health-care professionals per year. Clearly, the compelling nature of the topic has been established. No fewer than 30 hospitals and rehabilitation centers have opened specialized head-injury units within the past 5 years.

A second motivating force for producing this book has been the dearth of previous texts or articles directed toward educating the rehabilitation professional about head injury. The last book of this type was published in 1969. Drs. Walker and Caveness edited a book entitled *The Late Effects of Head Injury*, which was a compilation of papers from a symposium. At each meeting about head injury, rehabilitation professionals posed the question, "Why doesn't someone publish a book about rehabilitation and head injury?" Finally, we decided to answer this question by compiling the current volume.

Since this book is the first text on head-injury rehabilitation in many years, we have attempted to be as comprehensive as possible. The attempt to adequately cover such a broad topic is fraught with perils. By presenting a comprehensive overview of the subject, we have not been able to provide as much depth on some topics as we would like. Thus, the physician may be disappointed at the relatively few chapters devoted exclusively to medical assessment and management. Yet other texts may fulfill this need, such as the recently published book by Bryan Jennett and Graham Teasdale, *Management of Head Injuries* (F.A. Davis, 1981). Certain rehabilitation professionals may feel that their specialty area,

such as nursing or physical therapy, has not been given adequate space. Regrettably, the field of head injury encompasses so many disciplines that the volume would have exceeded 1000 pages if material was presented for every group of professionals involved with brain injury—for example, nutrition, law, recreational therapy, education, psychiatry, and orthopedic surgery. Nonetheless, we are of the opinion that the content of the book will be valuable for all those concerned with head injury, regardless of their specific area.

Another difficulty in writing this book was to strike a balance between an academic and a clinical point of view. Predictably, the point of view varies depending on each chapter's author. We have designed the book not only to highlight important research advances of the past decade but to allow clinicians to find it useful as a guide to clinical practice. It is our sincere hope that each reader will find something of value that will generalize to his or her clinical practice.

This book owes its existence to a great many people. First and foremost, we are indebted to our contributors, whose long and hard labors have resulted in this text. I am personally grateful to the indefatigable efforts of my co-editors, Drs. Griffith, Bond, and Miller. Without their assistance, the book would likely still be in the planning stages. The support and editorial assistance provided by Mr. Bob Martone has been exceedingly valuable. I would like to express my deep appreciation to my colleagues who had a major role in planning and running the series of head-injury courses that led to the volume, especially Richard and Christi Eisenberg, Linda Diehl, Rita Riani, Robin McNeny, Jean Cerny, and others at the Medical College of Virginia. I also appreciate the support and encouragement provided by my colleagues at the Department of Rehabilitation Medicine, Tufts-New England Medical Center—especially my chairman, Dr. Bruce Gans. My thanks are also extended to Dr. Roberta Trieschmann, Dr. Cynthia Dember, and Dr. Paul Karoly, all of whom were important influences in my early career as a graduate student. The assistance of Mrs. Sarah McGillowey in typing the final manuscript is gratefully acknowledged. Finally, I express my heartfelt appreciation to my wife Peggy, daughter Michelle, and parents Morris and Edythe for their love, support, and encouragement.

Mitchell Rosenthal

CONTRIBUTORS

John D. Banja, Ph.D.
Associate Professor
Department of Rehabilitation Medicine
Emory University School of Medicine
Coordinator of Clinical Ethics Education
Emory University Hospital
Atlanta, Georgia

Jeffrey T. Barth, Ph.D.
Chief, Medical Psychology/Neuropsychology
University of Virginia Medical School
Charlottesville, Virginia

Yehuda Ben-Yishay, Ph.D.
Professor, Clinical Rehabilitation Medicine
Director, Brain Injury Day Program
New York University Medical Center, Rusk
  Institute
New York, New York

Sandra E. Black, M.D., FRCP(C)
Head, Division of Neurology
Director, Cognitive Neurology Unit
Sunnybrook Health Science Center
Associate Professor, Neurology
University of Toronto
Toronto, Ontario, Canada

Sarah Blanton, M.P.T.
Staff Physical Therapist
Center for Rehabilitation Medicine
Division of Rehabilitation Services
Emery University Hospital
Atlanta, Georgia

Jean L. Blosser, Ed.D.
Professor
School of Speech-Language Pathology
University of Akron
Akron, Ohio

Jennifer A. Bogner, Ph.D.
Assistant Professor, Physical Medicine and
  Rehabilitation
The Ohio State University
Columbus, Ohio

Margaret Brown, Ph.D.
Director, Dissemination, Research, and
  Training
Center on the Community Integration of
  Individuals with TBI
The Mount Sinai Medical Center
Department of Rehabilitation Medicine
New York, New York

Maureen Campbell-Korves
President, Brain Injury Association of New
  York State
Coordinator, Consumer Involvement,
  Research, and Training
Center on the Community Integration of
  Individuals with TBI
The Mount Sinai Medical Center
Department of Rehabilitation Medicine
New York, New York

Anna J.L. Chorazy, M.D.
Clinical Associate Professor, Pediatrics
Children's Hospital of Pittsburgh
University of Pittsburgh School of Medicine
Medical Director
The Rehabilitation Institute of Pittsburgh
Pittsburgh, Pennsylvania

David X. Cifu, M.D.
Interim Chairman and Associate Professor,
Medical Director, Rehabilitation and Research
  Center
Co-Director, NIDRR Model System for TBI
  and SCI
Medical College of Virginia
Virginia Commonwealth University
Richmond, Virginia

John D. Corrigan, Ph.D.
Professor, Physical Medicine and
  Rehabilitation
Director, Ohio Valley Center for Brain Injury
  Prevention and Rehabilitation
The Ohio State University
Columbus, Ohio

Roberta DePompei, Ph.D.
Professor and Clinical Supervisor
School of Speech-Language Pathology and
    Audiology
University of Akron
Akron, Ohio

Paul T. Diamond, M.D.
Associate Professor, Physical Medicine and
    Rehabilitation
Department of Neurological Surgery
University of Virginia School of Medicine
Charlottesville, Virginia

Madeline C. DiPasquale, Ph.D.
Clinical Neuropsychologist, Drucker Brain
    Injury Center
MossRehab Hospital
Research Associate, Moss Rehabilitation
    Research Institute
Philadelphia, Pennsylvania

Ann-Christine Duhaime, M.D.
Associate Professor, Neurosurgery
University of Pennsylvania School of Medicine
Associate Neurosurgeon
Division of Neurosurgery
The Children's Hospital of Philadelphia
Philadelphia, Pennsylvania

Elie Elovic, M.D.
Clinical Assistant Professor
UMDNJ-Robert Wood Johnson School of
    Medicine
Director, Spasticity Clinic
Associate Medical Director
Center for Head Injury
JFK-Johnson Rehabilitation Institute
Edison, New Jersey

Jeffrey Englander, M.D.
Director of Brain Injury Rehabilitation and TBI
    Model System of Care
Department of Physical Medicine and
    Rehabilitation
Santa Clara Valley Medical Center
San Jose, California
Clinical Assistant Professor
Department of Functional Restoration
Stanford University School of Medicine
Stanford, California

Alberto Esquenazi, M.D.
Associate Professor, Physical Medicine and
    Rehabilitation
Temple University Health Sciences Center
Director, Gait and Motion Analysis Laboratory
MossRehab Hospital
Philadelphia, Pennsylvania

Timothy J. Feeney, Ph.D.
Assistant Professor
Department of Education
The Russell Sage Colleges
Troy, New York

Norman L. Fichtenberg, Ph.D.
Assistant Professor
Wayne State University School of Medicine
Rehabilitation Institute of Michigan
Detroit, Michigan

Steven Flanagan, M.D.
Assistant Professor
Mount Sinai School of Medicine
Medical Director, TBI Program
The Mount Sinai Hospital
New York, New York

Amy Herstein Gervasio, Ph.D.
Assistant Professor, Psychology
University of Wisconsin—Stevens Point
Stevens Point, Wisconsin

Wayne A. Gordon, Ph.D.
Professor, Rehabilitation Medicine
Mount Sinai School of Medicine
Project Director, Research and Training
Center on the Community Integration of
    Individuals with TBI
The Mount Sinai Medical Center
Department of Rehabilitation Medicine
New York, New York

D.I. Graham, Ph.D., M.B., B.Ch., F.R.C.Path.
Neuropathology Department
Institute of Neurological Science
Southern General Hospital
University of Glasgow
Glasgow, Scotland, United Kingdom

Ernest R. Griffith, M.D.
Private Practice, Physical Medicine and
    Rehabilitation
Associate Medical Director
HealthSouth Meridian Point Rehabilitation
    Hospital
Medical Director, Outpatient Rehabilitation
Sun Grove Village Care Center
Scottsdale, Arizona

Michael E. Groher, Ph.D.
Professor/Chief of Speech Pathology
Department of Communicative Disorders
College of Health Professions
Health Science Center
University of Florida
Gainesville, Florida

Karyl M. Hall, Ed.D.
Director of Rehabilitation Research
TBI/SCI Model System Grants Co-Director
Santa Clara Valley Medical Center
San Jose, California

Flora M. Hammond, M.D.
Director, Brain Injury Research
Charlotte Institute of Rehabilitation
Charlotte, North Carolina

Mary R. Hibbard, Ph.D.
Associate Professor, Rehabilitation Medicine
Mount Sinai School of Medicine
Director of Research
Research and Training
Center on the Community Integration of
    Individuals with TBI
New York, New York

Harvey E. Jacobs, Ph.D.
Psychologist
Center for Neurorehabilitation Services
Richmond, Virginia

Kenneth M. Jaffe, M.D.
Professor, Rehabilitation Medicine, Pediatrics,
    and Neurology Surgery
University of Washington School of Medicine
Director, Rehabilitation Medicine
Children's Hospital and Regional Medical
    Center
Seattle, Washington

Angela Johnson, M.A.Ed.
Research Associate
Rehabilitation Research and Training Center on
    Supported Employment
Virginia Commonwealth University
Richmond, Virginia

Douglas I. Katz, M.D.
Associate Professor, Neurology
Boston University School of Medicine
Boston, Massachusetts
Director, Neurorehabilitation
HealthSouth Braintree Rehabilitation Hospital
Braintree, Massachusetts

Mary Ann E. Keenan, M.D.
Professor, Physical Medicine and
    Rehabilitation
Temple University Health Sciences Center
Director, Neuro-Orthopaedics Program
Albert Einstein Medical Center
MossRehab Hospital
Philadelphia, Pennsylvania

Mary R.T. Kennedy, Ph.D.
Assistant Professor
Department of Communications Disorders
University of Minnesota
Minneapolis, Minnesota

Jess F. Kraus, Ph.D., M.P.H.
Director
Southern California Injury Prevention Research
    Center
School of Public Health
University of California Los Angeles
Los Angeles, California

Jeffrey S. Kreutzer, Ph.D., A.B.P.P.
Professor and Director, Rehabilitation ,
    Psychology, and Neuropsychology
Department of Physical Medicine and
    Rehabilitation
Medical College of Virginia
Virginia Commonwealth University
Richmond, Virginia

Andrea Laborde, M.D.
Assistant Professor
Temple University Medical School
Attending Physician
Drucker Brain Injury Center
MossRehab Hospital
Philadelphia, Pennsylvania

**Gary L. Lamb-Hart, M.Div., C.C.D.C. III,
    I.C.A.D.C.**
Center Manager
Ohio Valley Center for Brain Injury Prevention
    and Rehabilitation
Department of Physical Medicine and
    Rehabilitation
The Ohio State University
Columbus, Ohio

Stephen N. Macciocchi, Ph.D.
Director, Neuropsychology Division
Sheperd Center
Atlanta, Georgia

Catherine A. Mateer, Ph.D.
Professor
Department of Psychology
University of Victoria
Victoria, British Columbia, Canada

**Jane D. Mattson, Ph.D., O.T.R., C.C.M.,
    C.R.C.**
President
Jane Mattson Associates, Inc.
East Norwalk, Connecticut

Nathaniel H. Mayer, M.D.
Professor, Physical Medicine and
    Rehabilitation
Temple University Health Sciences Center
Director, Motor Control Analysis Laboratory
Director, Drucker Brain Injury Center

MossRehab Hospital
Philadelphia, Pennsylvania

David L. McArthur, Ph.D., M.P.H.
Adjunct Assistant Professor, Epidemiology
Southern California Injury Prevention
  Research Center
School of Public Health
University of California Los Angeles
Los Angeles, California

James T. McDeavitt, M.D.
Medical Director
Charlotte Institute of Rehabilitation
Charlotte, North Carolina

William W. McKinlay, Ph.D.
Director, Case Management Services Ltd.
Balerno, Edinburgh
Consultant Neuropsychologist
ScotCare National Brain Injury Rehabilitation
  Unit
Murdostoun Castle
Winshaw, Scotland, United Kingdom

Robin McNeny, O.T.R.
Supervisor, Occupational Therapy and
  Therapeutic Recreation
Rehabilitation and Research Center
Medical College of Virginia Hospitals
Virginia Commonwealth University
Richmond, Virginia

Linda J. Michaud, M.D.
Associate Professor, Clinical Physical
  Medicine
University of Cincinnati College of Medicine
Director, Pediatric Rehabilitation
Children's Hospital Medical Center
Cincinnati, Ohio

W. Jerry Mysiw, M.D.
Associate Professor, Physical Medicine and
  Rehabilitation
Medical Director, Brain Injury Program
Ohio State University College of Medicine
Columbus, Ohio

Michael O'Dell, M.D.
Associate Professor, Rehabilitation Medicine
Albert Einstein College of Medicine
New York, New York
Medical Director
Regional Center for Traumatic Brian Injury
Southside Hospital
Bayshore, New York

**Brian Pentland, M.B., Ch.B., F.R.C.P.,
  F.R.C.S.L.T.**
Edinburgh Healthcare
Scottish Brain Injury Rehabilitation Service

Astley Ainslie Hospital
Edinburgh, Scotland, United Kingdom

Linda Picon-Nieto, M.C.D., C.C.C.
Speech Language Pathologist
Traumatic Brain Injury Program
James A. Haley Veterans Hospital
Co-Investigator
Defense and Veterans Head Injury Program
Tampa, Florida

Susan Popek-Boeve, C.T.R.S.
DMC Rehabilitation Center-Novi
Novi, Michigan

Lisa Porter, M.O.T., O.T.R.
Staff Occupational Therapist
Grady Memorial Hospital
Physical Therapist
Center for Rehabilitation Medicine
Emory University School of Medicine
Atlanta, Georgia

George P. Prigatano, Ph.D.
Chairman, Clinical Neuropsychology
Barrow Neurological Institute
St. Joseph's Hospital and Medical Center
Phoenix, Arizona

Steven H. Putnam, Ph.D.
Assistant Professor
Wayne State University School of Medicine
Rehabilitation Institute of Michigan
Detroit, Michigan

Sarah Raskin, Ph.D.
Associate Professor
Department of Psychology
Trinity College
Hartford, Connecticut

Mitchell Rosenthal, Ph.D.
Professor and Associate Chair
Department of Physical Medicine and
  Rehabilitation
Wayne State University
Administrator, Research and Education
Rehabilitation Institute of Michigan
Detroit, Michigan

Mary Louise Russell, M.D.
Director, Children's Rehabilitation Services
Children's Hospital of Pittsburgh
Pediatric Physiatrist
The Rehabilitation Institute
Pittsburgh, Pennsylvania

Angelle M. Sander, Ph.D.
Assistant Professor
Department of Physical Medicine and
  Rehabilitation

Baylor College of Medicine
Houston, Texas

Donna Smith, P.T.
Physical Therapist
Center for Rehabilitation Medicine
Division of Rehabilitation Services
Emory University Hospital
Atlanta, Georgia

Thomas Watanabe, M.D.
Assistant Professor
University of Cincinnati
College of Medicine
Medical Director Neurorehabilitation
Drake Center, Inc.
Cincinnati, Ohio

Anna J. Watkiss, B.Sc.
Psychologist
Case Management Services, Ltd.
Edinburgh, Scotland, United Kingdom

Paul Wehman, Ph.D.
Professor, Physical Medicine/Rehabilitation
Director, Rehabilitation Research and Training
    Center on Supported Employment
Medical College of Virginia
Virginia Commonwealth University
Richmond, Virginia

Michael West, Ph.D.
Assistant Professor
Rehabilitation Research and Training Center on
    Supported Employment
Medical College of Virginia
Virginia Commonwealth University
Richmond, Virginia

**Ian R. Whittle, M.D., Ph.D., F.R.A.C.S.,
    F.R.C.S.E.**
Department of Clinical Neurosciences
Western General Hospital
Edinburgh, Scotland, United Kingdom

John Whyte, M.D., Ph.D.
Professor
Department of Physical Medicine and
    Rehabilitation
Temple University School of Medicine
Director
Moss Rehabilitation Research Institute
Attending Physiatrist
Drucker Brain Injury Center
MossRehab Hospital
Philadelphia, Pennsylvania

Adrienne D. Witol, Psy.D.
Neuropsychologist
Glenrose Rehabilitation Hospital
Edmonton, Alberta, Canada

Steven Wolf, Ph.D., P.T., F.A.P.T.A.
Professor and Director of Research
Department of Rehabilitation Medicine
Professor of Geriatrics
Department of Medicine
Associate Professor
Department of Cell Biology
Emory University School of Medicine
Director, Program in Restorative Neurology
Emory University Clinic
Atlanta, Georgia

Mark Ylvisaker, Ph.D.
Associate Professor
Department of Communication Disorders
College of Saint Rose
Albany, New York

Kathryn M. Yorkston, Ph.D.
Professor
Department of Rehabilitation Medicine
University of Washington
Seattle, Washington

Ross D. Zafonte, D.O.
Associate Professor and Associate Chairman
Department of Physical Medicine
Wayne State University
Chief of Staff
Senior Medical Director
Rehabilitation Institute of Michigan
Medical Director
Traumatic Brain Injury Program
Rehabilitation Institute of Michigan
Detroit, Michigan

**Nathan D. Zasler, M.D., FAAPM&R, FAADEP,
    CIME**
Fellow, American Academy of Physical
    Medicine and Rehabilitation
Fellow, American Academy of Disability
    Evaluating Physicians
Certified Independent Medical Examiner
Medical Director, Concussion Care Centre of
    Virginia, Ltd.
Chief Executive Officer and Medical Director
Tree of Life Living Centers, Inc.
Chief Executive Officer and Medical Director
National NeuroRehabilitation Consortium, Inc.
Glen Allen, Virginia

TABLE OF CONTENTS

Acute Aspects of Brain Injury

BRIAN PENTLAND,
MB, CHB, FRCP, FRCSLT

Incidence and Prevalence of, and Costs Associated with, Traumatic Brain Injury

JESS F. KRAUS, MPH, PHD
and DAVID L. McARTHUR, PHD, MPH

□ OBJECTIVES AND GLOSSARY

Scope, Limitations, and Technical Concerns

This chapter synthesizes findings from a variety of published research papers describing the incidence, prevalence, severity, outcomes, and costs of brain injury. A comparison of results among papers requires a level of uniformity among definitions of terms, variables, and measurement techniques that is rarely present. Therefore, although it is possible to report such findings and to draw an overall picture of brain injury in some regions of the world, such a portrayal is not without its limitations.

Epidemiological Terms and Meanings

Epidemiological terms in this chapter include *incidence* (the number of new instances or cases of TBI during a given period in a specified population; *prevalence* (the number of all instances) of TBI in a population at a designated time, which includes new cases and existing cases found during the specified period; *E-codes* (external causes of injury) using rubrics found in the ninth revision of the *International Classification of Diseases* (ICD), published by the World Health Organization[1]; *outcome*, the sequelae, consequences, end point, or specific findings that result from TBI.

The term *brain injury* itself is often defined differently across different published reports (Table 1–1). Although many writers use the term to mean acute damage to the central nervous system, others use the term *head injury*,[2,3] which allows for inclusion of patients with skull injuries, fracture, or soft-tissue damage to the face or head without any neurological consequences.

Case inclusion criteria vary from study to study. Research populations may comprise patients referred to neurological intensive care units[4–6] or treated in emergency departments (EDs) and released for outpatient observations.[7,8] In several studies,[9] those with immediate death or death on arrival at the ED are excluded. In some studies,[10–12] analyses focused on computerized hospital discharge data sets and death certificate review. These variations suggest caution in comparing findings across all studies.

Work on this chapter was supported by the Southern California Injury Prevention Research Center, which in turn is funded by the U.S. Centers for Disease Control and Prevention (Grant #CCR903622). In addition, support was provided by the UCLA Brain Injury Research Center, NIH PO5 #NS30308.

TABLE 1–1. Brain Injury Case Definitions and Severity Criteria in Selected U.S. Incidence Studies

Study Location (listed alphabetically by author)	Study Years	Case Definition	Severity Criteria
Olmstead County, MI (Annegers, et al.)[2]	1965–1974	Head injury with evidence of presumed brain involvement, i.e., concussion with loss of consciousness (LOC), post-traumatic amnesia (PTA), neurological signs of brain injury, skull fracture	1. Fatal: <28 days 2. Severe: intracranial hematoma, contusion, or LOC >24 h or PTA >24 h 3. Moderate: LOC or PTA 30 min–24 h, skull fractures, or both 4. Mild: LOC or PTA <30 min without skull fracture
San Diego County, CA (Klauber et al.)[36]	1978	ICD Codes (1986) 800, 801, 804, 806, 850–854 with hospital admission diagnosis or cause of death with skull fracture, LOC, PTA, neurological deficit, or seizure; no gunshot wounds	Glasgow Coma Scale (GCS) (categories formed from scores of 3, 4–5, 6–7, 8–15)
San Diego County, CA (Kraus et al.)[13]	1981	Physician-diagnosed physical damage from acute mechanical energy exchange resulting in concussion, hemorrhage, contusion, or laceration of brain	Modified GCS ■ Severe = ≤8 ■ Moderate = 9–15 *and* hospital stay of 48 h *and* brain surgery, *or* abnormal CAT, *or* GCS = 9–12 ■ Mild = all others
Maryland (MacKenzie, et al.)[10]	1986	ICD Codes 800, 801, 803, 804, 850–854	ICDMAP: converts ICD codes to Abbreviated Injury Severity Scores
Central Virginia (Rimel, et al.)[23]	Oct 1977–June 1979	CNS referral patients with significant head injury admitted to neurosurgical service	GCS ■ Severe = ≤8 ■ Moderate = 9–12 ■ Mild = 13–15
Chicago area (Whitman, et al.)[3]	1979–1980	Any hospital discharge diagnosis of ICD Codes 800–804, 830, 850–854, 873, 920, 959.0. Injury within 7 days prior to hospital visit and blow to head/face with LOC, or laceration of scalp/forehead	1. Fatal 2. Severe = intracranial hematoma, contusion, LOC/PTA >24 h 3. Moderate = LOC/PTA 30 min to ≤24 h 4. Mild = LOC/PTA <30 min 5. Trivial = remainder
Massachusetts (Schuster)[11]	1989–1991	Uniform Hospital Discharge Data ICD codes 850–850.9, 800–801.9, 803–804.9, 851–854.1, and 873; nonresidents and late effects cases were excluded	Not reported
Colorado, Missouri, Oklahoma, Utah (Thurman)[19]	1991–1993 1992–1993 1990–1993	Any hospital discharge diagnosis of ICD codes 800.0–801.9, 803.0–804.9, 850.0–854.1 plus death certificate review	Not reported

CAT = computerized axial tomography; CNS = central nervous system; GCS = Glasgow Coma Scale; ICD = International Classification of Diseases; LOC = loss of consciousness; PTA = post-traumatic amnesia.

☐ ESTIMATES OF INCIDENCE AND PREVALENCE

Fatal Incidence

The worldwide mortality from TBI is not known, but if an average mortality rate of 20 per 100,000 (Fig. 1–1) is applied to the world population of 5.3 billion, then about 1,060,000 die yearly with an associated TBI. In the United States in 1994, more than 147,500 persons died of traumatic injury—about 6.5 percent of all deaths in the United States. The exact percentage involving significant brain injury is not known, and mortality estimates vary. Findings from Minnesota[2] and California[13] suggest that about 50 percent of traumatic injury deaths are due to brain injury. The U.S. National Center for Health Statistics's multiple-cause-of-death data, analyzed by the U.S. Centers for Disease Control and Prevention,[12] indicate that about 51,000 of all injury deaths each year involve significant brain trauma. This figure is based on a case-finding process that involved an extensive list of possible TBI injury diagnoses including ICD-9 code 873 ("other wound to the head"). This code has been shown to include a substan-

tial percentage of gunshot wounds, but it is routinely excluded from ICD-9 codes used for case finding.[14,15]

The reported brain injury mortality rate varies from 14 to 30 per 100,000 population per year (Fig. 1–1). This range in rates probably reflects a variation in specificity of diagnosis on some death certificates, as well as changes in brain injury recognition across regions over the past 25 or so years.

Nonfatal Incidence

The only national estimate of all hospitalized and nonhospitalized nonfatal brain injury is from the United States and was derived from the National Health Interview Survey[16] (NHIS) for 1985 through 1987. Extrapolated to the 1990 U.S. Census population of about 249 million residents, the NHIS reports about 1.975 million head injuries per year. Unfortunately, this estimate probably includes head injuries in which no brain injury occurred. The extent of ED and non-ED diagnosis and treatment of brain injury is not known, but Fife,[17] on reexamination of the NHIS data base, concluded that only 16 per-

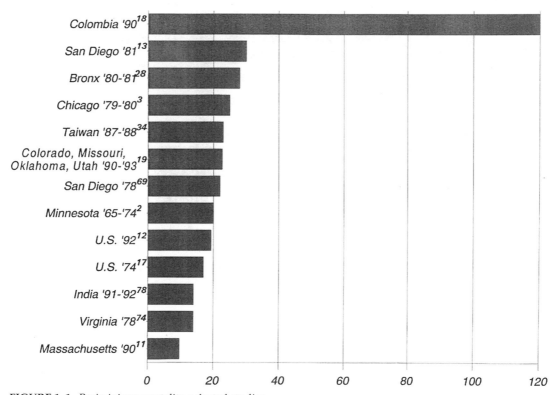

FIGURE 1–1. Brain injury mortality, selected studies.

cent of all head injuries resulted in an admission to a hospital. Fife concluded that only 1 of 6 persons with head (not necessarily brain) injuries has injuries severe enough to be admitted to a hospital. Because the number of individuals who seek some form of medical care from non-ED facilities is unknown, the figure of 1.975 million injuries from the NHIS remains an uncertain estimate of the true incidence of brain injury for an entire population.

Incidence data summarized in Figure 1–2 include brain injury rates from a variety of places. The rates range from a low of 96 per 100,000 in Massachusetts for 1990[11] to a high of 676 per 100,000 in Cali, Colombia, in the same year.[18] Despite some important differences that limit comparison among the studies cited, it is possible to estimate an average rate of fatal plus nonfatal hospitalized brain injuries reported in all studies of about 235 per 100,000 persons per year. When restricted to U.S. reports published in the last 20 years, the estimated rate is about 150 per 100,000 per year, which is used later in this chapter for purposes of disability estimation.

An estimate derived from published U.S. sources[12] is that about 373,000 persons were discharged from a hospital in 1992 with one or more brain injury diagnoses—a hospital admission rate of about 150 per 100,000 per year. The hospital discharge rate is useful for estimating the annual disability rate from injury. The difference in estimates between average incidence values in aggregate U.S. studies and data from hospital discharges or clinic visits may be due to definitional variation.

Some evidence suggests that TBI incidence is declining in the United States. Early reports from the 1970s and 1980s typically recorded TBI rates of about 200 to 250 per 100,000 population per year. Studies in recent years[11,19] suggest a decline in annual incidence, and a recent report by investigators from the U.S. Centers for Disease Control and Prevention demonstrated a slow decline in TBI mortality rates from 1979 through 1992 (Fig. 1–3).[12] Reasons for these changes are not known but may include more vehicles with air bags and wider use of seat belts in cars.

Another view on brain injury occurrence is provided by Figure 1–4, in which brain injury is compared with other leading diagnoses involving the head for 1983, 1988, and 1992. The most frequent first-listed diagnoses upon discharge (implying the primary reason for admission) from the National Hospital Discharge data are

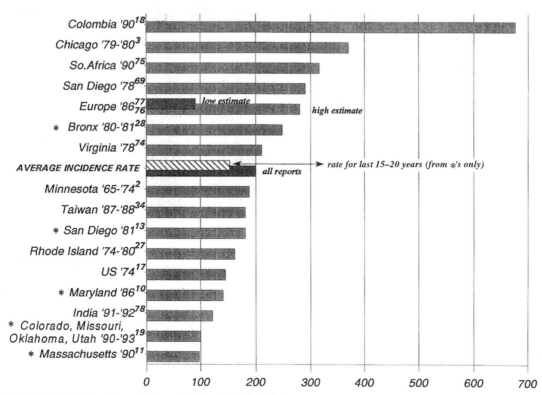

FIGURE 1–2. Brain injury incidence rates, selected studies.

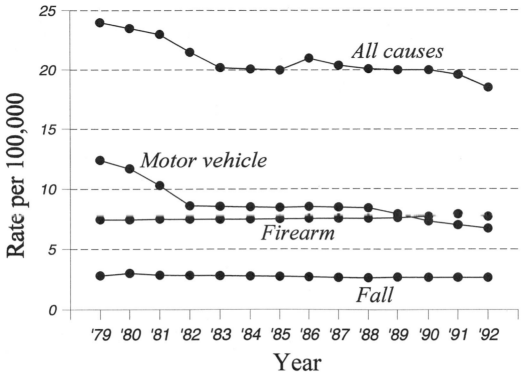

FIGURE 1–3. Injury mortality by selected causes, 1979–1992. (From Sosin, D, Sniezek, J, and Waxweiler, R: Trends in death associated with traumatic brain injury, 1979 through 1992. JAMA 273:1778–1780, 1995, with permission.)

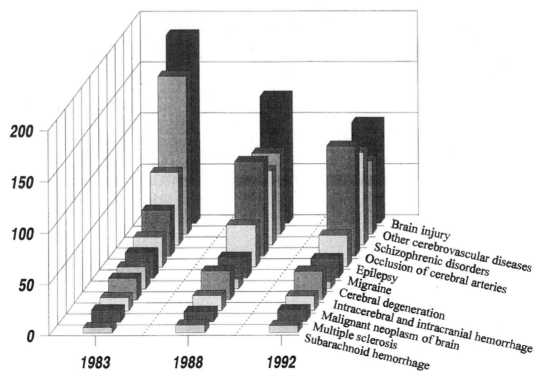

FIGURE 1–4. Incidence rates for leading injury diagnoses, 1983, 1988, and 1992.

presented as population rates. Many of the leading causes of neurological hospitalization occur at no more than one-fifth the rate for brain injury. Although the rates are not totally independent and are subject to the usual range of problems involving diagnostic bias, they illustrate the relative magnitudes of the various disorders affecting the brain. Information on brain injury occurrence allows monitoring of changes in incidence in the population, evaluation of effects of specific prevention measures or treatments, and identification of high-risk or hazardous exposure circumstances.

There appears to be a substantial decline from 1983 to 1992 in hospital admission rates for TBI as the first-listed diagnosis. The basis for this decline is not known. Note that, with a few exceptions, admission rates for most other neurological disorders have also declined. The ratios of TBI fatalities to hospital admissions and to emergency department visits for mild or trivial injury suggest that for every TBI death there are about 5 hospital admissions and 27 ED visits.[20]

Prevalence

The extent of TBI in the population is difficult to determine. Although the number of independent new hospitalized cases can be enumerated and the number of deaths attributable to TBI can be gauged, the number of persons with continuing neurological, behavioral, or cognitive impairment as a direct result of brain injury (current or in the past) is very difficult to ascertain. In some respects, TBI prevalence is a measure of residual impairment or disability. The U.S. national estimates of these conditions are not specific to a TBI etiology. Long-term population-based studies are infrequently reported, and when such studies are undertaken, the time course is highly variable.

Although the precise number of people with residual complications or impairments from TBI is not known, it is possible to estimate the annual number of new cases that will be part of the total prevalence pool of affected individuals. This estimate requires certain assumptions on the annual incidence rate, case fatality, and proportion with neurological impairments according to hospital admission severity assessment. If we assume an annual hospitalized TBI rate of 150 per 100,000 per year; a 1995 U.S. population of 265 million; hospitalized TBI severity proportion of 80 percent mild, 10 percent moderate, and 10 percent severe; hospital live discharge rates of 100 percent for mild TBI, 93 percent for moderate cases, and 42 percent for severe cases; and, finally, that 100 percent of se-

vere cases, 66.7 percent of moderate cases, and 10 percent of mild cases have some level of impairment, then the annual prevalence number for TBI can be represented as:

$$BID = Hn \sum_{i=1}^{k} p_i (1 - F_i) P_i$$

where BID = number with brain-injury disability

n = population base (265 million)

H = hospital admission rate (0.0015/year)

p_i = proportion in severity groups (mild 0.8, moderate 0.1, severe 0.1)

F_i = hospital case fatality rate for each severity group (mild 0.0, moderate 0.07, severe 0.58)

P_i = posthospital proportion of disability in each severity group (mild 0.1, moderate 0.667, severe 1.0)

or

$$BID = 0.0015 (265,000,000) [0.8 (1 - 0) (0.1) + 0.1 (1 - 0.07) (0.667) + 0.1(1 - 0.58) (1)]$$
$$= 73,152$$

According to this estimating model, the total number of new cases of disability from brain injury in the United States in 1995 was about 73,152, a rate of about 28 per 100,000 population.

❑ RISK FACTORS FOR TRAUMATIC BRAIN INJURY

High-Risk Groups

AGE

All studies of brain injury occurrence in the United States show that people 15 to 24 years old are at the highest risk. Patterns in age-specific rates (Fig. 1–5) illustrate, in all studies, two general high rates. The rates generally peak after age 15, decline after age 24, and continue to decline in the middle-aged years. The rates increase again beginning in the 60- to 65-year age range. (Composites in Fig. 1–5 were assembled from extant data covering the 1970s and 1980s.[20])

---

*References 2, 3, 10, 11, 13, 19–23.

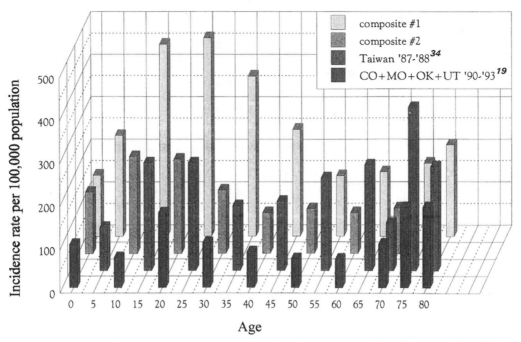

FIGURE 1–5. Age-specific brain injury rates, selected studies. CO = Colorado; MO = Missouri; OK = Oklahoma; UT = Utah.

SEX

All incidence reports agree that brain injury rates are higher for males than for females, with a rate ratio* from approximately 2.0 to 2.8. Although variation in rate ratios exists, the higher rates for males may reflect different exposure levels in the population studied. Injuries from motor vehicle crashes, contact sports, and interpersonal violence are all more common among males, who also show a higher rate of alcohol abuse.

RACE AND ETHNICITY

Although a few studies report that brain injury incidence is higher in nonwhites than in whites, there is justifiable concern over the quality of the information used to derive the rates. Hospital data vary widely in noting ethnicity or race in medical records; hence the true differences in brain injury rates by race or ethnic groups have yet to be determined accurately.

SOCIOECONOMIC STATUS

Socioeconomic status as measured by a number of indicators is a risk marker for certain populations with high incidence rates of brain injury. The National Health Interview Survey for 1985 through 1987[16] shows that the estimated aver-

age annual number of injuries and the rates per 100 persons per year are highest in families with the lowest income levels. Kraus et al.[24] observed this same finding from their study in San Diego County. Whitman et al.[3] reported the same conclusions in two socioeconomically different Chicago communities. In the San Diego County report, the surrogate for individual socioeconomic status was median family income per census tract. Findings did not change when the rates were adjusted by race or ethnicity. Hence, using race or ethnicity as a proxy for socioeconomic status may be inappropriate; other aspects of exposure within the "socioeconomic environment" should be explored.

High-Risk Exposures

ALCOHOL

The positive association between the blood alcohol concentration (BAC) and risk of injury is well established for almost every type of external cause of injury, including motor vehicle crashes, general aviation crashes, drownings, and violence.[25] Kraus et al.[26] found that 56 percent of adults with a brain injury diagnosis who were tested had a positive BAC. The BAC level was positively associated with physician-diagnosed neurological impairment and with length of hospitalization. Others have shown that drinking at the time of injury was associated with increased respiratory complications.[27] Dikmen et al.[28] have emphasized the importance of preinjury alcohol use in brain injury and the opportunity to intervene postinjury.

EXPOSURE TO ENERGY TRANSFER

The most frequent exposure associated with fatal and nonfatal brain injury is transport[2,3,10,13,17,28–30] (Fig. 1–6). This category includes automobiles, trucks, bicycles, motorcycles, pedestrians, aircraft, watercraft, and even farm equipment. Second in frequency are falls, usually among the elderly, and assaults are third.

Sports and recreation are a significant source of brain injury.[31] Although numerous studies indicate a significant proportion of fatal and nonfatal serious brain injuries are related to formal and informal recreation, there has been little attempt to evaluate this form of human activity with regard to incidence of TBI. Baker et al.[31] used data from the U.S. Consumer Product Safety Commission (CPSC) as well as data on hospitalized or fatally injured children younger than 16 years of age and other data from four states or counties to estimate TBI in recreational activities. The information available related to specific populations, and gross aggregate estimates from these data are difficult because of, again, wide differences in reporting features, injured population characteristics, case-finding techniques, and related methodological concerns. Also, the amount of exposure time among individuals in roller skating, horseback riding, or other activities was not known, and hence rates use general population denominators. According to CPSC data, of 758,000 persons with a recreational injury, approximately 11 percent (82,000) had a head injury; of 31,000 admitted to a hospital, 6200 had head injuries.

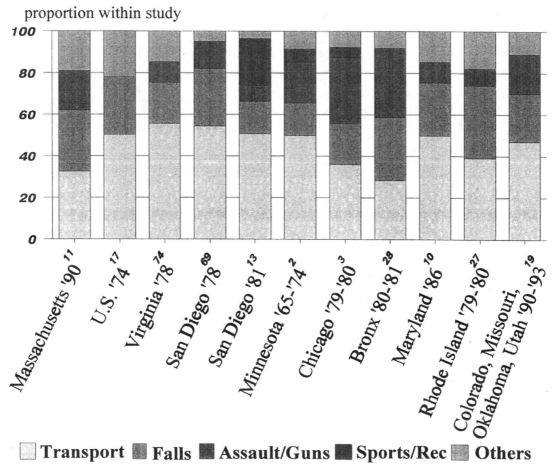

FIGURE 1–6. Relative proportions of brain injury by leading cause, selected studies.

A rough estimate of the number of U.S. fatalities due to recreational activities is 750 annually. About half of all head injuries treated in EDs were related to playground equipment. Ten percent of head injuries treated in EDs were related to horseback riding, and 25 percent of the concussions observed in EDs were related to this activity. Recreation or informal sports-related activities had highest rates of head injury for those under age 14. Finally, activities notable because of the large numbers of head injuries as a proportion of all injuries were horseback riding, skateboarding, skiing, sledding, and the use of playground equipment or children's toys. The authors concluded by suggesting that helmet use for many recreational activities should be explored, particularly horseback riding, skateboarding, in-line skating, sledding, and skiing.

The dominant type of transport exposure, motor vehicle crashes (Fig. 1–7), can be subdivided into three broad groups: vehicle occupants, riders on motorcycles, and pedestrians and bicyclists. Because most studies failed to stipulate occupant location, it is not possible to characterize driver versus passenger status, but vehicle occupants as a whole are the group most frequently brain injured. Risk of brain injury within different types of transport appears to differ dramatically across reports and is currently the subject of intense study (e.g., the contribution of seat belt use and motorcycle helmet use to the prevention of head injuries and fatalities).

OTHER PREINJURY EXPOSURES

A number of authors have asked if various conditions predispose children to exposures resulting in brain injury. Goldstein and Levin[32] reported that children with premorbid factors such as behavioral problems exhibit a greater tendency to incur brain injuries. However, Klonoff[33] could not show any relationship be-

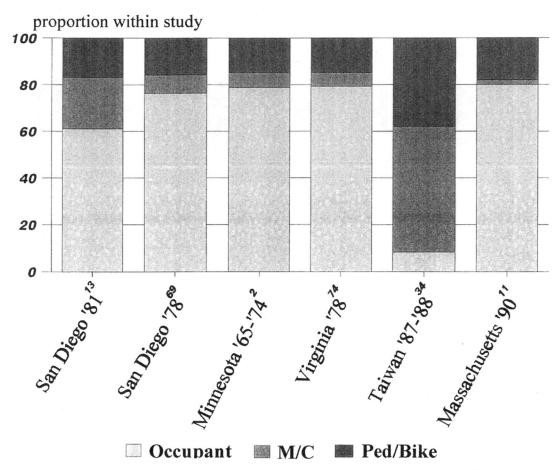

FIGURE 1–7. Relative proportions of brain injury by transportation-related causes, selected studies.

tween injury repetition and such factors as lower income or crowded housing that might alert public health authorities to target populations for prevention measures. A recent report by Dowd et al.[34] from New Zealand suggests that people hospitalized with an injury are at higher risk of a subsequent hospitalized injury within 1 year. This finding has implications for prevention via patient counseling during the hospital stay.

☐ OUTCOMES OF TRAUMATIC BRAIN INJURY

Gross Measures

Level of consciousness, the most common evaluation of brain injury severity, is measured by the Glasgow Coma Scale (GCS). The GCS is not without controversy, however. Prasad,[35] after careful examination of the sensitivity, reliability, validity, and responsiveness of the scale, concluded that the GCS is an established discriminative instrument, but that its validity, particularly as a predictive instrument, was not adequately studied. It has been widely observed by other investigators that the GCS is inappropriate for young children, those with severe facial injuries, those under the influence of alcohol or drugs, and those unfamiliar with the ED language.

The distribution of the severity of brain injury, as assessed by the GCS in a number of different studies, is shown in Figure 1–8. Brain injuries, as found in all studies, are generally classified as "mild" (i.e., a GCS score of 13–15). (Unfortunately, "mild" connotes an imprecise description of brain trauma and is differentially conceived by various researchers.) One study[29] reported a higher proportion of moderate and severe cases, probably because the study hospital was a referral institution to which serious injuries were more likely to be sent from the surrounding catchment area.

Although the literature is replete with reports describing brain trauma, few epidemiological studies have addressed the question of the nature and severity of the brain lesion. In the San

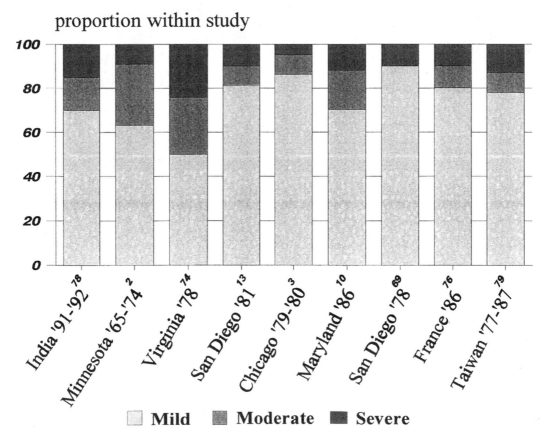

FIGURE 1–8. Relative proportion of brain injury by GCS severity group, selected studies.

Diego County cohort study,[13] however, clinical information was uniformly recorded and coded from the physicians' notes in the medical record. The data are population-based, as they refer to a single period from all hospitals in the region covering a specific enumerated population.

Figure 1–9 shows the distribution of brain injury lesions according to presence of fracture and location. Slightly less than half of all hospital-admitted persons with brain injuries have concussions without a concurrent fracture. Nearly 11 percent of those with a laceration or contusion of the brain do not have a concurrent fracture. Among those with brain hemorrhage, half do not have a concurrent skull fracture. In all of the major brain lesion categories, at least half of the cases do not have a concurrent fracture of the skull. Fracture is much less common among patients with a diagnosis of concussion or other cranial injury than among patients with a diagnosis of contusion, laceration, or hemorrhage.

Although the general mortality rate expressed per 100,000 population provides an idea of the level or magnitude of severe brain injury in the general population, the case fatality rate following hospital admission measures the immediate gross consequences of the trauma and has been used to assess treatment countermeasures.

Case fatality data are available from seven U.S. population-based incidence studies and three studies from two other countries (Fig. 1–10). Case fatality rates range from about 3 per 100 patients in Rhode Island[21] to about 17 per 100 hospitalized patients in Taiwan in 1987 and 1988.[35] Despite the temptation, comparisons across these studies would not be appropriate because their rates were not adjusted for severity.

Implications of Risk Markers on Outcomes

Over the last couple of decades, the search for relationships between early markers and late outcomes of brain injury has resulted in a diverse and sometimes contradictory literature. Age has been linked to mortality in many studies, but the shape of that relationship is subject to debate. In general, mortality increases with age,[36,37] but at least one study[38] found that children under the age of 5 either died or had good

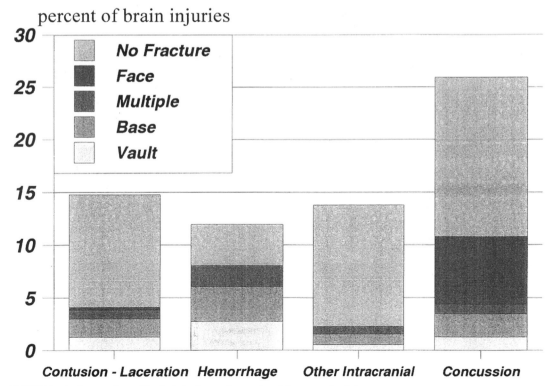

FIGURE 1–9. Proportion of brain injuries and associated fractures by injury type.

fatalities per 100 hospitalized persons

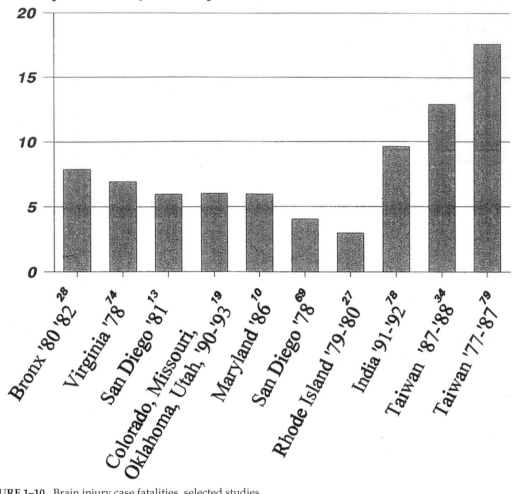

FIGURE 1–10. Brain injury case fatalities, selected studies.

recovery; that is, few recovered with disability. Brain injury after age 60, in contrast, leads either to death or to disability. Some researchers[39,40] have found that younger age groups have better outcomes according to the Glasgow Outcome Scale (GOS), but one recent study[41] found that increasing age was related to improved functional recovery.

Gender has a possible contribution to severity of injury and to long-term recovery. Mac Kenzie et al.[10] reported greater levels of injury severity in males but others did not.[42] Animal studies have also provided conflicting results. Reduced magnesium concentration and estrogen cycle have been related to poor outcome,[43] whereas increased progesterone levels have been associated with better recovery in female rats.[44] These findings, however, have yet to be demonstrated in humans.

Effects of the severity of the brain injury on outcome have long been appreciated. Glasgow Coma Scale (GCS) scores obtained soon after the injury have been appraised frequently for their usefulness in predicting long-term outcomes as assessed by the GOS.[39,45–49] Notably, the prediction appears to hold whether the GOS is obtained 1 week[50] or 1 year[46,51] later. Specific inquiries into the timing of administration of the GCS to the patient have found that outcomes for those persons assessed 6 hours after hospital admission were more accurately predicted than outcomes for those whose GCS was scored at the point of admission.[45] When combined with data from computed tomography (CT) scans, GCS scores gathered 48 hours after admission were better related to long-term outcomes than were admission GCS scores alone.[52] When combined with level of oxygenation, GCS scores obtained 72 hours after admission were the best-fitted predictors of long-term disability.[41] Information from the GCS has also been shown to have a good correlation with neurobehavioral outcomes.[46]

Post-traumatic amnesia (PTA) has been used widely as a measure of brain injury severity. PTA has been found to correlate well with GOS scores taken at both 6 and 12 months after injury[47] and with verbal and performance IQ at both 3 and 6 months.[53] Additionally, PTA has been shown to predict results of psychiatric disorders[54,55] and of the patient's capacity to return to work.[56] However, whereas one study found a relationship of PTA to general cognitive functioning after hospital discharge,[57] another found they were only weakly related,[7] and yet a third found no relationship at all.[58] Duration of unconsciousness following injury, which has been used frequently in studies of cognitive functioning in follow-up, has been found to relate to outcomes in intelligence, memory, language,[59] facial recognition,[60] personality change,[61] ability to return to work, and motor function.[62] At least one investigator,[58] however, has reported finding no relationship between duration of unconsciousness and general cognitive functioning during follow-up.

Various aspects of physiological and medical condition during hospitalization have been assessed for their link to outcomes. Among them are elevations in intracranial pressure (ICP), which has been seen to correlate with GOS scores obtained early in follow-up[63] and 6 months after discharge,[49] although one author cautions that age may be an important confounder.[40] Elevated ICP has been shown to increase long-term patient mortality.[64] The CT findings have been seen to predict long-term GOS scores in some studies[6,45] but not all.[38] Oculovestibular reflex deficits[39] and the size of mass lesions[40,63,65] have also been found to be good predictors of long-term GOS scores. Hemorrhage and fracture appear to play an important role in predicting death, unfavorable GOS scores, and long-term neurological deficits.[24] One study exploring delayed or secondary brain injury found that it predicted higher mortality, slower recovery, and poorer outcomes 6 months after injury.[66]

The strong possibility that one or more multivariate analytic solutions might better predict long-term outcomes than predictors considered singly has been studied by several investigators. For example, a high degree of predictability of the GOS at 1 year has been found by using a combination of six variables (age, GCS score, pupillary reactivity, surgical mass lesion, eye movements, and motor posturing).[67] Electroencephalography (EEG) and GCS together have

been seen to account for more than 95 percent of the variance of those outcomes assessed as either good outcome or death.[68] A composite EEG score alone was found to be moderately good in predicting 6-month GOS scores and better than other neurophysiological assessments.[69]

Age, PTA, and the worst neurological response during the early stages of treatment after injury have been shown to be good predictors of cognitive outcome 10 or more years later.[70] One of the more detailed multivariate analyses has shown that intracranial injury severity, extracranial injury severity, and pupillary response in the ED were predictive of patient survival, and GCS 72 hours following injury, intracranial injury severity, and extracranial injury severity were predictive of long-term disability.[41] Additionally, chest injuries and oxygenation levels were predictive of greater mortality and morbidity. Toward the development of a statistically based model easy enough for practical use, Mamelak et al.[71] conducted a retrospective records review and developed an ordered, weighted composite score that used best motor response, pupillary reactivity, and extraocular motility. When this composite was computed by using data at admission, it was shown to possess fairly good properties for prediction of survival at 6 months; when computed by using data 24 hours after admission, predictability improved greatly.

Unfortunately, a number of issues preclude a definitive general listing of predictors of short-term or long-term outcome following brain injury. Based on the evidence to date, the most stringent set of predictor variables suitable for all classes of TBI is not yet clear. Additionally, the course of outcome, especially coma type, can vary considerably over the course of the first year or more after injury.[42] Many of the existing studies have used noncomparable patient populations, different lengths of follow-up after hospital discharge, nonoverlapping sets of predictor variables, widely different definitions of outcome, dissimilar research designs, and nonequivalent statistical techniques. Also a long-standing problem is that many of the more widely used measures of outcome after brain injury are relatively crude instruments with unclear scaling properties. A thorough study of prediction of outcome will be highly data-intensive and require expensive repetitions of detailed physical, medical, and functional assessments throughout each patient's course of treatment and recovery. Because of wide variations in patient populations and injury severity distributions at any one treatment facility, multiple replications of the identical study design and multisite cooperation will be critical to establish the generalizability of any single prediction schema for brain injury outcome.

□ COSTS

Very little information on actual costs of brain injury was available until Max et al.[72] undertook large-scale analyses of data collected in the United States through 1985. They showed that the average lifetime cost per person for head injury across all levels of severity was approximately $85,000. For those who survived their initial injury, distinctions between minor, moderate, and relatively severe injury did not appear to result in large differences in medical care costs. However, very severe TBI and fatal injuries to the brain increased the overall lifetime cost by a factor of 4 to a combined total exceeding $300,000 per person. Loss of productivity over a lifetime showed dramatically higher overall costs for those injured between the ages of 15 and 44 than for those under 15 or over 44.

Miller et al.[73] used workers' compensation data from the late 1980s to evaluate injury costs across a wide variety of injuries. Comprehensive medical costs for brain injury amounted to more than $300,000 per person across all levels of injury severity. Miller et al.[74] included quality of life in cost calculations involving brain injury by global injury severity and showed that the most seriously injured persons (who survive their initial injuries) have projected acute-phase expenses of up to $2.4 million (in 1992 dollars), more than 18 times higher than mild brain injury. Because more brain injured individuals are surviving their initial injuries

now than in earlier years because of steady advances in neurosurgical intensive care, expenses have been increasing more rapidly for those who require high levels of long-term supportive care.

Recent insurance data, although based on smaller samples, indicate that costs can be very dissimilar across different degrees of TBI severity. Table 1–2 depicts five separate categorizations of injury and their estimated costs as of 1993.[75] With moderate confidence, the data can be extrapolated over the patient's expected life span to show the total financial demand anticipated (Table 1–2, last row). In constant dollars, severely injured individuals (who survive the acute phase of injury) require almost 40 times as much financial support over their life span as those with mild injuries, and those with moderate injuries require about 11 times as much financial support.

Using these figures, the total annual financial cost of brain injury in the United States can be roughly estimated at about $6.5 billion for care of new brain injury patients each year, plus another $13.5 billion for the annual continuing medical care for prior years' patients with TBI. None of these estimates, of course, can begin to do justice to the inescapable losses, both personal and financial, incurred by the patients' families.

REFERENCES

1. Commission on Professional and Hospital Activities: The International Classification of Diseases, 9th Revision, Clinical Modification (ICD.9.CM). Commission on Professional and Hospital Activities, Ann Arbor, Mich, 1986.
2. Annegers, JF, et al: The incidence, causes and secular trends of head trauma in Olmstead County, Minnesota, 1935–74. Neurology 30:91, 1980.

TABLE 1–2. Predicted Survival and Estimated Costs per Person by Severity of TBI

	Deep Persistent Coma	Persistent Vegetative State	Severe	Moderate	Mild
Survival[75]	Not exceeding 12 weeks	3 to 30 years	Normal (e.g., 44 years)	Normal	Normal
Acute care[75]	$49,000 to $376,000	$292,000	$578,750	$280,400	$500 to $15,800
Annual medical care[75]	$0	$185,100	$32,250 to $84,950	$6,700 to $23,340	$1,000 to $2,500
Extrapolated average lifetime cost*	$212,500	$3,346,150	$3,157,150	$941,280	$85,150

*Acute care plus (mean annual care × mean anticipated life span), constant dollars.

3. Whitman, S, Coonley-Hoganson, R, and Desai, BT: Comparative head trauma experiences in two socioeconomically different Chicago-area communities. A population study. Am J Epidemiol 119:570, 1984.

4. Auer, LM, et al: Predicting lethal outcome after severe head injury. A computer-assisted analysis of neurological symptoms and laboratory values. Acta Neurochir (Wien) 52:225, 1980.

5. Bruce, DA, et al: Outcome following severe head injuries in children. J Neurosurg 48:679, 1978.

6. Rimel, RW, et al: Moderate head injury: Completing the clinical spectrum of brain trauma. Neurosurgery 11:344, 1982.

7. Gronwall, SL, and Wrightson, P: Delayed recovery of intellectual function after minor head injury. Lancet 2:605, 1974.

8. Plaut, MR, and Gifford, RRM: Trivial head trauma and its consequences in a perspective of regional health care. Mil Med 141:244, 1976.

9. Jennett, B, et al: Head injuries in three Scottish neurosurgical units. BMJ 2:955, 1979.

10. MacKenzie, EJ, Edelstein, SL, and Flynn, JP: Hospitalized head-injured patients in Maryland: Incidence and severity of injuries. Md Med J 38:725, 1989.

11. Schuster, M: Traumatic Brain Injury in Massachusetts. Massachusetts Department of Public Health, Boston, 1994.

12. Sosin, D, Sniezek, J, and Waxweiler, R: Trends in death associated with traumatic brain injury, 1979 through 1992. JAMA 273:1778, 1995.

13. Kraus, JF, et al: The incidence of acute brain injury and serious impairment in a defined population. Am J Epidemiol 119:186, 1984.

14. Sosin, DM, Nelson, DE, and Sacks, JJ: Head injury deaths: The enormity of firearms. JAMA 268:791, 1992.

15. Nelson, DE, et al: Sensitivity of multiple-cause of mortality data for surveillance of deaths associated with head or neck injuries. MMWR CDC Surveill Summ 42:29, 1993.

16. Collins, JG: Types of injuries by selected characteristics: United States, 1985–1987. (National Center for Health Statistics) Vital Health Stat 10:175.

17. Fife, D: Head injury with and without hospital admission: Comparisons of incidence and shortterm disability. Am J Public Health 77:810, 1987.

18. Gutierrez, MI, Velasquez, M, and Levy, A: Epidemiology of head injury in Cali, Colombia. In Chiu, W-T, et al (eds): Epidemiology of Head and Spinal Cord Injury in Developing and Developed Countries. Proceedings of the First International Symposium of the Epidemiology of Head and Spinal Cord Injury. Taipei, Taiwan ROC, December 13–14, 1991 (publication date 1994), pp 113–120.

19. Thurman, D: Surveillance of Traumatic Brain Injury—Colorado, Missouri, Oklahoma, and Utah, 1990–93. CDC, Atlanta, GA, unpublished material, 1996.

20. Kraus, JF, and Sorenson, SB: Epidemiology. In Silver, JM, Yudofsky, SC, and Hales, RE (eds): Neuropsychiatry of Traumatic Brain Injury. American Psychiatric Press, Washington, DC, 1994, pp 3–41.

21. Fife, D, et al: Incidence and outcome of hospital-treated head injury in Rhode Island. Am J Public Health 76:773, 1986.

22. Lee, L-S, et al: Epidemiological study of head injuries in Taipei City, Taiwan. In Chiu, W-T, et al (eds): Epidemiology of Head and Spinal Cord Injury in Developing and Developed Countries. Proceedings of the First International Symposium of the Epidemiology of Head and Spinal Cord Injury. Taipei, Taiwan ROC, December 13–14, 1991 (publication date 1994), pp 129–136.

23. Rimel, RW, et al: Disability caused by minor head injury. Neurosurgery 9:221, 1981.

24. Kraus, JF, et al: The relationship of family income to the incidence, external causes, and outcomes of serious brain injury, San Diego County, California. Am J Public Health 76:1345, 1986.

25. Smith, G, and Kraus, J: Alcohol and residential, recreational, and occupational injuries: A review of the epidemiologic evidence. Annu Rev Public Health 9:99, 1988.

26. Kraus, J, et al: Alcohol and brain injuries: Persons blood-tested, prevalence of alcohol involvement, and early outcome following injury. J Public Health 79:294, 1989.

27. Gurney, JG, et al: The effects of alcohol intoxication on the initial treatment and hospital course of patients with acute brain injury. J Trauma 33:709, 1992.

28. Dikmen, SS, et al: Alcohol use before and after traumatic head injury. Ann Emerg Med 26:167, 1995.

29. Jagger, J, et al: Epidemiologic features of head injury in a predominantly rural population. J Trauma 24:40, 1984.

30. Cooper, JD, Tabaddor, K, and Hauser, WA: The epidemiology of head injury in the Bronx. Neuroepidemiology 2:70, 1983.

31. Baker, SP, et al: Head injuries in non-motorized informal recreation. Johns Hopkins University School of Public Health Injury Prevention Center, Baltimore, unpublished material, 1992.

32. Goldstein, FC, and Levin, HS: Epidemiology of pediatric closed head injury: Incidence, clinical characteristics, and risk factors. Journal of Learning Disabilities 20:518, 1987.

33. Klonoff, H: Head injuries in children: Predisposing factors, accident conditions, accident proneness and sequelae. Am J Public Health 61:2405, 1971.

34. Dowd, MD, et al: Hospitalizations for injury in New Zealand: Prior injury as a risk factor for assaultive injury. Am J Public Health 86:929, 1996.

35. Prasad, K: The Glasgow Coma Scale: A critical appraisal of its clinimetric properties. J Clin Epidemiol 49:755, 1996.

36. Klauber, MR, et al: Determinants of head injury mortality: Importance of the low risk patient. Neurosurgery 24:31, 1989.

37. Luerssen, TG, Klauber, MR, and Marshall, LF: Outcome from head injury related to patient's age: A longitudinal prospective study of adult and pediatric head injury. J Neurosurgery 68:409, 1988.

38. Waxman, K, Sundine, MJ, and Young, RF: Is early prediction of outcome in severe head injury possible? Arch Surg 126:1237, 1991.

39. Teasdale, G, and Jennett, B: Assessment and prognosis of coma after head injury. Acta Neurochir (Wien) 34:45, 1976.

40. Alberico, AM, et al: Outcome after severe head injury: Relationship to mass lesions, diffuse injury, and ICP course in pediatric and adult patients. J Neurosurg 67:648, 1987.

41. Michaud, LJ, et al: Predictors of survival and severity of disability after severe brain injury in children. Neurosurgery 31:254, 1992.

42. Klauber, MR, et al: Prospective study of patients hospitalized with head injury in San Diego County, 1978. Neurosurgery 9:236, 1981.

43. Emerson, CS, Headrick, JP, and Vink, R: Estrogen improves biochemical and neurologic outcome following traumatic brain injury in male rats, but not in females. Brain Res 608:95, 1993.

44. Roof, FF, et al: Gender-specific impairment on Morris water maze task after entorhinal cortex lesion. Behav Brain Res 57:47, 1993.

45. Levin, HS, et al: Severe head injury in children: Experience of the Traumatic Coma Data Bank. Neurosurgery 31:435, 1992.

46. Levin, HS, et al: Neurobehavioral outcome one year after severe head injury: Experience of the Traumatic Coma Data Bank. J Neurosurgery 73:699, 1990.

47. Bishara, SN, et al: Post-traumatic amnesia and Glasgow Coma Scale related to outcome in survivors in a consecutive series of patients with severe closed-head injury. Brain Inj 6:373, 1992.

48. Lokkeberg, AR, and Grimes, RM: Assessing the influence of non-treatment variables in a study of outcome from severe head injuries. J Neurosurg 61:254, 1984.

49. Marmarou, A, et al: Impact of ICP instability and hypotension on outcome in patients with severe head trauma. J Neurosurg 75:S59, 1991.

50. Wassertheil-Smoller, S, et al: Factors affecting short-term outcome of head trauma patients. Neuroepidemiology 1:154, 1982.

51. Wagstyl, J, Sutcliffe, AJ, and Alpar, EK: Early prediction of outcome following head injury in children. J Pediatr Surg 22:127, 1987.

52. Young, B, et al: Early prediction of outcome in head-injured patients. J Neurosurg 54:300, 1981.

53. Mandleberg, IA: Cognitive recovery after severe head injury. J Neurol Neurosurg Psychiatry 39:1001, 1976.

54. Bond, MR: Assessment of the psychosocial outcome of severe head injury. Acta Neurochir (Wien) 34:57, 1976.

55. Brown, G, et al: A prospective study of children with head injuries: III. Psychiatric sequelae. Psychol Med 11:63, 1981.

56. VanZomeren, AH, and VanDenBurg, W: Residual complaints of patients two years after severe head injury. J Neurol Neurosurg Psychiatry 48:21, 1985.

57. Bennett-Levy, JM: Long-term effects of severe closed head injury on memory: Evidence from a consecutive series of young adults. Acta Neurol Scand 70:285, 1984.

58. Barth, JT, et al: Neuropsychological sequelae of minor head injury. Neurosurgery 13:529, 1983.

59. Brooks, DN: Wechsler Memory Scale Performance and its relationship to brain damage after severe closed head injury. J Neurol Neurosurg Psychiatry 39:593, 1976.

60. Levin, HS, Grossman, RG, and Kelly, PJ: Impairment of facial recognition after closed head injuries of varying severity. Cortex 13:119, 1977.

61. Winogron, HW, Knights, RM, and Bawden, HN: Neuropsychological deficits following head injury in children. Journal of Clinical Neuropsychology 6:269, 1984.

62. Brink, JD, Imbus, C, and Woo-Sam, J: Physical recovery after severe closed head trauma in children and adolescents. J Pediatr 97:721, 1980.

63. Berger, MS, et al: Outcome from severe head injury in children and adolescents. J Neurosurg 62:194, 1985.

64. Miller, JD, et al: Significance of intracranial hypertension in severe head injury. J Neurosurg 47:503, 1977.

65. Robertson, CS, et al: Cerebral blood flow, arteriovenous oxygen difference, and outcome in head injured patients. J Neurol Neurosurg Psychiatry 55:594, 1992.

66. Stein, SC, et al: Delayed and progressive brain injury in closed-head trauma: Radiological demonstration. Neurosurgery 32:25, 1993.

67. Narayan, RK, et al: Improved confidence of outcome prediction in severe head injury. A comparative analysis of the clinical examination, multimodality evoked potentials, CT scanning, and intracranial pressure. J Neurosurg 54:751, 1981.

68. Thatcher, RW, et al: Comprehensive predictions of outcome in closed head-injured patients. Ann N Y Acad Sci 620:82, 1991.

69. Rae-Grant, AD, et al: Outcome of severe brain injury: A multimodality neurophysiologic study. J Trauma 40:401, 1996.

70. Lewin, W, Marshall, TFD, and Roberts, AH: Long-term outcome after severe head injury. BMJ 15:1533, 1979.

71. Mamelak, AN, Pitts, LH, and Damron, S: Predicting survival from head trauma 224 hours after injury: A practical method with therapeutic implications. J Trauma 41:91, 1996.

72. Max, W, MacKensie, E, and Rice, D: Head injuries: Costs and consequences. J Head Trauma Rehabil 6:76, 1991.

73. Miller, TR, et al: Databook on Nonfatal Injury: Incidence, Costs and Consequences. Urban Institute, Washington, DC, 1995.

74. Miller, TR, et al: Costs of head and neck injury and a benefit-cost analysis of bicycle helmets. In Society of Automotive Engineers: Head and Neck Injury. Society of Automotive Engineers, Warrendale, Pa, 1994, pp 211–240.

75. American Re-Insurance Company: Guidelines for Reserving Traumatic Brain Injury. American Re-Insurance Co, Princeton, NJ, 1993.

CHAPTER 2

Pathophysiological Aspects of Injury and Mechanisms of Recovery

D. I. GRAHAM, MB, BCH, PHD, FRCPATH

A considerable amount of literature now clearly shows that, singly or in combination, various processes may damage the brain after trauma and that mild, moderate, and severe categories of injury may be separated not so much by the nature of the lesion as by its amount and distribution. If this literature is correct, then there is likely to be a clinical and neuroradiological continuum from mild to severe damage, the structural basis of which can be inferred from postmortem studies on patients who have died with varying degrees of disability after brain injury.

☐ CLASSIFICATION AND MECHANISMS OF BRAIN DAMAGE

Any postmortem classification of brain damage after trauma to the head must take into account the full spectrum of clinical presentation and outcome: from the patient who remains in a coma from the moment of injury until death to the patient who is apparently normal after the initial injury but who, as a result of a complication, subsequently relapses into a fatal coma. Given that some structural damage is likely in all forms of traumatic brain injury, an important determinant of outcome is the preinjury condition of the brain. In other words, a good recovery is more likely in the healthy individual whose brain is normal than in an individual

with a similar level of injury whose brain, because of either preexisting developmental or acquired disorders, is abnormal. Even after a relatively minor head injury, the outcome in an individual who has already experienced cerebrovascular disease or head injury is likely to be much worse than in a person in whom premorbid conditions were not present.

Earlier classifications based on clinicopathological correlations helped to identify potentially preventable complications in patients after head injury, particularly those who "talked and died"[1] or "talked and deteriorated."[2] Under these circumstances, the fact that the patient had talked, only to deteriorate or subsequently die, is taken as evidence that the initial structural damage was minimal, although the head injury had initiated a progressive sequence of events that led subsequently to a fatal outcome or a persisting disability. Injury to the brain was therefore considered either primary (induced by mechanical forces), occurring at the moment of injury, or secondary or delayed (not mechanically induced) and therefore superimposed on an already mechanically injured brain. Secondary damage could be caused by complications either initiated by or independent of the primary damage.[3] These pathophysiological processes are not unique to the patient with brain injury but are commonly found in patients with other types of intracranial disease (Table 2–1).

We wish to thank Mrs. Marisa Hughes for typing this manuscript.

TABLE 2–1. Classification of Brain Damage after Head Injury

Primary	Secondary
Injury to scalp	Hypoxia ischemia
Fracture of skull	Swelling/edema
Surface contusions/ lacerations	Raised intracranial pressure
Intracranial hematoma	Meningitis
Diffuse axonal injury	Neurochemical changes

TABLE 2–3. Classification of Brain Damage after Head Injury

Focal	Diffuse
Injury to scalp	Hypoxia-ischemia
Fracture of skull	Diffuse axonal injury
Surface contusions/ lacerations	Diffuse brain swelling
Intracranial hematoma	Diffuse neurochemical changes
Raised intracranial pressure	Meningitis

Although the circumstances under which the brain can be injured after trauma are diverse and complex, major advances have been made in understanding the mechanisms by which brain damage occurs after head injury. There are two principal mechanisms: contact and acceleration-deceleration.[4] The conditions at the time of injury largely determine the associated pathology, reflecting, among other things, the amount of mechanical loading, the way in which it is distributed, and the time over which it has been applied[5] (Table 2–2).

Lesions caused by contact tend to result from either an object striking the head or contact between brain and skull. Acceleration-deceleration brain injury results from unrestricted movement of the head that leads to shear, tensile, and compressive strains. The principal structural damage in this type of accident is acute subdural hematoma from tearing of bridging veins and widespread damage to axons or blood vessels.

Another classification is based on the clinical and neuroradiological appreciation that the structural brain damage after trauma can be

categorized as either focal or diffuse (multifocal)[6] (Table 2–3).

From these considerations, it should be clear that in any given patient the outcome is the product of many factors. However, it is generally agreed that the focal pathologies associated with contact are likely to be sustained from a fall, whereas diffuse pathologies are more commonly associated with acceleration-deceleration in a traffic accident. Only understanding the biomechanical, molecular, and cellular events associated with brain injury after trauma allows specific mechanisms to be targeted in the hope of improving outcome.

The following account of the pathology of brain damage after trauma is based on autopsy studies, for which the brain must be properly fixed before dissection and appropriate histological studies carried out. This rule applies to both blunt injuries, which are by far the more common in civilian practice, and an account of which follows, and missile injuries, which are not discussed here.

□ BRAIN DAMAGE IN FATAL (BLUNT) NONMISSILE HEAD INJURY

Focal Brain Injury

LESIONS OF THE SCALP, SKULL, AND DURA

Lesions of the scalp, skull, and dura often provide a clue to the site and nature of the injury and alert the clinician to potential complications. For example, bruising at the back of the scalp is often associated with severe contusions of the frontal lobes; bruising of the mastoid process may be associated with traumatic subarachnoid hemorrhage; and bruising in the temple may be associated with a fracture and the subsequent development of an extradural hematoma. In many instances, laceration of the scalp is not of any great significance, but if there is severe bleeding, the patient may become hypotensive, thereby adding a secondary

TABLE 2–2. Classification of Brain Damage after Head Injury

Contact	Acceleration- Deceleration
Lesions of scalp	Tearing of bridging veins with formation of subdural hematoma
Fracture of skull with or without an associated extradural hematoma	Diffuse axonal injury
Surface contusions	Acute vascular injury Neurochemical changes
Intracerebral hemorrhage	

insult to the damaged brain. Furthermore, if there is an associated open depressed fracture of the skull, a laceration of the scalp may be a potential route for intracranial infection.

In general, the more severe the head injury, the more likely a skull fracture is. For example, the frequency of skull fracture is 3 percent in patients who are taken to emergency departments (EDs), 65 percent in patients admitted to a neurosurgical unit, and 80 percent in fatal cases.[7] Fractures of the skull may be limited to the vertex or to the base of the skull, or they may affect both. The majority are linear, affecting the vault of the skull in 62 percent of cases, with extension into the base of the skull in 17 percent. The fracture is said to be *depressed* if the fragments of the inner table of the skull are displaced inward by at least the thickness of the diploë, and such lesions are found in some 11 percent of patients. A depressed fracture is said to be *compound* if there is an associated laceration of the scalp and *penetrating* if there is also a tear in the dura.

Quite reasonably, one would anticipate that a fracture of the skull is necessarily associated with underlying brain damage, but this is not always so. For example, a crush injury may result in extensive fractures of the skull with little underlying brain damage, and the patient often remains conscious. More localized injury, for example, after an assault by a blunt object, may produce brain damage limited to the site of impact. Even under these circumstances, the fracture may be depressed and yet brain function remains intact, with only brief or limited loss of consciousness.

Similarly, the absence of a skull fracture does not necessarily mean that the brain has not been injured. Indeed, skull fracture is absent in about 20 percent of fatal cases. In pediatric practice, the capacity of a child's skull to bend may prevent the development of fracture, despite a considerable amount of underlying structural brain damage.

There is a strong association between skull fracture and the development of an intracranial hematoma,[8,9] particularly if, after the injury, the patient had a depressed level of consciousness. For example, only 1 in 6000 patients in EDs who did not have any of these features subsequently developed an intracranial hematoma, whereas the risk becomes 1 in 4 when these clinical features were present. The site of the fracture is also important. If the fracture affects the squamous part of the temporal bone, an extradural hematoma may develop.

SURFACE CONTUSIONS AND LACERATIONS OF THE BRAIN

By definition, the pia-arachnoid is intact over surface contusions and torn in lacerations. Con-

tusions have been considered the hallmark of brain damage caused by head injury and are present in 94 percent of fatal cases. They are most severe on the crests of gyri, and they have a very characteristic distribution affecting the poles of the frontal lobes, the inferior aspects of the frontal lobes including the gyri recti, the cortex above and below the operculum of the Sylvian fissures, the temporal poles, and the lateral and inferior aspects of the temporal lobes (Fig. 2–1). Less commonly, they are seen on the lower aspects of the cerebellar hemispheres.

Contusions occur at the crests of gyri and are invariably associated with some bleeding into the subarachnoid space. More severe lesions may extend into white matter, comprising a mixture of hemorrhage and necrosis, at the margin of which is an area of edema. Particularly when there has been extensive damage, an actual hematoma may develop within the affected gyrus, and if laceration of the pia-arachnoid has taken place, there may be bleeding into the subdural space. The combination of extensive contusion and an associated subdural hematoma is referred to as a *burst lobe*. Depending on the location of the lesion, there may or may not be an associated neurological deficit.

The surface contusions or lacerations and associated swelling may be sufficient to act as a mass lesion, with the subsequent sequela of raised intracranial pressure. Indeed, such a sequence of events was attributed to contusional

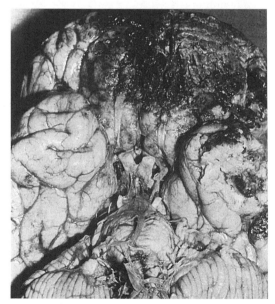

FIGURE 2–1. Acute surface contusions. There are hemorrhagic defects on the orbital surfaces of the frontal lobes and at the pole and on the undersurface of the left temporal lobe.

injury alone in 6 of 66 patients who "talked and died," 25 percent of whom did not have significant intracranial hematoma.[1] With survival, the contusions and lacerations heal and may be found in 2.5 percent of all autopsies in general hospitals.

Various types of contusion have been described. Reference has already been made to fracture contusions, which occur at the site of a fracture and are particularly severe in the frontal lobes and in association with fractures of the anterior fossae; *coup* contusions occur at the site of contact in the absence of a fracture, and *contrecoup* contusions occur in brain tissue diametrically opposite the point of contact.[10]

The development of a contusion index has allowed the depth and extent of contusions in different parts of the brain to be expressed quantitatively.[11] This index has shown that severe contusions are present in 10 percent of fatalities, moderately severe contusions in 78 percent, and mild contusions in 6 percent. The index has confirmed that contusions occur most commonly in the frontal and temporal lobes, are more severe in patients with a fracture of the skull than in those without a fracture, are less common in patients with diffuse brain injury than in those with focal brain injury, and are more severe in patients who do not experience a lucid interval than in those who do. More recently, a hemorrhagic lesion score has been derived that provides a finer discrimination of the distribution and severity of injury by including hemorrhagic lesions involving the corpus callosum and deep gray and white matter.[12]

INTRACRANIAL HEMATOMA

Intracranial hematoma is the most common cause of clinical deterioration and death in patients who experience a lucid interval—that is, those who "talk and die" or "talk and deteriorate" after injury.[1,13–15] Indeed, late recognition and treatment of intracranial hematoma are among the most—if not the most—important avoidable factors. Regardless of the severity of the head injury, there is always the possibility that an intracranial hematoma may complicate the injury. The bleeding usually begins at the time of injury, and by the time of admission to the hospital some 3 to 4 hours later there is a hematoma in between 30 and 60 percent of patients admitted in coma.

If the injury is mild, loss of consciousness may be limited to a few minutes, but a secondary loss of consciousness may develop because of an expanding intracranial hematoma. This textbook description of a lucid interval followed by coma occurs in only a minority of cases; many more patients are in coma from the time of injury, and in them a hematoma progressively develops.

Traumatic intracranial hematomas are usually classified according to the anatomic compartment in which they develop (Table 2–4).

Extradural (Epidural) Hematoma

An extradural (epidural) hematoma consists of an ovoid mass of clotted blood that lies between the bone of the vault or the base of the skull and the dura (Fig. 2–2). It is present in 5 to 15 percent of fatal head injuries[16,17] and in 85 percent of adult patients there is an associated fracture.[18] In children, a fracture is commonly absent.

In 70 percent of cases reported by Lewin[19] and McKissock et al.,[20] the extradural hematoma was caused by a fracture in the squamous part of the temporal bone that damaged an underlying branch of the middle meningeal artery. In the remaining cases, the hematoma may have developed in relation to the frontal and parietal parts of the brain or even within the posterior fossa, and occasionally they are multiple. Because the source of the bleeding is usually arterial, the hematoma enlarges fairly rapidly, gradually stripping the dura from the scalp to form a circumscribed ovoid mass that progressively indents and flattens the adjacent brain. In many cases, there is very little associated underlying brain damage.

Small hematomas may become completely organized; larger ones may undergo partial organization, their centers becoming cystic and filled with dark, viscous fluid. After about 2 weeks, the hematomas become smaller, and in the majority of patients are completely resolved by the fourth to sixth week after the injury.[21]

Intradural Hematomas

Subarachnoid Hematoma. There is a degree of subarachnoid hemorrhage in any serious brain injury, mostly occurring in association with sur-

---

TABLE 2–4. Classification of Intracranial Hematomas

1. Extradural (epidural) hematoma
2. Intradural hematoma
   a. Subdural hematoma
   b. Subarachnoid hematoma
   c. Discrete intracerebral or intracerebellar hematoma, not in continuity with the surface of the brain, and the burst lobe, an intracerebral or intracerebellar hematoma in continuity with the related subdural hematoma

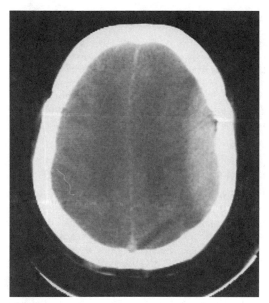

FIGURE 2–2. CT scan showing the characteristic bi-convex density of an extradural (epidural) hematoma. Reproduced with permission.

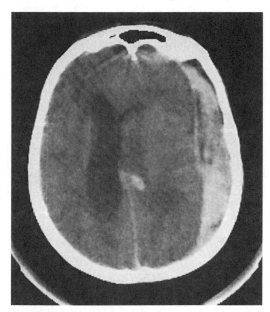

FIGURE 2–3. CT scan showing an extensive acute subdural hematoma, concave-convex in shape, and of mainly increased radiodensity, confirming its composition of solid clotted blood. The contralateral ventricle is shifted and dilated, indicating that intracranial pressure will be high. Reproduced with permission.

face contusions. In many cases, there is a thin layer of blood clot over the lateral and inferior aspects of the frontal and temporal lobes, but in 10 to 15 percent the amounts are larger and may constitute a subarachnoid hematoma. Under these circumstances, there may be associated constriction (vasospasm) of the cerebral arteries, and, if large amounts of subarachnoid hemorrhage are present in the posterior fossa, acute obstructive hydrocephalus may develop. In forensic (medicolegal) medicine, the entity of traumatic subarachnoid hemorrhage is well recognized as a result of damage to blood vessels in the posterior fossa,[22] often in association with a fracture of the base of the skull.[23,24]

Subdural Hematomas. Small amounts of hemorrhage within the subdural space are common in fatal brain injury. Because this blood can spread freely throughout the subdural space, it tends to cover the entire hemisphere, with the result that a subdural hematoma is usually larger than an extradural hematoma. The great majority of subdural hematomas are caused by rupture of veins that bridge the subdural space, where they connect the upper surface of the cerebral hemisphere to the sagittal sinus. Occasionally they are arterial in origin.

Subdural hematomas large enough to act as significant mass lesions have been variously reported in 26 to 63 percent of blunt head injuries[16,17] (Fig. 2–3). In 8 to 13 percent of cases, the hematomas are pure, with very little evidence of other brain damage. However, most are associated with considerable brain damage,

and therefore the mortality and morbidity are greater in subdural than in extradural hematomas, particularly in patients with a burst frontal or temporal lobe.

The current literature classifies a subdural hematoma as acute if it is composed of clot and blood (usually within the first 48 hours after injury), subacute if there is a mixture of clotted and fluid blood (developing between 2 and 14 days after injury), and chronic if the hematoma is fluid (developing more than 14 days after injury).[15] Chronic subdural hematoma occurs weeks or months after what may appear to have been a trivial head injury. However, a history of head injury is present in 25 to 50 percent of cases.[25,26] The hematoma becomes encapsulated, slowly increases in size, and may become sufficiently large to produce distortion and herniation of the brain (as discussed later). Chronic subdural hematoma is more common in the older age group than in younger patients and also more common in alcoholics.

Intracerebral and Intracerebellar Hematomas. Present in 16 to 20 percent of fatal cases, intracerebral and intracerebellar hematomas are often multiple and occur most commonly in the frontal and temporal lobes[15] (Fig. 2–4); less commonly, they occur in the cerebellum. Sometimes traumatic intracerebral hematomas develop several days after the injury, and the

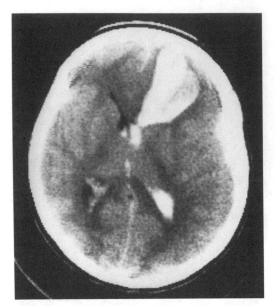

FIGURE 2–4. CT scan showing an extensive traumatic intracranial hematoma in the subfrontal region. There is also intraventricular hemorrhage. The patient had impairment of the blood clotting mechanisms. Reproduced with permission.

recognition of this possibility may have important medicolegal implications if the patient dies.[27,28] Relatively small hematomas deeply seated in the brain are now more commonly recognized by computed tomographic (CT) scanning and magnetic resonance imaging (MRI); many hematomas are often rather small and centered on midline structures, including parasagittal white matter (so-called gliding contusion), corpus callosum, structures in the walls of the third ventricle, and in the striatum (so-called basal ganglia hematomas). In the majority of these cases, the patients are in a coma, and the small hematomas are part of the clinicopathological entity of diffuse (multifocal) axonal injury.[29,30]

Sometimes patients are admitted to the hospital with a history of possible head injury. In these patients a solitary hematoma should be considered a result of either nontraumatic hypertensive bleeding or the rupture of a saccular aneurysm. Interpretation of the autopsy findings can be difficult, and much depends on the site of the hematoma. For example, a hematoma in the subfrontal or temporal region is more likely than not to be traumatic. The risk factors for the development of intracerebral hematoma include tumor, vascular malformation, and substance abuse. Patients receiving thrombolytic therapy are also at risk, and those who are receiving anticoagulants are at particular risk of developing intracerebral hemorrhage related to contusions.

"Burst" Lobe. A "burst" lobe is an intracerebral or an intracerebellar hematoma that is continuous with a subdural hematoma. It is presumed to be caused by damage to or laceration of superficial brain tissue. It is present in some 25 percent of fatal cases and occurs most commonly in the frontal and temporal lobes.

BRAIN DAMAGE CAUSED BY RAISED INTRACRANIAL PRESSURE

It is not surprising that intracranial pressure (ICP) is frequently elevated in patients after brain injury, given the mass effects of contusions or lacerations and intracranial hematomas within an essentially enclosed space.

In the normal adult, the ICP is usually in the range of 0 to 10 mmHg. Pressures over 20 mmHg are abnormal; when the ICP is greater than 40 mmHg, there is neurological dysfunction and impairment of brain electrical activity. As the ICP continues to rise, the ability of the cerebral circulation to maintain autoregulation and the normal cerebral perfusion become compromised. An ICP greater than 60 mmHg is invariably fatal, and there is increasing evidence that even pressures between 20 and 40 mmHg may be associated with increased morbidity.

If unchecked, an increase in the ICP is likely to kill the patient as a result of deformation of tissue, shift, the development of internal hernias, and secondary damage to the upper brain stem. This mechanism is the commonest cause of death in the neurosurgical intensive care unit; it is present in 75 percent of severely brain injured patients who die.[31]

A unilateral mass lesion causes distortion of the brain, a reduction in the volume of cerebrospinal fluid (CSF), and, in the closed skull, the formation of internal hernias (Fig. 2–5). Principal among these hernias is the displacement of the cingulate gyrus under the free edge of the falx (a subfalcine or supracallosal hernia) and the medial temporal gyrus downward through the incisura (a tentorial hernia) (Fig. 2–6). A mass lesion in the posterior fossa may result in herniation of the cerebellar tonsil through the foramen magnum (a tonsillar hernia). As these hernias develop, CSF spaces are obliterated, and pressure gradients begin to develop between the various intracranial compartments. Further progression is likely to mechanically deform blood vessels enough to cause vascular complications such as hemorrhage or infarction in the upper brain stem and variable degrees of ischemic damage within the territories of one or both posterior cerebral arteries. Less commonly, there is infarction of

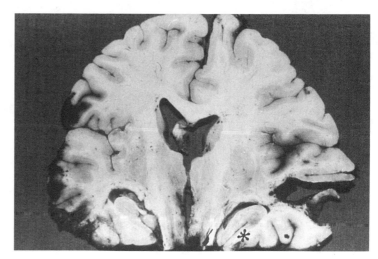

FIGURE 2–5. Lateral shift. There is displacement of the midline structures to the left, a supracallosal hernia, enlargement of the contralateral ventricle, and hemorrhagic pressure necrosis in relation to a tentorial hernia on the right (*asterisk*).

brain tissue supplied by the anterior cerebral, anterior choroidal, and the superior cerebellar arteries.[31] Infarction has also been recorded in

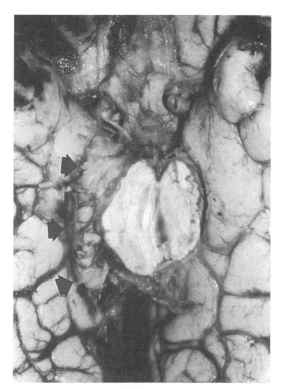

FIGURE 2–6. Tentorial hernia. There is a deep groove (*arrows*) in the right parahippocampal gyrus and hemorrhage in both the midline and the contralateral peduncle of the midbrain. Note the hemorrhage contusions on the lower aspects of the frontal and temporal lobes. An acute subdural hematoma had been removed surgically from the right side.

the anterior lobe of the pituitary gland in some 45 percent of cases.[32]

In certain categories of patients, there are strong indications for monitoring the ICP in the intensive care unit. During the initial phase of compensation with expansion of a mass lesion, there is obliteration of the subarachnoid space and a reduction in the size of the lateral ventricle ipsilateral to the mass lesion. If the lesion progresses in size, the ability of the brain to compensate for further expansion of the mass lesion becomes compromised. This period of decompensation occurs at the same time as internal herniation is developing. Eventually the hernias become impacted against the free edge of the falx, tentorium cerebelli, and foramen magnum, and a pressure differential is established between the intracranial compartments. Blood vessels normally present at the sites of internal herniation are at risk from compression by the hernias. The tentorial hernia, which consists of a mass lesion that herniates through the gap between the midbrain and the free edge of the tentorium cerebelli, is probably the most important. It distorts the upper brain stem, causing progressive motor dysfunction of the opposite limbs; hemorrhage into or infarction of the gray matter of the midbrain, causing a loss of consciousness; and compression of the ipsilateral oculomotor nerve between the posterior cerebral and the superior cerebellar arteries, causing a third nerve palsy. Further development of the process causes downward axial displacement of the brain stem, leading to impairment of respiration and ultimately apnea and, in a certain number of patients, the development of a Cushing response, identified by elevation of the blood pressure and bradycardia. The end result is vascular damage to the brain stem, often in the form of midline hemorrhages in the midbrain and pons. These vascular complications are thought to be a result of downward traction on the central perforating branches of the basilar artery, causing either direct rupture of the blood vessels or bleeding into areas of ischemic necrosis.

Death from secondary damage to the brain stem may be the result of one or more intracranial pathologies, such as contusion, brain swelling, and intracranial hematoma.

OTHER TYPES OF FOCAL BRAIN INJURY

In accidents that cause hyperextension of the head on the neck, traumatic separation of the pons and medulla is a well-recognized cause of death.[33,34] In many cases, there is an associated ring fracture at the base of the skull or dislocation and/or fracture of the first or second cervical vertebra. Although complete tears are immediately fatal, patients with small or incomplete tears at the pontomedullary junction may survive for some time after injury.[35–37]

Almost any of the cranial nerves may be damaged at the time of injury. The frequency with which injury to the cranial nerves occurs has been underestimated; MRI now provides a much more sensitive means of identifying damage than was previously possible with CT.[38]

Damage can also occur in the hypothalamus and pituitary gland. Occasionally the pituitary stalk is torn at the time of brain injury, but more frequently the stalk is intact, although there is infarction in the anterior lobe of the pituitary. A number of potential mechanisms have been put forward to explain this type of damage, including a fracture at the base of the skull that extends into the sella turcica, elevation of ICP that leads to distortion and compression of the pituitary stalk, and hypotensive shock analogous to postpartum necrosis of the pituitary.

Damage to blood vessels may also occur. It is now possible to identify by angiography various vascular lesions, including dissection or occlusion of the internal carotid or vertebral arteries, traumatic pseudoaneurysm, traumatic arteriovenous fistula, and venous thrombosis, and to assess vasospasm.

Imaging techniques after brain injury have shown that many patients have multiple lesions in the brain, some of which are hemorrhagic. The MRI is particularly useful in the detection of these lesions, the principal neuropathological correlates of which are lesions in lobar white matter, in the corpus callosum, and in the dorsolateral portions of the rostral brain stem adjacent to the superior cerebellar peduncles. These areas have since become known as the "shearing injury triad." However, such lesions are not restricted to these areas and are also found in periventricular structures, the hippocampal formation, the internal capsule, and occasionally deep within the cerebellar hemispheres.

Multiple petechial hemorrhages are not uncommonly found when patients die from severe brain injury. Although many of them may indeed have histological evidence of diffuse axonal injury (as discussed later), there are many other injuries, including diffuse vascular injury (also discussed later), in which the hemorrhages can be ascribed to a number of causes such as ischemic damage in the territory supplied by the pericallosal arteries—usually secondary to a supracallosal hernia, fat embolism, and a host of vascular and hematological abnormalities that constitute some of the medical complications of brain injury.

Diffuse Brain Injury

The term *diffuse brain injury* describes a number of pathologies, some of which are a consequence of acceleration-deceleration applied to white matter, others in which the injury is vascular in nature, and yet others that are secondary to hypoxia. Although these pathologies are widely distributed and in some instances are diffuse, the overall generic term *diffuse brain injury* is somewhat of a misnomer because in the majority of cases the pathology is multifocal.

DIFFUSE AXONAL INJURY

Diffuse axonal injury (DAI) has many synonyms and was first described under the heading of *diffuse degeneration of white matter.*[39] Since then, a variety of terms have been used that have helped to further characterize the entity (1) by mechanism, *shearing injury*[40,41]; (2) by location of the underlying pathology, *inner cerebral trauma*[42]; or (3) by combination of mechanism and the location of the principal path-

---

TABLE 2–5. Features of Diffuse Axonal Injury

1. A focal lesion in the corpus callosum and other midline structures involving the parasagittal white matter, the interventricular septum, and the walls of the third ventricle, with some intraventricular hemorrhage
2. A focal lesion in one or both dorsolateral sectors of the rostral brain stem
3. Microscopic evidence of widespread damage to axon

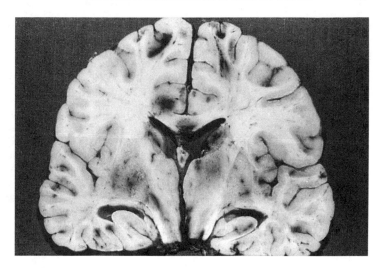

FIGURE 2–7. Diffuse axonal injury. Note the small hemorrhages in midline structures, including the parasagittal white matter ("gliding contusions"), the corpus callosum and intraventricular septum, and the cingulate gyrus.

ology, *diffuse damage of immediate impact type*[43] or *diffuse white matter shearing injury.*[44] There is now international recognition for the term *diffuse axonal injury.*[45,46]

In severe cases of diffuse axonal injury (Table 2–5), the hemorrhages in midline structures, including the brain stem, can usually be seen at the time of brain cutting (Fig. 2–7), in contrast to the widespread damage to axons that can be identified only microscopically. The histological appearances of the lesions depend on the length of survival after injury. If the patient survives for only a few days, midline structure lesions are usually hemorrhagic, but over time these result in shrunken, often cystic scars. However, the appearance of the important axonal lesions varies considerably over time. Thus, if survival is short (days), there are numerous axonal swellings and axonal bulbs,

which can be readily identified either as argyrophilic swellings in silver-stained preparations or by immunohistochemistry (Fig. 2–8). The swellings and bulbs are most commonly seen in deep structures and, in particular, the white matter of the parasagittal cortex, the corpus callosum, the internal capsule, and the long tracts of the brain stem. If survival extends to a number of weeks, the bulbs become less prominent, their site of formation now characterized by the development of clusters of microglia and macrophages. With even longer survival (months and years), neither bulbs nor microglia clusters can be seen, and axonal damage is recognized by the identification of the breakdown products of myelin. Therefore, in patients who survive severely disabled or in a vegetative state, abnormalities in the brain may be limited to small, healed, superficial contusions and exten-

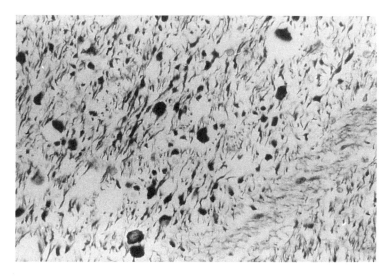

FIGURE 2–8. Diffuse axonal injury. Axonal swellings and bulbs in the brain stem. Palmgren ×320.

sive degeneration in the white matter. Coronal sections of such specimens reveal the characteristic features of relatively intact gray matter, a greatly reduced amount of central white matter, and compensatory enlargement of the ventricular system (Fig. 2–9). In most cases, it is still possible to identify the telltale focal lesions in the corpus callosum and the rostral brain stem.

Clinical and Pathological Grades of Diffuse Axonal Injury

With increasing experience it is apparent that DAI forms a distinct clinicopathological entity and is probably the principal pathological substrate that produces a continuum of neurological deficits from mild to severe brain injury. The entity was originally described in a series of patients in whom there was diffuse brain injury without an associated intracranial mass lesion (Fig. 2–10) and who accounted for about 35 percent of all deaths after brain injury.[4] Such patients were usually deeply comatose from the time of injury, with abnormal motor function consisting most frequently of extensive posturing of both the upper and lower limbs either spontaneously or in response to painful stimulation. The patients remained in this state for many weeks, during which time spontaneous eye opening returned, although in general they did not show an organized response to the environment, and recovery was limited to a severe disability or vegetative state. Under these circumstances, death was usually attributed to intercurrent infection. Evidence for a continuum was suggested in the late 1960s, when it was shown that occasional clusters of microglia can be found in patients dying from some unrelated cause soon after minor head injury.[47] These findings were confirmed by Clark,[48] who also drew attention to the frequent occurrence of clusters of microglia in the white matter of patients dying as a result of head injury, and Pilz[37] described the occurrence of axonal swellings in human brain injuries of varying severity. Further support for the concept of varying degrees of DAI was provided by Blumbergs et al.[49] In 1989 Adams et al.[50] introduced a new grading system. In grade 1, abnormalities were limited to histological evidence of axonal damage throughout the white matter with no focal accentuation in any of the midline structures. Cases were designated grade 2 if, in addition to the widely distributed axonal injury, there was also a focal lesion in the corpus callosum. Grade 3 DAI, the most severe, was characterized by diffuse damage to axons in the presence of focal lesions in both the corpus callosum and the brain stem. Further refinement of this grading system introduced subdivisions of grades 2 and 3 in which M indicated that the focal midline lesion could be seen macroscopically and m indicated that it could be identified only histologically. Associated clinicopathological correlations indicated that the lesser degrees of axonal injury could be associated with either a complete or partial lucid interval. Indeed, of the 122 cases studied by Adams et al.[50] there were two patients with a completely lucid interval who had grade 1 injury and 15 with grade 2 DAI with a partially lucid interval. In contrast, none of the patients with grade 3 DAI talked. The use of immunohistochemistry has further clarified the situation in that by using antibodies against amyloid precursor protein (APP) evidence of axonal damage has been found in a small series of patients who died from causes other than those associated with a previously sustained mild brain injury.[51] Immunohistochemistry has also provided greater

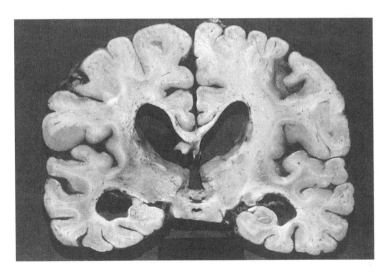

FIGURE 2–9. Diffuse axonal injury. Enlargement of the ventricular system in a patient who survived in a vegetative state for 21 months after a brain injury.

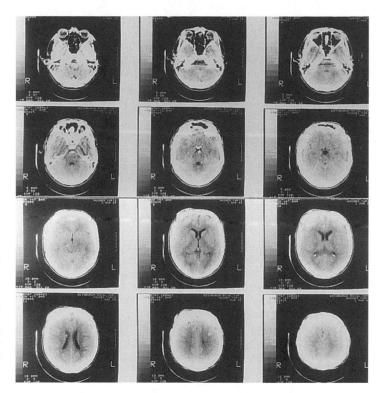

FIGURE 2–10. CT series in a patient with diffuse brain damage. The patient was rendered immediately and deeply unconscious (E_1, M_2, V_1) by a high-speed traffic accident. Small hemorrhages are scattered widely in the brain, but the ventricular system shows no compensation or shift, indicating that ICP is not increased. Reproduced with permission.

insight into the distribution of axonal damage after brain injury, and Blumbergs et al.[52] have derived a sector scoring method, the sensitivity of which allows the identification of variable amounts of axonal injury (and other pathologies) in patients with a wide range of Glasgow Coma Scores.

Even if it takes between 15 and 18 hours for axonal bulbs to be identified with certainty by using silver impregnation techniques in the human brain after injury, it is likely that, as revealed by the more sensitive technique of immunohistochemistry, the incidence of DAI is higher than the published figures would suggest. Indeed, a recent study shows that axonal injury of varying amounts is almost a universal finding in cases of fatal brain injury[53,54] and that, furthermore, damage to axons can now be identified in those whose survival has been as short as 3 hours.[55,56] However, at present a definitive diagnosis cannot be made in patients who survive for less than 3 hours, although DAI may be strongly suspected, particularly if there are focal lesions in the corpus callosum and in the brain stem.

Mechanisms of Axonal Injury

There have been considerable advances in the understanding of the nature and time course of axonal injury in the last 5 years.[57–59] The classi-cal view that axons are torn at the moment of injury—primary axotomy (immediate axonal disruption)—no longer appears to be true in most cases, although it does occur under conditions of high mechanical loading, such as a pontomedullary rent. In contrast, in conditions of mild to moderate brain injury, it is now apparent that there are processes of delayed axotomy, in which the affected axons become lobulated after 6 to 12 hours, and secondary axotomy, which occurs between 24 and 72 hours. Recent experimental work suggests that the time course of secondary axotomy is influenced by the species, the injury model, and the intensity of the injury.[59–62] In general, the time taken for secondary axotomy to occur in cats and pigs is longer than in rats and is longest in humans.

A well-recognized feature of axonal injury is Wallerian degeneration. Not until recently has the importance of deafferentation of various target sites been recognized,[63] one consequence of which is a phase of excitation.[64–67] Such changes might provide a possible explanation not only for the immediate morbidity but also for subsequent adaptive plasticity and associated recovery.

It has been suggested that physical stretch—mechanoporation at the time of injury—results in damage to the axolemma and related axoplasm at the injured node of Ranvier.[68,69] This change in membrane structure disrupts the capability of axons to maintain physiological ionic gradients and results in changes in concentrations of calcium, potassium, sodium, and chloride within the axoplasm. These changes in ion concentration in certain fibers may activate neutral proteases, which, in turn, denature the axonal cytoarchitecture. However, this hypothesis has not been universally accepted, an alternative view being that traumatic brain injury can either mechanically or functionally disturb the neurofilament subunits, thereby impairing axoplasmic transport.[62,70] Although changes in all three neurofilament subunits were identified, it was found that antibodies to the 68 kd subunit were particularly useful, in that within 60 minutes of brain injury there was a highly localized degradation of this subunit. These views are not necessarily incompatible or irreconcilable because it is increasingly apparent that the changes are complex, that there are both direct and indirect consequences of mechanical loading, and that ensuing functional impairment is a product of many factors,[71] which may not include morphologic abnormality.[72]

ISCHEMIC BRAIN DAMAGE

Neuropathological studies in the 1970s suggested that irreversible brain damage as a result of ischemia was common not only after fatal blunt brain injury, in large measure could be attributed to a critical reduction in regional cerebral blood flow (CBF), and therefore was potentially avoidable. An early study showed that irreversible damage was present in more than 90 percent of cases: It was classified as severe in 27 percent, moderately severe in 43 percent, and mild in 30 percent.[73] The lesions occurred more frequently within the hippocampus (>80%) and in the basal ganglia (about 80%) than in the cerebral cortex (46%) and in the cerebellum (44%). Clinicopathological correlations reported associations with episodes of hypoxia and raised ICP. Because much of this damage was considered avoidable or preventable, this study led to the reappraisal of the management and organization of patient care, with increased attention to recognition and treatment of hypoxia and hypotension at the scene of the accident, during interhospital transfer, and in critical care units and to the detection and release of brain compression by traumatic intracranial hematoma. Reappraisal of the amount of distribution of ischemic damage in a second cohort of fatal blunt brain injuries was carried out by Graham et al.[74] and in the same group some 10 years later, in which it was found that ischemic brain damage was still common (88% of cases), and there was no statistical difference in the amount of moderately severe and severe ischemic damage between the two groups of patients—55 percent (1968–1972) and 54 percent (1981–1982) respectively. There was an increase in the proportion of cases with diffuse damage in the cortex of the type seen in global cerebral ischemia, which was rather surprising, as it would have been expected that the greater use of resuscitative measures would have reduced this type of brain damage to some extent. Likely explanations were that the critical events responsible for these changes may have occurred almost immediately after the injury, before admission to a hospital, and even before the arrival of skilled personnel at the scene of the accident. Further explanation lay in the fact that the admission policy to the department of neurosurgery had changed, with more patients with an intracranial mass lesion being admitted for investigation and treatment, some of whom under previous guidelines would probably have died either in the ED or in the primary surgical ward.

Early clinical studies of acute brain injury had failed to demonstrate any evidence of cerebral ischemia.[75] However, subsequent work showed that CBF was reduced to threshold levels (≤ 18 mL/100 g/min) in one-third of patients within the first 6 hours of injury and that a significant correlation existed between motor score and cerebral blood flow in the first 8 hours after injury.[76] Further work using xenon-CT CBF measurements showed that during the first 4 hours after brain injury, patients without a surgical mass lesion showed a trend toward low initial flow with subsequent increases in CBF at 24 hours and that CBF in the first 24 hours after injury was significantly correlated with a low initial Glasgow Coma Score. Such studies suggest that reductions in either regional or global CBF with subsequent ischemia may occur within the first hours after severe injury and that a decreased perfusion might have important effects on brain viability and the subsequent outcome.

Although the suggested presence of true ischemia in the acute post-traumatic period remains rather controversial, it seems likely that the early postinjury period is associated with concomitant alterations of brain metabolism that may create a relative ischemia in vulnerable brain areas.[77–81] Under these conditions, it is postulated that there is an acute increase in glucose utilization and energy demand, coupled with a global hypoperfusion or oligemia, and that this may therefore reflect a state of relative ischemia that may adversely affect ion homeostasis, membrane function, and neuronal survival.

Several mechanisms may contribute to posttraumatic reduction in CBF that may ultimately lead to cerebral ischemia and infarction: the stretching and distortion of brain vessels as a result of mechanical displacement of brain structures, such as brain shift or herniation caused by intracranial mass lesion (as discussed earlier); arterial hypotension in association with multiple injuries; vasospasm of blood vessels in the circle of Willis; and post-traumatic changes in small blood vessels.[82–84] The role of vasospasm as a potential mechanism underlying the development of post-traumatic hypoperfusion has been emphasized recently by the use of transcranial Doppler ultrasonography.[85–87]

Secondary Insults

There is little doubt now that primary traumatic damage to the brain may be made worse by the superimposition of so-called secondary insults occurring soon after the injury, during transfer to the hospital, and during the subsequent treatment of the brain injured patient. Such insults may be of either intracranial or systemic origin and may actually arise during initial management or later in the intensive care unit. The full extent of these secondary insults became apparent between 1970 and 1985, when a number of researchers reported that in severely brain injured patients hypoxia was found in 30 percent and arterial hypotension in 15 percent on arrival in the ED. Largely because of better on-site resuscitation and transport arrangements, there has been a reduction of these early insults, attention now being directed toward the increasing awareness that such events after brain injury may actually occur within the intensive care unit. This awareness has largely been a result of continuous monitoring during intensive care and the correlations that exist between the adverse influences of these secondary insults and the clinical outcome. Current experience suggests that secondary insults occur more frequently and last longer than previously had been thought and that the duration of these insults is as important as their severity. Even the lowest grade of insult severity has been shown to have an adverse effect on outcome, although apparently the most relevant predictors of mortality at 12 months after injury have been the durations of hypotension, pyrexia, and hypoxemia.

DIFFUSE (MULTIFOCAL) VASCULAR INJURY

A form of acute brain injury after trauma is characterized by a series of multiple small hemorrhages that are particularly conspicuous in the white matter of the frontal and temporal lobes, in and adjacent to the thalamus, and in the brain stem. Small hemorrhages may also be seen in parasagittal white matter and in the corpus callosum. This pattern of brain damage is seen in patients who die either instantly or at the scene of the accident, although a number may survive for up to 24 hours. It is thought to represent a severe form of brain injury in which, as a result of acceleration-deceleration, tearing has occurred in small blood vessels. The relationship between this entity and that of diffuse (multifocal) axonal injury has yet to be defined.

SWELLING OF THE BRAIN

Swelling of the brain may be either localized or generalized and may occur either alone or in combination with other pathologies. In general, brain swelling is caused by an increase in the cerebral blood volume (congestive brain swelling) or in the water content of the brain tissue (cerebral edema). Brain swelling may contribute to an elevation of the ICP and death from secondary damage to the brain stem.

Swelling of the Brain Adjacent to Contusions, Lacerations, or an Intracerebral Hematoma

As a result of damage to the blood-brain barrier, water, electrolytes, and protein leak into brain tissue and spread into the adjacent white matter to form vasogenic edema readily detected within 24 to 48 hours of injury by CT or MRI. In many cases it reaches its peak between 4 and 8 days after injury, but it is largely caused by a combination of vascular damage, inadequate cerebral perfusion, and retention of fluid within the extracellular space. Therefore, this type of swelling is easy to understand when it occurs adjacent to contusions and lacerations.

Swelling of One Cerebral Hemisphere

Swelling of one cerebral hemisphere is most often seen in association with an ipsilateral acute subdural hematoma. When the hematoma is evacuated, the brain expands to fill the space (Fig. 2–11). The pathogenesis of this entity has not been fully determined, but it is probably caused by reperfusion of a vascular bed that has lost its physiological tone as a result of the mass effect of a subdural hematoma. When this vascular bed is reperfused, the blood vessels dilate, the blood-brain barrier becomes leaky, and there is diffuse swelling of one cerebral hemisphere, which in large measure is a consequence of vasogenic edema.

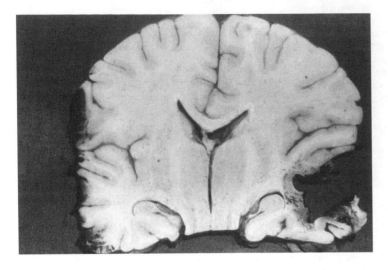

FIGURE 2–11. Unilateral brain swelling. There are bilateral superficial contusions and diffuse swelling of the right cerebral hemisphere on the same side as an acute subdural hematoma that had been evacuated.

Diffuse Swelling of Both Cerebral Hemispheres

This is a feature seen in children and young adults. If it is fatal, the brain is swollen diffusely and the ventricles are small and symmetrical. In a detailed neuropathological study of 63 fatally brain injured children aged from 2 to 15 years, diffuse brain swelling was found in 17 percent of cases. In a few, the swelling was associated with widespread hypoxic brain damage, secondary to post-traumatic status epilepticus or cardiorespiratory arrest. In most cases it was idiopathic, with the assumption that, like diffuse swelling of one cerebral hemisphere, the main etiology was reperfusion of a vascular bed that had become unresponsive to physiological stimuli after brain injury.[88] At first, vasodilatation induces a defective blood-brain barrier, leading to true vasogenic edema. However, neuroimaging has produced inconsistent results.

NEUROCHEMICAL AND CELLULAR CHANGES

Post-traumatic neurochemical alterations are likely to involve changes in the synthesis and/or release of both endogenous "neuroprotective" and "autodestructive" compounds. The identification of these compounds from the timing of the pathological cascade after brain injury provides a window of opportunity for treatment with pharmacological agents designed to modify gene expression, synthesis and release of transmitters, receptor binding, or the physiological activity of these factors with subsequent prevention or attenuation of neuronal damage. Some of the more important changes are described in the following paragraphs.

Acetylcholine

An increase in the concentration of acetylcholine in the brain has been reported after experimental traumatic brain injury. Other studies have shown a decrease in the binding of cholinergic receptors, and fluid percussion brain injury in the rat significantly decreases the affinity of muscarinic cholinergic receptor binding in both hippocampus and brain stem, changes that may last as long as 15 days after injury.[89,90] These and other data have led to the suggestion that activation of muscarinic cholinergic systems in the rostral pons mediates behavioral suppression associated with traumatic brain injury and that lasting behavioral deficits result from pathological excitation of forebrain structures induced by the release of acetylcholine. More recently, controlled cortical impact in the rat has been shown to cause an impairment of cholinergic neurons, which produces enhanced vulnerability to disruption of cholinergically mediated cognitive function, and previous studies have shown that administration of the anticholinergic compound scopolamine reduces neurobehavioral dysfunction after experimental brain injury in rats. In a recent preliminary study of presynaptic and postsynaptic markers of cholinergic transmission in human postmortem brain from patients who died after brain injury and matched controls, the mean value of choline acetyltransferase activity was reduced by about 50 percent in the brain injured group. In contrast, there was no difference between the brain injured and control groups in the levels of M1 or M2 receptor binding.[91] Given the involvement of acetylcholine in cognitive function, reduced cholinergic acetyltransferase activity may be associated with cognitive impairment in patients who survive a brain injury.

Arachidonic Acid Cascade

Damage to the cell membrane by calcium-activated proteases and lipases induces the production of a variety of potentially pathogenic agents from a breakdown of endogenous intracellular fatty acids. The formation of such compounds such as arachidonic acid activated to phospholipase A_2 lipo-oxygenase, cyclo-oxygenase, and various agents such as leukotrienes, thromboxanes, free fatty acids, and other breakdown products with arachidonic acid cascade have now been associated with neuronal death and poor outcome in models of experimental brain injury.[92–98]

Catecholamine and Monoamine Neurotransmitters

Laboratory studies have shown that circulating levels of epinephrine and norepinephrine increase with increasing severity of injury and that there are regional changes in the tissue concentration of them and of dopamine after experimental fluid percussion and controlled cortical impact brain injury in rats.[99,100] Other studies have shown changes in α_1-adrenergic receptor binding in damaged cortex and hippocampus after experimental lateral fluid percussion in the rat.[101]

It has also been suggested that activation of the serotonergic (5-HT) system plays a role, and an increase in 5-HT has been shown to be closely associated with the depression of local cerebral glucose utilization in regions showing extensive histological damage.[102,103]

Cytokines

The number of immunocompetent cells is increased in the plasma of brain injured patients, and it is possible that, because the blood-brain barrier is opened often for long periods, these cells may enter the injured brain and exert a neurotoxic effect.[104] Polymorphonuclear leukocytes accumulate within 24 hours in injured brain,[105] which correlates with the onset of post-traumatic brain swelling in rats.[106] However, experimentally induced neutropenia does not appear to influence the development of post-traumatic edema or reduce cortical lesion volume, although a decrease in volume after occlusion of the middle cerebral artery in immunosuppressed (neutropenic) rats has been described.[107] Macrophages undoubtedly play an important role in wound healing, and many of them secrete soluble factors, including cytokines that may influence post-traumatic neuronal survivability and outcome. Moreover, injured neuronal and nonneuronal cells within the central nervous system (CNS) can synthe-

size and secrete inflammatory cytokines that may mediate further brain damage. Among the cytokines implicated in this additional damage are tumor necrosis factor and the interleukin family of peptides. For example, after mechanical trauma to the brain, there is a large increase in the regional brain concentration of interleukin-1, interleukin-6, and tumor necrosis factor, suggesting that the CNS-derived cytokines may play a role in the pathophysiological cascade of brain damage after trauma.[108–111]

Endogenous Opioid Peptides

The regional immunoreactivity of the endogenous opioid dynorphin increases after a fluid percussion brain injury, which has been shown to correlate with structural brain damage and reductions in regional CBF.[112,113] Furthermore, both the intracerebroventricular and intraparenchymal microinjection of dynorphin and other κ-agonists worsens neurological injury, suggesting that, indeed, dynorphin has a pathogenic effect after brain injury.[114] However, pharmacological studies suggest that the effect is indirect and that it may be mediated by other neurotransmitter or neurochemical systems, including the excitatory amino acids glutamate and aspartate, an effect that can be reversed by both competitive and noncompetitive N-methyl-D-aspartate (NMDA) antagonists.[115] Although the mechanisms by which dynorphin induces NMDA receptor-mediated activity remain speculative, recent studies suggest that opioids may modulate the presynaptic release of excitatory amino acid neurotransmitters, thereby contributing to regional neuronal damage during the acute post-traumatic period.[116]

Excitatory Amino Acids

The extracellular excitatory amino acids (EEAs) glutamate and aspartate increase markedly after traumatic brain injury.[66,117–119] Although the amount varies in different models of traumatic brain injury, there is a close association between the increased intracellular concentration and total tissue concentrations of sodium and calcium.[120,121] The exact mechanisms underlying EAA-mediated cell death are not well understood, but it has been postulated that the sustained release of glutamate with prolonged postsynaptic excitation causes the early accumulation of intracellular sodium. This, in turn, leads to acute neuronal swelling and delayed calcium influx, which cause a cascade of metabolic disturbances within neurons that may lead eventually to cell death. These findings suggest that post-traumatic cognitive deficits may result partly from excitotoxic events, specifically targeting the hippocampus and inducing overt neuronal cell loss, cellular stress, and/or dysfunction, thereby disrupting normal synaptic transmission.[122]

Growth Factors

The potential of neurons and glial cells to recover after traumatic brain injury depends on both the post-traumatic ionic-neurotransmitter environment and the presence of neurotrophic substances (growth factors). They support nerve cell survival, induce the sprouting of neurites (plasticity), and facilitate the guidance of neurites to their proper target sites. The best-characterized neurotrophic factors include nerve growth factor (NGF), basic fibroblast growth factor (FGF), brain-derived neurotrophic factor, glial-derived neurotrophic factor, and NT-3. Some recent studies have suggested that these factors are synthesized or released after traumatic CNS injury and that their concentration increases during the first few days after a number of experimental procedures.[123,124] Relatively little is known about the neurotrophic factor response in experimental traumatic brain injury,[125] but NGF and FGF-like neurotrophic activity has been observed to increase in the CSF of brain injured patients.[126] The intraparenchymal infusion of NGF over 14 days after injury has also been reported to reduce septohippocampal cellular damage and improve neurobehavioral motor and cognitive function after fluid percussion brain injury in rats.[127] A neuroprotective effect of FGF has also been found in a rodent model of cortical contusion.[128]

Ion Changes

The principal ion changes are in calcium, magnesium, and potassium. Changes in calcium ion homeostasis are believed to be pivotal in the development of neuronal cell death. For example, total brain tissue calcium concentrations have recently been found to be significantly elevated in injured areas after both experimental fluid percussion brain injury and cortical contusion in rats,[129] and a significant increase in regional calcium accumulation has been shown to persist for at least 48 hours after fluid percussion brain injury in rats.[130] In support of this hypothesis is the finding of increased expression of some of the immediate early genes after fluid percussion injury; these genes are known to be activated by increase in intracellular calcium.[110]

Magnesium is involved in a number of critical cellular processes, and alterations in tissue magnesium impair maintenance of normal intracellular sodium and potassium gradients. After traumatic injury to the CNS, there is a reduction in brain magnesium, which is hypothesized to impair glucose utilization, energy metabolism, and protein synthesis, thereby reducing both oxidative and substrate level phosphorylation.[131,132] Because magnesium has an important regulatory role with respect to calcium transport and accumulation and to cerebrovascular contractility, changes in intracellular magnesium could potentially contribute to post-traumatic calcium-mediated neurotoxicity and/or the regulation of regional post-traumatic blood flow.

After experimental brain injury, there is a rapid and massive increase in the release of potassium into the extracellular space, which can be associated with burst discharges, depolarization, and spreading depression.[133,134] The increase in extracellular potassium has been thought to contribute to disruption of energy homeostasis, cerebral vasoconstriction, changes in cerebral glycolysis, and loss of consciousness.[135] The excess extracellular potassium is rapidly taken up by astrocytes, which may result in astrocytic edema, and this, in turn, may impair neuronal oxygen transport.

Oxygen-Free Radicals and Lipid Peroxidation

Hypoperfusion of brain tissue may stimulate the generation of oxygen-free radicals, principal among which is superoxide. Superoxide may arise from a number of sources that include the arachidonic acid cascade, the autooxidation of amine neurotransmitters, mitochondria leakage, xanthine oxidase activity, and oxidation-extravasated hemoglobin.[136,137] Additional sources, at least in the first few hours and days after trauma, may be activated microglia, infiltrating neutrophils, and macrophages. Within the injured nervous system, where pH is lowered, conditions are also favorable for the potential release of iron, which may then participate in the formation of hydroxy radicals. Iron also promotes the process of lipid peroxidation. Multiple studies have now shown that cats subjected to fluid percussion injury have early generation of superoxide radicals in the injured brain and that the degeneration of these radicals occurs in parallel with secondary injury to the brain and its microvasculature, including the formation of vasogenic brain edema.[135–137]

□ EXPERIMENTAL MODELS OF FOCAL AND DIFFUSE TRAUMATIC BRAIN INJURY

Although our understanding of traumatic brain injury has been greatly enhanced by the use of physical, computer, and cell culture models, it has been necessary to provide biologic validation of them by parallel animate models, in which the studies are designed to replicate certain aspects of human brain injury. Such models have been used extensively to investigate the precise mechanisms leading to the various sequelae of brain injury that may have an origin in focal, diffuse, or both types of brain injury. However, there is an increasing appreciation that, although the various pathologies may be described and characterized as either focal or diffuse and pure examples of each exist in clinical practice, there is considerable overlap between them.

Models of Focal Traumatic Brain Injury

In general, three techniques are commonly used to produce experimental focal brain injury: weight drop,[138,139] fluid percussion,[140–142] and rigid indentation.[143–145] Each of these techniques may be adjusted to generate a reproducible spectrum of injury severity.[146]

All three models typically produce focal contusion of the cortex, which histologically appears as hemorrhagic foci of necrosis that undergo changes characterized by absorption of the dead tissue, scarring, and development of a cavity. A further feature of the contusion is local disruption of the blood-brain barrier, but change is also seen well beyond the immediate vicinity of the contusion. This disruption facilitates formation of vasogenic edema, decreases in regional CBF, and an increase in glucose metabolism. Although blood flow from the contusion may not be at critical levels, it is now apparent that oligemia, in association with a hypermetabolic response to trauma, creates an injury-induced vulnerability; following traumatic injury, the brain may be at risk to even minor changes in CBF, increases in ICP, and apnea (as discussed previously).

With survival, there is a cellular response to the traumatic injury. For example, neutrophil polymorphs increase in number by 24 hours and migrate into the necrotic tissue. This process is followed by activation of microglia and the development of macrophages, which are particularly prominent at the sites of contusion. However, activation of microglia is also present throughout regions demonstrating disruption of the blood-brain barrier, including the hippocampus and thalamus. The cellular changes herald expression of cytokines and other markers of injury, including heat shock protein and immediate early genes. A very rapid and florid astrocytic response defines the margins of the contusion with the establishment of a glial limitans.

Many of the models show evidence of more widely distributed pathology. Changes include tissue tears in the dentate gyrus of the ipsilat-

eral hemisphere and axonal swellings and bulb formation in the white matter of both the ipsilateral and contralateral hemispheres.

Reference has been made to the concept of primary and secondary brain damage, with the implication that the latter is not restricted to brain injury but is the consequence of a further insult to an already damaged brain. Additional evidence is the identification of changes in various neuronal populations remote from the site of contusion. A number of mechanisms might account for these lesions, and their importance has been demonstrated by the finding that lesions in the CA-3 subfield and hilum of the dentate gyrus correlate with the severity of post-traumatic memory dysfunction.[145]

Models of Diffuse Traumatic Brain Injury

Typically, these models attempt to replicate the human clinicopathological entity of DAI, in which there is widespread microscopic evidence of damage to the axons. Damage to axons under these conditions has been shown to be produced primarily by high-strain rotational or angular acceleration, not necessarily associated with impact. Until relatively recently, only one animal model replicated all of the clinical features of DAI, the Penn-2 model, using nonhuman primates.[45,46] This model enabled a spectrum of pathology, the exact nature of which depended on the biomechanical profile of the injury. For example, rapid rotation acceleration in the sagittal plane produced subdural hematomas, whereas a slower acceleration in the coronal plane produced DAI.[147]

A porcine model of rotational acceleration brain injury was developed recently,[148] but, although axonal injury has been produced in subcortical white matter, it has not been possible to induce tissue tears or gliding contusions, and this injury is associated with only brief loss of consciousness.[149]

A rat model of impact acceleration brain injury, in which a weight is dropped onto a plate fixed to the cranium, has been shown to produce widely distributed axonal damage.[150] Unlike most brain injury models, the head is not fixed in place, and is allowed to rotate downward. It has been suggested that this motion, in combination with impact, results in the overt widespread damage to axons.

☐ OUTCOME AFTER BLUNT HEAD INJURY

The early and long-term neurobehavioral sequelae of mild to moderate blunt head injury are well known.[151-153] More recently, the role of behavioral outcome after severe head injury has also been studied, with particular emphasis on the relationship to structural and functional imaging.[154] In particular, predictors of recovery are duration of coma, resolution of post-traumatic amnesia, and long-term recovery of cognitive function, including memory. Although the precise structural basis of these various deficits is not known, they are more likely to be caused by diffuse or multiple foci of damage than by single focal lesions.

Many patients who sustain a blunt head injury make a good recovery. Others remain moderately or severely disabled or remain in the vegetative state.[155,156] The rapid growth of resuscitation and intensive care has now made the survival of patients with severe brain damage commonplace, with its medical, ethical, and legal implications.[157]

Severe Disability and Vegetative State

The neuropathology of severe disability after blunt head injury has been well studied,[158-161] with particular emphasis on the frequency of structural abnormalities in the rostral brain stem, intracranial mass lesions, brain swelling, and systemic hypoxia, in the belief that post-traumatic encephalopathy is, on the whole, due to secondary traumatic lesions and their sequelae. However, these conclusions were at variance with those of Strich,[162] who had earlier placed particular emphasis on the presence of diffuse brain damage in patients who remained vegetative after blunt head injury and on the failure to identify any cases of prolonged post-traumatic coma in which damage was confined to the brain stem.

The relative importance of focal versus diffuse pathology in the genesis of severe disability and the vegetative state became apparent after a comprehensive neuropathological analysis of 25 patients who had survived for more than 4 weeks after a blunt head injury.[163] Diffuse axonal injury was found in 22 cases. In 10 of these there was also moderate to severe ischemic brain damage, and in 2 there were midline lesions in the brain stem of the type associated with raised intracranial pressure and tentorial herniation. There was moderate to severe ischemic brain damage in 12 of the 25 cases, and in 8 of them there was also damage of the secondary type in the brain stem. In only one case was damage confined to the brain stem. These findings suggest that patients with intracranial expanding lesions who develop tentorial herniation and other secondary types of brain damage rarely survive for more than a few weeks.

This whole subject remains somewhat controversial, not only because there are problems of nomenclature but also in the interpretation of the pathogenesis of lesions in the brain stem, although the structural abnormalities indicative of DAI are the most common. Therefore, there seems to be increasing evidence from clinicopathological studies that the commonest causes of the vegetative state and severe disability after blunt head injury are DAI and diffuse ischemic brain damage. In a comprehensive recent review of the neuropathology of the persistent vegetative state after acute brain injury, three main patterns of damage were identified: widespread bilateral damage to the neocortex, diffuse damage to white matter, and bilateral damage to the thalamus.[164]

Hydrocephalus

In the acute phase, hydrocephalus is likely to be caused by large amounts of blood within the subarachnoid space, whereas, with survival, ventricular enlargement is probably secondary to fibrosis and hemosiderosis of the meninges. In each case, the basic problem is an impairment of absorption of CSF by the arachnoid granulations into the superior sagittal sinus. However, in patients who survive a blunt head injury, ventricular enlargement, whether symmetrical or not, is likely to be caused by a number of other pathological conditions. For example, in patients with DAI or severe ischemic brain damage, the ventricles enlarge, usually symmetrically as a result of widespread or multifocal brain damage, whereas the enlargement is asymmetrical if the pathology is focal, such as after healed contusions, intracerebral hematoma, or infarction.

Progressive Neurological Disease

Post-traumatic epilepsy is discussed in Chapters 4 and 6. Although there are reports of a possible connection between history of brain injury and Alzheimer's disease,[165-168] Pick's disease,[169] Parkinson's disease,[170] motor neuron disease (in U.K. and Europe; known as amyotrophic lateral sclerosis in the U.S.), and Creutzfeldt-Jakob disease,[171] a direct correlation between any of these disorders and a previous brain injury has not yet been established.

It is well recognized that repeated concussive or subconcussive blows as experienced by various athletes and particularly by boxers sometimes induces the development of neurological signs and progressive dementia.[172–175] This condition, known as *dementia pugilistica,* may develop some years after the last injury and is most likely to develop in boxers with long careers who have been dazed, if not knocked out, on many occasions. In a detailed study of the brains of 15 ex-boxers,[176] one of the characteristic patterns of damage was the presence of many neurofibrillary tangles diffusely throughout the cerebral cortex and the brain stem. These tangles broadly conform to the topographical pattern found in Alzheimer's disease. Further support for the possible association between a history of previous brain injury and Alzheimer's disease has been found after a further examination of the original cohort of patients studied by Corsellis et al.,[176] supplemented by material obtained from patients subjected to domestic violence,[177,178] in which it has been possible to demonstrate large numbers of diffuse plaques composed of β-amyloid. These studies suggest a similarity between the molecular neuropathology of dementia pugilistica and Alzheimer's disease.[179]

Diffuse plaques of β-amyloid have also been found in some 30 percent of fatal brain injuries.[180] Although they do not colocalize with the various pathologies of blunt head injury, they are found in association with an increased immunoreactivity of the precursor protein APP.[181] Sustained or repeated increased expression might trigger a sequence of events culminating in Alzheimer's disease by the overproduction or sustained production of APP, a subsequent increase in β-amyloid, and its deposition after cleavage as diffuse plaques, perhaps mediated through glial cytokines.[182–184]

The recent demonstration of an association between apolipoprotein E ε4 allele and the deposition of β-amyloid after brain injury[185] has provided a better understanding of the influence of genetic factors that may underlie the varying susceptibilities; in particular, there is an apo E genotype influence on both the immediate acute phase response and possibly the long-term pathological outcome after brain injury.[186] These findings suggest that apo E genotype influences the outcome after brain injury, and the mechanism underlying this relationship is as yet unclear. Of likely relevance is the observation that apo E binds to β-amyloid, promoting the formation of amyloid fibrils, and that the ε4 isoform of apo E is most efficient in this process.[187,188] The first clinical studies to look at the influence of the apo E genotype on outcome after acute brain injury suggest that it plays a significant role. In a recent study, for example, a higher frequency of apo E ε4 was reported in patients who did not recover from post-traumatic coma than in those who did recover consciousness.[189] These findings suggest a potential for predicting outcome based on apo E genotype,[190] either as a potential risk factor in certain occupations or leisure pursuits or as an index of likelihood of recovery after brain injury. No doubt the apo E genotype is but one of a host of factors that determine the ultimate outcome after head injury.

REFERENCES

1. Reilly, PL, et al: Patients with head injury who talk and die. Lancet 2:375, 1975.
2. Marshall, LF, Toole, BM, and Bowers, SA: The national coma data bank: Patients who talk and deteriorate: Implications for treatment. J Neurosurg 59:285, 1983.
3. Graham, DI, et al: Pathology of brain damage in head injury. In Cooper, PR (ed): Head Injury, ed 3. Williams & Wilkins, Baltimore, 1993, p 91.
4. Gennarelli, TA: Head injury in man and experimental animals: Clinical aspects. Acta Neurochir Suppl (Wien) 32:1, 1983.
5. Gennarelli, TA, and Thibault, LE: Biological models of head injury. In Becker, JP, and Povlishock, JT (eds): Central Nervous System Trauma Status Report. NINCDS, Bethesda, Md, 1985, p 591.
6. Graham, DI, and Gennarelli, TA: Trauma. In Graham DI, and Lantos PL (eds): Greenfield's Neuropathology, ed 6. Edward Arnold, London, 1997.
7. Jennett, JB, and Teasdale, G (eds): Management of Head Injuries. FA Davis, Philadelphia, 1981.
8. Mendelow, AD, Teasdale, G, and Jennett, B: Risks of intracranial haematoma in head injured adults. BMJ 287:1173, 1983.
9. Cooper, PR: Post traumatic intracranial mass lesions. In Cooper, PR (ed): Head Injury, ed 3. Williams & Wilkins, Baltimore, 1993, p 275.
10. Adams, JH: Head injury. In Adams, JH, and Duchen, LW (eds): Greenfield's Neuropathology, ed 5. Edward Arnold, London, 1992, p 106.
11. Adams, JH, et al: The contusion index: A reappraisal in human and experimental non-missile head injury. Neuropathol Appl Neurobiol 11:299, 1985.
12. Ryan, GA, McLean, AJ, and Vilenius, ATS: Brain injury patterns in fatally injured pedestrians. J Trauma 36:469, 1994.
13. Rockswold, GL, Leonard, PR, and Nagib, ME: Analysis of management in thirty-three closed injury patients who "talked and deteriorated." Neurosurgery 21:51, 1987.
14. Klauber, MR, et al: Determinants of head injury mortality: Importance of the low risk patient. Neurosurgery 24:31, 1989.
15. Bullock, R, and Teasdale, G: Surgical management of traumatic intracranial hematomas. In Braackman, R (ed): Handbook of Clinical Neurology, vol 15, Head Injury. Elsevier, Amsterdam, 1990, p 249.
16. Freytag, E: Autopsy findings in head injuries from blunt forces. Arch Pathol 75:402, 1963.
17. Maloney, AJF, and Whatmore, WJ: Clinical and pathological observations in fatal head injuries: A 5-year study of 172 cases. Br J Surg 56:23, 1969.
18. Jamieson, KG, and Yelland, JDN: Extradural hematoma: Report of 167 cases. J Neurosurg 29:13, 1968.
19. Lewin, W: Acute subdural and extradural haematoma in closed head injury. Ann R Coll Surg Engl 5:240, 1949.
20. McKissock, W, et al: Extradural haematoma: Observations on 125 cases. Lancet 2:167, 1960.
21. Bullock, R, Smith, RM, and van Dellen, JR: Nonoperative management of extradural hematoma. Neurosurgery 16:602, 1985.

22. Harland, WA, Pitts, JF, and Watson, AA: Subarachnoid haemorrhage due to upper cervical trauma. J Clin Pathol 36:1335, 1983.

23. Vanezis, P: Techniques used in the evaluation of vertebral trauma at post mortem. Forensic Sci Int 13:159, 1979.

24. Vanezis, P: Vertebral artery injuries in road-traffic accidents: A post-mortem study. J Forensic Sci Soc 26:281, 1986.

25. Fogelholm, R, and Waltimo, O: Epidemiology of chronic subdural haematoma. Acta Neurochir (Wien) 32:247, 1975.

26. Marshall, LF, Toole, BM, and Bowers, SA: The national traumatic coma data bank. Part 2: Patients who talk and deteriorate: Implications for treatment. J Neurosurg 59:285, 1983.

27. Nanassis, K, Frowein, RA, and Karimi, A: Delayed post-traumatic intracerebral bleeding. Neurosurg Rev 12 (suppl 1):243, 1989.

28. Elsner, H, et al: Delayed traumatic intracerebral hematomas. J Neurosurg 72:813, 1990.

29. Macpherson, P, et al: The significance of traumatic haematoma in the region of the basal ganglia. J Neurol Neurosurg Psychiatry 49:29, 1986.

30. Adams, JH, et al: Deep intracerebral (basal ganglia) haematomas in fatal non-missile head injury in man. J Neurol Neurosurg Psychiatry 49:1039, 1986.

31. Graham, DI, et al: Brain damage in non-missile head injury secondary to a high ICP. Neuropathol Appl Neurobiol 13:209, 1987.

32. Harper, CG, et al: Analysis of abnormalities in the pituitary gland in non-missile head injury. J Clin Pathol 39:769, 1986.

33. Lindenberg, R, and Freytag, E: Brainstem lesions of traumatic hyperextension of the head. Arch Pathol 90:509, 1970.

34. Simpson, DA, et al: Pontomedullary tears and other gross brainstem injuries after ventricular accidents. J Trauma 29:1519, 1989.

35. Britt, RH, et al: Traumatic lesions of the pontomedullary junction. Neurosurgery 6:623, 1980.

36. Pilz, P, Strohecker, J, and Grobovschek, M: Survival after pontomedullary tear. J Neurol Neurosurg Psychiatry 45:422, 1982.

37. Pilz, P: Axonal injury in head injury. Acta Neurochir Suppl (Wien) 32:119, 1980.

38. Gean, AD (ed): Imaging of Head Trauma. Raven Press, New York, 1994, p 497.

39. Strich, SJ: Diffuse degeneration of the cerebral white matter in severe dementia following head injury. J Neurol Neurosurg Psychiatry 19:163, 1956.

40. Strich, SJ: Shearing of the nerve fibres as a cause of brain damage due to head injury. Lancet 2:443, 1961.

41. Peerless, SJ, and Rewcastle, NB: Shear injuries of the brain. Can Med Assoc J 96:577, 1967.

42. Grcevic, N: The concept of inner cerebral trauma. Scand J Rehabil Med Suppl 17:25, 1988.

43. Adams, JH, et al: Diffuse brain damage of immediate impact type. Brain 100:489, 1977.

44. Zimmerman, RA, et al: Computed tomography of shearing injuries of the cerebral white matter. Radiology 127:393, 1978.

45. Gennarelli, TA, et al: Diffuse axonal injury and traumatic coma in the primate. Ann Neurol 12:564, 1982.

46. Adams, JH, et al: Diffuse axonal injury due to non-missile head injury in humans: An analysis of 45 cases. Ann Neurol 12:557, 1982.

47. Oppenheimer, DR: Microscopic lesions in the brain following head injury. J Neurol Neurosurg Psychiatry 37:463, 1968.

48. Clark, JM: Distribution of microglial clusters in the brain after head injury. J Neurol Neurosurg Psychiatry 37:463, 1974.

49. Blumbergs, PC, Jones, NR, and North JB: Diffuse axonal injury in head trauma. J Neurol Neurosurg Psychiatry 52:838, 1989.

50. Adams, JH, et al: Diffuse axonal injury in head injury: Definition, diagnosis and grading. Histopathology 15:49, 1989.

51. Blumbergs, PC, et al: Staining of amyloid precursor protein to study axonal damage in mild head injury. Lancet 344:1055, 1994.

52. Blumbergs, PC, et al: Topography of axonal injury as defined by amyloid precursor protein and the sector scoring method in mild and severe closed head injury. J Neurotrauma 12:565, 1995.

53. Gentleman, SM, et al: β-amyloid precursor protein (β-APP) as a marker for axonal injury after head injury. Neurosci Lett 160:139, 1993.

54. Gentleman, SM, et al: Axonal injury: A universal consequence of fatal closed head injury? Acta Neuropathol (Berl) 89:537, 1995.

55. Sherriff, FE, Bridges, LR, and Sivaloganathan, S: Early detection of axonal injury after human head trauma using immunocytochemistry for β-amyloid precursor protein. Acta Neuropathol (Berl) 87:55, 1994.

56. McKenzie, KJ, et al: Is β-APP a marker of axonal damage in short-surviving head injury? Acta Neuropathol (Berl) 92:608, 1996.

57. Povlishock, JT: Traumatically induced axonal injury: Pathogenesis and pathobiological implications. Brain Pathol 2:1, 1992.

58. Maxwell, WL, et al: Ultrastructural evidence of axonal shearing as a result of lateral acceleration of the head in non-human primates. Acta Neuropathol (Berl) 86:136, 1993.

59. Povlishock, JT, and Christman, CW: The pathobiology of traumatically induced axonal injury in animals and humans: A review of current thoughts. J Neurotrauma 12:555, 1995.

60. Povlishock, JT, et al: Axonal change in minor head injury. J Neuropathol Exp Neurol 42:225, 1983.

61. Erb, DE, and Povlishock, JT: Axonal damage in severe traumatic brain injury: An experimental study in the cat. Acta Neuropathol (Berl) 76:347, 1988.

62. Yaghmai, A, and Povlishock, JT: Traumatically induced reactive change as visualized through the use of monoclonal antibodies targeted to the neurofilament subunits. J Neuropathol Exp Neurol 51:158, 1992.

63. Erb, DE, and Povlishock, JT: Neuroplasticity following traumatic brain injury: A study of GABAergic terminal loss and recovery in the cat dorsal lateral vestibular nucleus. Exp Brain Res 83:253, 1991.

64. Hayes, RL, et al: Pretreatment with phencyclidine, an N-methyl-D-aspartate antagonist, attenuates long-term behavioral deficits in the rat produced by traumatic brain injury. J Neurotrauma 5:259, 1988.

65. Jenkins, LW, et al: Combined pre-trauma scopolamine and phencyclidine attenuates post-traumatic increased sensitivity to delayed secondary ischemia. J Neurotrauma 5:303, 1988.

66. Faden, AI, et al: The role of excitatory amino acids and NMDA receptors in traumatic brain injury. Science 244:798, 1989.

67. Hayes, RL, Jenkins, LW, and Lyeth, BG: Neuropharmacological mechanisms of traumatic brain injury: Acetylcholine and excitatory amino acids. J Neurotrauma 8:S173, 1991.

68. Adams, JH, et al: Diffuse axonal injury in non-missile head injury. J Neurol Neurosurg Psychiatry 54:481, 1991.

69. Gennarelli, TA: The spectrum of traumatic axonal injury. Neuropathol Appl Neurobiol 22:509, 1996.

70. Povlishock, JT, and Jenkins, LW: Are the pathobiological changes evoked by traumatic brain injury immediate and irreversible? Brain Pathol 5:415, 1995.

71. Maxwell, WL, Povlishock, JT, and Graham, DI: A mechanistic analysis of non-disruptive axonal injury. J Neurotrauma 14:419, 1997.

72. Tomei, G, et al: Morphology and neurophysiology of focal axonal injury experimentally induced in the guinea pig optic nerve. Acta Neuropathol (Berl) 80:506, 1990.

73. Graham, DI, Adams, JH, and Doyle, D: Ischaemic brain damage in fatal non-missile head injuries. J Neurol Sci 39:213, 1978.
74. Graham, DI, et al: Ischaemic brain damage is still common in fatal non-missile head injury. J Neurol Neurosurg Psychiatry 52:346, 1989.
75. Muizelaar, JP: Cerebral blood flow, cerebral blood volume, and cerebral metabolism after severe head injury. In Becker, DP, and Gudeman, SK (eds): Textbook of Head Injury. WB Saunders, Philadelphia, 1989, p 221.
76. Bouma, GJ, et al: Ultra-early evaluation of regional cerebral blood flow in severely head-injured patients using xenon-enhanced computerized tomography. J Neurosurg 77:360, 1992.
77. Miller, JD: Head injury. J Neurol Neurosurg Psychiatry 56:440, 1993.
78. Doberstein, CE, Hovda, DA, and Becker, DP: Clinical considerations in the reduction of secondary brain injury. Ann Emerg Med 22:933, 1993.
79. Hovda, DA, et al: Concussive brain injury produces a state of vulnerability for intracranial pressure perturbation in the absence of morphological damage. In Avezaat, CJJ, et al (eds): Intracranial Pressure VIII. Springer-Verlag, New York, 1993, p 469.
80. Jones, PA, et al: Measuring the burden of secondary insults in head-injured patients during intensive care. J Neurosurg Anesthesiol 6:4, 1994.
81. Hovda, DA: Metabolic dysfunction. In Narayan, RK, Wilberger, JE, and Povlishock, JT (eds): Neurotrauma. McGraw-Hill, New York, 1996, p 1459.
82. Maxwell, WL, et al: Response of cerebral microvasculature to brain injury. J Pathol 155:327, 1988.
83. Maxwell, WL, et al: The microvascular response to stretch injury in the adult guinea pig visual system. J Neurotrauma 8:271, 1991.
84. Dietrich, WD, Alonso, O, and Halley, M: Early microvascular and neuronal consequences to traumatic brain injury: A light and electron microscopic study in rats. J Neurotrauma 11:289, 1994.
85. Weber, M, Grolimund, P, and Seiler, RW: Evaluation of post traumatic cerebral blood flow velocities by transcranial Doppler ultrasonography. Neurosurgery 27:106, 1990.
86. Chan, K-H, Miller, JD, and Dearden, NM: Intracranial blood flow velocity after head injury: Relationship to severity of injury, time, neurological status and outcome. J Neurol Neurosurg Psychiatry 55:787, 1992.
87. Chan, K-H, Dearden, NM, and Miller, JD: Transcranial Doppler sonography. Acta Neurochir Suppl (Wien) 59:81, 1993.
88. Graham, DI, et al: Fatal head injury in children. J Clin Pathol 42:18, 1989.
89. Lyeth, BG, et al: Muscarinic cholinergic receptor binding in rat brain following traumatic brain injury. Brain Res 640:240, 1994.
90. Jiang, JY, et al: Muscarinic cholinergic receptor binding in rat brain at 15 days following traumatic brain injury. Brain Res 651:123, 1994.
91. Dewar, D, and Graham, DI: Depletion of choline acetyltransferase activity but preservation of M1 and M2 muscarinic receptor binding sites in temporal cortex following head injury: A preliminary human postmortem study. J Neurotrauma 13:181, 1996.
92. Wei, EP, Lamb, RG, and Kontos, HA: Increased phospholipase C activity after experimental brain injury. J Neurosurg 56:695, 1982.
93. Hall, E: Beneficial effects of acute intravenous ibuprofen on neurologic recovery of head-injured mice: Comparison of cyclooxygenase inhibition with inhibition of thromboxane A2 synthetase or 5-lipoxygenase. J Neurotrauma 2:75, 1985.
94. DeWitt, DS, et al: Experimental traumatic brain injury elevates brain prostaglandin E2 and thromboxane B2 levels in rats. J Neurotrauma 5:303, 1988.
95. Shohami, E, et al: Head injury induces increased prostaglandin synthesis in rat brain. J Cereb Blood Flow Metab 7:58, 1987.
96. Ellis, EF, et al: Increased plasma PGE2, 6-keto-PGF1a and 12-HETE levels following experimental concussive brain injury. J Neurotrauma 6:31, 1989.
97. Yergey, JA, and Heyes, MP: Brain eicosanoid formation following acute penetration injury as studied by *in vivo* microdialysis. J Cereb Blood Flow Metab 10:143, 1990.
98. Nakashima, T, et al: Phospholipase C activity in cerebrospinal fluid following subarachnoid hemorrhage related to brain damage. J Cereb Blood Flow Metab 13:255, 1993.
99. McIntosh, TK, Yu, T, and Gennarelli, TA: Alterations in regional brain catecholamine concentrations after experimental brain injury in the rat. J Neurochem 63:1426, 1994.
100. Prasad, MR, et al: Regional levels of lactate and norepinephrine after experimental brain injury. J Neurochem 63:1086, 1994.
101. Prasad, MR, et al: Decreased alpha-adrenergic receptors after experimental brain injury. J Neurotrauma 9:269, 1992.
102. Pappius, HM: Local cerebral glucose utilization in thermally traumatized rat brain. American Journal of Neurology 9:484, 1981.
103. Tsuiki, K, et al: Synthesis of serotonin in traumatized rat brain. J Neurochem 64:1319, 1995.
104. Zhuang, J, et al: The association of leukocytes with secondary brain injury. J Trauma 35:415, 1993.
105. Biagas, KV, et al: Assessment of post-traumatic polymorphonuclear leukocyte accumulation in rat brain using tissue myeloperoxidase assay and vinblastine treatment. J Neurotrauma 9:363, 1992.
106. Schoettle, RJ, et al: Early polymorphonuclear leukocyte accumulation correlates with the development of post-traumatic cerebral edema in rats. J Neurotrauma 7:207, 1990.
107. Chen, H, et al: Sequential neuronal and astrocytic changes after transient middle cerebral artery occlusion in the rat. J Neurol Sci 118:109, 1993.
108. Shohami, E, et al: Closed head injury triggers early production of TNFα and IL-6 by brain tissue. J Cereb Blood Flow Metab 14:615, 1994.
109. Fan, L, et al: Experimental brain injury induces expression of interleukin-1β mRNA in the rat brain. Molecular Brain Research 30:125, 1995.
110. Mocchetti, I, and Wrathall, JR: Neurotrophic factors in central nervous system trauma. J Neurotrauma 12:853, 1995.
111. Raghupathi, R, McIntosh, TK, and Smith DH: Cellular responses to experimental brain injury. Brain Pathol 5:437, 1995.
112. McIntosh, TK, et al: Endogenous opioids may mediate secondary damage after brain injury. Am J Physiol 253:E565, 1987.
113. McIntosh, TK, Head, VA, and Faden, AI: Alterations in regional concentrations of endogenous opioids following traumatic brain injury in the cat. Brain Res 425:225, 1987.
114. McIntosh, TK, et al: Central and systemic κ-opioid agonists exacerbate neurobehavioral response to brain injury in rats. Am J Physiol 267:R665, 1994.
115. Isaac, L, et al: MK-801 blocks dynorphin A (1-13)-induced loss of the tail-flick reflex in the rat. Brain Res 531:83, 1990.
116. Faden, AI: Dynorphin increases extracellular levels of excitatory amino acids in the brain through a nonopioid mechanism. J Neurosci 12:425, 1992.
117. Katayama, Y, et al: Massive increases in extracellular potassium and the indiscriminate release of glutamate following concussive brain injury. J Neurosurg 73:889, 1990.
118. Nilsson, P, et al: Changes in cortical extracellular levels of energy-related metabolites and amino acids follow-

ing concussive brain injury in rats. J Cereb Blood Flow Metab 10:631, 1990.

119. Palmer, AM, et al: Traumatic brain injury–induced excitotoxicity assessed in a controlled cortical impact model. J Neurochem 61:2015, 1993.

120. Olney, JW, et al: MK-801 powerfully protects against N-methyl aspartate neurotoxicity. Eur J Pharmacol 141:357, 1987.

121. Rothman, SM, and Olney, JW: Excitotoxicity and the NMDA receptor. Trends Neurosci 10:288, 1987.

122. Smith, DH, and McIntosh, TK: Traumatic brain injury and excitatory amino acids. In Narayan, RK, Wilberger, JE, and Povlishock, JT: Neurotrauma. McGraw-Hill, New York, 1996, p 1445.

123. Varon, S, Hagg, T, and Manthorpe, M: Nerve growth factor in CNS repair and regeneration. Adv Exp Med Biol 296:267, 1991.

124. Conner, JM, Fass-Holmes, B, and Varon, S: Changes in nerve growth factor immunoreactivity following entorhinal cortex lesions: Possible molecular mechanism regulating cholinergic sprouting. J Comp Neurol 345:409, 1994.

125. Leonard, JR, Maris, DO, and Grady, SM: Fluid percussion injury causes loss of forebrain choline acetyltransferase and nerve growth factor receptor immunoreactive cells in the rat. J Neurotrauma 11:379, 1994.

126. Patterson, SL, Grady, SM, and Bothwell, M: Nerve growth factor and a fibroblast growth factor-like neurotrophic activity in cerebrospinal fluid of brain injured human patients. Brain Res 605:43, 1993.

127. Sinson, G, Voddi, M, and McIntosh, TK: Nerve growth factor (NGF) administration attenuates cognitive but not neurobehavioral motor dysfunction or hippocampal cell loss following fluid-percussion brain injury in rats. J Neurochem 65:2209, 1995.

128. Dietrich, WD, et al: Post treatment with intravenous basic fibroblast growth factor reduces histopathological damage following fluid-percussion brain injury in rats. J Neurotrauma 13:302, 1996.

129. Shapira, Y, et al: Accumulation of calcium in the brain following head trauma. Neurol Res 11:169, 1989.

130. Hovda, DA, et al: Intracellular calcium accumulates for at least 48 hours following fluid percussion brain injury in the rat. Proceedings of the American Association of Neurological Surgeons 1:452, 1991.

131. Vink, R, and McIntosh, TK: Pharmacological and physiological effects of magnesium on experimental traumatic brain injury. Magnes Res 3:163, 1990.

132. Vink, R, et al: Opiate antagonist nalmefine improves intracellular free Mg^{2+}, bioenergetic state and neurological outcome following traumatic brain injury in rats. J Neurosci 10:3524, 1990.

133. Katayama, Y, et al: Massive increases in extracellular potassium and the indiscriminate release of glutamate following concussive brain injury. J Neurosurg 73:889, 1990.

134. DeSalles, AF, et al: Intra- and extracellular pH and extracellular potassium following mechanical brain injury in the cat. J Cereb Blood Flow Metab 7:S627, 1987.

135. Siesjo, B, and Wieloch, T: Brain injury: Neurochemical aspects. In Becker, DP, and Povlishock, J (eds): Central Nervous System Trauma Status Report. National Institutes of Health, Bethesda, Md, 1985, p 513.

136. Kontos, HA, and Povlishock, JT: Oxygen radicals in brain injury. Central Nervous System Trauma 3:527, 1986.

137. Hall, ED: Free radicals and lipid peroxidation. In Narayan, RK, Wilberger, JE, and Povlishock, JT (eds): Neurotrauma. McGraw-Hill, New York, 1996, p 1405.

138. Feeney, DM, et al: Responses to cortical injury. I. Methodology and local effects of contusions in the rat. Brain Res 211:67, 1981.

139. Shapiro, Y, et al: Experimental closed head injury in rats: Mechanical pathophysiologic and neurologic properties. Crit Care Med 16:258, 1989.

140. Dixon, CE, et al: A fluid percussion model of experimental brain injury in the rat: Neurological, physiological, amd histopathological characteristics. J Neurosurg 67:110, 1987.

141. McIntosh, TK, et al: Traumatic brain injury in the rat: Characterization of a lateral fluid percussion model. Neuroscience 28:233, 1989.

142. Toulmond, S, et al: Biochemical and histological alterations induced by fluid percussion brain injury in the rat. Brain Res 620:24, 1993.

143. Dixon, CE, et al: A controlled cortical impact model of traumatic brain injury in the rat. J Neurosci Methods 39:1, 1991.

144. Soares, HD, et al: Development of prolonged focal cerebral edema and regional cation change following experimental brain injury in the rat. J Neurochem 58:1845, 1992.

145. Smith, DH, et al: A model of parasagittal controlled cortical impact in the mouse: Cognitive and histopathologic effects. J Neurotrauma 12:169, 1995.

146. Gennarelli, TA: Animate models of human head injury. J Neurotrauma 11:357, 1994.

147. Gennarelli, TA, and Thibault, LE: Biomechanics of acute subdural hematoma. J Trauma 22:680, 1982.

148. Meaney, DF, Smith, DH, Ross, DT, Gennarelli, TA: Biomechanical analysis of experimental diffuse axonal injury in the miniature pig, J Neurotrauma 12:689, 1995.

149. Smith, DH, et al: Persistent memory dysfunction is associated with bilateral hippocampal damage following experimental brain injury. Neurosci Lett 168:151, 1994.

150. Marmarou, A, et al: A new model of diffuse brain injury in rats. J Neurosurg 80:291, 1994.

151. Rimel, RW, et al: Disability caused by minor head injury. Neurosurgery 9:221, 1981.

152. Rimel, RW, et al: Moderate head injury: Completing the clinical spectrum of brain trauma. Neurosurgery 11:344, 1982.

153. Levin, HS: Neurobehavioral outcome of mild to moderate head injury. In Hoff, JT, Anderson, TE, and Cole, TM (eds): Mild to Moderate Head Injury. Blackwell Scientific, Boston, 1989, p 153.

154. Levin, HS: Prediction of recovery from traumatic brain injury. J Neurotrauma 12:913, 1995.

155. Jennett, B, and Plum, F: Persistent vegetative state after brain damage. Lancet 1:734, 1972.

156. Jennett, B, and Bond, M: Assessment of outcome after severe brain damage. Lancet 1:480, 1975.

157. The Multi-Society Task Force on PVS: Medium aspects of the persistent vegetative state. N Engl J Med 330:1499, 1994.

158. Grcevic, N: Neuropathological correlates of supratentorial lesions in traumatic and nontraumatic apallic syndrome. In Ore, GD, et al (eds): The Apallic Syndrome. Springer Verlag, Berlin, 1977, p 109.

159. Jellinger, K, and Seitelberger, F: Protracted post-traumatic encephalopathy: Pathology, pathogenesis and clinical implications. J Neurol Sci 10:51, 1970.

160. Jellinger, K: Pathology and pathogenesis of apallic syndromes following closed head injuries. In Ore, GD, et al (eds): The Apallic Syndrome. Springer Verlag, Berlin, 1977, p 88.

161. Peters, G, and Rothemund, E: Neuropathology of the traumatic apallic syndrome. In Ore, GD, et al (eds): The Apallic Syndrome. Springer Verlag, Berlin, 1977, p 78.

162. Strich, SJ: The pathology of brain damage due to blunt head injuries. In Walker, AE, Caveness, WF, and Critchley, M (eds): The Late Effects of Head Injury. Charles C Thomas, Springfield, Ill, 1969, p 501.

163. McLellan, DR, et al: Structural basis of the vegetative state and prolonged coma after non-missile head injury. In Papo, I, Cohadon, F, and Massarotti, M (eds): Le Coma Traumatique. Liviana Editrice, Padova, 1986, p 165.

164. Kinney, HC, and Samuels, MA: Neuropathology of the persistent vegetative state: A review. J Neuropathol Exp Neurol 53:548, 1994.

165. Corsellis, JAN, and Brierley, JB: Observations on the pathology of insidious dementia following head injury. Journal of Mental Science 105:714, 1959.
166. Hollander, D, and Strich, SJ: Atypical Alzheimer's disease with congophilic angiopathy presenting with dementia of acute onset. In Wolstenholme, GEW, and O'Connor, M (eds): Alzheimer's Disease and Related Conditions, Ciba Foundation Symposium. Churchill, London, 1970, p 105.
167. Mortimer, JA: The epidemiology of Alzheimer's disease: Beyond risk factors. In Iqbal, K, et al (eds): Research Advances in Alzheimer's Disease and Related Disorders. John Wiley & Sons, Chichester, 1995, p 3.
168. Mayeux, R, et al: Genetic susceptibility and head injury as risk factors for Alzheimer's disease among community-dwelling elderly persons and their first-degree relatives. Ann Neurol 33:494, 1993.
169. McMenemey, WH, Grant, HC, and Behrman, S: Two examples of "presenile dementia" (Pick's disease and Stern-Garcin syndrome) with a history of trauma. Archiv für Psychiatrie und Nervenkrankheiten 208:162, 1965.
170. Grimberg, L: Paralysis agitans and trauma. J Nerv Ment Dis 79:14, 1934.
171. Behrman, S, Mandybur, T, and McMenemey, WH: Un cas de maladie Creutzfeld-Jakob à la suite d'un traumatisme cerebrale. Rev Neurol (Paris) 107:453, 1962.
172. Martland, HS: Punch drunk. JAMA 91:1103, 1928.
173. Critchley, M: Medical aspects of boxing particularly from a neurological standpoint. BMJ 1:357, 1957.
174. Mawdsley, C, and Ferguson, FR: Neurological disease in boxers. Lancet 2:795, 1963.
175. Corsellis, JAN: Boxing and the brain. BMJ 298:105, 1989.
176. Corsellis, JAN, Bruton, CJ, and Freeman-Browne, D: The aftermath of boxing. Psychol Med 3:270, 1973.
177. Roberts, GW, Allsop, D, and Bruton, CJ: The occult aftermath of boxing. J Neurol Neurosurg Psychiatry 53:373, 1990.
178. Roberts, GW, et al: Dementia in a punch-drunk wife. Lancet 335:918, 1990.
179. Gentleman, SM, Graham, DI, and Roberts, GW: Molecular pathology of head injury: Altered β-APP metabolism and the aetiology of Alzheimer's disease. Prog Brain Res 96:237, 1993.
180. Roberts, GW, et al: βA4 amyloid protein deposition in brain after severe head injury: Implications for the pathogenesis of Alzheimer's disease. J Neurol Neurosurg Psychiatry 57:419, 1994.
181. Graham, DI, et al: Distribution of β-amyloid protein in the brain following severe head injury. Neuropathol Appl Neurobiol 21:27, 1995.
182. Griffin, WST, et al: Brain interleukin-1 and S100 immunoreactivity elevated in Down's syndrome and Alzheimer's disease. Proc Natl Acad Sci U S A 86:7611, 1989.
183. Griffin, WST, et al: Microglial interleukin-1α expression in human head injury: Correlations with neuronal and neuritic β-amyloid precursor protein expression. Neurosci Lett 176:133, 1994.
184. Griffin, WST, et al: Interleukin-1 expression in different plaques in Alzheimer's disease: Significance in plaque evolution. J Neuropathol Exp Neurol 54:276, 1995.
185. Nicoll, JAR, Roberts, GW, and Graham, DI: Apolipoprotein E ε4 allele is associated with deposition of amyloid β-protein following head injury. Nature Medicine 1:135, 1995.
186. Mayeux, R, et al: Synergistic effects of traumatic head injury and apolipoprotein-ε in patients with Alzheimer's disease. Neurology 45:555, 1995.
187. Ma, J, et al: Amyloid-associated proteins α₁-antichymotrypsin and apolipoprotein E promote assembly of Alzheimer β-protein into filaments. Nature 372:45, 1994.
188. Strittmatter, WJ, et al: Binding of human apolipoprotein E to synthetic amyloid beta peptide: Isoform-specific effects and implications for late-onset Alzheimer disease. Proc Natl Acad Sci U S A 90:8098, 1993.
189. Sorbi, S, et al: ApoE as a prognostic factor for post-traumatic coma. Nature Medicine 1:852, 1995.
190. Nicoll, JAR: Genetics and head injury. Neuropathol Appl Neurobiol (in press).

Acute Management of Brain Injury

BRIAN PENTLAND, MB, CHB, FRCP, FRCSLT
and IAN R. WHITTLE, MD, PHD, FRACS, FRCSE

The principal components of brain injury management in the acute—or, indeed, any—phase are assessment, interventions directed at encouraging recovery and preventing complications, and evaluation of outcome. The last represents a reassessment that begins the cycle of management again with readjustment of the treatment program. In reality, of course, the process is not neatly compartmentalized but consists of continuous monitoring of the patient's state, with adjustment of the treatment approach accordingly. However, the concept of repeated evaluation, action, and reevaluation provides a useful framework that is applicable from the roadside to the latest stages of rehabilitation. Throughout the course of recovery from brain injury, the combined skills of a wide range of disciplines are required to ensure optimal recovery and resettlement.

□ ASSESSMENT OF BRAIN INJURY

Diagnosis

The diagnosis of acute brain injury is not usually in doubt. Nevertheless, occasions arise in which a person is found comatose or confused at home or in the street, and it is uncertain whether brain trauma has occurred. Doubt is particularly likely when alcohol or drugs are invoked as possible causes of a patient's coma. In such circumstances, the correct procedure is to treat patients as if they have sustained a significant brain injury. Alcohol is considered to be a contributory factor in between 32 and 62 percent of brain trauma cases in men.[1–3] The association with drug use is less well established.[4] The altered behavior or reduced consciousness that may accompany drug abuse, alcohol intoxication, or suicidal drug overdose can cloud the clinical picture and conceal life-threatening intracranial hematoma.

Epilepsy is another common source of confusion in patients who have sustained a brain injury. The sudden onset of coma caused by the rapid enlargement of an intracranial hematoma may be wrongly attributed to a seizure in which the clonic phase has been absent or has occurred unobserved. Valuable time may be wasted awaiting return of consciousness in a patient who is, in fact, continuing to deteriorate rapidly because of progressive brain compression. Other medical conditions, such as diabetes, myocardial infarction, or stroke, are occasionally the precipitating factor in brain injury. Especially in older people admitted with reduced levels of awareness or consciousness attributable to such conditions, the possibility of associated brain injury should be considered.

Clinical Evaluation

The aims of initial assessment are twofold: discovering how badly the patient is injured and determining the risk that further deterioration might supervene. Primary brain damage occurs at the time of injury, before the patient is first seen, and needs to be identified to determine the nature and extent of the damage incurred. However, the early detection and correction, as well as prevention, of secondary insults demand particular care. These insults are summarized in Table 3–1.

Patients who are conscious and able to converse should have a history taken and be examined in the standard way. If there has been no loss of consciousness and the individual can give an account of events, the primary damage is not likely to have been serious. The aim is to ensure that any secondary expanding lesion is recognized promptly. Headaches are common after brain injury, irrespective of severity, but a complaint of progressively worsening headache is suggestive of an expanding lesion, as is repeated vomiting. It is important to make an adequate examination of cognitive functions, such as attention and orientation, in those with apparently minor injury. Whenever possible, confirmation of events should be obtained from a witness, as the brain injured person's own testimony may be unreliable. Clearly, in those with impaired consciousness, the account of a witness is invaluable, and information from relatives or others of relevant past medical history and substance abuse may prove vital.

The first priorities in patients with impaired consciousness are to check for an obstructed airway, inadequate ventilation, or shock and to correct them if present. Full neurological examination is a valid index of brain damage only when the patient is adequately oxygenated and the blood pressure is restored to within normal range. The neurological evaluation of the comatose patient must be brief and objective.[5] In addition to assessing vital function, therefore, the assessment at the scene of the accident and during transfer to the hospital must include determining the Glasgow Coma Scale (GCS) score.[6]

The GCS consists of three elements of response: eye opening, motor responses, and verbal responses to standard stimuli. The initial stimulus is always verbal. If there is no response, the preferred pain stimulus consists of application of heavy pressure on the nailbed of the little finger or large toe. This stimulus should be done on each side to identify cases of hemiplegia. If no response occurs, pain should be applied to the sternal area and also above the neck, such as to the supraorbital area or the mastoid process, to identify the patient who is quadriplegic from concomitant cervical spinal cord injury.

The GCS has been extensively tested for interrater reliability and shows a high level of agreement, an issue of obvious importance when multiple observers may be sequentially observing the same patient. Based on the GCS score, patients may be rapidly assigned to the categories of severe, moderate, and minor brain injury, which determines the urgency of subsequent investigation and treatment. The summation of the scores for eye opening and motor and verbal responses ranges from 3 to 15. Conventionally, scores of 8 or less signify severe injury, 9 to 12 are classified as moderate, and 13 to 15 as minor. Patients who are hypoxic, in shock, or inebriated may have a GCS that does not accurately reflect the degree of brain damage. In children under 4 years of age, the Advanced Trauma Life Support (ATLS) modifications of the GCS should be used for the verbal component.[8] Both the GCS and the ATLS modification are summarized in Table 3–2.

The only other essential elements of the neurological examination in the immediate stage after injury are inspection of the pupils, the pupillary response to light, eye position, and presence of eye movement. The size and symmetry of the pupils should be recorded and a bright light shone into each eye in turn to observe the direct response in the ipsilateral eye and the consensual reflex in the opposite eye. A magnifying glass or a magnifying lens of the ophthalmoscope can detect weak pupillary responses to light or the presence of a response in miotic pupils. With optic nerve damage, light shone into the affected eye fails to produce a reflex response in either eye. This is termed an *afferent pupillary defect*, in contrast with the *efferent pupillary defect*, which occurs with third

---

TABLE 3–1. Secondary Systemic and Intracranial Insults in the Injured Brain

Systemic	Intracranial
Arterial hypoxemia	Hematoma: extradural, subdural, intracerebral
Arterial hypotension	Raised intracranial pressure (ICP): brain swelling and edema, acute
Hypercapnia	hydrocephalus
Anemia	Infection: meningitis, abscess/empyema
Pyrexia	Epilepsy
Hyponatremia	Vasospasm
Hypoglycemia	

TABLE 3–2. Glasgow Coma Scale: Adults and Children

	Examiner's Test	Response	Score
Eye opening	Spontaneous	Opens eyes on own	E4
	Speech	Opens eyes on request in a loud voice	E3
	Pain	Opens eyes on nailbed pressure	E2
	Pain	Has no eye opening	E1
Best motor response	Command	Follows simple commands	M6
	Pain	Pulls examiner's hand way	M5
	Pain	Pulls a limb away (flexion)	M4
	Pain	Has abnormal flexion (decorticate posturing)	M3
	Pain	Has extension (decerebrate posturing)	M2
	Pain	Makes no response	M1
Best verbal response	Speech	Converses with examiner and is oriented	V5
	Speech	Speaks in confused sentences or is disoriented	V4
	Speech	Speaks words but makes no sense	V3
	Speech	Makes sounds only, no words	V2
	Speech	Makes no noise	V1
Advanced Trauma Life Support Modification of best verbal response (children <4 yr)		Appropriate words or social smile, fixes and follows	V5
		Cries, but is consolable	V4
		Persistently irritable	V3
		Restless and agitated	V2
		No response	V1

cranial nerve damage. If the oculomotor nerve is injured, light shone into either eye fails to produce a response in the eye on the affected side, whereas light shone into the affected eye produces constriction of the opposite pupil. Asymmetry of pupil size may result from localized direct damage to the optic or oculomotor nerves or their pathways or from interruption of the cervical sympathetic pathways, called Horner's syndrome. Unilateral pupillary dilatation is, however, a well-recognized sign of transtentorial herniation that is due to an expanding ipsilateral intracranial mass (usually a traumatic hematoma). A slight difference in the size of pupils, so-called physiological anisocoria, occurs in about 15 to 30 percent of normal individuals, but response to light is present in these individuals. Bilateral loss of the pupillary light response is present in 20 to 25 percent of comatose patients with brain injury and indicates a lesion of the upper brain stem.[9] Bilateral small, particularly pinpoint, pupils in a comatose patient are usually an indication of a destructive lesion in the pons. Widely dilated pupils that are unreactive to light occur in end-stage cerebral hypoxia or ischemia. It is vital to remember, however, that opiate drugs can produce pinpoint pupils and high blood alcohol levels can cause dilated and sluggishly reactive pupils that can be misinterpreted as nonreactive.[10]

Checks of the airways, breathing, pulse, blood pressure, GCS, and pupil size and reactions should be carried out assiduously at least every 10 to 15 minutes during the first hour and regularly at a rate determined by progress thereafter.

In the emergency department (ED), after resuscitation, a more thorough assessment should be possible, in addition to the key measures of vital signs, level of consciousness, and pupil signs. Nonneurological signs of head injury, including abrasions, contusions, or swelling of the scalp that may indicate an underlying fracture, should be specifically looked for. Care must be taken not to manipulate any depressed fractures until the patient is in the operating theater. Bleeding from the ear or mouth, particularly if the blood is mixed with cerebrospinal fluid (CSF), may indicate a basal skull fracture. If, when such blood-stained fluid is allowed to drip onto filter paper or a piece of gauze, a pale halo surrounds the drop, the presence of CSF should be suspected. The presence of CSF otorrhea or rhinorrhea is proof not only that the patient has sustained a basal skull fracture but also that the dura and arachnoid maters surrounding the brain have been torn. Telltale bruising in the periorbital areas and behind the ears (Battle sign) takes several hours to appear and is not usually present on initial assessment in the ED. When present, however, these signs provide indications of fractures; "raccoon eyes" are associated with anterior fossa fracture, and bruising behind the ear (Battle sign) points to middle cranial fossa fracture.

All patients who are confused or in coma must be examined thoroughly from head to toe for extracranial injuries, especially when the brain injury has resulted from an automobile accident or a fall from a height. Particular care must be taken to detect spinal cord injury and to prevent further damage at the site of any such spinal injury by injudicious handling during examination. Urinary retention is rarely attributable to brain injury and is suggestive of spinal or pelvic injury. Similarly, flaccid paralysis of both legs should lead one to suspect spinal cord damage. The possibility of occult hemorrhage in the chest or abdomen should be remembered, and both regions should be carefully examined. Soft-tissue injuries around joints, skeletal fractures, and associated peripheral nerve damage should also be diligently sought. Concomitant orthopedic and other injuries are described in more detail in Chapter 4. In the case of the restless or agitated patient, in addition to intracranial causes, particular thought should be given to an underlying extracranial cause, such as an undetected fracture, other injury, or a full bladder.

The other important elements of the initial neurological examination, in addition to the GCS and pupillary responses, are the resting eye position and eye movement, which are tested primarily to indicate brain stem dysfunction. In the conscious, cooperative patient, eye movements and examination for ptosis, strabismus, and nystagmus can be done in the standard way. When the patient cannot obey commands, testing reflex eye movements becomes necessary. These tests cannot be done when there is suspicion of damage to the cervical spine or any other factor that impedes mobility of the head and neck. The oculocephalic, or "doll's eye," maneuver is carried out with the patient's head at 30 degrees from supine by moving the head rapidly from side to side to elicit lateral eye movements. The normal position of the eyes is central, and when the head is moved quickly to one side, the eyes swing back to regain this normal orientation. Thus, if the head is moved to the left, the normal response is for the eyes to move to the right to resume the central position. A similar phenomenon occurs when the examiner moves the patient's head up and down (the vertical oculocephalic reflex), provoking compensatory vertical movement of the eyes. These responses result from stimulation of the labyrinth and vestibular system, so that this system, as well as the central and peripheral oculomotor apparatus, must be intact to get a normal response. The oculovestibular reflexes depend on stimulating the vestibular system by applying cold or warm water to the tympanic membrane on either side. In the comatose patient, it is usual to restrict such caloric tests to cold stimuli by the application of ice cold water by syringe in the external auditory meatus. The normal response is conjugate devi-

ation of the eye toward the irrigated ear. Simultaneous irrigation of both ears should produce a vertical movement of both eyes, the vertical oculovestibular reflex. Absence of response or a dysconjugate response indicates a lesion of the vestibular and/or oculomotor apparatus, which may be peripheral or central in the brain stem.

In the belief that there is an anatomic and pathophysiological hierarchy of brain stem reflexes indicating the caudal extent of traumatic dysfunction in the brain stem, Born et al. proposed the addition of a fourth element—the brain stem reflex scale—to the three elements of the GCS.[11] This Glasgow-Liege Scale has been rigorously tested for reliability and prognostic power and has been shown to amplify the information provided by the standard GCS in comatose patients. The brain stem reflexes used in this system, in descending order, are the front-orbicular reflex, the vertical oculocephalic or oculovestibular reflex, the pupillary light reflex, the horizontal oculocephalic or oculovestibular reflex, and the oculocardiac reflex. The fronto-orbicular (or orbicularis oculi) reflex refers to orbicularis oculi contraction on percussion of the glabella; the oculocardiac reflex is bradycardia induced by increasing pressure on the eyeball.

The resting eye position should also be noted. Whereas in brain stem lesions, conjugate deviation of the eyes may occur, with the eyes deviating to the opposite side, conjugate deviation to the same side as the lesion is seen with posterior frontal cortical contusions. Roving eye movements may occur in the unconscious patient because of loss of volitional central fixation.

Papilledema is rare in the acute stage after brain injury, despite the fact that raised intracranial pressure is frequent.[12] It should still be checked for, however, as fundoscopy may reveal loss of venous pulsations or the presence of venous engorgement or subhyaloid or intravitreal hemorrhage. It is also relevant to look for the signs of meningism, neck stiffness, and Kernig's sign, particularly if the history of injury is vague or occurred several hours prior to presentation and the differential diagnosis of viral meningoencephalitis or meningitis apply. Movement of the neck must be done only after concomitant spinal cord injury has been excluded. Meningism is most likely to be the result of traumatic subarachnoid hemorrhage and usually takes several hours to develop. It is, however, necessary to consider secondary meningitis, especially in high-risk groups. In the conscious patient who is able to cooperate, a full neurological examination should be done. Focal signs in the cranial nerves or limbs may develop with an expanding intracranial lesion in a patient whose initial radiological examination has been unremarkable.

Radiological Evaluation

The initial assessment of the brain injured patient is completed in most cases only when plain x-rays of the skull and lateral cervical spine have been taken. Occasionally this is unnecessary in the fully conscious, alert patient, but plain films are mandatory for a history of loss of consciousness or amnesia; neurological symptoms or signs; blood or CSF leakage from the nose or ear; or scalp laceration, bruising, or swelling that raises the suspicion of a penetrating injury.[13] Skull radiographs can sometimes be omitted from the initial assessment if computed tomographic (CT) brain scan is to be carried out.[14]

The importance of detecting skull fractures is twofold: their potential association with intracranial hematoma and with the risk of infection. The discovery of a fracture of the vault of the skull in a fully conscious patient raises the risk of intracranial complications more than tenfold[15] and is therefore an indication for recommending CT scan.[16,17] The finding of a fluid level in the sphenoid sinus or the presence of intracranial air is indicative of basal skull fracture. Intracranial air is always an abnormal finding associated with dural tearing and the presence of communication between the outside (usually the paranasal sinuses) and the subarachnoid space. Such abnormalities and the presence of a depressed skull fracture or penetrating injury with evidence of intracranial foreign bodies are all associated with an increased risk of intracranial infection.

The x-ray films of the cervical spine should be scrutinized not only for fractures, subluxations, or dislocations of the spine but also for loss of disk height, widening of the interspinous spaces, distraction of disk spaces, and swelling of the prevertebral soft tissues. The latter may be the only clue that the patient has a severe spinal axial injury and that there may be an unstable cervical spine that happens to be aligned in the normal position while the patient is either recumbent or in a collar. Particularly in the comatose patient, plain radiographs should also be taken of the chest and thoracic spine. Other parts of the body in which bony or ligamentous injuries are suspected should also be x-rayed.

When these preliminary examinations and investigations have been concluded, and provided that the patient is in stable condition— with a good airway, adequate oxygenation, and normal blood pressure—it is safe to transfer the patient from the ED for further diagnostic or therapeutic measures. By far the most important further diagnostic measure is CT. Not every case of brain injury should undergo CT because the radiation exposure is twice that of a skull radiograph and the cost may be 4 times greater.[14] However, these considerations should not deter proceeding in all cases in which a skull fracture is present, the GCS score is below 15 for 24 hours or more, seizures have occurred, or a focal neurological deficit has been found.[17,18]

This noninvasive method of imaging the skull and brain has represented a major advance in brain injury care. CT makes it possible to detect intracranial hematomas and to delineate those lying outside the brain in the epidural or subdural spaces from intracerebral hematomas, which lie entirely within the substance of the brain.[19] Occasionally, the hematoma may be difficult to distinguish from brain substance on CT. Nevertheless, the mass effect of the hematoma is detectable by the distortion of the ventricular system and the shift of calcified or identifiable midline structures, such as the choroid plexus, the septum pellucidum, and the pineal gland. CT may also show parenchymal hemorrhage and contusions as regions of increased or mixed density. Brain edema and infarcts appear as regions of low density, although they become evident only after 2 or more days in most instances. Intracranial foreign bodies, intracranial air, and vault or basal fractures of the skull are other findings that may be revealed by CT. Finally, CT permits identification, with a high degree of reliability, of those patients in whom raised intracranial pressure (ICP) will be a problem. Midline shift on CT greater than 10 mm, effacement of the ipsilateral ventricle and dilatation of the contralateral ventricle, or loss of the image of the third ventricle and perimesencephalic cisterns indicates the likelihood of raised ICP.[20]

The urgency with which CT is obtained depends on the grade of severity of the brain injury. In severely brain injured patients (GCS 8 or less), the incidence of intracranial hematoma detected on CT is at least 40 percent.[15] There are no clinical signs that allow the clinician to distinguish reliably between comatose patients with intracranial hematoma and those with diffuse brain injury and swelling. In all severely brain injured patients, therefore, CT should be carried out as soon as the patient is judged safe to be moved from the ED. In cases of moderate injury (GCS 9 through 12), CT should be carried out soon after admission and immediately if the patient (1) has a linear or depressed skull fracture, (2) has focal neurological deficits, or (3) has had seizures. In cases of minor head injury (GCS 13 through 15), CT should also be carried out early if the patient has a skull fracture, has focal neurological deficit, or has had seizures. Even if these factors are absent, CT should be carried out if the patient does not regain the full GCS score of 15 points within 24 hours of admission to the hospital.

In a small number of patients, an epidural hematoma or other intracranial mass lesion develops only after the individual has been admitted to the hospital and after the first CT scan has been negative.[15] In any patient who suffers neurological deterioration or exhibits features suggestive of intracranial hypertension, such as persistent or worsening headache, vomiting, or continued drowsiness in the ward, a repeat CT scan should be carried out. If the original CT scan was performed within 6 hours of injury, an intracranial problem is much more likely to be the cause than a systemic complication, whereas if the original CT scan was done more than 6 hours after injury, the converse is true.[21]

Although magnetic resonance imaging (MRI) is more sensitive than CT in demonstrating brain abnormalities after brain injury and often yields positive findings in those patients classified as having minor brain injury, CT is undeniably the initial diagnostic test. It has the advantages of speed and accessibility, and it reliably detects significant hematomas.[22,23]

Angiography is seldom done nowadays in trauma cases, except when there is a suspicion that a spontaneous intracerebral or subarachnoid hemorrhage preceded the fall or automobile accident that caused the brain injury. It may also be performed following penetrating brain injury if damage to a major artery, a post-traumatic aneurysm, or a caroticocavernous fistula is suspected.

□ ACUTE TREATMENT OF BRAIN INJURY

Early Measures at the Scene of the Accident and in Transit

The most important single objective at this early stage is the establishment and maintenance of a clear airway. The mouth and throat must be cleared of blood, secretions, dentures, and any foreign bodies. All patients with brain injury should be considered as potentially having concomitant injuries to the cervical spine. The patient must be moved into the ambulance with extreme care to avoid unrestrained motion of the head and neck. If circumstances dictate that the patient be transported lying supine, an adequate artificial airway must be in position to prevent the tongue and lower jaw from falling back and occluding the airway. An oral or esophageal occlusive airway is adequate for

this purpose. If the patient does not have to be transported lying supine, the preferred position is three-quarters-prone because in this position the tongue does not fall back, the airway is kept clear, and, if vomiting occurs during transit, the risk of aspiration of vomitus or blood into the airway is much less. In the three-quarters-prone position, the patient is put on his or her side, then turned more face down, with the uppermost leg drawn up to prevent the patient from rolling entirely onto the face. The head is turned slightly to one side, and the tongue and lower jaw tend naturally to fall forward. If oxygen is available, it should be administered during transport to the hospital. Suction should be available in the ambulance to clear the mouth and nasopharynx of blood, vomitus, or secretions. Arterial blood pressure and heart rate should be checked. Systemic hypotension is virtually always due to excess blood loss from associated systemic injuries rather than to the brain injury. Low arterial blood pressure aggravates cerebral hypoxia and further reduces the cerebral perfusion. The presence of systemic hypotension in cases of severe head injury is associated with a twofold increase in mortality.[24] It is therefore imperative in such cases to establish an intravenous line and give crystalloid fluids. Bleeding from the scalp can be arrested by firm pressure and temporary bandaging.

The patient's level of consciousness should be checked by using the GCS and the pupillary findings noted, especially as local swelling around the eyes may make this step more difficult later. If possible, this information should be relayed to the ED staff at the receiving hospital before the arrival of the ambulance.

Management in the Emergency Department

At this stage, the goals of management are to provide normal levels of arterial oxygen tension and arterial blood pressure with adequate peripheral circulation while assessment of neurological status and extent of injuries proceeds. In the comatose patient, an endotracheal tube should be inserted as soon as possible and the cuff inflated. This action provides the best possible security for the airway against aspiration. As the cervical spine may be unstable because of injury, excessive extension of the neck must be avoided during insertion of the endotracheal tube. It may be necessary to perform nasotracheal intubation, a technique requiring expert skills. If intravenous lines have not already been established, this should be done, and blood specimens should be taken to check complete blood count, coagulation profile, serum electrolytes, and blood sugar and alcohol levels and for storage for estimation of drug levels and the like, if indicated. The bladder should be catheterized and careful fluid balance charting instituted.

The ED physician must decide whether it is safe to move the patient for further diagnostic or therapeutic measures. If the patient is to be artificially ventilated, sedative and muscle relaxant drugs are given, but only after an adequate examination of level of consciousness and neurological status.

The location, extent, and severity of all injuries should be carefully documented, preferably via a chart with outlines of the body. The vital signs, GCS score, and pupillary findings, together with any early laboratory results, should be noted on the chart. The neurological examination should be repeated every 10 to 15 minutes so that any trend toward deterioration or improvement can be detected. If the patient has suffered seizure(s) and the decision has been made to give anticonvulsant therapy with intravenous phenytoin, it should be infused slowly with continuous electrocardiographic (ECG) monitoring to guard against cardiac arrhythmias.

Because more brain injuries seen in EDs are minor, a major consideration is whom to admit and whom to allow to go home. All patients with any degree of mental confusion, even if ascribed to alcohol or drugs, and with a post-traumatic amnesia of more than 5 minutes should be admitted for observation, at least for a few hours. The presence of neurological symptoms or signs of a skull fracture are clear indications for admission. Those allowed to go home should receive written advice about changes that would require an urgent return to the hospital.[13]

Operative Management of Brain Injury

There are three main indications for surgical treatment of patients with brain injury. The first is to relieve brain compression due to either an intracranial hematoma or swollen contused and hemorrhagic brain tissue. This situation is virtually always an emergency, and decompressive surgery must be performed as soon as possible by a neurosurgeon with neuroanesthetic support. In comatose patients, it is common practice to administer a bolus of mannitol solution (0.5–1 g/kg) intravenously while the patient is still in the CT imaging suite prior to transfer to the operating theater.[25] The operation entails a craniotomy with exposure of the pertinent brain region(s). All large extracerebral

hematomas should be evacuated. Occasionally, when subdural hematomas are evacuated, it is also necessary to excise necrotic, hemorrhagic, and swollen brain tissue. However, neurosurgeons' opinions are divided concerning the precise indications for surgery and the appropriate approach to small hematomas, contusions, and intracerebral hematomas. Some advocate early surgical treatment, but a growing number prefer aggressive medical management with careful, continuous monitoring of both arterial and intracranial pressure and of jugular venous oxygen saturation. It is essential that CT be repeated as indicated by this monitoring because some intracranial hemorrhages considered initially to be too small to warrant evacuation may expand considerably over a relatively short time.[15]

The second broad indication for surgery is the prevention of infection after compound depressed or penetrating wounds. These procedures include debridement of penetrating wounds to the scalp, elevation of skull fragments, and repair of the dura. The bone fragments can be cleaned and the skull reconstituted with fragments. Removal of foreign, dead, or devitalized tissue from the brain and reconstitution or repair of the dura are the important steps to prevent late infection. Although surgical measures for the prevention of infection from compound wounds must be carried out relatively quickly, in general, exploration of isolated nonmissile compound depressed or penetrating injuries is not an emergency procedure. It may be preferable to wait until the patient has been adequately ventilated and other measures taken to reduce brain swelling and decrease ICP prior to the surgical procedure. Such measures improve the operative conditions by reducing brain hernia and consequently minimize the amount of brain tissue lost at the time of the surgical debridement. If surgery is delayed for much more than 24 hours, however, the risk of intracranial infection is increased. The exception is basal skull fracture, repair of which is usually postponed until any associated CSF leakage has persisted for several days and frontal lobe swelling has subsided.[14]

There is no evidence that surgical treatment of depressed skull fractures or penetrating injuries of the brain affects the incidence of epilepsy at a later date. Prevention of post-traumatic epilepsy is not, therefore, an indication for surgical treatment.

The third and most common surgical indication is to insert a device for monitoring the ICP. All methods, including intracerebral fiber-optic-tipped transducers and subdural or intraventricular catheters connected to an external transducer, require insertion via a burr or twist drill hole, usually in the right frontal bone. The indications for insertion of a monitoring device are shown in Table 3–3. Monitoring generally should continue for 2 to 3 days after severe brain injury to cover the expected duration of post-traumatic brain edema and swelling. It can, however, be continued as long as episodes of intracranial hypertension occur.

There is a trend toward early surgery in cases of craniofacial injury to obtain ideal correction of deformities, but, if the brain injury is severe with an expanding hematoma and problematic intracranial hypertension, surgery for these problems must take precedence. In selected cases of complex disruption of the craniofacial skeleton with associated cerebral and ophthalmologic problems, a single-stage craniofacial repair needs to be done early.[26] In such circumstances, comprehensive multiplanar neuroradiology is necessary preoperatively, and the neurosurgeon, maxillofacial surgeon, and ophthalmologist work as a team.

Nonoperative Management of Severe Head Injury

In the comatose patient, the underlying principles are to optimize cerebral homeostasis and prevent further neurological deterioration due to secondary brain insults. Because the potential causes of such secondary brain damage include hypoxemia, hypotension, fluid and electrolyte imbalance, intracranial hypertension, infection, and hyperthermia, indicators of these complications must be monitored carefully and continuously in the intensive care unit, where adverse trends can be recognized and corrected as rapidly as possible.

VENTILATION

Assisted respiration should be provided for all patients who exhibit any evidence of abnormal respiration. Hypoxia and hypercapnea ($Paco_2$ >35 mmHg or 5 kPa) must be avoided. The aims should be to keep arterial oxygen saturation as close as possible to 100 percent and to maintain arterial CO_2 tension at normal or slightly subnormal levels (circa <30 mmHg or 4 kPa).

In some centers, artificial ventilation via an endotracheal tube is used in all comatose patients for periods of 3 days to 3 weeks after injury. Despite some variation in practice, most would agree to its use in patients who have been comatose (GCS 8 or less) prior to the evacuation of an intracranial hematoma, in patients without hematomas who score GCS 6 or less, and in noncomatose patients in whom CT indicates severe brain injury or potential raised ICP. In addition, patients with less severe brain injuries who have significant facial, chest, or other systemic injuries may require ventilation.

For all patients in whom artificial ventilation and ICP monitoring are employed, arterial pressure should be monitored continuously via an indwelling intra-arterial catheter, which is also used for intermittent withdrawal of blood samples for measurement of arterial blood gases. In addition, a transcutaneous pulse oximeter is used to provide continuous information about tissue oxygenation, jugular venous oxygen saturation ($JVSo_2$) is monitored to detect cerebral ischemia, brain electrical activity is monitored by electroencephalography (EEG) or cerebral function monitor, core temperature is measured via a rectal probe, and blood volume is measured by central venous pressure lines or a Swan-Ganz catheter.

TREATMENT OF RAISED INTRACRANIAL PRESSURE

Raised ICP (defined as ICP >20 mmHg for more than 5 min) is common after severe brain injury. In one recent series of 215 patients who were comatose after brain injury, 53 percent had raised ICP.[27] Raised ICP is associated with a poor outcome, mainly because of brain shifts, herniation, and cerebral ischemia. Until recently, the major emphasis was on controlling ICP to keep it below 25 mmHg. However, what is now considered more important is maintenance of cerebral perfusion pressure (CPP), which is the mean arterial pressure (MAP) minus ICP. When CPP becomes less than 60 to 70 mmHg, cerebral ischemia can become a problem. This lowering of CPP and any elevation of ICP that appears to be accompanied by signs of uncal herniation (e.g., pupillary dilatation) are indications for measures to reduce the ICP.[28] After exclusion of systemic factors, such as airway obstruction or pyrexia, hyperventilation is used first to bring $Paco_2$ down to 4 to 3 kPa, but these

---

TABLE 3–3. Indications for Artificial Ventilation and for Continuous Recording of Intracranial Pressure

1. After evacuation of intracranial hematoma if patient in coma (GCS <8) beforehand
2. No hematoma but patient in deep coma (GCS <6)
3. Patient in coma (GCS <8) and CT signs of raised ICP (absence of third ventricle and of perimesencephalic CSF cisterns)
4. Combination of moderate/severe head injury (GCS <12) and severe chest or facial injuries

levels ideally should be used only briefly in that relative brain hypoxia results because of cerebral vasoconstriction and shifting of the oxygen-hemoglobin dissociation curve. If this effort is unsuccessful in reducing ICP, a choice must be made between (1) the administration of osmotic or hypnotic therapy and (2) vasopressor support to elevate the MAP.

Osmotic therapy consists of a 10- to 15-minute intravenous administration of mannitol (0.5 g/kg), usually followed by a diuretic, such as furosemide (20–40 mg), and then 100 mL stable plasma protein solution to preserve plasma volume. Sedative or hypnotic drug therapy consists of administration of barbiturates, such as thiopental, or agents like propofol that reduce cerebral blood flow (CBF) and cerebral metabolic rate and thereby reduce ICP and brain oxygen requirements. If jugular oxygen saturation monitoring reveals ischemia, vasopressor therapy is indicated because decreasing the CBF further with barbiturates merely aggravates the ischemia. It may also be necessary to monitor not only central venous pressure but also pulmonary artery and pulmonary capillary wedge pressure to ensure that there is no degree of hypovolemia present prior to giving osmotic or sedative drugs.

GENERAL AND METABOLIC CARE

The comatose patient after brain trauma requires full intensive care nursing attention to maintain optimal function and prevent avoidable complications. This care includes specific attention to management of excretory functions, skin care, positioning, chest care, and nutritional needs.

An indwelling urinary catheter is necessary to allow accurate monitoring of urinary output in the acute phase, but, as soon as is practical thereafter, it should be removed to reduce the risk of infection. Serum electrolyte levels should be checked daily and any tendency toward hyponatremia speedily corrected because it can cause osmotic brain edema. Similarly, if osmotic therapy has been used, hypernatremia and hyperosmolality, which can impair renal function, should be avoided. Bowel care usually consists of the regular use of laxative suppositories, and attention to this matter in the earliest stages can prevent troublesome problems from severe constipation later.

The comatose patient requires frequent changes of position and attention to skin care. The regular passive movement of the limbs may prevent subsequent musculoskeletal discomfort when recovery occurs and reduce the risk of contractures and deep venous thrombosis. These range-of-motion exercises should be performed by nurses as well as by therapists. Attention to positioning of the limbs is also important both to avoid contractures and to prevent aggravating spasticity.

Chest care includes humidified air to prevent crusting of sputum and aspiration of secretions from the airway, with vigorous physiotherapy to keep the lung fields clear and prevent atelectasis. Respiratory therapy should include vibration, percussion, and postural drainage within the restrictions imposed by ICP changes.

The cornea must be protected from drying and abrasion in the unconscious patient whose eyes are open. This protection may be achieved by administering lubricant eyedrops and carefully taping the eyelids closed.

For the first few days after severe brain injury, the nasogastric tube is used to keep the stomach empty so as to minimize the risk of aspiration of gastric contents into the lungs. Once bowel sounds return, usually after 72 hours, nasogastric tube feeding begins with half-strength milk at first and gradually working up to the full caloric requirement. In brain injured patients, the required caloric intake is surprisingly high, averaging 3000 kcal/day for an adult. Spontaneous abnormal motor activity increases this requirement. Metabolic responses to injury involve increased sympathetic tone and neuropeptide release mediated by the hypothalamus. Insulin secretion is inhibited, and levels of adrenaline, glycogen, growth hormone, antidiuretic hormone (ADH), cortisol, and aldosterone are increased. These changes result in an elevated basal metabolic rate with energy stores of glycogen and lipids consumed and 200 to 300 g of protein catabolized per day. Because alcohol abuse is a common contributory factor in brain injury, administration of thiamine should be considered to reduce the risk of the Wernicke-Korsakoff syndrome.[29]

A high temperature that develops soon after injury may be due to damage to the hypothalamic temperature-regulating centers, but it may arise from other common accompaniments of brain injury, including infection, the presence of blood in the CSF, and epileptic seizures. Respiratory infection is probably the most common infective cause, followed by urinary tract infection. In cases of transient or permanent CSF fistula, the possibility of meningitis, brain abscess, or subdural empyema must be borne in mind. Other causes of fever that should be considered and checked for are thrombophlebitis, pulmonary embolism, heterotopic ossification, and, of course, wound infection. The hypermetabolic state that can occur as a result of tonic extensor spasms, opisthotonos, and generalized spasticity may also lead to febrile episodes.

Control of body temperature may help to lower ICP by decreasing CBF and cerebral metabolism. Temperatures above 38°C must be avoided because they increase CBF and cerebral blood volume, both of which complicate ICP control. Pyrexia constitutes a common and major secondary brain insult.[15] Treatment approaches include adequate hydration, antipyretic agents (frequently by suppository), alcohol sponging, and cooling blankets. Care must, however, be taken not to induce generalized shivering, which, by increasing systemic and central venous pressures, can elevate ICP.

□ DRUG TREATMENT IN THE ACUTE STAGE

There is considerable controversy and limited consensus about the role of putative neuroprotective drugs in the early stages after brain injury. Much current interest relates to the potential of some agents to afford some protective effect in the damaged brain either biochemically or at a cellular level. Such possible neuroprotective drugs include calcium ion channel blockers, glutamate receptor blockers, and antioxidants.[30,31] Most have significant effects on cardiovascular and neurological function and currently should be used only under strict clinical trial conditions.

The debate over the prophylactic use of anticonvulsants after brain trauma has raged for many years and continues with evidence presented from both sides.[32,33] The increasing evidence of the danger of a detrimental effect on cognitive function from commonly used drugs such as phenytoin and carbamazepine[34] should perhaps encourage a commonsense caution to reserve the use of anticonvulsants to those who have actually had a seizure.

Opinions are similarly divided about the prophylactic use of antibiotics in patients who have CSF rhinorrhea or otorrhea or intracranial air on x-ray. Some neurosurgeons consider the risk of meningitis such that antibiotics must be used; others consider that doing so without evidence of actual infection does not prevent infection and runs the risk of encouraging the development of antibiotic-resistant strains of bacteria. Possibly, as is often the case regarding opinions that are polarized, the wise course is to treat according to the specific findings in individual cases.[35] Thus paralyzed, intubated, and ventilated patients in whom there are no signs of meningism should be given prophylaxis, whereas those who are clinically accessible with no features of meningism should not. The role of lumbar puncture in these groups of patients is determined by the level of ICP, presence of mass lesion, and overall clinical status.

In the acute or emergency setting, medications may have to be given to sedate patients to achieve CT or other investigations and to afford pain relief from associated injuries. Particularly in the case of elderly people who have sustained significant brain injury, other medical disorders may require drug treatment to be maintained or instituted during early care. In all such instances, the principal concerns should be constant review of the medication given and vigilance for potential adverse effects. Careful consideration should be given to all prescriptions because animal studies—and, increasingly, clinical experience—suggest that many agents given in the acute stage may have detrimental effects on the recovering brain.[36]

□ THE FAMILY DURING THE ACUTE STAGE

Brain injury can have profound consequences for the partner or spouse, parents, and others close to the patient. It is never too early to involve the family and wrong to exclude them except in extreme emergency situations. Investment of time in speaking to those close to the patient can pay dividends in that they may give helpful details of the preinjury medical history and, if they were present at the time of injury, useful information on the probable mechanism of injury. It can be easier to manage a confused or agitated individual when a familiar face is present, and the patient emerging from coma often responds first to a relative or friend rather than to professional staff.

Those closest to the patient also have their own problems at this stage. Feeling informed and involved from the earliest times can help them come to terms with the aftermath of serious brain injury. Consideration of their needs is just as central to rehabilitation as caring for the person who has sustained the injury. The management of the caregiver comprises the same fundamental process of assessment of individual needs, provision of support, and prevention of avoidable stress, followed by review and evaluation of their understanding and adaptation to the situation.

REFERENCES

1. Edna, T: Alcohol influence and head injury. Acta Chirurgica Scandinavica 148:209, 1982.
2. Gordon, WA, Mann, N, and Willer, B: Demographic and social characteristics of the traumatic brain injury model system database. J Head Trauma Rehabil 8:26, 1993.

3. Galbraith, S, et al: The relationship between alcohol and head injury and its effect on the conscious level. Br J Surg 63:128, 1976.
4. Corrigan, JD: Substance abuse as a mediating factor in outcome from traumatic brain injury. Arch Phys Med Rehabil 76:302, 1995.
5. Fisher, CM: The neurological examination of the comatose patient. Acta Neurol Scand 45:5, 1969.
6. Teasdale, G, and Jennett, B: Assessment of coma and impaired consciousness: A practical scale. Lancet 2:81, 1974.
7. Teasdale, G, Knill-Jones, R, and Vander Sande, JP: Observer variability in assessing impaired consciousness and coma. J Neurol Neurosurg Psychiatry 41:603, 1978.
8. American College of Surgeons: Advanced Trauma Life Support Student Manual, ed 5. American College of Surgeons, Chicago, 1993.
9. Miller, JD, et al: Further experiences in the management of severe brain injury. J Neurosurg 54:289, 1981.
10. Meyer, S, Gibb, T, and Jurkovich, GJ: Evaluation and significance of the pupillary light reflex in trauma patients. Ann Emerg Med 22:125, 1993.
11. Born, JD, et al: Relative prognostic value of best motor response and brain stem reflexes in patients with severe brain injury. Neurosurgery 16:595, 1985.
12. Selhorst, JB, et al: Papilledema after acute head injury. Neurosurg 16:357, 1985.
13. Briggs, M, et al: Guidelines for initial management after head injury in adults. BMJ 288:983, 1984.
14. Teasdale, GM: Head injury. Neurosurg Psychiatry 58:526, 1995.
15. Miller, JD: Evaluation and treatment of head injury in adults. Neurosurgery Quarterly 2:28, 1992.
16. Miller, JD: Minor, moderate and severe head injury. Neurosurg Rev 9:135, 1986.
17. Teasdale, GM, et al: Risks of acute traumatic intracranial haematoma in children and adults: Implications for managing head injuries. BMJ 300:363, 1990.
18. Servedei, F, et al: Extradural haematomas: An analysis of the changing characteristics of patients admitted from 1980–1986. Diagnostic and therapeutic implications in 158 cases. Brain Inj 2:87, 1988.
19. Robertson, FC, et al: The value of serial computerised tomography in the management of severe brain injury. Surg Neurol 12:161, 1979.
20. Marshall, LF, et al: A new classification of head injury based on computerised tomography. J Neurosurg 75:S14, 1991.
21. Knuckey, N, Gelbard, S, and Epstein, MH: The management of asymptomatic extradural hematomas: A prospective study. J Neurosurg 70:392, 1989.
22. Levin, HS, et al: Magnetic resonance imaging and computerised tomography in relation to the neurobehavioral sequelae of mild and moderate head injuries. J Neurosurg 66:706, 1987.
23. Orrison, WW, et al: Blinded comparison of cranial CT and MR in closed head injury evaluation. American Journal of Neuroradiology 15:351, 1994.
24. Chestnut, RM, et al: The role of secondary brain injury in determining outcome from severe brain injury. J Trauma 34:216, 1993.
25. Miller, JD: Head injury. J Neurol Neurosurg Psychiatry 56:440, 1993.
26. Lang, D: Management of head injury. In Johnson, CD, and Taylor, I (eds): Recent Advances in Surgery 17. Churchill Livingstone, Edinburgh, 1994, p 135.
27. Miller, JD, Piper, IR, and Dearden, NM: Management of intracranial hypertension in head injury: Matching treatment with cause. Acta Neurochir Suppl (Wien) 57:152, 1993.
28. Miller, JD: ICP monitoring: Present position and future directions. Acta Neurochir (Wien) 85:80, 1987.
29. Ferguson, RK, Soryal, IN, and Pentland, B: Thiamine deficiency in head injury: A missed secondary insult? Alcohol Alcohol 32:493, 1997.
30. Faden, A, and Salzman, C: Pharmacological strategies in CNS trauma. Trends Pharmacol Sci 13:29, 1992.
31. White, BC, and Krause, GS: Brain injury and repair mechanisms: The potential for pharmacologic therapy in closed-head trauma. Ann Emerg Med 22:970, 1993.
32. Young, B, et al: Failure of prophylactically administered phenytoin to prevent late posttraumatic seizures. J Neurosurg 58:236, 1983.
33. Temkin, NR, et al: A randomised double-blind study of phenytoin for the prevention of post-traumatic seizures. N Engl J Med 323:497, 1990.
34. Smith, KR, et al: Neurobehavioral effects of phenytoin and carbamazepine in patients recovering from brain trauma: A comparative study. Arch Neurol 51:653, 1994.
35. Eljamel, MS: Antibiotic prophylaxis in unrepaired CSF fistulae. Br J Neurosurg 7:501, 1993.
36. Goldstein, LB: Prescribing potentially harmful drugs to patients admitted to hospital after head injury. J Neurol Neurosurg Psychiatry 58:753, 1995.

Medical and Orthopedic Complications

FLORA M. HAMMOND, MD,
and JAMES T. McDEAVITT, MD

The medical management of patients with traumatic brain injury remains complex for weeks, months, and even years beyond the initial injury. The brain has a direct impact on every physiological function of the body, and potential medical complications arising from damage to this most ubiquitous organ are myriad. Management is further complicated by altered levels of consciousness, resulting in atypical presentation of common clinical problems. The clinician involved in the management of these individuals must maintain a comprehensive view of their condition so that secondary disability is minimized and functional outcome enhanced.

This chapter reviews clinical problems encountered in the care of patients with brain injury in the acute care setting and beyond. Space does not permit detailed discussion of every possible syndrome encountered. Rather, conditions are emphasized that are common, preventable, treatable, or particularly concerning to patients and their families.

☐ COMPLICATION BY ORGAN SYSTEM

Integument

The individual with traumatic brain injury (TBI) may suffer concurrent lacerations and abrasions requiring medical attention. Immobility may cause pressure sores to develop, particularly in the acute recovery period. The regions at greatest risk for breakdown include the occiput, sacrum, sacral cleft, hips, knees, heels, and malleoli. Those dependent for mobility require turning every 2 to 3 hours, attention to sitting posture and wheelchair fit, appropriate padding, and frequent skin monitoring.

Another common dermatologic complication is post-traumatic acne vulgaris, which may be related to endogenous or exogenous corticosteroids. Treatment of this condition is the same as with nontraumatic cases: oral antibiotic, topical antibiotic ointment, benzyl peroxide, or tretinoin, as appropriate for the individual. Allergic rash may develop, with anticonvulsant agents and antibiotics the most common culprits.

Head, Ears, Eyes, Nose, and Throat

AIRWAY MANAGEMENT

Over the past three decades, mechanical ventilation and tracheostomy have become standard care for patients with severe brain injuries.[1] In the acute care setting, airway control is necessary to provide hyperventilation, manage secretions, and prevent aspiration. Initial airway management is accomplished via endotracheal tube. However, the complication rate of endotracheal intubation increases after 7 to 10 days,

The authors would like to express our gratitude for the assistance provided by Lawrence Horn, MD, in reviewing this chapter.

at which point a tracheostomy is usually performed.[2] The procedure can be performed bedside in the intensive care unit and is generally safe and effective.[3-5] Decannulation is usually considered when the patient no longer requires hyperventilation, effectively manages secretions, and is judged to be at low risk for aspiration. A variety of laryngeal and tracheal pathologies may complicate removal of the device.

Tracheal granulomas occur in up to 56 percent of TBI patients with tracheostomies for longer than 1 month.[6] The exuberant overgrowth of epithelial tissue is the result of irritation by the appliance and usually occurs on the anterior portion of the trachea. It can be readily treated by direct excision or laser ablation.[6] Tracheal stenosis may also occur and lead to laryngeal obstruction in about 12 percent of patients.[6-8] Tracheal malacia, or thinning and incompetence of the tracheal wall, is infrequently observed with routine laryngoscopy[7,8]; When provocative maneuvers are employed, however, the reported incidence is 23 percent. Even in the presence of significant pathology, survivors of TBI may not exhibit symptoms of airway obstruction. In an otherwise neurologically intact individual, early symptoms of upper airway obstruction include dyspnea on exertion and diminished exercise tolerance. Patients with severe brain injury may not be able to exercise strenuously enough to elicit symptoms. Additionally, stridor, the hallmark of upper airway disease, may not be present until the severity of the stenosis reaches 90 percent.

Laryngeal pathologies, occurring less frequently, present with dysphonia and a "breathy" vocal quality. Vocal cord paralysis is usually due to direct trauma or damage to the recurrent laryngeal nerve; it is seen in approximately 3.3 to 6 percent of patients with long-term tracheostomies.[6-8]

There is no standardized, universally accepted process by which a patient is decannulated. Many clinicians sequentially downsize the tracheostomy tube when an uncuffed tube is tolerated. Once a small-diameter tube is in place, which allows air movement around the appliance, the opening is plugged. If the patient remains asymptomatic, has an effective cough, and appears able to manage secretions safely, the tube is removed and an occlusive dressing placed.[9]

Decannulation carries a potential risk of airway obstruction and pneumonia and should not be undertaken in a cavalier fashion. Nowak et al.[7] decannulated 72 patients with brain injuries, long-term tracheostomies, and various levels of cognitive functioning. All patients underwent laryngoscopy and, if necessary, treatment of laryngeal pathology prior to appliance removal. Ten patients (14%) died from pneumonia, two in the immediate pericannulation period and the remainder within 1 year. All of the deaths save one occurred in patients functioning at a Rancho level III, or poorer. The authors recommend that low-functioning patients not be decannulated. However, the study is flawed by the absence of a control group, and it is not clear that the mortalities were directly attributable to decannulation.

Many authors[6,7] recommend performing laryngoscopy of all patients prior to making a decannulation decision, based on the high incidence of pathological findings. Others[9] advocate direct visualization of the upper airway only in high-risk patients or those with respiratory distress. No study to date defines the frequency with which anatomic visualization alters care of the patient. For now, prudence dictates that laryngoscopy be performed on all symptomatic or unresponsive (Rancho level III or below) patients before decannulation is considered.

BRUXISM

Bruxism, the rhythmic grinding of teeth, is present in 5 to 20 percent of the general population[10,11] and may result in widening of the periodontal ligaments, increased alveolar bone loss, loose dentition, diffuse bone resorption in the anterior mandible, severe wearing of occlusive surfaces, and infection. In one study of comatose patients with bruxism, the phenomenon was present only in concert with significant neurological improvement.[11]

The etiology of neurogenic bruxism remains unclear. Stereotypical mouth movements have been reproduced in experimental animals with stimulation of the motor cortex or limbic system. The loss of cortical inhibition may also be a factor, as bruxism may be produced by hypothalamic lesions. The dopaminergic system may be important in the production of the syndrome, as dopamine increases gnawing behavior in rats and dopamine agonists have been known to precipitate bruxism in humans. Alternatively, serotonin may play a causative role. A case series[12] of four depressed patients developed bruxism with the initiation of a serotonin selective reuptake inhibitor (SSRI); all improved with either reduction in dosage of the antidepressant or with the addition of buspirone.

The treatment of neurogenic bruxism consists primarily of good oral hygiene. Bite guards may be useful to prevent dental damage. Botulinum toxin injections to the masseter muscles have been advocated[13] but are not performed for this purpose at most centers. Dopamine-depleting agents are of theoretical benefit, but these agents are generally avoided in patients with brain injury. Fortunately, more than half the cases resolve spontaneously.

Gastrointestinal

STRESS ULCERS

Gastrointestinal bleeding occurs in up to 80 percent[14] of survivors of major trauma and traumatic brain injury. Brain injury is a well-recognized major risk factor for the development of stress-related gastric ulcers. The incidence of clinically significant bleeding has declined over the past decade, presumably because of widespread prophylaxis with histamine H_2 receptor antagonists. Although these agents may not decrease the incidence of asymptomatic gastric erosions,[15] they are highly effective in the reduction of clinically significant bleeding.[15–17] It is less clear how long prophylaxis should continue; generally, agents are continued until the period of maximal physiological stress has passed.

Adverse reactions to H_2 receptor antagonists are rare but reported. Histamine receptors are present in mammalian brains and appear to exert an inhibitory effect on parts of the cerebral cortex.[18] Although agents in use clinically do not cross the blood-brain barrier readily, a variety of case reports document lethargy, mental status changes,[19] and psychosis[20,21] with both cimetidine and ranitidine, consequences of dopamine blockade. A single study[22] attempts to document cognitive effects of ranitidine in a controlled fashion. Patients undergoing elective surgery were given placebo, ranitidine, metoclopramide, or a combination of the two agents intravenously. Those receiving the H_2 antagonist alone experienced rare subjective complaints of drowsiness (5/32) or restlessness (1/32). Of note, one-third of patients receiving both agents developed akathisia.

HEPATIC DYSFUNCTION

Liver function tests are elevated after brain injury in up to 43 percent of patients in a rehabilitation setting.[23] Benign induction of hepatic enzymes by anticonvulsant medications is usually the culprit. However, other potential causes of hepatic dysfunction must be considered, including infectious hepatitis and biliary obstruction. Hepatic necrosis following cardiovascular shock with prolonged resuscitation is not uncommon.

It has long been recognized that all common anticonvulsant medications can produce asymptomatic elevations in hepatic enzymes measured in the serum.[24–27] Elevations of more than twice normal are not unusual and generally not an indication to withdraw therapy in the absence of symptoms.[28] γ-Glutamyl transferase (GGT) and alanine transaminase (ALT) are most commonly affected.[28] Aspartate transaminase and serum alkaline phosphatase may also be elevated, although perhaps no more so than in healthy age–matched controls.[29]

Significant hepatic damage is a rare but important side effect of all anticonvulsant medications. Although liver function tests are routinely monitored by many clinicians,[30] no literature demonstrates the ability of routine laboratory monitoring to predict the development of severe, life-threatening drug reactions.[31] There is a growing consensus in the literature that routine laboratory testing is not indicated[28,31]; rather, patients should be educated regarding the signs and symptoms of hepatic failure and evaluated immediately for nausea, fatigue, malaise, right upper quadrant pain, jaundice, bruising, abnormal bleeding, or change in seizure frequency.

NUTRITION AND FEEDING

The lack of validity of the Harris-Benedict equation in predicting the caloric requirements of survivors of brain injury in the acute setting is well documented. Patients display increased energy expenditure and protein catabolism. Multiple factors have been proposed to explain changes in nutritional needs, including the administration of steroids and mobility. However, the injury to the brain itself has a direct effect on nutritional needs.

Phillips et al.[32] evaluated children and adolescents from admission to 2 weeks after injury. Measured energy expenditure (MEE) was 1.3 times the Harris-Benedict predicted value for energy expenditure, with the equation becoming more predictive by the end of the second week. Sunderland and Heibrun[33] further evaluated the predictive value of a variety of energy expenditure formulas. A hundred and two patients were evaluated in an acute care setting. The best formula predicted the MEE within 75 to 125 percent of the true value in only 56 percent of measurements. Borzotta et al.[34] also measured energy expenditure directly and found that in 48 patients energy expenditure was 135 to 141 percent of the predicted MEE during the first 4 weeks of injury.

The majority of research has been performed in acute care environments. The literature shows that the Harris-Benedict equation consistently underestimates the caloric needs of individuals in this setting. However, the time course of return to normal energy homeostasis has not been well described. The nutritional status of survivors of brain injury, especially severe brain injuries, must be carefully monitored to avoid inappropriate weight loss or gain.

Enteral feeding is generally established as quickly as possible following the injury. Percutaneous endoscopic gastrostomy tubes are often placed and have the relative advantage of allowing bolus feeding. However, patients with severe brain injuries may display reduction in lower esophageal sphincter tone that may contribute to aspiration pneumonitis with gastric feeding.[35] Jejunal feedings should be considered in these patients.

Ongoing nutritional assessment is necessary. Even with continuous enteral feeding, patients may not receive the prescribed quantity of feeding because of interruptions for therapies, medication administration, and the like.[36,37]

Cardiovascular

CARDIAC DYSFUNCTION

Electrocardiographic (ECG) abnormalities and myocardial damage have been documented after TBI, subarachnoid hemorrhage, and cerebrovascular accident.[38–41] In a retrospective study of 180 individuals in an inpatient rehabilitation setting after TBI, Kalisky et al.[23] found a 21 percent occurrence of ECG abnormalities. McLeod et al.[42] prospectively studied 7 previously healthy young men following severe TBI and noted the development of sinus tachycardia in 5, ST depression indicative of progressive myocardial ischemia in 3, ventricular arrhythmia in 1, and 2 deaths. Cardiac isoenzyme elevation and myocardial necrosis have been observed in association with TBI.[43] The etiology of these findings may be related to the massive catecholamine release associated with TBI,[44] direct myocardial trauma, increased cardiac work and oxygen consumption, intracellular overload,[45] or increased intracranial pressure.[41,46]

Hypertension

Arterial hypertension is a frequently observed phenomenon in the acute and subacute periods following TBI, with an estimated incidence of 11 to 25 percent.[23,47] Post-traumatic hypertension usually resolves spontaneously, and long-term management with antihypertensive agents is rarely necessary. Labi and Horn,[48] in a retrospective study of 80 individuals with TBI discharged from a rehabilitation facility, found that of those who required antihypertensive medication, only 45 percent required treatment at the time of rehabilitation discharge, with all others successfully tapered off antihypertensive agents at subsequent follow-up.

Post-traumatic hypertension is frequently associated with a hyperadrenergic state of tachycardia, hyperhidrosis, temperature elevations, and increased cardiac output, suggesting the source to be central autonomic dyscontrol.[49] This sympathetic hyperactivity is correlated with findings of high elevations in plasma and urine catecholamine levels, particularly in severe TBI.[49–52] The hypothalamus is thought to be a key regulator of this phenomenon. However, other sources of autonomic control may be responsible, such as the orbital frontal cortex, septal complex, amygdala, thalamus, pituitary, locus ceruleus, nucleus tractus solitarius, nucleus ambiguus, dorsal vagal nucleus, and reticular activating system.[53] Other important potential etiologies of arterial hypertension should also be considered in the traumatically injured individual with sympathetic hyperactivity, including autonomic dysreflexia resulting from occult spinal cord injury, renal contusion, adrenal hemorrhage, and pheochromocytoma.[53] In addition, iatrogenic causes such as methylphenidate or ephedrine should be considered.

Arterial hypertension and its management are of particular interest because of the potential impact on cerebral blood flow, intracranial pressure, cerebral perfusion pressure, and pressure-volume index in the acute and subacute settings. In normal circumstances, cerebral blood flow (CBF) remains constant during changes in arterial pressure between 60 and 150 mmHg, accomplished through cerebral autoregulation. However, cerebral autoregulation is frequently impaired after TBI, resulting in passive changes in CBF in response to changes in arterial pressure. CBF is defined by the following formula:

$$CBF = K \frac{CPP \times d^4}{8 \times l \times v}$$

where K is a constant, CPP is cerebral perfusion pressure, d is blood vessel diameter, l is blood vessel length, and v is blood viscosity.[54] Cerebral perfusion pressure (CPP) is the difference between mean arterial pressure and intracranial pressure (ICP). From these definitions, it can be seen that CPP and CBF are augmented by increasing arterial pressure or decreasing ICP and that CBF is largely influenced by even small changes in blood vessel diameter. Many studies have investigated the effects of inducing reductions and elevations in arterial blood pressure on cerebral parameters.[55–58] Reductions in arterial blood pressure may decrease CBF and increase ICP. Bouma et al.[56] found that, in those with intact autoregulation, reducing blood pressure resulted in profound increases in ICP, whereas, in those with impaired autoregulation, ICP varied directly with blood pressure. Current data suggest that reductions in blood pressure should be avoided, as concurrent decrease in CBF may invoke cerebral ischemia. Then again, many emphasize the potential detrimental effects of hypertension.[58,59]

Hypertension may cause increased capillary hydrostatic pressure when arterial blood pressure exceeds the limits of autoregulation, leading to increased CBF and CPP and thereby increasing the risk of brain swelling,[59] cerebral edema, rebleeding, or continued hemorrhage. In the case of impaired autoregulation, even moderate elevations in arterial hypertension may result in increased capillary hydrostatic pressure. Studies regarding induced increases in arterial blood pressure for potential therapeutic benefit have failed to demonstrate consistent beneficial effects.[56]

Because of the critical balance between the detrimental effects of elevated blood pressures and the risk of inducing ischemia by lowering blood pressure, the optimal management of post-traumatic hypertension is controversial. If the choice has been made to administer an antihypertensive agent(s), the following points should be considered. Vasodilating agents, such as diazoxide, hydralazine, nitroprusside, and nitroglycerin, risk further increasing CBF despite lowering systemic blood pressure.[60] In addition, after TBI, hydralazine may increase cardiac work, increase myocardial oxygen demand, increase myocardial damage, and worsen pulmonary ventilation-perfusion inequality.[61] Propranolol has been recommended in TBI based on its observed effects on decreasing plasma catecholamines, cardiac index, myocardial oxygen demand, and heart rate, with improved pulmonary ventilation-perfusion inequality.[61] Central-acting antihypertensive agents may be sedating and thus should be avoided in this population.

THROMBOEMBOLIC DISEASE

Venous thromboembolism (VTE) is a well-recognized complication of major trauma, accountable for much morbidity and mortality. Estimates of its incidence vary widely. Geerts et al.[62] reported an incidence of 58 percent radiographically detectable lower extremity deep venous thrombosis (DVT) after major trauma, with 54 percent incidence in those with major brain trauma and 69 percent with lower extremity orthopedic injuries. In those detected to have DVT on venogram, only 1.5 percent (3/201) had clinical evidence suggestive of VTE. VTE is often clinically silent, with sudden death from pulmonary embolus as the first clinical sign in 70 to 80 percent.[63] Risk factors common to the trauma patient include venous stasis (because of immobility, hemiplegia, congestive heart failure, or previous VTE), trauma, surgery, lower extremity fractures, and age older than 40 years. Considering the high incidence of silent VTE, methodologies for early detection and prophylaxis are critical.

There is currently no available means to absolutely prevent VTE. The ideal prophylactic instrument should be effective, easy to administer and monitor, cost-efficient, and of minimal risk. At present, a number of prophylactic regimens are available, including graded-compression elastic stockings, intermittent pneumatic compression, unfractionated heparin, low-molecular-weight heparin, warfarin, or vena cava filter. Clinical studies have supported graded-compression elastic stockings as an inexpensive means of reducing the incidence of DVT in conjunction with other prophylactic measures. Intermittent pneumatic compression is an effective means of lessening DVT risk, particularly in those at risk of bleeding complications from pharmacological methods. However, lower extremity fractures and wounds may preclude the use of this device. Prophylactic anticoagulation in TBI is generally achieved with low-dose unfractionated heparin at a dose of 5000 units every 8 or 12 hours or low-molecular-weight heparin. Anticoagulant therapy in the individual with TBI is controversial because of the associated risk of intracranial hemorrhage and wound hematoma. The choice to use such agents in this population is made on a case-by-case basis by weighing the foreseen risks of developing VTE and incurring anticoagulation complications. In the individual at high risk for VTE in whom anticoagulants and intermittent pneumatic compression devices are contraindicated, a vena cava filter may be inserted prophylactically to reduce the risk of pulmonary embolism.

The methods available for the detection of DVT include ^{125}I-fibrinogen scanning, impedance plethysmography (IPG), doppler ultrasonography, B-mode ultrasonography, and contrast venography. The sensitivity of these measures, however, is greatly reduced when they are utilized as a screening tool for asymptomatic VTE. ^{125}I-fibrinogen scanning is more than 90 percent effective in detecting acute calf thrombi, with only 60 to 80 percent detection of proximal thrombi.[64] The utility of ^{125}I-fibrinogen scanning is in serial screening for calf thrombi or, diagnostically, in conjunction with IPG to detect proximal thrombi undetected by ^{125}I-fibrinogen scanning. IPG is associated with 90 to 93 percent sensitivity and 94 percent specificity for proximal thrombi.[65] False-negative results may occur from calf thrombi; small, nonocclusive proximal thrombi; and proximal thrombi with well-developed collaterals. Katz and McCulla[66] reported a false-negative rate of 4 to 10 percent in using IPG for asymptomatic rehabilitation inpatients, which demonstrates its limited efficacy as a screening device. False-positive findings may also result from improper positioning, failure to relax lower extremity musculature, and nonthrombotic outflow obstruction. Doppler ultrasonography is reported to have 95 percent sensitivity and 99 percent specificity for symptomatic proximal DVT[65]; it detects approximately 50 percent of symptomatic calf thrombi.[64] Interpreting doppler ultrasonography results is highly dependent upon skill and experience. B-mode ultrasonography, like IPG and doppler ultrasonography, has high sensitivity and specificity for symptomatic proximal thrombi, with limited ability to detect calf thrombi. Contrast venography remains the gold standard for the diagnosis of clinically suspected DVT. However, this procedure has several limitations, including contrast-induced thrombosis, contrast allergy, and patient discomfort.

Thromboembolism is initially treated with intravenous heparin or adjusted-dose subcutaneous heparin for 5 to 10 days.[67] Oral anticoagulation should overlap with heparin administration for 4 to 5 days; the heparin is discontinued once oral anticoagulation is therapeutic. Anticoagulation is continued for 3 to 6 months, with the prothrombin time prolonged to an INR of 2.0 to 3.0.[67] While the patient is on heparin, the platelet count should be monitored for the potential development of heparin-induced thrombocytopenia. Timing and safety of anticoagulation in TBI are uncertain. With TBI and multiple traumas, many individuals are at great risk for intracranial hemorrhage. In addition, TBI may predispose the individual to falls, further increasing the risk of bleeding with anticoagulation. If anticoagulation is contraindicated, or pulmonary emboli or VTE recur despite adequate anticoagulation, vena cava interruption is the appropriate treatment.[67] The most common complication of vena cava interruption is lower extremity edema.

Thromboembolic disease remains a serious problem, with no consensus regarding management. Available diagnostic tools are suboptimal as screening tools for asymptomatic VTE. Prophylactic methods must be tailored to the individual's clinical setting to limit complications. TBI poses unique complications to anticoagulation. Alternative treatment with vena cava interruption may be necessary in selected individuals.

Genitourinary System

NEUROGENIC BLADDER

Survivors of brain injury are frequently incontinent. Patients usually display a disinhibited type of neurogenic bladder, in which the bladder volume is reduced but empties completely with normal intravesicular volumes. However, other forms of urinary incontinence may be present. Urinary retention during the acute care phase may lead to stretching of the detrusor muscle and then to a myotonic bladder with inadequate emptying and overflow incontinence. Additionally, an upper or lower motor neuron voiding pattern may be present in the presence of an occult spinal cord injury. Finally, the presence of an outflow obstruction should be considered, especially in older men who may have a degree of prostatic hypertrophy. These problems are generally excluded with the demonstration of low postvoid residual urine volumes.

If the voiding pattern is consistent with a disinhibited type bladder, a "time void" program is usually initiated, in which the patient is offered the urinal or commode at a regular interval. Occasionally more elaborate behavioral programs may be necessary.[68,69]

PREGNANCY

Although pregnancy in the acute stages of traumatic brain injury is not common, a high index of suspicion must be maintained to ensure the health of the mother and a potentially viable fetus. Insemination may occur prior to the injury; during conjugal visits in a rehabilitation setting, or after discharge home or to a long-term care facility. Pregnancy should be ruled out in the acute period by laboratory testing in all women of child-bearing age. Pregnancy in a survivor of a brain injury poses several challenges. The relative importance of numerous radiological examinations to assess intracranial status and to detect and monitor fractures needs to be carefully considered. Attention must also be paid to the teratogenic potential of medications. Hypertension, a common sequela of TBI, may actually be a sign of preeclampsia. In addition, cognitive and physical deficits may interfere with the individual's ability for child care.

Irregularities in the menstrual cycle, especially amenorrhea, occur after significant trauma or brain injury. Menses usually return within 6 months of the injury. Neuroendocrine disorders may follow TBI, as the pituitary and hypothalamus are particularly susceptible to injury. If amenorrhea persists, laboratory evaluation of the pituitary-gonadotropin axis may be necessary. Patients and their families frequently assume amenorrhea following TBI assures infertility, but it most certainly does not. Education should be provided to all involved parties regarding the potential for fertility and appropriate birth control techniques to prevent unwanted pregnancy while the patient is still in the recovery process.

Endocrine

HYPONATREMIA

Hyponatremia may occur after TBI or subarachnoid hemorrhage. An acute drop in serum sodium may result in mental status changes, lethargy, coma, psychosis, seizures, cramps, or nausea. However, acute hyponatremia may be masked by symptoms of the primary brain injury. Laboratory monitoring may be necessary to detect the condition. The development of symptoms is largely dependent on the rate and magnitude of plasma osmolality decline, so patients with chronic hyponatremia may be entirely asymptomatic.

Hyponatremia has numerous recognized etiologies, all of which may occur concurrently with traumatic brain injury. Potential causes include cerebral salt wasting (CSW) syndrome, osmotic diuresis, salt-losing nephropathy, proximal renal tubular acidosis, hyperaldosteronism, vomit-

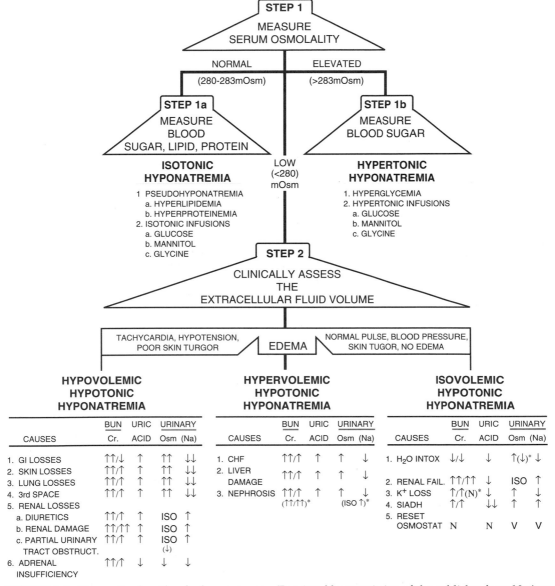

FIGURE 4–1. Diagnostic algorithm for hyponatremia. (Reprinted by permission of the publisher from Narins: Diagnostic strategies in disorders of fluid, electrolyte and acid-base homeostasis. American Journal of Medicine 72:498–501. Copyright 1982 by Excerpta Medica Inc.)

TABLE 4–1. Treatment Approaches for Hyponatremia

Tonicity and Extracellular Volume Status	Cause	Treatment
Hypotonic, hypervolemic	Renal failure Nephrotic syndrome Cirrhosis Heart failure	▪ Treat underlying disorder ▪ Water restriction
Hypotonic, euvolemic	SIADH	*Acute:* ▪ Loop-active diuretics ▪ Replacement of lost sodium *Chronic:* ▪ Water restriction ▪ Demeclocycline to induce free water excretion
	Hypothyroidism	▪ Thyroxine replacement ▪ Water restriction
	Water intoxication	▪ Psychiatric counseling ▪ Water restriction
Hypotonic, hypovolemic	*Extrarenal loss:* Vomiting Diarrhea Third space sequestration	▪ Correct underlying disorder ▪ Volume re-expansion
	Renal loss: Cerebral salt-wasting syndrome Diuretics Salt-losing nephropathy diuretics Proximal renal tubular acidosis Adrenal insufficiency	▪ Correct underlying disorder ▪ Volume re-expansion with isotonic saline
Isotonic hyponatremia	Pseudohyponatremia Isotonic infusions	▪ No specific treatment needed ▪ Treat the abnormality of lipid or protein metabolism
Hypertonic hyponatremia	Hyperglycemia Hypertonic infusions	▪ Correct underlying disorder

ing, diarrhea, third space sequestration, sodium potassium shift, syndrome of inappropriate secretion of antidiuretic hormone (SIADH), hypothyroidism, water intoxication, hyperglycemia, hyperlipidemia, infusion of excessive free water, renal failure, nephrotic syndrome, heart failure, and cirrhosis. Hyponatremia may also be iatrogenic from such common culprits as diuretics, carbamazepine, hypoglycemic agents (chlorpropamide, tolbutamide), narcotics (morphine, barbiturates), psychotropic agents (phenothiazine derivatives), antineoplastic agents (cyclophosphamide, vincristine), indomethacin, acetaminophen, clofibrate, nicotine, and oxytocin.[70] Accurate diagnosis depends upon appropriate measurement of serum tonicity and extracellular fluid volume status, as outlined in Figure 4–1. Establishing the correct etiology enables implementation of the appropriate treatment regimen (Table 4–1). Care must be taken not to correct hyponatremia too rapidly, as rapid increases in serum sodium can cause serious neurological damage, pontine myelinolysis, or congestive heart failure.

Hyponatremia associated with TBI is generally present in a hypotonic setting with either euvolemic (SIADH) or hypovolemic (CSW) volume status. In the early 1950s, hyponatremia associated with intracranial lesions was considered predominantly the consequence of CSW, which refers to renal sodium loss in the presence of intracranial disease, leading to progressive depletion of serum sodium and extracellular volume. In 1957, Schwartz et al.[71] reported SIADH, water retention resulting from excessive antidiuretic hormone (ADH), was responsible for two cases of hyponatremia associated with bronchogenic carcinoma. Subsequent studies appeared to support this observation. More recently, however, investigations have demonstrated 10 percent or greater plasma volume decrement in the majority of cases of hyponatremia associated with TBI,[72–74] excluding the diagnosis of SIADH in such cases. Volume depletion of this magnitude is a known physiological stimulus to ADH secretion. Thus, the frequent observation of ADH elevation may actually be appropriate rather than inappropriate. It appears that hyponatremia associated with TBI is more commonly the result of CSW if hypovolemia induces an appropriate release of ADH. Distinguishing between these two entities is crucial to the proper treatment of hyponatremia, as well as to general medical management of the individual with TBI. Accepted treatment of SIADH incorporates fluid restriction; in the case of CSW, however, fluid restriction may further deplete the extracellular volume. Following TBI or subarachnoid hemorrhage, this hypovolemic status may induce vasospasm, which may lead to additional brain tissue damage. Thus, suitable treatment of hyponatremia clearly requires accurate diagnosis of the underlying etiology.

HYPERNATREMIA

Hypernatremia may also complicate TBI. Common causes include central diabetes insipidus (DI), medications (e.g., phenytoin, lithium, demeclocycline), inability to obtain water, impaired thirst, sodium overload from endogenous or exogenous causes, or volume contraction with inadequate water replacement, as might occur with diarrhea, sensible or insensible losses, or osmotic diuresis. The diagnosis is determined by extracellular fluid volume status, as outlined in Figure 4–2.[69] DI, the most common cause of hypernatremia in TBI, is the result of ADH deficiency due to hypothalamic or pituitary damage. Treatment of central DI includes replacing ongoing water loss, slow correction of free water deficit, and ADH replacement through adminis-

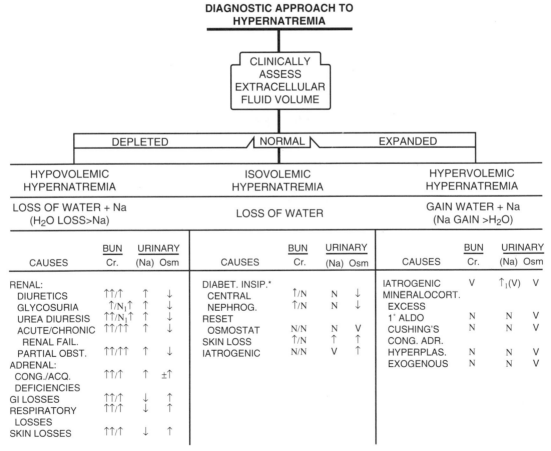

FIGURE 4–2. Diagnostic algorithm for hypernatremia. (Reprinted by permission of the publisher from Narins: Diagnostic strategies in disorders of fluid, electrolyte and acid-base homeostasis. American Journal of Medicine 72:498–501. Copyright 1982 by Excerpta Medica Inc.)

tration of aqueous vasopressin, lysine vasopressin nasal spray, or desmopressin acetate nasal drops (DDAVP).

ANTERIOR PITUITARY DISEASE

Symptomatic endocrine dysfunction after brain injury is relatively rare, occurring in only 4 percent of patients with brain injuries.[23] The signs and symptoms of anterior pituitary dysfunction relate to the multiple target organs involved but is often insidious. Hyperprolactinemia from loss of hypothalamic dopamine inhibition may produce gynecomastia, galactorrhea, impotence, and anovulation. Growth hormone deficiency is occult in adults but may have dramatic effects on growth in children. Although ACTH deficiency is seldom life threatening, it may become manifest during stress, producing fatigue, fever, hypotension, and mental aberrations. Thyroid-stimulating hormone (TSH) deficiency, with resultant hypothyroidism, can result in mental dullness, cold intolerance, and anemia. Lack of gonadotropins impairs libido, potency, and gametogenesis, with amenorrhea in women. Failure to achieve puberty may also occur, and precocious puberty has been reported.[75] Screening for anterior pituitary endocrine dysfunction should be considered in the presence of:

1. Signs or symptoms of endocrine dysfunction
2. Persistent amenorrhea
3. Evidence of posterior pituitary dysfunction (see hyponatremia and hypernatremia discussions)
4. Documented basilar skull and/or facial fractures
5. Poor neurological improvement or regression
6. History of severe hypotension or shock

Musculoskeletal

FRACTURES

Fractures are commonly associated with TBI and may lead to increased morbidity, mortality, and disability. Because of acute medical needs, altered consciousness, and impaired communication, diagnosis of fractures may be delayed. When Garland and Bailey[76] prospectively investigated 254 individuals with TBI admitted to a rehabilitation facility, they discovered an 11 percent incidence of undiagnosed fractures at the time of rehabilitation admission. Most concerning is the potential for undiagnosed spine fracture. A cervical spine injury must be assumed to be present until proven otherwise in every unconscious individual. The rehabilitation professional must maintain a high level of suspicion for axial and long-bone fractures, particularly looking for swelling, painful joint ranging, deformity, or unexplained neurological deficits. Screening radiographs are recommended, as appropriate for the injury mechanism and examination limitations. In comatose individuals who have sustained high-velocity injury, at a minimum, screening films should include the cervical and thoracic spine, pelvis including both hips, and bilateral knees, and bone scan may be necessary.[77] Treatment decisions must assume eventual good neurological recovery to ensure minimal disability. Early fracture fixation is generally the preferred mode of treatment considering the agitation, confusion, and increased muscle tone frequently present, as well as the need to avoid prolonged immobilization. Early fracture stabilization is associated with fewer pulmonary complications, improved nursing care, decreased use of pain medications, fewer joint contractures, decreased mortality, shortened hospital stay, and facilitation of rehabilitation efforts.[77] Casts must be applied in positions of function and checked regularly for neurovascular compromise, particularly in patients with impaired communication and altered consciousness.

PERIPHERAL NERVE INJURIES

Peripheral nerve injuries (PNI) are common, caused by trauma, improper positioning, postoperative complications, iatrogenic causes, and heterotopic ossification. The estimated incidence of PNI in cases of severe TBI is 34 percent. In Garland and Bailey's series,[76] 11 percent of patients presented with an undiagnosed PNI at the time of admission to a rehabilitation unit. Thus, particular attention is needed to the signs of PNI, including motor and sensory deficits, asymmetric hyperreflexia, muscle atrophy, and fasciculations. A flail extremity following trauma should be considered a plexus injury until proven otherwise. Electromyography and nerve conduction studies may be utilized to confirm the diagnosis, define the location and nature of nerve injury, and assess prognosis. Orthotic devices may be needed for contracture prevention, support, and increased function.

Understanding common mechanisms of PNI is important for effective prevention. Positioning the upper extremity in a flexed elbow, pronated forearm position increases susceptibility to ulnar neuropathy. Cubital tunnel capacity is maximized in elbow extension when the arcuate ligament is slack, and compromised in elbow flexion when the arcuate ligament is taut with medial ligament bulging. The cubital tunnel is brought closer to the surface with forearm pronation, and further from the surface with supination. The individual with TBI may be at risk for median nerve injury as a consequence of increased wrist flexion muscle tone or repetitive use in transfers and wheelchair propulsion. The radial nerve is frequently injured as a result of midshaft humerus fracture, extended pressure on bedrails or operating tables, or traction injury. The peroneal nerve risks injury from lateral decubitus positioning, frog-legged positioning (external hip rotation, knee flexion, and foot inversion, causing full stretch on the peroneal nerve), leg straps, improper cast fit, ankle sprain, and femoral fracture.

HETEROTOPIC OSSIFICATION

Heterotopic ossification (HO), the formation of mature lamellar bone in soft tissue, is a well-recognized complication of TBI, with 11 to 76 percent incidence. The variability in reported incidence is caused by differences in study design, study population, and diagnostic measure(s). The incidence of clinically significant cases is 10 to 20 percent, with joint ankylosis in less than 10 percent of HO lesions.[79] HO most commonly results in pain and limited range of motion but may be complicated by bony ankylosis, peripheral nerve compression (with particular susceptibility of the ulnar and femoral nerves), vascular compression, or lymphedema.[80] The development of such complications may greatly increase the disability and care needs beyond that resulting from the brain injury itself.

Identified risk factors include prolonged coma (>2 weeks), immobility, and limb spasticity. The presence of prolonged post-traumatic unconsciousness for 1 month or longer is associated with 61 to 77 percent incidence of HO as detected by screening radiographs.[81] The period of greatest risk for HO development is during the first 3 to 4 months after injury.

The etiology and pathophysiology of HO are uncertain. It is thought that fibroblasts inappropriately differentiate into bone-forming cells. An interaction between local and systemic factors is suspected to be a key factor in this conversion. Bone morphogenic protein has been isolated and shown to induce this transformation of undifferentiated mesenchymal cells to osteoblasts in vivo. The initial development phase is associated with inflammation and increased blood flow to the intended soft tissue. This phase is followed by bone matrix formation, with eventual crystallization to produce mature osseous bone. Histological studies of HO tissue have revealed true metabolically active bone, containing greater numbers of osteoblasts and osteoclasts than normal bone. HO maturation is generally completed by 6 to 18 months after injury. Unfortunately, this process is well underway long before clinical signs and symptoms become evident. Consequently, effective HO treatment strategies should be aimed at early initiation of prophylactic efforts.

HO affects large joints in the periarticular region and does not occur intra-articularly. The hips are most frequently involved, followed in frequency by the elbows, shoulders, and knees. Clinically, HO may present with limited range of motion (the most common sign), pain (the most common symptom), local swelling, erythema, warmth, muscle guarding, or low-grade fever. HO shares many signs and symptoms with other serious, potentially life-threatening disorders, earning description as "the benign disease with a malignant differential diagnosis."[82] The differential diagnosis includes deep venous thrombosis, tumor, septic joint, hematoma, cellulitis, and fracture.

Available diagnostic measures vary widely in cost, sensitivity, and specificity. The choice of diagnostic test depends on the time since injury, as well as the clinical presentation. Although specificity is poor, serum alkaline phosphatase (SAP) elevation may be the earliest and least expensive means of detection. In general, SAP begins rising within 2 weeks after injury, exceeds normal values by 3 weeks, and remains elevated for 5 months following injury.[83] However, alkaline phosphatase may be elevated for other reasons, such as fracture and hepatic dysfunction. Triple-phase bone scan (TPBS) is a sensitive means of early HO detection. Phase I (blood flow phase) and phase II (blood pool phase) become positive within the first 2 to 4 weeks after injury, and phase III (static phase) is positive by 4 to 8 weeks postinjury, with normalization by 7 to 12 months.[79] Positive TPBS may necessitate further assessment to differentiate HO from other processes such as bone tumor, metastasis, and osteomyelitis. Plain radiographs lag behind TPBS, taking 3 weeks to 2 months postinjury to reveal evidence of HO. Thus, the usefulness of plain radiographs for early detection is limited. Radiographs may be useful to confirm the presence and maturity of established HO, evaluate bony ankylosis, and detect occult fractures.

Therapeutic interventions for HO need to be considered in terms of prophylaxis and management. The primary goal should be prevention, as currently available treatment methods are suboptimal, with great potential disability resulting from HO. Individuals anticipated to be in prolonged coma with increased muscle tone are at highest risk for HO development and should be targeted with prophylactic measures. To maximize efficacy, prophylactic efforts must be started immediately.

Range of motion (ROM) exercises are utilized prophylactically and also as an essential treatment for developing HO. The goals of ROM are to maintain joint range, prevent ankylosis, and maximize eventual function. To prevent bony ankylosis in developing HO, forceful manipulation may be utilized, often performed under anesthesia. However, controversy exists as to whether aggressive ROM may cause microtrauma and local hemorrhage, predisposing the patient to HO development. Studies in animal models have suggested that forceful joint ranging may cause or aggravate HO. However, human studies have demonstrated good maintenance of joint range, with no detected increase in HO development.

Control of muscle tone is an important, often overlooked intervention in both prophylaxis and treatment. Joint ranging, icing, casting, and dantrolene sodium may assist in providing adequate control of abnormal muscle tone. Techniques for spasticity management are discussed further in Chapter 30.

Nonsteroidal anti-inflammatory drugs (NSAIDs) are effective in preventing HO after total hip arthroplasty[84-86] and after surgical resection of HO.[87] Whether these agents prevent the development of neurogenic HO is undetermined. The mechanism is thought to be through inhibited prostaglandin synthesis that leads to suppressed inflammatory response and inhibited mesenchymal cell proliferation. NSAIDs may also alter bone formation. Reduction of pain is an additional beneficial effect. Potential concerns about NSAIDs include risk of gastrointestinal bleeding, renal damage, and poor fracture healing. Patients should be screened for history of peptic ulcer disease and presence of renal disease. Dosages of agents studied include three daily doses of 25 mg indomethacin, 400 mg ibuprofen, or 1 g aspirin. To provide effective prophylaxis, these agents must be started as soon as possible.

Prophylaxis with etidronate disodium (EHDP) has also been proposed. The long-term effectiveness of this medication has not been proven and is the subject of much controversy. The physiological influence of EHDP upon bone is important to understanding this debate. The extracellular fluid is abundant with calcium pyrophosphate, which may precipitate on protein bone matrix to induce ossification. Bone calcification is regulated by circulating inorganic pyrophosphate and alkaline phosphatase. Pyrophosphate inhibits calcium deposition, as opposed to alkaline phosphatase, which destroys pyrophosphate and allows calcium deposition. EHDP is an inorganic pyrophosphate that is absorbed enterally and is stable to chemical and enzymatic degradation. This agent causes inhibition of calcium pyrophosphate precipitation, transformation of amorphous calcium pyrophosphate into crystalline hydroxyapatite, aggregation of hydroxyapatite crystals, and crystal growth. However, EHDP does not influence bone matrix formation, the initial phase of HO development. This causes concern as to whether EHDP only delays the crystallization of the osteoid matrix until the medication is discontinued. In addition, EHDP impairs the function of osteoblasts and osteoclasts. Upon cessation of EHDP, the osteoblastic bone-forming capacity returns before osteoclastic resorption recovers. Thus, with EHDP cessation, ossification may occur unopposed by bone resorption. However, in the individual with TBI, many improve neurologicaly during the period of EHDP treatment and are at less risk of functional limitations if ossification is delayed several months. EHDP has no use once the heterotopic tissue is ossified. Thus, EHDP should be started as soon after injury as possible.

Only one study has investigated the efficacy of EHDP following TBI. In this investigation by Speilman et al.,[88] a prospective group of 10 subjects with severe TBI who were in coma for longer than 2 weeks and were receiving EHDP (20 mg/kg/day for 12 weeks, followed by 10 mg/kg/day for 12 weeks) was compared with a retrospective control group. Clinically significant HO was present in 20 percent of those who received EHDP and 70 percent in the nontreatment group. Further investigation with randomized, controlled studies of the long-term effectiveness of EHDP for HO prevention in the TBI population is needed. *Physician's Desk Reference* does not mention the use of EHDP in association with TBI.

Given the uncertainty regarding EHDP effectiveness, the risk-benefit profile for EHDP use should be considered individually. The most common side effects are nausea, vomiting, diarrhea, and abdominal distress, generally resolved by dividing the daily dose. Less common serious side effects include osteomalacia associated with prolonged EHDP use (>6 months) and rickets when EHDP is administered to children. Many still question whether EHDP inhibits fracture healing, although studies have shown no evidence of altered healing of long-bone and spine fractures associated with EHDP use. EHDP may interfere with nutrition because tube feedings must be held a minimum of 30 minutes prior to and following EHDP dosing. These concerns must be weighed against the potential risk of worsened disability.

Other agents may hold promise for effective HO prophylaxis. Verapamil and warfarin have been proposed, but further investigation is needed to determine the effectiveness of these medications. Low-dose irradiation prevents HO development by blocking the conversion of mesenchymal cells to bone precursor cells. This effective prophylactic technique is commonly performed immediately following total hip arthroplasty. However, it is not practical following TBI, when multiple joints are at risk for HO development. Irradiation is generally ineffective once HO is detected.

Surgical resection of HO is frequently employed when severely limited ROM results in functional limitations, difficulty with hygiene or sitting, or pressure sores. Recurrence is common, particularly in the face of severe neurological compromise. Best results are obtained when resection is postponed 12 to 18 months to allow maturation of heterotopic bone and optimal neurological recovery. Prior to excision, spasticity should be controlled. Postoperative prophylaxis is critical and may include low-dose irradiation, EHDP for a minimum of 3 months, indomethacin, and ROM. Varghese[89] recommends initiating active and active-assisted ROM exercises as soon as the drains are removed, with progression to ambulation and functional training 10 to 14 days after surgery.

In summary, ROM, spasticity management, NSAIDs, and EHDP have roles in preventing HO following TBI. Once HO formation occurs, available treatment options are suboptimal and limited to forceful manipulation and surgical resection. HO may lead to complications that increase functional limitations resulting from TBI. Prophylaxis should target those at highest risk to get them through the most susceptible time period and allow neurological recovery prior to ossification.

REFLEX SYMPATHETIC DYSTROPHY SYNDROME

Reflex sympathetic dystrophy syndrome (RSDS) is a clinical complex of pain, swelling, vasomotor instability, trophic skin changes, joint contracture, and limited function. The most characteristic finding is diffuse distal limb pain, generally of burning quality. Allodynia (pain to touch) and hyperpathia (pain to light pressure) may also be present. Tenderness is generalized but greatest in periarticular regions.[90] The most common finding is localized swelling, although it may be mild and difficult to detect. A precipitating event generally precedes the onset of RSDS, such as trauma, fracture, central nervous system injury, peripheral nerve injury, myocardial infarction, or immobilization. However, in 25 to 30 percent of RSDS cases, no precipitating event is identified.[91]

The diagnosis of RSDS is primarily a clinical diagnosis. Several clinical diagnostic criteria have been proposed to increase consistency between clinicians and researchers. However, no standard definition has been established. The ad hoc committee of the American Association for Hand Surgery defines RSDS as diffuse pain out of proportion to the initial event, loss of function, and objective evidence of autonomic dys-

function.[92] Criteria proposed by Kozin[91] grade the presence of clinical findings according to diagnostic certainty. Because atypical and partial forms of RSDS are common and often fail to meet any specified diagnostic criteria, it is helpful to consider the sensitivity and specificity of various clinical findings. Reported sensitivity is 95 percent for hand and wrist swelling, 86 percent for metacarpal tenderness, 57 percent for wrist tenderness, 38 percent for interphalangeal tenderness, 38 percent for vasomotor change, and 33 percent for shoulder pain and tenderness.[93] Specificity is 100 percent for metacarpal tenderness, 95 percent for interphalangeal tenderness, 95 percent for vasomotor changes, 86 percent for wrist tenderness, 85 percent for shoulder pain and tenderness, and 17 percent for hand and wrist swelling.[93] Thus, metacarpal tenderness may be considered the single best clinical indicator, with 86 percent sensitivity and 100 percent specificity.

In the individual with TBI and altered consciousness or impaired communication, clinical assessment and diagnosis may be challenging. Several diagnostic tools are available to aid in the diagnosis including TPBS, roentgenography, and sympathetic blockade. TPBS is often helpful to confirm clinical suspicions and may detect RSDS prior to clinical presentation. Sensitivity of TPBS is reported to be 44 percent to 100 percent, and specificity, 60 percent to 92 percent.[94,95] The classic finding on TPBS is increased periarticular reuptake in multiple joints of the affected extremity, presumed a consequence of decreased sympathetic vasoconstriction that leads to hyperemia and increased bone metabolism. For detection with plain radiographs, demineralization of 30 to 50 percent is needed, which makes it a poor study for early diagnosis. Negative radiographs were reported by Kozin[91] in 20 percent of cases with definite RSDS. Thus, roentgenography may help identify more established cases with findings of patchy osteopenia, soft-tissue swelling, or surface erosions. Patchy osteopenia is supportive but not pathognomonic of RSDS, as it may also result from disuse atrophy. Sympathetic blockade associated with pain decrement is indicative of RSDS.

The natural course of RSDS is described as a continuum of three stages: acute, dystrophic, and atrophic. Stage I (acute) is associated with pain, edema, local hyperthermia or hypothermia, and increased hair and nail growth. In stage II (dystrophic), characteristic findings include constant pain, brawny edema, joint stiffness, subcutaneous tissue atrophy, livedo reticularis, brittle nails, and skin that is indurated, cool, and hyperhydrotic. Plain radiographs may reveal patchy osteoporosis in this stage. Entrance into stage III (atrophic) marks the onset of irreversible tissue damage with atrophy of skin, muscle, and bone that results in tapered digits and flexion contractures. Presence of pain in this stage is variable. Blood flow is generally decreased, causing the involved area to be cool and cyanotic. Plain radiographs reveal patchy demineralization characterized as having a ground glass appearance.

Initiating treatment early is crucial to preventing morbidity. Thus, a high index of suspicion is needed to avoid delay in diagnosis and treatment. Therapeutic goals are aimed at obtaining pain control, diminished sympathetic activity, and increased function. Several treatment methodologies may be required before relief is finally achieved. Techniques commonly used in the rehabilitation setting that are critical to the treatment of RSDS include passive and active range of motion, limb elevation, retrograde massage, desensitization, compression garments, local heat or cold, contrast baths, transcutaneous electrical nerve stimulation, ultrasound, biofeedback, functional training, and psychological intervention. Improved pain control may be needed to enhance participation in such programs. Sympathetic blockade provides relief for many inflicted with RSDS, with positive response rates of 49[96] to 63 percent.[97] Response to sympathetic blockade is frequently only transient, and serial blocks are generally required. Oral corticosteroids have demonstrated benefit. Kozin et al.[90] documented both clinical and symptomatic improvement in all subjects when 11 individuals with definite RSDS were given 60 mg prednisone daily for 3 to 4 days, followed by a tapering schedule (40 mg daily for 4 days, and then decreasing the daily dose by 10 mg every 3 days). Unless contraindicated, prednisone often provides effective, rapid relief, particularly for individuals unable to tolerate sympathetic blockade. However, a rebound of symptoms may occur when the prednisone is discontinued. Other therapeutic options may be required, including tricyclic antidepressants, calcitonin, phenoxybenzamine, propranolol, nifedipine, surgical sympathectomy, dorsal column stimulation, thalamotomy, acupuncture, or hypnosis. Prolonged use of splints in the presence of RSDS should be avoided because immobilization may exacerbate RSDS.

Central Nervous System

POST-TRAUMATIC EPILEPSY

Post-traumatic seizures (PTS) are an important complication of TBI. *Seizures* are defined as discrete clinical events reflecting temporary, physiological brain dysfunction, characterized by excessive hypersynchronous cortical neuron dis-

charge.[98] PTS are designated as immediate, early, or late according to the time from injury to seizure onset. Seizures during the first 24 hours after injury are immediate, those during the remainder of the first week are early PTS, and those after the first week are late PTS. Seizures are also classified by the location of cerebral origin, with partial seizures originating in a localized area of one hemisphere, whereas generalized seizures have a bilateral, symmetrical origin. Partial seizures are further subclassified as simple if consciousness remains intact and as complex if consciousness is impaired. Absence seizures rarely occur following TBI.

TBI is associated with 5 percent late seizure rate, with higher rates in those with penetrating head injury (33–50%), intracranial hematoma (25–30%), early seizure (25%), depressed skull fracture (3–70%), and prolonged coma or posttraumatic amnesia (35%).[99] Of those who develop PTS, onset occurs within 1 year postinjury in 50 to 66 percent and by 2 years in 75 to 80 percent. Approximately 50 percent of those who experience one seizure endure no further seizure activity, and 25 percent have no more than three episodes.[98]

The onset of seizure activity in an individual with no prior seizure history warrants thorough evaluation to assess for potential precipitating causes, such as infection, tumor, electrolyte disturbance, uremia, hypoglycemia, hypoxia, drug use, or alcohol intoxication. Assessment generally includes thorough clinical examination, serum electrolytes, complete blood count, serum calcium and magnesium levels, computed tomography, and magnetic resonance imaging (MRI). Confirming that the episode was indeed seizure activity may be challenging in the TBI patient with motor and cognitive deficits. Observation of the questioned activity may provide the most valuable information. Electroencephalography (EEG) with detection of seizure activity (spike and sharp waves) supports the diagnosis of PTS. However, EEG records the brain's activity at only one point in time. Thus, seizure activity may occur, and subsequent EEG provides no such evidence. Serum prolactin level, when elevated, is supportive of true seizure activity. However, normal serum prolactin levels do not exclude the possibility of seizure.[100]

Prophylactic use of anticonvulsants has not been proven effective in prospective, randomized, controlled studies.[101–103] Temkin et al.[103] compared phenytoin to placebo for seizure prophylaxis over a 2-year period. In this well-controlled study, phenytoin was effective during the first week postinjury. However, after 1 week, there was no significant difference in the two groups. Considering the questionable prophylactic efficacy, combined with high side effect profiles and risk of drug allergy, anticonvulsant agents should be reserved for the treatment of symptomatic seizures. Practice parameters for antiepileptic drug use proposed by a subcommittee of the Brain Injury Special Interest Group of the American Academy of Physical Medicine and Rehabilitation recommend that phenytoin, carbamazepine, valproic acid, or phenobarbital not be used for prophylaxis against late PTS but that such agents to prevent early PTS may be an appropriate treatment option.[104] When the decision is made to use anticonvulsant medication, an effort should be made to balance potential side effects and benefits, as illustrated in Table 4–2.

TABLE 4–2. Anticonvulsant Medications: Uses and Adverse Reactions

Medication	Uses	Adverse Reactions
Carbamazepine	• Partial seizures • Tonic-clonic, generalized seizures • Stabilization of agitation and psychotic behavior • Bipolar affective disorder • Neuralgia	• Acute: stupor or coma, hyperirritability, convulsions, respiratory depression • Chronic: drowsiness, vertigo, ataxia, diplopia, blurred vision, nausea, vomiting, aplastic anemia, agranulocytosis, hypersensitivity reactions (dermatitis, eosinophilia, splenomegaly, lymphadenopathy), transient mild leukopenia, transient thrombocytopenia, water retention with decreased serum osmolality and sodium, transient elevation of hepatic enzymes
Gabapentin	• Partial seizures	• Somnolence, dizziness, ataxia, fatigue
Lamotrigine	• Partial seizures • Absence seizures	• Dizziness, ataxia, blurred or double vision, nausea, vomiting, rash, Stevens-Johnson syndrome, disseminated intravascular coagulation
Phenobarbital	• Partial seizures • Tonic-clonic, generalized seizures	• Sedation, irritability and hyperactivity in children, agitation, confusion, rash, exfoliative dermatitis, hypothrombinemia with hemorrhage in newborns whose mothers took phenobarbital, osteomalacia, megaloblastic anemia • Nystagmus and ataxia at toxic doses
Phenytoin	• Partial seizures • Tonic-clonic, generalized seizures • Neuralgia	• Intravenous administration: cardiac arrhythmias, hypotension, CNS depression • Oral administration: disorders of the cerebellar and vestibular systems (such as nystagmus, ataxia, and vertigo), cerebellar atrophy, blurred vision, mydriasis, diplopia, ophthalmoplegia, behavioral changes (such as hyperactivity, confusion, dullness, drowsiness, and hallucinations), increased seizure frequency, gastrointestinal symptoms, gingival hyperplasia, osteomalacia, megaloblastic anemia, hirsutism, transient liver enzyme elevation, decreased antidiuretic hormone secretion leading to hypernatremia, hyperglycemia, glycosuria, hypocalcemia, Stevens-Johnson syndrome, systemic lupus erythematosus, neutropenia, leukopenia, red cell aplasia, agranulocytosis, thrombocytopenia, lymphadenopathy, hypothrombinemia in newborns whose mothers received phenytoin, reactions indicative of drug allergy (skin, bone marrow, liver function)
Valproic acid	• Partial seizures • Tonic-clonic, generalized seizures • Myoclonic seizures • Absence seizures • Stabilization of agitation and psychotic behavior	• Transient gastrointestinal symptoms such as anorexia, nausea, and vomiting; increased appetite; sedation; ataxia; tremor; rash; alopecia; hepatic enzyme elevation, fulminant hepatitis (rare, but fatal); acute pancreatitis; hyperammonemia

Anticonvulsant medication is generally initiated once a late seizure occurs. The goal is to control seizures with a single medication. An agent should be selected that meets the individual's needs according to seizure type, dosing frequency, route of administration, and beneficial effects, while minimizing side effects (Table 4–2). In the TBI population, carbamazepine and valproic acid are often preferred to more sedating medications such as phenobarbital and phenytoin. However, all anticonvulsant agents may cause some degree of sedation and cognitive deficits.[105] Further investigation into the effects of anticonvulsant medication in TBI is needed. The initially administered agent may not be the ideal agent for long-term use. Phenobarbital and phenytoin are commonly utilized acutely because of the need for parenteral delivery. More appropriate agents may later be substituted to meet the individual's needs. Wroblewski et al.[106] demonstrated carbamazepine substitution to be associated with comparable or improved seizure control. During anticonvulsant treatment, patients should be monitored for side effects and toxicity (Table 4–2), and potential drug interactions should be considered when new medications are prescribed (Table 4–3). The exact treatment duration needed is uncertain. It is sensible to consider anticonvulsant withdrawal following a 2-year seizure-free period. Callaghan et al.[107] prospectively studied anticonvulsant cessation after 2 years without seizures. In this study, a 34 percent relapse rate was observed. Relapse rates were highest when EEG findings were abnormal both prior to treatment and prior to anticonvulsant withdrawal. Other studies, however, have questioned the utility of EEG in predicting relapse.[108]

HYDROCEPHALUS

Ventriculomegaly is common after traumatic brain injury, and true hydrocephalus is relatively

---

TABLE 4–3. Anticonvulsant Medications: Common Drug Interactions

Medication	Drug Interactions
Carbamazepine	▪ Increased metabolism of carbamazepine (decreased levels) with phenobarbital, phenytoin, and valproic acid ▪ Enhances metabolism of phenobarbital ▪ Enhances metabolism of primidone into phenobarbital ▪ Reduces concentration and effectiveness of haloperidol ▪ Carbamazepine metabolism inhibited by propoxyphene and erythromycin
Lamotrigine	▪ When used concurrently with carbamazepine, may increase levels of 10,11-epoxide (an active metabolite of carbamazepine) ▪ Half-life of lamotrigine is reduced to 15 h when used concurrently with carbamazepine, phenobarbital, or primidone ▪ Reduces valproic acid concentration
Phenobarbital	▪ Increased levels (as much as 40%) of phenobarbital when valproic acid administered concurrently ▪ Phenobarbital levels may be increased when concurrently administering phenytoin ▪ Phenobarbital has a variable reaction with phenytoin levels
Phenytoin	▪ Phenytoin levels may increase with concurrent use of chloramphenicol, cimetidine, dicumarol, disulfiram, isoniazid, and sulfonamides ▪ Free phenytoin levels may increase with concurrent use of valproic acid and phenylbutazone ▪ Decreased total levels of phenytoin may occur with sulfisoxazole, salicylates, and tolbutamide ▪ Decreased phenytoin levels with concurrent use of carbamazepine ▪ Decreased carbamazepine levels with concurrent use of phenytoin ▪ Increased or decreased levels of phenytoin when concurrently administered with phenobarbital ▪ When concurrently used with theophylline, phenytoin levels may be lowered and theophylline metabolized more rapidly ▪ May decrease effectiveness of oral contraceptives ▪ Enhances metabolism of corticosteroids
Valproic acid	▪ Increases levels of phenobarbital ▪ Inhibits metabolism of phenytoin ▪ Rare development of absence status epilepticus associated with concurrent use of clonazepam

rare. As many as 72 percent of individuals with severe brain injuries display enlarged ventricles,[109] and an incidence of 23 percent has been reported in a rehabilitation setting.[110] However, most ventriculomegaly is due to cerebral atrophy and ex vacuo changes. Older literature,[111] which relied on pneumoencephalography for diagnosis, placed the incidence of true hydrocephalus after TBI at 1 to 2 percent. A more accurate estimate is in the range of 3.9[112] to 8 percent.[113]

Hydrocephalus is caused by the disruption of normal flow and/or absorption of cerebral spinal fluid through the ventricular system. The abnormal enlargement of the ventricles is traditionally classified into noncommunicating and communicating subtypes, the former suggesting an obstruction within the ventricular system and the latter an obstruction within the subarachnoid space. Alternative systems of classification have recently been proposed, in part because careful imaging and CSF flow studies often fail to identify an obstruction in many noncommunicating cases.[114]

Hydrocephalus in TBI is generally of the communicating type, secondary to arachnoiditis and impaired resorption through the pacchionian (arachnoid) granulations. Transependymal and transpial absorption directly into the white matter venous system may also be important.[114,115] On occasion, hemosiderin deposits may be evident in the subarachnoid space on MRI,[115] suggesting a possible role of intraventricular subarachnoid blood in the development of the problem.

It has been suggested that traumatic subarachnoid hemorrhage (SAH), a rare (<5%)[116,117] sequela of TBI, may place individuals at risk to develop communicating hydrocephalus. A very high incidence of hydrocephalus following spontaneous SAH has been well documented, in the range of 20[118] to 23 percent.[119] However, development of true hydrocephalus following traumatic SAH is much lower, between 2[117] and 7[116] percent.

Although the incidence is low, the identification of post-traumatic hydrocephalus is important as one of the few potentially treatable causes of neurological dysfunction after TBI. Vigilance must continue into the subacute and chronic phases of care because significant improvement has been noted after shunting as long as 2 years after the initial injury.[120,121] Others[110] have reported poor response after shunting TBI patients.

Differentiation between hydrocephalus and ex vacuo changes is a common clinical problem. Although diagnostic algorithms have been proposed,[122] there is no universally accepted test to identify hydrocephalus with adequate specificity. The diagnosis is often made on the basis of multiple factors, including history, physical findings, laboratory testing, and clinical judgment.

Hydrocephalus of rapid onset is readily detected clinically and often associated with nausea, vomiting, headache, papilledema, and obtundation. A more insidious form of normal pressure hydrocephalus was originally described in the mid-1960s, presenting with the now well-known triad of dementia, gait ataxia, and urinary incontinence.[122] These symptoms remain one of the strongest indicators of normal pressure hydrocephalus. Unfortunately, they are often of little utility in the diagnosis of suspected hydrocephalus in TBI because many patients with brain injuries exhibit baseline impairments in their sensorium, gait, and sphincter control. When compared with TBI survivors without hydrocephalus,[112] those with the condition exhibit longer duration of coma, more significant impairment of motor control, more behavioral problems, and poorer vocational outcomes. Clearly, any functional change following TBI should alert the clinician to the possibility of hydrocephalus, even after months or years.[121]

Computed tomography (CT) and MRI of the brain reveal nonspecific ventriculomegaly. Factors that favor the diagnosis of post-traumatic hydrocephalus over ex vacuo changes defined by Barkovich and Edwards[115] include (1) commensurate dilatation of the temporal horn with the lateral ventricles, (2) enlargement of the anterior or posterior recesses of the third ventricle, (3) narrowing of the mamilopontine distance, (4) narrowing of the ventricular angle, (5) widening of the frontal horn radius, and (6) effacement of the cortical sulci. Other measurements have been proposed as well.[123,124] In addition, true hydrocephalus is associated with transependymal extravasation of CSF into the periventricular white matter. This fluid is often apparent as a periventricular hypodense region on CT and is also well visualized on MRI.[115]

Radioisotope cisternography has been in clinical use for three decades.[125] A radioactive tracer is injected via lumbar puncture into the lumbar cistern. Delay of greater than 24 hours in appearance of the tracer over the cortical convexities indicates poor flow, consistent with hydrocephalus. Although used commonly in many centers,[122] one retrospective analysis demonstrates cisternography does not improve clinical decision making over using clinical and CT findings alone.[124] Of note, CSF flow information can now be more directly measured by utilizing commonly available MRI scanners.[126]

Lumbar puncture has been used successfully to treat acute hydrocephalus after SAH.[119] A favorable neurological response to a lumbar puncture has been proposed as a potential predictor of neurological improvement following shunting procedures. Wikkelso et al.[127] studied 24 symptomatic patients with presumed normal pressure hydrocephalus; they withdrew 50 mL of CSF from each patient and tested memory, perceptual functions, reaction time, and ambulation prior to and immediately following the lumbar puncture. All tests were helpful in identifying those with a favorable response to shunting. Ambulation alone was the strongest predictor, explaining 92 percent of the variance between responders and nonresponders. However, the "tap test" appears to be specific but not very sensitive; a significant number of shunt responders were predicted to be nonresponders. Therefore, although a positive result may be helpful, a negative test does not assure that the patient will not benefit from ventricular decompression.

In the future, single-proton emission tomography (SPECT), a technique to measure CBF, may also have a role in the evaluation of hydrocephalus. Anecdotally, increase in flow to the basal ganglia has been noted in patients who respond to shunting.[122] Shinoda et al.[128] performed SPECT scans on five infants and children prior to shunting and concluded that those with slower appearance of radioactivity in specific areas of white matter responded favorably to a shunt. The authors postulate that the areas of slow filling represent potentially salvageable areas of low perfusion.[129]

In conclusion, post-traumatic hydrocephalus should be considered in any patient with a brain injury who deteriorates functionally or neurologically. The diagnosis should also be entertained in those who fail to show improvement. Specific neuroradiographic signs help to distinguish atrophy from hydrocephalus, but the absence of these signs does not ensure a correct diagnosis. Additional testing may be useful, but there is no commonly accepted diagnostic algorithm. The diagnosis often relies heavily on clinical judgment.

CAROTID CAVERNOUS FISTULA

Carotid cavernous fistula formation is a rare complication of brain trauma. However, its recognition is of paramount importance because of the availability of definitive treatment and its potential for blindness if it is unrecognized. A carotid cavernous fistula is an abnormal vascular connection between the cavernous sinus and carotid artery, associated with basilar skull fracture.[127] Symptoms include headache, conjunctival injection, visual changes, pulsatile proptosis, and epistaxis. Cranial bruits may be present. Although the fistula may form in the early stages following injury, presentation may be delayed for several months.[130]

Bacterial meningitis may also follow brain injury. However, the incidence is low (<2%) and also associated with basilar skull fractures.[131]

CENTRAL VENOUS THROMBOSIS

Central venous thrombosis (CVT) is a rare but serious complication of TBI, with numerous causes or predisposing factors identified. Those factors most pertinent to TBI are head trauma, neurosurgical procedures, infection, inflammatory processes, oral contraceptives, and idiopathic. The superior sagittal sinus (SSS), lateral sinus, and cerebral veins are the most frequently involved structures, with cavernous sinus and cerebellar veins involved less commonly. Its clinical presentation is highly variable, mimicking other processes associated with TBI, which makes the diagnosis challenging. Signs and symptoms may include headache, papilledema, increased intracranial pressure, nausea and vomiting, motor or sensory deficit, bilateral cortical signs, alteration of consciousness, psychotic disturbance, nuchal rigidity, multiple cranial nerve palsies, dysphasia, cerebellar incoordination, nystagmus, visual disturbance, hearing loss, and gait abnormalities. In a retrospective review of 795 cases of SSS thrombosis, Schell and Rathe noted the following symptoms: severe headache (53%); seizures (49%); hemiplegia, tetraplegia, or paraparesis (48%); elevated cerebral spinal fluid pressure (46%); coma (38%), papilledema (33%); visual disturbances (25%); and nuchal rigidity (18%).[132] Common findings of cavernous sinus thrombosis are chemosis, proptosis, painful ophthalmoplegia, and abducens nerve palsy. CT scan imaging with and without injected contrast is important both to establish the diagnosis of CVT and to exclude other processes such as hemorrhage, abscess, and tumor. CT scan findings suggestive of CVT include the empty delta sign (posterior SSS thrombosis), cord sign (thrombosed cortical vein), dense triangle (freshly congealed blood in the SSS), contrast enhancement of falx or tentorium, small ventricles, enlarged ventricles, gyral enhancement, hypodensity, spontaneous hyperdensity, and hemorrhagic venous infarcts.[133] CT scan imaging may fail to reveal the diagnosis of CVT with normal findings in 10 to 20 percent, necessitating MRI or angiography in some cases. Therapeutic needs may include regimens to lower intracranial pressure, anticonvulsant medication, antibiotics, and antithrombotic agents. Treatment of the thrombotic process is controversial because of risk of cerebral hemorrhage. With the advent of antibiotics and improved diagnostic methods, outcome has improved for this previously lethal process.

◻ SUMMARY

TBI is associated with multiple medical problems. These complications may be the result of the trauma itself, manifestations of the brain injury, iatrogenic causes, or exacerbations of premorbid conditions. The recent trend of shortened length of stay in acute medical facilities has been associated with increasing medical acuity in the rehabilitation setting.

The rehabilitation professional must bear in mind that 11 to 30 percent of medical and musculoskeletal disorders may not have been identified at the time of transfer to a rehabilitation facility.[134] Standard physical examination is often incomplete because of altered consciousness, poor comprehension or cooperation, or communication deficits. It is therefore crucial to use the appropriate screening technologies available. In addition, the clinician must maintain a high index of suspicion and perform frequent examinations as the individual's neurological status progresses. Awareness of the potential medical and orthopedic complications for these disorders may prevent unnecessary disability and enhance eventual outcome.

REFERENCES

1. Jennett, B, et al: Treatment for severe head injury. J Neurol Neurosurg Psychiatry 43:289, 1980.
2. Lanza, D, et al: Predictive value of the Glasgow Coma Scale for tracheotomy in head-injured patients. Ann Otol Rhinol Laryngol 99:38, 1990.
3. Schachner, A, et al: Percutaneous tracheostomy: A new method. Crit Care Med 17:1052, 1989.
4. Lanza, D, et al: Early complications of airway management in head-injured patients. Laryngoscope 100:958, 1990.
5. Moore, F, et al: Percutaneous tracheostomy/gastrostomy in brain-injured patients: A minimally invasive alternative. J Trauma 33:435, 1992.
6. Law, JH, et al: Increased frequency of obstructive airway abnormalities with long-term tracheostomy. Chest 104:136, 1993.
7. Nowak, P, Cohn, A, and Guidice, M: Airway complications in patients with closed-head injuries. Am J Otolaryngol 8:91, 1987.
8. Citta-Pietrolungo, TJ, et al: Complications of tracheostomy and decannulation in pediatric and young patients with traumatic brain injury. Arch Phys Med Rehabil 74:905, 1993.
9. Klingbeil, G: Airway problems in patients with traumatic brain injury. Arch Phys Med Rehabil 69:493, 1988.
10. Gallagher, S: Diagnosis and treatment of bruxism: A review of the literature. General Dentist 28:62, 1980.
11. Pratap-Chand, RP, et al: Bruxism: Its significance in coma. Clin Neurol Neurosurg 87:113, 1985.
12. Ellison, JM, and Stanziani, P. SSRI-associated nocturnal bruxism in four patients. J Clin Psychiatry 54:432, 1993.
13. Van Zandijcke, M, and Marchau, MM: Treatment of bruxism with botulinum toxin injections. J Neurol Neurosurg Psychiatry 53:530, 1990.
14. Watts, C, and Clark, K: Gastric acidity in the comatose patient. J Neurosurg 30:107, 1969.
15. Halloran, L, et al: Prevention of acute gastrointestinal complications after severe head injury: A controlled trial of cimetidine prophylaxis. Am J Surg 139:44, 1980.
16. Metz, C, et al: Impact of multiple risk factors and ranitidine prophylaxis on the development of stress-related upper gastrointestinal bleeding: A prospective, multicenter, double-blind randomized trial. Crit Care Med 21:1844, 1993.
17. Burgess, P, et al: Effect of ranitidine on intragastric pH and stress-related upper gastrointestinal bleeding in patients with severe head injury. Dig Dis Sci 40:645, 1995.
18. Kanof, P, and Greengard, P: Brain histamine receptors as targets for antidepressant drugs. Nature 272:329, 1978.
19. Rosse, R: Cimetidine and mental status changes. J Clin Psychiatry 47:99, 1986.
20. Miller, M, Perry, C, and Siris, S: Psychosis in association with combined cimetidine and imipramine treatment. Psychosomatics 28:217, 1987.
21. Lesser, I, et al: Delusions in a patient treated with histamine H2 receptor antagonists. Psychosomatics 28:501, 1987.
22. Schroeder, J, et al: The effect of intravenous ranitidine and metoclopramide on behavior, cognitive function, and affect. Anesth Analg 78:359, 1994.
23. Kalisky, A, et al: Medical problems encountered during rehabilitation of patients with head injury. Arch Phys Med Rehabil 66:25, 1985.
24. Rosalki, S, Tarlow, D, and Rau, D: Plasma gamma-glutamyl transpeptidase elevation in patients receiving enzyme-inducing drugs. Lancet ii:376, 1971.
25. Andreasen, P, Lyngbye, J, and Trolle, E: Abnormalities in liver function tests during long-term diphenylhydantoin therapy in epileptic out-patients. Acta Med Scand 194:261, 1973.
26. Aiges, H, et al: The effects of phenobarbital and diphenylhydantoin on liver function and morphology. J Pediatr 97:22, 1980.
27. Porter, R, and Kelley, K: Antiepileptic drug and mild liver function elevation. JAMA 253:22, 1985.
28. Wall, M, et al: Liver function tests in persons receiving anticonvulsant medications. Seizure 1:187, 1992.
29. Mendis, G, Gibberd, F, and Hunt, H: Plasma activities of hepatic enzymes in patients on anticonvulsant therapy. Seizure 2:319, 1993.
30. Rivey, MP, and Stone, JD: Carbamazepine hypersensitivity reaction. Brain Inj 5:57, 1991.
31. Pellock, JM, and Willmore, LJ: A rational guide to routine blood monitoring in patients receiving antiepileptic drugs. Neurology 41:961, 1991.
32. Phillips, R, et al: Nutritional support and measured energy expenditure of the child and adolescent with head injury. J Neurosurg 67:846, 1987.
33. Sunderland, PM, and Heibrun, MP: Estimating energy expenditure in traumatic brain injury: Comparison of indirect calorimetry with predictive formulas. Neurosurgery 31:246, 1992.
34. Borzotta, AP, et al: Enteral versus parenteral nutrition after severe closed head injury. J Trauma 37:459, 1994.
35. Saxe, JM, et al: Lower esophageal sphincter dysfunction precludes safe gastric feeding after head injury. J Trauma 37:581, 1994.
36. Stechmiller, J, et al: Interruption of enteral feedings in head injured patients. J Neurosci Nurs 26:224, 1994.
37. Kiel, M: Enteral tube feeding in a patient with traumatic brain injury. Arch Phys Med Rehabil 75:116, 1994.
38. Burch, GE, Meyers, R, and Abildskov, JA: A new electrocardiographic pattern observed in cerebrovascular accidents. Circulation 9:719, 1954.
39. Fentz, V, and Gormsen, J: Electrocardiographic patterns in patients with cerebrovascular accidents. Circulation 15:22, 1962.
40. Hammer, W, Luessenhop, A, and Weintraub, A: Observation on the electrocardiographic changes associated with subarachnoid hemorrhage with special reference their genesis. Am J Med 59:427, 1975.

41. Jachuck, SJ, et al: Electrocardiographic abnormalities associated with raised intracranial pressure. BMJ 1:242, 1975.
42. McLeod, A, et al: Cardiac sequelae of acute head injury. Br Heart J 47:221, 1982.
43. Hackenberry, LE, et al: Biochemical evidence of myocardial injury after severe head trauma. Crit Care Med 10:641, 1982.
44. Haft, J: Cardiovascular injury induced by sympathetic catecholamines. Prog Cardiovasc Dis 17:73, 1974.
45. Fleckenstein, A: Myocardial fiber necrosis due to intracellular Ca overload: A new principle in cardiac pathophysiology. In Dhalla, NS (ed): Myocardial Biology. University Park Press, Baltimore, 1974, p 4:563.
46. Shanlin, R, et al: Increased intracranial pressure elicits hypertension, increased sympathetic activity, electrocardiographic abnormalities and myocardial damage in rats. JACC 12:727, 1988.
47. Jennett, B, and Teasdale, G: Management of Head Injuries. Contemporary Neurology Series, vol 20. FA Davis, Philadelphia, 1981.
48. Labi, MC, and Horn, LJ: Hypertension in traumatic brain injury. Brain Inj 4:365, 1990.
49. Clifton, G, et al: Cardiovascular response to severe head injury. J Neurosurg 59:447, 1983.
50. Rosner, M, Newsome, H, and Becker, D: Mechanical brain injury: The sympathoadrenal response. J Neurosurg 61:76, 1984.
51. Hortnagl, H, et al: The activity of the sympathetic nervous system following severe head injury. Intensive Care Med 6:169, 1980.
52. Wortsman, J, et al: Hyperadrenergic state after head injury. JAMA 243:1459, 1980.
53. Sandel, ME, Abrams, P, and Horn, L: Hypertension after brain injury: Case report. Arch Phys Med Rehabil 67:469, 1986.
54. Muizelaar, JP, and Schroder, ML: Overview of monitoring of cerebral blood flow and metabolism after severe head injury. Can J Neurol Sci 21:S6, 1994.
55. Bouma, G, et al: Cerebral circulation and metabolism after severe traumatic brain injury: The elusive role of ischemia. J Neurosurg 75:685, 1991.
56. Bouma, G, et al: Blood pressure and intracranial pressure-volume dynamics in severe head injury: A relationship with cerebral blood flow. J Neurosurg 77:15, 1992.
57. Rosner, M, and Daughton, S: Cerebral perfusion pressure management in head injury. J Trauma 30:933, 1990.
58. Shalit, MN, and Cotev, S: Interrelationship between blood pressure and regional cerebral blood flow in experimental intracranial hypertension. J Neurosurg 40:594, 1974.
59. Marshall, WJ, Jackson, JLF, and Lagnfitt, TW: Brain swelling caused by trauma and arterial hypertension: Hemodynamic aspects. Arch Neurol 21:545, 1969.
60. Simard, JM, and Bellefleur, M: Systemic arterial hypertension in head trauma. Am J Cardiol 63:32C, 1989.
61. Robertson, C, et al: Treatment of hypertension associated with head injury. J Neurosurg 59:455, 1983.
62. Geerts, W, et al: A prospective study of venous thromboembolism after major trauma. N Engl J Med 331:1601, 1994.
63. Rubinstein, I, Murray, D, and Hoffstein, V: Fatal pulmonary embolism in hospitalized patients. Arch Intern Med 148:1425, 1988.
64. Hirsh, J: Diagnosis of venous thrombosis and pulmonary embolism. Am J Cardiol 65:45C, 1990.
65. Dawson, N, Reid, J, and Brosseuk, D: IPG compared with duplex ultrasonography for detection of deep vein thrombosis. Journal of Vascular Technology 16:146, 1992.
66. Katz, R, and McCulla, M: Impedance plethysmography as a scanning procedure for asymptomatic deep venous thrombosis in a rehabilitation hospital. Arch Phys Med Rehabil 76:833, 1995.
67. Hyers, T, Hull, R, and Weg, J: Antithrombotic therapy for venous thromboembolic disease. Chest 108:225S, 1995.

68. Garcia, JG, and Lam, C: Treating urinary incontinence in a head-injured adult. Brain Inj 4:203, 1990.
69. Youngson, HA, and Alderman, N: Fear of incontinence and its effects on its community-based rehabilitation programme after severe brain injury: Successful remediation of escape behavior using behavior modification. Brain Inj 8:23, 1994.
70. Narins, R, et al: Diagnostic strategies in disorders of fluid, electrolyte and acid-base homeostasis. Am J Med 72:498, 1982.
71. Schwartz, WB, et al: Syndrome of renal sodium loss and hyponatremia probably resulting from inappropriate secretion of antidiuretic hormone. Am J Med 23:529, 1957.
72. Nelson, PB, et al: Hyponatremia in intracranial disease: Perhaps not the syndrome of inappropriate secretion of antidiuretic hormone (SIADH). J Neurosurg 55:938, 1981.
73. Wijdicks, EFM, et al: Volume depletion and natriuresis in patients with a ruptured intracranial aneurysm. Ann Neurol 18:211, 1985.
74. Poon, WS, et al: Secretion of antidiuretic hormone in neurosurgical patients: Appropriate or inappropriate? Aust N Z J Surg 59:173, 1989.
75. Blendonohy, PM, and Philip, PA: Precocious puberty in children after traumatic brain injury. Brain Inj 5:63, 1991.
76. Garland, D, and Bailey, S: Undetected injuries in head injured adults. Clin Orthop 155:162, 1981.
77. Garland, D, and Rhoades, M: Orthopedic management of brain-injured adults: Part II. Clin Orthop 131:111, 1978.
78. Stone, L, and Keenan, MA: Peripheral nerve injuries in the adult with traumatic brain injury. Clin Orthop 233:136, 1988.
79. Garland, D: A clinical perspective on common forms of acquired heterotopic ossification. Clin Orthop 263:13, 1991.
80. Varghese, G, et al: Nonarticular complication of heterotopic ossification: A clinical review. Arch Phys Med Rehabil 72:1009, 1991.
81. Sazbon, L, et al: Widespread periarticular new-bone formation in long-term comatose patients. J Bone Joint Surg Br 63:120, 1981.
82. Goldman, AB: Myositis ossificans circumscripta: A benign lesion with differential diagnosis. AJR Am J Roentgenol 126:32, 1976.
83. Orzel, J, and Rudd, T: Heterotopic bone formation: Clinical laboratory, and imaging correlation. J Nucl Med 26:125, 1985.
84. Ritter, MA, and Gioe, TJ: The effect of indomethacin on para-articular ectopic ossification following total hip arthroplasty. Clin Orthop 167:113, 1982.
85. Kjaersgaard-Anderson, P, and Schmidt, SA: Indomethacin for prevention of ectopic ossification after hip arthroplasty. Acta Orthop Scand 57:12, 1986.
86. Schmidt, SA, et al: The use of indomethacin to prevent the formation of heterotopic bone after total hip replacement. J Bone Joint Surg Am 70:834, 1988.
87. Mital, M, Garber, J, and Stinson, J: Ectopic bone formation in children and adolescents with head injuries: Its management. J Pediatr Orthop 7:83, 1987.
88. Speilman, G, Gennarelli, TA, and Rogers, CR: Disodium etidronate: Its role in preventing heterotopic ossification in severe head injury. Arch Phys Med Rehabil 64:539, 1983.
89. Varghese, G: Heterotopic ossification. Physical Medicine and Rehabilitation Clinics of North America 3:407, 1992.
90. Kozin, F, et al: The reflex sympathetic dystrophy syndrome I. Clinical and histological studies: Evidence for bilaterality, response to corticosteroids and articular involvement. Am J Med 60:321, 1976.
91. Kozin, F: Reflex sympathetic dystrophy syndrome. Bull Rheum Dis 36:1, 1986.
92. Amadio, PC, et al: Reflex sympathetic dystrophy syndrome: Consensus report of an ad hoc committee of the American Association for Hand Surgery on the defini-

tion of reflex sympathetic dystrophy syndrome. Plast Reconstr Surg 87:371, 1991.

93. Tepperman, P, et al: Reflex sympathetic dystrophy in hemiplegia. Arch Phys Med Rehabil 5:93, 1984.

94. Weiss, L, et al: Prognostic value of triple phase bone scanning for reflex sympathetic dystrophy in hemiplegia. Arch Phys Med Rehabil 74:716, 1993.

95. Davidoff, G, et al: Predictive value of the three-phase technetium bone scan in the diagnosis of reflex sympathetic dystrophy syndrome. Arch Phys Med Rehabil 70:135, 1989.

96. Steinbrocker, O, Neustdt, D, and Lapin, L: Shoulder-hand syndrome: Sympathetic block compared with corticotropin and cortisone therapy. JAMA 153:788, 1946.

97. Shumacker, HB, and Abramson, DI: Posttraumatic vasomotor disorders: With particular reference to late manifestations and treatment. Surg Gynecol Obstet 88:417, 1949.

98. Yablon, SA: Posttraumatic seizures. Arch Phys Med Rehabil 74:983, 1993.

99. Ludwig, B: Post-traumatic seizures. Physical Medicine and Rehabilitation: State of Art Reviews 7:461, 1993.

100. Hammond, FM, Yablon, SA, and Bontke, CF: Potential role of serum prolactin measurement in the diagnosis of late posttraumatic seizures. Am J Phys Med Rehabil 75:1996.

101. Young, B, et al: Failure of prophylactically administered phenytoin to prevent late post-traumatic seizures. J Neurosurg 58:236, 1983.

102. McQueen, JK, et al: Low risk of late post-traumatic seizures following severe head injury: Implications for clinical trials of prophylaxis. J Neurol Neurosurg Psychiatry 46:899, 1983.

103. Temkin, N, et al: A randomized, double-blind study of phenytoin for the prevention post-traumatic seizures. N Engl J Med 323:497, 1990.

104. Brain Injury Special Interest Group of the American Academy of Physical Medicine and Rehabilitation: Practice parameter: Antiepileptic drug treatment of post-traumatic seizures. Arch Phys Med Rehabil 79:594, 1998.

105. Massagli, T: Neurobehavioral effects of phenytoin, carbamazepine, and valproic acid: Implications for use in traumatic brain injury. Arch Phys Med Rehabil 72:219, 1991.

106. Wroblewski, BA, et al: Carbamazepine replacement of phenytoin, phenobarbital, and primidone in a rehabilitation setting: Effects on seizure control. Brain Inj 3:149, 1989.

107. Callaghan, N, Garrett, A, and Goggin, T: Withdrawal of anticonvulsant drugs in patients free of seizures for two years. N Engl J Med 318:942, 1988.

108. Overweg, J, et al: Prediction of seizure recurrence after withdrawal of antiepileptic drugs. In Dam, M, Gram, L, and Penry, JK (eds): Advances in epileptology: Twelfth Epilepsy International Symposium. Raven Press, New York, 1981, p 503.

109. Levin, H, et al: Ventricular enlargement after closed head injury. Arch Neurol 38:623, 1981.

110. Timming, R, Orrison, W, and Mikula, J: Computerized tomography and rehabilitation outcome after severe head trauma. Arch Phys Med Rehabil 63:154, 1982.

111. Granholm, L, and Svendgaard, N: Hydrocephalus following traumatic head injuries. Scand J Rehabil Med 4:31, 1972.

112. Groswasser, Z, et al: Incidence, CT findings and rehabilitation outcome of patients with communicative hydrocephalus following severe head injury. Brain Inj 2:267, 1988.

113. French, B, and Dublin, A: The value of computerized tomography in the management of 1000 consecutive head injuries. Surg Neurol 7:171, 1977.

114. Mori, K: Current concept of hydrocephalus: Evolution of new classifications. Child Nerv Syst 11:523, 1995.

115. Barkovich, AJ, and Edwards, MS: Applications of neuroimaging in hydrocephalus. Pediatr Neurosurg 18:65, 1992.

116. Lipper, M, et al: Computed tomography in the prediction of outcome in head injury. AJNR Am J Neuroradiol 6:7, 1985.

117. LeRoux, P, et al: Intraventricular hemorrhage in blunt head trauma: An analysis of 43 cases. Neurosurgery 31:678, 1992.

118. Demircivl, F, et al: Traumatic subarachnoid hemorrhage. Analysis of 89 cases. Acta Neurochir (Wien) 122:45, 1993.

119. Hasan, D, Lindsay, K, and Vermeulen, M: Treatment of acute hydrocephalus after subarachnoid hemorrhage with serial lumbar puncture. Stroke 22:190, 1991.

120. Seliger, G, et al: Late improvement in closed head injury with a low-pressure valve shunt. Brain Inj 6:71, 1992.

121. Sheffler, L, et al: Shunting in chronic post-traumatic hydrocephalus: Demonstration of neurophysiologic improvement. Arch Phys Med Rehabil 75:338, 1994.

122. Kopniczky, Z, et al: Our policy in diagnosis and treatment of hydrocephalus. Child Nerv Syst 11:102, 1995.

123. Adams, R, et al: Symptomatic occult hydrocephalus with "normal" cerebrospinal fluid pressure. N Engl J Med 273:117, 1965.

124. Vanneste, J, et al: Normal-pressure hydrocephalus: Is cisternography still useful in selecting patients for a shunt? Arch Neurol 49:366, 1992.

125. Heinz, ER, and Karp, HR: Abnormal isotope cisternography in symptomatic occult hydrocephalus: A correlative isotopic-neuroradiological study in 130 subjects. Radiology 95:109, 1970.

126. Bradley, W Jr, et al: Flowing cerebrospinal fluid in normal and hydrocephalic states: Appearance on MR images. Radiology 159:611, 1986.

127. Wikkelso, C, et al: Normal pressure hydrocephalus: Predictive value of the cerebrospinal fluid tap-test. Acta Neurol Scand 73:566, 1986.

128. Shinoda, M, et al: Single photon emission computerized tomography in childhood hydrocephalus. Child Nerv Syst 8:219, 1992.

129. Robertson, JM: Carotid-cavernous sinus fistula accompany facial trauma. Br J Oral Surg 14:195, 1977.

130. Dubov, WE, and Bach, JR: Delayed presentation of a carotid-cavernous sinus fistula in a patient with traumatic brain injury. Am J Phys Med Rehabil 70:178, 1991.

131. Baltas, I, et al: Posttraumatic meningitis: Bacteriology, hydrocephalus, and outcome. Neurosurgery 35:1994.

132. Schell, C, and Rathe, R: Superior sagittal sinus thrombosis: Still a killer. West J Med 149:304, 1988.

133. Ameri, A, and Bousser, M: Central venous thrombosis. Neurol Clin 10:87, 1992.

134. Bontke, CF: Medical complications related to traumatic brain injury. Physical Medicine and Rehabilitation: State of the Art Reviews 3:43, 1989.

Cognitive and Behavioral Effects of Brain Injury

WILLIAM W. McKINLAY, PHD,
and ANNA J. WATKISS, BSC

Traumatic brain injury (TBI) may result in a broad range of deficits and changes that affect both physical and mental status. It is unusual, even for survivors of significant TBI who make a good physical recovery, to escape changes in cognition and emotional/behavioral adjustment. Moreover, in the long run, mental changes contribute more than physical changes to overall disability.[1,2] They are certainly key factors affecting return to work[3-5] and, in many cases, the need for care and supervision.[6]

This chapter deals with the following topics:

1. The early effects of injury on cognition and behavior in the days and weeks after injury
2. The emergence, over weeks and months, of the cognitive deficits that are characteristic of such injury, a process linked to the demands placed on the individual
3. The development of insight into limitations
4. The emergence, also over weeks and months, of emotional and behavioral changes
5. Key factors that may mediate outcome
6. Some implications of these cognitive and emotional/behavioral changes for future adjustment

☐ EARLY EFFECTS

The extent of mental changes is not fully apparent at the outset after severe TBI; indeed, it usu-ally takes many months for the nature and extent of these changes to make themselves known. An immediate cognitive effect, which is usually apparent, is loss of memory (amnesia) for the period around the time of the accident.[7]

Retrograde Amnesia

What usually happens is as follows: Suppose the injury is sustained by Mr. X in a traffic accident at 2 P.M. on a Wednesday soon after he left his office. His memories for events *prior to* 2 P.M. on Wednesday are lost. His last memory may be of being in the car minutes before the accident, or it may be of leaving the office, or of breakfast or lunch, or of some other event in the course of the day. It may—usually in more severely injured patients—be an event days, months, or even longer before the accident. This time is the period of retrograde amnesia (RA). Early after the injury, the period of RA may be relatively long. As time passes, the injured person usually starts to recall a little more, and RA no longer extends so far back in time.[8,9] In general, the shrinkage of RA does not continue indefinitely but reaches a minimum. Usually the accident (or assault or other incident) is not fully recalled.

Occasionally the "shrinkage" of RA is not entirely genuine. The injured person may have constructed an image of what probably happened based on information from others and find it hard to distinguish memories from others' descriptions.

In some cases, RA is very long. Some investigators suspect that psychological rather than organic factors are responsible.[9] Recent evidence gives grounds for caution in assuming that long RA, even when other aspects of memory impairment are not so marked, is psychogenic. Squire[10] and Alvarez and Squire[11] have argued that the hippocampus has a temporary role in drawing together information from various cortical sites to produce a "whole" memory and that memories initially dependent on this system gradually become established elsewhere in the cortex. This might suggest that hippocampal damage is related to RA. Kapur et al.,[12] however, have reported a case of long RA with mild, patchy impairment of other aspects of memory in which magnetic resonance (MR) scanning failed to show evidence of hippocampal, thalamic, or other medial limbic-diencephalic damage but did show bilateral anterior temporal lobe damage. The exploration of the causes of RA continues, and the precise underlying structures implicated remain uncertain; it is important to recognize that organic factors may well be at work, even with long RA in the absence of other severe memory deficit.

Post-Traumatic Amnesia

There is also a period of loss of memory after the injury—that is, post-traumatic amnesia (PTA). To continue with the same example, Mr. X (who was injured at 2 P.M. on Wednesday) may have his first memory of a hospital visit that took place on the Friday afternoon after injury. He might have isolated memories before then, but if his memory returned on the Friday afternoon and was reasonably continuous thereafter, then that would amount to a period of PTA of about 2 days. In the classical definition, the period of post-traumatic amnesia *includes* any periods of coma and unconsciousness.[7,13] Toward the end of the period of post-traumatic amnesia, patients may appear quite lucid but have no recall of what they are saying or doing or of what is said or done around them.

THE USEFULNESS OF POST-TRAUMATIC AMNESIA IN PREDICTING OUTCOME

As described in Chapter 1, duration of PTA is often used to categorize severity of injury, according to the following criteria[7,13]:

Less than 5 minutes: very mild

5 to 60 minutes: mild

1 to 24 hours: moderate

1 to 7 days: severe

1 to 4 weeks: very severe

More than 4 weeks: extremely severe

Van Zomeren and van den Burg[14] suggest that a cutoff of 13 days provides a better dividing line between severe and very severe injury. Their reasoning is that those with PTA of fewer than 13 days had markedly fewer reported impairments and a much better chance of return to work than those above this cutoff. The same study[14] draws our attention to the fact that outcome is not a global matter but has different components, only some of which may reflect injury severity. These authors studied 57 severely brain injured adults 2 years after injury. What they describe as "complaints" or "intolerances" (items such as irritability, fatigue, and headache) were not related to severity or to return to work. Reports of "impairment" (items such as poor concentration, forgetfulness, slowness, and inability to divide attention), however, were related to severity (as measured by PTA duration) and also to return to work.

There are two further important caveats to be noted in predicting outcome from PTA (or other indices of severity). First, severity does not tell the whole story of TBI, and other factors, including preinjury factors, exact nature and location of brain injury, and social supports, are also important. Second, there are questions as to the adequacy of initial management and the extent to which a well-planned and comprehensive package of rehabilitation is available to the individual, both of which are likely to affect the eventual outcome.

However, based on present knowledge, the best guide we can give to the significance of PTA is Table 5–1, which is based on and adapted from a previous summary by Brooks and McKinlay.[15]

PTA is becoming increasingly difficult to assess accurately because of modern methods of neurosurgical management. Patients are often intubated, ventilated, and sedated.[16] Nevertheless, it usually remains possible to assess PTA in broad bands, and PTA remains a useful index of severity.[17]

Most civilian traumatic brain injuries are "closed" head injuries; that is, the injury is produced by sudden acceleration-deceleration forces that concuss the brain.[13] If such injury is significant, there is virtually always RA (the "signature" of significant closed-head injury, according to Jennett[18]) and PTA. Exceptions are head injury produced by a penetrating wound (e.g., gunshot or shrapnel) or by a depressed fracture (e.g., when the head was struck by an object such as a hammer or axe). In such cases, provided that there is *not also* a significant element of acceleration-deceleration injury, the injured person may recall the injury, although memory and consciousness are often lost soon

TABLE 5–1. A Classification of Post-Traumatic Amnesia

Length of PTA	Likely Outcome
1 Day or less	Expect quick and full recovery with appropriate management. (A few may show persisting disability.)
More than 1 day, less than 1 wk	Recovery period more prolonged—now a matter of weeks or months. Full recovery possible, for most of these cases, with good management.
1 To 2 wk	Recovery a matter of many months. Many patients are left with residual problems even after the "recovery" process has ended, but one can be reasonably optimistic about functional recovery with good management.
2 To 4 wk	Process of recovery is very prolonged—1 year or longer is not unusual. Permanent deficits are likely. There must be increasing pessimism about functional recovery when PTA reaches these lengths.
More than 4 wk	Permanent deficits, indeed significant disability, now certain. It is not just a matter of "recovery" but of long-term retraining and management.

Source: Adapted from Brooks, DN, and McKinlay, WW: Evidence and Quantification in Head Injury: Seminar notes. Unpublished material, 1989, with permission.

after, as brain swelling, bleeding, and other secondary results of injury start to exert their influence.[13] This sequence of events means that the durations of RA and PTA are less useful in gauging the severity of such injuries than they are in relation to acceleration-deceleration injuries.

COMPLICATIONS OF MEMORY LOSS AND AMNESIA

The existence of RA and PTA may, of course, later give rise to some difficulty. There may be difficulties in relation to court proceedings, given that the injured person has a memory gap for the event. Moreover, survivors of TBI are sometimes, understandably, intensely curious about this gap.[19] They have undergone a major, life-changing event, yet cannot recall how it happened; the usual control that people hope to have over their lives is lost.

Recall of the Injury and Post-Traumatic Stress Disorder

Many take the view that this gap in memory is a blessing in disguise because the injured party has no recollection of the injury or its immediate aftermath. There has been some controversy as to whether post-traumatic stress disorder (PTSD) may arise in conjunction with brain injury. Boake and Bontke[20] have suggested that they cannot coexist or at least that they do so only rarely; Rattok[20] suggests that they can coexist but do so rather rarely. PTSD after brain injury is more likely after milder injuries than after more severe injuries. The gap in memory produced by RA and PTA is, of course, shorter in milder injuries than in severe ones, and more of the circumstances surrounding the trauma are recalled. Sbordone and Liter's study,[21] which failed to find any cases of PTSD alongside brain injury, was based on 70 cases, a fairly small number to detect a rare phenomenon. McMillan[19] found 10 cases with PTSD from a total of 312 minor and severe TBI cases, supporting the idea that the conditions can, indeed, coexist but so do only rarely. McMillan and other authors[19,22] have raised the possibility that patients may develop PTSD as a reaction to the traumatic sequelae of the injury, even if they do not have a direct memory of the event itself. McMillan[19] notes:

> Some of the cases reported here remembered little before wakening in a hospital bed, but found this in itself distressing having little understanding of what had befallen them, why they should be in hospital and receiving medical treatment, or of how they sustained physical injuries. Nightmares and intrusive recollections were related to these experiences. . . . (p. 757)

Emergence of Further Deficits: Agitation and Restlessness

Apart from the *very* early cognitive effects noted (i.e., RA and PTA), the most evident psychological or mental effect may be a period of agitation and restlessness.[23–25]

Control of agitation and restlessness may be achieved by a variety of means, including adjustment to milieu (alterations in environment and staff or family behavior), physical and chemical restraints, and behavioral and self-monitoring methods.[26] Gualtieri[27] and Bell and Cardenas[28] have recently reviewed neuropharmacological treatments in the treatment of agitation and aggression.

A less common but distressing problem is emotional lability or emotional incontinence, comprising involuntary and inappropriate periods of weeping, grimacing, or laughing. Treatment with serotonin reuptake inhibitors such as fluoxetine have been reported as effective in controlling emotionalism.[29,30]

☐ COGNITIVE DEFICITS

The cognitive effects of the injury may include a range of deficits. These deficits often take some time to make themselves felt, although they can be uncovered by testing. Patients who are not attempting to work or to carry out their normal day-to-day activities may be quite unaware of the extent of their limitations. The topics for discussion in this section are:

1. Emergence of cognitive deficits
2. Language and communication difficulties
3. Intellectual deficits
4. Memory and learning deficits
5. Attentional deficits
6. Deficits in executive function

Emergence of Cognitive Deficits

Studies that involve sequential assessment show that improvement occurs fairly rapidly at the outset and gradually slows until a plateau is reached.[31,32] There is, however, something of a paradox regarding cognitive limitations: although deficits decrease on testing as recovery proceeds, to patient and family they may appear subjectively to become more obtrusive with the passage of time. In the early stages of recovery, few "normal" cognitive demands are made of TBI survivors, so that they, in fact, experience few memory failures. However, when they attempt to resume normal everyday life and, in particular, social and work activities, their cognitive and memory deficits are liable to become exposed.[33] Studies of elderly people show that having fewer appointments to keep and being engaged in less demanding activities are relevant to having fewer failures of prospective memory.[34]

In a more general sense, there are also differences between memory function as formally assessed and memory problems as reported in "everyday life." Sunderland et al.[35,36] reported that scores on formal test measures did not nec-essarily correlate closely to patients' and relatives' reports on questionnaires and checklists of memory failures. Among the implications are that assessment of everyday memory adds further information to formal assessment and that this aspect takes better account of the interaction between deficits and the memory demands that arise from the interests and occupation of the individuals.[37]

The assessment of cognitive function after brain injury is a matter for other chapters. Note at this point, however, the range of difficulties that may arise and that it is important to assess *change* in function rather than simply to assess the ability level without reference to likely premorbid capacities.[38] The assessment of premorbid ability, although important, can, of course, be difficult because it virtually always has to be assessed retrospectively.[39,40]

Language and Communication Difficulties

Frank dysphasia is relatively uncommon after TBI, which is not surprising, given the predominantly diffuse nature of the pathology. However, communication difficulties in a broader sense are by no means rare.

Heilman et al.[41] reported aphasia in only 13 of 750 (1.7%) consecutive TBI hospital admissions. Recently, Gil et al.[42] reported dysphasia in 11.1 percent of a group of 351 TBI patients who were consecutive admissions to a rehabilitation hospital. The group had a median coma duration of 15.2 days, so that, as a whole, the group had injuries of considerable severity. In contrast, when subtler aspects of language and communication are studied, as in two reports by Hartley and Jensen,[43,44] problems are much more common. All 11 of their subjects (mean coma duration 32 days) showed difficulty, most commonly with conversational fluency and naming, although only 5 were classified as having dysphasia, and all of them had mild anomic dysphasia.

Increasingly, attention is moving from dysphasia as such toward a range of communication-relevant skills, including pragmatics. For example, Linscott et al.[45] have proposed a scale to assess a broad range of aspects of communication after TBI. Aspects assessed include clarity of expression, social style, and appropriateness of subject matter.

Intellectual Deficits

Intellectual deficits (assessed by performance on IQ-type measures) have been described in the literature.[31,32,46] These deficits tend to be found in performance (nonverbal) aspects more than in verbal aspects of intelligence, probably because performance items require integration of a number of functions and because they are usually speeded tasks.[31] Intellectual measures show recovery over time, with rapid initial improvement slowing to an eventual plateau and producing a characteristic recovery curve. The more severe the injury (as assessed by PTA duration), the lower the scores on intellectual tests.[46]

However, the main and most characteristic deficits after TBI are not in intellectual level. For example, Johnstone et al.,[38] in a study of cognitive decline after TBI, found intelligence the least affected of a range of abilities considered—for example, in the Glasgow studies of Brooks et al.,[31,32,46] in which the median PTA was about 14 to 21 days (depending on which study), corresponding to very severe TBI—the extent of intellectual deficit was not particularly great. By 1 year after injury, differences in IQ between the TBI groups and the comparison groups were fairly modest, amounting to between 5 and 9 IQ points. Although this difference was statistically significant in these group studies, in trying to infer change in an individual case, a difference of that size is, in fact, rather modest.[47]

Memory and Learning Deficits

Memory loss immediately before and after injury (i.e., RA and PTA) has already been discussed. The discussion of memory here concerns the later problems encountered by those suffering a brain injury, which tend to come sharply into focus when they try to return to day-to-day life. Memory deficits are among the most commonly reported deficits after brain injury; they are reported in 54 to 87 percent in four studies of very severe TBI carried out 1 or 2 years after injury.[1,14,48,49] It is in memory that some of the most telling cognitive deficits after brain injury lie. Such deficits are a major reason for failure to return to work[3,5,50] and to a broad range of daily activities.[36]

Very short-term memory (memory lasting a few seconds, such as that assessed in the verbal mode by forward digit span) is usually not impaired even after very severe injury.[51] Memory for events that happened well before the injury, sometimes referred to as *remote memory*, usually seems to be relatively unaffected.[8]

However, what is common is difficulty learning new information, retaining it, and subsequently retrieving it, although it is not always

clear at just which of these stages the failures occur. TBI survivors experience this as failures of memory for day-to-day events, including forgetting to pass on messages, repeating questions, forgetting recent events, and having difficulty studying or learning new information.[36] Such difficulties can persist for many years and probably indefinitely in many cases.

Various authors have reviewed the memory difficulties that arise after head injury, and consideration has been given to the various modalities (e.g., verbal and visuo-spatial) and stages (registration, storage, and recall) in which failures may occur. While a detailed review of all of these matters is beyond the scope of this chapter, there are some particular aspects that are especially pertinent in rehabilitation. Brooks[52] noted that:

"... any clinician has seen the motivationally impaired patient who does not care about learning; or the frontally damaged patient who cannot make appropriate action plans for efficient learning; or the attentionally impaired patient who cannot sustain attention long enough for effective information encoding." (p. 164)

Poor performance in memory tasks can therefore arise for a variety of reasons, and moreover failures may occur at various stages of the memory process (registration, storage, and retrieval). Careful assessment of both memory and other possible related reasons for failure needs to be made. It is also important to remember that even the most severe memory deficits may be, to some extent, capable of amelioration, as is suggested by study of amnesic patients.[53,54]

Attentional Deficits

Attention is a notoriously difficult term to define and is apt to be interpreted to mean different things by different people. However, consistent themes in the literature on brain injury are a reduction in the capacity to sustain attention, especially on speeded tasks, and "divided attention." Van Zomeren and Brouwer,[55] who have researched and reviewed the topic, say that slowness in information processing leads to deficits in divided attention, the capacity to keep the mind on more than one task at a time—in other words, to multitask or to keep a number of balls in the air. Sometimes this deficit takes an extreme form after TBI, and some patients cannot even read the newspaper if there is the distraction of a conversation or a TV program in the background. Deficits in this area are common; for example, "poor concentration" was reported in 33 to 62 percent in four studies of very severe TBI that were carried out 1 or 2 years after injury.[1,14,53,54]

Executive Function

Executive problems, which are often associated with frontal lobe damage, are also common after brain injury. This area has always been particularly difficult to assess.[56] In extreme cases, the signs may be obvious. Patients find it difficult to move flexibly from task to task, perhaps either doing very little or alternatively persisting with a task long beyond the point at which they need to engage in it.

However, frontal lobe difficulties may be both subtle and pervasive: Difficulties may arise with planning, initiation, and overall control of various cognitive functions.[57] Therefore, frontal lobe damage may also influence a wide range of cognitive abilities, including memory and other aspects of cognition.[58]

□ ADJUSTING TO THE EFFECTS OF BRAIN INJURY

The cognitive difficulties that have been described—and, indeed, other problems, tend to emerge during rehabilitation as increasing demands are made of the TBI survivor. Many of these difficulties tend to come into particularly sharp focus at or soon after discharge home, or at least when "normal" social and other demands start to be made of the TBI survivor.

Prigatano has used the phrase "the problem of lost normality."[33] He notes that most patients want to return to work or school as soon as possible and are inclined to believe that professionals are overstating their problems. When they return to work or school, however, Prigatano notes, they are likely to "fail unexpectedly." The resumption of other normal activities, such as activities of daily living or social obligations, is also liable to expose the difficulties, both to patients and to those around them.

It is perhaps not surprising, therefore, that what have come to be called "psychosocial difficulties," particularly emotional and behavioral changes, should appear to increase during the first year after injury.[1] Organic reasons for the increase seem unlikely, given that brain injury is not a degenerative disorder and that there tends to be recovery in other aspects of function, including cognition.

Alternative explanations have been proposed: Either these problems "increase" because family members stop making allowances and bring them more sharply into focus with the passage of time, or the patient increasingly exhibits these problems as a secondary reaction to limitations.[59]

Insight and Denial

An important aspect of adjustment to the effects of injury has to do with awareness of deficit. Unawareness of deficit, sometimes referred to as *anosognosia*, or lack of insight, is sometimes found in TBI survivors[60] and has its parallel in denial on the part of relatives.[61]

Lack of or limited insight is a problem that has received particular comment in relation to brain injury.[60,62–64] It has proved difficult to measure, although a recent approach by Fleming et al.[60] provides a promising way of assessing it and a good description of the stages in the development of insight. In the early stages, when insight is very limited, the TBI survivor's focus is apt to be upon a particular physical disability, if such is present. Not only is the focus confined to that disability in disregard of others but also the implications of it are not worked through. Patients often say that there is nothing else wrong with them, that their memory is as good as ever, and that they have no psychosocial problems. Insight then advances, often in stages, so that the implications of the physical limitation begin to be accepted, as is the presence of other problems such as memory difficulties or personality changes. Eventually, the implications of these problems also are accepted, and the final stage in the achievement of insight is the adaptation of future life plans to aim for a degree of rehabilitation and recovery but also an accommodation to limitations.

The parallel phenomenon in relatives, that of denial, was described by Romano,[61] who gave some extreme examples. She noted that the "massive shock" of a family member who is suddenly reduced to a state of severe disability would prompt fantasies such as "she will get well because, after all, she has three children." Sometimes in less severe form, this, too, is a phenomenon familiar to those who work with brain injured patients and their relatives, especially in the early stages of recovery.

In many ways, denial can be seen as a positive coping mechanism in relatives who simply do not take in, all at once, the full extent of the changes in the injured person and the lifestyle adaptations that are required as a result. It may be part of the process of coming to accept these changes that leads relatives to report increasing frequency of changes in the patient in the months and years after injury.

Although some studies have compared the accounts given by patients and relatives,[65,66] it is difficult to conclude which is likely to be more accurate. It is perhaps naive to suppose that one or the other could be relied on for "the truth" and better to regard the perspective of each as part of the overall picture.

In relation to memory, however, Sunderland et al.[35] did find evidence that the accounts of relatives tended to be more reliable and to provide a more valid indication of the extent of the memory deficits present. The same authors also note that asking clients to report on memory failures is a memory test in itself and that failure to reveal problems may not be entirely a matter of insight. They increased the accuracy of patients' accounts by asking participants to fill in a checklist, reporting a memory failure as it happened rather than estimating retrospectively.

☐ EMOTIONAL AND BEHAVIORAL CHANGES

As the initial effects of injury settle, there emerges in the weeks and months after severe TBI a set of changes, particularly in emotional adjustment and behavior, which have come to be included under the term *psychosocial changes*.[1,6,14,48,49,67,68] Much of the research in this area has relied on the accounts of relatives, given concerns about patients' limited insight, especially soon after injury.[59]

The most frequently reported psychosocial changes are similar across TBI follow-up studies. The most common changes in four studies are shown in Table 5–2. Particularly common problems in all these studies are irritability and impatience, poor memory, slowness, and tiredness. The frequency with which problems arise varies according to injury severity and who was reporting (patient or relative).[1,14,59,67] In interpreting and comparing such studies, the timing of follow-up and the extent of access to rehabilitation services are also relevant. The studies of the Glasgow group[1,69] provide an example of how problems vary over time. Some problems became less common over time; for example, slowness dropped from 86 percent at 3 months to 67 percent at 12 months, although at 5-year follow-up slowness was still reported in 67 percent of cases. However, the opposite is liable to happen with emotional and behavioral changes; indeed, personality change, reported in 49 percent at 3 months and 60 percent at 12 months, had risen to 74 percent at 5 years. Possible reasons for such changes were discussed earlier.

Whether rehabilitation affects the frequency of emotional and behavioral problems remains to be seen. The most encouraging studies of rehabilitation outcome (reviewed by Cope[70]) concentrate on improvements in functional competence (activities of daily living, work, level of dependence) rather than on emotional and behavioral problems as such, and it is not neces-

TABLE 5–2. The Six Most Frequently Reported Problems Following TBI: A Comparison of Four Studies

		McKinlay et al[1]		Van Zomeren and van den Burg[14]		Gray et al[49]		Ponsford et al[48]	
Years after injury		1		2		1		2	
Severity		median PTA = 21 days		median PTA = 22 days		median GCS = 8 or less		median PTA = about 28 days	
Reporter and number		Relatives (*n* = 55)		Patients (*n* = 57)		Relatives (*n* = 47)		Patients (*n* = 175)	
		THE SIX PROBLEMS MOST FREQUENTLY REPORTED IN PERCENTAGES							
	1	Irritability	71	Forgetfulness	54	Memory problems	87	Memory problems	74
	2	Impatience	71	Irritability	39	Impatience	74	Fatigue	72
	3	Tiredness	69	Slowness	33	Slowness	74	Word-finding difficulties	68
	4	Poor memory	69	Poor concentration	33	Tiredness	72	Irritability	67
	5	Slowness	67	Fatigue	30	Poor balance	67	Speed of thinking	64
	6	Bad temper	67	Dizziness	26	Word-finding difficulties	66	Concentration	62

sarily true that functional gains are echoed by gains in all other areas.

The overall picture of emotional and behavioral change after TBI that emerges is that relatives of the TBI survivor are likely to feel that the brain injury has changed the person they knew. Personality change is a common report and, indeed, the most common long-term emotional-behavioral change reported in Brooks et al.'s study.[69] The presence of personality change is associated with a wide range of emotional and behavioral problems, although the particular features of reduced self-reliance, disliking company, unhappiness, excitability, childishness, and unreasonableness have been particularly associated with those patients judged to show personality change.[71]

The broad range of emotional and behavioral changes that may follow TBI has proved difficult to categorize, and different authors have tried to do so in different ways. The following is only one possible way of grouping these difficulties.

Lack of Insight

At its worst, lack of insight or reduced insight may make it very difficult to work with patients in the rehabilitation setting and interfere with their striving toward attainable goals.[63] Moreover, the fact that it sometimes exists—and the need, therefore, to gather information from relatives as well as patients—requires of rehabilitation professionals a delicate balancing act whereby they try to obtain all the necessary information while respecting the TBI survivor's desire to be "normal" and self-determining.

Undercontrol

Various commonly reported changes after TBI reflect what has been termed *undercontrol*, basically a reduced capacity to control both temper and mood state.[1] It results in a short temper with frequent inability to shrug off minor annoyances and sometimes frank violence against others, especially members of the family.[69]

Although few would argue against an organic cause of disinhibited behavior, especially in a patient with bilateral frontal lobe damage, nonorganic factors also seem likely to contribute to temper problems; given that they become more frequent at later follow-ups,[1,59] they may be at least in part an expression of frustration with current limitations. Difficulties of this sort are especially difficult for relatives to cope with and are closely associated with the degree of "burden" or stress in caregivers.[1,72,73]

Undercontrol may also affect patients' ability to regulate mood, and rapid mood swings and other forms of emotional lability, such as tearfulness or overwhelming emotional experiences, may arise. Moreover, lack of control may extend to sexual disinhibition, which may take such forms as invasion of body space, inappropriate kissing, or exposure.

Apathy and Tiredness

Whereas the problems of undercontrol might be said to lead to positive disorders of behavior, the problems of apathy and tiredness lead to negative behavior problems. TBI survivors may appear depressed yet deny depressive mood. "Get up and go" is lacking, and the patient may seem prepared to sit and do nothing at all. If left alone, in fact, many simply watch television all day. Motivation has "gotten up and gone."

Sufficiently prompted by someone else, they may perform adequately until distracted, the situation changes, or some problem is encountered, when they just stop. This sort of behavior is a severe impediment to rehabilitation and can be very difficult for family members to tolerate.

Extreme tiredness is also, in effect, a sort of reduced behavior in which the patient has great difficulty staying awake. Indeed, tiring easily is one of the most common sequelae[1,14,48,49] and tiredness is apt to exacerbate all difficulties (physical, cognitive, and emotional). A more general, prolonged difficulty in staying awake probably results from damage to the structures in the brain stem that control arousal. The problem of fatigue can be a very limiting factor. Many people are simply not able to live life as fully as they would wish because of their limited resources of energy.

Depressed and Anxious Mood

Depressed mood is common, although just how common varies from study to study. For example, it was reported in about 60 percent of TBI survivors in the Glasgow follow-up studies[1,69] up to 5 years after injury and in a similar number in Ponsford et al.'s 2-year follow-up.[48] In both studies, relatives' accounts were the source. Lower prevalence rates (of around 20 percent) have been reported from surveys of patients themselves.[14,74] For most patients, the depression they suffer seems to be low mood rather than a full depressive disorder, but it is nonetheless important. Nearly one patient in five is reported to have contemplated suicide at some stage during the first 5 years, although few make an attempt.[69] Of course, some people who have suffered a brain injury are not in the least depressed; because of limited insight, they do not realize the extent of their limitations.

Feelings of tension and anxiety are also common and reported by relatives in around 60 percent of TBI survivors up to 5 years after injury.[1,48,69] As with depression, patients themselves reported such problems in fewer instances—18 to 25 percent.[14,74] Again, like depressed mood, anxiety does not necessarily diminish over time. It can arise as a secondary reaction to brain injury. Many people find that, as a result of specific impairments, they can no longer go out to work, and they now require help in day-to-day living. As a result, they lose confidence and develop low self-esteem.

A smaller proportion of patients present with other neurotic symptomatology. For example, increased obsessional checking behavior is seen, albeit only occasionally. Phobic anxiety may develop, perhaps associated with how the injury was sustained. For example, in the case of an assault, a patient may be anxious in an environment similar to that in which the injury was sustained, for example, crowded places at night.

Social Behavior

Some of those who suffer brain injuries demonstrate a marked change in social behavior. A loss of social skills may affect relationships and friendships.[75] People with brain injury may show impaired perception of, and use of, body language, making them socially awkward. For example, in a follow-up study 2 to 7 years after injury,[65] relatives reported that 38 percent of TBI survivors talked excessively, 38 percent behaved in a socially embarrassing way, and 30 percent tended to withdraw from social interaction; 22 percent of family members reported that patients had become more intrusive or prying. Generally, in many cases the brain-injured person changed from being a companion or confidant to being someone who needs to be watched and managed.

Withdrawal from social interaction is a particularly serious problem. TBI survivors often seem to lose the ability to "read" others' social behavior. Among the many factors that may contribute to this phenomenon are trouble remembering names, inability to remember information about the people they are talking to, inability to cope if more than one person speaks at a time because of divided attention deficits, and loss of self-confidence. As a result, TBI survivors often become socially isolated, depressed, and overly dependent on family members and fail to reintegrate into society.[76,77]

Psychiatric Diagnoses

So far in this chapter and, indeed, in much of the literature, the psychosocial changes following brain injury have been dealt with in a descriptive way. The question arises as to whether particular psychiatric syndromes can be diagnosed. There has recently been some interest[78] in using the *Diagnostic and Statistical Manual of Mental Disorders,* fourth edition (DSM-IV)—one of the principal diagnostic schemes.[79]

Many of the changes after brain injury do not fit psychiatric syndrome criteria. Despite the high frequency of some of these problems, formal psychiatric disorders have generally been considered relatively uncommon (although not all agree[78]).

A useful example of the difficulty in applying such diagnostic criteria is depression. Several of the defining symptoms, in terms of DSM-IV, may arise after TBI for reasons other than depression. Fatigue and diminished concentration after TBI may result from physical weakness or damage to frontal lobes and arousal centers, for example, and weight loss or gain is common after any severe injury as a direct result of injury or forced changes in activity levels.

◻ MEDIATING FACTORS

Severity

Injury severity is obviously of possible importance in determining the extent of cognitive, emotional, and behavioral changes. In the early stages after injury, it does seem that severity measures such as depth of coma (Glasgow Coma Scale) and PTA duration do help in predicting the extent of the difficulties.[80,81] With the passage of time, social support seems to become more important, and severity effects are less pronounced.[76,77,82–84]

Recent articles suggest that outcome—in the sense of community reintegration (employment and independent living) and psychosocial adjustment—is determined by having a social support structure in place and by maintaining adequate social networks rather than being predominantly determined by severity.

It would be wrong, of course, to exclude severity entirely. Plainly, the great majority of people who suffer only mild injury make a good recovery, and the likelihood of severe disability is much greater after severe injury. This finding is borne out by studies that look at a wide range of severities.[85] Within individual studies, severity effects are often attenuated because some studies confine themselves to a fairly narrow range of severity. However, very fine gradations as regards predicted outcome cannot be made on the basis of severity alone; a broad approach is all that can be achieved.

Predicting outcome of brain injury is not just a matter of how severe the injury was. Secondary effects can also have particular importance; for example, subdural hematoma has been identified as a feature associated with poor prognosis independent of severity of injury.[86]

Age at Injury and Premorbid Factors

Another factor that has received attention is age. The Kennard principle[87] suggests that children are more resilient and make better recoveries after brain injury. Recent evidence, however, suggests that the outcome may be worse in persons injured in childhood. There are good reasons for arguing from first principles that to go through childhood and adolescence with a deficit is likely to have a negative effect on the normal pattern of development, especially of more complex skills.

Asikainen et al.[85] studied 508 Finnish patients at an average of 12 years after injury and looked at social and employment outcome, among other things. Those injured at 7 years of age or younger had worse outcomes on the Glasgow Outcome Scale[88] and were less often capable of employment than those injured at ages 8 to 16. Those aged 17 to 25 at the time of injury had better outcomes than those who were younger or older at the time of injury.

At the same time, studies that have concentrated on the older adult have been emerging, and it seems that those in old age are also more vulnerable and have poorer outcomes.[85,89–93]

Various other premorbid factors have been suggested to be relevant to outcome, such as preinjury education, work history, and alcohol use.[82] However, because the effect of these variables is not always straightforward, caution should be exercised in considering the probable impact of such factors in rehabilitation practice.

□ IMPLICATIONS FOR FUTURE ADJUSTMENT

Return to Work

Rates of return to work are often low, and cognitive and emotional-behavioral changes are key factors.[3,94,95] Brooks et al.[3] in their sample of 98 severely injured patients, seen 2 to 7 years after severe injury, report that the rate of employment dropped from 86 percent before injury to 29 percent after injury. These figures may represent an overly gloomy picture because vocational rehabilitation was not usually available in this study. However, there are key behavioral and cognitive problems that need to be overcome to return to work successfully.[3,94,96]

Problems with verbal memory and mental speed and concentration have been reported as especially associated with difficulty reentering employment.[3,4] Moreover, among patients who fail to achieve consistent return to work, there is a higher incidence of cognitive and emotional-behavioral problems, including lack of insight.[3,76,77,82–84,94,96,97]

Family Burden and Social Isolation

Family burden, or stress on caring relatives, has received a good deal of attention and is also associated with particular changes in TBI survivors, especially emotional and behavioral changes.[1,69,72,73,77] Role changes are common after brain injury, with the spouse becoming less a life partner and more a caregiver or supervisor. Not surprisingly, spouses of brain injured persons have been reported to suffer higher levels of stress than parents caring for offspring with a brain injury,[73,98,99] which, of course, is not to say that parents are unaffected by the effects of caring for their brain injured children.

High stress levels experienced by caregivers are especially related to emotional and behavioral disturbances in the injured patient.[1,69,72,73,77] Overall personality change in the patient—including poor emotional control (quick temper, changeability), reduction in energy (being lifeless and listless), and difficult or unreasonable behavior—is associated with burden on relatives.[71] Other factors, however, are also relevant; for example, relatives who had difficulty in dealing with life stresses before the brain injury are more vulnerable thereafter.[100]

The finding that many brain injured patients become lonely and socially isolated is increasingly noted. Mooney[101] and Morton and Wehman[77] have reviewed this topic. Mooney[101] especially notes the role of personality change in leading to social isolation; Morton and Wehman's review[77] emphasizes the rehabilitation implications.

□ CONCLUSIONS

Of the deficits that may follow TBI, cognitive and emotional-behavioral difficulties are particularly important. They contribute greatly to overall disability and present a challenge to rehabilitation.

The very early cognitive effects (RA and PTA) and the very early behavioral effects (agitation and restlessness) generally resolve, and the characteristic picture of cognitive deficit and emotional-behavioral change after brain injury starts to emerge.

Memory deficits are perhaps the most characteristic and widespread cognitive problems of all after TBI, but attentional deficits and executive dysfunction are also important. Although they show a degree of resolution on testing, paradoxically it is often not until the recovery process is well under way that patients (and, indeed, relatives) become aware of them, prompted by the experience of cognitive failures as normal activities are resumed.

This process of gradual adjustment is also seen in relation to emotional and behavioral problems. Patients' insight into them often develops in stages, and only as the months after injury pass do patients and relatives realize the nature and extent of these problems. Undercontrol (quick temper, changeable moods), apathy and tiredness, depressed and anxious mood, and changes in social behavior are all common.

Cognitive and behavioral changes play a part in various long-term problems of the TBI survivor, especially vocational reentry, burden on caregivers, and social isolation. Minimizing the extent and the effects of such problems is therefore a key challenge for all involved in rehabilitation—practitioners, TBI survivors, and their families and friends.

REFERENCES

1. McKinlay, WW, et al: The short term outcome of severe blunt head injury as reported by relatives of the injured persons. J Neurol Neurosurg Psychiatry 44:527, 1981.
2. Jennett, B, et al: Disability after severe head injury: Observations on the use of the Glasgow Outcome Scale. J Neurol Neurosurg Psychiatry 44:285, 1981.
3. Brooks, DN, et al: Return to work within the first seven years of severe head injury. Brain Inj 1:5, 1987.
4. Lam, CS, Priddy, DA, and Johnson, P: Neuropsychological indicators of employability following traumatic brain injury. Rehabilitation Counselling Bulletin 35:68, 1991.
5. Ruff, RM, et al: Predictors of outcome following severe head trauma: Follow-up data from the Traumatic Coma Data Bank. Brain Inj 7:101, 1993.
6. Dikmen, S, Machamaer, J, and Temkin, N: Psychosocial outcome in patients with moderate to severe head injury: 2-Year follow-up. Brain Inj 7:113, 1993.
7. Russell, WR: The Traumatic Amnesias. Oxford University Press, New York, 1971.
8. Schacter, DL, and Crovitz, HF: Memory function after closed head injury: A review of the quantitative research. Cortex 13:150, 1977.
9. Teasdale, G, and Brooks, N: Traumatic amnesia. In Fredriks, JAM (ed): Handbook of Clinical Neurology, Vol 1: Clinical Neuropsychology. Elsevier, Amsterdam, 1984.
10. Squire, LR: Memory and the hippocampus: A synthesis from findings with rats, monkeys, and humans. Psychol Rev 99:195, 1992.
11. Alvarez, P, and Squire, LR: Memory consolidation and the medial temporal lobe: A simple networks model. Proc Nat Acad Sci USA 91:7041, 1994.
12. Kapur, N, et al: Focal retrograde-amnesia following bilateral temporal-lobe pathology: A neuropsychological and magnetic-resonance study. Brain 115:73, 1992.
13. Jennett, B, and Teasdale, G: Management of Head Injuries. FA Davis, Philadelphia, 1981.
14. Van Zomeren, AH, and van den Burg, W: Residual complaints of patients two years after severe head injury. J Neurol Neurosurg Psychiatry 48:21, 1985.
15. Brooks, DN, and McKinlay, WW: Evidence and Quantification in Head Injury: Seminar notes. Unpublished material, 1989.
16. Teasdale, GM: Head injury. J Neurol Neurosurg Psychiatry 58:526, 1995.
17. Wilson, JTL, et al: Posttraumatic amnesia: Still a valuable yardstick. J Neurol Neurosurg Psychiatry 57:198, 1994.
18. Jennett, B: The best yardstick we have. Lancet 2:1445, 1961.
19. McMillan, TM: Post-traumatic stress disorder following minor and severe closed head injury: 10 single cases. Brain Inj 10:749, 1996.
20. Rattok, J, Boake, C, and Bonthke, CF: Do patients with mild brain injuries have posttraumatic stress disorder too? J Head Trauma Rehabil 11:95, 1996.
21. Sbordone, RJ, and Liter, JC: Mild traumatic brain injury does not produce post-traumatic stress disorder. Brain Inj 9:405, 1995.
22. Ohry, A, Rattok, J, and Solomon, Z: Post-traumatic stress disorder in brain injury patients. Brain Inj 10:687, 1996.
23. Levin, HS, and Grossman, RG: Behavioral sequelae of closed head injury. Arch Neurol 35:720, 1978.
24. Reyes, RL, Bhattacharyya, AK, and Heller, D: Traumatic head injury: Restlessness & agitation as prognosticators of physical and psychological impairment in patients. Arch Phys Med Rehabil 62:20, 1981.
25. Brooke, M, et al: Agitation and restlessness after closed head injury: A prospective study of 100 consecutive admissions. Arch Phys Med Rehabil 73:320, 1992.
26. Gervasio, AJ, and Matthies, BK: Behavioral management of agitation in the traumatically brain-injured person. Neurorehabilitation 5:309, 1995.
27. Gualtieri, CT: Review: Pharmacotherapy and the neurobehavioural sequelae of traumatic brain injury. Brain Inj 2:101, 1988.
28. Bell, KR, and Cardenas, DC: New frontiers of neuropharmacologic treatment of brain injury agitation. Neurorehabilitation 5:233, 1995.
29. Sloan, RL, Brown, KW, and Pentland, B: Fluoxetine as a treatment for emotional lability after brain injury. Brain Inj 6:315, 1992.
30. Seliger, GM, et al: Fluoxetine improves emotional incontinence. Brain Inj 6:267, 1992.
31. Mandleberg, IA, and Brooks, DN: Cognitive recovery after severe head injury, 1. Serial testing on the Wechsler Adult Intelligence Scale. J Neurol Neurosurg Psychiatry 38:1121, 1975.
32. Brooks, DN, and Aughton, ME: Cognitive recovery during the first year after severe blunt head injury. International Rehabilitation Medicine 1:166, 1979.
33. Prigatano, GP: 1994 Sheldon Berrol, MD, Senior Lectureship: The problem of lost normality after brain injury. J Head Trauma Rehabil 10:87, 1995.
34. Maylor, EA: Older people's memory for the past and the future. Psychologist 9:456, 1996.
35. Sunderland, A, Harris, JE, and Baddeley, AD: Do laboratory tests predict everyday memory? A neuropsychological study. Journal of Verbal Learning and Verbal Behavior 22:341, 1983.
36. Sunderland, A, Harris, JE, and Gleave, J: Memory failures in everyday life following severe head injury. Journal of Clinical Neuropsychology 6:127, 1984.
37. Hickox, A, and Sunderland, A: Questionnaire and checklist approaches to assessment of everyday memory problems. In Crawford, JR, Parker, DM, and McKinlay, WW

(eds): A Handbook of Neuropsychological Assessment. Lawrence Erlbaum, Hove, England, 1992.

38. Johnstone, B, Hexum, CL, and Ashkanazi, G: Extent of cognitive decline in traumatic brain injury based on estimates of premorbid intelligence. Brain Inj 9:377, 1995.

39. Ruff, RM, Mueller, J, and Jurica, P: Estimation of premorbid functioning after traumatic brain injury. Neurorehabilitation 7:39, 1996.

40. O'Carroll, R: The assessment of premorbid ability: A critical review. Neurocase 1:83, 1995.

41. Heilman, KM, Safran, A, and Geschwind, N: Closed head trauma and aphasia. J Neurol Neurosurg Psychiatry 34:265, 1971.

42. Gil, M, et al: Vocational outcome of aphasic patients following severe traumatic brain injury. Brain Inj 10:39, 1996.

43. Hartley, LL, and Jensen, PJ: Narrative and procedural discourse after closed head injury. Brain Inj 5:267, 1991.

44. Hartley, LL, and Jensen, PJ: Three discourse profiles of closed head injury speakers: Theoretical and clinical implications. Brain Inj 6:271, 1992.

45. Linscott, RJ, Knight, RG, and Godfrey, HPD: The Profile of Functional Impairment in Communication (PFIC): A measure of communication impairment for clinical use. Brain Inj 10:397, 1996.

46. Brooks, DN, and Aughton, ME: Psychological consequences of blunt head injury. International Rehabilitation Medicine 1:160, 1979.

47. Miller, E: Some basic principles of neuropsychological assessment. In Crawford, JR, Parker, DM, and McKinlay, WW (eds): A Handbook of Neuropsychological Assessment. Lawrence Erlbaum, Hove, England, 1992.

48. Ponsford, JL, Olver, JH, and Curran, C: A profile of outcome: 2 Years after traumatic brain injury. Brain Inj 9:1, 1995.

49. Gray, JM, et al: Negative symptoms in the traumatically brain-injured during the first year postdischarge, and their effect on rehabilitation status, work status and family burden. Clinical Rehabilitation 8:188, 1994.

50. Schacter, DL, Glisky, EL, and McGlynn, SII: Impact of memory disorder on everyday life: Awareness of deficits and return to work. In Tupper, DE, and Cicerone, KD (eds): Neuropsychology of Everyday Life: Assessment and Basic Competencies. Kluwer, Boston, 1990.

51. Brooks, DN: Long and short term memory in head injured patients. Cortex 11:329, 1975.

52. Brooks, DN: Cognitive deficits. In Rosenthal, M, et al (eds): Rehabilitation of the Adult and Child with Traumatic Brain Injury. FA Davis, Philadelphia, 1990.

53. Brooks, DN, and Baddeley, AD: What can amnesic patients learn? Neuropsychologica 14:111, 1976.

54. Godfrey, HPD, and Knight, RG: Interventions for amnesics: A review. Br J Clin Psychol 26:83, 1987.

55. Van Zomeren, AH, and Brouwer, WH: Attention deficits after closed head injury. In Deelman, BG, Saan, RJ, and van Zomeren, AH (eds): Traumatic Brain Injury: Clinical, Social and Rehabilitational Aspects. Swets & Zeitlinger, Amsterdam, 1990.

56. Parker, DM, and Crawford, JR: Assessment of frontal lobe dysfunction. In Crawford, JR, Parker, DM, and McKinlay, WW (eds): A Handbook of Neuropsychological Assessment. Lawrence Erlbaum, Hove, England, 1992.

57. Perecman, E: The Frontal Lobes Revisited. Lawrence Erlbaum, Hillsdale, New Jersey, 1985.

58. Stuss, DT, and Benson, DF: The frontal lobes and control of cognition and memory. In Perecman, E: The Frontal Lobes Revisited. Lawrence Erlbaum, Hillsdale, New Jersey, 1985.

59. McKinlay, WW, and Brooks, DN: Methodological problems in assessing psychosocial recovery following severe head injury. J Clin Neuropsychol 6:87, 1984.

60. Fleming, JM, Strong, J, and Ashton, R: Self-awareness of deficits in adults with traumatic brain injury: How best to measure? Brain Inj 10:1, 1996.

61. Romano, M: Family response to traumatic brain injury. Scand J Rehabil Med 6:1, 1974.

62. McGlynn, SM, and Schachter, DL: Unawareness of deficits in neuropsychology syndromes. J Clin Exp Neuropsychol 11:143, 1989.

63. Langer, KG, and Padrone, FJ: Psychotherapeutic treatment of awareness in acute rehabilitation of traumatic brain injury. Neuropsychological Rehabilitation 2:59, 1992.

64. Malia, KB, Torode, S, and Powell, GE: Insight and progress in rehabilitation after brain injury. Clinical Rehabilitation 7:23, 1993.

65. Brooks, N, et al: The effects of severe ⟨…⟩ on patient and relative within 7 years of injury. ⟨…⟩ Head Trauma Rehabil 2:1, 1987.

66. Tepper, S, Beatty, P, and DeJong, G: Outcomes in traumatic brain injury: Self-report versus report of significant others. Brain Inj 10:575, 1996.

67. Oddy, M, et al: Social adjustment after closed head injury: A further follow-up seven years after injury. J Neurol Neurosurg Psychiatry 48:564, 1985.

68. Thomsen, IV: Late outcome of very severe blunt head trauma: A 10–15 year second follow-up. J Neurol Neurosurg Psychiatry 47:260, 1984.

69. Brooks, DN, et al: The five year outcome of severe blunt head injury: A relative's view. J Neurol Neurosurg Psychiatry 49:764, 1986.

70. Cope, DN: The effectiveness of traumatic brain injury rehabilitation: A review. Brain Inj 9:649, 1995.

71. Brooks, DN, and McKinlay, WW: Personality and behavioural change after severe blunt head injury: A relative's view. J Neurol Neurosurg Psychiatry 46:336, 1983.

72. Kreutzer, JS, Gervasio, AH, and Camplair, PS: Primary caregivers' psychological status and family functioning after traumatic brain injury. Brain Inj 8:197, 1994.

73. Kreutzer, JS, Gervasio, AH, and Camplair, PS: Patient correlates of caregivers' distress and family functioning after traumatic brain injury. Brain Inj 8:211, 1994.

74. O'Carroll, RE, Woodrow, J, and Maroun, F: Psychosexual and psychosocial sequelae of closed head injury. Brain Inj 5:303, 1991.

75. Spence, SE, et al: First impressions count: A controlled investigation of social skill following closed head injury. Br J Clin Psychol 32:309, 1993.

76. Finset, A, et al: Self-reported social networks and interpersonal support 2 years after severe traumatic brain injury. Brain Inj 9:141, 1995.

77. Morton, MV, and Wehman, P: Psychosocial and emotional sequelae of individuals with traumatic brain injury: A literature review and recommendations. Brain Inj 9:81, 1995.

78. Van Reekum, R, et al: Psychiatric disorders after traumatic brain injury. Brain Inj 10:319, 1996.

79. Diagnostic and Statistical Manual of Mental Disorders, ed 4 (DSM-IV). American Psychiatric Association, Washington, DC, 1994.

80. Cowen, TD, et al: Influence of early variables in traumatic brain injury on FIM scores and rehabilitation length of stay and charges. Arch Phys Med Rehabil 76:797, 1995.

81. Dikmen, S, and Machamer, JE: Neurobehavioral outcomes and their determinants. J Head Trauma Rehabil 10:74, 1995.

82. Webb, CR, et al: Explaining quality of life for persons with traumatic brain injuries 2 years after injury. Arch Phys Med Rehabil 76:1113, 1995.

83. Brzuzy, S, and Corrigan, JD: Predictors of living independently after moderate to severe traumatic brain injury: A comparison study. J Head Trauma Rehabil 11:74, 1996.

84. Kendall, E, and Terry, DJ: Psychosocial adjustment following closed head injury: A model for understanding individual differences and predicting outcome. Neuropsychological Rehabilitation 6:101, 1996.

85. Asikainen, I, Kaste, M, and Sarna, S: Patients with traumatic brain injury referred to a rehabilitation and re-employment programme: Social and professional outcome

for 508 Finnish patients 5 or more years after injury. Brain Inj 10:883, 1996.

86. Gennarelli, TA, et al: Influence of the type of intracranial lesion on outcome from severe head injury. J Neurosurg 56:26, 1982.

87. Kennard, MA: Age and other factors in motor recovery from precentral lesions in monkeys. Am J Physiol 115:138, 1936.

88. Jennett, B, and Bond, M: Assessment of outcome after severe brain damage. Lancet 1:480, 1975.

89. Donders, J, and Ballard, E: Psychological adjustment characteristics of children before and after moderate to severe traumatic brain injury. J Head Trauma Rehabil 11:67, 1996.

90. Webb, C, et al: Age and recovery from brain injury: Clinical opinions and experimental evidence. Brain Inj 10:303, 1996.

91. Goldstein, FC, and Levin, HS: Neurobehavioral outcome of traumatic brain injury in older adults: Initial findings. J Head Trauma Rehabil 10:57, 1995.

92. Reeder, KP, et al: Impact of age on functional outcome following traumatic brain injury. J Head Trauma Rehabil 11:22, 1996.

93. Rakier, A, et al: Head injuries in the elderly. Brain Inj 9:187, 1995.

94. McMordie, WR, Barker, SL, and Pauolo, TM: Return to work (RTW) after head injury. Brain Inj 4:57, 1990.

95. Sander, AM, et al: A multicenter longitudinal investigation of return to work and community integration following traumatic brain injury. J Head Trauma Rehabil 11:70, 1996.

96. Ponsford, JL, et al: Prediction of employment status 2 years after traumatic brain injury. Brain Inj 9:11, 1995.

97. Melamed, S, Grosswaser, Z, and Stern MJ: Acceptance of disability, work involvement and subjective rehabilitation status of traumatic brain-injury (TBI) patients. Brain Inj 6:233, 1991.

98. Thomsen, IV: The patient with severe head injury and his family. Scand J Rehabil Med 6:180, 1974.

99. Leathem, J, Heath, E, and Woolley, C: Relatives' perceptions of role change, social support and stress after traumatic brain injury. Brain Inj 10:27, 1996.

100. Livingston, MG: Head injury: The relatives' response. Brain Inj 1:33, 1987.

101. Mooney, GF: Relative contributions of neurophysical, cognitive, and personality changes to disability after brain injury. Cognitive Rehabilitation 6:14, 1988.

Specialized Assessment Techniques

JEFFREY S. KREUTZER, PHD

Neurological and Neuroradiological Evaluation

DOUGLAS I. KATZ, MD,
and SANDRA E. BLACK, MD, FRCP(C)

☐ PURPOSE OF THE NEUROLOGICAL EVALUATION

The neurological evaluation of patients with traumatic brain injury (TBI) may serve several purposes. For patients in rehabilitation, the purpose of the evaluation may be to address specific neurological impairments or complications such as spastic hemiparesis or seizures, to provide a general survey of the neurological system as part of the team evaluation, or to establish a neurological diagnosis and prognosis to help guide rehabilitative management. This last purpose uses neurological assessment to establish a neuropathologically based diagnosis as the foundation for understanding a patient's neurological impairments and disabilities and for projecting the course of recovery and outcome. This chapter addresses the components of a neurological evaluation that serves all of these purposes, with particular emphasis on formulating a neurological diagnosis and prognosis.

☐ NEUROLOGICAL EVALUATION AND TEAM MANAGEMENT

How the neurological assessment is performed and how it is incorporated into rehabilitation team management may vary. Because the principal problems affecting patients with TBI are neurological, clinicians from each discipline perform some aspects of a neurological evaluation as part of their routine assessment procedures. For instance, the physical therapist assesses motor strength and coordination, and the speech therapist looks at attention, memory, and other mental functions as part of an evaluation. The complete neurological evaluation is usually compiled by a physician with neurological expertise (e.g., neurologist or physiatrist), but other physician or nonphysician specialists, such as neuropsychologists, may be involved. This specialist may function as a consultant or an integral member of the rehabilitation team. Some familiarity with the natural history and neurobehavioral syndromes associated with TBI is necessary to translate neurological information into a form useful for rehabilitative management. This expertise is usually beyond the typical residency training and experience of neurologists and physiatrists.

Neurological questions depend on the phase of recovery during which the patient is evaluated. In the acute phase, for instance, issues of survival and neurosurgical intervention predominate. The emphasis is on recognizing lesions, such as subdural hematomas, that may require surgical intervention or managing life-threatening complications, such as brain swelling. For patients assessed in the acute rehabilitation setting, questions involve clarifying the type and severity of brain damage, recognizing neurobehavioral syndromes, distinguishing impairments related to the brain injury from those that are related to other factors (e.g., heterotopic ossification, premorbid developmental disorders), characterizing specific elemental neurological impairments that require follow-up evaluation or treatment (e.g., anosmia, ophthalmoplegia), recognizing delayed complications (e.g., hydrocephalus, seizures, chronic subdural collections), and establishing prognosis. At later stages, in postacute rehabilitation settings, neurological questions might involve characterizing and managing residual neurological syndromes and conditions (e.g., aphasia, spastic paresis, movement disorders, seizures), ruling out late neurological complications that may throw recovery off course, and fine-tuning the long-term prognosis.

Neurological assessment and diagnosis in *rehabilitation* settings are somewhat different than in *acute* settings (Table 6–1). Acute neurological diagnosis begins with clusters of neurological symptoms and signs (syndromes) to formulate an anatomic diagnosis leading to an etiologic or pathological diagnosis. Functional diagnosis is usually a later, secondary concern. Neurological assessment and diagnosis for the rehabilitation setting are almost the reverse of this process. The etiologic diagnosis is not the end point but the starting point. By the time a patient reaches a rehabilitation setting, the cause, type, and, to a large extent, severity of brain injury are already known. Neurological signs and symptoms (syndromic diagnosis) may be rapidly changing and emerging, particularly as patients resume conscious, purposeful behavior or their attentional disturbances wane with resolving confusion. Functional diagnosis is central to the assessment. The neurological assessment should help to elaborate functional diagnosis in the context of the pathological, anatomic, and syndromic diagnoses. These clinical and pathophysiological formulations should lead to prognostication regarding the time course of recovery and probabilities of long-term outcome. Therefore, to provide useful information in the rehabilitation setting, the neurological evaluation should promote an understanding of a patient's clinical presentation in relation to the type and severity of brain damage. Further, when viewed in the context of natural history, evaluation of a patient's functioning can be seen as part of a dynamic neurological recovery process and not simply a static listing of neurological impairments and disabilities at a single point in time. This evaluation provides a framework for setting appropriate goals in a realistic time frame; it should help in the selection of proper treatment strategies at the appropriate stage of recovery, and in avoiding unnecessary treatment for problems that may resolve spontaneously or those that will not recover even with direct, restorative treatment strategies. This type of assessment also promotes early recognition of treatable complications (e.g., hydrocephalus, medication side effects) when natural history appears to be violated for a given patient. The neurological evaluation must also account for the interaction of neurological problems with nonneurological factors such as age, premorbid problems and assets, psychosocial issues, and environmental influences.

□ NEUROPATHOLOGICALLY BASED DIAGNOSIS

It is useful to divide the pathological consequences of TBI into *focal* and *diffuse* categories for the purposes of constructing the neurological evaluation and formulating neurological diagnosis and prognosis. Table 6–2 outlines an organization of traumatic neuropathology into primary and secondary events within focal and diffuse categories. (A full discussion of the pathophysiol-

TABLE 6–1. Steps to Neurological Diagnosis in Acute and Rehabilitation Settings

Steps	Acute Setting	Rehabilitation Setting
I	■ Begins with *symptoms* and *signs* based on history and examination	■ Begins with *impairments* and *disabilities* to formulate *functional diagnosis*
II	■ Formulate *syndromic diagnosis*	■ *Etiologic diagnosis* usually known
III	■ Correlate with *anatomic diagnosis*	■ Reformulate *anatomic* and *neuropathological diagnosis*
IV	■ Develop *etiologic* or *neuropathological diagnosis*	■ Recast *syndromic diagnosis* based on symptoms and signs in context of neuropathological diagnosis
V	■ May formulate *functional diagnosis* but usually secondary	■ Elaborate *functional diagnosis* with respect to syndromic diagnosis, neuropathological diagnosis, and natural history to formulate *prognosis*

TABLE 6–2. Focal and Diffuse, Primary and Secondary Traumatic Neuropathologies

	Focal	Diffuse
Primary injury	• Focal cortical contusion • Large, deep cerebral hemorrhage (extracerebral hemorrhage)	• Diffuse axonal injury • Petechial white matter hemorrhages
Secondary injury	• Delayed neuronal injury • Microvascular injury • Focal hypoxic-ischemic injury • Herniation	• Delayed neuronal injury • Microvascular injury • Diffuse hypoxic-ischemic injury

ogy of TBI is provided in Chapter 2.) The principal diffuse pathology is *diffuse axonal injury* (DAI); other vascular phenomena and secondary effects, such as excitotoxicity, may accompany DAI.[1] The principal focal pathology is *focal cortical contusion* (FCC), which may also have a host of secondary effects, including herniation from mass effect. Other forms of primarily focal injury include deep hemorrhages (not involving cortical surface) and focal ischemic damage (strokes), commonly posterior cerebral artery territory infarcts resulting from temporal lobe herniations. Extracerebral hemorrhages (subdural and epidural hematomas) usually exert clinical effects by way of secondary mass effect (herniation, ischemia) or associated pathologies (underlying contusion, concomitent, DAI). Often patients with TBI have various combinations of different pathological entities, and it is a challenge to sort their independent or interacting clinical effects. A system of neurological evaluation as outlined in this chapter can help sort out how the mix of pathologies produces the patient's clinical picture and how recovery may evolve.

Natural History

DIFFUSE INJURY

Patients with diffuse pathology (DAI and associated secondary injury) follow a generally recognizable pattern of recovery that occurs in a similar fashion across the spectrum of severity. The pattern may be described within the context of three major epochs of recovery (Fig. 6–1). The first is immediate unconsciousness, without lucid interval. The next epoch is a proportionally longer period of emerging consciousness and confusion, closely linked to dense anterograde amnesia (post-traumatic amnesia [PTA]). Following resolution of confusion and PTA is a yet proportionally longer epoch of postconfusional restoration of function. The duration of these epochs and the severity of impairments within each epoch largely correspond to the severity of diffuse injury and form

much of the basis for predicting the time course of recovery and the outcome (e.g., depth of coma by Glasgow Coma Scale, duration of unconsciousness, duration of PTA, neuropsychological measures at particular times postinjury). Patients with the least severe diffuse injuries (mild concussion) evolve through the epoch of unconsciousness (if unconsciousness occurs at all) in seconds to minutes and through the epoch of confusion usually in minutes to hours, followed by a postconfusional recovery period typically lasting days to weeks. The transition through the earliest stages may be brief, unwitnessed, and difficult to recognize. Patients with severe TBI may require days to weeks to evolve through unconsciousness, weeks to months to resolve confusion and PTA, and months to years to evolve through the residual recovery period (see Fig. 6–1). Those with the most severe diffuse injuries may stall at some stage in this recovery process. These epochs of recovery appear to be proportionally related, each subsequent epoch severalfold longer than the previous one.[2] The proportionality in the duration of these epochs can be useful for clinical planning and prognosis. Research has provided evidence of a predictable relationship between the duration of unconsciousness (LOC) and duration of confusion (PTA) in a series of patients with diffuse injury defined by a linear regression model[2]:

$$\text{PTA (weeks)} = 0.4 \times \text{LOC (days)} + 3.6$$

This pattern of recovery has been further described according to various schemas; the most widely used is the Rancho Los Amigos levels of cognitive functioning[3] (Table 6–3). Another schema, modified from one proposed by Alexander,[4] better follows neurological nomenclature (Table 6–4). The first stage, *coma* (corresponding to Rancho level I), refers to unconsciousness, without spontaneous eye opening. The depth of coma early in this stage is one of the key indices of injury severity. Almost all survivors progress to the next stage, *vegetative state–wakeful uncon-*

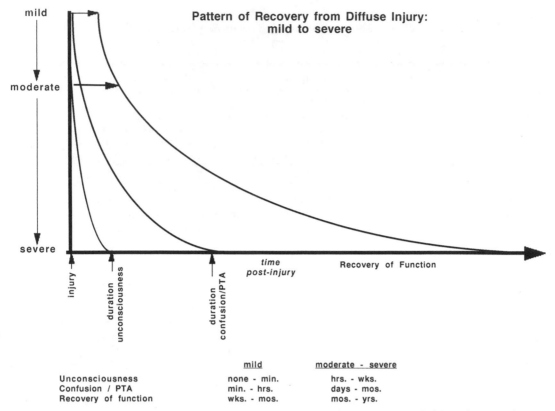

FIGURE 6–1. Pattern of recovery associated with diffuse traumatic brain injury divided into three epochs: unconsciousness, confusion–post-traumatic amnesia (PTA), postconfusional recovery. Epochs of recovery vary in duration based on injury severity.

sciousness (Rancho level II), within 3 to 4 weeks, defined by spontaneous eye opening and sleep-wake cycles, without conscious awareness. A small proportion of very severely injured patients remain vegetative (designated *permanent vegetative state*, if prolonged over 1 year),[5] but most progress to a stage of erratic, inconsistent purposeful responsiveness and low-level cog-

---

TABLE 6–3. Rancho Los Amigos Levels of Cognitive Functioning

I.	No response
II.	Generalized responses
III.	Localized responses
IV.	Confused—agitated
V.	Confused—inappropriate
VI.	Confused—appropriate
VII.	Automatic—appropriate
VIII.	Purposeful and appropriate

Source: Hagen, C, Malkmus, D, and Durham, P: Levels of Cognitive Functioning. Ranchos Los Amigos Hospital, Downey, Calif, 1972.

---

nitive awareness, termed *minimally conscious state* (Rancho level III). Patients are typically mute or hypoverbal at this stage. Transition to this stage designates the resolution of unconsciousness (frequently referred to as the *duration of coma*), often marked by the ability to follow commands. The time to reach this stage (duration of unconsciousness) is another key index of injury severity.

As cognitive responses become more consistent and patients begin to communicate, they enter the stage designated *confusional state* (Rancho levels IV, V, and partly VI). Agitated, poorly modulated, and, less commonly, hypokinetic behavioral disturbances are common during this stage. Disturbances in basic attention and dense anterograde amnesia (PTA) define this stage. Despite the severe effect on explicit learning and episodic memory (day-to-day experience), patients can learn specific motor or cognitive tasks (implicit or procedural learning) even while lacking explicit knowledge of the experience.[6] The resolution of this stage is marked by restoration of continuous day-to-day memory and orientation, as well as vast improvements in

---

TABLE 6–4. Stages of Recovery from Diffuse Injury

1. *Coma:* unresponsive, eyes closed
2. *Vegetative state–wakeful unconsciousness:* no cognitive responsiveness, gross wakefulness, sleep-wake cycles
3. *Minimally conscious state:* some purposeful responsiveness, inconsistent responses to commands, often mute
4. *Confusional state:* recovered speech, amnesic (PTA), severe attentional deficits, agitated, hypoaroused, or labile behavior
5. *Postconfusional–evolving independence:* resolution PTA, cognitive improvement, achieving independence in daily self-care, improving social interaction; developing independence at home
6. *Intellectual and social competence:* recovering cognitive abilities, goal-directed behaviors, social skills, personality; developing independence in community; returning to academic or vocational pursuits

Source: Alexander, MP: Traumatic brain injury. In Benson, DF, and Blumer, D (eds): Psychiatric Aspects of Neurologic Disease. Grune & Stratton, New York, 1982, p 231.

---

directed and sustained attention. Time to the end of this stage is also an important index of injury severity: *duration of PTA.*

In the next stage, *postconfusional–evolving independence* (Rancho levels VI and VII) patients begin to develop functional independence in basic activities of daily living (ADLs), but they still have cognitive problems, particularly in higher-level attention, speed of processing, memory efficiency, and executive functions. Most hospitalized rehabilitation patients return home at this stage. Although basic insight and safety awareness return, patients usually require some level of supervision because of impairments in reasoning and judgment, often compounded by impulsivity and forgetfulness. Although severe behavioral disturbances usually resolve, disinhibition and impaired social awareness are common continuing problems. Impairments in specific cognitive modalities can be better characterized at this stage.

The next stage, termed *intellectual-social competence* (Rancho levels VII and VIII), tracks later recovery and is somewhat arbitrarily marked by resumption of household independence. As higher-level cognitive capacities and social functioning improve, patients can begin to return to previous social roles and activities. Return of higher levels of self-awareness is an important part of the evolution through this stage. It deserves emphasis again that not all patients progress through all these stages of recovery, in large part related to severity of diffuse injury, secondary complication, or, possibly, the residual effects of focal damage.

FOCAL INJURY

The natural history of focal pathology is largely dependent on lesion characteristics: location, size and depth, bilaterality (especially involving homologous areas), and secondary damage. The usual location of FCCs, the principal form of focal pathology, in the limbic and heteromodal association areas of the anterior frontal and temporal lobes, defines their typical cognitive and behavioral effects: impairments in executive function, higher-order attention, and behavior modulation. (These same problems can occur with diffuse injuries in the absence of FCC.) Other locations may present different problems. For instance, lesions extending more posteriorly in the left temporal association areas may cause language disorders, characteristically anomic or transcortical sensory aphasia.

Small differences in the depth of the lesion, involving a greater proportion of white matter pathways as they converge at deeper levels, can make enormous differences with respect to clinical effects and recovery. Further, bilateral involvement may portend a much worse prognosis; conversely, patients with unilateral lesions, particularly involving less lateralized neural systems (e.g., prefrontal), can have considerable recovery.[7]

The time course of recovery of focal lesions such as FCC is probably identical to focal hemorrhagic lesions of other causes. Recovery probably evolves more rapidly than equivalent problems of similar severity caused by diffuse injuries (e.g., executive functions). It also deserves emphasis that the specific clinical effects of focal pathology are often embedded in the evolving clinical recovery process of diffuse injuries. Detection of particular localizing syndromes may be difficult until unmasked with the resolution of attention problems as confusion clears. Further difficulties in distinguishing effects of focal lesions are presented because neurobehavioral syndromes may be identical to those related to diffuse injury (e.g., dysexecutive syndrome; behavioral dysregulation).

The following sections discuss the components of the neurological evaluation: neurological history, neurological examination, neuroradiological assessment, and neurophysiological assessment. The discussion includes some of the typical neurological impairments and syndromes of patients with TBI. Next, the discussion centers on how this information can be used to formulate a neurological diagnosis and prognosis that is meaningful for rehabilitation.

◻ ELEMENTS OF THE NEUROLOGICAL ASSESSMENT

As with any clinical evaluation, the neurological assessment consists of a history and an examination. The examination is composed of the mental status and physical components. Ancillary studies usually include neuroradiological evaluation, particularly an acute computed tomography (CT) scan. Follow-up magnetic resonance imaging (MRI) or CT scans may be ordered later, and supplemental studies may include electrophysiological evaluation (electroencephalography [EEG], evoked responses, quantitative EEG) and perhaps functional imaging studies (single-photo emission tomography [SPECT], functional MRI). Any use of ancillary studies should be tied to specific clinical questions or management decisions at the appropriate times postinjury.

History

The history is an essential part of the evaluation of any disorder, and it is particularly important for precise diagnosis after TBI. For patients with TBI, the challenge is compounded because patients are usually unable to give an account of the injury and its immediate aftermath themselves because of PTA. The patient's own account of the effects of the injury, even after PTA has resolved, may be limited because of reduced awareness of deficits at earliest phases of recovery. It is necessary to construct the history from various other sources, such as witnesses, family, and acute hospital and emergency medical services (EMS) records. Once confusion and PTA have cleared, some recovery information can be gleaned from the patient's earliest recall (e.g., duration of PTA). It cannot be overemphasized, however, that rehabilitation clinicians must go back to the earlier records to obtain essential information for neurological diagnosis.

Several points in the history are key to the complete TBI diagnosis.

1. *Mechanism of injury* to distinguish those associated with primarily contact forces (e.g., assault with blunt object, fall from standing [<6 feet]) from those involving significant acceleration-deceleration forces (e.g., motor vehicle accident, fall of significant height [>6 feet]), or both; seatbelt restraint, helmets, deployment of airbags, ejection from the vehicle, and windshield head impact damage may give important clues as to the nature of the injury mechanics.

2. *Loss of consciousness* and whether immediate or delayed (immediate LOC attributable to diffuse axonal injury; delayed LOC associated with expanding mass lesion, such as subdural, epidural, or intracerebral hematoma).

3. *Depth of coma,* including range of Glasgow Coma Scale scores (Table 6–5) in the hours postinjury, especially poststabilization (the lowest postresuscitation GCS score probably carries the most prognostic information, but the highest attained score, any nonneurologic confounds, and the early progression in scores should be considered).

4. Early *hemodynamic or respiratory instability* (indicating potential for secondary hypoxic-ischemic injury).

TABLE 6–5. Glasgow Coma Scale

Response	Points
Eye Opening	
Spontaneous	4
To speech	3
To pain	2
None	1
Best Motor Response	
Obeys commands	6
Localized to pain stimuli	5
Withdraws from pain stimuli	4
Decorticate flexion	3
Decerebrate extension	2
None	1
Verbal Response	
Oriented	5
Confused conversation	4
Inappropriate words	3
Incomprehensible sounds	2
None	1

Score: 3–15 points.

Source: Teasdale, G, and Jennett, B: Assessment of coma and impaired consciousness: A practical scale. Lancet 2:81, 1974.

5. Early *brain stem abnormalities,* such as pupillary dilatation and third nerve palsy resulting from temporal herniation.

6. *Neuroimaging,* acute and subacute CT and MRI scans (these should be obtained for direct viewing, but often only radiologists' reports or secondary reports are available).

7. *Course of early recovery* including emergence from unconsciousness: Time to first follow commands is a principal criterion, but other signs of early purposeful behavior such as willful movements, specific discrimination of stimuli, and attempt at verbalization are also signs of emergent consciousness.

8. Resolution of *post-traumatic amnesia* (PTA) can be estimated retrospectively by patient's reports of first postinjury memories, first reports of full orientation, or family's perception of the patient's resumption of continuous episodic memory. The patient's self-report of "coma" or "unconsciousness" is often an experience of amnesia, so it can be used to estimate PTA. The examiner needs to be clear whether the patient is offering somebody else's observation of the period of unconsciousness or the patient's own subjective account of the restoration of episodic memories. PTA will usually not have resolved for most patients admitted to inpatient rehabilitation and can be determined prospectively by such instruments as the Galveston Orientation Amnesia Test (GOAT).[9]

9. *Secondary neurological complications* such as seizures are important elements of the neurological history.

10. *Other injuries,* apart from the brain injury, including fractures and injury to other organ systems (e.g., liver laceration, spleen rupture, pneumothorax, cardiac contusion) should be described.

11. *Other medical problems* in the acute and subacute period (e.g., infections) should be elaborated because all may affect the rate of neurological recovery. The history should include a review of other organ systems for contribution problems.

12. Account for *medications* or other treatments that may act on the central nervous system or confound neurological evaluation (e.g., benzodiazepines and neuroleptics for agitation, narcotic pain medication, sedative sleeping medications, some antihypertensives, chemical paralytics at the time of intubation).

13. *Past medical history* should pay particular attention to previous neurological, psycho-logical, or developmental disturbances. Previous history of TBI, depression, psychosis, learning disabilities, attention deficit/hyperactive disorders, or alcohol or other substance abuse may be potent issues in recovery and interpretation of cognitive and behavioral problems.

14. *Social history* should include an accounting of the patient's living situation, physical home environment, family, principal supports and caretakers, education history, vocational history, hobbies and interests, premorbid personality, and habits.

The Neurological Examination of the Patient with Traumatic Brain Injury

MENTAL STATUS

The mental status examination is the most important component of the neurological examination of patients with TBI. Paradoxically, it is the portion of the examination with which neurologists and others are often least comfortable. Further, some of the most prevalent cognitive and behavioral problems following TBI—inframodal cognitive functions, including arousal and attention, and supramodal operations, such as executive functions and behavioral regulation[10–12]—are the most difficult to characterize. Direct disruption of particular cognitive modalities, such as language, praxis, or visuospatial ability, is also common, but modalities are frequently disrupted secondarily as a result of impairments in attention, processing speed, or other governing mental operations. Memory is one of the most commonly affected modalities after TBI.[13] Different components of memory may be separately affected (e.g., anterograde versus retrograde, implicit versus explicit, procedural versus declarative, verbal versus nonverbal), and memory may be secondarily affected by impairments in other cognitive spheres.

The mental status examination should be approached in the same manner as other aspects of the physical examination, employing structured probes of various areas of mental functioning. A full discussion of the mental status examination merits at least chapter-length importance itself, and the reader is referred to Chapter 9 in this text and to other texts on the subject.[14] The survey of cognitive functions should include assessments of arousal, attention, memory, language, visuospatial capacity, emotional state, reasoning, executive functions, insight, and thought content. More specific probes and standardized assessment tools may be used to elaborate specific impairments in the same way the clinician might expand the evaluation of dysfunction in a particular organ system in the physical examination.

Mental Status Evaluation Based on Stage of Recovery

The nature of the mental status examination should be guided by the stage of recovery at which the patient is encountered. In the earlier stages (*coma, vegetative state, minimally conscious state*), when arousal is the overwhelming problem, the mental status examination is centered on determining the depth of unconsciousness and the nature of the patient's responses. The Glasgow Coma Scale (GCS)[15] is often employed as an assessment tool to evaluate the patient's responses to verbal, tactile, and noxious stimulation (Table 6–5). Eye opening, limb movements, and vocalizations are the scored responses. (See Chapter 3 for further discussion of the Glasgow Coma Scale.) Patients in coma achieve GCS scores up to 8: eyes not spontaneously open (eyes, ≤3 points); no localized motor responses, at best, withdrawal (motor, ≤4 points); no purposeful vocalizations (verbal, 1 point). Patients in vegetative states may score up to 9 points (eyes, 4 points for spontaneous eye opening). Patients who are emerging from unconsciousness but are not fully wakeful or responding to command or vocalizing reach GCS scores of 9 to 12. Patients who are conscious but confused have GCS scores of 13 or 14. The evaluation may be confounded by a number of factors such as a tracheotomy tube, severe periorbital swelling, or paralytic agents.

The mental status examination at this level of recovery aims to determine whether a patient's responses are reflexive and automatic or purposeful and cognitively mediated. The ability to follow commands is usually the first unequivocal sign of conscious behavior. Sometimes response to command is ambiguous because of inconsistency or unclear specificity. The transition to fully conscious behavior is not abrupt, especially in patients with more severe injuries. Responses are often erratic in patients who are emerging from unconsciousness. The examiner should assure adequate warm-up time for arousal and a reasonable interstimulus interval to avoid perseveration and fatigue. In patients who are not clearly following commands, the examiner should search for other signs of cortically mediated responses, including purposeful motor behavior such as visual tracking, localized movements toward stimuli, or manipulation of objects. Sometimes a change in frequency of a stereotyped response (especially in a patient with a limited repertoire of movements be-

cause of severe motor impairment) specified to a stimulus is the first sign of cognition (e.g., facial expression or crying in response only to photograph of patient's children). The examiner should use various manipulations of stimuli, choose the best response modalities, and observe the nature of the patient's spontaneous and reflex movements to avoid misinterpretation of purposefulness. The next step in the mental status assessment of the low arousal states is the patient's communication abilities, usually yes or no responses at first.

In the next phase of recovery (*confusional state*), when conscious behavior is established, attention and anterograde memory deficits are the main targets of assessment. The bedside mental status exam should focus on the nature of attentional disturbance by observing the patient's ability to focus, sustain, and shift attention and the level of distractibility. Tasks such as digit span forward and reverse, serial subtractions of varying difficulty, reverse spelling, recitation of months backward, and mental calculation may be used to track attentional capacity. Level of arousal is another important component of the evaluation to distinguish patients who are underaroused, slow to respond, and hypokinetic from those who are hyperarousable, with rapid escalations to agitation and restlessness. The bedside evaluation of memory should focus on the patient's orientation, anterograde loss including the presence of personal episodic memories (e.g., recall of visitors, meals, day's activities, hospital course, current events) and ability to learn new information (e.g., word lists, facts, examiner's name, figures, location of hidden objects), retrograde loss (biographical information, historical events, presidents), and semantic knowledge (basic facts and fund of knowledge). Detailed, overelaborative evaluations of these and other cognitive domains are useless at this stage because arousal and attentional disturbances limit performance in all spheres, and cognitive capacity is usually highly variable and rapidly changing.

In the postconfusional stages of recovery (*emerging independence; intellectual and social competence*), the mental status examination should characterize the extent of continuing impairments, albeit higher level, in attention and memory. It should look at function in other higher-level cognitive spheres, such as executive functions, and clarify impairments in particular modalities, such as those that may be attributed to focal damage (e.g., aphasia). It should track the patient's self-awareness and insight, particularly in the realm of judgment and safety. At this phase of recovery, more elaborate neuropsychological evaluation begins to be useful as the confounding effects caused by basic attentional deficits wane.

The bedside or office mental status exam should include evaluations of attention and concentration at progressively greater levels of complexity. Speed of processing should be assessed by timing various concentrated tasks. The patient's mental control and ability to divide attention between two tasks or two sets of stimuli might be evaluated by multistep mental calculations or performance of a simple motor task while counting backward. Patients with diffuse brain injury and focal frontal lesions may have difficulty sustaining performance, and word list generation tasks (semantic and single-letter categories) are sensitive, reliable measures.

After PTA has resolved, memory may be assessed by more difficult explicit learning tasks. The examiner may present a list of words (at least greater than the patient's auditory or digit span, e.g., 9 or more) and evaluate immediate recall over repeated trials and with delayed recall (spontaneous and cued). Nonverbal memory can be assessed by using immediate and delayed recall of figures and topographical recall of hospital landmarks. Episodic memory can be assessed by recall of the patient's recent experience or recounting of current events, pushing the patient for specific details.

The examiner should assess language with an evaluation of spontaneous output (fluency, content, grammar, paraphasias), naming, comprehension, repetition, reading, and writing. Praxis is evaluated by having the patient pantomime oral, limb, and whole-body movements to command or by imitation.

Visuospatial capacity may be assessed by having the patient draw a clock, copy designs, and bisect an array of lines. These tests may demonstrate hemispatial neglect and use of segmental strategies (such as with right hemisphere focal lesions) and poor planning (such as with diffuse and focal frontal injury).

The examiner should assess higher-level reasoning, abstract thinking, judgment, and problem solving. Interpretation of proverbs and idioms (especially those less familiar) and judgment of similarities of paired items (e.g., river and lake, eye and ear, poem and sculpture) are commonly employed tests. The examiner might also ask a patient to recount the steps of common or less familiar tasks (e.g., changing a tire, preparing scrambled eggs, planning to see a movie, managing an emergency situation such as a traffic accident or burglary).

Insight should be judged by the patient's awareness of his or her injury, disabilities, and capability of returning to premorbid activities. Patients usually recount the facts of their injuries and physical incapacities before demonstrating full awareness of cognitive deficits or inability to resume activities.

Evaluation of emotional state includes assessment of affect and mood by observation and direct questioning. Behavior and social awareness are judged by the patient's interaction during the examination and by historical information regarding the patient's premorbid personality.

ELEMENTAL NEUROLOGICAL EXAMINATION

The elemental neurological examination includes an assessment of motor and sensory capacities, traditionally divided into cranial nerves, motor function, coordination, reflexes, sensory function, gait, and stance (Table 6–6). (The reader is referred to other texts for a complete description of the elemental neurological examination.[16]) The following discussion highlights some of the common elemental neurological problems that occur in patients after TBI. Cognitive and behavioral problems are more consistent and predictable than motor and sensory problems. In general, the more severe the injury, the more likely are motor and other elemental neurological problems,[17–19] but there is not a clear proportional relationship.[20,21]

Cranial Nerves

Patients develop cranial nerve dysfunction either as a result of peripheral injury, usually related to fracture or other localized cranial nerve injury, or as a result of central injury, resulting from brain stem damage or secondarily from cerebral damage ("pseudobulbar"). The most common problems are described below and include anosmia (cranial nerve I), visual loss (cranial nerve II), ocular dysmotility (cranial nerves III, IV, and VI), facial weakness (cranial nerve VII), and hearing and vestibular dysfunction (cranial nerve VIII).[22] Cranial nerves V and IX through XII are less commonly affected directly.

Damage to the *olfactory nerve* (I) occurs in about 7 percent of patients with TBI.[22,23] The site of injury is not clear, but injury is often associated with anterior fossa basilar skull fractures or large orbital frontal contusions.[23] Although anosmia can occur with even mild injuries, the olfactory filaments are relatively protected against shear strain in the cribriform plate.[23] Recovery occurs in a third to half of patients, usually within the first 3 months, but late recoveries, up to 5 years, have been reported.[22] Evaluation should be performed by having the patient identify common smells while avoiding noxious, volatile substances that also stimulate the trigeminal (V) nerve.

Injury to the *optic nerve* (II) occurs in up to 5 percent of patients with head trauma[23] and can

TABLE 6–6. Elemental Neurologic Examination: Usual Areas of Evaluation

Cranial Nerves

1. Olfactory nerve
   - Identify common smells
2. Optic nerve
   - Pupillary response (afferent)
   - Acuity
   - Visual fields
3, 4, 6. Oculomotor, trochlear, and abducens nerves
   - Eye movements
   - Pupillary response (efferent)
   - Lid elevation
5. Trigeminal nerve
   - Facial sensation
   - Corneal response (afferent)
   - Jaw closure
7. Facial nerve
   - Facial movement and strength
   - Taste
   - Corneal response (efferent)
8. Auditory and vestibular nerve
   - Hearing low amplitude sounds, Rinne and Weber tuning fork tests
   - Nystagmus, with and without provocative maneuvers
9, 10. Glossopharyngeal and vagus nerves
   - Gag reflex, palate elevation
11. Spinal accessory nerve
   - Shoulder shrug (trapezius) and head turning (sternomastoid)
12. Hypoglossal nerve
   - Tongue protrusion

Motor evaluation

- Tone (spasticity, rigidity, hypotonia)
- Power (muscle strength testing)
- Isolated movement (quality of motor isolation and control)
- Involuntary movements (tremor, choreoathetosis, dystonic posturing)
- Coordination (heel-knee-shin and finger-nosefinger tests, rapid alternating movements)

Reflexes

- Deep tendon reflexes
- Plantar responses
- Disinhibited primitive reflexes

Gait, stance, balance

- Static balance, challenges (e.g., unilateral or tandem stance)
- Gait (base, stride, symmetry, posture), stressed gait (e.g., tandem walking)

Sensation

- Temperature, pain
- Light touch, position sense, vibration
- Romberg sign (loss of balance with eyes closed)

occur with damage to the globe, the intraorbital portion of the nerve, and the most vulnerable part, within the optic canal.[22] Injury to the intracranial portion is less common. The mechanisms are focal contusion, ischemia, and shear strain; optic nerve damage is sometimes associated with large frontal contusions. Recovery occurs in up to a third of patients.[22] Other retrochiasmal visual disturbances also occur in patients with TBI owing to focal damage or, perhaps, concentrated DAI within visual pathways or the occipital cortex. Posterior cerebral artery territory infarction after herniation is a common cause. The retrochiasmal injuries are distinguished from optic nerve injuries in that they cause corresponding visual field defects in both eyes rather than visual impairment in one eye. Evaluation of vision should include pupillary response, acuity, and visual field testing.

Injury to the *oculomotor* (III), *trochlear* (IV), or *abducens* (VI) nerves occurs in up to 4 percent of patients,[22] most frequently in the third and sixth nerves. The site of injury may be the orbit, the cavernous sinus, or an intracranial locus. The third nerve is often injured at the point it exits through the dura or may suffer compression with temporal lobe herniation. Hemorrhages in the fourth nerve where it wraps around the brain stem can sometime be observed on MRI scans.[24] The sixth nerve may be affected by raised intracranial pressures or may be damaged along with cranial nerves VII and VIII, associated with petrous bone fractures. Complete recovery of oculomotor problems is reported in about 40 percent of patients,[22] but functional recovery probably occurs in the majority of patients, most within 6 to 12 months.

Ocular motility problems also commonly result from brain stem dysfunction in the internuclear and supranuclear pathways. Deficits in upgaze, convergence, and accommodation (focusing on near objects) are frequent, probably owing to the effects of DAI on the upper midbrain. Vestibular dysfunction may also affect eye movements, causing nystagmus and skew deviation.

Neurological evaluation of ocular motility should involve tracking objects in the six cardinal positions, convergence on near targets, pursuit movements, saccades, pupillary function, and eyelid elevation. Difficulty in moving the eye inward, or upward and downward, with preserved outward movement suggests third nerve dysfunction (often with pupillary dilatation and ptosis); difficulty intorting or moving an eye down and in indicates a fourth nerve problem (often associated with compensatory head tilt to the side opposite the affected eye); difficulty moving the eye outward suggests sixth nerve dysfunction.

The *facial nerve* (VII) is vulnerable to injury along its long course through the temporal bone, which occurs with fractures in approximately 3 percent of patients with TBI.[22] This type of injury causes a peripheral pattern of facial weakness involving the upper face and eye closure, in addition to the lower face. (It is distinct from hemifacial weakness with central lesions, which usually spares the upper face.) The more proximal the lesion in the temporal bone, the more likely is ipsilateral loss of taste (chorda tympani nerve), hyperacusis (nerve to stapedius muscle), or impaired lacrimation. Prognosis for recovery of facial nerve function is favorable in most cases, unless complete transection has occurred.[23] Eye protection and lubrication are important to prevent corneal abrasion and ulceration.

Damage to the *auditory* and *vestibular nerves* (VIII) or their end organs may occur with or without temporal bone fractures. Damage at the internal auditory meatus commonly involves both the seventh and eighth cranial nerves. Labyrinthine concussion may result in auditory or vestibular symptoms. Peripheral vestibular symptoms frequently occur as a result of dislodgment of the otoliths from the utricle into the posterior semicircular canal or cupula (cupulolithiasis or canalolithiasis) or disruption of the oval or round window of cochlea (perilymph fistula). Vestibular dysfunction also occurs with central nervous system injury, usually in association with DAI and sometimes combined with peripheral vestibular injury. Central causes of hearing loss are rare. Bedside evaluation includes tests of hearing (low-amplitude sounds and Rinne and Weber tuning fork tests) and vestibular function (examining for nystagmus, with or without provocative maneuvers, such as head shaking, Hallpike-Dix posterior-lateral head tilt test). More elaborate tests such as audiometry, electronystagmography, and rotational chair testing may be necessary. Prognosis depends on the site of damage. There is usually compensatory recovery of vestibular function, using the undamaged contralateral side, even before recovery of the injured side.

Motor Disorders

A variety of motor problems, including hemiparesis, spasticity, incoordination, imbalance, dysequilibrium, gait disturbance, dysarthria, dysphagia, and movement disorders, may be observed in patients with TBI.[17,21] Patients often present with a mix of these motor deficits, particularly patients with diffuse injuries that may cause bilateral disruption of multiple motor systems. Again, motor problems are more likely with more severe injuries[17–19] as determined by lower GCS score,[17] longer coma,[19] or longer

PTA.[18] The depth of lesion[17] and signs of brain stem injury[18] are other factors predictive of more severe motor problems. Patients with more severe diffuse injuries (DAI) have more concentrated amounts of axonal loss deeper in the neuraxis (e.g., brain stem), where converging motor pathways are more likely to be involved.[25,26]

Recovery of motor functions can be quite variable[27,28] but seems to follow certain predictable functional sequences: recovery of equilibrium reactions, followed by protective reactions; rolling before sitting and standing; climbing stairs before hopping and jumping.[28] Recovery of motor function occurs over a more rapid time course than recovery of cognitive functions. For instance, of those who recover isolated movement after arm paresis, the vast majority do so by 4 months postinjury.[29]

Several patterns of motor dysfunction may occur. In patients with diffuse injuries, motor impairments are usually bilateral and often asymmetrical. Combinations of spastic paresis, incoordination, balance and gait disorders, eye motility problems, dysarthria, and dysphagia are common early in recovery.[21] Significant postural dyscontrol and spastic paresis occur in about one-third of patients with severe TBI.[17,21] Balance and gait disorders may result from disruption of one or more motor or sensory systems: vestibular, visual, proprioceptive, and postural motor responses that keep the center of body mass within defined limits.[30,31] Various forms of movement disorders may occur, although less commonly than the preceding disorders. Tremors, dystonia, myoclonus, chorea, athetosis, ballismus, tics, and parkinsonism have all been described in patients with TBI[32] (see also Chapter 30).

Aside from central motor system disturbance, motor function may be affected by abnormalities in superordinate processes and peripheral control. Patients with problems such as apraxia or akinesia may have significant motor disability, even without a specific elemental motor disturbance. Peripheral nerve injuries (e.g., brachial plexus), musculoskeletal injuries, contractures, and joint limitations (e.g., heterotopic ossification) may also limit motor functioning.

There is no single pattern of motor impairment after TBI. Mixed bilateral, multisystem deficits related to diffuse injury or secondary brain stem injury are more common than localized deficits related to primarily focal lesions. Indeed, the typical locations of focal lesions (FCC in frontal and temporal areas) usually spare motor systems.

Evaluation of motor disorders should encompass assessments of the various interrelated motor and sensory systems. The physical neurological examination includes assessments of tone, strength, and movement. Passive movement across various joints can distinguish the various disorders of tone. *Spasticity* is defined as a velocity-dependent increase in resistance to passive movement. With cerebral damage, spasticity is greatest in antigravity muscle groups, flexors of the upper extremities and extensors of the lower extremities. Head and neck position and degree of recumbency may produce significant variability of tone. *Rigidity* is an increase in passive resistance independent of velocity, and *cogwheel rigidity* occurs when rigidity is superimposed on tremor. *Paratonia* refers to the inability of a patient to voluntarily relax, often attributed to bilateral prefrontal brain damage. *Hypotonia* and *flaccidity* can be seen in early stages of central nervous system (CNS) motor paralysis, with cerebellar lesions, or with peripheral nerve injuries. Contractures may also limit range, superimposed on tone problems. The degree of contractures can sometimes be assessed by passive ranging when a patient is asleep, when most tone is eliminated, or by using temporary anesthetic nerve blocks. Muscle power and the quality of active movement can be assessed by rating the patient's active resistance and observing spontaneous and directed movements. The examiner should observe patterns of movement in the limbs, head, neck, and trunk, including the degree of flexor or extensor synergies and the patient's ability to isolate movement out of synergistic patterns. The stages of recovery from hemiplegia described by Brunnstrom[33] are useful in describing the typical evolution of tone, strength, and movement from flaccidity, through increasing tone, through synergistic movements, to waning tone and beginning isolated movement. The ability to isolate movement reflects the integrity of the primary motor cortex and cortical spinal pathways.

Coordination can be evaluated by having the patient direct limb movements at targets or along a specific path (e.g., finger to nose and heel to shin tests). Rapid alternating movements between agonists and antagonists are another useful test. Disruption of various motor and sensory systems can affect coordination, but cerebellar system damage causes characteristic dysmetria (overshooting and undershooting), dyssynergia, dysdiadochokinesia (abnormal rapid alternating movements), and intention tremor.

Peripheral nerve injury that causes motor and sensory loss commonly occurs in patients with TBI. Peripheral motor impairment can be distinguished from central motor impairment in that it causes hypotonia, hyporeflexia, and, eventually, muscle wasting. The distribution of weakness and sensory loss corresponds to the locus of nerve damage: nerve root, brachial or lumbosacral plexus, or peripheral nerve. Electromyography and nerve conduction studies may supplement the physical examination to help localize the lesion and assess degree of denervation or renervation.

Vestibular and *postural control* problems are also common. Disruption of postural control may result from damage to one or more of the neural components.[31] The neural components include sensory systems (visual, vestibular, and somatosensory), motor systems (generating ankle, hip, and step strategies), and central integrating and adaptive systems.[30,31] Patients may experience vertigo, disequilibrium, and motion sickness as a result of central or peripheral vestibular system damage.

Physical examination consists of evaluation of gait and stance, including stance with eyes open and closed (Romberg test), and more challenging tasks, such as tandem stance, unilateral stance, hopping, tandem walking, and perturbations to stance. Additionally, evaluation of eye movements, especially for spontaneous nystagmus (with fixation blocked by Fenzel lenses), provoked nystagmus (head shaking and Hallpike-Dix maneuvers), vestibular occular reflex (maintaining fixation on distant object with head oscillations), suppression of the vestibular occular reflex (fixation on patient's own thumb with whole body rotation), and smooth pursuits (observing for catch-up saccades), is helpful in evaluating the vestibular system. The assessment may be supplemented by more sophisticated laboratory tests such as rotary chair testing, which assesses the integrity of the vestibular occular reflex, and dynamic posturography,[30] which analyzes the organization of the sensory components of balance.

Swallowing and *articulation* disorders are important motor control problems in patients with TBI. They may occur separately, and dysarthria is usually more persistent than dysphagia.[34] Risk of aspiration is the main concern. Swallowing evaluation includes bedside assessment of oral motor and sensory functions, observation of swallowing and protective mechanisms (e.g., cough), direct examination of laryngeal movement, and videofluorographic barium swallow examination.[35]

◻ NEUROIMAGING IN TRAUMATIC BRAIN INJURY

The advent of CT in the 1970s revolutionized diagnosis, management, and prognostication of TBI. CT has its limitations, however, and newer neuroimaging techniques such as MRI,[36] positron emission tomography (PET),[37] and SPECT,[38] available since the 1980s, have made possible better understanding of pathophysiological mechanisms and more accurate prediction of outcome in TBI.

Contribution of Computed Tomography

Because of its wide availability, brevity of examination, and sensitivity to blood even in the early hours after injury, CT scanning is still the investigation of first choice in TBI. CT depends on the absorption of x-rays by various tissues to display anatomy and pathological alterations caused by brain injury. Beam-hardening artifacts from high-density adjacent bone and partial-volume effects can obscure superficial brain anatomy, particularly in the inferior frontal and temporal regions and in the posterior fossa, which are sites of predilection in TBI, as discussed in Chapter 2. CT is best for the timely detection of extradural and intradural blood collections that may require surgical evacuation. CT can also indirectly reveal increased intracranial pressure through obscuration of brain stem cisternae, compression of the ventricles, midline shifts, and loss of gray-white matter differentiation.

The heterogeneity of TBI and differential outcome in relation to pathophysiology has now been well established by two decades of experience with CT scanning in this population. The early CT series[39–41] verified the high incidence of CT abnormalities in severe brain injury and the correlation of clinical severity with the extent of damage demonstrated on CT. Later studies demonstrated that CT added predictive value to clinical assessment in TBI.[42–45] One early large (*n* = 1107) prospective multicenter study of severe TBI (GCS <8) further demonstrated the heterogeneity of pathophysiological mechanisms in TBI and their different implications for outcome.[46] Depending on the lesion category, mortality ranged from 9 to 74 percent (41 percent overall), and patients with good outcome ranged from 6 to 68 percent (overall 20%). For example, subdural hemorrhage with GCS of 3 to 5 had a 74 percent mortality with only 8 percent good recovery, whereas DAI with a GCS of 6 to 8 had a 9 percent mortality and 68 percent good recovery.[46] The importance of both clinical severity and type of pathology for understanding TBI outcome was further illustrated in another prospective series (*n* = 277) in which multiple unilateral or bilateral brain contusions, extracranial fluid collections with postoperative swelling, and DAI had a poorer prognosis than single contusions, extracerebral hematomas without swelling, brain swelling alone, or a normal scan.[47] Serial CT demonstrated dynamic changes after injury, for example, the appearance or enlargement of contusions (Fig. 6–2) and the development of secondary effects of injury such as mass effect and brain swelling with increased intracranial pressure (ICP).[47]

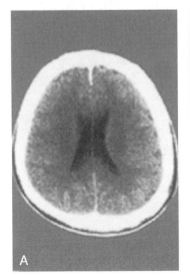 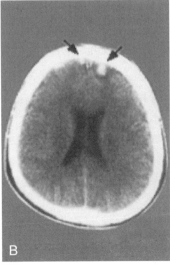 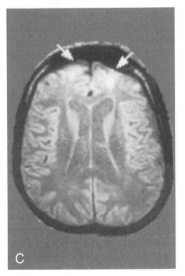

FIGURE 6–2. Evolving frontal contusions in a 42-year-old man who fainted and fractured his right parietal bone in a bathroom at work. GCS was 15, but PTA lasted 4 days. The initial CT scan was negative (*A*), and a scan at 3 days showed frontal hemorrhagic contusions (*B, black arrows*). T$_2$-weighted MRI 1 year later showed hyperintensity at the frontal poles bilaterally (*C, white arrows*). This patient has significant frontal cognitive defects and has been unable to return to any employment.

Other studies further demonstrated that CT could indirectly index increased ICP. Mortality was shown to be related to obscuration of basal cisterns on CT, particularly in patients with admission GCS between 6 and 8: Mortality was 22 percent with normal cisterns, 39 percent with compression, and 77 percent when cisterns were absent because of herniation effects.[48] In 753 consecutive patients with GCS lower than 8, effacement of cisterns carried 3 times the risk of mortality.[49]

Different classification systems have been proposed for TBI.[45–47,50] The need for multicenter studies with standardized data collection protocols, including CT analysis to study outcome in different types of injury systematically, prompted the organization of the National Traumatic Coma Data Bank.[51] Most classifications differentiate between diffuse and focal damage, as illustrated in Table 6–7, which also lists secondary effects of injury, such as territorial infarction from mass effect and herniation, and hypoxic-ischemic injury from hypotension and/or hypoxia. The usefulness of a classification system depends on its purpose—that is, whether it

is being used for acute management decisions and prediction of short-term survival or whether long-term functional and neuropsychological sequelae are the focus.[45] Although most classifications differentiate between focal and diffuse injury, the reality is that both types of insults are frequently combined in many TBI victims, and no consensus has yet been achieved for a common classification system.[52]

Focal injury includes epidural, subdural, and intracerebral hematomas and contusions. Mass effect from these lesions can lead to herniation and/or focal territorial infarction caused by compression of the brain arteries, most commonly the posterior cerebral artery. DAI can be inferred on CT from small hemorrhagic lesions at the gray-white junction of the cerebral cortex (Fig. 6–3) and in the corpus callosum (Fig. 6–4), deep nuclei, and brain stem (Fig. 6–5), depending on the severity of injury. In addition, DAI is frequently associated with diffuse brain swelling. Hypoxic injury, particularly to vulnerable medial temporal structures, can occur because of respiratory or cardiac dysfunction at the time of injury or sustained hypotension associated with shock.

TABLE 6–7. Neuroimaging and Traumatic Brain Injury Neuropathology

Neuropathology	CT/MRI Findings
Primary Effects	
Diffuse axonal injury (DAI) (shearing from acceleration-deceleration injury)	*Acute:* Diffuse swelling and/or subarachnoid and/or intraventricular hemorrhage and/or hyperintensities and/or hemorrhages in white matter, corpus callosum, brain stem. Imaging may also be negative. *Late:* Cortical atrophy and ventricular enlargement.
Focal cortical contusion or parenchymal hematoma	*Acute:* Hemorrhage/edema extending from cortical surface. *Late:* Necrosis and cavitation, hyperintense on T_1 and hypointense on T_2.
Deep cerebral hematoma	Basal ganglia or thalamic hemorrhage (caused by same mechanism as DAI, but hemorrhage is ≥ 1 cm³ acutely).
Extracerebral hematoma	Extradural or subdural blood collections.
Secondary Effects	
Hypoxic-ischemic injury	
▪ Diffuse	May see borderzone ischemic change, bilateral basal ganglia lesions, and/or hippocampal atrophy.
▪ Focal	Infarction in vascular territories or associated with mass lesions.
Herniation	Loss of perimesencephalic cisternal markings on side of mass lesion. Midline shift. Downward displacement of upper brain stem. Ischemic change in lower diencephalon. Posterior cerebral artery territory infarction.

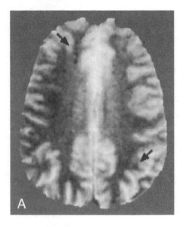
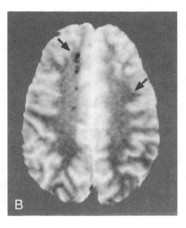

FIGURE 6–3. Hemorrhagic shear injuries appear as small black dots (*black arrows*) on two slices of this gradient echo MRI scan. This 19-year-old university student was thrown from a car and was unconscious for a few hours. Two years later, he still had problems in attention, had developed significant depression, and was unable to continue his education.

These latter injuries are less easily detectable on structural imaging and are usually inferred by clinical documentation of hypotension or hypoxia or by the persistence of neuropsychological sequelae suggestive of these additional insults. Figure 6–6 shows both of these mechanisms of secondary injury.

Despite severe injury, some TBI patients have no abnormalities on CT scanning, presumably reflecting diffuse injury for which this technique is relatively insensitive. In a series of 448 patients with GCS below 8, 70 subjects had a normal CT scan on the day of admission and 46 of these remained normal with serial scanning.[53] This number represented 25 percent of those with DAI. Although 76 percent of those with normal scans made a good recovery, 19 percent had coma persisting longer than 2 weeks with subsequent severe disability. Brain atrophy at 6 months was a common sequela, despite the initial normal CT, implying diffuse injury.[53] Delayed lesions (usually contusions) occurred in 24 patients, 9 of whom had no clinical deterioration. In summary, although an initially normal scan generally bodes well in severe TBI, evolving abnormalities may be noted if subjects are serially imaged even in the absence of clinical deterioration, and atrophy is a frequent long-term sequela.

Just as a normal CT may be found with severe TBI, abnormalities on CT scanning may accompany mild TBI (Fig. 6–7). That mild concus-

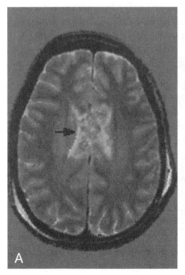
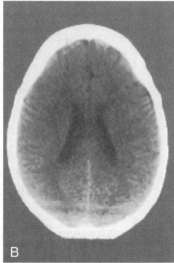
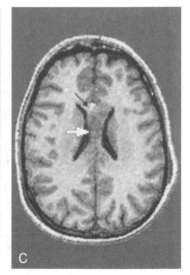

FIGURE 6–4. Severe corpus callosum injury caused by a motor vehicle accident in a 21-year-old woman. On axial MRI, the lesions are hyperintense on T_2-weighted images (*A, black arrow*) and hypointense on T_1-weighted images (*C, white arrow*). A small hemorrhage in the genu is also present (*C, small black arrow*). Note that the CT obtained the day before showed no lesions in the corpus callosum.

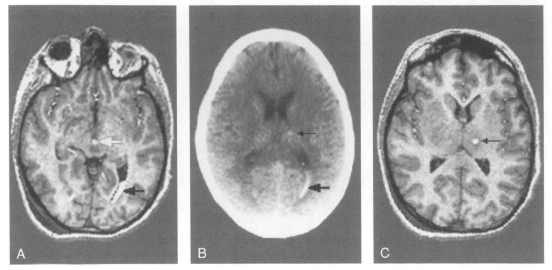

FIGURE 6–5. Findings indicative of DAI in the same 21-year-old woman depicted in Fig. 6–4. The large black arrow shows intraventricular blood on both MRI (*A*) and CT (*B*). Small, deep intraparenchymal hemorrhages are also seen in the midbrain (*A, white arrow*) and thalamus (*B* and *C, small black arrow*). Admission GCS was 4, with minimal improvement by 10 weeks.

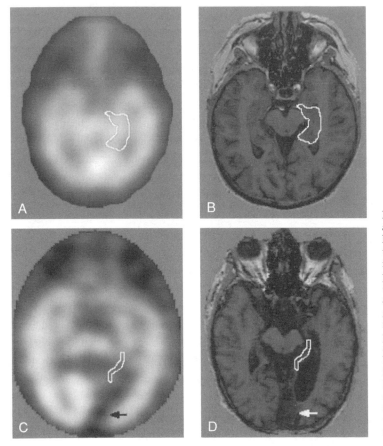

FIGURE 6–6. Coregistered SPECT and T_1-weighted MRI show the left hippocampal region as a white tracing on SPECT (*A*) and MRI (*B*) in a normal control subject compared with the SPECT (*A*) and MRI (*B*) of a TBI patient, whose severe anterograde and complete retrograde memory deficits have never resolved. Note the shrunken hippocampal formation on the right and its virtual absence on the left, both on structural and functional imaging. The patient also suffered left occipital infarction because of compression of the left posterial cerebral artery from herniation in the acute phase (*C, black arrow; D, white arrow*).

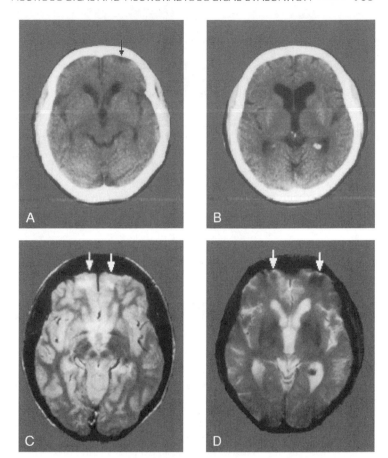

FIGURE 6–7. Possible residual of left frontal contusion is seen in *A* but not *B* of this follow-up CT in a 60-year-old lawyer who was hit by a car. She did not lose consciousness and continued to work successfully over the next 10 years, until she developed progressive memory loss, prompting the MRI scan. The T_2-weighted image (*C*) shows bilateral inferior frontal hyperintensities appearing as low signal on the gradient echo sequence (*D*), indicating that these were hemorrhagic. The minimal neuropsychological consequences of her injuries contrast with those depicted in Fig. 6–2 and demonstrate that neuroimaging must always be interpreted in the clinical context.

sion can result in DAI has been suggested in experimental animal models of trauma[54] and neuropathologically in humans.[55] In one series of 658 TBI patients who experienced amnesia or a brief loss of consciousness (>5 min) and were admitted with a GCS of 13 to 15, 18 percent showed abnormalities on CT (40% at GCS 13, 18% at GCS 14, 12% at GCS 15).[56] Twenty-one had skull fractures, 19 had hematomas, and 1 had an epidural. These authors recommend routine CT scanning, even for patients with mild brain injury.

Contribution of Magnetic Resonance Image Scanning

MRI scanning offers several advantages over CT, especially for longer-term prognostication in TBI. MRI utilizes computer processing of radiofrequency-induced excitations of protons aligned in a strong magnetic field. This technique is more sensitive to pathology than x-ray attenuation; because bone has a very low signal

on MRI, extracerebral blood collections and pathology in the posterior fossa, inferior frontal, and temporal regions are better seen. Furthermore, imaging can be conducted in all three planes without moving the patient, and the better contrast between gray and white matter reveals anatomic detail more readily. Sulci can be seen even if they are compressed by extradural collections. Small, chronic subdural hematomas can be discerned and distinguished from a hygroma (cerebrospinal fluid collection without blood). (See Gean, 1994,[36] for a comprehensive treatise, amply illustrated, on imaging of brain trauma.) Unfortunately, hemorrhage within 72 hours can sometimes be isointense on MRI and therefore difficult to detect. Thus CT continues to be the investigation of choice in the acute TBI because recognition of hemorrhage is clinically important. Within a few days, blood becomes hyperintense on T_1-weighted images and hypointense on T_2-weighted images, at which point MRI becomes more sensitive than CT in detection of intracranial blood.[57] The main disadvantages of MRI are the longer imaging times, the incompatibility of many life-support systems with the magnetic field, and lack of availability in many centers, especially outside the United States. The introduction of new, faster imaging sequences and of MRI-compatible life-support systems has overcome some of these problems, but MRI has not replaced the need for CT in acute TBI.

COMPARISON WITH COMPUTED TOMOGRAPHY

When MRI became available in the early 1980s, a number of comparison studies with MRI and CT were undertaken. As expected, CT was superior to MRI in detecting hemorrhagic lesions, such as subarachnoid and parenchymal hemorrhages in the first 72 hours[58,59]; however, MRI did detect lesions not demonstrated on CT, such as small, nonsurgical subdural and epidural hematomas and nonhemorrhagic contusions.[58,60] MRI had a clear advantage in characterizing lesions of all types in the subacute and chronic recovery period.[57] Gradient echo imaging sequences can help detect postacute hemorrhages, emphasizing magnetic susceptibility effects of old blood (hemosiderin)[61] (see Fig. 6–3).

With regard to specific lesion types, the superiority of MRI has been unequivocal for brain stem lesions (82% vs. 18%)[59,62] and deep lesions, such as petechial hemorrhages seen in patients with DAI.[57,62,63]

With regard to location and type of pathology, a large prospective series demonstrated findings consistent with DAI in 48 percent, and lesions (petechial hemorrhages) were most often in the cortical-subcortical junction (50%), the corpus callosum (21%), or corona radiata (19%).[62] Focal parenchymal lesions (contusions) were found in 44 percent, 46 percent in temporal areas, and 31 percent in frontal areas.

MRI also has an advantage in imaging the corpus callosum (see Fig. 6–4), which may be the site of small hemorrhages and also reflects the extent of white matter atrophy.[64] Cross-sectional corpus callosum area on sagittal MRI correlated with ventricular brain ratio (VBR).[64]

MAGNETIC RESONANCE IMAGING FINDINGS IN RELATION TO OTHER SEVERITY MEASURES

The number of deep lesions on MRI appears to correlate with the severity of injury (see Fig. 6–4). There was a relationship between the number of deep lesions and level of consciousness,[63] duration of unconsciousness, and PTA.[65] Even so, some patients with relatively mild injuries also had deep lesions, some involving the brain stem.[66,67] The corpus callosum cross-sectional area did not correlate with GCS or duration of unconsciousness,[64] even though it is a reflection of overall brain atrophy. The number of brain regions in which focal cortical lesions were found did correlate with PTA.[65] The conclusion from these studies was that CT is still essential for blood clot detection in acute TBI but that MRI provides much more information than CT on the location, severity, and pathophysiology of TBI in the acute and chronic phase of injury and therefore provides a better tool for determining brain-behavior correlations and for predicting clinical-neurobehavioral outcome. Research in the last several years, therefore, has turned to investigation of the clinical value of MRI in understanding neurobehavioral outcome.

MAGNETIC RESONANCE IMAGING AND NEUROPSYCHOLOGICAL OUTCOME IN TRAUMATIC BRAIN INJURY

The relationship of imaging with neuropsychological outcome has centered on two main areas: correlations of neuropsychological measures with atrophy and depth of lesion, largely indices of diffuse injury; and correlation of focal lesion location with particular neuropsychological impairments. The heterogeneity of recovery patterns may be partly explained by the variable mix of pathophysiology, yet few studies have investigated the neuropsychological outcome based on CT or MRI classification of the type of injury, and none has clearly accounted for interaction of different pathologies. In one such study, neuropsychological testing was performed on two occasions within 1 year in 30 conscious survivors who had DAI, focal damage, and/or diffuse swelling.[68] Learning difficulties were found in all types of injury, but IQ and visual-motor recovery did not differ between the groups. DAI survivors performed less well on neuropsychological testing at 6 months than the other two groups, but their deficit profile was similar to those with diffuse swelling at the 1-year follow-up.[68]

Studies that have examined the relationship between neuropsychological impairments and lesion localization have been disappointing. These results may be the result of the confound of interacting pathologies (i.e., diffuse injury), the heterogeneity of focal lesion localization (not all frontal lesions are the same), or the insensitivity of the neuropsychological measures employed for the focal lesions typically studied (heteromodal and limbic areas of the frontal and temporal lobes). Levin et al.[69] found little correlation of memory or executive functions with frontal or temporal lesion localization in 50 patients with mild to moderate TBI studied with serial MRI and neurobehavioral testing up to 3 months postinjury. Of interest in this study, 80 percent of patients with mild to moderate TBI (defined by GCS scores) had focal lesions on acute MRI (only 10% detected by acute CT), and 30 percent of these lesions did not show up on 3-month follow-up MRI. Five of these patients still had behavior deficits. (Thus, if the early scan had not been obtained, these lesions would have been missed.) There was better correlation of neurobehavioral findings and focal lesions in a group of children studied by the same group, in that frontal lesion volume predicted performance on frontal lobe tasks and other aspects of cognitive performance [70,71] Wilson et al.[52] demonstrated only weak correlations of tests of short-term visual and verbal learning with specific lesion sites. Wilson and Wyper[72] pointed out that the weak relationship between lesion localization and neuropsychological measures may result from the effects of diffuse brain damage statistically overwhelming focal effects and that the typical neurobehavioral problems after TBI—memory, attention, and executive functions—have widely distributed cerebral representations.

The relationship between measures of atrophy or depth of lesion and neuropsychological functioning has been more clearly demonstrated. One of the earliest studies on brain-behavior correlations in TBI examined the relationship between ventricular enlargement on CT obtained 30 days postinjury and neuropsychological outcome.[73] Enlargement of the ventricles expressed as a VBR occurred in 72 percent of the TBI subjects and correlated to duration of coma, IQ, and memory performance (see also Meyers et al.[74]). In a longer-term rehabilitation outcome study of severe TBI, patients with enlarged ventricles on CT had the poorest outcome.[75] One group of investigators established that a greater than 50 percent increase in VBR correlated with poor memory performance but not with IQ.[76] Ventricular enlargement from atrophy needs to be distinguished from obstructive hydrocephalus. Later onset of ventriculomegaly (e.g., 3 mo postinjury)[72] and proportionality of ventricular and sulcal enlargement support the diagnosis of atrophy. In other MRI studies, poor cognitive outcome was associated with increased VBR[52] and with deep location of lesions.[52,77] Deep lesions were regarded as indexing severe injury and, in turn, correlated with increased VBR.[52] The association of deep lesions with severity supports a centripetal model of diffuse injury (greater concentration of DAI in deeper structures with more severe injuries), but the relationship between lesion depth and functional measures is not very strong.[72]

Just when brain atrophy can be detected after TBI has been addressed in more recent studies,

which have begun to take advantage of computerized techniques for quantitative volumetric measurement of brain regions on MRI.[78] In two opportunistic single-case studies, in which subjects had a preinjury scan and then suffered TBI, it was shown that the day-of-injury CT scan could be used as a baseline index of premorbid ventricular size, thereby allowing recognition of the timing and extent of ventricular enlargement.[79,80] In one case, 50 percent ventricular dilatation had already occurred by day 15, with little change thereafter. In the other case, reimaged at day 42, ventricular enlargement was evident and remained unchanged on repeat scanning at 6 months. The time to stability in VBR is somewhat earlier than might be expected for atrophic changes to be complete. The concept that day-of-injury CT can be used as an index of premorbid ventricular size with quantitative MRI scanning in follow-up opens the way for routine quantification of brain atrophy as a clinically feasible procedure, which could be important in assessing rehabilitation potential, understanding outcome, and documenting effects of injury for medical-legal purposes.

Measures of atrophy in specific brain cortical or subcortical regions are now available and could provide better measures of severity or more precise brain-behavior correlations. For example, the cross-sectional area of the fornix is readily measurable as a fornix brain ratio (FBR) on axial MR. The lowest FBR, implying deep white matter disruptions, correlated with the poorest performance on memory measures.[81] The best predictors of the Wechsler Memory Quotient in a subsequent study were the VBR and GCS.[82]

In summary, CT scanning remains a necessary emergency maneuver in moderate to severe brain injury. It is sensitive to hematomas acutely and can demonstrate ventricular enlargement and atrophy in the longer term. MRI is more sensitive to pathology and has revealed patterns of injury that have enhanced appreciation of the heterogeneity of TBI, while demonstrating its complexities and the limitations of simplistic classifications. A simple dichotomy into focal and diffuse injury may be misleading because combinations of pathology are likely the general rule. MRI has underlined the importance of diffuse injury, which contributes to a varying degree to effects of focal injury and also complicates the search for correspondence between particular localization of injury and neuropsychological deficits. Generally, in TBI, anterior predominates over posterior damage, deeper lesions are associated with more severe injury, and bilateral damage causes more severe deficits than unilateral damage. MRI is also more able to detect secondary effects of injury, and longer-term outcome is better quantified by MRI. In particular, the extent of diffuse injury can be indexed by corpus callosum atrophy, regional brain volume measurements, and ventricular enlargement. There is a pressing need for follow-up studies to better understand the predictive value of structural imaging in the acute stage of TBI and the correlations between brain pathology and clinical neurobehavioral outcome in the chronic phase of TBI.

Contribution of Single-Photon Emission Computed Tomography Imaging

Although more sensitive than CT, standard structural MRI can reveal only macroscopic changes. Newer MR applications, including MR spectroscopy,[83] diffusion weighted MRI,[84] and MR angiography,[85] have potential to further elucidate mechanisms and location of injury, but further studies are needed. The functional impact of TBI may also be discerned, however, as changes in regional cerebral blood flow, which are usually coupled to local metabolism and neuronal function. For this reason, functional imaging techniques may have utility in detecting brain dysfunction in TBI in correlation with behavioral outcome. PET is the gold standard of functional imaging,[37] but it is an expensive procedure requiring a cyclotron, not readily available in most centers and not generally to large consecutive series. Cerebral blood flow (CBF) measurement using xenon inhalation techniques has poor spatial resolution and likewise has been confined to a few research centers.[86] Functional MRI takes advantage of differences in magnetic properties in deoxygenated versus oxygenated hemoglobin in response to activation to map regional cerebral blood flow.[87] This rapidly developing technology has great potential, especially in the chronic phase of TBI, to demonstrate online deficits in information processing.

An alternative approach has been SPECT, which utilizes conventional nuclear medicine instrumentation.[88] A disadvantage of SPECT in comparison with PET, however, is that it does not allow absolute measures of blood flow. Regional counts must be normalized to a brain region relatively free of injury, which can be problematic in TBI. PET also has superior spatial resolution, although hardware improvement (e.g., three-headed cameras for SPECT) are closing this gap. The development of SPECT was initially hampered by the lack of appropriate radiopharmaceuticals. Initially, ^{123}I-labeled amines were used in a few centers, but they were costly and had limited availability. In the late 1980s, a

[99m]T-labeled tracer, hexamethylpropyleneamineoxine (HM-PAO) or Ceretec became available for use with rotating gamma cameras available in most nuclear medicine departments. It has rapid brain uptake and is retained in cerebral structures for several hours.[88] More recently ECD (Neurolyte), an alternative tracer, has been introduced. Several published studies have described the use of SPECT in TBI,[38,89,90] and a few have also used PET.

In a few small PET series, metabolic deficits correlated with neuropsychological impairments where CT lesions did not.[91,92] The functional abnormality seen on PET tends to be larger than the structural lesion, and abnormalities can be seen that are not evident on structural imaging techniques.[93,94] In subjects who had normal MR and CT but persisting neuropsychological abnormalities, PET revealed deficits in the frontal and anterior temporal region.[95]

A number of studies have compared HM-PAO SPECT to CT and/or MRI in both the acute and chronic phase of TBI. All these studies report more lesions on SPECT than on structural imaging, and, when focal lesions are present on both types of imaging, the blood flow deficit seen on SPECT is frequently larger.[96–103] Although SPECT may be more sensitive to focal injury, it is relatively insensitive to brain swelling.[100] Furthermore, even though SPECT showed lesions not seen on CT in 39 percent in one study ($n = 15$), in 20 percent some abnormalities, including contusions and subarachnoid and subdural hemorrhages, were seen only on CT.[100]

On semiquantitative analysis of SPECT, frontal to posterior hemispheric perfusion ratios are usually lower than normal, and in one study the anterior-posterior ratio correlated to performance on six of eight neuropsychological tests, whereas VBR correlated with only two.[102] In this study, SPECT was particularly useful in minor brain injury because it revealed abnormalities not seen on CT and MRI; 43 percent of the SPECT abnormalities were seen in the frontal region (illustrated in Fig. 6–8), and 40 percent in the temporal region. VBR was normal in the minor brain injury group, whereas the anterior-posterior ratio was abnormal in both major and minor brain injury.[102] Other groups have also shown that SPECT may be particularly useful in documenting abnormality in mild brain injury. In a study of 20 subjects with initial GCS of 13 to 15, 88 percent had abnormal SPECT and 38 percent had abnormal CT.[99] Fifty percent of those with a normal CT had abnormalities on SPECT. In eight subjects with skull fractures and a normal CT, five had decreased perfusion at the site of the fracture, and two had other abnormalities. CT was superior in detecting extra-axial lesions. SPECT in this

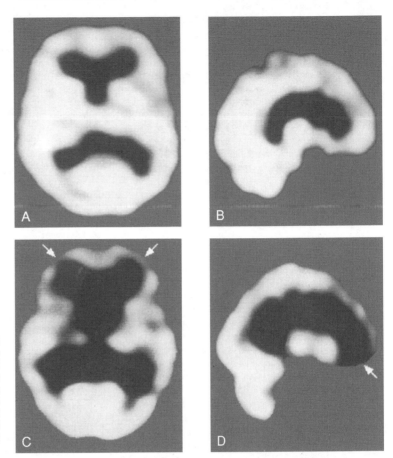

FIGURE 6–8. Axial (*A*) and sagittal (*B*) SPECT shows the pattern of uptake in a normal control subject in comparison to the scan of the lawyer with frontal contusions described in Fig. 6–7. Note the significant frontal hypoperfusion evident on the axial view bilaterally (*C*) and on the sagittal view (*D*).

series, however, correlated poorly with the severity of injury. Furthermore, 6 percent of controls in one study showed abnormalities on SPECT,[99] reflecting the nonspecific nature of this technique.

Other studies have shown that SPECT correlates better than structural imaging to neuropsychological outcome[104] and to specific neuropsychological deficits.[105] SPECT can also be useful in acute TBI for the prediction of poor outcome. For example, the degree of hypoperfusion can predict clinical deterioration in patients with hemorrhage.[106] Patients in a prolonged vegetative state had a global reduction in cerebral perfusion on SPECT, which was associated with a poor outcome.[107] However, the presence of focal deficits alone did not always predict a good outcome, and some patients with a poor outcome did not show global hypoperfusion.[107] In a study of mild (*n* = 25) and moderate (*n* = 42) TBI, 51 percent showed perfusion deficits on SPECT, primarily in the frontal and temporal regions.[103] In the patients with abnormal scans, 26 percent normalized over time, and 80 percent of these made a good recovery; in those with persisting signs and symptoms, SPECT remained abnormal in 95 per-

cent.[103] In 19 subjects in another study, the number of lesions seen and relative CBF correlated to the Glasgow Outcome Scale.[108] In a larger series of TBI patients (*n* = 36) imaged a mean of 3 years postinjury and compared with 29 controls, decreased thalamic uptake on SPECT was the best predictor of poor neuropsychological outcome.[109] The authors suggested that thalamic decrease may be an indicator of severe DAI with multiple cortical-cortical and subcortical-cortical disconnections. A study that evaluated social and emotional behavior as well as cognitive outcome revealed that social withdrawal and isolation correlated with decrease in left hemisphere flow, aggressive behavior correlated with decrease in right hemisphere flow, and disinhibition correlated with decreased flow bifrontally.[107] As in the previous study, overall psychological impairment correlated best with the thalamic flow.[107] Evidence is accumulating to suggest, therefore, that SPECT may be a useful adjunct to clinical assessment in prognostication of TBI.[89,90] Still lacking are prospective, serial studies of SPECT in TBI in correlation with both structural imaging and neurobehavioral measures.

In summary, lack of standardization in acquisition parameters and subjectivity in interpretation have led many to be skeptical about the findings on SPECT in TBI. The prognostic significance of high and low flow, if any, is unclear, and the nonspecific nature of SPECT abnormalities requires that interpretation be done in relation to structural imaging such as CT or MRI. Nevertheless, SPECT appears to be more sensitive in the detection of abnormalities in TBI than structural imaging with CT or MRI and may correlate better with neuropsychological profiles both cross-sectionally and longitudinally.

□ ELECTROPHYSIOLOGICAL EVALUATION

Electrophysiological studies that may be used in the evaluation of patients with TBI include routine electroencephalography (EEG), quantitative EEG, and evoked potentials: brain stem auditory (BAEP), visual (VEP), somatosensory (SSEP), multimodal (MEP), and event-related evoked potentials. These tools provide a window on physiological brain function and are another means of evaluating clinical functioning. For patients with TBI who are in rehabilitation, electrophysiological studies may aid in following a patient's course of recovery, especially in early stages when patients are unable to interact with the examiner. They may provide additional information for establishing prognosis and may contribute to the diagnosis of post-traumatic seizures. Electrophysiological studies are not as sensitive as functional neuroimaging in localizing the area of dysfunction.

A full discussion of electrophysiologic evaluation is beyond the scope of this chapter. The reader is referred to the review by Newlon[110] and other sources[111–121] for more information on this topic.

□ DIAGNOSIS AND PROGNOSIS

The steps outlined next are important considerations in formulating a specific neurologically based diagnosis and prognosis consistent with the system of evaluation in this chapter.

1. Diffuse Brain Injury

The first question is to establish the presence and severity of diffuse injury, principally DAI. Because there is as yet no direct in vivo biologic measure of DAI, diagnosis rests on indirect clinical criteria: a significant acceleration-deceleration mechanism (e.g., for severe DAI, motor vehicle accident or fall of >6 ft), immediate loss of consciousness (no lucid interval), and supportive neuroimaging findings (diffuse swelling, petechial hemorrhages, small subarachnoid and intraventricular hemorrhages). The neurological examination confirms the patient's stage of recovery and particular neurobehavioral profile. Severity is determined by clinical measures (e.g., GCS at acute hospital admission, duration of unconsciousness, and PTA) and neuroimaging criteria (e.g., degree of atrophy or depth of small hemorrhages),[73,122] From this, one can construct broad probabilities of outcome based on information from large series of patients. Chapter 8 includes information on how some of the variables relate to outcome. Figure 6–9 illustrates probabilities of outcome in a group of patients with DAI based on duration of unconsciousness and PTA according to a relatively nonspecific measure, the Glasgow Outcome Scale.[123] Of the three clinical variables, PTA is the best predictor of outcome, followed by duration of unconsciousness, followed by GCS.[2]

2. Focal Brain Injury

The next major question is the extent of any focal injury: focal cortical contusion, large deep cerebral hemorrhages, focal hypoxic-ischemic injury, extracerebral hematomas (subdural and epidural). Neuroimaging studies make the diagnosis. Clinical evaluation will characterize neurobehavioral syndromes that may relate to focal damage. Lesion location, size and depth, bilaterality, and secondary damage from mass effect are important variables that predict clinical recovery. Later imaging studies are essential to project longer-term effects because the residual damage may be quite different than the extent of lesion and secondary processes on early scans.

3. Secondary Injury

The next step involves questions about factors that may influence recovery and outcome expectations. Diagnosis of the extent of secondary injury is difficult because there is usually no means of direct diagnosis, unless focal ischemic changes are observed on CT or MRI. Two routinely recorded parameters may indicate a high probability of secondary hypoxic-ischemic diffuse injury: a critical drop in systemic blood pressure (i.e., <90 mm systolic) or persistent increase in intracranial pressure (>20 cm H_2O).[124]

Herniation, a shift of brain tissue out of its normal compartment when mass effect of a focal lesion is excessive, may cause local and distal secondary damage. Neuroimaging can dem-

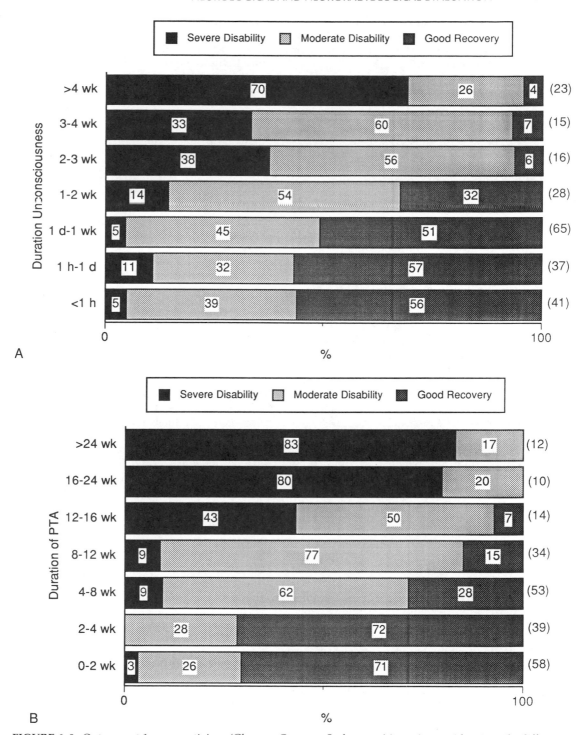

FIGURE 6–9. Outcome at 1-year postinjury (Glasgow Outcome Scale scores) in patients with primarily diffuse injury admitted to inpatient rehabilitation related to (*A*) duration of unconsciousness (*n* = 225) and (*B*) duration of PTA (*n* = 220).

onstrate these shifts, and clinical signs, such as ipsilateral pupillary dilatation from brain stem compression with temporal herniations, help make the diagnosis.

Secondary focal hypoxic-ischemic injury may result from perfusion defects of various causes (mass lesions, vasospasm). Temporal herniation, causing compression of the posterior cerebral artery, is one common cause. Neuroimaging supports the diagnosis (Fig. 6–6).

4. Late Secondary Complications

Late secondary complications may throw recovery off course and cause regression or early plateauing of recovery. Hydrocephalus resulting from obstruction in cerebrospinal fluid circulation or absorption may occur in about 4 percent of patients with severe TBI.[125] It must be distinguished from ventricular enlargement resulting from atrophy. Recognition of hydrocephalus is important because it is potentially treatable with shunting.

Other late complications include chronic extracerebral fluid collection such as chronic subdural hygromas (CSF collections) and chronic subdural hematomas, abscesses, and seizures.

5. Seizures

Events are classified as immediate, early, or late, depending on whether seizures occur within minutes, within the first week, or after the first week postinjury. Immediate seizures are frequent among children[126] and have little prognostic significance for the development of post-traumatic epilepsy. Early seizures have an incidence of about 5 percent and present a 20 to 30 percent risk of late seizures.[127,128] The risk of late post-traumatic epilepsy is much higher after a late seizure, perhaps as high as 70 percent.[129] The overall incidence of post-traumatic epilepsy is 4 to 7 percent[128] but is highly dependent on such factors as severity, age (higher in children), and type of pathology. Annegers et al.[126] graded severity based on presence of focal hemorrhage and duration of PTA or coma and reported incidence of late seizures in 11.5 percent of patients with severe injuries (contusion, hemorrhage, or PTA or coma >24 h), 1.6 percent in those with moderate injuries (skull fracture or 30 min to 24 h PTA or coma), and only 0.6 percent in those with mild injuries (<30 min coma or PTA). (Recognize that the synonymous use of coma and amnesia does mix two nonequivalent severity measures.) This study indicates a relatively trivial risk of seizures in patients with mild TBI. Penetrating injury presents a high risk of late seizures (35 to 50%[130]),

and focal hemorrhagic lesions of any sort indicate a higher risk (35%[123]). More than half of patients with post-traumatic seizures experience onset within the first year and 75 to 80 percent by the second year. At 5 years, the risk is probably back to preinjury levels, but seizure onset after 5 years is known to occur.[126,128,130]

Seizures are diagnosed mainly by history and clinical observation. Because patients may be unaware of the episode if consciousness is altered (generalized or complex-partial seizures), eyewitness observations are key to the diagnosis. EEG merely supports the clinical suspicion and is never the only diagnostic modality. The routine EEG rarely records the event itself. Interictal (between events) findings such as spikes, sharp waves, or spike wave complexes may suggest a risk of seizures, but a diagnosis of epilepsy is not based on interictal abnormalities. Likewise, a normal EEG does not rule out epilepsy. Repeated studies, sleep-deprived studies, and longer-term monitoring (inpatient video EEG or outpatient ambulatory EEG) may increase the chance of capturing a seizure or interictal abnormalities. EEG is not a good prognostic tool for predicting either risk of epilepsy or rate of remission.

Seizures are usually stereotypical and generally last from a few seconds to a few minutes. Longer seizures and status epilepticus are rare, especially in adults. Focal motor seizures are common (about 40% of late seizures), and the majority go on to secondary generalization, with loss of consciousness and possibly bilateral tonic-clonic movements.[131] Complex-partial seizures are another common form of late seizures. When consciousness is affected, there is usually a period of postictal confusion and drowsiness. Seizures sometimes arise out of sleep, and incontinence may accompany the episode. Seizures must be distinguished from other paroxysmal episodes such as syncope, transient ischemic attacks, migraine headaches, sleep disorders, transient metabolic disturbances, and pseudoseizures. (See Chapter 4 for a discussion of treatment and prophylaxis.)

6. Medical Comorbidities

Factors such as centrally acting medications (e.g., sedatives, narcotic pain medications), infections, respiratory distress syndrome, and metabolic abnormalities may slow the course of recovery, particularly in early phases. (See Chapter 4.)

7. Noninjury Factors

Age is one of the most important factors. The influence of advancing age on recovery is ap-

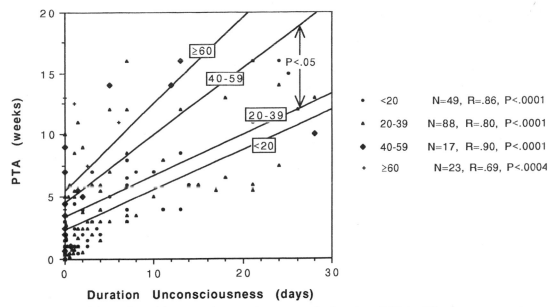

FIGURE 6–10. Relationship of duration of unconsciousness to the duration of PTA in different age groups in patients with primarily diffuse TBI. There was a significantly prolonged PTA for any given duration of unconsciousness for older patients (over age 40). (Reprinted with permission from Katz, DI, and Alexander, MP: Predicting course of recovery and outcome for patients admitted to rehabilitation. Arch Neurol 51:661, 1994. Copyright 1994, American Medical Association.)

parent as early as 40; the complex effect is apparent in higher mortality, prolonged PTA at any given severity (Fig. 6–10), slowed recovery, and worse overall outcome.[2,131,132]

Finally, the neurological diagnosis needs to be viewed in the context of personal characteristics and environmental and social influences, both premorbid and postinjury. These other noninjury influences take on more proportional influence than neurological factors in shaping recovery as time from the injury progresses.

These steps can enable construction of a neuropathologically based diagnosis that establishes injury type and severity and a clinical profile that clarifies stage of recovery and neurobehavioral syndromes. Combining this information with secondary, medical, and noninjury factors, as well as knowledge about natural history, can lead to recovery profiles projected for individual patients. This process can provide valuable information for goal setting and long-term planning.[133]

❑ CONCLUSION

In this chapter we have attempted to highlight the components of neurological, neuroradiological, and neurophysiological evaluation useful in assessing patients with TBI who are in rehabilitation. The chapter included discussions

of common neurological problems relevant to particular areas of neurological assessment. Various types of neuroradiological assessment were considered in terms of their sensitivity, specificity, and contribution to clinical assessment. Based on the neuropathological effects of TBI and the natural history of TBI, we have provided a framework with which to guide the neurological evaluation and to interpret information from the assessment. The culmination of the complete neurological evaluation should be a neurological diagnosis and prognosis that can help guide rehabilitation management. We have outlined the important elements of information that should go into formulating a diagnosis and prognosis. As pointed out, the purpose and form of neurological evaluation vary, depending on the makeup of the rehabilitation team and the roles of clinicians with neurological expertise. In any case, the challenge to the clinician performing neurological assessment is to provide information in a context that is useful for rehabilitation management and the rehabilitation team, including the patient and her or his family.

REFERENCES

1. Faden, AP, et al: The role of excitatory amino acids and NMDA receptors in traumatic brain injury. Science 244:798, 1989.

2. Katz, DI, and Alexander, MP: Predicting course of recovery and outcome for patients admitted to rehabilitation. Arch Neurol 51:661, 1994.
3. Hagen, C, Malkmus, D, and Durham, P: Levels of Cognitive Functioning. Ranchos Los Amigos Hospital, Downey, Calif, 1972.
4. Alexander, MP: Traumatic brain injury. In Benson, DF, and Blumer, D (eds): Psychiatric Aspects of Neurologic Disease. McGraw-Hill, New York, 1982, p 251.
5. Multisociety Task Force on PVS: Medical aspects of the persistent vegetative state. N Engl J Med 330:1499, 1994.
6. Ewart, J, et al: Procedural memory during post-traumatic amnesia in survivors of closed head injury: Implications for rehabilitation. Arch Neurol 46:911, 1989.
7. Geschwind, N: Late changes in the nervous system: An overview. In Stein, D, Rosen, J, and Butters, N (eds): Plasticity and Recovery of Function in the Central Nervous System. Academic Press, New York, 1974, p 467.
8. Levin, HS, Gary, HE Jr, and Eisenberg, HM: Neurobehavioral outcome one year after severe head injury: Experience of the traumatic coma data bank. J Neurosurg 73:699, 1990.
9. Levin, HS, O'Donnell, VM, and Grossman, RG: The Galveston Orientation and Amnesia Test: A practical scale to assess cognition after head injury. J Nerv Ment Dis 167:675, 1979.
10. Stuss, DT, et al: Fatigue, divided and focused attention and consistency of performance. J Neurol Neurosurg Psychiatry 52:742, 1989.
11. Shallice, T, and Burgess, PW: Deficits in strategy application following frontal lobe damage in man. Brain 114:727, 1991.
12. Ponsford, J, and Kinsella, G: Attentional deficits following closed head injury. J Clin Exp Neuropsychol 14:822, 1992.
13. Levin, HS: Memory deficit after closed head injury. J Clin Exp Neuropsychol 12:129, 1989.
14. Strub, RL, and Black FW: The Mental Status Examination in Neurology. FA Davis, Philadelphia, 1983.
15. Teasdale, G, and Jennett, B: Assessment of coma and impaired consciousness: A practical scale. Lancet 2:81, 1974.
16. Mayo Clinic and Mayo Foundation: Clinical Examinations in Neurology, ed 6. St Louis, Mosby, 1991.
17. Wober, C, et al: Posturographic measurement of body sway in survivors of severe closed head injury. Arch Phys Med Rehabil 74:1151, 1993.
18. Thomsen, IV: Late outcome of very severe blunt head trauma: A 10–15 year second follow-up. J Neurol Neurosurg Psychiatry 47:260, 1984.
19. MacPherson, V, Sullivan, SJ, and Lambert, J: Prediction of motor status 3 and 6 months post severe traumatic brain injury. Brain Inj 6:489, 1992.
20. Wong, PP, et al: Re-examining the concept of severity in traumatic brain injury. Brain Inj 8:509, 1994.
21. Katz, DI, Roberts, MB, and Alexander, MP: Motor problems after traumatic brain injury: Relationship to length of hospitalization and disability. Arch Phys Med Rehabil 76:592, 1995.
22. Keane, JR, and Baloh, RW: Post-traumatic cranial neuropathies. Neurol Clin 10:849, 1992.
23. Rovit, RL, and Murali, R: Injuries of the cranial nerves. In Cooper, PR (ed): Head Injury, ed 3. Baltimore, Williams & Wilkins, 1993.
24. Mernoff, ST, Katz, DI, and Alexander, MP: Evaluation of IV cranial nerve palsies after closed head injury. Neurology (suppl)44:313, 1994.
25. Gennarelli, TA, et al: Diffuse axonal injury and traumatic coma in the primate. Ann Neurol 12:564, 1982.
26. Blumbergs, PC, Jones, NR, and North, JB: Diffuse axonal injury in head trauma. J Neurol Neurosurg Psychiatry 52:838, 1989.
27. Cohadon, F, et al: Recovery of motor function after severe traumatic coma. Scand J Rehabil Med (suppl)17:75, 1988.

28. Swaine, BR, and Sullivan, SJ: Longitudinal profile of early motor recovery following severe traumatic brain injury. Brain Inj 10:347, 1996.
29. Katz, DI, Alexander, MP, and Klein, RB: Recovery of arm function in patients with paresis after traumatic brain injury. Arch Phys Med Rehabil 79:488, 1998.
30. Newton, RA: Balance abilities in individuals with moderate and severe traumatic brain injury. Brain Inj 9:445, 1995.
31. Shumway-Cook, A, and Olmscheid, R: A systems analysis of postural dyscontrol in traumatical brain-injured patients. J Head Trauma Rehabil 5:51, 1990.
32. Koller, WC, Wong, GF, and Lang, A: Post-traumatic movement disorders: A review. Mov Disord 4:20, 1989.
33. Brunnstrom, S: Recovery stages and evaluation procedures. In Brunnstrom, S (ed): Movement therapy in hemiplegia. Harper & Row, Philadelphia, 1966, p 34.
34. Yorkston, KM, et al: The relationship between speech and swallowing disorders in head-injured patients. J Head Trauma Rehabil 4:1, 1989.
35. Logemann, JA: Evaluation and treatment planning for the head injury patient with oral intake disorders. J Head Trauma Rehabil 4:24, 1989.
36. Gean, AD: Imaging of Head Trauma. Raven Press, New York, 1994.
37. Cherry, SR, and Phelps, ME: Imaging brain function with positron emission tomography. In Toga, AW, and Mazziotta, JC (eds): Brain Mapping: The Methods. Academic Press, Toronto, 1996, p 191.
38. Tikofsky, RS, and Van Heertum, RL: Trauma. In Van Heertum, RL, and Tikofsky, RS (eds): Cerebral SPECT Imaging. Raven Press, New York, 1995, p 171.
39. Merino-deVillasante, J, and Taveras, JM: Computerized tomography (CT) in acute head trauma. AJR Am J Roentgenol 126:765, 1976.
40. French, BN, and Dublin, AB: The value of computerized tomography in the management of 1000 consecutive head injuries. Surg Neurol 7:171, 1977.
41. Zimmerman, RA, Bilaniuk, LT, and Gennarelli, T: Computerized tomography of shear injury of the cerebral white matter. Radiology 127:393, 1978.
42. Narayan, RK, Greenberg, RP, and Miller, JD: Improved confidence of outcome prediction in severe head injury. J Neurosurg 54:751, 1984.
43. Van Dongen, KJ, Braakman, R, and Gelpke, GJ: The prognostic value of computerized tomography in comatose head injured patients. J Neurosurg 59:951, 1983.
44. Lipper, MH, Kishore, PRS, and Enas, GG: Computed tomography in the prediction of outcome in head injury. AJR Am J Roentgenol 144:483, 1985.
45. Teasdale, G, Teasdale, E, and Hadley, D: Computed tomographic and magnetic resonance imaging classification of head injury. J Neurotrauma (suppl 1)9:S249, 1992.
46. Gennarelli, TA, et al: Influence of the type of intracranial lesion on outcome from severe head injury. J Neurosurg 56:26, 1982.
47. Lobato, RD, et al: Outcome from severe head injury related to the type of intracranial lesion. J Neurosurg 59:762, 1983.
48. Toutant, SM, et al: Absent or compressed basal cisterns on first CT scan: Ominous predictors of outcome in severe head injury. J Neurosurg 61:691, 1984.
49. Eisenberg, HM, et al: Initial CT findings in 753 patients with severe head injury: A report from the NIH traumatic coma data bank. J Neurosurg 73:688, 1990.
50. Marshall, LF, et al: The diagnosis of head injury requires a classification based on computed axial tomography. J Neurotrauma (suppl 1)9:S287, 1992.
51. Marshall, LF, et al: The national traumatic coma data bank, Part 1: Design, purpose, goals, and results. J Neurosurg 59:276, 1983.
52. Wilson, JTL, et al: Early and late magnetic resonance imaging and neuropsychological outcome after head injury. J Neurol Neurosurg Psychiatry 51:391, 1988.

53. Lobato, RD, et al: Normal computerized tomography scans in severe head injury: Prognostic and clinical management implications. J Neurosurg 65:784, 1986.

54. Jane, JA, Steward, O, and Gennarelli, T: Axonal degeneration induced by experimental noninvasive minor head injury. J Neurosurg 62:96, 1985.

55. Pilz, P: Axonal injury in head injury. Acta Neurochir Suppl (Wien) 32:119, 1983.

56. Stein, SC, and Ross, SE: The value of computed tomographic scans in patients with low-risk head injuries. Neurosurgery 26:638, 1990.

57. Zimmerman, RA, et al: Head injury: Early results of comparing CT and high-field MR. AJR Am J Roentgenol 147:1215, 1986.

58. Snow, RB, et al: Comparison of magnetic resonance imaging and computed tomography in the evaluation of head injury. Neurosurgery 18:45, 1986.

59. Gentry, LR, et al: Prospective comparative study of immediate-field MR and CT in the evaluation of closed head trauma. AJR Am J Roentgenol 9:91, 1988.

60. Groswasser, Z, et al: Magnetic resonance imaging in head injured patients with normal late computed tomography scans. Surg Neurol 27:331, 1987.

61. DeRosier, C, et al: MRI and cranial traumas in the acute phase. J Neuroradiol 18:309, 1991.

62. Gentry, LR, Godersky, JC, and Thompson, B: MR imaging of head trauma: Review of the distribution and radiopathic features of traumatic lesions. AJR Am J Roentgenol 150:663, 1988.

63. Jenkins, A, et al: Brain lesions detected by magnetic resonance imaging in mild and severe head injuries. Lancet 2:445, 1986.

64. Levin, HS, et al: Corpus callosal atrophy following closed head injury: Detection with magnetic resonance imaging. J Neurosurg 73:77, 1990.

65. Wilson, JTL, et al: Post-traumatic amnesia: Still a valuable yardstick. J Neurol Neurosurg Psychiatry 56:198, 1993.

66. Wong, CW: The MRI and CT evidence of primary brain stem injury. Surg Neurol 39:37, 1993.

67. Hadley, DM, et al: Magnetic resonance imaging in acute head injury. Clin Radiol 39:131, 1988.

68. Uzzell, BP, et al: Influence of lesions detected by computerized tomography on outcome and neuropsychological recovery after severe head injury. Neurosurgery 20:396, 1987.

69. Levin, HS, et al: Serial MRI and neurobehavioural findings after mild to moderate closed head injury. J Neurol Neurosurg Psychiatry 54:255, 1992.

70. Levin, HS, et al: Cognition in relation to magnetic resonance imaging in head-injured children and adolescents. Arch Neurol 50:897, 1993.

71. Levin, HS, et al: Tower of London performance in relation to magnetic resonance imaging following closed head injury in children. Neuropsychologia 8:171, 1994.

72. Wilson, JTL, and Wyper, D: Neuroimaging and neuropsychological functioning following closed head injury: CT, MRI, and SPECT. J Head Trauma Rehabil 7(2):29, 1992.

73. Levin, HS, et al: Ventricular enlargement after closed head injury. Arch Neurol 38:623, 1981.

74. Meyers, CA, et al: Early versus late lateral ventricular enlargement following closed head injury. J Neurol Neurosurg Psychiatry 46:1092, 1983.

75. Timming, R, Orrison, WW, and Mikula, JA: Computerized tomography and rehabilitation outcome after severe head trauma. Arch Phys Med Rehabil 63:154, 1982.

76. Anderson, CV, and Bigler, ED: Ventricular dilation, cortical atrophy, and neuropsychological outcome following traumatic brain injury. Journal of Neuropsychiatry and Clinical Neurosciences 7:42, 1995.

77. Godersky, JC, et al: Magnetic resonance imaging and neurobehavioural outcome in traumatic brain injury. Acta Neurochir Suppl (Wien) 51:311, 1990.

78. Hohne, KH, and Pommert, A: Volume visualization. In Toga, AW, and Mazziotta, JC (eds): Brain Mapping: The Methods. Academic Press, Toronto, 1996, p 423.

79. Bigler, ED, et al: Degenerative changes in traumatic brain injury: Post-injury magnetic resonance identified ventricular expansion compared to pre-injury levels. Brain Res Bull 28:651, 1992.

80. Bigler, ED, et al: Day-of-injury CT as an index to pre-injury brain morphology: Degree of post-injury degenerative changes identified by CT and MR neuroimaging. Brain Inj 7:125, 1993.

81. Gale, SD, et al: Fornix degeneration and memory in traumatic brain injury. Brain Res Bull 32:343, 1993.

82. Gale, SD, et al: Nonspecific white matter degeneration following traumatic brain injury. Journal of the Neuropsychological Society 1:17, 1995.

83. Naruse, S, et al: 1H- and 31P-CSI of head injury in chronic stage. Proceedings of the Society of Magnetic Resonance in Medicine 3:1485, 1993.

84. Hanstock, CC, et al: Diffusion-weighted imaging differentiates ischemic tissue from traumatized tissue. Stroke 25:843, 1994.

85. Sklar, EML, et al: Magnetic resonance application in cerebral injury. Radiol Clin North Am 30:353, 1992.

86. Obrist, WD, et al: Cerebral blood flow and metabolism in comatose patients with acute head injury: Relationship to intracranial hypertension. J Neurosurg 61:241, 1984.

87. Cohen, MS: Rapid MRI and functional applications. In Toga, AW, and Mazziotta, JC (eds): Brain Mapping: The Methods. Academic Press, Toronto, 1996, p 223.

88. Van Heertum, RL, and Tikofsky, RS: Cerebral SPECT Imaging. Raven Press, New York, 1995.

89. Tikofsky, RS: Evaluating traumatic brain injury: Correlating perfusion patterns and function. J Nucl Med 35:227, 1994.

90. Tikofsky, RS: Predicting outcome in traumatic brain injury: What role for rCBF/SPECT. J Nucl Med 35:947, 1994.

91. Rao, N, et al: 18F positron emission computed tomography in closed head injury. Arch Phys Med Rehabil 65:780, 1984.

92. Roberts, MA, et al: Neurobehavioral dysfunction following mild traumatic brain injury in childhood: A case report with positive findings on positron emission tomography (PET). Brain Inj 9:427, 1995.

93. Langfitt, TW, et al: Computerized tomography, magnetic resonance imaging, and positron emission tomography in the study of brain trauma. J Neurosurg 64:760, 1986.

94. Tenjin, H, et al: Positron emission tomographic studies on cerebral hemodynamics in patients with cerebral contusion. Neurosurgery 26:971, 1990.

95. Ruff, RM, et al: Selected cases of poor outcome following a minor brain trauma: Comparing neuropsychological and positron emission tomography assessment. Brain Inj 8:297, 1994.

96. Abdel-Dayem, HM, et al: Changes in cerebral perfusion after acute head injury: Comparison of CT with Tc-99m HM-PAO SPECT. Radiology 165:221, 1987.

97. Reid, RH, et al: Cerebral perfusion imaging with technetium-99m HMPAO following cerebral trauma. Clin Nucl Med 15:383, 1990.

98. Gray, B, et al: Technetium-99m-HMPAO SPECT in the evaluation of patients with remote history of traumatic head injury: A comparison with x-ray computed tomography. J Nucl Med 33:52, 1992.

99. Nedd, K, et al: 99m-TC-HMPAO-SPECT of the brain in mild to moderate traumatic brain injury patients compared with CT: A prospective study. Brain Inj 7:469, 1993.

100. Roper, SN, et al: An analysis of cerebral blood flow in acute closed-head injury using technetium-99m-HM-PAO SPECT and computed tomography. J Nucl Med 32:1684, 1991.

101. Masdeu, JC, et al: Early single-photon emission computed tomography in mild head trauma. J Neuroimaging 4:177, 1994.
102. Ichise, M, et al: Technetium-99m-HMPAO SPECT, CT and MRI in the evaluation of patients with chronic traumatic brain injury: A correlation with neuropsychological performance. J Nucl Med 35:217, 1994.
103. Jacobs, A, et al: Prospective evaluation of technetium-99m-HMPAO SPECT in mild and moderate traumatic brain injury. J Nucl Med 35:942, 1994.
104. Weidmann, KD, et al: SPECT cerebral blood flow, MR imaging and neuropsychological findings in traumatic head injury. Neuropsychologia 3:267, 1989.
105. Goncalves, JM, et al: HM-PAO SPECT in head trauma. Acta Neurochir Suppl (Wien) 55:11, 1992.
106. Choksey, MS, et al: TC-HMPAO SPECT studies in traumatic intracerebral haematoma. J Neurol Neurosurg Psychiatry 54:6, 1991.
107. Oder, W, et al: Behavioral and psychosocial sequalae of severe closed head injury and regional cerebral blood flow: A SPECT study. J Neurol Neurosurg Psychiatry 55:475, 1992.
108. Newton, MR, et al: A study comparing SPECT with CT and MRI after closed head injury. J Neurol Neurosurg Psychiatry 55:92, 1992.
109. Goldenberg, G, et al: Cerebral correlates of disturbed executive function and memory in survivors of severe closed head injury: A SPECT study. J Neurol Neurosurg Psychiatry 55:362, 1992.
110. Newlon, PG: Electrophysiological monitoring in head injury. In Narayan, RK, Wilberger, JE, and Povtishock, IT (eds): Neurotrauma. McGraw-Hill, New York, 1996, pp 563–575.
111. Gutling, E, et al: EEG reactivity in the prognosis of severe head injury. Neurology 45:915, 1995.
112. Courjon, J, and Scherzer, E: Traumatic disorders. In Remond, A, Magnus, O, and Courjon, J (eds): Handbook of Electroencephalography and Clinical Neurophysiology. Elsevier, Amsterdam, 1972.
113. Hakkinen, VK, Kaukinen, S, and Heikkila, H: The correlation of EEG compressed spectral array to Glasgow Coma Scale in traumatic coma patients. Int J Clin Monit Comput 5:97, 1988.
114. Epstein, CM: Computerized EEG in the courtroom. Neurology 44:1566, 1994.
115. Hume, AL, and Cant, BR: Central somatosensory conduction after head injury. Ann Neurol 10:411, 1981.
116. Cusumano, S, et al: Assessing brain function in posttraumatic coma by means of bit-mapped SEPs, BAEPs, CT, SPECT and clinical scores: Prognostic implications. Electroencephalogr Clin Neurophysiol 84:499, 1992.
117. Keren, O, et al: Follow-up studies of somatosensory evoked potentials and auditory brainstem evoked potentials in patients with post-coma unawareness (PCU) of traumatic brain injury. Brain Inj 8:239, 1994.
118. Rappaport, M, Hall, K, and Hopkins, K: Evoked brain potentials and disability in brain-damaged patients. Arch Phys Med Rehabil 58:333, 1977.
119. Rumpl, E, et al: Central somatosensory evoked potentials in posttraumatic coma. Electroencephalogr Clin Neurophysiol 56:583, 1983.
120. Newlon, PG, Greenberg, RP, and Hyatt, MS: The dynamics of neuronal dysfunction and recovery following severe head injury assessed with serial multimodal evoked potentials. J Neurosurg 57:168, 1982.
121. Olbrich, HM, et al: Evoked potential assessment of mental function during recovery from severe head injury. Surg Neurol 26:112, 1986.
122. Levin, HS, et al: Relationship of depth of brain lesions to consciousness and outcome after closed head injury. J Neurosurg 69:861, 1988.
123. Jennett, B, and Bond, M: Assessment of outcome after severe brain damage. Lancet 1:480, 1975.
124. Marmarou, A, et al: Impact of ICP instability and hypotension on outcome in patients with severe head trauma. J Neurosurg (suppl)75:59, 1991.
125. Grosswasser, Z, et al: Incidence, CT findings and rehabilitation outcome of patients with communicating hydrocephalus following severe brain injury. Brain Inj 2:267, 1988.
126. Annegers, JF, et al: Seizures after head trauma: A population study. Neurology 30:683, 1980.
127. Jennett, B: Early traumatic epilepsy: Incidence and significance after non-missile injuries. Arch Neurol 30:394, 1974.
128. Yablon, SA: Posttraumatic seizures. Arch Phys Med Rehabil 74:983, 1993.
129. Jennett, B: Epilepsy after non-missile head injuries. Scott Med J 18:8, 1973.
130. Salazar, AM, et al: Epilepsy after penetrating head injury: I. Clinical correlates. Neurology 35:1406, 1985.
131. Jennett, B, and Teasdale, G: Management of Head Injuries. FA Davis, Philadelphia, 1981.
132. Vollmer, DG, et al: Age and outcome following traumatic head injury. The influence of advancing age. Neurology (suppl)40:276, 1991.
133. Katz, DI: Traumatic brain injury. In Mills, VM, Cassidy, JW, and Katz, DI (eds): Neurologic Rehabilitation: A Guide to Diagnosis, Prognosis and Treatment Planning. Blackwell Science, Boston, 1998.

CHAPTER 7

Physiatric Assessment in Traumatic Brain Injury

NATHAN D. ZASLER, MD, FAAPM&R, FAADEP, CIME

◻ ROLE OF THE PHYSIATRIST

There continues to be some controversy, even among physiatrists themselves, regarding the role of this medical specialty in the care of people with traumatic brain injury (TBI). In general, physiatrists are the best-suited physicians to direct brain injury rehabilitation programs not only because of the specifics of their training but also because of their functionally oriented holistic treatment approach, as opposed to the traditional disease-oriented medical model of assessment and treatment. This major philosophical difference in patient care has numerous practical ramifications that support the physiatrist as the primary care physician for people with acquired neurological disability, including problems related to traumatic brain injury.[1] In the long run, the skilled physiatrist can assist the patient, family, and society by improving the likelihood of community and vocational reentry and ultimately the overall quality of life of all those affected by what is often a catastrophic life event.[2]

There are not many physicians who are interested in and/or capable, based on either training or experience, of working within the structure of an interdisciplinary team model of care. Clinical training experience should ideally include adequate exposure to associated relevant fields such as neuropsychopharmacology, neuropsychiatry, neurology, neurosurgery, neuro-orthopedics, neuro-otology, neuro-ophthalmology, internal medicine, basic neural sciences, and neuropsychology.[3]

Deficiencies in training may result in physiatrists who are not adequately prepared to assess and therefore treat persons with TBI. Specifically, in many physical medicine and rehabilitation residency training programs, there is a general dearth of clinical rotations and experience in brain injury rehabilitation. Some residencies have neither a specific specialized program or unit for patients with TBI, in particular, traumatic brain injury (TBI), nor a physiatrist dedicated to this subspecialty area. There is currently no requirement for training in brain injury rehabilitation mandated for board certification in the United States by the American Board of Physical Medicine and Rehabilitation, a fact that may need to be looked at with greater scrutiny to augment the quality of physicians completing such training programs.

It is hoped that this chapter provides all readers—and not just specialists in physical medicine and rehabilitation—with an overview of the physiatric assessment process as germane to a variety of clinical issues, including the role of diagnostic testing, caveats regarding prognostication, differential diagnostic dilemmas, causality determination, and interactional issues with patients and their families.

◻ CLINICAL ASSESSMENT ISSUES

Nomenclature

One of the biggest problems in our field is the continued disparity in nomenclature used by physiatrists as well as by other medical specialists. A problem exists when three physicians examine the same patient and each one "labels" what is seen differently. Terms such as *coma, vegetative state,* and *persistent/permanent vegetative state* (PVS) are commonly misused, as are terms like *brain injury* and *head injury.* If even we do not know what we mean, we cannot expect others to understand what we are saying in the context of clinical assessment. We need to make a concerted effort to agree on a common nomenclature, and the place to start is obviously within our own field.[4]

Use of Outcome Measures

As rehabilitationists, we have an obligation to critically assess our interventional efficacy. If we are not using objective, valid, and reliable outcome measures that have been standardized, we are falling short of what should be a standard of care within the field for assessment of treatment responses. Understanding what measures to use and when to use them is beyond the scope of this chapter; however, it is critical to understand that each measure has inherent liabilities and benefits. An appreciation for each measure's pros and cons, sensitivity, and specificity is paramount to using outcome measures properly.[5]

Appropriately used outcome measures, preferably functionally based, can assist clinicians in multiple ways, including assessment of program or interventional efficacy, documentation of rehabilitation course and outcome, assessment of need for specific services and interventions, and adjuvant discharge or admission criteria for specific programmatic levels (see Chapter 8).

Standardization of Assessment and Treatment Protocols

At present, there are few nationally accepted protocols in our field for dealing with the scope of observed impairment and functional disability in TBI. Everyone has different ways of approaching the same clinical problems for assessment and maybe even more so from a treatment standpoint.[5] Sometimes this disparity in approach leads to the same clinical outcomes and sometimes not. Part of the problem stems from the lack of a consolidated research foundation for our field. Another component derives from the historical lack of cooperative efforts in research across providers to improve the state of the field at large. A major agenda item for brain injury rehabilitation over the next decade should be to standardize the clini-

cal assessment and care provided to survivors of TBI.[3]

Assessment Overview

Rehabilitative evaluation of this patient population should include a thorough history and physical examination to define global impairments and a good functional evaluation to determine disabilities and, as appropriate and practical, functional handicaps. The well-trained physiatrist is uniquely qualified among physician specialists to evaluate people with TBI because of their knowledge of how neurological and musculoskeletal impairments potentially affect functional capabilities. More important, the physiatrist, by training and use of a holistic approach to patient care, understands what can potentially be offered to optimize functional disability associated with such impairments.[1,3,6]

The context of the evaluation dictates, to some extent, the scope and detail of the assessment process. The examining physiatrist should understand ahead of time the purpose of the clinical evaluation, which is germane to the amount of time and scope of the assessment. The physiatrist may be asked to answer a specific referral question, such as how a person with hemiparesis secondary to brain injury can ambulate better, or be requested to perform a comprehensive impairment and disability evaluation. Without question, the source and type of evaluation requested dictate the time spent on the assessment, the areas of assessment focus, and the form and content of the report provided. A medicolegal evaluation or a workers' compensation independent medical examination (IME) is likely much broader in scope than an inpatient consultation for consideration of the patient for transfer to an acute rehabilitation program. The level of ability of the patient or examinee to participate in the evaluation and the degree of general neurological impairment also affect the degree of examination detail that the physiatrist is able to achieve. For example, a mental status exam on a patient in a low-level neurological state is more limited than the same type of exam in a high-functioning individual following a concussion, who may be able to participate in more comprehensive cognitive testing by the examining physician. To some extent, the location of the evaluation within the clinical continuum of care also dictates the type of note or report generated by the examining physiatrist. Therefore, in an inpatient setting, the consultative report on any given patient likely has much more neuromedical detail than a consultative report for an individual in a community-based transitional program.

The language of the evaluation in terms of medical terminology also varies, depending on the requesting party. In a clinical setting, medical terminology may be understandable by all who may review the evaluation or note, including nurse case managers. In the context of providing evaluations for a nonclinician such as a family member, patient, lawyer, or insurance company, the clinician must either use more common lay terms or explain technical terms within the body of the report.

Depending on the context of the evaluation, the report may need to address potentially delicate issues, including the capacity of a given examinee to drive, live independently, handle finances, or take care of children. A report may also address other issues that may have adverse effects on the examinee who is made aware of the findings or reads the report. Such issues include a diagnosis of severe psychiatric and/or behavioral disturbance or notation that the exam findings were of a nonorganic nature. Possibilities for such nonorganic presentations may include psychoemotional or psychiatric factors such as factitious disorder, somatoform disorders, and malingering. In any of these scenarios, the examining clinician may need to consider stipulating who can read the report because disclosure of the information directly to the patient or examinee may not be in his or her best interest, emotionally or otherwise. Certainly, the manner in which statements are made or couched can sometimes address such concerns wholly or at least in part.

In the context of an IME, it must be clear to the examinee at the outset of the assessment that the clinician is not there to develop a "physician-patient" rapport or convey clinical impressions. Rather, the clinician's role in this context is to provide an unbiased opinion or report to the party requesting the evaluation.

The physiatrist must also take into consideration a number of variables in the context of evaluating any person with TBI relative to how issues such as fatigue, time of day, positioning (including upright posture), medications or lack thereof (including recent general anesthesia), and intercurrent illness may affect reported symptoms and exam findings at a given evaluation as well as across time.[7]

Through experience, the physiatrist learns the frequency with which particular types of patients require long-term follow-up. Without question, this determination is made to a great extent based on the scope of neuromedical care that is being provided by the treating physiatrist for that particular patient. There are many physiatrists who espouse a primary care role for themselves for people with TBI and others with acquired or congenital disabilities. Other physiatrists, although not interested in performing a primary care role per se, do provide relatively comprehensive neuromedical and rehabilitative care, typically management of all sequelae related to the brain injury, including nonsurgical treatment of functional, neurological, and behavioral residua, which may encompass prescription and monitoring of psychotropic medications as well as anticonvulsants, performance of various therapeutic blocks for intra-articular pathology, and nerve and myofascial pain and spasticity, and more traditional physiatric interventions. Still other physiatrists see their role as confined in the strictest sense to traditional physical medicine and rehabilitation interventions. In this case, more frequent follow-up is clearly less necessary than when more comprehensive care is provided.

In the context of follow-up assessments, the physiatrist should inquire about progress and changes since the last evaluation, response to specific treatment interventions whether pharmacological or nonpharmacological, and compliance with the recommended treatment regimen. If the patient is in active rehabilitation, the physiatrist should review therapy and neuropsychological progress notes to determine specific areas of ongoing functional difficulty. Corroborative information from sources other than the patient, particularly if patient insight may be suboptimal, should be sought, including family, treatment team, and employer, as applicable. As medically indicated, follow-up laboratory work should be ordered to monitor drug compliance, rule out drug-induced side effects, and determine therapeutic thresholds relative to the clinical symptoms being treated.

When declines in functional status are noted by the examiner or reported by the family or patient, the physiatrist should assess the etiology of the observed decline. Neurological complications to consider in such a context include post-traumatic epilepsy, communicating hydrocephalus, late extra-axial collections, and late-onset movement disorders. Affective issues including neuropsychiatric sequelae of TBI and secondary psychoemotional responses, particularly depression, must also be considered when a patient presents with unexpected functional decline following brain injury. Musculoskeletal and peripheral neurological complications of chronic physical impairments should also be kept in mind as sources of late functional decline. Certainly, the physiatrist should also be aware of neurological, medical, and psychoemotional issues that are not related to TBI that may compound or complicate existing TBI-related disability. The treating physiatrist who concludes that the problem is outside his or her purview of expertise and/or experience is professionally obliged to refer the patient to an appropriate medical specialist for further evaluation and treatment.

Access to subspecialists such as neuro-otologists, neuro-ophthalmologists, and neuropsychiatrists may be critical in patient diagnosis and treatment. The primary treating physician must have a "subspeciality" knowledge base and sufficient breadth of clinical experience in dealing with this patient population to truly optimize patient care. Ideally, a continuum of clinical services, both neuromedical and rehabilitative, should be available.

History

Historical information should include accident circumstances; presence of acute alteration in consciousness (dazed versus loss of consciousness); pressure and duration of coma, vegetative state, and retrograde and anterograde amnesia; blood alcohol level and drug screen (if available); and initial Glasgow Coma Scale score. Additionally, any other information that may have prognostic significance should be reviewed, including early intracranial pressures, presence of early hypoxemia or hypotension, and early seizures.

Of additional significance is any information pertaining to the initial evaluation, including neurological status and any neurodiagnostic information such as brain computed tomography (CT) or magnetic resonance imaging (MRI), evoked potentials, and electroencephalograms. Nonneurological related diagnostics are also important in the review process, in part to exclude occult injuries, and might include cervical spine films, skull films, extremity x-rays, chest x-rays, and electromyographic studies.[4,5]

Any pertinent preinjury information should be elicited that may negatively affect rehabilitation potential, including prior psychological and/or psychiatric problems, history of learning disability, prior substance abuse, criminal record, and any history of prior loss of consciousness or traumatic brain injury. An adequate history should also delve into such issues as the person's developmental history; hand, eye, and foot dominance; educational history and performance, including evidence of learning disability or attention deficit disorder; military service; vocational history; legal record, including prior arrests and litigation, as applicable; cultural and language background; religious and sexual preferences; and marital history.

The patient's past medical history should be thoroughly explored, including major hospitalizations and surgeries, prior health problems including any neurological symptoms such as headache and dizziness as relevant to current symptoms, and prior mental health treatment and/or diagnoses. It is also paramount to inquire about current and recent life stressors, both before and after TBI, such as deaths in the family, marital discord or divorce, financial problems, academic failure, and/or vocational difficulties, among other possibilities.[5,8]

Family history should be elicited, particularly as germane to neurological and/or psychiatric problems, as well as alcoholism and inherited family disorders. The health status of first-degree relatives, their age of death, and their cause of death should all be explored.

Physical Examination

Comprehensive assessment should include a physical examination with particular focus on neurological and musculoskeletal systems. Further testing, including referral for neuropsychological examination, therapy evaluations, neurodiagnostic workup, and/or functional evaluation, can be done as needed once the initial assessment is complete.

The physical exam should include a thorough general assessment of all relevant body systems. The neurological evaluation should be particularly thorough, given the emphasis on brain injury related impairments and their importance in understanding the patient's present status and functional prognosis. The cranial nerves should be evaluated systematically, 1 through 12. Given the frequency of cranial nerve injuries in TBI, clinicians should be familiar with in-depth assessment techniques of each nerve's function.

Deep tendon reflexes including evaluation of any pathological reflexes suggesting upper motor neuron dysfunction should be conducted. So-called frontal release signs and soft signs (e.g., palmomental reflexes, glabellar reflex, jaw jerk and snout), tests of presumptive frontal lobe status such as maneuvers for motor praxis (fist-side of palm-palm; also called the *Mandrake maneuver*), frontal motor sequencing tasks involving bilateral motor coordination activities, and such exams as the Luria suppression test can also be included.

Sensory evaluation should ideally encompass ability to perceive light touch, temperature, proprioception, vibration, pain, and visual stimuli, the last to confrontation and visual threat. Tests of parietal sensory function such as tactile gnosis, graphesthesia, and testing for extinction to simultaneous stimulation should also be included as part of the sensory testing battery.

Cerebellar testing should consist of assessment for nystagmus, dysmetria, dysdiadochokinesia, ataxia, check, and rebound. The Romberg exam, as well as Sharpened Romberg (one foot in front of the other, thereby further narrowing the base of support), should be done, if the patient can stand unassisted, to assess balance capabilities. The Romberg exam was originally designed to assess proprioceptive impairment caused by posterior column dysfunction but can be used to detect deficits in the vestibular and cerebellar systems as well, as related to balance function. Gait should always be assessed if possible, as should functional mobility skills in general, both with and without assistive devices.

The motor examination should assess muscle strength, tone, presence of spasticity, limitations in range of motion caused by tone or contracture (which adversely affect ability to rate motor strength), motor activity level, abnormal posturing or movements, and motor control.[9]

Cognitive-linguistic function should ideally be evaluated in a comprehensive manner. Standardized assessment tools such as the Folstein Mini–Mental State Exam (MMSE) are acceptable screening techniques; however, the limitations of such testing must be acknowledged by the examining clinician. Such tests as the MMSE should not substitute for a more comprehensive assessment, particularly of patients with milder neurological impairment. Level of consciousness should be assessed, as well as attention, vigilance, comprehension (verbal and written), expression (verbal and written), prosody (expressive and receptive), memory (verbal and visual), orientation, learning, constructional abilities, mathematical skills, concept formation, and abstract thought processes. Related cortical functions should be assessed as part and parcel of a thorough neurobehavioral exam, including praxis (e.g., ideomotor and ideational), right-left orientation, gnostic functions (e.g., finger, stereognosis, and visual), topographical orientation, perseveration, denial, and neglect.

The examining physiatrist should have an intimate knowledge of neurobehavioral syndromes commonly encountered after acquired brain injury, including orbitofrontal, dorsolateral frontal, anterior bitemporal (Klüver-Bucy syndrome), limbic syndromes, and temporolimbic syndromes such as predicament irrelevant anxiety, temporolimbic epilepsy (TLE), and episodic dyscontrol. Affect and mood should be fully described as part of the behavioral assessment, which should also include inquiry and/or observation of neurovegetative symptoms, homicidal or suicidal ideation, disordered thought (e.g., paranoia, delusions, hallucinations), pressured speech, tangentiality, denial of deficit, and circumlocution.[10,11] One should also be aware in the assessment context of the array of psychoemotional sequelae that may follow trauma, including post-traumatic stress disorder, acute stress reactions, dissociative reactions, acute psychoses, depression, and adjustment disorder, to name a few. Psychological problems associated with non–central nervous system injuries seen concurrently with TBI, such as panic attacks, anxiety disorders, and agoraphobia associated with vestibulopathy, must also be well understood by the assessing physiatrist.

Concurrent administration of psychological testing in the form of personality inventories such as the Minnesota Multiphasic Personality Inventory can be very helpful in more fully appreciating the scope and etiology of claimed impairment and functional disability. One cannot, however, apply traditional psychiatric interpretations to such psychological testing in this patient population. Minimally, the physiatrist should refer for appropriate neuropsychological and/or psychological testing to assist, when clinically indicated, with appropriate apportionment of clinical symptoms to neurological versus nonneurological factors.

Other Assessment Issues

It is critical for the physiatrist to be familiar with the associated musculoskeletal and "peripheral" neurological (both somatic and autonomic) sequelae of cranial (head) trauma, as well as cervical spine flexion/extension injuries—so-called whiplash—to adequately diagnose and treat people with traumatic brain injury.[12] Adequate and timely recognition of myofascial pain disorders related to traumatic injury to the neck or cranium is critical in this patient population because of the array of symptoms (both somatic and autonomic) that can be related to referred pain from trigger points in the facial, cranial, cervical, and upper back musculature.[13] The differentiation of cervical and cranial trauma sequelae from true brain injury sequelae is critical in proper diagnosis and treatment of injury-related problems. Many so-called postconcussional symptoms purportedly secondary to brain injury may actually be related to injury to the head or neck. Clinicians need to understand that after any significant physical trauma, particularly motor vehicle accidents and falls, an individual may have symptoms related to "whiplash" (cervical acceleration-deceleration [CAD] injury), head or cranial trauma (structures outside the brain), and/or brain injury.[12,14–16] Differentiation of the underlying etiology of reported symptoms is critical in assessing causality and apportionment, determining the appropriate treatment, enabling accurate impairment rating, and facilitating prognostication.

Many different factors must be considered to assess an examinee in a holistic fashion. When it

---

TABLE 7–1. Comprehensive Assessment of Acquired Brain Injury

History

Accident-related facts
Initial neurological presentation
Preinjury information
    Past medical and surgical history
    Substance abuse
    Developmental history
    Educational history
    Military and legal record
    Vocational history
    Psychosocial history
    Life stressors
Family history

Physical

Comprehensive when possible, with primary
    focus the neuromusculoskeletal systems
Neurological
    Cranial nerves I–XII
    Deep tendon and pathological reflexes
    Sensory exam
    Cerebellar exam
    Motor exam
    Cognitive linguistic exam
    Behavioral assessment
    Consideration of psychoemotional testing
    Consideration of dissimulation testing
Musculoskeletal
    Head
    Face and temporomandibular joints
    Extremities
    Axial structures
        Neck
        Back
        Pelvis
        Chest/thorax

---

comes to cognitive functioning, there is still a lot that is not well understood relative to the impact of conditions such as depression, pain, sleep disturbance, anxiety, post-traumatic stress disorder (PTSD), and vestibular (as well as other sensory) dysfunction on neuropsychological testing. It is therefore critical for the treating or examining physiatrist to look critically at all testing, including neuropsychological evaluation(s), to determine if there is evidence to support any contention of cognitive impairment on the basis of TBI or, if the cognitive dysfunction noted is as a result of other factors, in part or total (Table 7–1).

□ ROLE OF DIAGNOSTIC EXAMS IN ASSESSMENT

For neurodiagnostic testing, static and functional imaging (single-photon emission computed tomography [SPECT] and positron emission to-

mography [PET]), electrographic monitoring via electroencephalography (EEG, with or without compressed spectral analysis), evoked potentials including but not limited to brain stem auditory evoked responses (BAERs) and cognitive evoked potentials (so-called P-300s), quantitative EEG, electronystagmography with calorics, posturographic evaluation, polysomnography, and olfactory-gustatory evaluation may all provide useful clinical and medicolegal information in this patient population.

Clinicians should be aware of the anticipated neurodiagnostic findings in patients who have had mild forms of TBI. For example, the vast majority of static imaging tests including brain MRI and CT are normal (whether performed early or late), as are the majority of standard electrophysiological measures such as EEG, in patients with mild TBI. Newer techniques including but not limited to quantitative EEG (QEEG), magnetic source imaging (MSI), and functional imaging via such modalities as SPECT and functional MRI hold promise of providing more objective evidence of brain dysfunction in people with TBI[15] (see Chapter 6). At the same time, however, it must be acknowledged that tests such as QEEG and functional imaging are not generally diagnostic—that is, pathognomonic—of traumatic brain injury and can be abnormal in association with a variety of different conditions such as depression, post-traumatic stress disorder, alcoholism, and dementia.

A variety of other tests—including balance assessment via posturography, electronystagmography, chemosensory evaluation, and audiologic evaluation—may assist in the differentiation between brain and nonbrain impairments. The discretionary use of special procedures—such as differential blocks for pain, amytal interviews for suspected conversion disorders, and manual medicine techniques—should also be considered when appropos.

□ PROGNOSTICATION ISSUES IN ASSESSMENT

There are few clinical conditions that follow TBI for which the prognosis is 100 percent certain early after the initial insult or, for that matter, within the first 1 to 2 years postinjury. Clinicians must remain aware of this fact and take it into consideration when they talk with patients and families. As rehabilitation physicians, we are often asked to make prognostic statements regarding patients after traumatic brain injury. Three main groups of factors can be used to aid in the overall postinjury prognostication of this patient population: preinjury, injury, and postinjury parameters. A significant amount of literature deals with acute injury and the prognostic implications of clinical and laboratory parameters,[17] but little methodologically sound information is available that does adequate justice to the role of preinjury and postinjury factors in the prognosis of either neurological or functional outcome.

Preinjury Parameters

Preinjury parameters that must be considered in analyzing a patient's prognosis include psychosocial background, history of learning disability, prior psychological and/or psychiatric problems, prior history of substance abuse, prior brain injury (regardless of etiology), and developmental history.[18,19] Available data support the conclusion that people with higher preinjury levels of function have better functional outcomes after TBI than individuals with suboptimal preinjury psychosocial and/or intellectual status. Factors such as the amount of neural reserve play at least some part, as yet poorly quantified, in determining how well an individual will recover following TBI. People with any significant prior injury may find an otherwise trivial neurological insult much more devastating than they would have, had they not had such a history. Research literature also supports the general contention that patients who are younger typically have a better outcome than patients who are older, both neurologically and functionally, regardless of injury severity, although this relationship does not appear to be linear.[20]

Injury Parameters

In the acute care setting, clinical parameters can be analyzed separately as well as multifactorially to assess both neurological and functional outcome prognosis. The best-known scale is probably the Glasgow Coma Scale (GCS) score developed by Jennett and Teasdale.[21] The scale basically provides clinicians with a standardized brief neurological assessment tool for use in the acute care setting. The GCS score has been shown to be highly correlated with acute morbidity and mortality, although not as strongly correlated with long-term functional outcome. Three clinical parameters—best motor response, verbal response, and visual response—make up the total GCS score, which ranges from 3 to 15. The scores are differentially weighted, with eye opening ranging from 1 to 4, best verbal response from 1 to 5, and best motor response from 1 to 6. Total GCS scores between 3 and 8 define severe neurological insult, scores between 9 and 12 are moderate, and

scores between 13 and 15 are mild. Although each of the three variables on the GCS holds prognostic utility in and of itself, the motor score has been found to be the most sensitive of the three measures relative to long-term outcome. The predictive validity, specificity, and sensitivity increase significantly when all three parameters are assessed conjointly. Variations of the GCS scores, such as the Glasgow-Liege Scale, allow more sensitive prediction of outcome by taking into consideration clinical evidence of brain stem dysfunction.[22]

Clinical findings that are useful in prognosticating outcome in the early setting include oculocephalic and oculovestibular reflex abnormalities, which may indicate significant brain stem damage. Longer durations of coma and posttraumatic amnesia have also been associated with poorer neurological and functional outcomes. Advances in neuroimaging have enabled correlations to be made between early static imaging, as well as functional imaging, and outcome. Electrophysiological assessment via multimodal evoked potentials (including visual evoked responses, auditory brain stem responses, and somatosensory evoked responses) and a variety of electroencephalographic modalities such as compressed spectral analysis and quantitative EEG have also been correlated either singly or in multifactorial analysis of outcome prognosis. A variety of cerebrospinal fluid markers including creatine kinase and lactate dehydrogenase have also been studied relative to their correlation with the severity of central neurological damage. Cerebrospinal fluid neurotransmitter and neurotransmitter metabolite levels have also been studied relative to their relation with acute neurological morbidity and mortality; levels tend to have a direct correlation with a higher degree of neurological morbidity.

Acute medical variables that have been associated with a worse outcome include mass lesions on imaging, protracted elevated intracranial pressure beyond 40 mmHg, and cardiopulmonary complications.[23] Concurrent hypoxic-ischemic injury, whether internal or external, must also be considered as a comorbidity that is associated with poorer short- and long-term neurological and functional prognosis. Hypoxic-ischemic insult may be focal or diffuse. The focal variety is generally the result of infarction of a vascular territory, quite commonly in the distribution of the posterior cerebral artery as a result of transtentorial temporal lobe herniation. Diffuse hypoxic insult, like diffuse axonal injury (DAI) as a result of trauma, has a predilection for damaging certain areas more so than others, including the medial temporal lobe structures (hippocampi), basal ganglia, and Purkinje fibers of the cerebellum. When very severe, hypoxic insult may result in diffuse cortical neuronal loss. Ischemic insult may also result in so-called watershed infarctions in parenchymal areas between major arterial vascular territories.[24]

Postinjury Parameters

Numerous studies have attempted to provide clinicians with information to aid them in prognosticating outcome and morbidity in the subacute and chronic phases after TBI. Once a patient has reached the rehabilitation phase of care, many clinicians may not be as in tune as they should be to specific clinical findings and/or functional impediments and their prognostic significance. The longer the duration of the vegetative state, the greater the likelihood that the individual will remain vegetative, all other things being equal. In patients who are minimally conscious, some researchers have correlated the presence of communicating hydrocephalus and central dysautonomia with poorer neurological and functional outcomes.[25] Agitation during the recovery phase has been theorized to be correlated with better than worse functional outcomes in comparison with psychomotorically slow or absent behavior. Anosognosia or denial of deficit can be a troublesome neurobehavioral sequela of TBI because of safety implications and the patient's inability to appreciate the need for further rehabilitative interventions. Lower extremity flexion synergy patterns are typically considered a poor prognostic sign for functional ambulation. Significant behavioral problems tend to indicate a poorer prognosis for successful independent community reentry. Further research is obviously necessary to clarify which specific impairments are poor prognostic indicators for specific functional goals and abilities (Table 7–2).

A physiatrist may be asked to make prognoses regarding a number of different issues, including impairments and disability related to the functional realms of cognition, behavior, and/or physical functioning (e.g., walking, driving, returning to competitive employment). Certainly, one may be asked to comment on the prognosis for persistent somatic complaints such as headache, dizziness, tinnitus, hearing loss, and alterations in taste or smell, among other subjective patient complaints. Other areas of potential commentary regarding prognoses include future medical complications and need for neuromedical as well as rehabilitative care as related to the TBI.

The last major area for physiatrist prognostication is life expectancy. There are generally no formulas per se to calculate life expectancy, and these determinations are based on an

---

TABLE 7–2. Prognostication in Acquired Brain Injury

Preinjury parameters

Psychosocial background
History of learning disability
Prior acquired brain injury
History of substance abuse
Developmental delay
Poor preinjury intellectual status
Low neural reserve
Age (younger generally better)

Injury parameters

Glasgow Coma Scale
Brain stem abnormalities
Coma duration
Duration of post-traumatic amnesia
Static imaging findings
Evoked potential data using MMEPs
Compressed spectral analysis EEG
Cerebrospinal fluid markers (e.g., creatine kinase, neurotransmitter metabolites, lactate dehydrogenase)
Elevated intracranial pressure
Concurrent hypoxic-ischemic injury

Postinjury parameters

Rate of neurological recovery
Neuromedical morbidity factors
Agitation/akathisia
Anosognosia
Pathological tone and flexion synergy patterns
Neurobehavioral dysfunction
Persistent somatic complaints in postconcussion disorder

---

analysis of morbidity factors and clinician experience with the particular type of patient. Literature on life expectancy in specific populations (e.g., vegetative state and post-traumatic epilepsy) should be interpreted with caution relative to its utility in determining case-specific life expectancies. Additionally, there are multiple concerns regarding methodological issues germane to statistical analysis, sample size limitations, and significant covariables that may not have been adequately factored into the overall data analysis with many of these studies.

One of the biggest problems in our field is the disparate nature of prognoses that are provided across medical disciplines to patients, families, case managers, other health care professionals, and insurance companies. There are various reasons for this problem. Surprising or not, many clinicians do not have an adequate understanding of the range of potential neurological or functional outcomes, and many do not have an adequate grasp of the historical and current literature pertaining to outcome predictors, both early and late. Yet, a large body of literature provides clinicians with guidelines for prognostication on a multitude of clinical issues, ranging from early mortality and morbidity to long-term functional outcome.

Another factor that sometimes negatively affects early predictions, particularly on the part of nonrehabilitation physicians, is that many, if not most, of these professionals never follow survivors of brain injury long term. They therefore have little perception of what happens either neurologically or functionally 1, 5, 10, or more years postinjury.

Ultimately, prognoses should be given when requested but couched in a philosophy of "realistic but optimistic" appraisal. In general, terms like *never* and *always* should be avoided, as there are seldom absolutes relative to predictive validity in our field. Instead, as the "prognosticating professionals," we should strive for presenting a range of outcomes, from the worst potential scenario to the best, with the most likely somewhere in the middle of that range. Prognoses must be made with specific impairments in mind. Each impairment typically has a different prognosis relative to time till maximal medical improvement (MMI).[6] Posttraumatic epilepsy has a very different prognosis than other potential neurological impairments following TBI, such as anosmia (smell loss), tremor, aphasia, or vascular headache. Functional prognoses must be considered separately from neurological prognoses. The presence of neurological impairment after TBI does not by any means rule out the possibility of full functional reentry into community, vocational, and avocational roles. Similarly, there are patients who are significantly disabled who have little demonstrable neurological impairment. In the latter cases, keep in mind unrelated conditions, including preexisting psychiatric problems, malingering, substance abuse, conversion disorders (or other somatoform disorders), and catastrophic emotional responses to injury. In general, negative prognostic factors for TBI include older age, poor preinjury psychoemotional adjustment, low preinjury intellectual status, preinjury significant substance abuse, and prior brain injury.[14,26] Generally, one should not make final neuromedical or functional prognoses in patients with established TBI until *at least* 18 to 24 months postinjury, if not longer in certain cases, given the experience of monitoring long-term outcome in this patient population. In patients with more severe injury and significant diffuse brain injury, ongoing neurological improvements can be seen well beyond 2 years postinjury.

Professionals should realize that it is acceptable to say we do not know exactly how well patients are going to do relative to their functional recovery—specifically, whether they will ever talk or walk again, or whether they will always have severe behavioral problems, as just a few examples.

☐ DIFFERENTIAL DIAGNOSTIC ISSUES IN PHYSIATRIC ASSESSMENT

Physiatrists should remain aware of the potential for secondary gain, malingering, chronic pain, and preinjury and postinjury psychological and psychiatric disorders to affect subjective symptoms and/or the recovery course. Clinicians should be aware that the majority of symptomatic patients following "concussions" are *not* malingerers and do have some sort of legitimate injury—but not necessarily TBI.[27] Careful scrutiny of all cases to assess for any contributing factors, conscious as well as unconscious, and methodical neuromedical assessment are highly recommended to differentiate sequelae secondary to brain injury from cranial/cranial adnexal and cervical trauma impairments.[27-30] Evaluating professionals often tend to overdiagnose mild TBI (MTBI) based on "abnormal" neuropsychological testing and/or nonspecific somatic complaints that are not necessarily pathognomonic of brain injury. Often the extent of secondary psychoemotional factors that may not necessarily be causally related to the accident in question are not adequately appreciated by the treating clinician. Finally, assessments for dissimulation (i.e., malingering, a conscious effort to appear bad) are grossly lacking in most physician and neuropsychological assessments of this patient population.[27,31,32] Unfortunately, the science and art of differential diagnosis often seem to be missing from the TBI and particularly the MTBI evaluation process.

Response styles need to be considered in the assessment of the veracity of examinee and claimant reports. Response styles can include malingering, defensiveness, irrelevant responding, random responding, honest responding, and hybrid responding (a combination of the aforementioned response variants). Examinees may present themselves as worse off than they actually are. This type of behavior is termed *dissimulation.* When patients present themselves in a better light than they actually are, then the term *simulation behavior* is used.[31]

The clinician must monitor a variety of response patterns, including whether there is resistance to assessment, violation of testing rules, explaining away of success, or admission of cue perception. Physicians must be familiar with exam strategies designed to evaluate nonorganic musculoskeletal and neurological disorders, including special bedside physical exam techniques and cognitive as well as physical "malingering tests."

Hoover's test may be used to garner further information about the organic basis of lower extremity weakness. Patchy sensory loss or sensory loss in a nondermatomal distribution, such as a midline sensory demarcation, generally implies nonorganicity. Physiatrists should remain aware of sensory complaints secondary to referred myofascial pain, which present with nondermatomal pain complaint patterns. People with feigned or nonorganic gait disturbances are best evaluated by requesting that they walk backward or sideways. Nonpronator drift in the absence of other findings consistent with upper motor neuron dysfunction, such as asymmetric deep tendon reflexes with hyperreflexia on the involved side, must be interpreted as suggesting proximal shoulder muscle weakness, malingering behavior, or a conversional symptom.[33]

A number of bedside tests can be given as screens of cognitive malingering or dissimulation behavior. These tests should not be used as definitive measures of malingering; rather, they should increase the examiner's index of suspicion regarding the presence of dissimulation behavior. Some of the bedside assessment strategies for cognitive dissimulation include the Rey Fifteen-Item Memory Test, the Rey Dot-Counting Test, the Portland Digit Recognition Test, and the Hiscock Forced Choice Test.[31] The MMPI also has validity measures that may be of assistance in garnering further information regarding patient response bias, consistency, and veracity. Some of the MMPI measures used for this purpose include the L, K, and F scales, Wiener Harmon Subtle-Obvious Scales, Gough Dissimulation Scale, Lachar and Wrobel Critical Items, TRIN and VRIN scales, and the Positive Malingering Scale[31,32] (see Chapter 9).

The only two ways to definitively know that people are malingering are for them to tell the examiner that they are faking or for the examiner to observe them doing something they previously said they could not (e.g., examinees who ambulate with significant impairment in your office but then walk to their cars without the previously noted impairments).

Evaluating clinicians should be familiar with factitious disorder, malingering, somatoform disorders (conversion disorders including nonepileptic seizures [pseudoseizures], somatoform pain disorder, somatization disorder, and undifferentiated somatoform disorder), and body dysmorphic disorder.[33,34] Factitious disorder involves the voluntary production of psychological and/or physical symptoms when the only reinforcer is the assumption of the "patient role"

without other identifiable secondary gain issues.[34] The presence of secondary gain issues, such as a legal settlement, avoidance of work or incarceration, or additional attention from family or spouse, distinguishes between factitious disorder and malingering.[35]

A conversion disorder is a disturbance suggesting a physical, typically neurological, disorder, such as hemiparesis or a visual field cut that is psychoemotionally based. If temporally related to an accident or other environmental stressor, a conversion disorder may be fully apportioned to the injury in question. A thorough history and physical examination, possibly augmented by an amytal interview, should allow an astute clinician to make a diagnosis of a conversion disorder. Conversional symptoms generally improve with administration of intravenous sodium amytal, whereas "true" organic neurological symptoms typically get worse. The utility of hypnosis is still relatively untested for diagnosis or treatment of conversion disorder and/or malingering. Hypnosis cannot assist in the detection of untruthfulness, particularly in that examinees can lie under hypnosis. Hypnosis can, however, assist in the recovery of lost memories.[33-35]

Somatization disorder involves a history of pain related to at least four different sites, generally begins before age 30 and occurs over a period of several years, and features recurring, multiple, clinically significant somatic complaints. Somatization disorder is more common in women than in men and has a relatively strong family pattern.[33,34]

Other disorders that may or may not be related to an injury per se but were claimed to have resulted in impairment and functional disability include hypochondriasis, post-traumatic stress disorder (PTSD), depression, and unconscious exaggeration of symptoms. Hypochondriasis is an overconcern for symptoms that persists longer than 6 months. Hypochondriasis does not apply when the concern is focused on body appearance; in such instances, a diagnosis of body dysmorphic disorder is more appropriate. When it is of delusional intensity, the clinician must differentiate a hypochondriacal type of concern from a catastrophic reaction. PTSD diagnostic criteria have actually been "softened" since the third revised edition of the *Diagnostic and Statistical Manual* (DSM-IIIR) and now are more subjective and prone to greater evaluator bias. Diagnostic criteria as defined in DSM-IV must be met to appropriately assign a diagnosis of PTSD.[33,34,36] Treatment strategies combining counseling, psychotherapy, and psychopharmacological management, as well as newer techniques such as eye movement desensitization reprocessing (EMDR), may all work well for treating PTSD. Modulation of sleep disturbance, depression, and intrusive phenomena should be the focus of psychopharmacological treatment.

Following traumatic injuries, some examinees may have post-traumatic anxiety disorders and phobias without PTSD per se. In a forensic context, one must keep in mind that any DSM-IV diagnosis, including PTSD and depression, has potential for malingering.[36] Post-traumatic depression, stress disorders, and anxiety conditions that receive timely and appropriate assessment and treatment generally have a good psychiatric and functional prognosis.

Symptom exaggeration may be related to multiple factors and serve a wide range of psychological needs, including but not necessarily limited to legitimizing latent dependency needs, resolving preexisting life conflicts, retaliating against employer or spouse, a "plea for help," and allaying anxiety and/or insecurity. One common reason for such behavior in people with postconcussive disorder is to assure acknowledgment on the part of the evaluating clinician that, indeed, something is wrong with them, given the fact that they have likely been seen by other clinicians who were unable to find "anything neurologically wrong."[37] Unfortunately, some patients with long histories of preexisting psychiatric and psychoemotional problems latch onto a specific injury and make it responsible for all their problems in life. Those individuals with significant negative prognostic indicators for TBI outcome tend to do worse when faced with real injury. In assessing patients with claims of being "totally disabled" following uncomplicated mild brain injury, clinicians should consider nonneurological and/or nonorganic contributors.[6] In the rehabilitation setting, it is not uncommon to see patients with depression, not necessarily related to an accident, and post traumatic stress disorder who are incorrectly diagnosed as having postconcussive disorder (PCD) or MTBI. Such errors in diagnostic accuracy only amplify and promulgate misperceptions, functional disability, and health care costs (Table 7–3).

□ CAUSALITY DETERMINATION

To establish causality between claimed impairments and a specific injury in time, one must analyze the influence of preexisting conditions on the current set of claimed postinjury residua. One must also assess whether the claimed impairments are truly neurological, as opposed to inadvertently labeled as such. A prime example is headache in PCD, which is more often than not cervicogenic in origin and associated with myofascial referred pain.[38] The temporal onset of subjective complaints, objective findings with the injury event, and the consistency of complaints with expectations for similar types of injuries are also of utmost importance. The time of symptom onset must be understood in relation to when one expects to see specific types of problems following brain injury. For example, both seizures and movement disorders can first be manifested months to years after any severity of TBI. Having corroborative information from family, acquaintances, and coworkers or supervisors is also important to further validate examinee complaints.

One of the most telling signs supportive of potential nonorganicity is an atypical recovery pattern evidencing a decline in function over time rather than an improvement. Such a pattern is particularly suggestive for nonneurological factors after an otherwise uncomplicated MTBI in the absence of other neurological explanations. The assessing physiatrist *must*, however, take into consideration potential neurological complications such as late subdural hematomas, epilepsy (clinical and subclinical), and communicating hydrocephalus, particularly after more severe brain injury, as possible explanations for a

---

TABLE 7–3. Differential Diagnostic Issues in Acquired Brain Injury

Psychological and/or psychiatric diagnoses associated with trauma

Depression
Anxiety disorders
Phobic disorders
Post-traumatic stress disorder
Malingering
Factitious disorders
Somatoform disorders
Hypochondriasis

Neurological disorders not related to acquired brain injury

Senile dementia, Alzheimer's type (SDAT)
Multiple sclerosis
Multi-infarct dementia
Acquired dementias secondary to infectious or nutritional etiologies
Cerebrovascular disease

Symptom magnification

Psychiatric disorders not related to acquired brain injury

Malingering
Factitious disorders
Somatoform disorders
Hypochondriasis

decrement in neuromedical or functional status.[39] Psychoemotional and psychiatric issues, secondary to the TBI or unrelated, must always be given consideration as potential etiologies of an atypical recovery pattern involving late decline. Additionally, one must consider the possibility of concurrent medical and/or neurological conditions in isolation or in conjunction with TBI that may complicate diagnosis and treatment. Such disorders include hypothyroidism, chronic fatigue syndrome, Lyme disease, and reversible and irreversible dementias.

From a diagnostic standpoint, to optimally critique whether an event is causally related to current problems reported by the examinee, the clinician must observe test-taking behaviors, analyze test performance patterns and performance in relation to test item difficulty, and assess both neuropsychological and physical examination findings in context.[29,31,32]

Clinicians must remain aware of the difficulties encountered in the clinical assessment of patients with TBI, particularly those with MTBI and potentially associated PCD. The likelihood for symptom magnification as well as malingering becomes more of an issue when a condition's diagnosis relies heavily on claimant subjective report and/or when the diagnostics typically done for such a condition are either expected to be "unremarkable" or may not be pathognomonic of the condition in question.[8,15] These latter issues are particularly true for MTBI and PCD diagnosis. When there are doubts, then clinicians with specific expertise in differential diagnosis in this patient population should be brought in to assist further with case analysis.

□ PHYSIATRIST INTERACTIONS WITH PATIENTS AND FAMILIES

The skills needed to develop good rapport with patients and their families are not learned by reading this or any other book chapter or article. Instead, as with many of the aspects of medical care, rapport is learned through experience and hands-on work. Physical medicine and rehabilitation—in particular, brain injury rehabilitation—is one of the few medical specialties that truly allow the physician to develop a long-term relationship with patients and their significant others. First impressions can go a long way in building long-lasting rapport and is certainly crucial in optimizing the assessment process.

Taking the extra time to let people know that you care about them—in a sense treating them as if each one was your only patient—helps further facilitate bonding among physician, patient, and family. Minimizing interruptions during discussions also lets individuals know that you are there for them and not just there to make a buck. Any measures that can be taken to fulfill special requests provide an additional basis for nurturing a trusting relationship.[40] The better the rapport with the person being assessed, the more likely the examining physiatrist is to get an accurate and complete history and optimal cooperation on the physical examination.

Appropriate and timely prognostic information should be provided, as previously discussed. "Threads of hope" are necessary for those with TBI and their families to maintain the motivation to facilitate ongoing rehabilitation efforts. Good rapport not only optimizes the working relationship between the involved parties but also enhances the quality of care, compliance with prescribed interventions, and the patient's ability to comprehend the treatment process.

As physicians working with survivors of TBI, we see them when they are extremely vulnerable, both individually and more globally. It is our duty to safeguard our patients' individual and civil rights as fellow human beings. All too frequently, we rehabilitation professionals lose sight of our commitment as health care professionals to guarantee our patient's rights of free choice when they have the capability of making the required decisions. If and when they do not have the capacity to make independent sound medical decisions, then appropriate measures should be taken to safeguard their rights by proceeding through established judicial measures such as guardianship. We should advocate on their behalf and, more important, facilitate their own abilities to advocate for themselves.[3]

Clinicians should be aware of respecting patients' rights of confidentiality and privacy, which so often do not receive the attention they deserve in rehabilitation settings. We tend to think we know best what to do for the patient, and our collective attitude may at times be paternalistic because of our training and perspective on patient care, as well as our self-perceived role as care "overseers." We should be more introspective about how providing health care, of any kind, may desensitize those providing the care to the needs of those receiving it.

Although physicians deal with capacity and competency issues on a daily basis in the field of brain injury rehabilitation, too few are familiar with the medical and legal aspects of determining capacity. Additionally, physicians should be familiar enough with the "functional" levels of capacity, thereby protecting patient rights against overly broad rulings regarding capacity. By advocating on behalf of patients and ensuring that the "least restrictive" environment that optimally guarantees their safety is provided, we can better avoid situations that result in restriction of constitutionally protected rights.[41]

Patients and family members should be given educational materials, and the clinician should take the time to explain the condition, natural history, and prognosis. The patient and family *must* understand the condition, the resultant impairments, the prognosis, and the treatment, as applicable, to optimize their own adjustment process. Physicians need to empower families to advocate for their loved one and themselves. By empowering families, we help facilitate the rehabilitation process and further enhance its efficiency. Educating families is paramount to maximizing compliance with prescribed programs as well as medications.

Being able to communicate with families in language they understand rather than medical jargon further facilitates the educational process. As physicians, we become so used to our scientific and technical language that we sometimes find it difficult to communicate at a level that is comprehensible to the average layperson. Being cognizant of how we communicate, rather than just being aware of what we communicate, is essential in helping families gain a better grasp on things as they are and things as they will be.

Brain injury, regardless of its etiology, can be a devastating event for not only the affected individual but also his or her family. Timely and adequate communication with both patients and families is paramount to facilitating the recovery process and assisting all concerned with optimizing their individual coping strategies. Maintaining a balance between optimism and realism is critical. Our role as physicians should be to inform families to the best of our capability but at the same time *never* remove hope. Ultimately, we should provide realistic appraisals of prognosis based on available literature, prognostic parameters, patient and family traits, and our own personal clinical experiences.[42–46]

As appropriate, referrals for counseling and support groups may help further facilitate the adjustment process. There are occasions when the information being conveyed may indeed not be good news. Regardless of when this occurs postinjury, it is many times difficult for physicians to convey such information to family members.[47]

Clinicians must deal with the fact that in most instances we are unable to "cure" and instead must settle for ameliorating the impact of neurological impairments on functional status. In many ways, this philosophical tenet is in contradistinction to values instilled in us throughout our medical education: Doctors make patients better. The aforementioned perspectives are often not appreciated by families, and one would question whether they should be. It is important for us as clinicians to remain sensitive to our own value system and inherent philosophies regarding the care that we render. By being more introspective, we can improve our ability to communicate, thereby not only maximizing adjustment and understanding but also facilitating ongoing recovery.

☐ CONCLUSIONS

For physiatrists to optimally assess persons with TBI, there must be a greater commitment to facilitating training in brain injury rehabilitation and related fields during and following physical medicine and rehabilitation residency. Physiatrists must remain committed to ongoing self-education and honing of their clinical assessment and diagnostic skills to enhance the medical rehabilitation care they are providing. Physiatrists should continue to distinguish themselves from other health care professionals in the way they relate to and develop rapport with people who are neurologically disabled, particularly with regard to taking a holistic approach to both assessment and treatment of impairments and associated functional disability. Most important, there is no substitute for thoroughness in performing the history and physical examination. A comprehensive assessment optimizes the accuracy of diagnostic impressions and ultimately the efficacy of all future treatment plans.

REFERENCES

1. Francisco, GE, Chae, JC, and DeLisa, JA: Physiatry as a primary care specialty. Am J Phys Med Rehabil 74:186, 1995.
2. Haig, AJ, et al: Outpatient planning for persons with physical disabilities: A randomized prospective trial of physiatrist alone versus a multidisciplinary team. Arch Phys Med Rehabil 76:341, 1995.
3. Zasler, ND: A medical perspective on physician training and brain injury rehabilitation. In Durgin, CJ, Schmidt, ND, and Fryer, LJ (eds): Staff Development and Clinical Intervention in Brain Injury Rehabilitation. Aspen, Gaithersburg, 1993.
4. Kreutzer, JS, Zasler, ND, and Wehman, PH: Neuromedical and psychosocial aspects of rehabilitation after traumatic brain injury. In Fletcher, G, et al (eds): Rehabilitation Medicine: State of the Art. Lea & Febiger, New York, 1992.
5. Zasler, ND: Catastrophic traumatic brain injury. In: Price, DR, and Lees-Haley, PR (eds): The Insurer's Handbook of Psychological Injury Claims. Claims Books, Seattle, 1995.
6. Zasler, ND: Impairment and disability evaluation in post-concussive disorders. In Rizzo, M, and Tranel, D

(eds): Head Injury and Post-Concussive Syndrome. Churchill Livingstone, New York, 1996, p 351.

7. Cope, DN: Physiatric assessment for rehabilitation. In Rosenthal, M, et al (eds): Rehabilitation of the Adult and Child with Traumatic Brain Injury. FA Davis, Philadelphia, 1990, p 253.

8. Sbordone, RJ, and Purisch, AD: Hazards of blind analysis of neuropsychological test data in assessing cognitive disability: The role of confounding factors. NeuroRehabilitation 7:15, 1996.

9. Nolan, MF: Introduction to the Neurologic Examination. FA Davis, Philadelphia, 1996.

10. Taylor, CA, and Price, TRP: Neuropsychiatric assessment. In Silver, JM, Yudofsky, SC, and Hales, RE (eds): Neuropsychiatry of Traumatic Brain Injury. American Psychiatric Press, Washington, DC, 1994, p 81.

11. Strub, RL, and Black, FW: The Mental Status Examination in Neurology. FA Davis, Philadelphia, 1993.

12. Zasler, ND: Mild traumatic brain injury medical assessment and intervention. J Head Trauma Rehabil 8(3):13, 1993.

13. Travell, JG, and Simons, DG: Myofascial Pain and Dysfunction: The Trigger Point Manual. Williams & Wilkins, Baltimore, 1983.

14. Zasler, ND: Neuromedical diagnosis and treatment of post-concussive disorders. In Horn, L, and Zasler, ND (eds): Rehabilitation of Post-Concussive Disorders. Hanley & Belfus, Philadelphia, 1992.

15. Zasler, ND: Neuromedical diagnosis and management of post-concussive disorders. In Horn, L, and Zasler, ND (eds): Medical Rehabilitation of Traumatic Brain Injury. Hanley & Belfus, Philadelphia, 1992, p 133.

16. Evans, RW: The postconcussion syndrome and the sequelae of mild head injury. Neurol Clin 10:1, 1992.

17. Jennett, B, et al: Head injury. In Evans, RW, Baskin, DS, and Yatsu, FM (eds): Prognosis of Neurological Disorders. Oxford University Press, New York, 1992, p 85.

18. Bond, MR: Assessment of psychosocial outcome of severe head injury. Acta Neurochir (Wien) 34:57, 1976.

19. Heiskanen, O, et al: Prognosis of depressed skull fractures. Acta Neurochirurgica Scand 139:605, 1973.

20. Choi, SS, et al: Chart for outcome prediction in severe head injury. J Neurosurg 59:294, 1983.

21. Jennett, B, and Teasdale, G: Assessment of coma and impaired consciousness: A practical scale. Lancet 2:74, 1972.

22. Born, JD: The Glasgow-Liege Scale. Prognostic value and evolution of motor response and brainstem reflexes after severe head injury. Acta Neurochir (Wien) 9:1, 1988.

23. Horn, LJ, and Cope, DN: Traumatic brain injury. State of the Art Reviews in Physical Medicine and Rehabilitation 3:1, 1989.

24. Katz, DI: Neuropathology and neurobehavioral recovery from closed head injury. J Head Trauma Rehabil 7(2):1, 1992.

25. Groswasser, Z, and Sazborn, L: Outcome in 134 patients with prolonged posttraumatic unawareness. J Neurosurg 72:81, 1990.

26. Binder, LM: Persisting symptoms after mild head injury: A review of the postconcussive syndrome. J Clin Exp Neuropsychol 8:323, 1986.

27. McCaffrey, FJ, et al: Forensic issues in mild head injury. J Head Trauma Rehabil 8(3):38, 1993.

28. Radanov, BP: Cognitive functioning after common whiplash. Arch Neurol 50:87, 1993.

29. Ruff, RM, Wylie, T, and Tennant, W: Malingering and malingering-like aspects of mild closed head injury. J Head Trauma Rehabil 8(3):60, 1993.

30. National NeuroRehabilitation Consortium (NNRC) Inc: Factors in Evaluating a Neuropsychological Report: A Neurophysiatric Perspective. NNRC Publications, Richmond, Va, 1994.

31. Niles, KJ, and Sweet, JJ: Neuropsychological assessment and malingering: A critical review of past and present strategies. Archives of Clinical Neuropsychology 9:501, 1994.

32. Millis, SR, and Putnam, SH: Evaluation of malingering in the neuropsychological examination of mild head injury. NeuroRehabilitation 7:55, 1996.

33. Weintraub, MI: Malingering and conversion reactions. Neurol Clin 13:2, 1995.

34. American Psychiatric Association: Diagnostic and Statistical Manual of Mental Disorders, ed 4. American Psychiatric Association, Washington, DC, 1994.

35. Rogers, R (ed): Clinical Assessment of Malingering and Deception. Guilford, New York, 1988.

36. Simon, RI (ed): Post-Traumatic Stress Disorder in Litigation: Guidelines for Assessment. American Psychiatric Press, Washington, DC, 1995.

37. Kay, T, et al: Toward a neuropsychological model of functional disability after mild traumatic brain injury. Neuropsychology 6:371, 1993.

38. Horn, L: Post-concussive headache. In Horn, L, and Zasler, ND (eds): Rehabilitation of Post-Concussive Disorders. Hanley & Belfus, Philadelphia, 1992, p 69.

39. Giacino, JT, and Zasler, ND: Outcome following severe brain injury: The comatose, vegetative and minimally responsive patient. J Head Trauma Rehabil 10(1):40, 1995.

40. Franke, J: Boning up on bedside manner: In an era of high-tech medicine and managed care, physician-patient communication is more important than ever. Tex Med 91:32, 1995.

41. Hart, T, and Nagele, D: The assessment of competency in traumatic brain injury. NeuroRehabilitation 7:27, 1996.

42. Blustein, J: The family in medical decisionmaking. Hastings Cent Rep 23:6, 1993.

43. Rizzo, M, and Tranel, D (eds): Head Injury and Postconcussive Syndrome. Churchill Livingstone, New York, 1996.

44. Horn, LJ, and Zasler, ND: Medical Rehabilitation of Traumatic Brain Injury. Hanley & Belfus, Philadelphia, 1996.

45. Becker, DP, and Gudeman, SK (eds): Textbook of Head Injury. WB Saunders, Philadelphia, 1989.

46. Giacino, JT, et al: Recommendations for use of uniform nomenclature pertinent to patients with severe alterations in consciousness. Arch Phys Med Rehabil 76:205, 1995.

47. Zasler, N: Advocacy in the physician-patient relationship. Headway: Virginia Head Injury Foundation Newsletter 12:2, 1994.

CHAPTER 8

Functional Assessment in Traumatic Brain Injury

KARYL M. HALL, EDD

The value of assessing the functional status and outcome of those with traumatic brain injury (TBI) has become increasingly evident. In past years, documentation of functional status was used to determine progress of patients in the clinical setting. The clinician is now being asked to document the effects of treatment not only for clinical purposes but also for justification to payers and for program evaluation and accreditation. In the face of managed health care, the importance of functional assessment of patients in the rehabilitation setting for conducting research on treatment effectiveness may become the means of justifying our very existence.[1,2]

A continuum of treatment intensities and/or programs—that is, "levels of care" from injury through community integration—is seen as a cost-effective means for managing individuals with TBI.[3–5] Providing levels of care presents new challenges for measuring function appropriate to the phase of recovery. Traditional inpatient measures become less sensitive and relevant as individuals return to the community.[5,6] In addition to insensitivity or substantial ceiling effects, these instruments may not be measuring the important functional goals for extended levels of care.

The definition of *function* in this context is the natural, required, or expected activity of a person. Functional measures can therefore apply in any of the three levels of the World Health Organization model of disablement: impairment, disability, and handicap.[7] *Impairment* is defined as "any loss or abnormality of psychological, physiological, or anatomical structure or function" (p. 47), that is, organic disablement. Those in the acute injury phase of recovery and those in coma are functioning at the impairment level. *Disability* is defined as any restriction or lack (resulting from an impairment) of ability to perform an activity in the manner or within the range considered normal for a human being" (p. 143), typically the phase of recovery while a person is in inpatient rehabilitation. *Handicap* is defined as "a disadvantage for a given individual, resulting from an impairment or a disability, that limits or prevents the fulfillment of a role that is normal (depending on age, sex, and social and cultural factors) for that individual" (p. 183). Handicap encompasses the individual's role in the family and community, a focus of nonresidential rehabilitation and long-term follow-up.

Recently, the handicap phase of recovery has been the focus of rehabilitation providers because it is the bottom line in terms of long-term costs of care, impact on society, and quality of life for the client and family.[8,9] The task of clinicians is to measure important functional performances of clients that will have significant implications for real life, while avoiding burdening the rehabilitation staff with extensive and redundant or meaningless documentation.

This chapter first defines the criteria by which to judge measures; second, describes measures currently used and their properties; and third, suggests a hypothetical minimal data set for TBI.

☐ CONSIDERATIONS IN CHOOSING MEASURES

Of the myriad available published scales,[10,11] this section reviews realistically brief TBI rehabilitation outcomes measures that, at the least, have evidence of validity and reliability. Most measures available address disabilities of individuals with TBI. Less available are seasoned tools to measure handicap in the community. Measuring individuals' general level of functioning in a rehabilitation setting, from acute to postacute, outpatient or residential settings, may require progressively different measurement tools. Setting new individual goals in concert with the patient and family at each major step in recovery is essential in any rehabilitation program. This approach can also be taken for choosing assessment tools.

There are several criteria used to determine whether a particular tool meets one's needs. Some of the guidelines here are dependent on the existence of other guidelines, are in apparent conflict, or overlap considerably. No one tool meets all of the following criteria, and all the criteria are not equal in importance.

Validity

Validity is established when a scale measures what it claims to measure. We are concerned with at least three kinds of validity in any scale.[12] The first is criterion-referenced validity, the extent to which a test score predicts an outcome or correlates with other information currently available that is external to the measure. The second is content validity, the extent to which items represent all facets of the factor being assessed. The third type of validity is construct validity, the degree to which the test scores relate to real-world effects, tying the measure to a group of theoretical assumptions. Validity, in its global definition, is an essential requirement of a measure.

Reliability

Reliability is the degree to which ratings on an instrument are consistent or reproducible when administered under similar circumstances. There are three types of reliability to consider. The first is test-retest reliability: the degree to which the scores remain stable upon retesting, all else being constant. The second is interrater reliability among raters—that is, that different raters can independently assign similar ratings to the client. The third type of reliability is internal consistency, in which all parts of the test are highly intercorrelated, so that the trait being measured is being measured by all items.

The most important of these for our purposes is interrater reliability. Unfortunately, a great deal of the literature has used correlations instead of the more appropriate Kappa coefficients to establish interrater reliability. Items rated on scales with few response alternatives, where there is the likelihood of agreement by chance, provide inflated interrater reliability statistics unless chance agreement is factored out, as it is in the Kappa coefficient.

Another concern is the reliability between client and caregiver or family member ratings. There have been conflicting results in the literature on this topic, depending in part on which scale is under investigation.[13,14] As a general principle, the more objective the subject matter, the higher the interrater reliability. For example, client employment status is highly reliable between raters. However, how much the consumer assists with tasks at home very much varies with the perspective of the rater; the client predictably rates this behavior more favorably than does the caregiver or family member.[15,16] Discrepancies in ratings may occur as often for the general population as for the TBI population, for example, between spouses or parent and child. A difficulty arises when the clinician must rely on more than one consistent source for information, which creates questionable reliability of responses.

Sensitivity or Precision

The scale must be sensitive enough to reflect clinically significant changes in function, an important factor to consider in choosing a scale.[6] Lack of sensitivity was a major complaint about the Glasgow Outcome Scale, the first well-known descriptor of function: Significant gains were not necessarily reflected.[17] Some scales may be sensitive at one end and not at the other. Generally speaking, those in extended coma or those longer postinjury require more sensitive scales to reflect less dramatic changes. These floor and ceiling effects are common problems in scaling and should be attended to, as they negatively affect conclusions regarding patient progress and program effectiveness.

Time Required to Complete the Measure (Brevity)

Often the best-planned program evaluation or research protocols have missing or unreliable data because the staff were remiss in completing the forms. Long and complicated rating scales are more justifiable in research studies, where data collection is the priority of dedicated staff. Numerous items often are highly correlated and provide little if any new information with which to predict outcomes or measure progress. For instance, the 13 motor items of the Functional Independence Measure

(FIM)™ are highly intercorrelated. However, brevity is a virtue only if the instrument will adequately answer the questions posed.

Expertise Required to Complete the Measure

Some scales require the specialized expertise of specific disciplines to complete each of the items. Other scales can be completed by a trained research assistant or other nonclinician. Ratings on some scales can be "captured" retrospectively from medical chart review or extrapolated from other ratings. Others require in-depth knowledge of the individual. Demanding measurement tools require time, money, and dedicated staff.

Comparability

Is the scale used at other centers, and is it recognized by other professionals in the field? It is becoming increasingly critical that we all speak the same language. Findings can best be compared across centers when the assessment tools are the same. We do not want to accept a tool simply because it is in common use, but the task then becomes to offer a better alternative and convince others to use it.

Continuity

An ideal scale would adequately capture change from injury through long-term follow-up. However, we run the risk of giving up sensitivity by gaining breadth. Many good scales were not constructed for such a broad purpose, and ultimately continuity may need to be sacrificed for sensitivity in programs focusing on a specific window in the rehabilitation process.

Phone Capability

For practical purposes, phone assessments are generally required for follow-up, unless we are resigned to a great deal of missing data and a biased sample. In-person interviews are generally thought to be more desirable when possible, but they are often impractical. The reliability between in-person and phone interview ratings in the literature is high, especially for less severely injured individuals.[18,19] However, phone interviews restrict options for assessment of handicap. Any tool that requires studied observation for reliability and tools that require more than several minutes to complete obviously would not be feasible. Self-assessment measures with several options for answers, as in multiple choice, are also not amenable to phone interview. Questions need to be brief and formatted for yes-no or simple response answers.

Other considerations to reduce follow-up sample bias include (1) services for finding and/or contacting "lost" patients, such as EQUIFAX and TRW, (2) payment or other incentives offered to clients for their time spent answering questions, and (3) interviewing the family member or caregiver when the client is unavailable or unable to respond. Mail requests typically have a poor yield unless followed by phone or personal contact.

Standardization

Measures have usually been standardized on norms appropriate for the population being tested (patient versus normal). This is generally not an issue for functional assessment scales because the assumption is that "normal" is the baseline "perfect" score. Beyond that, it is difficult to establish norms for the brain injured population because severity of injury varies across subjects (patient versus other like patients). Assessing test-retest reliability on the individual is also often inappropriate during recovery, as change (improvement) is expected. What is often important is whether the scale was developed with individuals with TBI in mind, such that the content is appropriate (i.e., content validity).

Supportive Documentation

The scale should define terms, spell out limitations, and provide guidelines for rating. Training assistance and/or materials should be available. The longer and more difficult the scale, the more time and training materials are necessary. Even the simplest of scales benefits from definitions of terms. If applicable, specific instructions for phone interviews are helpful.

Age Limitations

This chapter focuses on tools appropriate for the adult population, but some of the tools can be adapted for younger age groups. Any in-house modifications, however, can affect established validity and reliability. Normal developmental variations add to the difficulties of assessing younger populations, and therefore justify more complex scales. The Wee-FIM,[20–23] the Pediatric Evaluation of Disability Inventory (PEDI),[24] and the Vineland Daily Living Skills Scale[25] are examples of better-known tools for use with children.

Comprehensiveness

A comprehensive functional assessment scale transcends individual therapy goals to reflect a global picture of the client. It may necessitate involvement by several disciplines to obtain accurate ratings across factors. Comprehensive tools completed in clinical conference can facilitate a team approach to treatment rather than individual discipline specialization.

Availability of Tool

If a scale is proprietary, it may have had less exposure and therefore be less recognized by the therapeutic community. Often facilities will not purchase a scale because they have not been able to pilot it or because the resources to do so are not available. This, in turn, negatively affects comparability.

The following sections address evaluation of (1) patients in coma, (2) those who have rehabilitation potential (i.e., at least emerging from coma), (3) handicap issues for those who have emerged from coma and are living in the community, and (4) mild brain injury.

□ INDICES OF IMPAIRMENT: SEVERITY OF INJURY

These scales are appropriate primarily in acute hospital settings early after injury. They are the most likely to be valued for their ability to predict gross outcome and are indicators of impairment. Because severity of initial injury is crucial to interpreting outcomes data—that is, making valid outcome comparisons by assuring equal initial severity between groups—it is imperative that programs uniformly assess severity-related factors.

Coma Measures

The best early indicators of severity are (1) the best and worst Glasgow Coma Scale (GCS) scores within 24 h of injury, (2) length of coma (duration of GCS <9), and (3) duration of posttraumatic amnesia (PTA).

The most universally recognized impairment measure in TBI is the GCS.[26] It has simple scoring for assessing depth of coma and is a necessary component of any TBI data set. The best and worst scores within the first 24 hours have been used as an indication of severity of injury,[27] although use of the best versus worst score is still debated. Rating 6 hours and beyond after injury reduces the likelihood of confounding factors such as temporary medical conditions.[28] If the Disability Rating Scale (DRS; discussed later) is used, the GCS (best score) can be easily obtained from it. A GCS of 3 to 8 has been defined as severe injury; 9 to 12, moderate; and 13 to 15, mild brain injury.

The GCS has been found to be a robust predictor of outcomes,[29–31] including costs and especially mortality, but with some exceptions. Of the three items in the scale (eye opening, communication ability, and best motor response), motor response has proven to be the most powerful predictor of early outcome.[32] In a study by Jennett et al.,[33] a first 24-hour best GCS score of 3 to 4 resulted in death or vegetative state in 87 percent of patients. Scores of 5 to 7 resulted in death or vegetative state in 53 percent and moderate or good recovery in 34 percent. Scores of 8 to 10 resulted in moderate or good recovery in 68 percent, and a score of 11 predicted moderate or good recovery in 87 percent.

An early DRS score represents exclusively the GCS if the patient is severely injured because higher-level items are held constant. DRS scores obtained on 128 individuals within 72 hours of cerebrovascular accident (CVA) or TBI were significantly correlated with acute hospital length of stay, DRS scores at discharge, and disposition at discharge.[34] The GCS (first 24 h, worse score) was found to be directly related to length of stay in rehabilitation, charges, and the discharge DRS.[35] Vogenthaler et al.[36] found that initial GCS predicted hours of assistance required at 4- to 7-year follow-up as well.

Length of coma (LOC) can be determined by using the GCS repeatedly (*coma* is defined as a score of ≤8 on the GCS). LOC is also a good predictor but more difficult to collect than the 24-hour GCS.[37] Ruff et al.[38] reported that those in coma less than 20 days were 2.7 times more likely to return to work (RTW) in the first 6 months than those with longer coma. McMordie et al.[39] reported that for those who had a LOC longer than 1 day, only 8 cases (5%) of the individuals had returned to full-time work an average of 6.7 years postinjury.

Investigators have attempted to improve on the sensitivity of the GCS by adding items. The longer scales are appropriate for consideration by programs that treat numbers of patients in extended coma or minimally responsive states. The Glasgow-Liege Scale, an extension of the GCS, assesses brain stem reflexes in craniocaudal order for deep coma.[40] Examples of other scales of enhanced sensitivity for use with those in coma and minimally conscious states are the Coma–Near Coma Scale,[41] the Coma Recovery Scale,[42] the Sensory Stimulation Assessment Measure,[43] and the Western Neuro-Sensory

Stimulation Profile.[44] Comparisons among these scales are discussed by O'Dell et al.[45]

Other Indicators of Severity of Injury

Emergence from PTA is defined by a Galveston Orientation and Amnesia Test (GOAT) score of 75 or higher for 2 consecutive days.[32] Length of PTA information is difficult to obtain because it requires close monitoring by staff to reliably determine when the GOAT score reaches 75.[46] Predictive validity of PTA has been recognized for many years,[32,47] but accurate data on length of PTA are difficult to obtain, especially by retrospective medical record review. PTA is commonly defined as the time between injury and recovery of full memory for day-to-day events. Jennett and Teasdale[48] found that if PTA was shorter than 14 days, the 6-month outcome was good in 83 percent of patients, moderate in 17 percent, and never severe. Even with PTA of 15 to 28 days, only 3 percent had a severe outcome and 66 percent a good recovery. A PTA of more than 28 days, however, yielded 6-month severe outcomes in 30 percent of patients and good recovery in 27 percent. Simple retrospective data on duration of PTA have repeatedly shown robust correlations with treatment costs and general outcomes. GOAT scores are not useful prognostic indicators in rehabilitation, as patients generally have emerged from PTA by time of admission.[49] Longer-term cognitive outcome at 12 months and beyond has not been shown to be consistently related to PTA. However, rate of cognitive recovery appears to have a strong relationship to PTA.[28]

☐ INDICES OF DISABILITY

Functional Assessment Measures

Disability scales are the most numerous of the scales available and are used in inpatient rehabilitation programs and, to a somewhat lesser extent, in postacute community programs. Disability scales typically address self-care, mobility, and, more variably, cognition, communication, and behavior. The following are some of the better-known tools.

The Functional Independence Measure (FIM; Table 8–1) is an 18-item scale with seven levels of independence per item. It is the product of an effort to resolve the long-standing problem of lack of uniform measurement of disability and rehabilitation outcomes. The FIM emerged from a national task force of rehabilitation professionals

TABLE 8–1. Functional Independence Measure and Functional Assessment Measure

Motor Items	Cognition Items
Self-care	*Communication*
Eating	Comprehension
Grooming	Expression
Bathing	Reading*
Dressing upper body	Writing*
Dressing lower body	Speech intelligibility*
Toileting	
Swallowing*	*Psychosocial adjustment*
Sphincter control	Social interaction
Bladder management	Emotional status*
Bowel management	Adjustment to limitations*
Mobility	Employability*
Bed, chair, wheelchair transfer	
Toilet transfer	*Cognitive function*
Tub, shower transfer	Problem solving
Car transfer*	Memory
Walking/wheelchair locomotion	Orientation*
Stairs	Attention*
Community access*	Safety judgment*

*FAM items.
FIM/FIM+FAM Scale Levels of Function scoring:
Independent:
7   Complete independence (timely, safe)
6   Modified independence (extra time, devices)
Modified dependence:
5   Supervision (cuing, coaxing, prompting)
4   Minimal assist (performs 75% or more of task)
3   Moderate assist (performs 50% to 74% of task)
Complete dependence:
2   Maximal assist (performs 25% to 49% of task)
1   Total assist (performs less than 25% of task)
Source: FIM™: Guide for the Uniform Data Set for Medical Rehabilitation, Version 5.0, Buffalo, NY 14214. SUNY-Buffalo, 1996. FAM: Santa Clara Valley Medical Center, 751 S. Bascom Avenue, San Jose, CA 95128 (PM & R). www.tbi-sci.org

and researchers.[50] The Uniform Data System for Medical Rehabilitation (UDS)[20] is a nationwide shared database that uses the FIM. It provides FIM training materials and certifies reliability of raters at more than 1000 participating facilities. The FIM requires training to rate reliably. It has become a proprietary measurement tool.

The FIM was intended to be sensitive to change in an individual over the course of a comprehensive inpatient medical rehabilitation program only. As a case in point, recent analysis of the FIM revealed that 49 percent of a TBI sample ($n = 133$) were independent (score of 6 or 7) by inpatient rehabilitation discharge and 84 percent by 1 year postinjury. The FIM is not diagnosis specific, as it was developed for use with all rehabilitation patients. It can be completed in 15 to 30 minutes in conference, by observation, or by telephone interview. Evaluation of the metric properties of the FIM have been reported extensively.[51–53] Rasch analysis of the FIM has identified two measurement dimensions: motor and cognitive function. Although it has been found to be reliable and key validity characteristics have been established,[53,54] the FIM has only five items directly addressing cognitive, behavioral, and communication issues, which limits its content validity for TBI. The FIM is so widely used that it has become almost a necessity for communication across inpatient programs. The rehabilitation admission FIM motor score has been found to be a powerful predictor of length of stay, charges, and discharge FIM and is more predictive than the FIM cognition score.[53,55] The clinician can therefore obtain a reasonable estimate of time required in rehabilitation and discharge functional status from this information.

The Functional Assessment Measure[6,56] (FAM; Table 8–1) was developed as an adjunct to the FIM to address the major functional areas in TBI that are less emphasized in the FIM. The FAM adds 12 items on cognitive, behavioral, communication, and community function to the FIM. The total 30-item combination is referred to as the FIM+FAM. Rasch analyses on FAM items at rehabilitation admission correlated significantly with indices of injury severity in a pattern very similar to FIM items.

The FAM does appear to add sensitivity beyond the FIM alone at inpatient rehabilitation discharge.[6] The FAM does not appear to contribute beyond the FIM in predicting length of inpatient stay or costs or to assist significantly in reducing the robust ceiling effect of the FIM 1 year after injury.[6] Preliminary data suggest that FAM items involving abstract concepts such as "attention" tend to be less reliable than directly observable behaviors. However, reliability of the FAM has been demonstrated to the extent that staff can be trained to 80 percent or better accuracy (K. Hall, unpublished data). In summary, the FAM items can be recommended only if the treating staff want to document specific areas that the FIM does not address directly and are willing to complete the additional items to do so.

The Disability Rating Scale (DRS; Table 8–2) was developed and tested in a rehabilitation setting with individuals who had sustained moderate and severe TBIs.[57] The purpose of the scale is to measure general functional status and reflect functionally significant changes over time. One advantage of the DRS is its ability to track an individual from coma to community, providing consistency of measurement baseline over time, because various items in this scale address all three WHO categories: impairment, disability, and handicap. The DRS has eight items: The first three items (eye opening, communication ability, and motor response) are a slight modification of the GCS and reflect impairment ratings. Items 4 through 6 (cognitive ability for feeding, toileting, and grooming) reflect level of disability. The level of functioning item is the modification of Scranton's scale[58] and reflects handicap, as does the last item, employability. The DRS is easy to use, both in its lack of complexity and its brevity (generally under 5 min). The fact that it can be scored from direct observation of the client, via interview, or by phone is also beneficial.[59]

Interrater reliability of the DRS has been established for the TBI population,[60,61] despite the rather inferential character of some of its items (e.g., the scoring of cognitive ability in self care activities of daily living [ADLs] rather than actual performance in self-care). Rasch analysis has confirmed that the DRS measures a wide range of disability with less sensitivity for mild injury. Validity characteristics have been established.[62,63] It is sensitive to patient improvement in inpatient TBI rehabilitation,[17] although the FIM is more sensitive for patients with a FIM score above 25.[64] Ceiling effects at discharge and 1 year postinjury are far lower for the DRS than for the FIM (6% vs. 49% and 47% vs. 84% of cases are independent, respectively).

Cope et al.[65] reported that 1 year after discharge from a postacute rehabilitation system 62 percent of those with an admission DRS of 1 to 3 (mild) were employed competitively or in school. In the group with an admission score of 4 to 6 (moderate), 39 percent were employed or in school, and for those with a DRS of 7 to 20 (severe), 11 percent were employed or in school. Only 6 of the 54 clients in the severe range on postacute rehabilitation admission were working competitively or in school 1 year later. Cope et al.[66] also found that admission DRS scores predicted length of stay in the postacute program and personal assistance required in the community.

Novack et al.[67] found that DRS scores higher than 15 on inpatient rehabilitation admission, higher than 7 on discharge, and higher than 4 at 3 months were incompatible with RTW 1 to 2 years postinjury. Rao and Kilgore[68] found that the rehabilitation admission and discharge DRS scores combined predicted return to work with 76 percent accuracy.

The drawbacks of the DRS include its assessment of general rather than specific functional changes and its relatively poor sensitivity to extreme functional levels of deficit: It is not particularly suited to functional evaluation of mild TBI or of very severe impairment (DRS greater than 22). Specialized coma scales are recom-

TABLE 8–2. Disability Rating Scale

1. *Eye opening*	2. *Communication*	3. *Motor response*
0 Spontaneous	0 Oriented	0 Obeying
1 To speech	1 Confused	1 Localizing
2 To pain	2 Inappropriate	2 Withdrawing
3 None	3 Incomprehensible	3 Flexing
	4 None	4 Extending
		5 None

4. *Feeding**	5. *Toileting**	6. *Grooming**
0.0 Complete	0.0 Complete	0.0 Complete
0.5	0.5	0.5
1.0 Partial	1.0 Partial	1.0 Partial
1.5	1.5	1.5
2.0 Minimal	2.0 Minimal	2.0 Minimal
2.5	2.5	2.5
3.0 None	3.0 None	3.0 None

7. *Level of functioning (physical and cognitive disability)*	8. *"Employability" (as full-time worker, homemaker, or student)*
0.0 Completely independent	0.0 Not restricted
0.5	0.5
1.0 Independent in special environment	1.0 Selected jobs, competitive
1.5	1.5
2.0 Mildly dependent–limited assistance (nonresident helper)	2.0 Sheltered workshop, noncompetitive
2.5	2.5
3.0 Moderately dependent–moderate assistance (person in home)	3.0 Not employable
3.5	
4.0 Markedly dependent–assist all major activities, all times	
4.5	
5.0 Totally dependent–24-hour nursing care	

*Cognitive ability only. Knows how and when to feed, toilet, or groom self.
Source: FAM: Santa Clara Valley Medical Center, 751 S. Bascom Avenue, San Jose, CA 95128 (PM&R). www.tbi-sci.org

mended for very low functioning patients. DRS authors have recommended half-unit increments on the rating scale rather than whole units for items 4 through 8 to increase sensitivity.

The Rancho Los Amigos Levels of Cognitive Functioning Scale (LCFS; Table 8–3), also known as the Rancho Scale, was not originally designed as a scale but as nomenclature for eight stages of cognitive function for brain injured patients.[69,70] The Rancho Scale has reached almost universal acceptance in the United States because of its simplicity and clinical utility. The LCFS is an asset to a data set for these reasons alone.

There are numerous other scales in the field, many of which have excellent characteristics, but may, for our purposes, be too long or too specific or lack experience in the rehabilitation community. The Patient Evaluation Conference System (PECS) is useful both for program evaluation and in team conferences.[71] It is proprietary but comprehensive, and its reliability and metric characteristics have been well researched. It con-

tains 79 functional assessment items pertinent to inpatient status. It has a number of items that assess instrumental activities of daily living, household, and community skills, providing the range that is needed in TBI outcome assessment. The PECS has been shown to predict RTW and other important outcomes.[72]

The Rehabilitation Institute of Chicago Functional Assessment Scale (RIC-FAS) has 66 items on a 7-point scale like the FIM and includes the 18 FIM items. Version III includes higher-level ADLs for application in cognitive retraining or other outpatient programs. All 66 items of the RIC-FAS are not intended for all diagnostic groups or all phases of recovery. The scale is being further refined and is available for a nominal fee.[73]

The Glasgow Outcome Scale[74] was commonly used before other scales were developed. As a brief descriptive outcome scale, it has been replaced by the DRS due to its poor sensitivity, although it is still seen occasionally in the literature, especially in studies investigating early

TABLE 8–3. Rancho Los Amigos Scale (Level of Cognitive Functioning Scale)

1. Level I: No response. Patient does not respond to external stimuli and appears asleep.

2. Level II: Generalized response. Patient reacts to external stimuli in nonspecific, inconsistent, and nonpurposeful manner with stereotypic and limited responses.

3. Level III: Localized response. Patient responds specifically and inconsistently with delays to stimuli but may follow simple commands for motor action.

4. Level IV: Confused, agitated response. Patient exhibits bizarre, nonpurposeful, incoherent, or inappropriate behaviors; has no short-term recall; attention is short and nonselective.

5. Level V: Confused, inappropriate, nonagitated response. Patient gives random, fragmented, and nonpurposeful responses to complex or unstructured stimuli. Simple commands are followed consistently, memory and selective attention are impaired, and new information is not retained.

6. Level VI: Confused, appropriate response. Patient gives context-appropriate, goal-directed responses, dependent upon external input for direction. There is carryover for relearned, but not for new tasks, and recent memory problems persist.

7. Level VII: Automatic, appropriate response. Patient behaves appropriately in familiar settings, performs daily routines automatically, and shows carryover for new learning at lower than normal rates. Patient initiates social interactions, but judgment remains impaired.

8. Level VIII: Purposeful, appropriate response. Patient oriented and responds to the environment, but abstract reasoning abilities are decreased relative to premorbid levels.

acute medical predictors of gross outcome. The five categories of the original scale are dead, vegetative, severely disabled, moderately disabled, and good recovery. An extended version of the scale divides each of the latter three categories in two, making eight categories.

Single-Concept Measures

Length of stay in an inpatient program provides an indirect measure of costs and amount of treatment, is easy to obtain, and requires no training. It is an essential component of any data set. Program interruptions (up to a maximum of 30 days)—for example, for surgery or extended home pass—should be excluded from length of program stay to accurately reflect time actually in treatment. Length of stay as an outcome measure is becoming less meaningful because of managed care; that is, patients are no longer being discharged only when they meet optimum goals or other clinical markers.

Hospital or rehabilitation *charges* excluding physician fees are easily accessed at most institutions. Information can range from a simple division of total charges by days to obtain a per diem rate or a capitation rate (division by numbers treated), to detailed billing information for each individual. Simple charges per patient are often easiest to obtain and are grossly applicable across subjects and centers. Actual costs are more difficult to obtain.

Time (intensity) and type of treatment are more difficult to obtain in a multidisciplinary setting than simple days in rehabilitation. However, service utilization information, conceivably obtained simultaneously with charges information, is essential in today's health care environment as a critical consideration in determining the effectiveness of rehabilitation generally and comparing outcomes given different treatments and treatment intensities.

Client Satisfaction with Services

Although it is not a functional assessment, some measure of *client or family satisfaction* is a Commission on Accreditation of Rehabilitation Facilities (CARF) minimum requirement. Feedback on client satisfaction is among the most potent and practical elements of a quality-outcome monitoring system if a mechanism is in place to provide feedback to supervisors *and* treating staff. Satisfaction is commonly queried using a 5- to 7-point scale. In the recent climate encouraging training across specialities, the scale should avoid discipline-specific questions. Suggested generic items are listed by Hall and Johnson.[75] Ware and Hayes recommend asking patients to rate on an "excellent" to "poor" scale.[76]

☐ INDICES OF HANDICAP

In the past, handicap issues have been the focus of behavior modification, cognitive remediation, and vocational readiness programs. Acute hospital and rehabilitation programs have typically been less concerned with handicap because they treat at the level of impairment and disability. With increased pressure to demonstrate the long-term outcomes from rehabilitation interventions, handicap issues are taking on greater significance for all rehabilitation programs.[1,77] Rehabilitation programs are having to assess clients after discharge from their program; follow-up assessment has become a CARF requirement. Phone interview techniques are the only practical method for data collection, translating to the need for brief, simple tools.

Options for measuring handicap are limited. Programs that have the interest, capacity, and/or requirement to follow clients in the community after program discharge may look to community integration scales to measure effectiveness of their programs. It is recommended that the individual with TBI be interviewed, assuming the individual is oriented and able to communicate.[78]

Community Integration

The Community Integration Questionnaire (CIQ) was developed for the assessment of community integration specifically for individuals with TBI.[79,80] The CIQ contains 15 items, including participation in household activities, shopping, errands, leisure activities, visiting friends, social events, and performance of productive activities. Factor analysis has supported the separation of these items into three dimensions: home integration, social integration, and productivity. The scale can be self-administered or obtained by personal or phone interview in 10 to 15 minutes. Agreement between survivor and family responses regarding the survivor is acceptable but not optimum. The home integration subscale provides the least agreement: The client rating is consistently more "optimistic" than the significant other. The productivity subscale has higher interrater agreement.[14] The CIQ discriminates between a TBI and control sample and among survivors with three different levels of independent living.[79]

A concern is with use of the tool without preinjury data for comparison. Corrigan and Deming[9] found significant mean CIQ differences for retrospectively obtained premorbid versus follow-up samples except on the home integration subscale. Appropriate community integration more likely means restoration of the person to his or her preinjury pattern than attainment of fixed outcomes. A retrospective preinjury assessment is optimal. This is probably true with any measure of handicap or community integration outcome. There are limited norms by which to compare scores.[79] However, it was found that by 1 year postinjury, individuals with TBI were scoring very close to the normative sample on home and social integration subscales.[6]

Considering the variation in interrater agreement, premorbid versus follow-up scores, and ceiling effects among the three subscales, a composite total score would be a questionable practice. It is recommended that each subscale retain its own identified score.

The Craig Handicap Assessment and Reporting Technique (CHART) was designed to mea-

sure handicap in individuals with spinal cord injury (SCI) in the community. Twenty-seven questions are divided into five dimensions: physical independence, mobility, occupation, social integration, and economic self-sufficiency. Psychometric properties, reliability, and validity of the CHART have been demonstrated for the SCI population.[81] It may have promise for TBI. The disadvantages are that it is longer than the CIQ and that the questions and scoring are more complex. A recent revision adding a cognitive/orientation dimension is currently undergoing reliability and validity testing across five impairment groups, including TBI. More work needs to be done to make the CHART appropriate to the TBI population.[79]

The Patient Competency Rating Scale (PCRS) is another tool worth mentioning. The PCRS is a 30-item self-report scale with responses from 1 (can't do) to 5 (can do with ease). The questions are easily understood. It asks about everything from ADLs to cognitive problems to anger and other inappropriate behaviors, apparently capturing the essence of "typical" problems for those with TBI in the community.[15,82] It is especially impressive in that a significantly handicapped person can score poorly on the PCRS but fairly well on the CIQ and CHART because the PCRS incorporates important behavioral and cognitive problems beyond community integration.

Single-Concept Handicap Measures

Employment is an indication of successful integration of the individual into society. Rating "productive activity" gives some credit for recreational and volunteer time, as measured in the CIQ and CHART. Employment and productive life activities are relatively easily documented. The FIM+FAM and DRS document work and school "employability." Ben-Yishay et al.[83] developed a detailed yet easily completed 10-item Employability Rating Scale, which distinguishes between part-time and full-time work.

The Occupational Status Scale is a 16-option scale that reflects hours of work, type of activity, and a comparison with preinjury employment status.[84] The Monthly Employment Ratio is an index capturing actual work behavior over time, derived by dividing the number of months the client was employed during an employment phase by the total possible months that he or she had an opportunity to be employed.[85] For further discussion of employment evaluation, see Vogelsberg[86] and Fraser.[87]

Living arrangement (disposition) provides some estimate of the level of dependence of the individual and cost to society. However, the fact that an individual lives at home may reflect the dedication of the family, cultural influences, or economic resources, rather than independence. Nevertheless, discharge to private residence is considered a good outcome, and transfer to a chronic care facility a poor outcome. Categories of residence used by the TBI Model Systems National Database[88] provide a comprehensive list of options. These categories are not ordinal in scaling or intended to be anything more than descriptive. Another interesting option that combines residence, "with whom living," and level of independence information into one 10-point scale is described by Ashley et al.[84]

Level of assisted care/supervision required is a direct method of determining global level of independence. Several factors may need to be considered, such as paid personal assistance versus unpaid assistance by family or friends, supervision versus physical assistance, the skill level and intensity of intervention required, whether the unpaid helper would be around anyway, and weekend versus weekday variations. A recently developed scale that rises above these concerns is the Supervision Rating Scale (SRS).[89] It is a single 13-option item from "independent" to "physical restraints needed."

Service utilization in the community is also an important factor to document in today's health care environment. One method for recording this information is shown in Table 8–4.

Psychosocial and Behavioral Adjustment

The assessment of psychosocial adjustment is often incorporated into a neuropsychological battery. We now have experience with a few scales in this domain.[90] The NeuroBehavioral Rating Scale (NRS) includes 27 cognitive and emotional disturbances rated on a 7-point scale. It was developed from a scale for psychiatric patients, requiring training, subjective judgment, and familiarity with the patient.[91] Interrater reliability is satisfactory, and validity has been established. Given the limited options, it has been the scale of choice for assessing behavioral changes following TBI in neurosurgical trials.

The lengthy Katz Adjustment Scale (KAS)[92,93] assesses personality and social adjustment from the client's and/or relative's perspective. Interrater reliability and concurrent validity have been established, and normative data are available. Bond's Social Scale is six simple, practical items on social outcomes, including work, leisure pursuits, family cohesion, legal offenses, sexual problems, and alcohol abuse on 3- to 5-point scales.[94] The PCRS, mentioned earlier, is also an option for psychosocial and behavioral dimensions, although it assesses more than these domains.

Scales that document more specific behavioral problems, for example, the Agitated Behavior Scale[95] and depression scales, are more focused than the scope of this review. There are many other factors that have relevance but for which assessment instruments are poorly validated or lengthy for practical use in routine outcome data collection, for example, measures of family burden and stress, or the Neurobehavioral Functioning Inventory (NFI).[96] The NFI is a new measure listing 83 brief complaints, such as "threatens to hurt self," "reads slowly," "back pain," rated on a 5-point scale from "never" to "always." Presently interrater reliability between client and family responses on the NFI is being evaluated (TBI Model Systems study).

Quality of life is arguably an ultimate aim of rehabilitation. Several methods of assessment of life satisfaction, a related concept, have been used in groups of persons with TBI. These include the Life Satisfaction Index-A,[97] the Satisfaction with Life Scale,[98] and the Quality of Life Scale.[99] Because of the dubious relationship between rehabilitation interventions and life satisfaction, it seems reasonable to restrict data collection in this area. Gill and Feinstein[100] reviewed a number of quality of life scales and concluded that data from two questions would meet most needs: (1) How would you rate your overall health over the last _____ on a 1 to 5 scale? and (2) How would you rate your overall quality of life over the last _____ on a 1 to 5 scale? (1 = very poor, 5 = excellent).

Mild Brain Injury (MBI) Assessment

People who sustain a MBI rarely experience inpatient rehabilitation, and therefore handicap issues are the focus of evaluation. Because of the mild nature of the injuries, sensitive measures are required to detect subtler problems. Neuropsychological testing can be appropriate for this diagnostic group, such as the Randt Memory Test (specified subtests: Five Item, Digit Span, and Story with Delay), Controlled Oral Word Association Test (COWAT), and Visual Search Test. Physicians often use a brief screening tool such as the Mini–Mental Status Exam or the Neurobehavioral Cognitive Status Exam to assess cognitive deficits.[101] Other measures for the MBI population generally involve self-assessments, such as subjective complaints scales.[96,102,103] Subjective scales are problematic in that the literature suggests that many enduring MBI symptoms may be attributed to psychological distress.[104,105] Another confounding issue is the functional status of the individual before the injury as compared with postmorbid status. A Psychosocial History Checklist[106] may assist the clinician in determining changes due to the MBI.

TABLE 8–4. Service Utilization

Since your discharge from the hospital (during the past _____ months), have you received any services, related to your brain injury, from:

Service	Yes	Number of months	Total number of visits	Group session or treatment?	No	Do not know	I declined service	Wanted but not recommended; reason?
Physician								
Physical therapist								
Occupational therapist								
Audiologist/optometrist								
Speech therapist or pathologist								
Case manager: helps get services								
Recreation therapist								
Psychology/mental health counselor								
Skilled nursing								
Visiting nurse								
Paid personal care attendant								
Reader or interpreter								
Adult day care/activity center								
Services for alcohol/drug abuse								
Center for independent living								
Respiratory therapist								
Social worker								
Transportation services								
Acute hospitalization								
Subacute hospitalization								
Nursing home								
Group Home								
Vocational rehabilitation								
Sheltered workshop								
Job coaching								
Financial public assistance								
Legal assistance (public)								
Other:								

The Mayo-Portland Adaptability Inventory (MPAI) rates emotional behavior, functional abilities, cognition, pain, and physical disabilities specifically for those with mild to moderate TBI in outpatient rehabilitation. Thirty items are rated on a 4-point scale.[107] It correlates well with the DRS, and the cognitive total score correlates highly with numerous neuropsychological tests of cognitive performance.

□ SUMMARY OF RECOMMENDATIONS BY TYPE OF PROGRAM

The WHO model is a straightforward method for determining the types of measures appropriate in a given program. That is, impairment measures as described previously in this chapter would be appropriate in acute inpatient care; coma measures would be applied for low-level patients in acute care or inpatient rehabilitation programs; disability measures for inpatient rehabilitation, subacute inpatient care, and skilled nursing facilities (unless very low level); and handicap measures in day programs and for any services where the client lives in the community, not an institution. Some measures appropriate to those with mild brain injury may also apply for those in postacute nonresidential programs and vice versa.

□ A MINIMAL DATA SET FOR TRAUMATIC BRAIN INJURY

Concept of a Minimal Uniform Data Set

There is no single right way of treating problems associated with TBI. A more adequate, uniform score-keeping system, however, is needed to help us identify strategies that provide the greatest long-term benefit to clients. How we can make intelligent decisions, and assist survivors and families to make intelligent decisions, must be based on objective analyses of large pools of information across treating facilities.[108] In recognition of this need in the field of rehabilitation, the concept of a national data system has been discussed in some detail.[109]

When contemplating both a national data set and one's local data set, several questions are raised, such as timelines for measurement, data content, tools appropriate for the functional level of the clientele, and measurement across levels of care. Regarding timelines for measurement, admission and discharge from a rehabilitation program are givens. However, rehabilitation admission and discharge alone do not provide enough information about the individual's likely recovery curve or the long-term stability of outcomes. Likewise, information from the acute hospitalization is needed to understand and adjust for severity of injury. General severity scales and time since injury can be factored to adjust or interpret outcomes in terms of severity of injury. This adjustment is key to a useful—as opposed to misleading—TBI outcomes database, in which programs with a similar clientele can be compared equitably. Severity of injury indicators predict survival and quality of life. The reader is referred to Zafonte et al.[28] for a coherent review of early medical predictors of outcome in severe TBI.

Additionally, the *preinjury* background factors (e.g., preinjury employment, family, social history) need to be assessed to understand handicap outcomes and to adjust them for preinjury and environmental factors. Clinical interventions take on new meaning when preinjury conditions are known, for example, teaching an individual to read "again" who was illiterate before the injury, or employment as a goal for an individual who was unemployed for years before the injury.

Follow-up is essential to assess real-world, as opposed to clinical, outcomes. Discharge does not represent maximum functional potential for most TBI clients. The traditional goal of *maximum* independence at discharge is now becoming the *minimum* independence required before transfer to a less expensive and intensive level of care. Because of early inpatient discharge, follow-up becomes even more essential to measure any impact on outcome.

Regarding choice of follow-up time, there is a trade-off between outcome caused by rehabilitation treatment and the desire to assess "final" outcomes. CARF states that evaluation should occur long enough after intervention for accurate assessment but soon enough to infer a causal relationship. Common points for follow-up in practice and in program evaluation are 6 and 12 months after injury.[110]

In the short term, and for local program evaluation efforts, the most practical course is probably to develop outcomes data systems based on program types, such as acute, subacute, and postacute programs (e.g., residential or day programs). In the longer term, this approach is unsatisfactory or at least limiting, as clients with similar problems may be treated in different settings. Only patient-driven data across the course of recovery can answer the most important questions of the relative cost-effectiveness and appropriateness of alternative placements.

TABLE 8–5. Suggested Minimal Data Set Content for Clinical Prediction and Documentation and Program Evaluation in Rehabilitation

Inpatient	Outpatient	Mild Brain Injury (GCS 13–15)	
X	X	X	Demographics*
X	X	X	Glasgow Coma Scale first 24 h
X	X		Length of coma/post-traumatic amnesia
X			Functional Independence Measure admission and discharge
X	X		Disability Rating Scale and Levels of Cognitive Functioning Scale
X	X	X	CAGE†
X	X		Supervision Rating Scale
X	X	X	Service utilizations, dates, and amount
	X		Patient Competency Rating Scale
		X	Subjective Complaint Scale
X	X	X	Client Satisfaction with Services
	X	X	Life Satisfaction (2 questions)

*Date of birth, injury, death, gender, ethnicity, dates of adm/dc, etiology, ICD9 codes, contact information, payer. Preinjury and postinjury employment/school (CIQ subscale), marital status, education, living setting, drug use, other significant preexisting conditions.
†Four questions to determine alcohol use. Has been modified for drug use as well.

Content of the Data Set

What basic information would give the clinician the tools to predict outcomes, document patient status and progress, and conduct program evaluation in the most parsimonious, cost-conscious manner, potentially consistent with what other centers are doing? Table 8–5 presents suggested content to achieve these goals.

The choice of content for any data set is always an evolutionary process, dependent in part on the objectives of the user. However, at some point we must come to consensus in the field. Common basic content across programs, with severity-adjusted outcomes and large sample populations, will facilitate communication and comparison of outcomes at a new and needed level of sophistication.

□ SUMMARY

This chapter has discussed a number of factors to consider in choosing measures to assess function in those having sustained a traumatic brain injury: validity, reliability, sensitivity, brevity, expertise required, comparability, continuity, phone capability, standardization, supportive documentation, age limitations, comprehensiveness, and availability. Measures that appear to have merit without being too cumbersome have been discussed. They are defined by the WHO classifications of impairment, disability, and handicap. Indices of impairment include measures of coma and other indicators of severity of injury, such as GCS and PTA. Indices of disability include functional assessment measures, such as FIM and DRS, and single-concept measures, such as length of stay, charges, treatment intensity or type, and client satisfaction with services. Handicap includes a review of community integration scales, productive activities, disposition, supervision required, service utilization, psychosocial and behavior adjustment, and measures appropriate for those with mild brain injuries. Those measures appropriate by type of program have been summarized.

Finally, it is proposed that a national data set be established or, at the least, that each center use a common template for measuring status and outcomes for the sake of communication, collaboration, and comparison. As more severely involved cases reach outpatient and subacute programs earlier after injury, it behooves us in the field to apply measures as appropriate to the functional level of an individual but defined within uniform parameters such as those outlined in this chapter, a challenge to which we must rise.

This work was supported by grant #H133A70018, National Institute on Disability and Rehabilitation Research, U.S. Department of Education. For copies of scales, further information, and updates, log on to: www.tbims.org/combi.

REFERENCES

1. Hall, K, Englander, J, and Wilmot, C: Commentary on model systems of care in neurotrauma: Clinical perspectives and future directions. NeuroRehabilitation 4:76, 1994.
2. Cope, D, and O'Lear, J: A clinical and economic perspective on head injury rehabilitation. J Head Trauma Rehabil 8:1, 1993.
3. Goka, RS, and Arakaki, AH: Brain injury rehabilitation: The continuum of care. Brain Injury Rehabilitation 26: 420, 1994–95.
4. Burke, D: Models of brain injury rehabilitation. Brain Inj 9:735, 1995.
5. Kilgore, KM: Measuring outcomes in the postacute continuum. Arch Phys Med Rehabil 76:SC21, 1995.
6. Hall, K: Functional measures after traumatic brain injury: Ceiling effects of FIM, FIM+FAM, DRS and CIQ. J Head Trauma Rehabil 11:27, 1996.
7. World Health Organization: International classification of impairments, disabilities, and handicaps: A manual of classification relating to the consequences of disease. World Health Organization, Geneva, 1990.
8. Whiteneck, GG: Measuring what matters: Key rehabilitation outcomes. Arch Phys Med Rehabil 75:1073, 1994.
9. Corrigan, JD, and Deming, R: Psychometric characteristics of the Community Integration Questionnaire: Replication and extension. J Head Trauma Rehabil 10:41, 1995.
10. Johnston, M, et al: Research in physical medicine and rehabilitation: XII. Measurement tools with application to brain injury. Am J Phys Med Rehabil 70:40, 1991.
11. Hall, K: Overview of functional assessment scales in brain injury rehabilitation. NeuroRehabilitation 2:98, 1992.
12. Hinderer, S, and Hinderer, K: Quantitative methods of evaluation. In DeLisa, J (ed): Rehabilitation Medicine Principles and Practice. JB Lippincott, Philadelphia, 1993.
13. Tepper, S, Beatty, P, and DeJong, G: Outcomes in traumatic brain injury: Self-report versus report of significant others. Brain Inj 10:575, 1996.
14. Sander, A, et al: Agreement between persons with traumatic brain injury and their relatives regarding psychosocial outcome using the Community Integration Questionnaire. Arch Phys Med Rehabil 78:353, 1997.
15. Prigatano, GP, and Altman, IM: Impaired awareness of behavioral limitations after traumatic brain injury. Arch Phys Med Rehabil 71:1058, 1990.
16. Goldstein, G, and McCue, M: Differences between patient and informant functional outcome ratings in head-injured individuals. International Journal of Rehabilitation and Health 1:25, 1995.
17. Hall, K, Cope, N, and Rappaport, M: Glasgow Outcome Scale and Disability Rating Scale: Comparative usefulness in following recovery in traumatic head injury. Arch Phys Med Rehabil 66:35, 1985.
18. Korner-Bitensky, N, et al: Health-related information postdischarge: Telephone versus face-to-face interviewing. Arch Phys Med Rehabil 75:1287, 1994.
19. Smith, P, et al: Intermodal agreement of follow-up telephone functional assessment using the functional independence measure in patients with stroke. Arch Phys Med Rehabil 77:431, 1996.
20. Uniform Data System for Medical Rehabilitation. SUNY, South Campus, Buffalo, NY, 1993. (716) 829-2076; Fax (716) 829-2080.
21. Msall, M, et al: The Functional Independence Measure for children (WeeFIM). Conceptual basis and pilot use in children with developmental disabilities. Clin Pediatr (Phila) 33:421, 1994.
22. Msall, M, et al: Wee-FIM. Normative sample of an instrument for tracking functional independence in children. Clin Pediatr (Phila) 33:431, 1994.
23. DiScala, C, et al: Functional outcome in children with traumatic brain injury. Agreement between clinical judgment and the Functional Independence Measure. Am J Phys Med Rehabil 71:145, 1992.
24. Haley, S, et al: Tufts Assessment of Motor Performance: An empirical approach to identifying motor performance categories. Arch Phys Med Rehabil 72:359, 1991.
25. Msall, M, et al: Functional status of extremely preterm infants at kindergarten entry. Dev Med Child Neurol 35:746, 1993.
26. Teasdale, G, and Jennett, B: Assessment of coma and impaired consciousness: A practical scale. Lancet 2:81, 1974.
27. Levin, H, et al: Neurobehavioral outcome one year after severe head injury: Experience of the Traumatic Coma Data Bank. J Neurosurg 73:699, 1990.
28. Zafonte, R, Hammond, F, and Peterson, J: Predicting outcome in the slow to respond traumatically brain injured patient: Acute and subacute parameters. NeuroRehabilitation 6:19, 1996.
29. Gensemer, I, et al: Psychological consequences of blunt head trauma and relation to other indices of severity of injury. Ann Emerg Med 18:9, 1989.
30. Rocca, B, et al: Comparison of four severity scores in patients with head trauma. J Trauma 29:299, 1989.
31. Young, B, et al: Early prediction of outcome in head-injured patients. J Neurosurg 54:300, 1981.
32. Bond, M: Standardized methods of assessing and predicting outcome. In Rosenthal, M, et al (eds): Rehabilitation of the Adult and Child with Traumatic Brain Injury. FA Davis, Philadelphia, 1990.
33. Jennett, B, et al: Prognosis in series of patients with severe head injury. Neurosurgery 4:283, 1979.
34. Eliason, M, and Topp, B: Predictive validity of Rappaport's Disability Rating Scale in subjects with acute brain dysfunction. Phys Ther 64:1357, 1984.
35. Lehmkuhl, LD, et al: Factors that influence costs and length of stay of persons with traumatic brain injury in acute care and inpatient rehabilitation. J Head Trauma Rehabil 8:88, 1993.
36. Vogenthaler, D, Smith, K, and Goldfader, P: Head injury, a multivariate study: Predicting long-term productivity and independent living outcome. Brain Inj 3:369, 1989.
37. Putnam, SH, and Adams, KM: Regression-based prediction of long-term outcome following multidisciplinary rehabilitation for traumatic brain injury. Clinical Neuropsychologist 6:383, 1992.
38. Ruff, R, et al: Predictors of outcome following severe head trauma: Follow-up data from the Traumatic Coma Data Bank. Brain Inj 7:101, 1993.
39. McMordie, W, Barker, S, and Paolo, T: Return to work (RTW) after head injury. Brain Inj 4:57, 1990.
40. Spittler, J, Langenstein, H, and Calabrese, P: Dir quantifizierung krank-hafter betwussteins-storungen: gutekritierien, zwecke, handichkeit (Quantifying pathological disorders of consciousness: Reliability criteria, aims, feasibility). Anasthesiol Intensivmed Notfallmed Schmerzther 28:213, 1993.
41. Rappaport, M, Doughtery, A, and Kelting, D: Evaluation of coma and vegetative states. Arch Phys Med Rehabil 73:628, 1992.
42. Giacino, J, et al: Monitoring rate of recovery to predict outcome in minimally responsive patients. Arch Phys Med Rehabil 72:897, 1991.
43. Rader, MA, and Ellis, DW: The Sensory Stimulation Assessment Measure (SSAM): A tool for early evaluation of severely brain-injured patients. Brain Inj 8:309, 1994.
44. Ansell, B, and Keenan, J: The Western Neuro Sensory Stimulation Profile: A tool for assessing slow-to-recover head-injured patients. Arch Phys Med Rehabil 70:104, 1989.
45. O'Dell, M, et al: Standardized assessment instruments for minimally-responsive, brain-injured patients. NeuroRehabilitation 6:45, 1996.
46. Forrester, G, Encel, J, and Geffen, G: Measuring posttraumatic amnesia (PTA): An historical review. Brain Inj 8:175, 1994.

47. Bishara, S, et al: PTA and GCS related to outcome in survivors in a consecutive series of patients with severe closed head injury. Brain Inj 6:373, 1992.
48. Jennett, B, and Teasdale, G: Management of Head Injuries. FA Davis, Philadelphia, 1981.
49. Kreutzer, J, et al: Neuropsychological characteristics of patients with brain injury: Preliminary findings from a multicenter investigation. J Head Trauma Rehabil 8:47, 1993.
50. Hamilton, B, et al: Interrater agreement of the seven-level Functional Independence Measure (FIM) (abstract). Arch Phys Med Rehabil 72:790, 1991.
51. Linacre, JM, et al: The structure and stability of the Functional Independence Measure. Arch Phys Med Rehabil 75:127, 1994.
52. Long, W, et al: Determining normative standards for Functional Independence Measure transitions in rehabilitation. Arch Phys Med Rehabil 75:144, 1994.
53. Heinemann, AW, et al: Measurement characteristics of the functional independence measure. Topics in Stroke Rehabilitation 1:1, 1994.
54. Emhoff, T, et al: Functional scoring of multitrauma patients: Who ends up where? J Trauma 9:1227, 1991.
55. Cohen, T, et al: Influence of early variables in traumatic brain injury on functional independence measure scores and rehabilitation length of stay and changes. Arch Phys Med Rehabil 76:797, 1995.
56. Hall, K, et al: Characteristics and comparisons of functional assessment indices: Disability Rating Scale, Functional Independence Measure, and Functional Assessment Measure. J Head Trauma Rehabil 8:60, 1993.
57. Rappaport, M, et al: Disability Rating Scale for severe head trauma: Coma to community. Arch Phys Med Rehabil 63:118, 1982.
58. Scranton, J, Fogel, M, and Erdman, WI: Evaluation of functional levels of patients during and following rehabilitation. Arch Phys Med Rehabil 51:1, 1970.
59. Rappaport, M, Herrero-Backe, C, and Winterfield, K: Head injury outcome up to ten years later. Arch Phys Med Rehabil 70:885, 1989.
60. Gouvier, W, Blanton, P, and LaPorte, K: Reliability and validity of the Disability Rating Scale and the Levels of Cognitive Functioning Scale in monitoring recovery from severe head injury. Arch Phys Med Rehabil 68:94, 1987.
61. Novack, T, et al: Primary caregiver distress following severe head injury. J Head Trauma Rehabil 6:69, 1992.
62. Fleming, J, Thy, BO, and Maas, F: Prognosis of rehabilitation outcome in head injury using disability rating scale. Arch Phys Med Rehabil 75:156, 1994.
63. Fryer, L, and Haffey, W: Cognitive rehabilitation and community readaptation: Outcomes from two program models. J Head Trauma Rehabil 2:51, 1987.
64. Bowers, D, and Kofroth, L: Comparison: Disability Rating Scale and Functional Independence Measure during recovery from traumatic brain injury. Arch Phys Med Rehabil 70:A58, 1989.
65. Cope, D, et al: Brain injury: Analysis of outcome in a post-acute rehabilitation system. Part 1: General analysis. Brain Inj 5:111, 1991.
66. Cope, N, et al: Brain injury: Analysis of outcome in a post-acute rehabilitation system. Part 2: Subanalyses. Brain Inj 5:127, 1991.
67. Novack, T, Bennett, G, and Berquist, T: Disability rating scale scores during recovery from head injury. Meeting of the American Academy of Physical Medicine and Rehabilitation (50th annual) and the American Congress of Rehab Medicine (65th annual), poster presentation, Seattle, 1988.
68. Rao, N, and Kilgore, K: Predicting return to work in traumatic brain injury using a variety of assessment scales. Arch Phys Med Rehabil 71:763, 1990.
69. Hagen, C: Language cognitive disorganization following closed head injury: A conceptualization. In Trexler, L (ed): Cognitive Rehabilitation: Conceptualization and Intervention. Plenum Press, New York, 1982, p 131.
70. Malkmus, D: Cognitive assessment and goal setting. In Rehabilitation of the Head Injured Adult: Comprehensive Management. Professional Staff Association of Rancho Los Amigos Hospital, Downey, Calif, 1979.
71. Harvey, R, and Jellienk, H: Functional performance assessment: A program approach. Arch Phys Med Rehabil 62:456, 1981.
72. Rao, N, and Kilgore, K: Predicting return to work in traumatic brain injury using assessment scales. Arch Phys Med Rehabil 73:911, 1992.
73. Cichowski, KC: Taking the FIM one step further. Hospital Rehab 93:91, 1995.
74. Jennett, B, et al: Disability after severe head injury: Observations on the use of the Glasgow Outcome Scale. J Neurol Neurosurg Psychiatry 44:285, 1981.
75. Hall, KM, and Johnston, MV: Part II: Measurement tools for a nationwide data system. Arch Phys Med Rehabil 75:SC10, 1994.
76. Ware, JJ, and Hays, R: Methods for measuring patient satisfaction with specific medical encounters. Med Care 26:393, 1988.
77. Hagen, C: Managed care: It may be an opportunity. NeuroRehabilitation 4:58, 1994.
78. Antonak, R, Livneb, H, and Antonak, C: A review of research on psychosocial adjustment to impairment in persons with traumatic brain injury. J Head Trauma Rehabil 8:87, 1993.
79. Willer, B, et al: Assessment of community integration following rehabilitation for traumatic brain injury. J Head Trauma Rehabil 8:75, 1993.
80. Willer, B, Ottenbacher, KJ, and Coad, ML: The community integration questionnaire. Am J Phys Med Rehabil 73:103, 1994.
81. Whiteneck, G, et al: Quantifying handicap: A new measure of long-term rehabilitation outcomes. Arch Phys Med Rehabil 73:519, 1992.
82. Fordyce, DJ, and Roueche, JR: Changes in perspectives of disability among patients, staff, and relatives during rehabilitation of brain injury. Rehabilitation Psychology 31:217, 1986.
83. Ben-Yishay, et al: Relationship between employability and vocational outcome after intensive holistic cognitive rehabilitation. J Head Trauma Rehabil 2:35, 1987.
84. Ashley, M, Persel, C, and Krych, D: Changes in reimbursement climate: Relationship among outcome, cost and payor type in the postacute rehabilitation environment. J Head Trauma Rehabil 8:30, 1993.
85. Wehman, P, et al: Employment outcomes of persons following traumatic brain injury: Pre-injury, post-injury, and supported employment. Brain Inj 3:397, 1989.
86. Vogelsberg, R: Quantifying consumer outcomes. In Wehman, P, and Kreutzer, J (eds): Vocational Rehabilitation for Persons with Traumatic Brain Injury. Aspen, Rockville, Md, 1990.
87. Fraser, R: Vocational evaluation. J Head Trauma Rehabil 6:46, 1991.
88. Harrison-Felix, C, et al: Descriptive findings from traumatic brain injury model systems national database. J Head Trauma Rehabil 7:1, 1996.
89. Boake, C: Supervision Rating Scale: A measure of functional outcome from brain injury. Arch Phys Med Rehabil 77:765, 1996.
90. Burton, L, and Volpe, B: Social Adjustment Scale assessments in traumatic brain injury. Journal of Rehabilitation 4:34, 1993.
91. Levin, H, et al: The neurobehavioral rating scale: Assessment of the behavioural sequelae of head injury by the clinician. J Neurol Neurosurg Psychiatry 50:183, 1987.
92. Katz, MM, and Lyerly, SB: Methods for measuring adjustment and social behavior in the community: I. Rationale, description, discriminative validity and scale development. Psychol Rep 13:503, 1963.
93. Jackson, H, et al: The Katz Adjustment Scale: Modification for use with victims of traumatic brain and spinal injury. Brain Inj 6:109, 1992.

94. Bond, M: Assessment of the psychosocial outcome after severe head injury. Acta Neurochir (Wien) 34:57, 1976.
95. Corrigan, J: Development of a scale for assessment of agitation following traumatic brain injury. J Clin Exp Neuropsychol 11:261, 1989.
96. Kreutzer, JS, et al: Validation of a Neurobehavioral Functioning Inventory for adults with traumatic brain injury. Arch Phys Med Rehabil 77:001, 1996.
97. McDowell, I, and Newell, C: Measuring health: A guide to rating scales and questionnaires. Oxford University Press, New York, 1987.
98. Diener, E, et al: The satisfaction with life scale. J Pers Assess 49:71, 1985.
99. Chubon, R: Development of a quality-of-life rating scale for use in health-care evaluation. Evaluation and the Health Professions 10:186, 1987.
100. Gill, TM, and Feinstein, AR: A critical appraisal of the quality of Quality-of-Life Measures. JAMA 272:619, 1994.
101. Kiernan, R, et al: The neurobehavioral cognitive status examination: A brief but differentiated approach to cognitive assessment. Ann Intern Med 107:481, 1987.
102. Englander, J, et al: Mild traumatic brain injury in an insured population: Subjective complaints and return to work. Brain Inj 6:161, 1992.
103. Jay, G, Goka, R, and Arakaki, A: Minor traumatic brain injury: Review of clinical data and appropriate evaluation and treatment. Journal of Insurance Medicine 27:262, 1996.
104. Andersson, S, et al: Amantadine in cognitive failure in patients with traumatic head injuries. Tidsskrift for Den Norske Lae ye forening 112:2070, 1992.
105. Karzmark, P, Hall, K, and Englander, J: Late-onset postconcussion symptoms after mild brain injury: The role of premorbid, injury-related, environmental, and personality factors. Brain Inj 9:21, 1995.
106. Hall, K, and Johnston, M: Outcomes evaluation in traumatic brain injury rehabilitation: Part 2: Measurement tools for a nationwide data system. Arch Phys Med Rehabil 75:10, 1994.
107. Malec, JF, and Thompson, JM: Relationship of the Mayo-Portland Adaptability inventory to functional outcome and cognitive performance measures. J Head Trauma Rehabil 9:1, 1994.
108. Johnston, MV, and Hall, KM: Part I: Overview and System Principles. Arch Phys Med Rehabil 75:SC2, 1994.
109. Hall, KM: Establishing a national TBI information system based upon a unified data set. Arch Phys Med Rehabil Supplement 78:S5, 1997.
110. Clifton, GL, et al: Outcome measures for clinical trials involving traumatically brain-injured patients: Report of a conference. Neurosurgery 31:975, 1992.

CHAPTER 9

Neuropsychological Examination of the Patient with Traumatic Brain Injury

STEVEN H. PUTNAM, PHD,
and NORMAN L. FICHTENBERG, PHD

This chapter addresses several issues particularly relevant to the neuropsychological examination of the patient with traumatic brain injury (TBI): (1) interpretive approaches to neuropsychological examination data; (2) preparation of the patient for examination; (3) examination of patients with special needs; (4) estimation of pre-TBI cognitive status; (5) practice effects associated with retesting; (6) TBI and litigation; (7) patient demographic, base rate, and normative considerations; (8) neuropsychological test findings in TBI; and (9) neuropsychological data and outcome prediction. This chapter does not contrast so-called qualitative and quantitative approaches to neuropsychological assessment. We concur with Adams[1]: "Such warm-fuzzy cold-prickly dichotomies are of no interest to the methodologically adept neuropsychologist, of limited guidance to the journeyman, and misleading to the novice" (p. 329). Similarly, the chapter does not enter into the "tiresome, food-fight debate concerning flexible, clinical approaches and rigid batteries"[1] (p. 329), despite the passion that has characterized this issue within the neuropsychological community in the past. There are, of course, many approaches to neuropsychological assessment that, along with geographic location and practice setting, have been associated with differences in fees for service and length of assessment time.[2] Whatever philosophical arguments have historically been put forth by those promoting one approach versus other approaches need to be reconsidered in light of the current economic environment and its impact on health care practices. Unfortunately, with the growing emphasis on cost-reduction policies, the pressure to perform briefer assessments may become increasingly difficult to withstand.[3]

Results of a national survey of members of the Division of Clinical Neuropsychology (Division 40) of the American Psychological Association[4] reported that 46 percent of the respondents' clinical time involved neuropsychological assessment, in contrast to only 13 percent for treatment activities. Furthermore, respondents indicated that 23 percent of their total clinical time was spent working with patients who had sustained TBI, which was well in excess of the time involved with other patient groups. Certainly, neuropsychological assessment of the patient with TBI comprises a significant component of the practice of the contemporary clinical neuropsychologist. For the profession at large, working with the TBI population represents a significant opportunity to distinguish itself in providing unique services to this very large and often complex clinical group.

ASSESSMENT

Clinicians working with patients in clinical settings must rely on their knowledge of the functioning of the living human brain via direct and indirect methods of examination. Direct methods such as computed tomography (CT) and magnetic resonance imaging (MRI) provide valuable information on the morphologic and pathological aspects of the brain, while electroencephalography (EEG) provides information about fluctuations in the electrical activity of the brain, particularly the cortex. The measurement of regional cerebral blood flow (rCBF) reflects the brain's metabolic activity as change in the magnitude of blood flow in different brain regions. Positron emission tomography (PET) and single-photon emission computed tomography (SPECT) permit visualization of brain function directly through administration of radiopharmaceuticals that emit decay signals indicating the level of brain activity in a given brain region.

Neuropsychological examination is an indirect and functional, albeit complementary, method of examining brain status by precisely measuring and observing behavior under controlled conditions. In this time of remarkable advances in neuroimaging and other criterion procedures, requiring a patient to remember a story, sequence a series of letters and numbers, or copy a design may seem antiquated to the lay observer. However, as Reitan and Wolfson[5] have stated, "Although neurological diagnosis can validly be established using many other techniques and methods (e.g., CT and MRI) the *psychological* consequences of cerebral damage are uniquely represented by neuropsychological evaluation" (p. 403). The data from these sophisticated neurodiagnostic procedures may furnish limited information that is instructive in the practical and functional aspects of how to rehabilitate the patient. For instance, how can the patient best learn? What are the functional strengths that can serve as a foundation for rehabilitation strategies? Considering the consequences of such practical issues, neuropsychological measurement will unquestionably continue to play a central role in the assessment and treatment of the patient with TBI. Despite the unique diagnostic contributions offered by the neuropsychological examination, in most clinical settings it represents one component of patient assessment. Indeed, the collaborative and synergistic power of the manifold procedures available has exponentially increased our understanding of brain processes and substrates in TBI. Langfitt et al.[6] have observed, "The continually evolving power of the methodologies of contemporary neuropsychology to localize brain dysfunction permits correlation of neurological, behavioral, and cognitive abnormalities with disturbed regional brain function measured by morphological and biochemical means" (p. 31).

THE NEUROPSYCHOLOGICAL EXAMINATION

Two pioneers in the field of neuropsychology whose contributions have shaped the practice of contemporary neuropsychological assessment are Arthur L. Benton and Ralph M. Reitan. Benton[7] has asserted, "The basic function of the neuropsychological assessment is to provide a valid description of the patient's mental status, covering both cognitive processes and affective state. Among the major cognitive processes that need to be assessed are attention-concentration, speed of information processing and decision making, memory, and communicative skills" (p. 112). Reitan and Wolfson[8] have elaborated on the essential components of the neuropsychological examination by emphasizing, "Any battery of tests which assesses human brain-behavior relationships must have three components: (1) content, or measurement of the types of psychological functions represented by the brain, (2) measurement strategies which permit application of the results to individual subjects, and (3) validation of the measurements through formal research procedures, with respect to clinical evaluations and applications." They state further that, ideally, "A neuropsychological test battery must be able to measure the full range of behavioral functions subserved by the brain" (p. 23).

The emphasis in this chapter on psychometric measurement in neuropsychological assessment accentuates the importance of accuracy and reliability in formally examining a patient's behavior. Russell[9] observes, "The advantage of scaled tests over the brief tests used in the neurological approach has the same advantage that using a thermometer has over feeling a person's forehead in order to tell whether there is a fever" (p. 53). However, it cannot be assumed that all measurements producing a quantitative value are of the same quality or necessarily have the same meaning. Although the topic is beyond the scope of this chapter, the procedures employed must, of course, meet accepted psychometric standards of reliability and validity.[10]

The usefulness of neuropsychological assessment is especially evident in the context of TBI. Benton[7] has suggested that neuropsychological assessment has, perhaps, played a more central role in the assessment of TBI than of other types of cerebral injury or disease. He proposed that this prominence was associated with the following factors: (1) Individuals with

TBI tend not to show classical signs of cerebral dysfunction (e.g., aphasia), and (2) postconcussion syndrome is frequently present. Benton[9] explained,

> Given the lack of hard evidence of brain injury, many clinicians viewed these behavioral deviations as reflecting neurosis or affective disorder, if not outright simulation or exaggeration . . . (neuro) psychological testing tended to disclose diverse deficits that were not evident in the clinical examination and its effect was to strengthen the proposition that the behavioral changes with mild or moderate closed head injuries were, in fact, produced by post-traumatic alterations in brain function. (pp. 111–112).

There has, indeed, been a virtual explosion of published data on the neuropsychological sequelae of TBI, some of which are reviewed later in this chapter.

❑ COMPLIMENTARY INFERENTIAL APPROACHES TO THE INTERPRETATION OF NEUROPSYCHOLOGICAL TEST DATA

Certain neuropsychological measures and test batteries are amenable to a multilevel method of clinical diagnostic inference involving both interindividual and intraindividual comparisons. This method permits a comparison of test performances relative to a cohort reference group as well as within the patient's own brain-behavior status, which, of course, implicates the importance of the utilization of a comprehensive battery of measures in the examination of the patient with TBI.[11] These established methods of inference, which are typically combined with clinical interview, history, and observation, are as follows: (1) level of performance, (2) comparison of right and left sides of the body on upper extremity sensory-perceptual and motor measures, (3) identification of pathognomonic signs, and (4) analysis of configurations and relationships of performance among various measures.

Level of Performance

Assessing a patient's performance requires a comparison of his or her score on any given test with the known distribution of scores for normal and/or pathological populations. This assessment can also be used to categorize a patient's performance as falling within the "normal" or "abnormal" range, provided that valid cut-off scores are available for the measure utilized. However, as Boll[12] and Reitan and Wolfson[8] have observed, this approach does present potential problems. The overlap in score distribution between normal and neurologically impaired individuals is frequently too great to apply this interpretive approach as the exclusive method for differential diagnosis. For instance, Dikmen et al.[11] report that 25 percent of their (non-TBI) trauma control group had Halstead Impairment Index scores of 0.3 or worse, whereas more than 25 percent of the TBI sample with coma length up to 2 weeks had scores of 0.3 or better.

In considering optimal cut-off scores for an expanded Halstead-Reitan Battery (HRB), Heaton et al.[13] report that only 10 percent of 455 normal subjects produced absolutely *no* impaired scores, and the median number of impaired scores across 40 different measures was 4. They emphasized, "It is a serious mistake to assume that one or more test scores beyond the accepted cut-off scores always indicate the presence of an acquired cerebral disorder" (p. 36). This point is particularly critical with regard to minimizing the false-positive error rate in diagnostic decisions. It is similarly important to emphasize that certain individuals demonstrate above-average performances despite having sustained cerebral damage and that some people deliver poor performances who, in fact, do not have cerebral damage. The level of performance approach is an interindividual inferential method that compares central tendency in relation to variability in two or more groups. Of course, as suggested, the biologic condition of the brain is not the only factor that influences performance on neuropsychological measures. Relevant sociodemographic variables, personality differences in approach to examination challenges, completeness of motivation, and other relevant factors (e.g., depression, pain, distraction, fatigue, and psychopharmacological effects) can have an impact on an individual's performance. Finally, the collection of tests employed to examine the patient with TBI should not be based solely on adequacy of performance but, rather, should also address potential intraindividual variations in performance.

Comparison of Performances Between the Two Sides of the Body

A number of measures, particularly those in the HRB, produce quantifiable comparisons on upper extremity sensory and motor measures that augment the standard neurological examination. Using the patient as his or her own control offers certain advantages to a comparison of performance relative to a normative group. The relative relationship between the dominant and nondominant upper extremities is predictable, and abnormal discrepancies may be associated with a neurological substrate, particularly if peripheral factors can be ruled out. As a general principle, increased celerity, strength, and dexterity are expected with dominant hand vis-à-vis nondominant hand performance on *motoric* measures (e.g., finger oscillation, strength of grip); however, interpretation must consider the frequency with which given differences occur in the neurologically normal population.[14,15] Symmetrical results are expected between the two sides of the body on sensory-perceptual measures (e.g., tactile finger recognition, fingertip number writing perception). The expected patterns of performance on more complex tasks involving sensory and motor processes may be less evident because of the auxiliary cognitive requirements involved.

Comparison of performances between the two sides of the body is less influenced by most of the factors that confound level of performance interpretations, such as age, education, and anxiety. These patient characteristics are less relevant with this approach, given the likelihood that both sides of the body would be affected equally. Certain neurological lesions may produce lateralized sensory, motor, or psychomotor discrepancies, and this method of inference may yield useful information about the hemispheric localization of such centrally mediated deficits. For instance, damage to the primary motor or premotor cortex often produces a dysfunction of fine motor movements in the contralateral hand. With regard to the effects of TBI, upper extremity motor skills are as predictive of postinjury employment as higher-level cognitive skills.[16,17] The motor programming requirements of a task such as finger oscillation, with its emphasis on speed and pacing, may be associated with information-processing deficits rather than motor dysfunction per se, making it useful in evaluating recovery course and outcome from TBI.[18] Although motor and sensory tasks are each differentially sensitive to brain-behavior dysfunction, procedures that involve sensory-motor integration (e.g., pegboard tasks) increase the sensitivity to cerebral changes.[19] In any event, diagnostic considerations in the individual case must consider the relationship across the various measures administered.

Pathognomonic Signs

Certain examination behaviors, by their very presence, may represent neurological dysfunction. This method typically requires a dichotomous decision as to the presence or absence of the pathognomonic behavior. This component is especially valuable because true-positive results are relatively rare but always highly predictive. Of course, the difficulties inherent in the pathognomonic sign approach include the relative subjectivity of the clinician's evaluation and the low base rate for positive responses, which may increase the likelihood of obtaining false-negative errors. It is similar to the standard neurological examination in which a sign, such as the Babinski reflex, is considered pathognomonic of an upper motor neuron lesion. A potential weakness of this inferential strategy is its failure to distinguish a significant proportion of individuals with bona fide brain-behavior dysfunction. Moreover, certain neurological diseases do not produce observable pathognomonic signs. Tension centers around the fact that it is necessary to administer relatively simple untimed tasks (e.g., naming common objects) to avoid complications associated with level of performance, and a brain impaired patient may perform in a normal manner, which, of course, increases the false-negative error rate. However, "a single defective performance, when it occurs, is still a valid indication of brain impairment"[8] (p. 153).

At present, there is no comprehensive or authoritative listing of pathognomonic signs. There are also no standard scoring criteria for determination of a pathognomonic sign. However, Reitan and Wolfson[8] provide useful guidelines along with patient examples to assist the process for certain pathognomonic signs. To a great extent, the successful application of this method of inference depends on the sophistication and experience of the clinician. Reitan[20] has emphasized, "As with interpretations of EEG tracings, it is necessary to teach recognition of these kinds of deficiencies by example" (p. 17).

Analysis of Configurations and Relationships of Performance

Heaton et al.[13] have stated, "What distinguishes the normals from persons with acquired brain disorders is not just the number or even the severity of deficits, but also the nature and *pattern* of those deficits" (p. 36). Indeed, an analysis of the configuration and relationship of performances across various measures can reveal more about a patient's brain-behavior status than how the patient performed on each test individually. This method represents an *intra*individual comparison procedure that is useful in identifying the uniqueness of an individual's cognitive ability structure. Of course, the necessity of considering base rates in the interpretation of the configurations and patterns produced by the patient is of particular importance. A simple example of this method of interpretation involves significant differences in Verbal and Performance IQ. Most clinicians administering the WAIS-R to acutely injured TBI patients have come to recognize the common pattern of a lower Performance IQ relative to Verbal IQ.[21,22] In part, it can be accounted for by a diminution in central processing speed commonly associated with diffuse brain injury, which interferes with performance efficiency on novel visually guided tasks for which expeditiousness is demanded. The rate at which this pattern resolves is often an indicator of recovery of overall cognitive efficiency.

Kaufman[23] provides useful base rate percentages for Verbal IQ–Performance IQ differences found in the WAIS-R standardization sample at different Full-Scale IQ levels. Finally, a potential weakness of this method—namely, practice effects from previous testing on relative score configurations—is discussed later.

The use of a comprehensive collection of neuropsychological measures allows use of most or all of these interpretive methods in the individual case. The relative emphasis on one approach versus another is often based on the patient, injury, and referral characteristics, as well as the measures administered.

Second-party ratings of the patient's behavior can be a useful adjunct to the formal neuropsychological examination, with its focus on the measurement of cognitive functioning. Although such methods are a relatively common component of assessments conducted with children, their application with adults is far more limited. The Neuropsychology Behavior and Affect Profile (NBAP) shows promise as a standardized and well-validated instrument specifically developed for use with brain impaired patients.[24-26] The individual (often a family member) completing the questionnaire responds to a variety of rationally derived items that pertain to behaviors and emotions as either present or absent, both preinjury and currently. This format permits a direct comparison of perceived changes and their magnitude relative to the patient's premorbid status. A parallel form is available for the patient to complete about himself or herself, providing another dimension of comparison of perceptions regarding the patient. These responses form the basis for a profile that includes four validity scales and the following five clinical scales: Indifference (anosognosia or denial of illness), Inappropriateness (unusual or bizarre behavior), Pragnosia (defects in the pragmatics of communicative style), Depression (apathy, withdrawal, crying behavior, and sadness), and Mania (impulsivity, irritability, and euphoria). Satz et al.[26] found the validity scales to be effective in differentiating trained simulators from informants of two groups of patients with TBI.

◻ PREPARING THE PATIENT FOR NEUROPSYCHOLOGICAL EXAMINATION

The goal of the neuropsychological examination is not to produce merely a *typical* performance but rather the *optimal* performance. Accordingly, a valid examination requires the expenditure of time in the preparation of the patient to facilitate the necessary intrapersonal and interpersonal conditions. Because behavior is sampled across a range of activities, and diagnostic inferences are made regarding the patient's brain-behavior status, it is imperative that the examiner inspires the patient to undertake an enthusiastic exploration of his or her cognitive abilities. Of course, there is no simple formula here, and clinical acumen regarding individual differences in personality and cultural background must dictate in the individual case. Analogies and metaphors can be presented in an attempt to explain the purpose and nature of the examination. For instance, certain patients find useful a weight-lifting analogy: To measure their physical strength, the number of plates on the bar will gradually be increased until the bar cannot be fully elevated. Some patients enjoy the opportunity to perform for the examiner, and others are self-conscious about being observed; both dispositions may relate to the patient's adaptation to current deficits as well as to a unique reinforcement history. With conscientious patients, simply indicating that the examination has been requested by their doctor is often sufficient to elicit complete cooperation. With many patients, references to "testing" should be avoided, inasmuch as this term may connote judgment and potential for failure. It may hold negative valence for individuals whose school experiences were inauspicious.

Referrals by attorneys often do not allow for subsequent follow-up and treatment or for doctor-patient privileges, issues that need to be clarified. In these cases, it may be useful to assure the patient that, if he or she delivers a full effort, the procedures employed are capable of identifying neuropsychological changes that may be present. This approach may also dissuade the apprehensive patient intending to "assist" the examiner by accentuating his or her difficulties in response to different examination challenges. Such sensitivities to the patient ultimately decrease their anxiety, suspicion, and resistance and increase the integrity of the data collected.

The presence of others in the examination room is to be avoided. Although this point seems intuitively obvious, this issue has recently come to the forefront of attention because of the frequent requests by those in the legal community for neuropsychological examination of litigants. Changes in performance associated with the presence of a third-party observer during examination have been demonstrated.[27] In this regard, McCaffrey et al.[28] have discussed the social psychological phenomenon of social facilitation (performing in the presence of another person) and its potential effects on performance in the neuropsychological examination. Binder and Johnson-Greene[27] conclude that "current knowledge suggests that unnecessary observers . . . should be excluded from the examination of adult patients because tests are standardized and validated without significant others present in the examination room" (p. 78).

The essential point in preparing the patient is that neuropsychological evaluation involves the collection of behavioral observations and measurements elicited from an injured person who is placed in a subordinate role. From the patient's perspective, they are required to perform activities with which they may have had no previous experience and do not fully understand and that require many hours of dedicated effort. In this latter respect, the neuropsychological examination is strikingly different from most neuromedical evaluations. From the neuropsychologist's perspective, the examination is an experiment in which samples of complex motivated human behavior are elicited, observed, measured, and interpreted across a wide range of neurocognitive domains. The emphasis on participatory behavior represents another critical distinction between the neuropsychological examination and certain medical procedures. During these latter procedures, the patient often is required to remain relatively passive; the only necessary behavior is compliance.

☐ EXAMINATION OF PATIENTS WITH SPECIAL NEEDS

Brain injured patients presenting with certain types of disabilities and levels of impairment may pose unique challenges in conducting a neuropsychological examination. Assessment modifications may be required when limitations in the patient's ability to respond interfere with standard test administration.

Such limitations may be associated with preexisting as well as traumatically induced defects in receptive or expressive neurobehavioral modalities. When a patient has significant difficulty seeing the test materials, hearing the examiner, speaking, or handling and manipulating objects, deviations from the standard administration of the test battery may be unavoidable.

However, decision making in these instances should, of course, strive to minimize departures from the standard protocol. Each step removed from standardized and normed procedures that have been validated with the brain injured population may challenge the reliability and validity of the obtained data as well as the degree of confidence that can be placed in their interpretation. Moreover, when a routine measure is replaced with another test, it may be the case that the substitute does not provide equivalent coverage of the neuropsychological functions of interest. (For example, a recognition memory paradigm may overcome a variety of limitations that interfere with the administration of standard memory batteries, but critical aspects of memory—such as multitrial learning, free retrieval, and delayed recall—will not be covered.)

Consideration should be given first to modification of procedures in a manner that allows standard measures to be employed. Examples include shifting the location of visual stimulus material to the unaffected hemispace for unilateral inattention or homonymous field cuts; writing instructions for the hearing impaired; permitting written responses, pointing, or use of augmentative communication devices for oral motor dysfunction; using the nondominant hand during visuomotor tasks for dominant-sided hemiparesis. When procedural modifications are inadequate, consideration may be given to the alteration of standard materials. Examples include rearranging visual stimulus arrays from horizontal to vertical for hemispatial inattention or hemianopsia and enlarging print for decreased visual acuity. Finally, alternative measures may be required. In this regard, Lezak's *Neuropsychological Assessment*[29] is a useful resource that describes a wide range of neuropsychological tests and clinical procedures.

Severely impaired patients in the acute phase of recovery also pose assessment challenges. As a general rule, data obtained while the patient is in an altered state of consciousness (i.e., post-traumatic amnesia; PTA) are of limited value because of the pervasive effects of the confusional state, and it is advisable to delay administration of comprehensive testing until PTA has sufficiently subsided.[30] The severity, course, and resolution of PTA may be tracked by daily administration of a brief measure of PTA. The Galveston Orientation and Amnesia Test[31] (GOAT) is widely employed in acute medical settings for such a purpose. When PTA has sufficiently resolved as indicated by a certain score threshold on the GOAT, administration of a standard battery may be precluded by profound cognitive impairment. In such cases, Lezak[29] recommends consideration of measures designed for younger patients that allow performances to be assessed in terms of age levels.

□ ESTIMATION OF STATUS BEFORE TRAUMATIC BRAIN INJURY

Babcock[32] and later Yates[33] reported that certain psychological tasks, such as vocabulary, were relatively resilient to the effects of cerebral damage, whereas performance on other tests—most notably memory, learning, and motor speed—were frequently diminished. This observation became a basis for the notion that premorbid functioning could, in fact, be estimated and used as a comparison with currently obtained results.

Various procedures have since been developed in an effort to provide some estimation of cognitive functioning prior to the TBI. These procedures include mathematical modeling of sociodemographic variables and current measure estimates such as word reading. Regression modeling of sociodemographic variables in approximating WAIS-R IQ values[34] is useful in providing general parameter estimates, but it frequently produces values within a restricted range complicated by large standard error of estimates (12 to 13 IQ points). If premorbid Full Scale IQ is above 115 or below 85 (i.e., one plus or minus standard deviation from the mean), this formula likely results in artifactual ceiling-floor effects. The inclusion of certain performance variables (WAIS-R Vocabulary and Picture Completion subtests) has been reported to attenuate the range problem while increasing the predictive validity of the Barona index.[35] Sweet et al.[36] reported that the Barona formula did not predict better than chance when employed with neurologically normal psychiatric patients and a heterogeneous sample of brain damaged patients. They concluded, "Although the formulas appear to be fairly reliable for *groups* of patients, there is no assurance that the estimates produced by the regression formulas will be accurate in individual cases. . . . In general, these formulas may be useful in research (i.e., matching subjects) or when cautiously used in conjunction with past records (e.g., school or military). However, they should not be used in isolation with individual patients" (p. 43). While limited, this approach does offer the advantage of applicability to a variety of patients; in fact, one need not actually examine the patient to apply the index.

Procedures requiring the correct pronunciation of irregularly spelled words (e.g., *colonel*, *debris*), which have little relationship to normal phonetics, can provide another estimate of a literate patient's premorbid intellectual functioning, based on two principal assumptions: (1) Accurate reading of such words requires previous familiarity (recognition), which is based on rote knowledge and past education rather than current ability to phonetically decode (process) the words; and (2) word reading ability in general is fairly resilient to intellectual decline.[37,38] Unfortunately, this procedure also produces a restricted range of scores with overestimates and underestimates. However, the inclusion of gender and education as predictor variables provided a superior estimate to either word reading measured with the National Adult Reading Test (NART) or demographics alone.[39] Race and parental education, when combined with performance on the Wide Range Achievement Test–Revised (WRAT-R), expanded the range of prediction of this method, which relies less on irregularly spelled words.[40] Word reading procedures such as the North American Adult Reading Test (NAART) produce much smaller standard errors of estimate than the Barona index, and a discrepancy of 15 points between estimated and obtained Verbal or Full Scale IQ identifies intellectual deterioration at the 95 percent confidence level.[37] Obviously, such procedures cannot be used with patients who are aphasic, have a preexisting reading disorder, or have a disturbance of visual acuity. Its use with people whose native language is not English needs to be done cautiously, if at all.

In spite of the need for the neuropsychologists to precisely infer premorbid cognitive status, at present there is no uniformly agreed upon method for doing so. Of course, a thoughtful review of all available school, medical, and occupational records continues to be essential in arriving at estimations in the individual case. Matarazzo[41] emphasizes,

> The assessment of intelligence, personality, or type or level of impairment is a highly complex operation that involves extracting diagnostic meaning from an individual's personal history and objectively recorded test scores. Rather than being totally objective, assessment involves a subjective component. . . . In the hands of a good clinician, the results of an examination of intelligence or personality, correlated with information from the person's history, are as useful as analogous information would be in the hands of a good surgeon, internist, accountant or plumber. (pp. 1000–1001)

Sbordone[42] asserts that many patients with TBI are unreliable historians and recommends interviewing collateral sources. He offers that a careful review of the patient's background information "will frequently uncover a history of preexisting neurological disease, psychological problems, prior head trauma, drowning episodes, seizures, hyperactivity, dyslexia, left-handedness, stuttering, sexual molestation and rape, alcoholism, criminal behavior, poor academic performance, or drug abuse" (p. 27). Such information can, of course, be probative in making necessary discriminations between preexisting functional limitations and those directly associated with TBI. Such determinations are of interest to those developing a treatment plan with realistic expectations, as well as to attorneys and third-party payers concerned about the issue of liability.

☐ PRACTICE EFFECTS ASSOCIATED WITH RETESTING

The need to reexamine patients can be related to monitoring recovery, evaluating treatment efficacy, or desiring a second opinion or as a part of the tactical position of an attorney seeking to have a client examined by a professional of their own choosing. In discussing this issue, Dikmen et al.[11] observe, "In clinical practice, it is nearly impossible to find a head-injured patient who has not been tested at least once during the year postinjury" (p. 87). *Practice effect* is a term associated with *artifactual* improvements in test scores related to familiarity with the testing procedures. Of course, certain kinds of improvement evidenced by patients in retesting are readily observable (e.g., reduction of hemiparesis), and other kinds of change may often be associated primarily with practice effects (e.g., quicker assembly of a puzzle). It is a relatively complex issue, and at present there is no uniformly agreed-upon time interval between initial testing and retesting to mitigate the influence of practice effects. Furthermore, a wide range of test batteries and procedures are used throughout the neuropsychological community,[29] and a given patient may be presented with a completely different array of measures at retesting, which would minimize practice effects.

One particularly troublesome aspect of the practice effect issue is the application of normative data (e.g., comprehensive norms[13]), which are based on a single administration of the respective tests to the reference sample. Given the differential sensitivity of many neuropsychological measures to retesting across different time intervals, application of these norms to an individual tested on a second or third occasion with the same instruments may produce further imprecision. Concerning abnormal intertest scatter in retest profiles (e.g., WAIS-R), the differential sensitivity of each subtest to practice effects needs thoughtful consideration in interpreting the test profile configurally.[43] Similarly, it is unknown if pathognomonic intratest scatter on

WAIS-R subtests is mitigated when the patient is retested.[44] A further complication is the effects of different types and severities of TBI and the length of time postinjury. Reitan and Wolfson[8] have asserted:

> There is no way to know that the amount of practice effect (improvement on successive testings) of a control group would be perfectly equivalent to the practice effect expected from brain injured subjects. It is entirely possible that subjects with a brain injury would not be able to profit as much or learn as much from previous exposure to the tests as control subjects. Variations might even be expected to occur differentially among brain damaged subjects, with more impaired persons being able to profit from earlier testing experience less well. (p. 366)

In any event, it will continue to remain a pressing issue in contemporary practice. As suggested by Putnam et al.,[45] "Learning to discriminate practice effects from actual behavioral change may well become the assessment challenge of the 1990s" (p. 316).

An interesting collateral of this issue has been the comparison of test-retest results in order to indirectly evaluate the representativeness of the patient's behavior. Cullum et al.[46] assert that "examination of performance reliability across testings may be a powerful means by which neuropsychologists can detect patients who are not consistently putting forth adequate effort on the examination" (p. 168). Based on this premise, Reitan and Wolfson[47] recently developed the Retest Consistency Index and Response Consistency Index, which utilize a comparison of difference scores from several WAIS subtests and HRB variables to form a Dissimulation Index. The authors reasoned, "If the subject was not putting forth maximum effort, the scores on the two testings would be more variable, and perhaps even worse on the second testing, because of the need to 'prove' one's impairment as the time of judgment came closer" (p. 575). They report this index differentially classified 100 percent of the litigating versus nonlitigating patients who sustained TBI; that is, the results demonstrated that the retest performances of the litigating TBI patients were significantly less consistent between the two testings. Such an approach to the assessment of motivation appears promising, having the advantage of using the patient as his or her own control while being unrelated to the patient's level of performance.

Sawrie et al.[48] have employed a method for determining meaningful change that computes a Reliable Change (RC) index score and employs a regression procedure to establish norms for expected change from baseline performances for each of the measures administered. Baseline scores were regressed on retest scores, with age, education, duration of illness, and the interval between the initial and second testing entered as predictors and the results standardized to a common metric to facilitate clinical application. Sawrie et al.[48] assert, "Through the use of the applied RC cutoff values and regression change norms, the clinician is able to evaluate both the significance and magnitude of change across various cognitive measures. . . . This offers a distinct advantage over previous arbitrary methods such as determining change on the basis of one standard deviation movement from baseline performance" (p. 563). Although the RC is an important step forward in addressing this issue, it will be necessary to apply these methods to local samples of patients who have sustained TBI to derive relevant change norms and cutoff values.

☐ TRAUMATIC BRAIN INJURY AND LITIGATION

A chapter on neuropsychological assessment and TBI would not be representative of contemporary practice without coverage of its application in legal proceedings. At present, neuropsychological assessment of the patient with TBI typically involves litigation. However, the presence of neuropsychologists in the court room is a relatively recent development, and not without controversy.[49,50] Schwartz[51] has discussed how neuropsychological assessment is a painless and non-life-threatening procedure that is deemed an acceptable method for determination of (1) presence or absence of brain damage, (2) preinjury and postinjury comparisons of changes in mental and emotional functioning, (3) an individual's standing in relation to normative groups to determine current level of ability and degree of deviation from the norm, (4) anatomic comparisons and contrasts with neurodiagnostic measures, and (5) the *type* of brain damage present. Schwartz[51] explains, "Since one or several of these matters is usually at issue in legal cases, neuropsychologists have had an obvious and expanded role in the legal arena" (p. 52). Lees-Haley[52] has elaborated on this matter by emphasizing, "The neuropsychological evaluation can substantiate causality . . . and may be able to explain troubling claims like reports of loss of memory for critical events . . . [and] apparent discrepancies in the claim (e.g., when some brain functions appear normal in someone claiming serious brain impairment" (pp. 84–85). Despite what appears to be a proliferating presence in the courtroom, a recent survey of 1521 neuropsychologists reported that half of the sample were not involved in forensic activities.[53]

This increase in forensic applications of neuropsychology has introduced dramatic changes into the examination milieu, such as requests for observers or recording devices in the examination room,[23] "an unfavorable motivational context [in which patients] are rewarded with financial compensation for poor performance,"[54] the accentuation and interference of psychosocial factors,[55] an adversarial role vis-à-vis the patient,[41] requests for raw test data to be sent to nonpsychologists,[56] the potential for malingering,[55,57] and even reports of attorneys who "coach" patients prior to a scheduled neuropsychological examination.[58] The insidious role of confirmatory bias has taken on a renewed emphasis in this adversarial and highly remunerative environment,[53,59] which, of course, underscores the considerable importance of recognizing that neuropsychological test scores alone do not indicate the presence or nature of residuals from a TBI but, rather, the interpretation of the data by the neuropsychologist. As expressed by Fastenau and Adams,[60] "Simple deviance from neurologically normal performances as a brainless . . . definition of impairment has simply gotten out of hand" (p. 448). Of course, professional competency is at the heart of the issue and relates directly to the training and credentialing necessary to perform neuropsychological examinations of patients.[61–63] As Lezak declared,[29] "The amount of additional knowledge that must be absorbed and the variety of additional clinical skills that must be learned and polished preclude any quick acquisition of neuropsychological expertise" (pp. 4–5). The proliferation of the inadequately trained practitioner appears to be precisely what Matthews[64] has referred to as the "malignant bloom nourished by the head injury industry" (p. 33).

☐ DEMOGRAPHIC ADJUSTMENTS, BASE RATES, AND THE SENSITIVITY-SPECIFICITY ISSUE

Adjustments of score values based on sociodemographic characteristics of the patient are a common practice in contemporary clinical neuropsychological assessment. Reitan and Wolfson[8] state, "It is well recognized that a person's chronological age, education, socioeconomic status, medical history, personality, specific skills, and the host of variables that determine human individuality are all factors that contribute to an individual's psychological performance" (p. 25). However, not all agree on the appropriate application of such normative data to individuals with neurological dysfunction.

Reitan and Wolfson[5] have recently protested, "The diminished significance of age and education among brain damaged subjects indicates that interpretation of neuropsychological data should depend on test results that are definite indicators of brain damage . . . rather than rely on scores adjusted for attribute variables" (p. 156). A consensus on this issue does not exist, but it will surely generate energetic debate within the profession. The application of demographically derived norms is much less complex in examining patients with milder-spectrum TBI, given the uncertainty of classifying these patients as "brain damaged subjects." As reported by Alves et al.,[65] Dikmen et al.,[11,66] and Levin et al.,[67] neuropsychological outcome from mild TBI is quite favorable, and the application of normative data based on samples without brain damage would appear to be without controversy.

Perhaps the most widely used normative data base in contemporary clinical neuropsychology has been developed by Heaton et al.[13] However, this system, with its companion software, has recently been criticized for producing 21 subdivisions (based on 10 age, 6 educational, and 2 gender levels) with an inadequate number of subjects represented in certain cells.[60] In part, this is a result of providing corrections for *all* 54 of the measures employed, even those for which no demographic influence had been demonstrated (e.g., age alone accounts for variance on Tactual Performance Test, dominant hand performance). Heaton et al.[68] respond that their demographic corrections employed only age and education, with three levels each, which produced 9 rather than 120 cells. Furthermore, they emphasize that the score transformations based on demographic characteristics were based on more than 350 subjects for the majority of measures in their battery. These authors conclude, "All available data strongly suggest that substantial demographic biases are eliminated or greatly reduced by using the demographically corrected norms" (p. 457). It is not a dichotomous decision to use or not use these norms. Rather, it is imperative that the clinician is informed about the limitations and appropriate application of the norms.

Even when demographic adjustments are available and appropriately applied, proper consideration must be given to (1) sensitivity (true positive rate), the proportion of patients with a condition (e.g., TBI) who are identified by a positive examination finding; and (2) specificity (true negative rate), the proportion of patients without a condition (e.g., TBI) who are correctly identified by a negative or normal examination. Of course, unequivocal confirmation that the patient has sustained a TBI is again

more complex when these statistical concepts are applied to milder severity cases. Moreover, even though a mild TBI may have occurred in the past, symptom resolution may be complete at the time of neuropsychological examination. In any event, the sensitivity and specificity of the measures utilized can overcome the limitations of between-group comparisons based strictly on statistical significance. However, these statistics cannot definitively determine if a given patient has the particular disorder that is the focus of the examination. This, of course, requires the calculation of the local base rate or prevalence of the condition in question. Awareness and use of diagnostic efficiency statistics of tests and, ideally, cutoff thresholds that are adjusted to local base rates may prevent clinicians from overinterpreting the significance of an isolated abnormal neuropsychological test score, thus resulting in a misdiagnosis. Base rates not only dictate an a priori probability that combines with diagnostic information to produce a clinical decision but also actually form the basis for the primary strategy that guides the production of hypotheses regarding the examination of the individual patient. Indeed, failure to properly consider base rate information is a critical source of diagnostic error in conducting neuropsychological examinations.[69] The importance of obtaining *local* diagnostic base rates can not be overstated; these data can be derived from clinical data bases, medical records, or epidemiological or clinical studies of comparable patient samples. It should be pointed out that patients examined at the request of an attorney may, in fact, represent a sample with different characteristics than individuals seen primarily for clinical or treatment purposes. Lees-Haley[70] has asserted, "Litigation is a special context that appears to have different base rates and different evaluation requirements than traditional therapeutic or clinical environments" (p. 387).

Because characteristics such as age, education, gender, and IQ are patient attribute variables believed to influence performance on certain neuropsychological measures, this issue must necessarily be considered in selecting tests. Published population base rates for impaired-range performance levels and the prevalence of differences in scores between independent measures also represent an important advantage in test score interpretation. Table 9–1 provides a nonexhaustive listing of neuropsychological tests and batteries and author sources for which various normative adjustments and base rates are currently available. However, the sample demographics from which the standard scores are derived may not be directly comparable across this listing of tests; that is, the conversion from a raw score to a stan-

**TABLE 9–1. Normative Information Available
for Selected Neuropsychological Tests and Batteries**

Test Name	Age	Education	Gender	IQ	Base Rates	References
Benton Visual Retention Test	X	X				Youngjohn et al.[72]
Boston Naming Test	X	X	X		X	Heaton et al.[13] Lichtenberg et al.[73] Ross et al.[74]
Buschke Selective Reminding Test	X		X			Larrabee et al.[75]
California Verbal Learning Test	X		X	X		Wiens et al.[76]
Continuous Visual Memory Test	X				X	Trahan and Larrabee[77]
Controlled Oral Word Association Test	X	X	X			Benton et al.[78] Ruff et al.[79]
Facial Recognition Test	X	X				Benton et al.[80]
Halstead-Reitan Battery	X	X	X		X	Heaton et al.[13] Warner et al.[81]
Hooper Visual Organization Test	X	X				Hooper[82]
Judgment of Line Orientation	X		X			Benton et al.[80]
Memory Assessment Scales	X	X			X	Williams[83]
Multilingual Aphasia Examination	X	X				Benton et al.[78]
Paced Auditory Serial Addition Task	X			X		Brittain et al.[84]
Peabody Individual Achievement Test	X	X	X		X	Heaton et al.[13]
Peabody Picture Vocabulary Test	X					Dunn and Dunn[85]
Recognition Memory Test	X					Warrington[86]
Rey Auditory Verbal Learning Test	X	X		X		Wiens et al.[87]
Ruff Figural Fluency Test	X	X				Ruff[88]
Stroop Neuropsychological Screening Test	X					Trenerry et al.[89]
Symbol Digit Modalities Test	X	X	X		X	Smith[90]
Thurstone Word Fluency Test	X	X	X		X	Heaton et al.[13]
Wechsler Adult Intelligence Scale–Revised	X	X	X		X	Heaton et al.[91] Warner et al.[81]
Wechsler Memory Scale–Revised	X					Wechsler[92]
Wide Range Achievement Test 3	X					Wilkinson[93]
Wisconsin Card Sorting Test	X	X	X			Heaton et al.[94]

dard score may be based on several variables (e.g., education, age, and gender) for some tests but only one or two variables on other tests (e.g., age only). Despite the use of a common metric (e.g., mean = 50, standard deviation = 10), the obtained scores may not be directly comparable. As declared by Axelrod and Goldman,[71] "Accurate interpretation of neuropsychological data is contingent on the professional's knowledge as to how demographic data are incorporated into each normative data set used" (p. 161).

❑ NEUROPSYCHOLOGICAL TEST FINDINGS ASSOCIATED WITH TRAUMATIC BRAIN INJURY

Dikmen et al.[95] have been instrumental in emphasizing the need to heed sample characteristics of studies in considering the expected course of neuropsychological recovery. In particular, studies based on *consecutive* samples of patients with TBI are most representative of the course of recovery following TBI.

Because outcome problems are the selection criteria for convenience samples, studies based on these samples permit only very limited generalizations. . . . A common error . . . is to arrive at conclusions regarding the nature, severity, and prevalence of problems in head-injured patients in general on the basis of these select samples. Because head-injured patients without permanent sequelae or with only mild persisting difficulties are simply not included, these conclusions are likely to overestimate problems in the head-injured population[96] (p. 75).

There is, of course, no invariable neuropsychological "fingerprint" pattern after TBI. Newcombe[97] has stated, "It cannot be assumed that closed head injury, resulting from a variety of different incidents and from different physical and spatial force-patterns, is a single clinical entity with a pathognomonic pattern" (p. 129). Furthermore, concerning "typical" neuropsychological findings, considerations must be given to TBI severity, time since TBI, and occurrence of secondary complications subsequent to the TBI. Reitan and Wolfson[8] point out,

> There is undoubtedly a wide range of variation among normal brains in both the level and structure of abilities. Imposed on this initial realization that normal brains vary considerably was the definite possibility that two brains sustaining similar damage may not demonstrate the exact same behavioral deficits. . . . Studies of persons with various types of lesions—located in different parts of the brain, and sustained at different times and at different ages—made it clear that brain damage showed a great deal of variability. (p. 24)

For instance, although Millis and Ricker[98] found that selective impairments in verbal learning were characteristic of all patients having sustained moderate to severe TBI, they identified four subgroups characterized by both quantitative and qualitative performance differences on the California Verbal Learning Test (CVLT). A recent replication of this study[99] supported the robustness of these subgroups while identifying distinctive patterns across several additional neuropsychological measures (e.g., Trail Making Test).

Among the most comprehensive studies providing data on patterns of neuropsychological recovery are the Traumatic Brain Injury Model Systems of Care,[100] studies from the Traumatic Coma Data Bank,[67] and a series of studies conducted by Dikmen et al. Kreutzer et al.[100] report findings from a sample of patients (n = 243) derived from five model systems centers initially

tested at an average of 48 days after moderate to severe TBI (admission Glasgow Coma Scale scores between 3 and 12). A large percentage of the sample performed in the impaired range across several attentional measures. Double Letter Cancellation Test (91 percent), Symbol Digit Modalities Test-Written and Oral (87 percent), and Trail Making Test, Part B (82 percent) and Part A (72 percent). More than three-quarters of the sample demonstrated impaired performances in fine hand-eye motor speed and dexterity in the Grooved Pegboard Test (73 percent) and verbal learning as evaluated with the Rey Auditory Verbal Learning Test (76 percent).

Equally interesting are the relatively small percentages of the sample producing impaired performances on Digit Span Backward (24%), Visual Memory Span–Backward (34%), Visual Memory Span–Forward (38%), Token Test (39%), WAIS-R Similarities (39%), Benton Visual Discrimination Test (43%), WAIS-R Block Design (47%), and Digit Span Forward (50%). The percentage of TBI patients performing acceptably on the Digit Span subtest is consistent with the findings reported by Crosson et al.[43] When the sample was retested at 1 year follow-up, significant improvements were found on 15 of 22 neuropsychological measures (68%). Changes were not found on measures of orientation (GOAT), nonverbal reasoning (Wisconsin Card Sort), and verbal concept formation (Similarities) at 1 year because in the initial testing a relatively small percentage of the sample produced impaired performances on these particular measures. Kreutzer et al.[100] state, "Improvements in test means can be misleading. . . . Patients may improve on some tests and show declines on others when tested at the same follow-up interval. . . . Declines and improvement may be differentially related to injury, age, treatment, and other factors" (p. 56).

Neuropsychological studies pertaining to early stages of recovery from TBI have focused largely on acutely injured patients in an inpatient setting. Neuropsychological assessment in an outpatient rehabilitation setting involves a postacute population in which (1) neurocognitive sequelae have demonstrated varying degrees of resolution with time and (2) the proportion of mild TBI (GCS = 13–15) cases—particularly those not requiring inpatient rehabilitation—is greater.

Tables 9–2 and 9–3 present information on the sensitivity of select neuropsychological measures and the WAIS-R in a postacute outpatient brain injury sample. The data were derived from 56 consecutive comprehensive evaluations for TBI neurorehabilitation services within the outpatient services of Rehabilitation Institute of Michigan. Sample characteristics were as follows: 64 percent of the sample was male; aver-

TABLE 9–2. Sensitivity of Select Tests to Postacute Traumatic Brain Injury (*n* = 56)

Neuropsychological Measures	Percentage Impaired*	Source of Normative Data for T-scores
Symbol Digit Modalities Test, oral	58.9	Smith[90]
Grooved Pegboard (dominant)	58.9	Heaton et al.[13]
Grooved Pegboard (nondominant)	57.1	
Symbol Digit Modalities Test, written	55.4	
MAS: List Acquisition	48.2	Williams[83]
MAS: List Recall	48.2	
MAS: Delayed List Recall	42.7	
Trailmaking Test, part B	35.7	Heaton et al.[13]
Trailmaking Test, part A	33.9	
Finger Tapping (nondominant)	30.4	Heaton et al.[13]
MAS: Verbal Memory	28.6	
Finger Tapping (dominant)	26.8	
Controlled Oral Word Association Test	26.8	Ruff et al.[79]
Visual Naming (MAE)	21.4	Benton et al.[78]
MAS: Global Memory	21.4	
MAS: Visual Memory	12.5	
MAS: Short-Term Memory	08.9	

*Impairment criterion: scores below 1.5 SD from the mean of a normative sample.

age age was 34.1 (SD = 12.7); mean years of formal education was 11.8 (SD = 2.2) and mean estimated premorbid Full Scale IQ, based upon the North American Adult Reading Test, was 93.3 (SD = 9.9); 52 percent of sample received initial emergency department GCS scores of 7 or less and 14 percent were given GCS ratings of

TABLE 9–3. Sensitivity of WAIS-R to Postacute Traumatic Brain Injury (*n* = 56)

WAIS-R Subtests and Indices	Percentage Impaired*†
Information	28.6
Object Assembly	26.8
Verbal Scale IQ	26.8
Full Scale IQ	23.2
Digit Symbol	21.4
Performance Scale IQ	19.6
Vocabulary	19.6
Block Design	17.9
Comprehension	17.9
Arithmetic	16.1
Picture Arrangement	16.1
Picture Completion	08.9
Similarities	07.2
Digit Span	05.4

*T-scores based upon normative data from Heaton et al.[91]
†Impairment criterion: scores below 1.5 SD from the mean of a normative sample.

15; mean and median time postinjury were, respectively, 7.6 (SD = 13.2) and 3 months; motor vehicle accidents were the cause of injury in 72 percent of the cases; and 36 percent of the cases involved litigation or workers' compensation.

Although the overall sensitivity of all the neuropsychological measures to brain injury was lower for the postacute group than for the more acute population, the rank ordering of neurocognitive tasks from most to least sensitive was, in fact, quite similar. Challenges requiring manual dexterity, complex attention, executive control, and auditory-verbal learning exhibited the highest sensitivity; measures of psychomotor speed, immediate memory span, linguistic functioning, and general intellectual abilities were least sensitive. Certain tests—specifically, the WAIS-R Digit Span, Similarities, and Picture Completion subtests—appeared to be strikingly insensitive to brain injury at the postacute level.

Dikmen et al.[11] have stressed the importance of conducting a neuropsychological examination that provides comprehensive information about brain-behavior relationships in TBI. They studied a large representative sample with varying degrees of TBI severity across a wide range of neuropsychological measures. Minimum selection criteria consisted of a period of loss of consciousness or post-traumatic amnesia for at least 1 hour and hospitalization. A control group of 132 individuals (matched for age, sex, and education) had sustained various bodily traumas not including the head. This prospective study of 436 TBI patients examined at 1 year postinjury found a clear dose-response relationship between length of coma (time to follow commands) and neuropsychological test performance. Dikmen et al.[11] state,

> Even with a single index of severity (duration of coma or time to follow commands) there is essentially a continuum, with small differences in severity being reflected in small differences in outcome . . . more reliable differences between head-injured and the controls are on measures of simple motor (e.g., Finger Tapping Test) and psychomotor problem-solving speed (Tactual Performance Test) and overall neuropsychological performance (Impairment Index) rather than on more specific measures of attention and memory. (p. 84)

As severity of the TBI increased, diminution of upper extremity motor speed became more evident. For instance, as coma length increased from the level of 7 to 13 days to the level of 14 to 28 days, dominant-hand finger-tapping speed declined from an average of 44 to 36 taps per 10-second periods. Marked decrements in neuropsychological test performance also became more prominent in other cognitive domains as TBI severity increased. Across the same coma length interval, the number of errors on the Halstead Category Test, a measure of abstract and conceptual reasoning, increased from an average of 50 to 78, and Trail Making Part B time increased from an average of 101 to 165 seconds.

Toward the other end of the severity continuum, no differences were found on these measures between the control group and the patients sustaining the mildest TBIs at 1 year follow-up. In fact, Dikmen et al.[11] declare, "Significant neuropsychological impairment due to a mild head injury is as unlikely as is escaping an impairment in the case of a very severe head injury" (p. 87). A particular strength in the Dikmen et al.[11] study is the inclusion of a comprehensive neuropsychological test battery, which revealed considerable variability in performance, especially apparent among the more severe TBI groups. However, a general pattern was reported for patients experiencing 2 weeks or more of coma to display more significant impairments on all measures administered at 1 year than groups with less severe TBI.

□ NEUROPSYCHOLOGICAL EXAMINATION AND OUTCOME PREDICTION

Thus far, the focus of the chapter has been directed toward assessing a patient's current neurocognitive status. The remaining sections address the application of neuropsychological data in anticipating common postacute challenges. The *predictive* use of these data is of paramount importance to the treatment team, the patient, and the family. Specifically, neuropsychological data are an integral element in the determination of prognosis of potential vocational status, level of functional independence within the home and community, and identification of cognitive impairments.

□ VOCATIONAL OUTCOME

The ability of neuropsychological test data to forecast vocational outcome has been relatively well established in the TBI literature.[101-105] Crepeau and Scherzer[102] reviewed the vocational outcome literature, including the predictive power of neuropsychological test variables. Subjecting 41 studies that met rigorous inclusion criteria to meta-analysis, they found a constellation of neurocognitive domains associated with vocational outcome. Executive functioning measures, such as the Wisconsin Card Sorting Test and the Trail Making Test, correlated highly with employment outcome. Measures of language, visually oriented cognitive domains, and global cognitive status (e.g., intellectual test scores and Halstead Impairment Index) were moderately associated with employment status.

Recent studies have demonstrated that neuropsychological data obtained relatively soon after TBI are useful in predicting later vocational outcome. Baseline measures of motor speed, selective attention, prose memory, visuoconstruction, and mental flexibility were associated with job or school status at 6 months postinjury in a study of 93 cases from the Traumatic Coma Data Bank.[106] The Halstead Impairment Index, a summarical value derived from seven variables in the HRB, computed at 1 month postinjury proved to be a powerful predictor of employment status during the first year for 366 TBI cases reported by Dikmen et al.[104]

As the interval of time between injury and administration of neuropsychological testing increases, the predictive power of the test data becomes attenuated. In the Traumatic Coma Data Bank study, predictors of later job and school status were more limited and largely confined to motor speed, selective attention, and visuoconstruction at 6 months postinjury compared with baseline testing.[106] Fraser et al.[16] report that neuropsychological data at both 1 month and 1 year postinjury were predictive of employment outcome; however, the predictive power of test scores gathered at 1 year was notably weaker than that collected at 1 month. Neuropsychological test data gathered 4 years after TBI did not prove to predict vocational or academic status.[107]

Taken as a whole, the research literature indicates that neuropsychological measurement can serve as a valuable tool in the process of vocational planning and decision making. Patients and their families need guidance in developing reasonable expectations as to when the patient can work again and at what level of proficiency. Providers also require reliable prognostic data to plan for the rehabilitation and vocational needs of TBI patients. Bowman[101] recently found, "In terms of occupational functioning and everyday activities, scores on tests of cognitive and emotional functioning provided more accurate guidance as to what might be expected of a discharged patient in comparison with biomedical indicators" (p. 390).

Global severity of neurocognitive impairment indices and the pattern of deficits provide a basis for estimating time frames for the initiation of prevocational rehabilitation and subsequent return to work.

The importance of conducting a *comprehensive* neuropsychological evaluation very *early* after the injury is clearly demonstrated with respect to vocational considerations. Intuitively, it may seem as though the benefits of administering a lengthy battery of tests during the first couple of months will be more than offset by the challenge of such an undertaking or that early testing simply will not provide helpful data. We would assert the contrary. The research reviewed here demonstrates that the information derived from assessments conducted soon after the injury, particularly a comprehensive evaluation at 1 month postinjury,[104] is more powerful than later neuropsychological data or any other clinical variables[102] with respect to forecasting vocational needs and outcome.

When neuropsychological data are interpreted and communicated to others for vocational planning purposes, it is important to avoid statements that preclude a return to meaningful, productive activity. The experience of Wehman et al.[108] in returning patients with severe TBI to work has led them to conclude that, even for difficult vocational cases, positive outcomes are, in fact, attainable, although admittedly less frequent.[109]

Identifying the circumstances under which a brain injured person will be able to work requires more than a simple review of test scores. Both the nature of the job held prior to the injury and the nature of the deficits produced by the injury must be carefully considered. For example, the more a job entails overlearned skills involving routines and procedures, with less demand for independent decision-making and executive organizational capacities, the better the prognosis for a successful return to the premorbid work position. At the same time, consideration must be given to the nature of the neurocognitive sequelae, particularly those aspects of cognition that have proven to be critical vocational indicators—namely, motor speed, complex attention and executive control, memory, visuoconstructional skills, and global cognitive status. The greater the severity of deficits in these neurocognitive domains, the more likely it is that vocational rehabilitation will require extensive preparation and job coaching, a modified work situation, or supported employment. The task of the neuropsychologist is to analyze the test data with particular attention to the "fit" between the job demands and the patient's repertoire of measured skills.

The analysis of neuropsychological data for vocational purposes also involves the integration of test findings with other factors related to vocational outcome, including the preinjury sociodemographic variables of age, level of education, work history and type of occupation, and socioeconomic status. Moreover, probative peri-injury variables such as GCS score, duration of coma, length of hospitalization, severity of physical limitations, and presence of significant psychosocial impairment must be reviewed.[102,104,106,108,110–112] An understanding of the relative contribution of each of these personal and injury-related variables to the prediction of vocational outcome is essential.

❑ PSYCHOSOCIAL OUTCOME

A fundamental marker of recovery and rehabilitation outcome is the degree to which individuals regain their premorbid level of independence within the home and community. This category, often referred to as *psychosocial outcome,* typically subsumes a conglomeration of endeavors: both basic and advanced activities of daily living (ADLs), management of household role functions, community involvement, and management of transportation within the community, including safe operation of a motor vehicle. Data that forecast the probable level of independence a TBI patient will eventually reach provide a necessary framework for allocating resources and planning for the future needs of the patient.

Recent literature addressing the relationship between neuropsychological test data and psychosocial outcome[101,103,113] has found grounds for, in the view of Rosenthal and Millis,[113] "cautious optimism." Although data have, on the whole, been encouraging, the quantity of research in this area has been relatively modest, and the quality has been hampered by shortcomings in the selection of measures pertaining to neuropsychological status and psychosocial outcome. Unfortunately, as noted by Kreutzer et al.,[100] "There is a dearth of longitudinal data regarding changes in cognitive functioning beyond the acute phase of injury" (p. 57).

Nevertheless, significant relationships between the status of specific neurocognitive domains and various aspects of household and community functioning have been reported. Baseline scores (obtained on an inpatient unit within the first 4 mo postinjury) on executive control and memory measures were predictive of overall level of independence within the home and community at 1 year postinjury.[114] Information-processing proficiency at 5 months postinjury correlated significantly with level of independence in ADL functioning at 12 months postinjury.[115] Late neuropsychological testing (i.e., approximately 2 to 3 yr postinjury) compared with even later psychosocial outcome (approximately 4 yr after neuropsychological testing) revealed a positive association between memory, executive control, visuoperceptual, and global cognitive performance levels and psychosocial status.[116]

Studies measuring concurrent neuropsychological and psychosocial functioning have found motor speed, complex attention and executive control, memory, visuoconstructional skills, and psychometric intelligence to correlate with level of independence.[17,31,117–120]

The underlying theme in these studies is that certain aspects of cognition, particularly complex attention and executive control, memory, and global cognitive functioning, are related to psychosocial status regardless of whether the neuropsychological measures are administered early or late in the recovery or prospectively versus concurrently with functional outcome. Thus, neuropsychological test data can be used to provide direction in decision making about the current and future needs of patients with TBI. It is worth noting here that test scores obtained at 1 month postinjury are highly predictive of later neuropsychological status, exceeding the predictive power of neurological severity indices, such as duration and depth of coma.[103] Therefore, early measurement of neuropsychological status permits formulation of rehabilitation treatment in advance as well as long-term aftercare planning within the first weeks and months postinjury.

A specific aspect of functional independence that deserves mention is the operation of a motor vehicle. An individual's readiness to drive after TBI is usually of considerable interest and has vocational as well as quality-of-life implications. It is also a community safety concern. Un-fortunately, research in this area has produced mixed results, and evidence supporting the predictive validity of neuropsychological testing is sparse. Positive correlations between test scores and driving outcome have been obtained for the WAIS-R FSIQ,[121] WAIS-R Picture Completion and Picture Arrangement subtests,[122] and the oral portion of the Symbol Digit Modalities Test.[123] In their driving fitness literature review, however, van Zomeran et al.[124] conclude that the ability of traditional measures to determine driving proficiency and safety is inadequate, noting that a number of studies had failed to find an association between neuropsychological test scores and driving outcome. This issue is ripe for research. The current state of knowledge is based on studies that have typically examined subject groups containing a mixture of diagnoses, employed truncated batteries, and failed to construct valid measures of driving ability.

☐ TREATMENT RECOMMENDATIONS

Neuropsychological examination data may mistakenly be viewed as an end product rather than the basis for the construction of treatment strategies and action plans. To provide TBI patients with tailored interventions, rehabilitation teams often look to the neuropsychological examination for practical guidance and direction. It allows the team to address specific areas of impairment while building on the relative neurocognitive strengths profiled in the neuropsychological examination.

☐ COGNITIVE REHABILITATION

The patient's need for modification of conventional treatment protocols can be gauged by very basic neuropsychological functions, such as level of arousal and orientation. Participation in traditional rehabilitation therapies requires a minimal capacity to maintain alertness and to register new information. Addressing the issue of deficit awareness may become an initial focus of treatment. In this regard, it is important to clarify the nature of the problem because different levels of awareness may be involved and treatment strategies can vary accordingly.[125] Deaton[126] recommends participation in patient-peer groups as an important component of intervention for deficient self-awareness. Cicerone[127] favors community-based activities and efforts to increase self-observation, such as checklists, self-monitoring procedures, and videotapes. Of particular importance is the use of neuropsychological test data in the modification of treatment strategies.

□ PSYCHOTHERAPY

The formulation of recommendations from the neuropsychological data is not complete until the issue of psychotherapeutic intervention has been addressed. The importance of treating psychological and emotional sequelae of brain injury as an integral part of the rehabilitation process has gained greater acceptance and appreciation in recent years.[109,128–132]

The selection of appropriate therapeutic modalities in each case may be guided by the severity of global cognitive impairment, the configuration of impaired and relatively spared cognitive capacities, and the nature of premorbid personality functioning.[133] As a general rule, the greater the global impairment, the more pharmacological and/or environmental interventions, such as behavior modification strategies, are required. The greater the compromise of executive functions, particularly those involved in self-organization and response inhibition, the more active the therapist must be and the more structure the therapist must impose on the sessions.

Expressive and insight-oriented psychotherapeutic approaches require "minimal" verbal skills (e.g., WAIS-R VIQ >75),[134] some preservation of the capacity to express personal needs and comprehend ideas put forth by the therapist,[135] and a basic awareness of cognitive deficits and behavioral problems.[136] Group therapy may be appropriate for patients who possess good receptive and, at least, minimal expressive language skills, do not evidence psychotic symptoms, and are not physically dangerous.[134] Patients who appear to be poor group therapy candidates because of their deficient appreciation for or tolerance of the group process may benefit from highly structured "discussion" groups.[127] For patients with a history of very mild brain insult who produce excessive polysymptomatology, psychotherapy may serve as the core intervention, with traditional rehabilitation therapies occupying an ancillary role.[137–141] Putnam and Millis[141] have recently proposed that stress inoculation training interventions, as developed by Meichenbaum,[142] may hold promise for these unusual but challenging cases.

□ CONCLUSIONS

The issues and challenges inherent in the neuropsychological assessment of the patient with TBI are dynamic rather than static. Remarkable advances in emergency medical procedures, neuroimaging and functional imaging techniques, and invitations to assist the trier of fact have affected how we practice, as have continuing developments in psychometrics and behavioral neurology. The discipline of clinical neuropsychology indeed has much to offer via its ability to measure and understand brain-behavior relationships. When integrated with a thoughtful understanding of a patient's abiding personality characteristics and psychosocial context, the neuropsychological examination is a principal contributor to the diagnostic and rehabilitation process for the patient with TBI.

REFERENCES

1. Adams, KM: Will the real handbook of clinical neuropsychology please stand? J Clin Exp Neuropsychol 7: 327, 1985.
2. Putnam, SH, and DeLuca, JW: The *TCN* professional practice survey: Part I: General practices of neuropsychologists in primary and private practice settings. Clinical Neuropsychologist 4:199, 1990.
3. Sweet, JJ, Westergaard, CK, and Moberg, PJ: Managed care experiences of clinical neuropsychologists. Clinical Neuropsychologist 9:214, 1995.
4. Putnam, SH, and DeLuca, JW: The *TCN* professional practice survey: Part II: An analysis of the fees of neuropsychologists by practice demographics. Clinical Neuropsychologist 5:103, 1991.
5. Reitan, RM, and Wolfson, D: Influence of age and education on neuropsychological test results. Clinical Neuropsychologist 9:151, 1995.
6. Langfitt, TW, et al: Regional structure and function in head-injured patients: Correlation of CT, MRI, PET, CBF, and neuropsychological assessment. In Levin, H, Grafman, J, and Eisenberg, HM (eds): Neurobehavioral Recovery from Head Injury. Oxford University Press, New York, 1987, p 30.
7. Benton, A: Thoughts on the application of neuropsychological tests. In Levin, H, Grafman, J, and Eisenberg, HM (eds): Neurobehavioral Recovery from Head Injury. Oxford University Press, New York, 1987, p 111.
8. Reitan, RM, and Wolfson, D: The Halstead-Reitan Neuropsychological Test Battery (ed 2). Neuropsychological Press, Tuscon, 1993.
9. Russell, EW: The psychometric foundation of clinical neuropsychology. In Filskov, SB, and Boll, TJ (eds): Handbook of Clinical Neuropsychology, vol 2. John Wiley, New York, 1986, p 45.
10. Anastasi, A: Psychological Testing (ed 5). Macmillan, New York, 1982.
11. Dikmen, S, et al: Neuropsychological outcome at 1 year post head injury. Neuropsychology 9:80, 1995.
12. Boll, TJ: The Halstead-Reitan Neuropsychological Battery. In Filskov, SB, and Boll, TJ (eds): Handbook of Clinical Neuropsychology. John Wiley, New York, 1981.
13. Heaton, R, Grant, I, and Matthews, C: Comprehensive Norms for an Expanded Halstead-Reitan Battery. Psychological Assessment Resources, Odessa, Fla, 1991.
14. Bornstein, RA: Normative data on intermanual differences on three tests of motor performance. J Clin Exp Neuropsychol 8:12, 1986.
15. Thompson, LL, et al: Comparison of preferred and non-preferred hand performance on four neuropsychological motor tasks. Clinical Neuropsychologist 1:324, 1987.
16. Fraser, R, et al: Employability of head injury survivors: First year post-injury. Rehabilitation Counseling Bulletin 31:276, 1988.
17. Klonoff, P, Costa, L, and Snow, W: Predictors and indicators of quality of life in patients with closed-head injury. J Clin Exp Neuropsychol 8:469, 1986.

18. Haaland, KY, et al: Recovery of simple motor skills after head injury. J Clin Exp Neuropsychol 16:448, 1994.

19. Haaland, KY, Harrington, DL, and Yeo, RA: The effects of task complexity on motor performance in left and right hemisphere stroke patients. Neuropsychologia 25: 783, 1987.

20. Reitan, RM: Theoretical and methodological bases of the Halstead-Reitan Neuropsychological Test Battery. In Grant, I, and Adams, KM (eds): Neuropsychological Assessment of Neuropsychiatric Disorders. Oxford University Press, New York, 1986, p 3.

21. Mandleberg, IA: Cognitive recovery after severe head injury: II: Wechsler Adult Intelligence Scale during post-traumatic amnesia. J Neurol Neurosurg Psychiatry 38:1127, 1975.

22. Mandleberg, IA, and Brooks, DN: Cognitive recovery after severe head injury: I: Serial testing on the Wechsler Adult Intelligence Scale. J Neurol Neurosurg Psychiatry 38:121, 1975.

23. Kaufman, AS: Assessing Adolescent and Adult Intelligence. Allyn & Bacon, Boston, 1990.

24. Nelson, LD, et al: Development and validation of the neuropsychology behavior and affect profile. Psychological Assessment: A Journal of Consulting and Clinical Psychology 1:266, 1989.

25. Nelson, LD, et al: Cross-validation of the Neuropsychology Behavior and Affect Profile in stroke patients. Psychological Assessment: A Journal of Consulting and Clinical Psychology 5:374, 1993.

26. Satz, P, et al: Development and evaluation of validity scales for the Neuropsychology Behavior and Affect Profile. Psychological Assessment: A Journal of Consulting and Clinical Psychology 8:115, 1996.

27. Binder, LM, and Johnson-Greene, D: Observer effects on neuropsychological performance: A case report. Clinical Neuropsychologist 9:74, 1995.

28. McCaffrey, RJ, et al: Presence of third parties during neuropsychological evaluations: Who is evaluating whom? Clinical Neuropsychologist 10:435, 1996.

29. Lezak, MD: Neuropsychological Assessment, 3 ed. Oxford University Press, New York, 1995.

30. Hannay, HJ, et al: Outcome measures for patients with head injuries: Report of the Outcome Measures Subcommittee. J Head Trauma Rehabil 11(6):41, 1996.

31. Levin, H, et al: Long-term neuropsychological outcome of closed head injury. J Neurosurg 50:412, 1979.

32. Babcock, H: An experiment in the measurement of mental deterioration. Arch Psychol (Frankf) 117:35, 1930.

33. Yates, AJ: The use of vocabulary in the measurement of intellectual deterioration: A review. Journal of Mental Science 102:409, 1956.

34. Barona, A, Reynolds, C, and Chastain, R: A demographically based index of premorbid intelligence for the WAIS-R. J Consult Clin Psychol 52:885, 1984.

35. Krull, KR, Scott, JG, and Sherer, M: Estimation of premorbid intelligence from combined performance and demographic variables. Clinical Neuropsychologist 9:83, 1995.

36. Sweet, JJ, Moberg, PJ, and Tovian, SM: Evaluation of Wechsler Adult Intelligence Scale–Revised premorbid IQ formulas in clinical populations. Psychological Assessment 2:41, 1990.

37. Blair, J, and Spreen, O: Predicting premorbid IQ: A revision of the National Adult Reading Test. Clinical Neuropsychologist 3:129, 1989.

38. Nelson, HE, and McKenna, P: The use of current reading ability in the assessment of dementia. Br J Soc Clin Psychol 14:259, 1975.

39. Willshire, D, Kinsella, G, and Prior, M: Estimating WAIS-R IQ from the National Adult Reading Test: A cross-validation. J Clin Exp Neuropsychol 13:204, 1991.

40. Kareken, DA, Gur, RC, and Saykin, AJ: Reading on the Wide Range Achievement Test–Revised and parental education as predictors of IQ: Comparison with the Barona formula. Archives of Clinical Neuropsychology 10:147, 1995.

41. Matarazzo, JD: Psychological assessment versus psychological testing: Validation from Binet to the school, clinic, and courtroom. Am Psychol 45:999, 1990.

42. Sbordone, RJ: Ecological validity: Some critical issues for the neuropsychologist. In Sbordone, RJ, and Long, CJ (eds): Ecological Validity of Neuropsychological Testing. GR Press/St. Lucie Press, DelRay Beach, Fla, 1996.

43. Crosson, B, et al: WAIS-R pattern clusters after blunt-head injury. Clinical Neuropsychologist 4:253, 1990.

44. Mittenburg, W, Hammeke, TA, and Rao, SM: Intratest scatter on the WAIS-R as a pathognomonic sign of brain injury. Psychological Assessment 1:273, 1989.

45. Putnam, SH, Adams, KM, and Schneider, A: One day test-retest reliability of neuropsychological tests in a personal injury case. Psychological Assessment: A Journal of Consulting and Clinical Psychology 4:312, 1992.

46. Cullum, C, Heaton, RK, and Grant, I: Psychogenic factors influencing neuropsychological performance: Somatoform disorders, factitious disorders, and malingering. In Doerr, HO, and Carlin, AS (eds): Forensic Neuropsychology: Legal and Scientific Bases. Guilford, New York, 1991.

47. Reitan, RM, and Wolfson, D: The question of validity of neuropsychological test scores among head-injured litigants: Development of a dissimulation index. Archives of Clinical Neuropsychology 11:573, 1996.

48. Sawrie, SM, et al: Empirical methods for assessing meaningful change following epilepsy surgery. Journal of the International Neuropsychological Society 2:556, 1996.

49. Faust, D: The art of practicing a science that does not yet exist. Neuropsychol Rev 2:205, 1991.

50. Adams, KM, and Putnam, SH: Coping with professional skeptics: Reply to Faust. Psychological Assessment: A Journal of Consulting and Clinical Psychology 6:5, 1994.

51. Schwartz, ML: Limitations on neuropsychological testimony by the Florida Appellate Decisions: Action, Reaction, and Counteraction. Clinical Neuropsychologist 1:51, 1987.

52. Lees-Haley, P: Mild brain injury: Proving lost earnings. Trial November:83, 1987.

53. Putnam, SH, DeLuca, JW, and Anderson, C: The Second TCN salary survey: A survey of neuropsychologists, Part 2. Clinical Neuropsychologist 8:245, 1994.

54. Youngjohn, JR, Burrows, L, and Erdal, K: Brain damage or compensation neurosis? The controversial post-concussion syndrome. Clinical Neuropsychologist 9:112, 1995.

55. Putnam, SH, Millis, SR, and Adams, KM: Mild traumatic brain injury: Beyond cognitive assessment. In Grant, I, and Adams KM (eds): Neuropsychological Assessment of Neuropsychiatric Disorders, ed 2. Oxford University Press, New York, 1996, p 529.

56. Naugle, RI, and McSweeny, AJ: On the practice of routinely appending neuropsychological data to reports. Clinical Neuropsychologist 9:245, 1995.

57. Nies, KJ, and Sweet, JJ: Neuropsychological assessment and malingering: A critical review of past and present strategies. Archives of Clinical Neuropsychology 9:501, 1994.

58. Youngjohn, JR: Confirmed attorney coaching prior to neuropsychological evaluation. Assessment 2:279, 1995.

59. Faust, D, Ziskin, J, and Hiers, JB: Brain Damage Claims: Coping with Neuropsychological Evidence. Law and Psychology Press, Los Angeles, 1991.

60. Fastenau, PS, and Adams, KM: Heaton, Grant, and Matthews' Comprehensive Norms: An overzealous attempt. J Clin Exp Neuropsychol 18:444, 1996.

61. Bornstein, RA: Entry into clinical neuropsychology: Graduate, undergraduate, and beyond. Clinical Neuropsychologist 2:213, 1988.

62. Report of the Division 40 Task Force on Education, Accreditation, and Credentialing. Guidelines for doctoral training programs in clinical neuropsychology. Clinical Neuropsychologist 1:29, 1987.

63. Report of the Division 40 Task Force on Education, Accreditation, and Credentialing. Professional issues: Defi-

64. Matthews, C: They asked for a speech. Clinical Neuropsychologist 4:327, 1990.
65. Alves, W, Macciocchi, SN, and Barth, JT: Postconcussive symptoms after uncomplicated mild head injury. J Head Trauma Rehabil 8(3):48, 1993.
66. Dikmen, S, McLean, A, and Temkin, N: Neuropsychological and psychosocial consequences of minor head injury. J Neurol Neurosurg Psychiatry 49:1227, 1986.
67. Levin, HS, et al: Neurobehavioral outcome following minor head injury: A three center study. J Neurosurg 66:234, 1987.
68. Heaton, RK, et al: Demographic corrections with comprehensive norms: An overzealous attempt or good start? J Clin Exp Neuropsychol 18:449, 1996.
69. Rourke, BP, and Brown, GG: Clinical neuropsychology and behavioral neurology: Similarities and differences. In Filskov, SB, and Boll, TJ (eds): Handbook of Clinical Neuropsychology, vol 2. John Wiley, New York, 1986, p 3.
70. Lees-Haley, PR: Neuropsychological complaint base rates of personal injury claimants. Forensic Reports 5:385, 1992.
71. Axelrod, BN, and Goldman, RS: Use of demographic corrections in neuropsychological interpretation: How standard are standard scores? Clinical Neuropsychologist 10:159, 1996.
72. Youngjohn, JR, Larrabee, G, and Crook, T: New adult age- and education-corrected norms for the Benton Visual Retention Test. Clinical Neuropsychologist 7:155, 1993.
73. Lichtenberg, PA, Ross, T, and Christensen, B: Preliminary normative data on the Boston Naming Test for an older urban population. Clinical Neuropsychologist 8:109, 1994.
74. Ross, TP, Lichtenberg, PA, and Christensen, BK: Normative data on the Boston Naming Test for elderly adults in a demographically diverse medical sample. Clinical Neuropsychologist 9:321, 1995.
75. Larrabee, G, et al: Neuropsychology 2:173, 1988.
76. Wiens, A, Tindall, A, and Crossen, J: California Verbal Learning Test: A normative study. Clinical Neuropsychologist 8:75, 1994.
77. Trahan, D, and Larrabee, G: Continuous Visual Memory Test Professional Manual. Psychological Assessment Resources, Odessa, Fla, 1988.
78. Benton, A, Hamsher, deS, and Sivan, A: Multilingual Aphasia Examination. University of Iowa, Iowa City, 1994.
79. Ruff, RM, et al: Benton Controlled Oral Word Association Test: Reliability and updated norms. Archives of Clinical Neuropsychology 11:329, 1996.
80. Benton, A, et al: Contributions to Neuropsychological Assessment. Oxford University Press, New York, 1983.
81. Warner, MH, et al: Relationships between IQ and neuropsychological measures in neuropsychiatric populations: Within laboratory and cross-cultural replications using WAIS and WAIS-R. J Clin Exp Neuropsychol 9:545, 1987.
82. Hooper, HE: Hooper Visual Organizational Test (VOT) Manual. Western Psychological Services, Los Angeles, 1983.
83. Williams, JM: Memory Assessment Scales Professional Manual. Psychological Assessment Resources, Odessa, Fla, 1991.
84. Brittain, J, et al: Effects of age and IQ on Paced Auditory Serial Addition Task (PASAT) performance. Clinical Neuropsychologist 5:163, 1991.
85. Dunn, L, and Dunn, L: Peabody Picture Vocabulary Test-Revised Manual. American Guidance Service, Circle Pines, 1981.
86. Warrington, E: Recognition Memory Test Manual. NFER-Nelson, Windsor, UK, 1984.
87. Wiens, A, McMinn, M, and Crossen, J: Rey Auditory-Verbal Learning Test: Development of norms for healthy young adults. Clinical Neuropsychologist 2:67, 1988.
88. Ruff, R: Ruff Figural Fluency Test Administration Manual. Neuropsychological Resources, San Diego, 1988.
89. Trenerry, M, et al: Stroop Neuropsychological Screening Test Manual. Psychological Assessment Resources, Odessa, Fla, 1989.
90. Smith, A: Symbol Digit Modalities Test Manual. Western Psychological Services, Los Angeles, 1992.
91. Heaton, RK, Grant, I, and Matthews, CG: Comprehensive Norms for an Expanded Halstead-Reitan Battery: A Supplement for the Wechsler Adult Intelligence Scale–Revised. Psychological Assessment Resources, Odessa, 1992.
92. Wechsler, D: Wechsler Memory Scale–Revised. Psychological Corporation, New York, 1987.
93. Wilkinson, G: The Wide Range Achievement Test Administration Manual. Wide Range, Wilmington, 1993.
94. Heaton, R, et al: Wisconsin Card Sorting Test Manual. Psychological Assessment Resources, Odessa, Fla, 1993.
95. Dikmen, S, et al: Minor and severe head injury emotional sequelae. Brain Inj 6:477, 1992.
96. Dikmen, S, and Temkin, N: Determination of the effects of head injury and recovery in behavioral research. In Levin, H, Grafman, J, and Eisenberg, HM (eds): Neurobehavioral Recovery from Head Injury. Oxford University Press, New York, 1987, p 73.
97. Newcombe, F: Psychometric and behavioral evidence: Scope, limitations, and ecological validity. In Levin H, Grafman, J, and Eisenberg HM (eds): Neurobehavioral Recovery from Head Injury. Oxford University Press, New York, 1987, p 129.
98. Millis, SR, and Ricker, JH: Verbal learning patterns in moderate and severe traumatic brain injury. J Clin Exp Neuropsychol 16:498, 1994.
99. Deshpande, SA, et al: Verbal learning subtypes in traumatic brain injury: A replication. J Clin Exp Neuropsychol 18:836, 1996.
100. Kreutzer, JS, et al: Neuropsychological characteristics of patients with brain injury: Preliminary findings from a multicenter investigation. J Head Trauma Rehabil 8(2):47, 1993.
101. Bowman, ML: Ecological validity of neuropsychological and other predictors following head injury. Clinical Neuropsychologist 10:382, 1996.
102. Crepeau, F, and Scherzer, P: Predictors and indicators of work status after traumatic brain injury: A meta-analysis. Neuropsychological Rehabilitation 3:5, 1993.
103. Dikmen, S, and Machamer, J: Neurobehavioral outcomes and their determinants. J Head Trauma Rehabil 10(1):74, 1995.
104. Dikmen, S, et al: Employment following traumatic head injuries: Archives of Neurology 51:177, 1994.
105. Fraser, R, and Wehman, P: Traumatic brain injury rehabilitation: Issues in vocational outcome. NeuroRehabilitation 5:39, 1995.
106. Ruff, R, et al: Predictors of outcome following severe head trauma: Follow-up data from the Traumatic Coma Data Bank. Brain Inj 7:101, 1993.
107. Walker, M, Hannay, H, and Davidson, K: PAI and the prediction of level of vocational/academic outcome. J Clin Exp Neuropsychol 14:29, 1992.
108. Wehman, P, et al: Return to work for persons with severe traumatic brain injury: A data-based approach to program development. J Head Trauma Rehabil 10(1):27, 1995.
109. Putnam, SH, and Adams, KM: Regression based prediction of long-term outcome following multidisciplinary rehabilitation for traumatic brain injury. Clinical Neuropsychologist 6:383, 1992.
110. McMordie, W, Barker, S, and Paolo, T: Return to work (RTW) after head injury. Brain Inj 4:57, 1990.
111. Prigatano, G, Klonoff, P, and O'Brien, K: Productivity after neuropsychologically oriented milieu rehabilitation. J Head Trauma Rehabil 9(1):91, 1994.
112. Vogenthaler, D, Smith, K, and Goldfader, P: Head injury, a multivariate study: Predicting long-term productivity and independent living outcome. Brain Inj 7:28, 1989.

113. Rosenthal, M, and Millis, S: Relating neuropsychological indicators to psychosocial outcome after traumatic brain injury. NeuroRehabilitation 2:1, 1992.

114. Millis, S, Rosenthal, M, and Lourie, I: Predicting community integration after traumatic brain injury with neuropsychological measures. Int J Neurosci 79:165, 1994.

115. Van Zomeren, A: Reaction Time and Attention after Closed Head Injury. Swets & Zeitlinger, Lisse, Netherlands, 1981.

116. Acker, M, and Davis J: Psychology test scores associated with late outcome in head injury. Neuropsychology 3:123, 1989.

117. Baum, B, and Hall, K: Relationship between constructional praxis and dressing in the head injured. Am J Occup Ther 35:438, 1981.

118. Jennett, B, et al: Disability after severe head injury: Observations on the use of the Glasgow Outcome Scale. J Neurol Neurosurg Psychiatry 44:285, 1981.

119. Malec, J, Zweber, B, and DePompolo, R: The Rivermead Behavioral Memory Test: Laboratory neurocognitive measures and everyday functioning. J Head Trauma Rehabil 5(3):60, 1990.

120. Schretlen, D: Accounting for variance in long-term recovery from traumatic brain injury with executive abilities and injury severity. J Clin Exp Neuropsychol 14:77, 1992.

121. Hopewell, C, and Price, R: Driving after head injury. J Clin Exp Neuropsychol 7:148, 1985.

122. Sivak, M, et al: Driving and perceptual/cognitive skills: Behavioral consequences of brain damage. Arch Phys Med Rehabil 62:476, 1981.

123. Gouvier, W, et al: Psychometric prediction of driving performance among the disabled. Arch Phys Med Rehabil 70:745, 1989.

124. Van Zomeran, A, Brouwer, W, and Minderhoud, J: Acquired brain damage and driving: A review. Arch Phys Med Rehabil 68:697, 1987.

125. Crosson, B, et al: Awareness and compensation in postacute head injury rehabilitation. J Head Trauma Rehabil 4(3):46, 1989.

126. Deaton, A: Denial in the aftermath of traumatic head injury: Its manifestations, measurement, and treatment. Rehabilitation Psychology 31:231, 1986.

127. Cicerone, K: Psychotherapeutic interventions with traumatically brain-injured patients. Rehabilitation Psychology 34:105, 1989.

128. Haynes, S: The experience of grief in the head-injured adult. Archives of Clinical Neuropsychology 9:232, 1994.

129. Klonoff, P, and Lage, G: Narcissistic injury in patients with traumatic brain injury. J Head Trauma Rehabil 6(4):11, 1991.

130. Miller, L: Psychotherapy of the Brain Injured Patient. Norton, New York, 1993.

131. Mittenberg, W, Zielinski, R, and Fichera, S: Recovery from mild head injury: A treatment manual for patients. Psychotherapy in Private Practice 12:37, 1993.

132. Prigatano, G: Disordered mind, wounded soul: The emerging role of psychotherapy in rehabilitation after brain injury. J Head Trauma Rehabil 6(4):1, 1991.

133. Lewis, L: A framework for developing a psychotherapy treatment plan with brain-injured patients. J Head Trauma Rehabil 6(4):22, 1991.

134. Prigatano, GP: Psychotherapy after brain injury. In Prigatano, GP, et al (eds): Neuropsychological Rehabilitation after Brain Injury. Johns Hopkins University Press, Baltimore, 1986.

135. Lewis, L, and Rosenberg, SJ: Psychoanalytic psychotherapy with brain-injured adult psychiatric patients. J Nerv Ment Dis 178:69, 1990.

136. Bennett, T: Individual psychotherapy & minor head head injury. Cognitive Rehabilitation 7:20, 1989.

137. Cicerone, K: Psychotherapy after mild traumatic brain injury: Relation to the nature and severity of subjective complaints. J Head Trauma Rehabil 6(4):30, 1991.

138. Conboy, T, Barth, J, and Boll, T: Treatment and rehabilitation of mild and moderate head trauma. Rehabilitation Psychology 31:203, 1986.

139. Kay, T: Neuropsychological treatment of mild traumatic brain injury. J Head Trauma Rehabil 8(3):74, 1993.

140. Novack, T, Roth, D, and Boll, T: Treatment alternatives following mild head injury. Rehabilitation Counseling Bulletin 31:313, 1988.

141. Putnam, SH, and Millis, SR: Psychosocial factors in the development and maintenance of chronic somatic and functional symptoms following mild traumatic brain injury. Advances in Medical Psychotherapy 7:1, 1994.

142. Meichenbaum, D: Stress Inoculation Training. Pergamon, New York, 1985.

CHAPTER 10

Emotional, Behavioral, and Personality Assessment after Traumatic Brain Injury

ADRIENNE D. WITOL, PSYD,
JEFFREY S. KREUTZER, PHD,
and ANGELLE M. SANDER, PHD

For the past two decades, researchers and clinicians have endeavored to describe the complete spectrum of traumatic brain injury (TBI) sequelae. The physical and cognitive changes resulting from TBI have been well documented.[1] Less is known about the emotional, behavioral, and personality problems often described as more distressing to family members and a greater detriment to long-term adjustment.[2–5] These problems have the potential to exacerbate physical and cognitive difficulties. Levin et al.[1] were among the first to carefully delineate injury-related emotional, behavioral, and personality problems, which they labeled "neurobehavioral."

This chapter describes a systematic method of evaluating and describing neurobehavioral changes after TBI and a comprehensive approach to assessment. Information about referral questions, records review, observational and interview techniques, and quantitative assessment is presented. Finally, it discusses methods of synthesizing information to reach formal diagnostic conclusions. Philosophically, neurobehavioral assessment is portrayed as a complement to neuropsychological assessment (Chapter 9), which addresses cognitive and psychomotor functioning.

❑ AN OVERVIEW OF RESEARCH ON NEUROBEHAVIORAL FUNCTIONING

Most studies of neurobehavioral functioning have focused on relatively acute stages of injury. The earliest studies were conducted in Europe. At postinjury intervals ranging from 3 to 6 months, relatives of severely injured patients reported numerous emotional and behavioral changes, including irritability, decreased energy and enthusiasm, mood swings, fatigue, slowness, and aggression.[6–8]

Although many European researchers relied on relatives' reports, investigators in the United

This work was partly supported by Grants #G0087C0219 and #H133P2006 from the National Institute on Disability and Rehabilitation Research, United States Department of Education.

States used a clinician-completed inventory, the Neurobehavioral Rating Scale,[9] to describe emotional, personality, and behavioral sequelae. Studying a sample of 101 patients at 1 to 6 months postinjury, Levin et al.[9] reported a high incidence of conceptual disorganization, disinhibition, decreased insight and awareness, decreased initiative and motivation, and poor planning. Keyser et al.[10] found similar results. In a prospective, multicenter study, they reported on a sample of 295 acute rehabilitation patients with mild, moderate, and severe injury at an average of 47 days postinjury. Using the Neurobehavioral Rating Scale, the authors found a high incidence of memory deficits, inaccurate insight, inattention, reduced alertness, conceptual disorganization, poor planning, fatigue, and blunted affect. Few patients were reported as having problems with hallucinations, guilt, or unusual thought content.

Families and professionals may be tempted to ignore neurobehavioral problems and hope for spontaneous resolution. However, research examining long-term outcome has revealed that many difficulties persist or worsen at intervals ranging from 2 to 20 years postinjury.[3,11–16] For example, in a longitudinal investigation of severe brain injury patients, Thomsen[3] compared outcome at 2 to 5 years postinjury against outcome at 10 to 15 years postinjury. At both follow-up intervals, poor memory, loss of social contact, personality and emotional changes, and slowness were reported as problematic for a majority of patients. Lack of interests, poor concentration, aspontaneity, sensitivity, distress, and fatigue were also commonly reported. Thomsen commented on the variability of recovery, noting that some patients declined and others improved.

Kreutzer et al.[17] reported on a sample of 135 rehabilitation outpatients. Averaging 3.5 years postinjury, 55 percent were unemployed, and most had severe injuries. At least 88 percent reported problems related to confusion, fatigue, frustration, boredom, and difficulty in thinking of the right word. At least 75 percent of patients were reported as having problems with losing their train of thought, thinking slowly, having trouble in making decisions, and experiencing restlessness, impatience, poor concentration, and forgetfulness. Feeling sad and blue, lonely, and misunderstood by others was reported by at least 70 percent of the sample. In one of the longest-term follow-up to date, Witol et al.[18] provided information on a group of 37 unemployed, primarily male patients ranging from 10 to 34 years postinjury. Average age at the time of injury was 17.4, average age at follow-up was 33.2, and average duration of unconsciousness was 58.1 days. Most commonly reported were slowness and problems relating to mood. For example, frustration, impatience, boredom, and restlessness were among the most frequent problems. In addition to memory problems, slow reading, writing, moving, and thinking were also reported.

In summary, the literature suggests that many neurobehavioral problems are chronic. Similar problems have been encountered at times varying from 3 months to 34 years postinjury. Fatigue, irritability, frustration, memory loss, and slowness were among the most frequently reported neurobehavioral findings. Given the longevity of neurobehavioral sequelae, accurate evaluation, including determination of contributing and exacerbating variables, becomes increasingly important.

□ A COMPREHENSIVE APPROACH TO NEUROBEHAVIORAL ASSESSMENT

Given the variability and high incidence of neurobehavioral problems, their persistence, and their potential to influence rehabilitation efficacy, assessment is an important first step in developing an individualized treatment plan. Assessment begins with developing and clarifying the referral question. Assessment next involves collecting information from a variety of sources with different methods. Typically, clinicians rely on four sources of information: (1) records review, (2) behavioral observation, (3) clinical interviews, and (4) quantitative testing. Finally, the information is synthesized for diagnostic formulation, development of recommendations, and treatment planning. The quality of the information collected has an important impact on the value of diagnostic formulations and treatment planning.

Clarifying the Referral Question

The evaluation process is often instigated by a referral source or as part of the treatment team's standard assessment protocol. Many times referral sources have clearly conceptualized concerns that may or may not be directly communicated. Vague questions may lead to wasted effort and to the referral source presuming that the evaluator has failed to adequately complete the assignment. The examiner who is interested in providing an efficient and comprehensive assessment process needs to clarify the goals and suggest additional goals.

Referral questions typically fall into several categories. First, diagnostic and descriptive information about the patient is solicited (Table 10–1). Second, referral sources may request information about the functional implications of neurobehavioral problems (Table 10–2). Descriptions

---

TABLE 10–1. Referral Questions Pertaining to Emotional Status

1. How is the patient different since the injury?
2. Is there evidence of preexisting emotional difficulties?
3. Are present symptoms consistent with preexisting problems, related to brain injury, or a combination of both?
4. Is the patient depressed or simply lacking initiative because of frontal lobe injury?
5. Is the patient anxious or having difficulty with expression of anger? Is there evidence of post-traumatic stress disorder?
6. Is the patient at risk to harm self or others?
7. Do pain and unresolved physical symptoms contribute to emotional difficulties?
8. Is there evidence that emotional distress contributes to cognitive and functional impairments?
9. Describe and distinguish between psychological denial and anosognosia.

TABLE 10–3. Referral Questions Pertaining to Treatment Issues

1. What types of intervention will be most effective?
2. Indicate reasonable treatment goals and suggest priority areas.
3. What is the patient's potential for improvement?
4. Is the patient a good candidate for individual or group therapy?
5. Is training in social skills or assertiveness likely to be beneficial?
6. Provide pain management recommendations.

---

of the patient's ability to carry out specific responsibilities, comparison of preinjury and postinjury attributes, and consideration of postinjury progress are often important. Third, many professionals request treatment recommendations and inquire about a patient's potential to benefit from therapy (Table 10–3).

Records Review

A thorough review of records is invaluable. Although the task can be time-consuming, careful

---

TABLE 10–2. Referral Questions Pertaining to Functional Implications of Neurobehavioral Problems

1. Can the patient return to a previous position or an alternative position in a part-time or full-time capacity?
2. How will neurobehavioral difficulties affect social interactions with family, friends, customers, and colleagues?
3. Should an alternative academic or vocational placement be considered, given the patient's emotional difficulties?
4. How will the patient's emotional status affect parenting skills?
5. How does the patient normally respond to instruction? What feedback presentation style will most likely elicit the best response?
6. Can the patient live independently? If not, what level of supervision is recommended? Are social judgment, impassivity, and disinhibition a concern?

---

review saves time in the long run and provides direction for interviews, quantitative assessment, and needed treatment interventions. Table 10–4 lists categories of important information, documentation sources, and their potential relevance to neurobehavioral assessment. Clinicians should weigh the costs against the potential benefits for each individual case.

The following two scenarios highlight the need for comprehensive records review in making admission and treatment decisions. Both persons were referred for admission to a selective transitional living program that admits 7 to 10 clients each year.

Case 1 ■ At 26, John, a divorced father of five, sustained a severe brain injury and was admitted for hospitalization with a blood alcohol level more than twice the legal limit. Reportedly, he saw a counselor for "adjustment problems" when he was 17. Now 28, he boasted that he held seven different jobs before age 25. He attributed job changes to an interest in finding "a job with a future." When asked about alcohol consumption, John denied that he had a problem. Work performance evaluations that were obtained revealed that John had been disciplined and terminated for "explosive behavior" and "drinking on the job."

Case 2 ■ Mary, a 28-year-old mother of two young children who had been active in her church, sustained a "devastating" brain injury when she was thrown from a horse during a family outing. Prior to her injury, Mary worked as an accountant for a small data processing firm. Mary was reluctant to discuss preinjury difficulties. She explains, "My life before the injury was wonderful. Everything seemed to be going well." Talking by phone with her employer, you learn that she'd received several formal reprimands. Before her injury, she'd routinely missed Fridays and Mondays, calling in sick each time. Medical records revealed many vague somatic complaints (e.g., stomachache, head pains, bloating, numb-

TABLE 10–4. Sources of Documentation for Records Review and Potential Relevance to Neurobehavioral Findings

Information Category	Documentation Sources	Potential Relevance to Neurobehavioral Findings
Academic history	√ Grade transcripts and pattern of grades √ Attendance patterns √ Conduct reports	■ Response to authority figures ■ Ability to function in a structured environment ■ Social and emotional stability
Vocational history	√ Performance reviews √ Job applications, resume √ Salary and wage history; attendance patterns √ Grievances and disciplinary action	■ Response to authority figures ■ Work attitudes and habits ■ Ability to function in a structured environment ■ Social and emotional stability, interpersonal skills
Health and medical history	√ Preinjury and postinjury medical, rehabilitation, and mental health records √ Prior applications for disability benefits	Psychiatric and psychological disorders: ■ Somatization signs ■ Substance abuse ■ Depression and anxiety

Legal history	√ Arrests, incarcerations, including drunk driving
	√ Previous involvement in litigation
		■ Social judgment
		■ Preexisting personality and psychiatric disorders
		  □ Antisocial behavior
		  □ Substance abuse

ness). In almost every case, thorough diagnostic testing provided no substantiation for her claims of illness.

For both cases, review of medical and employment records dramatically improved clinicians' understanding of factors that could significantly influence progress in the rehabilitation program. John's history of job instability, substance abuse, and aggressive behavior had important implications for rehabilitation planning. Mary's history of somatization raises concerns about her motivation for treatment and her prognosis for recovery.

Although records are potentially helpful, their accuracy and completeness cannot be assumed. In some cases, incorrect information is transmitted from one record to another. In other situations, clinicians avoid recording information or asking about issues that might be uncomfortable for them or the patient. Careful validation of information sources and clinical interviews are important next steps.

Behavioral Observation

Observation is an important means of assessing behaviors that may not be easily tapped by quantitative assessment measures. Information about personal appearance, interpersonal skills, affect, and executive skills is often derived primarily from clinical observation (Table 10–5).

In many cases, patients are observed during the course of a structured evaluation, when they are "on their best behavior." Less formal situations typically provide the best representation of behavior in a variety of more realistic situations. Here, observation provides invaluable information about attributes unsuited to formal evaluation. For example, psychologists have traditionally had difficulty developing valid measures of initiative, social judgment, flexibility, and persistence.

Information tends to be most valuable when based on observations made at different times, in different settings, and by different people. Where possible, behavior should be observed during the course of interdisciplinary therapies and outings. Interviews in home settings provide excellent opportunities for observation; however, their use is often limited by constraints of time and distance.

The shortcoming of observation relate to the difficulty of accurately quantifying behavior, which may diminish interobserver reliability and challenge the validity of efforts to measure change over time or make comparisons between patients. Furthermore, observation alone does not provide information about the etiology and duration of neurobehavioral attributes. Interviews, records review, and history taking are often necessary to establish etiology and course. Formal behavioral analysis methods are more completely described in the work of Wood,[19,20] Eames,[21] Eames et al.,[22] and Jacobs.[23]

TABLE 10–5. Behavioral Observations Relevant to Neurobehavioral Assessment

Category	Specifically Assess:
Appearance	√ Physical condition √ Hygiene √ Clothing
Attitude toward testing	√ Cooperation √ Consistency of efforts √ Persistence and follow-through
Social interaction skills	√ Eye contact with examiner √ Spontaneous conversation or lack thereof √ Listening skills √ Tone of voice (e.g., sarcastic, monotonous, elated) √ Display of inappropriate behaviors (e.g., aggressive or sexual) √ Uncooperative or hostile
Spontaneity and initiative	√ Impulsivity √ Response rate √ Motor restlessness or psychomotor retardation
Thought patterns	√ Organization of ideas √ Evidence of delusions or hallucinations √ Ability to stay on topic √ Appropriate responses to questions
Affect	√ Range (full? appropriate to content?) √ Frustration tolerance √ Obvious anxiety √ Emotional lability √ Grief, tearfulness √ Emotional withdrawal √ Euphoria
Approach to testing	√ Flexibility in shifting between activities √ Problem-solving approach √ Response to failures and success √ Awareness of errors √ Initiative and follow-through

Clinical Interview

Medical and psychological professionals routinely rely heavily on interviews to gather information about behavior and emotional adjustment. Many clinicians use structured interviews to ensure the collection of comprehensive information. Several structured interviews have been designed to assess mental status, activity levels, and preinjury history in patients with TBI.[24] For example, the General Health and History Questionnaire (GHHQ)[25] solicits information on preinjury and postinjury demographics, work history, substance abuse, and criminal history. Other clinicians tailor their interview questions to meet the unique needs of individual patients. A combination of the two approaches is most likely to be effective. A structured interview can serve as a basis for all clients, with additional questions added as needed.

For assessment, interviewers should focus on symptom patterns, stresses, social functioning, coping strategies, and expectations to evaluate a patient's emotional and behavioral status. Table 10–6 shows global and open-ended sample questions, which are intended to serve only as a starting point for an interview. To make an accurate diagnosis, clinicians need to ask about symptoms in greater detail.

When possible, clinicians should interview family members as well as patients to get more than one perspective on functioning. However, confusion can result when information collected from family members is discrepant from that provided by patients. Researchers have shown that patients and family members often disagree about patients' emotional and personality functioning.[2,12,26,27] Disagreement has been attributed to commonly observed impairments in comprehension, memory, and self-awareness. Other researchers have found that family members and patients did not differ significantly in their perceptions of depression and aggression.[28] Differences may be partly attributable to the format and specificity of questions. For example, several researchers have found that patients' reports of difficulties were more consis-

TABLE 10–6. Suggested Areas of Inquiry during Clinical Interview

1. What problems or symptoms is the patient currently experiencing? Were any of these problems present before the injury? If so, have they worsened since the injury?
2. What are the perceived effects of symptoms on vocational, academic, and social functioning? Distinguish between preinjury and postinjury functioning.
3. What are the preinjury and postinjury stressors? Is a certain stressor perceived as triggering the onset of symptoms?
4. What types of coping strategies does the individual use? Do certain types of strategies appear to work better than others?
5. How do family members respond to the patient's symptoms (e.g., with anger, ignoring, offers of help or encouragement)?
6. What are the patient's feelings regarding the future? Does the patient expect symptoms to remain stable or change? Is the patient making plans for the future, or has the patient given up hope?
7. How was the patient's social functioning prior to injury? Has social functioning changed (e.g., more withdrawn, less interested in people)?

TABLE 10–7. Factors Indicating a Need for Emphasis on Caregiver Interviews

Emphasize Caregiver Interviews When the Patient . . .

1. Cannot respond reliably because of communication difficulties
2. Has severe memory deficits that seriously impede the ability to recall day-to-day activities
3. Does not acknowledge having *any* difficulties
4. Is unable to cooperate secondary to inability to understand or complete task
5. Is unwilling to cooperate

"area of expertise" concerning the patient. Although obtaining information from multiple sources can increase diagnostic accuracy, the extra time and effort must be carefully weighed against the information that is more readily available. Clinicians should also be careful to obtain the patient's consent to conduct such interviews.

Quantitative Assessment Approaches

Quantification of behavioral and emotional attributes offers at least four major advantages. First, quantification adds an element of objectivity by allowing clinicians to compare scores derived from individual patients with other groups of patients, over time, and with optimal scores. Second, in answering personally sensitive questions, some people are more comfortable, open, and honest on a questionnaire than in a face-to-face interview situation. Third, quantitative measures provide information on

tent with family members' when questions were specific rather than global.[29–31] Based on the research findings, clinicians are encouraged to use specific, behaviorally anchored questions when interviewing patients. For example, asking, "Do you feel sad a good deal of the time? Do you enjoy things the way you used to?" is more likely to elicit an accurate response than asking, "Do you feel depressed?"

Regardless of cognitive impairments, patients and family members, based on their unique experiences and personalities, often have different perspectives. Thus, clinicians are frequently faced with the challenge of integrating discrepant information to arrive at accurate conclusions. Tables 10–7 and 10–8 provide information to help examiners decide which viewpoint to emphasize. Consideration of all viewpoints develops rapport, ensures the collection of comprehensive information, and increases the likelihood of making an accurate diagnosis. Conveying respect for all points of view also increases compliance with treatment recommendations.

A final note concerns interviews with people other than the patient or family members. Some clinicians have the option of obtaining information from multiple sources, including employers, teachers, and counselors. In such cases, interview questions are tailored to fit the type and level of contact that each individual has with the patient—in essence, the informant's

TABLE 10–8. Factors Indicating a Need for Emphasis on Interviews with Patients

Emphasize Patient Interviews When	
The Patient . . .	**The Family . . .**
1. Is unable to identify someone familiar with his or her activities	1. Has difficulty identifying any positive areas of functioning
2. The patient's memory and communication skills are not severely impaired	2. Has a high level of conflict

attributes not readily observed during an interview. Fourth, questionnaires can be completed before the patient sees the examiner or as a supplement to the interview. During the interview, the examiner can then selectively focus on relevant issues.

Inflexibility is often cited as a limitation of quantitative measures. Asking everyone the same questions may exclude important information that might be gathered through observation or informal questioning. Also, some questionnaires have been described as too complex for persons with cognitive impairments or limited education.

Clinicians have available a wide variety of measures to quantify patients' problems, symptoms, or behaviors. Instrument selection depends on individual needs, the clinicians' theoretical orientation, time constraints, the mental status and educational level of respondents, and the attributes of available measures. Quantitative measures may be distinguished on the basis of:

- **Focus or content area.** Unidimensional measures focus on a single attribute (e.g., depression), whereas multidimensional measures delineate a variety of attributes (e.g., memory, physical symptoms, aggressiveness).
- **Ease of completion.** The complexity and language used may limit the feasibility of administration to respondents with cognitive impairments or limited education.
- **Relevance to brain injury population.** Measures vary with respect to their intent. Some were designed specifically to characterize persons with brain injury; others were developed to characterize psychiatric or medical populations.
- **Psychometric properties.**
  □ **Validity.** Validity refers to the extent to which statistical evidence supports the use for which the test was intended (e.g., as a measure of depression or aggression). With suitable factor analytic evidence, some tests allow computation and meaningful comparison of scale scores.
  □ **Reliability.** Test-retest reliability refers to the extent to which readministration of the measure yields a similar score. Test-retest reliability is applicable only if the attribute being measured is assumed to be stable over time. For example, depression may naturally fluctuate over time, and fluctuations in test scores would not necessarily indicate an unreliable measure. Interrater reliability reflects the extent to which two respondents describing the same attribute obtain similar scores.
  □ **Availability of normative data.** In select cases, patients' scores can be compared to those of normal people or of other people with similar types of injury.

A Review of Assessment Tools

The following section reviews commonly used quantitative assessment tools and the individual benefits and disadvantages of each in the brain injury population. It includes each tool's unique contributions, administration format, and the availability of alternative forms, availability of TBI norms, and susceptibility to impression management or motivational difficulties (Table 10–9). Rather than a comprehensive listing of all possible measures, we have selected examples of commonly used and practical measures with evidence of reliability and validity that are relevant to people with brain injury. The measures can be classified into two major categories: (1) questionnaires assessing mood and personality, developed originally for psychiatric populations; and (2) rating scales and inventories developed specifically for people with brain injury.

MOOD AND PERSONALITY QUESTIONNAIRE

Beck Depression Inventory

The Beck Depression Inventory[32] (BDI) is a 21-item, self-administered, multiple-choice questionnaire designed to detect the severity of depression in adolescents and adults. For each item, individuals must choose one of four responses that "best describes the way you have been feeling during the past week including today." Items correspond to such content areas as hopelessness, guilt, anhedonia, suicidal ideation, decreased initiative, appetite and sleep disturbance, emotional lability, and health concerns. Completion time is approximately 5 to 10 minutes. A 13-item short form is also available. Correlations between the short and long forms range from .89 to .97.[33]

Factor analytic studies of the BDI have supported the division of items into cognitive-affective (first 13 items), performance, and somatic subscales.[34,35] Concurrent validity has been demonstrated by high correlations with the Minnesota Multiphasic Personality Inventory (MMPI) Scale 2,[36] the Zung Self-Rating Depression Scale,[36] and the Hamilton Psychiatric Rating Scale for Depression.[37] Regarding content validity, the BDI has been determined to adequately assess six of the nine criteria for affective disorders in the third edition of the *Diagnostic and Statistical Manual* (DSM-III).[37] The adequacy of sleep and appetite disturbance assessment has been questioned.[37] For example,

TABLE 10–9. Brief Review of Test Highlights

Measure	Content Areas	Administration Time (min)	Versions	Comments
Beck Depression Inventory	Depression symptoms • Affective • Cognitive • Vegetative	5–15	Patient	1. Requires 6th-grade reading ability. 2. Strong emphasis on physical symptoms of depression. Symptoms of medical illness may be mistakenly attributed to depression. 3. Repeated administration allows measurement of treatment-related and spontaneous changes.
Brief Symptom Inventory	Emotional adjustment • Depression • Anxiety • Interpersonal skills • Anger • Somatization	45–75	Patient	1. Requires 6th-grade reading ability. 2. Uncertain validity for persons with brain injury; neurobehavioral symptoms may be mislabeled as "psychiatric."
Hamilton Depression Rating Scale	A. Depressive symptoms • Cognitive • Affective • Vegetative B. Participation in daily activities	15–30	Clinician	1. Brief screening inventory administered in the context of a clinical interview. 2. Useful for persons with limited reading and writing skills.
MMPI/MMPI-2	Emotional status • Emotional adjustment • Psychopathology • Social skills	75–120	Patient	1. MMPI-2 developed for ages 18 to adult 2. MMPI-2 requires 6th-grade reading ability. MMPI requires 8th-grade reading ability. 3. Audiotaped and computer-administered versions available.
Neurobehavioral Functioning Inventory	Frequency of neurobehavioral symptoms • Cognitive • Emotional • Somatic	15–30	Patient Caregiver	1. Specifically developed to assess problems common to traumatic brain injury 2. For persons with severe brain injury, responses may be susceptible to awareness limitations.
Neurobehavioral Rating Scale	Neurobehavioral symptoms • Affective • Cognitive • Behavioral	10–15	Clinician	1. Ceiling effects may limit usefulness in postacute settings.
Katz Adjustment Scale	Emotional status • Behavior • Social adjustment • Recreational and social activities	45–50	Caregiver	1. Provides information regarding the degree to which activities meet caregiver expectations. 2. Assesses behavior in the community. 3. Ratings susceptible to denial and unrealistic expectations.
Mayo-Portland Adaptability Inventory	Functional impact of neurobehavioral symptoms • Emotional adjustment • Social skills	20–30	Patient Caregiver Clinician	1. Specifically developed for use with TBI. 2. Preliminary evidence of reliability and validity.

the BDI asks about decreased sleep and appetite but not about the increases often associated with depression. Furthermore, the BDI does not assess psychomotor restlessness or retardation.

The BDI was originally developed to distinguish between depressed and nondepressed psychiatric patients. Items were generated by professionals based on clinical observations, including descriptions of symptoms frequently provided by depressed patients. BDI scores have been shown to reliably discriminate depressed psychiatric patients from those with dysthymia[38] and generalized anxiety disorder.[39] Although not intended as a screening instrument, the BDI has also been shown to discriminate between psychiatric patients and the normal population.[39,40] However, concern has been expressed regarding the accuracy of the BDI's detection of depression in the normal population.[41,42]

Despite the measure's popularity, relatively few studies have examined the BDI's effectiveness in detecting depression in people with TBI. Of concern is the fact that a third of the items relate specifically to many of the somatic complaints and performance problems commonly reported by persons with TBI (e.g., decreased initiation, fatigue); overlap between symptoms of TBI and depression decreases the BDI's utility with the brain injured population. The cognitive-affective subscale has been suggested as a means of detecting depression in medical patients whose scores on the performance and somatic subscales may be affected by physical illness. However, this distinction is not likely to be useful with the TBI population because brain injury causes cognitive and affective changes, as well as somatic and performance changes. In spite of difficulties, the BDI can be useful with brain injured patients as long as the results are interpreted cautiously, with careful consideration of the effects of organic dysfunction on symptoms.[43]

Brief Symptom Inventory

The Brief Symptom Inventory[44] (BSI) is a short form of the Symptom Checklist-90-R (SCL-90), which was developed to discriminate between psychiatric patients in different diagnostic groups. The BSI is a 53-item self-report measure to assess the severity of psychiatric symptoms. Items are rated on a 5-point Likert scale with regard to the severity of symptoms during the past week (0 = not at all; 4 = extremely). Completion of the BSI requires at least a sixth-grade reading level. Responses yield nine subscale scores: Somatization, Obsessive-Compulsive, Interpersonal Sensitivity, Depression, Anxiety, Hostility, Phobic Anxiety, Paranoid Ideation, and Psychoticism. Besides the nine subscale scores, there are three global indices: The Global Severity Index (GSI) is an indicator of the current overall level of distress, the Positive Symptom Total (PST) is a measure of the absolute number of endorsed symptoms, and the Positive Symptom Index (PSI) is a measure of severity adjusted for the number of symptoms endorsed.

The BSI has been used in outpatient and inpatient settings. Factor analytic procedures have revealed that the factor structure of the BSI is equivalent to that of the SCL-90.[44] Test-retest reliabilities range from .80 to .90 for the global indices and from .68 to .91 for the subscale scores.[45] Internal consistency coefficients range from .71 to .85.[45] For a sample of 501 forensic psychiatric inpatients and outpatients, Boulet and Boss[46] reported moderate convergent validity and poor discriminate validity for the BSI scales. Factor analysis yielded one factor that accounted for 71 percent of the variance. The authors concluded that the BSI was a promising global measure of psychological distress but that the subscale profiles were not valid. Individual subscale analyses of the BSI was not recommended.

Only a few studies have utilized the BSI with the TBI population. Landsman et al.[47] administered the BSI to 137 patients with TBI and documented significant levels of emotional distress. Hinkeldey and Corrigan[48] administered the BSI to 55 persons with severe TBI. Analysis revealed significant elevations on all three global distress indices. Examination of the individual subscale scores revealed elevations on the Depression, Obsessive-Compulsive, Phobic Anxiety, Paranoid Ideation, and Psychoticism scales.

The BSI's brevity makes it a useful tool for assessing emotional status in persons with TBI, who often have poor stamina or problems with distractibility. The BSI has been described as easier to administer than traditional measures, such as the MMPI or the Katz Adjustment Scale.[48] A further advantage is that extensive normative data for the general population are available.[45] The BSI lacks validity scales to help identify persons who are poorly motivated, malingering, or denying difficulties. Furthermore, as with other measures developed with psychiatric populations, the utility of the BSI to diagnosing emotional distress in persons with brain injury is suspect. Symptoms of brain injury frequently overlap with psychiatric symptoms (e.g., depression, anxiety), which may lead to a high number of false positives.

Hamilton Depression Rating Scale

The Hamilton Depression Rating Scale[49] (HDRS) is a 17-item scale designed to quantify the clinician's diagnostic observations. The clinician completes items through interviews with patients and relatives and review of medical records. The scale surveys cognitive, emotional, and somatic symptoms of depression, as well as their impact on daily activities. Scores range from 0 to 60, with higher scores reflecting greater levels of depression.

The HDRS has been used by several researchers to assess depression in persons with neurological disorders.[50–52] However, relatively few of the investigations focused on people with TBI. Leach et al.[52] utilized the HDRS to assess depression in a sample of 39 persons with TBI. Nearly three-quarters (73%) were identified as mildly depressed. Two patients were severely depressed, and 21 percent were classified as not depressed.

Research examining the validity of the HDRS in TBI populations has been relatively rare. Unfortunately, somatic (47%), behavioral (29%), and cognitive complaints (12%) make up a large proportion of the scale's items. Thus, more than three-fourths of the items may be attributable to neurobehavioral sequelae of TBI rather than depression.

Minnesota Multiphasic Personality Inventory

The MMPI and MMPI-2[53,54] are perhaps the most widely used means of assessing emotional functioning among most populations, including neurological patients. The original MMPI items were chosen for their ability to discriminate between various psychiatric diagnostic groups. The MMPI (566 items) and MMPI-2 (567 items) are self-administered questionnaires consisting of true-false items, with each item corresponding to a specific symptom. The items comprise 10 clinical scales and 3 validity scales. The MMPI-2 has three additional validity scales to assess response consistency throughout the test and to detect "true" or "false" response biases. The diagnostic utility of the MMPI and MMPI-2 for clinical psychiatric samples has been consistently demonstrated.[55] In the years since the instrument's development, numerous subscales have been developed to detect a variety of specific difficulties, ranging from alcoholism to post-traumatic stress disorder. The construct and predictive validity of most of these scales has not been confirmed. An advantage of the MMPI and MMPI-2 is their adaptability for various populations. For example, versions are available for non-English-speaking patients, and a tape-recorded version is available for those who cannot read or are visually handicapped.

The statistically sophisticated development process, popularity, and ease of administration of the MMPI and MMPI-2 have led to their adaptation for people with brain injury and other neurological disorders. However, concerns have been raised about the validity and accuracy of the MMPI in evaluating persons with TBI. The concerns focus on three main issues. First, the length of the MMPI and the complex wording of certain questions are inappropriate for patients with attentional or reading comprehension difficulties. Burke et al.[56] reported that people with TBI tend to respond inconsistently to items. The inclusion of response inconsistency scales on the MMPI-2 addresses this issue by allowing examiners to easily identify patients who respond inconsistently. However, the cost in time and energy for a brain injured person to complete the questionnaire must be carefully weighed against the possibility that the profile will be interpreted as invalid. A priori administration of reading comprehension measures can identify persons who are unsuited for the measure.

A second criticism is relevant to most self-report measures. Persons with brain injury often exhibit decreased awareness, which can affect their ability to respond accurately to questions. Again, inconsistencies in responding that result from awareness difficulties may be detected by the validity scale scores, but the potential for wasted time and energy should be carefully considered.

A third criticism of the use of the MMPI with the brain injured population concerns the overlap of symptoms between brain injury and many psychiatric diagnoses. Researchers have cautioned that use of the MMPI with people with TBI may result in a large number of false-positive diagnoses of psychiatric difficulties.[57–62] For example, the physical difficulties typically experienced following brain injury (e.g., headaches, dizziness, fatigue) result in elevations on scales 1 and 3. Clinicians who interpret these elevations as indicative of somatoform or conversion disorder, without considering the contribution of the brain injury, will draw erroneous conclusions. The MMPI and MMPI-2 scales that have been shown to be most elevated in patients with TBI are scales 1, 2, 3, 7, and 8.[59–63]

In an effort to factor out the impact of neurological symptoms on MMPI scale scores, some researchers have developed correction factors. For example, Cripe[58] reported on 85 MMPI items that could be diagnosed by neurological patients with no psychiatric difficulties. The items, labeled the Cripe Neurologic Symptoms, reflect difficulties that are commonly observed in patients with neurological disorders in the following categories: attention/mental control; sleep and appetite disturbance; regulation of emotions; fatigue/decreased energy; physical symptoms (e.g., headaches, blank spells, sensory disturbance), memory, motor control, pain, dizziness and nausea, sexual dysfunction, speech/language problems, and vocational difficulty. Cripe recommended that clinicians should, when interpreting the MMPI in populations with neurological problems, carefully investigate the types of items endorsed by patients, especially in these content areas.

Gass[61] found two factors that discriminated between patients with TBI and the MMPI-2 adult normative sample. Factor 1, labeled the Neurologic Complaints factor, consisted of items corresponding to cognitive, speech, and motor difficulties. Factor 2 consisted of five items that reflected psychiatric difficulties, including distrust of others, social discomfort, and unusual experiences. Gass recommended scoring profiles twice for TBI patients, once according to standard protocol and once after eliminating the factor 1 items.

RATING SCALES AND INVENTORIES DEVELOPED FOR TRAUMATIC BRAIN INJURY

Neurobehavioral Functioning Inventory

The Neurobehavioral Functioning Inventory (NFI) is an 83-item scale developed to assess the frequency of neurobehavioral difficulties following TBI.[25,64] NFI items were originally formulated and compiled based on interviews with patients who sustained traumatic brain injuries and their family members, as well as on extensive literature reviews. Based on confirmatory factor analysis with 520 respondents, the original 105-item questionnaire was reduced to 83 items loading on six factors: Depression, Somatic, Memory/Attention, Communication, Aggression, and Motor skills.[64]

The NFI can be administered orally or self-administered (e.g., completed at home in advance of evaluation or in the clinic). Two versions are available, one for completion by the patient and another by informants (e.g., family members). Each item is rated on a 5-point scale based on frequency of occurrence: never (1), rarely (2), sometimes (3), often (4), or always (5). A subset of items may also be rated as not applicable. Norms based on patients' age at time of injury and injury severity are available for both patient and significant other versions.[65]

Kreutzer et al.[64] provided evidence for the NFI's internal reliability. Cronbach's alpha coefficients for each scale were as follows: Depression (.93), Somatic (.86), Memory/Attention (.95), Communication (.88), Aggression (.89), and Motor (.87). Interrater reliability has

been demonstrated by high rates of concordance between patients' and family members' ratings on all scales except Communication.[28] On the Communication scale, patients endorsed more symptoms than did family members. Criterion-related validity was demonstrated by significant relationships between the Communication and Memory/Attention scales and scores on neuropsychological measures.[64] Criterion-related validity was also evidenced by relationship between the NFI factor scales and the MMPI clinical scales 1, 2, 3, 7, and 8. NFI Somatic and Motor scale scores were related to MMPI scales 1, 2, and 3. All six NFI scales were significantly related to MMPI Scale 2. Scores on MMPI scale 8 were related to the NFI Depression and Memory/Attention Scales, and scores on MMPI scale 7 were related to NFI Depression and Somatic scales.

The NFI has several advantages. First, the measure was designed specifically to assess the types of problems typically observed after TBI. Patients and family members can complete the NFI on their own and yield information about patients' problem areas that can be followed up during the clinical interview. Second, the NFI is multidimensional, assessing a wide range of difficulties and yielding six scale scores rather than a global measure of functioning. Third, the availability of both patient and significant other forms enables clinicians to obtain more than one perspective on patients' difficulties. Normative data for persons of similar age and injury severity are available for both patient and significant other versions. Fourth, the NFI has been translated into other languages, including Spanish, German, and French.

The limitations of the NFI relate primarily to lack of normative data on uninjured persons. Many of the items (e.g., headaches, feeling sad or blue) would likely be endorsed as occurring at least sometimes by people in the normal population. Thus, the ability of the NFI to discriminate between persons with TBI and those without is limited. Another limitation relates to the lack of validity scales to detect malingering or self-awareness problems.

The Neurobehavioral Rating Scale

The Neurobehavioral Rating Scale (NRS)[9] is a 27-item scale developed to assess emotional and behavioral difficulties exhibited by patients with brain injury. The NRS was devised to address concerns about the validity of self-report inventories regarding emotions and behavior during the early stages of recovery from brain injury. The measure was adapted from the Brief Psychiatric Rating Scale, a measure assessing emotional and behavioral problems in the psychiatric population. In addition to the traditional scales, items were added to assess attention, memory, insight, and disinhibition. The NRS is completed by clinicians based on an interview. Although a structured interview was used in the development of the measure, Levin et al.[9] reported that any interview assessing the issues addressed by the NRS would be acceptable. Items are rated on an ordinal 7-point scale (1 = not present; 7 = extremely severe).

Initial evidence of validity was reported by Levin et al.[9] based on a sample of 101 patients with nonmissile head injuries. Using principal components analysis, they identified four major factors: cognition/energy, metacognition, somatic concern/anxiety, and language. Construct validity was evidenced by the fact that persons with more severe injuries showed greater disturbance on three of the four factors (cognition/energy, metacognition, language). Also, the total score decreased from initial testing (1–3 mo postinjury) to a 6-month follow-up, indicating that the NRS was measuring behaviors affected by brain injury. A subsequent study conducted with a Taiwanese population revealed the presence of seven factors: Excitement, Cognition, Energy, Metacognition, Anxiety, Decreased Initiative/Motivation, and Speech.[16]

Adequate reliability has also been demonstrated for the NRS. Interrater reliability coefficients have ranged from .88 to .90 for an acute TBI sample[9] to 80 percent interrater agreement for an inpatient rehabilitation sample.[66] Adequate internal consistency was evidenced by Cronbach's alpha ranging from .87 to .89, using two different raters and two inpatient rehabilitation samples.[66]

The NRS appears to be the most useful tool available for monitoring behavior early after injury, including during acute hospitalization and rehabilitation. The measure has been shown to be sensitive to behaviors typically affected by brain injury, including memory, conceptual disorganization, poor planning, and inaccurate insight.[9,10,66] Completion by the clinician makes the NRS appropriate for patients who may have severe cognitive impairments, including lack of awareness and insight. The NRS has been validated for use as a rating tool based on observation during daily therapies in an inpatient setting; clinicians can save time by not having to conduct structured interviews.[66]

The NRS appears to be a less sensitive measure for people in later stages of recovery. Research has shown that most patients show minimal disturbance on most items at 6 to 8 months postinjury.[9,10] Because much research has documented the persistence of neurobehavioral problems at intervals ranging from 5 to 15 years postinjury,[3,12,18] the apparent inability of the NRS to detect long-term problems is a concern. A further criticism is its minimal reliance on the reports of family members, who may have greater knowledge of changes from the patient's preinjury functioning. Finally, concerns have been expressed that the standard interview procedure reduces the likelihood of observing daily problem behaviors.[10]

The Katz Adjustment Scale: Relative Form

The Katz Adjustment Scale Relative Form[67] (KAS-R) was originally developed to assess the adjustment of psychiatric patients who had returned to the community. Areas assessed include behavioral symptoms, social adjustment, recreational activities, and social role functioning. The questionnaire contains five subscales or forms that are completed by someone who has detailed knowledge of the patient's daily activities. Form R1 contains 127 items relating to a patient's emotional and behavioral adjustment. Each symptom (e.g., sleep disturbance) is rated on a Likert scale for frequency of occurrence (1 = almost never; 4 = almost always). Form R2 consists of 16 items regarding the patient's level of performance in socially expected activities (e.g., working, helping with household chores). Items are rated on a Likert scale (1 = not doing, 2 = doing some, 3 = doing regularly). Form R3 consists of the same items as R2, but relatives rate their expectations of a patient's activities rather than actual activity levels. Forms R4 and R5 contain 22 items regarding participation in specific leisure activities (e.g., watching television, shopping). Items on form R4 correspond to the patient's actual activity levels (1 = frequently, 3 = probably never); items on R5 ask about relatives' satisfaction with the patient's activity levels (1 = satisfied with what he does, 3 = would like to see him do less).

Factor analysis of form R1 has yielded three major factors: social obstreperousness, acute psychoticism, and withdrawn depression.[67] The three factors subsume 12 subacute scores. Good test-retest reliability, with an intertest interval of 8 weeks, has been demonstrated for all three factors.[68] Internal consistency has been demonstrated by Cronbach alpha coefficients ranging from .78 to .94 for the subscales.[69]

The areas measured by the KASR have been described as particularly relevant for patients with brain injury living in the community.[70] The instrument has been used in a number of studies investigating adjustment after brain injury. KASR scores have been shown to discriminate between patients with brain injury and uninjured patients.[71] Significant elevations for patients with brain injury have been documented on most scales, including Belligerence, Helplessness, Anxiety, General Psychopathology, Confusion, Bizarreness, Negativism, and Hyperactivity.[48,72,73] Klonoff et al.[73] found that scores at 2 to 4 years postinjury were related to injury severity, motor dysfunction, education, acuteness of injury, and the presence of seizure disorder and frontal lobe damage. Scores also showed diagnostic utility by predicting group membership for patients with mild TBI, severe TBI, spinal cord injury (SCI), and a combined SCI plus severe TBI group.

Mayo-Portland Adaptability Inventory

The Mayo Portland Adaptability Inventory[74] (MPAI) was adapted from the Portland Adaptability Inventory (PAI) developed by Lezak.[75] The original PAI consisted of 24 items to assess TBI patients' abilities in three areas: temperament and emotionality, activities and social behavior, and physical capabilities. The MPAI consists of 30 items reflecting typical problems after brain injury. Each item is rated on a 4-point scale (0 = no impairment, 3 = severe impairment). Emphasis is placed on the extent to which impairments interfere with everyday functioning. In the original standardization sample, consisting of 50 outpatients, six scales were used: physical/medical, cognition, emotion, everyday activities, social behaviors, and behavior.[74] Concurrent validity was evidenced by significant correlations with the Disability Rating Scale and with various neuropsychological measures. MPAI scores were able to discriminate between good and poor outcome groups based on Rancho Los Amigos Levels of Cognitive Functioning Scale ratings.

The results of a subsequent study supported a slightly different scale structure. Using a sample of 204 patients with mixed etiology (80% TBI, 12% cerebrovascular accident, 8% other), Bohac et al.[76] identified an eight-factor solution that best described the data, accounting for 64.4 percent of the variance in MPAI scores: activities of daily living, social initiation, cognition, impaired self-awareness/distress, social skills/support, independence, visuoperceptual, and psychiatric. Significant relationships between MPAI scores and neuropsychological measures were noted for all subscales except Social Initiation, Social Skills/Support, and Psychiatric. The authors concluded that the eight-factor structure better represents the multidimensional nature of problems associated with TBI and is more clinically useful.

Interrater reliability of the MPAI has been addressed by comparing staff ratings to those of patients and their family members.[77] The ratings of staff and family members were significantly related. A relationship between staff and patient ratings was noted for those patients who were depressed but not for nondepressed patients. Finally, family members' ratings were moderately related to staff and patient ratings. A relatively stronger relationship between family and staff versus family and patient ratings was noted for nondepressed patients.

The MPAI appears to be a promising tool for measuring the multidimensional nature of behavior and adjustment after brain injury. However, more research is needed on psychometric properties, including confirmatory factor analysis and cross-validation.

Diagnosis

In the final step of assessment, information collected from a variety of sources is integrated to formulate a diagnosis. The diagnosis provides information about the history, patterns of behavior, and symptoms. This label helps professionals communicate, allows record keeping on incidence, and guides treatment planning.

The *Diagnostic and Statistical Manual of Mental Disorders*, fourth edition[78] (DSM-IV) is the most commonly used classification system for behavioral, psychological, and biological disorders in the United States. The book provides extensive information about each diagnosis, including (1) diagnostic features; (2) associated features and disorders; (3) age, culture, and gender features; (4) course and prevalence; and (5) differential diagnosis. Assignment of a diagnosis requires that the condition distresses the individual and results in impairment of social or occupational functioning.

The DSM-IV is a multiaxial classification system developed primarily for persons with psychiatric disorders such as schizophrenia, anxiety and mood disorders, somatoform, and dissociative disorders. Labels for psychiatric, developmental, and personality disorders are listed on axes I and II. Medical diagnostic information (e.g., status after evacuation of subdural hematoma secondary to severe brain injury) is listed on axis III. Psychosocial stressors (e.g., unemployment, family conflict) that can affect psychological status are enumerated on axis IV. Axis V is the Global Assessment of Functioning Scale, which depicts overall psychological functioning. Values between 1 ("persistent danger of severely hurting self or others," p. 32) and 100 ("superior functioning in a wide range of activities and no symptoms," p. 32) are assigned, with higher values denoting better functioning levels. The DSM-IV does not require a distinction between preinjury and postinjury disorders. Nevertheless, such distinctions are helpful in formulating realistic treatment plans.

TABLE 10–10. DSM-IV Diagnoses Frequently Assigned following Brain Injury

Adjustment disorder

- Excessive distress in response to a normally stressful event
- Symptom onset within 3 mo of event and resolution within 6 mo; symptoms can extend beyond 6 mo with ongoing stress
- Depending on symptom constellation, may be labeled as (1) "with depressed mood," (2) "with anxiety," or (3) "with mixed anxiety and depressed mood"

Conversion disorder

- Motor or sensory dysfunction (e.g., paralysis, seizures, loss of vision) that mimics a neurological disorder, but symptoms cannot be explained by a medical cause
- Symptoms not intentionally feigned; onset preceded by stress or conflict

Major depressive disorder

- Sadness, loss of interest, or reduced pleasure in former activities for at least 2 wk; suicidal ideation
- Substantial change in sleep or appetite; decreased energy or fatigue
- Psychomotor agitation or retardation
- Decreased concentration, difficulty making decisions

Acute stress disorder and post-traumatic stress disorder (PTSD)

- Exposure to an event that is life-threatening to self or others
- Evokes extreme feelings of fear, horror, helplessness
- Intrusive thoughts regarding incident, substantial anxiety, increased arousal (e.g., hypervigilance)
- When symptoms persist beyond 1 mo, a diagnosis of PTSD is given

Psychological symptoms affecting medical condition

- Symptoms (e.g., anxiety, depression) do not meet criteria for an axis I or II disorder
- Substantial effects of symptom on medical condition (e.g., worries about disability exacerbate postinjury headaches and concentration problems)

Somatization disorder

- History of multiple physical complaints requiring treatment, beginning before age 30
- Symptoms relate to pain, gastrointestinal difficulties, sexual dysfunction, or pseudoneurological symptoms (e.g., paralysis, amnesia, impaired coordination)
- Symptoms not substantiated by thorough medical examination; symptoms not intentionally feigned

---

The DSM-IV system is generally adequate for people with brain injury and helps qualify pre-existing and concomitant psychiatric difficulties. Table 10–10 provides a listing of DSM-IV diagnoses commonly assigned after brain injury and the major attributes of each. The manual has more detailed information.

Caution must be used in applying DSM-IV criteria to the population with brain injury. Many symptoms of psychiatric diagnoses overlap with those of brain injury. For example, fatigue and decreased concentration are symptoms of both depression and brain injury. Further confusion is created by the myth that emotion and personality are affected by psychological rather than neurological causes.[59] Organic dysfunction can be a cause of both emotional and cognitive difficulties. Accurate diagnosis requires (1) careful review of medical records, including preinjury history; (2) neuropsychological evaluation to discern patterns of cognitive and psychomotor ability; and (3) psychological evaluation to discern levels of awareness and reaction to disability. One strategy to improve diagnostic accuracy is to first differentiate between the cognitive, behavioral, and emotional criteria of the diagnosis, then determine which of the patients' symptoms are specifically due to neurobehavioral changes (e.g., decreased concentration due to brain injury), and finally use this information to provide differing emphasis to diagnostically relevant symptoms.

The international classification of diseases (ICD-9) has also been used for classification.[79] Developed as a comprehensive listing of medical and mental health disorders, many of the ICD-9 mental health disorders are similar to those described in DSM-IV. Unfortunately, the ICD-9 does not provide detailed criteria or differential diagnostic information. As such, the manual is most useful for calculating incidence and prevalence.

□ SUMMARY

Accurate description and diagnosis of emotional and personality disorders are important first steps in treatment planning. Reliable information collected over time provides an index of change and a basis for formulating a prognosis. Accurate diagnosis requires a synthesis of information from a variety of sources, including records review, behavioral observation, clinical interview, and quantitative assessment. Formidable challenges to clinical efficiency and formulating reliable diagnoses remain. The neurological sequelae of brain injury are often complex. Also, many patients bring complicated preinjury and postinjury psychosocial histories.

The research on measurement of emotional and personality changes after brain injury has lagged behind investigation of cognitive changes. Future directions for research include (1) collection of normative data for brain injury and neurologically normal populations and (2) development of measures more specific to the needs of patients with brain injury. Multidimensional measures that tap a wide range of behaviors along a continuum of different stages of recovery should also be explored.

REFERENCES

1. Levin, H, Benton, AL, and Grossman, RG: Neurobehavioral Consequences of Closed Head Injury. Oxford University Press, New York, 1982.
2. Thomsen, IV: The patient with severe head injury and his family. Scand J Rehabil Med 6:180, 1974.
3. Thomsen, IV: Late outcome of very severe blunt head trauma: A 10–15 year second follow-up. J Neurol Neurosurg Psychiatry 47:260–68, 1984.
4. Lezak, MD: Living with the characterologically altered brain injured patient. J Clin Psychiatry 39:111, 1978.
5. Brooks, DN: The head-injured family. J Clin Exp Neuropsychol 13:155, 1991.
6. Oddy, M, Humphrey, M, and Uttley, D: Subjective impairment and social recovery after closed head injury. J Neurol Neurosurg Psychiatry 41:611–16, 1978.
7. McKinlay, WW, Brooks, DN, and Bond, MR: The short term outcome of severe blunt head injury as reported by the relatives of the injured person. J Neurol Neurosurg Psychiatry 44:527, 1981.
8. Brooks, DN, and McKinlay, W: Personality and behavioral change after severe blunt head injury: A relatives' view. J Neurol Neurosurg Psychiatry 46:336–44, 1983.
9. Levin, HS, et al: The Neurobehavioral Rating Scale: Assessment of the behavioral sequelae of head injury by the clinician. J Neurol Neurosurg Psychiatry 50:183–93, 1987.
10. Keyser, L, et al: A multi-center investigation of neurobehavioral outcome after traumatic brain injury. NeuroRehabilitation 5:255–67, 1995.
11. Goethe, K, and Levin, H: Behavioral manifestations during the early and long-term stages of recovery after closed head injury. Psychiatric Annals 14:540–46, 1984.
12. Oddy, M, et al: Social adjustment after closed head injury: A further follow-up seven years after injury. J Neurol Neurosurg Psychiatry 48:564–68, 1985.
13. Brooks, N, et al: The five year outcome of severe blunt head injury: A relative's view. J Neurol Neurosurg Psychiatry 49:764, 1986.
14. Brooks, N, et al: The effects of severe head injury on patient and relative within seven years of injury. J Head Trauma Rehabil 2:1, 1987.
15. Rappaport, M, et al: Head injury outcome up to ten years later. Arch Phys Med Rehabil 70:885–93, 1989.
16. Chiu, W, et al: Neurobehavioral manifestations following closed head injury. J Formos Med Assoc 92:255–62, 1993.
17. Kreutzer, JS, et al: Neurobehavioral outcome following traumatic brain injury: Review, methodology, and implications for cognitive rehabilitation. In Kreutzer, JS, and Wehman, PH (eds): Cognitive Rehabilitation for Persons with Traumatic Brain Injury: A Functional Approach. Paul H. Brookes Publishing, Baltimore, 1991.
18. Witol, AD, et al: Long term neurobehavioral characteristics after brain injury: Implications for vocational rehabilitation. Journal of Vocational Rehabilitation 7:159–67, 1996.
19. Wood, RL: Brain injury rehabilitation: A neurobehavioral approach. Aspen, Frederick, Md, 1987.
20. Wood, RL: Conditioning procedures in brain injury rehabilitation. In Wood, RL (ed): Neurobehavioral Sequelae of Closed Head Injury. Taylor and Francis, New York, 1990.
21. Eames, P: Behavior disorders after severe head injury: Their nature and causes and strategies for management. J Head Trauma Rehabil 3:1–6, 1988.
22. Eames, P, Haffey, WJ, and Cope, DN: Treatment of behavioral disorders. In Rosenthal, M, et al (eds): Rehabilitation of the Adult and Child with Traumatic Brain Injury (ed 2). FA Davis, Philadelphia, 1990.
23. Jacobs, H: Behavior Analysis Guidelines and Brain Injury Rehabilitation: People, Principles, and Programs. Aspen, Gaithersburg, Md, 1993.
24. Kay, T, et al: The head injury family interview: A clinical and research tool. J Head Trauma Rehabil 10:12–31, 1995.
25. Kreutzer, J, et al: General Health and History Questionnaire. Richmond, Virginia, Rehabilitation Research and Training Center on Severe Traumatic Brain Injury, Medical College of Virginia, 1987.
26. McKinlay, WW, and Brooks, DN: Methodological problems in assessing psychosocial recovery following severe head injury. Journal of Clinical Neuropsychology 6:87–99, 1984.
27. Prigatano, GP, Altman, IM, and O'Brien, KP: Behavioral limitations that traumatic brain-injured patients tend to underestimate. Clinical Neuropsychologist 4:163–76, 1990.
28. Seel, RT, Kreutzer, JS, and Sander, AM: Concordance of patients' and family members' ratings of neurobehavioral functioning after traumatic brain injury. Arch Phys Med Rehabil 78(11):1254–1259, 1997.
29. Gasquoine, PG: Affective state and awareness of sensory and cognitive effects after closed head injury. Neuropsychologia 4:187–96, 1992.
30. Sherer, M, et al: Awareness of deficits after traumatic brain injury: Comparison of patient, family, and clinician ratings (abstract). Journal of the International Neuropsychology Society 2:17, 1996.
31. Kinsella, G, et al: Emotional disorder and its assessment within the severe head injury population. Psychol Med 18:57–63, 1988.
32. Beck, AT, et al: Cognitive Therapy of Depression. Guilford, New York, 1979.
33. Beck, AT, Rial, WY, and Rickels, K: Short form of depression inventory: Cross validation. Psychol Rep 34:1184–86, 1974.
34. Cavanaugh, SV, Clark, DC, and Gibbons, RD: Diagnosing depression in the hospitalized medically ill. Psychosomatics 24:809–15, 1983.
35. Tanaka, JS, and Huba, GJ: Confirmatory hierarchical factor analysis of psychological distress measures. J Pers Soc Psychol 46:621–35, 1984.
36. Schaefer, A, et al: Comparison of the validities of the Beck, Zung, and MMPI depression scales. J Consult Clin Psychol 53:415–18, 1985.
37. Beck, AT, and Steer, RA: Beck Depression Inventory Manual. The Psychological Corporation and Harcourt Brace Jovanovich, San Antonio, 1987.
38. Steer, RA, et al: Self-reported depressive symptoms differentiating major depression from dysthymic disorders. J Clin Psychol 43:246–50, 1987.
39. Steer, RA, et al: Differentiation of depressive disorders from generalized anxiety by the Beck Depression Inventory. J Clin Psychol 40:475–78, 1986.
40. Byerly, EC, and Carlson, WA: Comparison among inpatients, outpatients and normals on three self-report depression inventories. J Clin Psychol 38:797–804, 1982.
41. Dobson, KS, and Breiter, HJ: Cognitive assessment of depression: Reliability and validity of three measures. J Abnorm Psychol 92:107–9, 1981.
42. Sacco, WP: Invalid use of the Beck Depression Inventory to identify depressed college-student subjects: A methodological comment. Cognitive Therapy Research 5:143–47, 1981.
43. Christensen, BK, et al: The role of depression in rehabilitation outcome during acute recovery from traumatic brain injury. Advances in Medical Psychotherapy 7:23–38, 1994.

44. Derogatis, LR: Brief Symptom Inventory. Clinical Psychometric Research, Baltimore, 1975.
45. Derogatis, LR, and Melisaratos, N: The Brief Symptom Inventory: An introductory report. Psychol Med 13:595–605, 1983.
46. Boulet, J, and Boss, MW: Reliability and validity of the Brief Symptom Inventory. Psychological Assessment 3:433–37, 1991.
47. Landsman, IS, et al: The psychosocial consequences of traumatic injury. J Behav Med 13:561–80, 1990.
48. Hinkeldey, NS, and Corrigan, JD: The structure of head injured patients' neurobehavioral complaints: A preliminary study. Brain Inj 4:115–33, 1990.
49. Hamilton, M: Development of a rating scale for primary depressive illness. Br J Soc Clin Psychol 6:278–96, 1967.
50. Robinson, RG: Mood disorders in left handed stroke patients. Am J Psychiatry 142:1424–29, 1985.
51. Lipsey, JR, et al: Mood change following bilateral hemisphere brain injury. Br J Psychiatry 143:266–73, 1983.
52. Leach, LR, et al: Family functioning, social support and depression after traumatic brain injury. Brain Inj 8:599–606, 1994.
53. Hathaway, SR, and McKinley, JC: The Minnesota Multiphasic Personality Manual (Revised). Psychological Corporation, New York, 1951.
54. Butcher, JN, et al: Minnesota Multiphasic Personality Inventory-2 (MMPI-2): Manual for Administration and Scoring. University of Minnesota Press, Minneapolis, 1989.
55. Greene, R: The MMPI-2/MMPI: An Interpretive Manual. Allyn & Bacon, Needham Heights, Mass, 1991.
56. Burke, JM, Smith, SA, and Imhoff, CL: The response styles of post-acute traumatic brain injured patients on the MMPI. Brain Inj 3:335–40, 1989.
57. Dikmen, S, and Reitan, RM: MMPI correlates of adaptive ability deficits in patients with brain lesions. J Nerv Ment Dis 165:247–53, 1977.
58. Cripe, LI: The clinical use of the MMPI with neurologic patients: A new perspective. Paper presented at the Army Medical Department Psychology Conference, Seattle, June 1988.
59. Cripe, LI: Personality assessment of brain-impaired patients. In Maruish, ME, and Moses, JA (eds): Clinical Neuropsychology: Theoretical Foundations for Practitioners. Lawrence Erlbaum, Mahwah, NJ, 1997.
60. Cripe, LI: The MMPI in neuropsychological assessment: A murky measure. Applied Neuropsychology 3:97–103, 1997.
61. Gass, CS: MMPI-2 interpretation and closed head injury. Psychological Assessment 3:27–31, 1991.
62. Leininger, BE, Kreutzer, JS, and Hill, MR: Comparison of minor and severe head injury emotional sequelae using the MMPI. Brain Inj 5:199–205, 1991.
63. Black, FW: Unilateral brain lesions and MMPI performance: A preliminary study. Percept Mot Skills 40:87–93, 1975.
64. Kreutzer, JS, et al: Validation of a neurobehavioral functioning inventory for adults with traumatic brain injury. Arch Phys Med Rehabil 77:116–24, 1996.
65. Kreutzer, JS, Seel, R, and Marwitz, JH: The Neurobehavioral Functioning Inventory–Revised: Manual for Administration and Scoring. Richmond, Va: Medical College of Virginia, 1997.
66. Corrigan, JD, et al: The Neurobehavioral Rating Scale: Replication in an acute, inpatient rehabilitation setting. Brain Inj 4:215–22, 1990.
67. Katz, MM, and Lyerly, SB: Methods for measuring adjustment and social behavior in the community. I. Rationale, description, discriminate validity and scale development. Psychol Rep 13:503–35, 1963.
68. Ruff, HM, and Niemann, H: Cognitive rehabilitation versus day treatment in head injured adults: Is there an impact on emotional and psychosocial adjustment? Brain Inj 4:339–47, 1990.
69. Goran, DA, and Fabiano, RJ: The scaling of the Katz Adjustment Scale in a traumatic brain injury rehabilitation sample. Brain Inj 7:219–29, 1993.
70. Lezak, M: Observational methods, rating scales, and inventories. In Lezak, K: Neuropsychological Assessment. Oxford University Press, New York, 1995.
71. Goodman, WA, Ball, JD, and Peck, E: Psychosocial characteristics of head-injured patients: A comparison of factor structures of the Katz Adjustment Scale (abstract). J Clin Exp Neuropsychol 10:42, 1988.
72. Fordyce, DJ, Roueche, JR, and Prigatano, GP: Enhanced emotional reactions in chronic head trauma patients. J Neurol Neurosurg Psychiatry 46:620–24, 1983.
73. Klonoff, PS, Costa, LD, and Snow, WG: Predictors and indicators of quality of life in patients with closed-head injury. J Clin Exp Neuropsychol 8:469–85, 1986.
74. Malec, JF, and Thompson, JM: Relationship of the Mayo-Portland Adaptability Inventory to functional outcome and cognitive performance measures. J Head Trauma Rehabil 9:1–15, 1994.
75. Lezak, MD: Relationships between personality disorders, social disturbances, and physical disability following traumatic brain injury. J Head Trauma Rehabil 2:57–69, 1987.
76. Bohac, DL, Malec, JF, and Moessner, AM: Factor analysis of the Mayo-Portland Adaptability Inventory: Structure and validity. Brain Inj 11:469–82, 1997.
77. Malec, JF, Machulda, MM, and Moessner, AM: Differing problem perceptions of staff, survivors, and significant others after brain injury. J Head Trauma Rehabil 12:1–13, 1997.
78. American Psychiatric Association. Diagnostic and Statistical Manual of Mental Disorders, ed 4. American Psychiatric Association, Washington, DC, 1994.
79. ICD-9-CM: International Classification of Diseases, Ninth Revision, Clinical Modification, ed 5. Medicode, Salt Lake City, 1995.

CHAPTER 11

Evaluation of Communication and Swallowing Disorders

MICHAEL E. GROHER, PHD,
and LINDA PICON-NIETO, MCD, CCC

❏ COMMUNICATION DISORDERS

Although it is difficult to separate communication disorders from the cognitive substrates that support communication, this chapter focuses on both formal and informal assessments of speech and language following brain injury. Additionally, it discusses the evaluation and management of oropharyngeal swallowing disorders as a consequence of brain injury.

The Importance of Assessment

The capacity to communicate with others allows us to interact with our environment. Loss of the ability to process language, motorically control speech output, or express thoughts meaningfully is a devastating but frequent finding secondary to traumatic brain injury (TBI). Assessing communication deficits that result from TBI often presents a challenge not only to the speech-language pathologist but also to those involved in the care and rehabilitation of the patient. For unresponsive patients who are not able to participate in or contribute to their care and for patients who communicate but whose words confuse, hurt, and alienate those around them, the challenges are tremendous. In fact, frequently it is not the obvious motor speech or language disorder that presents the problem. Of greater concern is the lack of response, the fluent and incoherent attempts to respond, or the inability to engage in socially appropriate conversation.

Brooks[1] found a relatively low frequency (20–30%) of formal language problems following TBI as reported by families and patients compared with reports of actual neuropsychological impairments. He concluded, however, that the number increased to almost half of those reporting (40–50%) if communication in general is considered. The most consistent complaints from patients and their families included word-finding deficits and difficulties in grasping the subtleties of a conversation.

Neurogenic Communication Disorders

We cannot discuss assessment of communication disorders in this population without first acknowledging that the task of differentiating problems in communication from cognitive dysfunction is, at best, a formidable task. On account of the variability of damage in TBI, it is not possible to associate it with any particular aspect of communication or a pathological process because some aspects of communication may be spared or impaired following insult to the brain.[2] Speech and language by themselves must be recognized as only parts of the communication process. Assessment strategies must account for the fact that deficient communication after brain trauma can range from complete inability to understand the spoken word or articulate thoughts to the inability to express any relevant thoughts or meaningful content in the presence of fluent and clearly articulated speech. As has been so eloquently pointed out, patients with aphasia communicate better than they talk, whereas patients who have sustained traumatic brain injury often appear to talk better than they communicate.[3,4]

Characteristics of Communication Deficits

Aphasic disorders are reported in 2 percent[5] and up to 32 percent[6-8] of the TBI population. Although frank aphasia is relatively rare, researchers have described deficits in language, communicative competence, and social behavior as some of the most penalizing and long-term outcomes of TBI. Such deficits frequently impede successful reentry into the community.[9-12] According to Holland,[13] the qualitative differences in language use differentiate this population from that with traditional language disorders.

Adamovich and Henderson[14] describe two general patterns of neurobehavioral sequelae that can be found after TBI. One, associated with focal lesions, may present communication disorder patterns similar to those found after stroke. The other is a consequence of more diffuse and widespread damage. Diffuse damage usually produces deficits that affect communicative competence in areas such as memory, attention, processing speed and capacity, and self-monitoring.

A variety of communication areas can be impaired or spared following TBI.[2] Communication deficits described in TBI patients include impaired auditory comprehension,[15] anomia,[13,16] verbal and literal paraphasias,[16] reduced word fluency,[17] impaired visual naming,[18] and associated impairments of reading and writing.[19] Others have described communication deficits attributable to cognitive-language disorganization resulting from impairments of attention, discrimination, sequencing, recall, categorization, association and integration, and analysis and synthesis of information.[20] These impairments are evident in the tangential, fragmented, and irrelevant communication efforts consistently described in this patient population.[16,21]

The Process of Evaluation

The assessment of communication deficits associated with cognitive dysfunction requires that the skilled clinician identify the underlying cognitive causes of communicative failure. The approach to evaluation is tied closely with the need to understand the components of speech and language as part of the patient's total cognitive-communication schema. A measure of the patient's cognitive and behavioral status, of which speech and language are only parts, should be highly correlated with the ability to be a successful communicator. In this context, it becomes important to gather data that describe not only the patient's motor speech and basic linguistic skills but also his or her ability to respond and relate to the environment. Adopting the philosophical approach of measuring the patient's communicative effectiveness, rather than just speech and language, allows the clinician to describe more accurately the wide range of potential disability in this patient population. Evaluation of communicative competence in patients with TBI includes more than the traditional speech and language approach we might take with other neurogenic disorders. The evaluation process must focus on the "total person" and how communicative effectiveness, or lack thereof, affects every aspect of the survivor's life. It must address not only the specific underlying processes that contribute to the deficits but also the functional limitations of ineffective communication.

Cognitive deficits and their assessment are discussed here as they relate to responsiveness and social communication. Evaluation of cognitive deficits following traumatic brain injury is discussed in Chapter 9.

The Initial Evaluation

The point in time when the speech-language pathologist is first consulted to assist in the assessment of the TBI patient may vary from setting to setting. Assessments take place in the neuro intensive care unit, an acute care or postacute care facility, a rehabilitation or subacute rehabilitation unit, or a chronic care facility. Regardless of when in the recovery process we are first consulted, some pieces of information are always critical to decisions on how to proceed with the patient. For this reason, a review of the case history is crucial for the process of evaluation. Although most of the necessary information to complete an initial assessment is contained in the medical record, it is imperative to recognize the need to interview the patient who is able to be interviewed, staff members already involved in the care of the patient, and any family members and significant others who are available. As important as the medical history, the course of hospitalization, and information regarding surgical or other interventions are to the initial evaluation process, the significance of a thorough interview cannot be underestimated in determining the patient's immediate communication needs and the appropriate course of assessment.

The clinician must be careful not to fall into the trap of confusing an initial evaluation with a comprehensive evaluation. Often patients are unresponsive or minimally responsive and not easily testable with a standard psychometric battery. Some clinicians do not realize that unresponsiveness to standard test questions does not mean that the patient is not "testable." Prior to initiation of an evaluation, clinicians should select test materials based on historical information and experience. Some clinicians, regardless of the individual historical characteristics of the patient, administer a "favorite" standard battery of tests. The patient's failure to participate in this standard battery creates the impression that he or she is "not testable." Clinicians need to develop the flexibility to move away from their standard test battery and focus on what the patient is able and unable to do. A "no response" to a programmed stimulus is a response that is worth noting. Failure to document the circumstances in which "no response" is elicited may result in wasted efforts in readministering tasks in hopes that the expected response is elicited. Such an approach is oriented more to treatment than to evaluation.

During the initial evaluation, it may be impossible for the clinician to obtain all of the necessary information to fully assess an individual's cognitive communication status or to make definite prognostic judgments, design treatment plans, and set outcome goals. The initial evaluation should be short, simple, highly functional, and aimed at uncovering the strengths and weaknesses necessary to facilitate the immediate communication needs of the patient. By determining the most salient strengths and weaknesses of the patient, the clinician can assist staff and family in capitalizing on the viable communication avenues while decreasing demands on the patient's areas of deficiency. The initial evaluation should provide guidance to staff and family to facilitate the patient's care. Ideally, it should help to determine the next step in the evaluation process and, although not comprehensive, it does need to be complete to be effective. Hartley[22] offers the following guidelines for an initial evaluation:

1. Review the records of the individual.
2. Obtain the individual's perspective on his or her abilities, areas of need, and goals.
3. Obtain input from the family or significant others regarding cognitive-communicative functioning.

4. Conduct standardized testing of cognitive-communicative processes and semantic knowledge, making use of clinical observations as well as standardized procedures.
5. Use checklists or rating scales to evaluate cognitive communication in unstructured, real-life activities.
6. Evaluate discourse comprehension and production.

All or some of these areas may be briefly explored during the initial evaluation. It should be followed by in-depth examination during the comprehensive assessment process. The specific areas to assess during the initial evaluation vary with the time frame available, the level or recovery stage of the patient, and her or his current medical or psychosocial situation.

The first aspect to consider during the initial evaluation, the reason for the request, can usually be settled by asking the referring physician, the patient, other staff, or family members. Then, the current means of communication must be identified. Individual variables such as age, gender, cultural and ethnic background, educational level, and premorbid communication style must be taken into account. In addition, knowledge of the type, site, and severity of the injury and the stage in the recovery process is critical in determining the direction of the initial evaluation and eventually of the comprehensive evaluation. All of this information alerts the examiner to the immediate communication needs of the patient and assists in counseling the patient, the health care team, and the family. Furthermore, analysis of this information should result in a prognostic impression. Relevant issues to consider during the initial evaluation are summarized in Table 11–1.

The immediate needs of TBI patients may be very different. For instance, the immediate needs of a low-level, recently injured hospital inpatient differ from those of an individual who has been unemployed since his injury and is living at home.

The focus of the initial evaluation in the early stages of recovery is basic issues of auditory and visual perception, attention and orientation, swallowing, and establishment of functional means of communication. Specifically, the goals are to assess (1) ability to follow directions and comprehend questions; (2) ability to communicate basic wants and needs; (3) ability to respond to the environment based on arousability, responsiveness, attentiveness, and awareness; (4) the need for coma management techniques; (5) the presence of swallowing difficulties; (6) the educational needs of the family regarding cognition, communication, and swallowing; and (7) the need for environmental management.[23] If appropriate, referral needs also must be addressed. For instance, referrals to gastroenterology, otolaryngology, neuro-ophthalmology or ophthal-

TABLE 11–1. Relevant Issues to Consider during the Initial Evaluation

Medical status

- Ventilator/oxygen dependency
- Tracheostomy
- Medications
- Nutritional status
  □ Feeding tubes
- Neurological status
  □ Hemorrhage/craniotomy
  □ Seizures
  □ Acute and chronic hydrocephalus/ventriculostomy
  □ Anoxia/hypoxia

Recovery status

- Time postonset
- Cognitive/behavioral
  □ Length of coma
  □ Length of post-traumatic amnesia
- Emotional

Lesion site

- Focal damage
- Diffuse damage

Communication status

- Verbal/nonverbal
- Effective/ineffective
  □ Presence and type of communication disorder
- Postmorbid/premorbid
- Augmentative
  □ Uses device
  □ Cannot use device

Psychosocial status

- Acute inpatient/chronic inpatient/chronic outpatient
- Living situation
  □ Independent
  □ Supervised
  □ Assisted
- Perceptions and expectations
  □ Patient
  □ Family
  □ Staff

Feeding/swallowing status

- Nutritional status
- Current method of nutrition/hydration
  □ Oral
  □ Nonoral
- Aspiration risk
- Advanced directives

Referrals indicated

- Gastroenterology
- Otolaryngologist (ear, nose, and throat)
- Ophthalmology/neuro-ophthalmology
- Rehabilitation/neurology
- Audiology
- Radiology
- Psychiatry

mology, radiology, audiology, rehabilitation medicine, neurology, or psychiatry often are indicated. During the later stages of recovery, the initial evaluation emphasizes high-level language processing and effective use of verbal expression, such as abstract language, verbal power, and speed.[4]

The Comprehensive Evaluation

The comprehensive evaluation, unlike the initial evaluation, is a time-consuming and involved process. The word *process* was chosen deliberately to characterize the comprehensive evaluation as an in-depth, ongoing series of actions as part of a prescribed procedure. At this point the clinician becomes an investigator who is no longer solely interested in immediate communication needs or basic communication strengths and weaknesses but in the underlying impairments. The goals of the comprehensive evaluation are (1) further explaining problems previously identified, (2) identifying new problems, (3) uncovering the causative factors and the conditions associated with those problems, (4) determining treatment candidacy and outcome measures, and (5) determining compensatory strategies that may be beneficial.

The comprehensive evaluation of cognitive communication deficits following TBI is one of the most complex and involved assessments the speech-language pathologist performs. First, it requires mastery in the assessment of traditional motor speech, language, voice, and fluency disorders. Second, it requires the ability to evaluate those in the context of associated cognitive deficits that may effect their "testability." Third, it may have to be performed with patients who are confused, unaware, or in denial of any functional limitations and/or the need for evaluation. Fourth, it should include an assessment of pragmatic skills, and the constructs that comprise pragmatic communication functions still have not achieved total consensus among the experts.

The outcome of an evaluation should be consistent with the assessment goal. The final objective should be to compile, analyze, and interpret all of the information gathered to answer the question from the referring source. In addition to those mentioned in the initial evaluation, relevant issues to consider during the comprehensive evaluation are summarized in Table 11–2.

The Minimally Responsive Patient

Baseline measures of communication are crucial to the evaluation of the low-level and slow-to-recover patient. A review of the most com-

---

TABLE 11–2. Relevant Issues to Consider during the Comprehensive Evaluation

- Changes in medical or neurological status since initial evaluation
- Premorbid and postmorbid factors
- Environmental factors
- Presence of family or significant other
- Psychosocial, social, educational, and employment history
- Psychological factors, including premorbid psychiatric history
- Adjustment issues
- Financial or legal considerations and how these might affect candidacy for treatment or follow-up and discharge planning
- Current patient and family goals and expectations
- Current standardized assessment data (cognitive, speech, language, linguistic); deviations from premorbid characteristics and from the norm
- Behavioral observations of the patient within the hospital setting and during ecologically valid, real-world tasks and situations; cognitive communication characteristics using rating scales by the patient, staff, and family
- Rehabilitation potential including treatment indicators, goals, and plans
- Prognostic indicators of rehabilitation potential and outcome
- Indication that results of the evaluation and management recommendations match the patient's and family's expectations, needs, and resources

---

monly used tools in medical settings after traumatic brain injury, such as the Glasgow Coma Scale[24] and the Rancho Los Amigos Scale of Cognitive Functioning,[25] reveals that language comprehension and expression are utilized as a gauge for recovery of function. Initial measures of recovery of function center on the patient's ability to focus on the environment and respond to it appropriately. Communication impairment is a crucial aspect of the post-traumatic recovery process. The path of assessing and restoring communicative function usually is long and difficult, with multiple evaluations at different levels of recovery.

Certain factors must be considered in the assessment of the low-level patient regardless of the tool used. The evaluation process must take into account (1) what has transpired before the evaluation, such as other evaluations, toileting, or multiple visitors; (2) the time of day; (3) the type of stimuli and structure provided; (4) the method and consistency of stimulus administration; (5) the input and output modalities being evaluated; (6) the variety, speed, and quality of the response; (7) the familiarity of the person administering the stimuli; and (8) other influencing factors, such as distracting environments. The clinician must be cautious in interpreting findings and assigning cognitive levels after the initial evaluation. Many such extraneous variables may vary from day to day and can alter the clinical picture.

At any point during the recovery process, particularly during the early stages, the clinician must be cognizant of the patient's medical status. Medical complications may persist outside the intensive care unit or after transfer to a rehabilitation unit. Of importance are complications that may affect the evaluation of communication and swallowing disorders, such as post-traumatic seizures, ventricular dilatation, delayed or recurrent hemorrhage, gastrointestinal problems, respiratory or airway problems, and cardiovascular problems.[26] It is not uncommon for the speech-language pathologist to be the one to alert the staff to neurological changes in the course of an evaluation.

Particularly in the early stages of recovery, assessment of communication and cognitive disorders is an ongoing process not easily differentiated from a sensory stimulation program. Not to be confused with a never-ending evaluation, the reassessment of the minimally responsive patient is indicative of changes since the initial evaluation and helps to determine readiness for a comprehensive evaluation. Generally, frequency of reassessments is dictated by individual patient variables. Reassessments of the minimally responsive patient may be performed daily, weekly, or even monthly, depending on the rate and pattern of recovery. In some cases, the reassessment uncovers additional deficits or strengths that may have been masked during the first evaluation attempt. In other cases, it verifies the presence or absence of change in ability, a skill that serves as a prognostic indicator.

While helping to detect deficits and monitor recovery of function, the outcome of the evaluation in the low-level patient population should provide information for maximizing such recovery. For instance, if the patient presents as a strong visual learner, the staff can be alerted to enhance their instructions with visual cues, such as models or pictures. If the patient presents with neglect or hemianopsia, recommendations can be made as to the preferred side to approach the patient or position the bed in the room.

Controversy exists as to when in the course of recovery the expertise of the speech-language pathologist should be sought, what type of evaluation or interventions, if any, should be administered, and whether early evaluation and treatment in this patient population are efficacious. Also, clinicians often are faced with insurance reimbursement issues that dictate which diagnoses can receive services and what type of interventions may be utilized. Therefore, the evaluation of the low-level, minimally responsive patient requires that the clinician is skilled in making a prompt determination of both cognitive and communication strengths to facilitate the care of the patient and have a functional impact on the recovery process. For the assessment to have such an impact on the recovery process, the clinician must use evaluation tools that clearly document changes in function.

A multitude of well-established formal assessment batteries are available to the speech-language pathologist. Unfortunately, most are not appropriate for minimally responsive patients because they require responses well above their level of functioning. Following are descriptions of some available measures of low-level cognitive communication.

THE WESTERN NEURO SENSORY STIMULATION PROFILE

One formal objective measure of cognitive function that can be used effectively with severely impaired TBI patients is the Western Neuro Sensory Stimulation Profile (WNSSP).[27,28] Designed to objectively assess and monitor behavior changes during the early stages of recovery, this tool consists of 33 items that assess (1) arousal/attention, (2) expressive communication, and response to (3) auditory, (4) visual, (5) tactile, and (6) olfactory stimulation. Utilizing the sensory stimulation paradigm of the Rancho Los Amigos Hospital Scale of Cognitive Function, the WNSSP provides a series of organized stimuli and input modalities that describe functional cognitive communication status, and assist in developing treatment plans, monitoring changes in performance, and documenting recovery patterns.[27]

The scoring method of the WNSSP is an adaptation of the well-known multidimensional scoring system developed by Porch[29] to capture the elements of cuing and response latency in a hierarchical manner. It is based on the premise that an accurate and immediate response is better than a cued or delayed response. In administering the WNSSP, the clinician is exploring (1) the presence or absence of response to a stimulus, (2) the type and appropriateness of response, (3) the amount of delay from stimulus presentation to response, and (4) whether a cue was necessary to elicit the response. The total score for the WNSSP is the sum of points attained on all 33 test items, with a maximum possible score of 113.

Unlike some other measures of cognitive communication recovery, the WNSSP has a variety of features that allow the clinician flexibility without altering the results of the examination. For instance, the scoring system provides a score for "missing value or not applicable" to distinguish a stimulus that received a poor score because of no response, from one to which the patient was not able to respond because of physical limitations (e.g., cranial nerve paralysis or intubation). Omitting those in the final total allows the clinician to assess the patient and monitor responses based on the patient's capabilities, rather than on predetermined values. The WNSSP also permits the clinician to score the "best response observed" when the patient does not respond to the test items; that is, if the patient does not respond to presentation of a sound source but is observed to respond appropriately to environmental sounds during the examination, that response may be scored. In a population that is well known for variable arousal and attention, this option allows the clinician to effectively document the patient's actual performance yet take into account other influencing factors. The WNSSP is fairly easy to administer and requires few materials. However, it may be too long and difficult for the patient who has fluctuating levels of alertness.

THE RAPPAPORT COMA/NEAR COMA SCALE

The Rappaport Coma/Near Coma (CNC) Scale[30] was developed to measure small clinical changes in patients with severe traumatic and nontraumatic brain injury. Designed for the evaluation of patients in coma and vegetative states, this tool helps the clinician identify even the smallest changes in clinical status, which may be predictive of outcome and indicative of the appropriate level of care for the patient. The CNC is unlike the WNSSP and rating scales such as the Glasgow Coma Scale, the Rancho Los Amigos Scale, and the Disability Rating Scale,[31] which evaluate low to high levels of functioning. The CNC provides a detailed assessment of lower-level cognitive functioning. The CNC scale has five levels of awareness and responsivity—no coma, near coma, moderate coma, marked coma, and extreme coma—and eight parameters: auditory, command responsivity, visual, threat, olfactory, tactile, pain, and vocalization. Eleven different tasks in each area define level of severity. The CNC scale is helpful in detecting which low-functioning patients are likely to demonstrate progress (usually those in near coma or better) and which are unlikely to improve. According to the authors, degree of recovery is closely tied to multiple factors, of which the CNC scale is only a part.

To the extent possible at this early stage, the evaluation also should include an assessment of the motor and sensory systems to determine the presence or absence of pathology in end organs, which clearly affects interpretation of the evaluation result. Often observation and comparison of the left and right sides of the body give the clinician valuable localizing information when a detailed oral-motor evaluation is impossible.

The Confused Patient

At this stage, the patient is awake, but behavior is often bizarre and disruptive. The patient may be verbal but incoherent and inappropriate. He or she may perform automatic motor activities such as sitting or reaching, but attention span and cooperation are often poor. Heightened awareness in a state of confusion often results in excessive emotional reactions.

Although evaluation of this type of patient involves discovering some of the same deficits as in the low-level patient, the confused and agitated patient presents new challenges. One challenge might be the use of physical or chemical restraints, which are often necessary in the management of the agitated TBI patient and present an obstacle to obtaining the most accurate information about a patient's response appropriateness and accuracy. Although it may be relatively easy to circumvent physical restraints, it is imperative that the clinician be familiar with chemical restraints. Chemical restraints, such as sedatives, and their effects on motoric and cognitive abilities may have a significant impact on the results of the evaluation by masking or producing deficits in communication and swallowing abilities.

Because of the characteristically short attention spans and uncooperative tendencies of these patients, the measures used must be designed to gather a maximum amount of information in a short time. In the patient with established verbal skills, the evaluation should not only sample linguistic skills but also focus on the cognitive prerequisites for effective language use. The tests or tasks chosen to evaluate the patient should be easy to administer and contain few props and/or test booklets to minimize distractions and overstimulation. Preferably, the evaluation should be administered in a quiet area that is familiar to the patient and with as few observers and interruptions as possible.

As the patient becomes more responsive, actual patterns of communication and communication disorders may become apparent. Descriptions of the communication disorders during these stages range from global involvement[32] to disorders of naming.[5] Because of the range of impairments in TBI and, in particular, the subtler linguistic and paralinguistic deficits to which standard aphasia batteries may be insensitive, selected portions of standardized language evaluation tools should be used. Administration of selected subtests from the Communicative Abilities of Daily Living,[33] the Western Aphasia Battery,[34] the Boston Diagnostic Aphasia Examination,[35] the Boston Assessment of Severe Aphasia,[36] or the Aphasia Diagnostic Profile,[37] may prove beneficial in identifying and outlining problems in basic language functions.[38,39] Scores on these batteries should be interpreted with caution. For instance, a low score on auditory comprehension tasks may be the result of confusion or shallow recall and not lack of comprehension of the spoken word. When there is a question, individual responses should be examined.

Early identification of language or linguistic disturbance is crucial in the management of the confused and agitated patient. Providing compensations for these deficits has a significant impact on other aspects of the recovery process. As Groher[16] pointed out in his study of speech and language characteristics of patients with TBI, improvement in language functions is directly related to a reduction in negative behavior patterns, such as striking out and uncooperativeness.

Assessment of the impact of cognitive abilities on communication impairments is important. One cannot provide an accurate description of a patient's language capacity without a thorough evaluation of the cognitive constructs of attention, memory, executive functions, and information processing. Additionally, the evaluation should help to discover which conditions in the environment facilitate the patient's communication with that environment. For instance, time of day, room lighting, number of visitors, and communication modality might affect the patient's response. Documentation of these conditions and education of the family and staff about them should facilitate the individual's recovery and behavior management. It also should provide data for treatment.

For the confused TBI patient who presents with a limited attention span and decreased physical stamina, various commercially available tools enable the clinician to assess cognitive and communicative abilities in a formal but brief manner. The following tests are appropriate cognitive-communication measures for the confused patient.

THE BRIEF TEST OF HEAD INJURY

The Brief Test of Head Injury (BTHI)[40] is a cognitive-communicative tool designed to quickly identify and measure cognitive and linguistic deficits manifested in TBI. Although administration time is approximately 30 minutes, it can be administered over several shorter sessions. The patient often can receive full credit for gestural responses, a unique feature of the BTHI. The BTHI is comprised of seven clusters: Orientation and Attention, Following Commands, Linguistic Organization, Reading Comprehension, Naming, Memory, and Visual-Spatial Skills. With the lower-level patient, it is very useful to track severity of impairment over time. As the patient moves to higher cognitive levels, the BTHI also may provide guidance for further testing based on subtest performance.

THE BARRY REHABILITATION INPATIENT SCREENING OF COGNITION

The Barry Rehabilitation Inpatient Screening of Cognition (BRISC)[41] takes about 30 minutes and is easy to administer at bedside. It is divided into eight functional categories: reading, copying, verbal concepts, orientation, mental imagery, mental control, word fluency (list generation), and delayed recall of graphic and verbal material. The clinician can sample a variety of cognitive-communication abilities; other abilities can be inferred from the patient's performance. The BRISC is sensitive to the subtle cognitive changes often demonstrated in the early stages of recovery. As with any other screening instrument, it should be used to formulate initial impressions and not to replace an in-depth battery.

THE SPEED AND CAPACITY OF LANGUAGE PROCESSING

The Speed and Capacity of Language Processing (SCOLP)[42] is a brief and easily administered tool designed to measure amount and rate of language processing. Slowness in cognitive processing is a common sequela of TBI. The SCOLP enables the clinician to differentiate between the individual who was premorbidly slow and one who is experiencing cognitive slowness as a result of brain damage. Accommodations may need to be made for the patient with visual impairment, as the test is normed only for visual administration.

THE SCALES OF COGNITIVE ABILITY FOR TRAUMATIC BRAIN INJURY

The Scales of Cognitive Ability for Traumatic Brain Injury (SCATBI)[43] provide a useful method to assess cognitive and linguistic deficits following TBI. It examines underlying cognitive processes necessary for communication, such as perception and discrimination, orientation, organization, recall, and reasoning.

The examination is completed by the average patient in approximately 2 hours, although the examiner may choose to administer it in multiple short sessions. For the low-level patient, one may choose to administer only the low-functioning subtests (perception and discrimination, orientation, and organization), which often yield the same severity score as the entire test in half the time.

INFORMAL TESTING

Informal assessment strategies frequently can be used to provide a setting to observe cognitive-communication behaviors without the obvious intent of a formal evaluation. One of the most valuable informal tools available to the speech-language pathologist is the art of conversation. Walking into a patient's environment without a test booklet or a clipboard enables one to simply observe the patient's natural communicative behaviors without the use of questions or tasks to elicit a structured response. Although an informal conversation in a naturalistic environment does not take the place of the formal evaluation, it should be considered an important part of data collection. It is particularly relevant when interpreting family member reports on the communication problems or successes of TBI survivors. Such reports usually are based on their own experiences with the patient during everyday conversation, not on formal assessment measures. Validation of family reports often can be accomplished if the clinician documents conversational exchanges with the patient during a variety of encounters and contexts.

RATING SCALES

Rating scales of cognitive and pragmatic communication behaviors also may be helpful during the nonagitated stages of recovery. Pragmatic scales, for instance, are frequently useful to evaluate a communication sample. One obtains a baseline measure by engaging the patient in several structured and unstructured conversation tasks designed to elicit various styles of discourse, such as narrative, procedural, and conversational. Further discussion of rating scales for pragmatic behaviors follows.

The Purposeful and Appropriate Patient

Evaluating the communication deficits of the high-level patient may not be an easy task because of the limitation of formal measures in capturing their deficits. Although linguistic impairments may be present, standard aphasia batteries fall short in the assessment of the subtleties and use of high-level language.[16] It has been recommended that the clinician utilize portions of traditional language batteries to tap into the areas desired and supplement them with other selected tests of language function.[4,38,39] In addition, limited normative data are available on pragmatic behaviors, particularly because of the significant variability in what is considered to be "normal." Normalcy often is influenced by situational, cultural, and social factors.[44] According to Sohlberg and Mateer,[4] the comprehensive evaluation of communication abilities in higher-level patients must include (1) observation of the brain-injured individual in a natural communication situation in which he or she is conversing with a discourse partner, (2) a list or taxonomy of pragmatic behaviors from which to judge performance, and (3) a method for translating information gleaned through observation into treatment goals and objectives.

Many of the evaluation tools discussed in the previous section continue to prove beneficial in the evaluation of basic cognitive-communication deficits. By their nature, however, these tools fall short in the evaluation of language use in everyday contexts and situations. In addition to linguistic assessment, the evaluation of language use and conversational skills is necessary in the purposeful and appropriate patient for the clinician to effectively document a patient's deficits. This evaluation may be accomplished through structured tasks, such as role-play situations, and unstructured tasks, such as everyday conversation.[22]

The depth and complexity of the pragmatic communication assessment may be dictated by a variety of factors, including the purpose of the evaluation, patient or family complaint, coexisting disorders, time constraints, and treatment or postevaluation plan. It must include formal, objective, and widely recognized tools for the evaluation of the cognitive-communication disorders of the TBI patient. Because of the evident shortcomings of conventional batteries, several models have surfaced for the evaluation of verbal and nonverbal quality of communicative behaviors in higher-level patients. These models address the significance of pragmatic communication skills as an inseparable variable of cognitive and communicative efficiency. Examples of these models include pragmatic rating scales, discourse analysis, communicative competence, and discourse comprehension.

PRAGMATIC RATING SCALES

Several commercially available pragmatic rating scales are intended to assess pragmatic communication behaviors. One is the Pragmatic Protocol,[45,46] which was designed to identify the communication problems of the brain-injured patient vis-à-vis a noninjured population. It provides a taxonomy of 30 communication behaviors in three main categories: verbal aspects (such as speech acts, topic initiation and cohesion, turn-taking, lexical selection, and stylistic variations), paralinguistic aspects (such as prosody, intelligibility, vocal intensity and quality, and fluency), and nonverbal aspects (such as body movement, personal distance, postures, and facial expressions). Utilizing a videotaped sample of unstructured conversation, communicative behaviors are judged as appropriate (the behavior facilitated the interaction or was neutral) or inappropriate (the behavior detracted from the interchange and penalized the speaker).[22]

Another scale of pragmatic behaviors is the Communication Performance Scale.[47] This scale, adapted from the Pragmatic Protocol, contains 13 pragmatic behaviors such as intelligibility and prosody, kinesthetic factors, lexical and grammatical factors, listening and attention, language and topic, and self-regulating behaviors such as initiation, repair, and interrupting. Each behavior is rated on a 5-point scale, with 1 the worst. This rating scale is more useful than the Pragmatic Protocol because the description of the disorder is more precise.

The Interaction Checklist for Augmentative Communication (INCH)[48] has been described as a useful taxonomy for the clinician rating pragmatic behaviors. Although developed as a checklist for use with the augmentative communication population, it provides the clinician with a structured set of behaviors to observe and rate in the TBI patient.

Other pragmatic checklists reported in the literature include the Profile of Communicative Appropriateness,[49] the Pragmatic Inventory for Brain Injury,[50] and the Rating Scale of Pragmatic Communication Skills (RICE).[51]

Traditionally, communication behaviors have been analyzed, judged, and rated by expert listeners for the evaluation of various communication disorders. For the most comprehensive assessment of pragmatic communication skills in the TBI patient, perceptions and ratings by others who interact with the individual should be included. Because of the variability in communication behaviors frequently seen in this patient population, the evaluation process must take into account a variety of scenarios. For instance, the social and communication behaviors that may be appropriate in communicating with a friend would not be appropriate in a formal situation, such as a medical appointment. Rating of various communication styles and their appropriateness to the situation is best accomplished by combining data from formally obtained communication samples and the impressions of all those interacting with the patient in a variety of environments.

DISCOURSE ANALYSIS

Some researchers have attempted to evaluate pragmatic communication by using a detailed analysis of discourse parameters. Thorough discourse analysis is labor intensive and time consuming. In that it usually involves extensive calculations and computations of each individual aspect of the communication sample, discourse analysis may not always be feasible.

Mentis and Prutting[52] developed a multidimensional topic analysis tool sensitive to the problems of topic management in the TBI population. They characterized the topic management skills of the brain-injured person as having limited discourse structure. They added that discourse is characterized by incoherent topic changes and ambiguous, unrelated, and incomplete ideational units during both conversation and monologue samples. The authors concluded that multidimensional topical coherence analysis has the potential to identify, quantify, and describe those aspects of topic management that have been globally described by others as tangential, fragmented, and irrelevant.[16,21]

Other proponents of discourse analysis, such as Hartley and Jensen,[53] advocate the use of specific measures of communication, such as productivity (quantity and rate), content (informational quality), and cohesion (how well discourse is tied together) to describe the communication deficits of the TBI patient. They feel that the value of discourse evaluation lies not in the ability to discover the underlying reasons for the impairment but in the ability to identify and describe it as it affects the person's communicative effectiveness in relation to normal production.

McDonald[54] and McDonald and Pearce[55] describe discourse analysis in terms of the number, type, and sequence of ideas expressed. In their study utilizing the "dice game" task as originally described by Flavell,[56] a control group and a group of brain injured patients were asked to explain the rules of a new game to a third "naive" listener. The elicited discourse was analyzed and summarized into the following categories: total number of propositions, number of repeated propositions, number of extra details, number of essential propositions that were mentioned or inferred, sequence in which the essential propositions were mentioned, and overall sequence in which all propositions were mentioned. Results revealed that, despite both groups producing similar quantities of information, the brain injured group mentioned fewer essential points and produced more irrelevant asides. Both features are consistent with the impoverished and tangential conversational style reported in the TBI population. The authors concluded that discourse evaluation of the dice game is a sufficiently reliable, relevant, and ecologically valid communication exercise that is more likely to elicit cognitive communication deficits than structured testing.

In an attempt to fill the void of linguistic assessments and pragmatic scales administered in isolation, newer assessment methods have emerged. Recent advances reported in the literature suggest the failure of pragmatic assessment tools to consider the evaluation of communication as an interactive rather than unitary process.[57,58] Most of the rating scales of pragmatic behaviors are designed to judge the communication act and the conversant's ability to meet his or her communicative intent. Although some scales include sociolinguistic sensitivity ratings,[49] most do not consider the communication partner.

COMMUNICATIVE COMPETENCE

One tool that attempts to consider the communication partner is the Behaviorally Referenced Rating System of Intermediate Social Skills (BRISS).[58] It consists of five scales that measure nonverbal aspects of communication and six dealing with verbal aspects of communication. In addition to the verbal and linguistic aspects of social skills described in the Pragmatic Protocol, the BRISS contains two scales that directly address the complex interactional skills of how "the conversant adapts to the social context": (1) the personal conversational style, with three subscales rating self-disclosure, humor, and social manners such as politeness, use of compliments and interruptions, and (2) partner-directed behavior. A useful feature of this tool, the Part-Dir scale, focuses on behaviors requiring awareness of and sensitivity to the communication partner and an understanding of how one's own behavior affects the communication partner. By expanding the focus from the static to the dynamic aspect of the communication situation, the authors claim the BRISS is sensitive to the most complex cognitive skills of attention, cognitive flexibility, analysis, and decision making. Also, the BRISS can provide qualitative as well as quantitative data. By providing a 7-point scale with behavioral referents, the rater has the option of marking behavioral referents such as "laughs inappropriately some of the time" and can assign a rating score, useful for documentation of changes over time. Despite that, the BRISS fails to detect subtle changes over time because of high within-subject variability, according to the authors. They conclude, however, that when combined with more global and subjective measures of change, such as improvement in social competence, the BRISS may provide a useful source of behavioral referents for treatment planning.

DISCOURSE COMPREHENSION

Discourse comprehension is indirectly evaluated in the patient's ability to manage conversation effectively. Without adequate comprehension, the individual would not be able to maintain a logical or coherent communication exchange with a partner. Few tools, however, evaluate discourse comprehension as an important and independent entity of conversation. Instead, they focus on the comprehension of sentence components. One tool that attempts to do this is the Discourse Comprehension Test (DCT).[59] Designed to assess the comprehension and retention of spoken narrative discourse of adults with aphasia, right brain injury, or traumatic brain injury, it taps into cognitive communication deficits that standard tests designed to assess comprehension of single words or isolated sentences cannot. The DCT consists of 10 stories presented on audiotape (or on paper for the reading comprehension portion of the test) and a set of yes-no questions for each story. The questions assess the patient's ability to comprehend and remember information that is either stated or implied. They provide the examiner with a format to evaluate language subtleties and provide indications of deficit patterns and beneficial compensatory strategies. Unlike standard batteries, the DCT allows the clinician to systematically examine the individual's auditory comprehension capacity in a familiar and naturalistic fashion.

In conclusion, although discourse analysis may be useful to clearly document treatment effects, it is time consuming and therefore may be inefficient. Rating scales, by contrast, are time efficient and provide the clinician with a list of baseline behaviors useful in development of treatment plans, but they sometimes leave the clinician feeling that a numerical rating may not be sufficient to functionally describe the pragmatic communication behavior patterns of the TBI patient.

Some pragmatic communication deficits, such as poor eye contact and topic management, may be a common finding in TBI. In our assessment experience, two general patterns of pragmatic communication deficits have emerged. One pattern of behaviors (hyperpragmatic) is seen in the patient who talks excessively, fails to yield speaking turns, jumps from topic to topic, makes multiple tangential and irrelevant comments, and may demonstrate laughter or other inappropriate behaviors. The other pattern (hypopragmatic) is seen in patients who do not initiate conversation, exhibit excessive response delay, fail to provide relevant details or information, and do not provide feedback to the communication partner.

The clinician may use rating scales or discourse analysis to quantify these often observable behaviors and formulate objective treatment goals. The hyperpragmatic and hypopragmatic categorizations can guide treatment planning but may be too subjective or broad in some circumstances. In the clinical setting, they also may prove beneficial when the expected functional outcome is a decrease in the patient's and family's subjective complaints and not a number change.

☐ SWALLOWING DISORDERS

The Importance of Swallowing

If the patient's cognitive status is severely compromised after TBI, oral ingestion is precluded. Enteral feedings by nasogastric tube or by gastrostomy tube provide the patient with nutritional needs. Nutritional demands following head injury are high, and the importance of maintaining adequate calories and hydration to facilitate postinjury recovery cannot be underestimated. Attempts at oral ingestion may be one of the first opportunities the patient has to return to a familiar, pleasurable activity. Family members frequently inquire about the timing of the resumption of oral ingestion because it signals a return to health. Return to familiar, overlearned processes such as those involved in feeding may help to reduce post-traumatic confusion. For these reasons, the health care team needs to develop a plan for the evaluation and management of the patient's swallowing disorder early in the post-traumatic phase.

Categories of Impairment

Impairment of oropharyngeal swallowing after TBI is found in as many as 30 percent of patients who enter a rehabilitation setting.[60] There are no available data documenting the incidence of dysphagia by levels of severity in the acute circumstance, but, if consciousness levels and mental status are severely affected, the patient can be considered at risk for oral ingestion. Assessment of swallow function following TBI should be focused on three major areas of potential impairment: (1) cognitive control over the eating circumstance, (2) loss of the neuromuscular control of the swallow sequence, and

(3) iatrogenic causes. The probability is high that these causative factors are present in all patients identified with oropharyngeal dysphagia following TBI.

Cognitive Controls

Generalized reduction of cognitive integrity after TBI may result in failure to understand the mechanics or importance of feeding, inability to maintain sufficient attention to the feeding process, and failure to cooperate with evaluative procedures that assess the integrity of the oropharyngeal swallow response.

Patients who are unable to recognize or execute the process of food transport may be at risk nutritionally or at risk for dysphagic complications. Those patients with visual-spatial disorders may not be able to consistently sequence the motor skills involved in utensil selection and utilization. Those patients with neglect may be unable to locate food items on their trays, and others may not be able to initiate the feeding process. Others, even in the absence of primary sensory loss, may not comprehend when food that requires additional processing is placed in the oral cavity. Such impairments in patients with varying levels of alertness may cause oral contents to fall unnoticed into the pharynx and airway. Impulsivity as a result of cognitive impairment may result in inappropriate selection of bite size, food selection, or rate of intake. These behaviors have the potential to decompensate the oral and pharyngeal swallow sequence. Identifying the risk of a lack of mental control over the feeding process is best accomplished by observations of the patient during mealtime. Observations should document the ability to select utensils and sequence the steps in their use, the ability to identify and select food items, the speed of transport and bolus preparation, and ability or interest in initiating and maintaining swallowing activity.

An inability to maintain sufficient attention to ingestion often limits not only oral intake but also swallowing safety. Documentation of the patient's ability to finish an entire meal is important in deciding if the patient who might be tube-fed can progress to full or partial oral alimentation. Environmental distractions may cause attention to be diverted from the swallowing process with resultant aspiration. Particular attention should be paid to the patient who, when distracted while eating, makes attempts at phonation. Opening and closing the airway to phonate while eating may result in tracheal penetration. In addition, patients who may have learned postural compensations or special swallowing maneuvers may not always be able to use them appropriately or consistently because of fluctuating or poor attentional skills, memory loss, or an unexpected interruption in the execution of a planned motor activity.

Cognitive disorders often result in the need for modification in physical assessment because of poor cooperation. For instance, valid results from videofluorography to assess the dynamic function of the swallow response requires a patient to remain relatively immobile. The unfamiliarity of the radiographic suite and the concomitant auditory and visual distractions of testing procedures render radiographic intepretation of swallowing events difficult. For this reason, observations of those cognitive components that affect swallow during feeding trials in familiar environments are recommended for patients whose cognitive status precludes consistent cooperation with physical or laboratory examination.

Neuromuscular Controls

Assessment of the integrity of the sensory and motor components of the pharyngeal swallow should be designed to differentiate levels of central nervous system involvement. Those with bilateral impairment of the upper motor neuron system evidence discoordination of the swallow response, usually more for liquids than for solids. Those with lower motor neuron and cranial nerve impairment have extensive weakness in the muscles subserving swallow, which results in poor bolus propulsion for both liquids and solids.[61] Patients with left unilateral hemispheric disease are more likely to have oral stage disorders, including delay in initiation and bolus formation, whereas those with right hemispheric impairment are more predisposed to pharyngeally focused abnormality.[62] Both groups are at risk for aspiration. Differentiation between unilateral and bilateral disease is accomplished by standard examination of neurological systems. In the acute circumstance of brain injury, diffuse signs are common but difficult to establish in the muscles that control the swallowing response. Inference of the control of the muscles for swallow often must be made from observations of the extremities because of the patient's inability to cooperate with the standard examination of the oral peripheral swallow mechanism.

Iatrogenic Causes

Iatrogenic causative factors that precipitate or exacerbate swallowing disorders in patients with TBI include intubation, tracheostomy with or without ventilator support, and medications.

In the acute stages of head injury, patients may require emergency intubation. Potential complications from intubation that affect the laryngopharynx and swallow competence include granuloma, webs, laryngeal subluxation, ulcerations, ankylosis, subglottic stenosis, tracheal malacia, and vocal fold paralysis.[63] Direct visualization of the laryngopharynx and trachea is accomplished best with fiberoptic endoscopy and may be necessary to rule out complications from intubation that decompensate the oropharyngeal swallow response. Patients who are intubated frequently are being fed enterally by nasogastric tube. The negative effect of nasogastric tubes on the swallow response is not known; however, prolonged use may lead to nasal ulceration, sinus infection, and fibrotic changes within the pharyngoesophageal segment. Agitated patients may pull them from both the nose and the stomach, necessitating restraints or the need to speed the planned schedule for oral alimentation. Insertion of feeding tubes through the upper and lower esophageal sphincter may predispose a bedfast patient with reduced consciousness levels to increased risk of aspiration because of interruption in the sphincter's response as a protective mechanism against gastric reflux. Acute medical management also may include tracheostomy, which predisposes the patient to tracheal aspiration by limiting the protective function of laryngeal elevation[64] and by diminishing the glottal closure reflex.[65] Tracheostomy tubes that have cuffs that are inflated severely restrict laryngeal elevation and may not always provide adequate airway protection.[66]

The effects of medications on an already compromised neurological system may result in either precipitation or exacerbation of oropharyngeal dysphagia. Of particular concern are the benzodiazepines, used primarily for sedative, relaxant, and anticonvulsant therapy. These classes of drugs in high doses may restrict the activity of the striated muscle controls needed for efficient swallow. Combined with their known side effects on cognition, benzodiazepines may significantly affect the pharyngeal swallow. Buchholtz et al.[67] described two patients with severe pharyngeal weakness and dysphagia, secondary to high doses of alprazolam, which resolved with the removal of the drug. Other classes of drugs such as antidepressants, anticholinergics, antispasmodics, and neuroleptics may reduce arousal and alertness levels and result in severe xerostomia. Without adequate moisture in the oral cavity, swallow initiation is impaired, with potential for unintentional spillage into the airway.

Assessment Approaches

Returning patients to oral ingestion in the early stages of brain injury should receive priority in the medical evaluation process. Return to the basic function of swallowing may help to minimize post-traumatic confusion because the patient can return to a familiar activity. However, assessment of swallow function in those patients with TBI may be limited by their inability to fully cooperate with formal testing. In some cases, instrumental assessment is not possible, and clinicians must rely on detailed observations of swallowing to make inferences about swallowing safety. Observations are best gathered at different times during the day to account for variability in cognitive status and fatiguability that may affect intake amount. Some patients are able to tolerate only 10 successful minutes of feeding per meal and therefore would be candidates for more frequent, smaller portions if oral ingestion is to be successful. These observations can be made by using a swallow evaluation tray that contains thin fluids such as water, thicker fluids such as nectars, semisolids such as yogurt and purees, ice chips, and ground meats. Various volumes of test items should be used, ranging from 5 to 20 mL. These trials are done only when patients are fully alert, can follow basic commands, manage their own secretions, are free of pulmonary complications or infections, and have an overall health status that is stable or markedly improved. Observations of failure in swallow initiation, choking and coughing, and changes in voice quality or respiratory rate should be noted as potential signs of swallow abnormality. Although the goal of assessment often is to rule out tracheal aspiration, the clinician also needs to establish which food or fluids are best tolerated. For instance, those patients with neurological impairment are more likely to aspirate liquids than semisolids.

Videofluorography remains the laboratory examination of choice to study pharyngeal swallow in patients who can not be examined physically with confidence, but it does require considerable patient cooperation. Those whose injury results in significant changes in upright posture are particularly difficult to evaluate by videofluorography.

Fiberoptic endoscopic evaluation of swallow (FEES)[68] is useful with this population because it combines direct visualization of the laryngopharynx and can be combined with an evaluation of swallow performance. Food and fluid items typically are dyed with food coloring for better visualization. The patient is asked to swallow selected food items, and observations of preswallow and postswallow events are videotaped for review. Because of the portability of examination equipment, this examination can be performed in the intensive care unit, at the bedside, or in a setting that is free of distraction and familiar to the patient.

Patients who are ventilator dependent with tracheostomy may require assessment at the bedside. The blue dye test is recommended to identify food or secretions in the airway or at the tracheotomy site. Aspiration also may be detected with deep tracheal suction after swallow attempts. This method may identify aspiration in some patients, but its validity in identifying aspiration has been questioned.[69]

Although computerized cervical auscultation is in the early stages of assessment development, it may provide an instrumental assessment of the pharyngeal swallow response and can be used as a tool to monitor ongoing swallow performance. Advantages include its noninvasive procedure and the potential for numerous repeat evaluations. Clinicians input the auditory swallow signal directly into the computer for sound and swallow pattern analysis.[70,71]

□ SUMMARY

The extent of communication and swallowing impairment following traumatic brain injury depends on the nature and severity of the insult. After the physical and psychometric evaluation, a distinction is made between the focal impairments and diffuse effects that impact the cognitive constructs necessary for efficient communication. The potential for the interaction of these disabilities should be acknowledged. Both focal and diffuse lesions also may affect swallowing performance at the peripheral and central levels of neural organization.

Assessment of communication should focus directly on the patient's motor and linguistic performance by using standardized and functional measures and on her or his ability to use communication strategies to relate to the environment. Those cognitive processes that subserve communication, such as attention, memory, and perception, require evaluation in the context of communicative effectiveness in numerous environments with differing communication requirements. Ideally, the assessment is tailored to the severity of impairment and to the patient's level of cognitive functioning. Initial assessment strategies should be guided toward achieving an understanding of the patient's communication strengths and weaknesses and toward establishing a viable communication system. It also should provide the health care team with specific, achievable communication

goals. The comprehensive evaluation that follows should lead toward a convergent thinking process. In this process, all information is gathered and analyzed with the intent of finding the common cognitive denominators that contribute most to the overall disability.

For patients with post-traumatic dysphagia, return to full oral alimentation is frequently achievable. Severe swallow impairment is best managed by gastrostomy. Concurrent with sensory and motor recovery, swallowing safety should be evaluated by bedside trials, dynamic radiography, or fiberoptic endoscopy. Because of the potential for loss of cortical controls over the eating circumstance, patients need to be observed and monitored for an entire meal. The decision to remove the patient's enteral feeding depends on sufficient oral intake without airway compromise. The effects of iatrogenic sources of dysphagia, such as medications and tracheostomy, are complicating factors to swallowing impairment in this population; swallowing often improves when they can be discontinued.

REFERENCES

1. Brooks, N: Closed Head Trauma: Assessing the Common Cognitive Problems. In Lezak, MD (ed): Assessment of the Behavioral Consequences of Head Trauma. Alan R Liss, New York, 1989, p 61.
2. Ylvisaker, M: Communication outcome following traumatic brain injury. Seminars in Speech and Language 13:239, 1992.
3. Holland, AL: Some practical considerations in aphasia rehabilitation. In Sullivan, M, and Kommers, MS (eds): Rationale for adult aphasia therapy. University of Nebraska Medical Center, Omaha, 1977.
4. Sohlberg, MM, and Mateer, CA: Introduction to Cognitive Rehabilitation: Theory and Practice. Guilford, New York, 1989.
5. Heilman, KM, Safran, A, and Geshwind, N: Closed head trauma and aphasia. J Neurol Neurosurg Psychiatry 34:265, 1971.
6. Sarno, MT: The nature of verbal impairment after closed head injury. J Nerv Ment Dis 168:685, 1980.
7. Sarno, MT: Verbal impairment after closed head injury: Report of a replication study. J Nerv Ment Dis 172:475, 1984.
8. Sarno, MT: Head Injury: Language and speech defects. Scand J Rehabil Med 17:55, 1988.
9. McKinlay, WW, et al: The short term outcome of severe blunt injury as reported by relatives of the injured persons. J Neurol Neurosurg Psychiatry 44:527, 1981.
10. Brooks, DN, and McKinlay, WW: Personality and behavioral change after severe blunt head injury: a relative's view. J Neurol Neurosurg Psychiatry 46:336, 1983.
11. Lezak, MD: Relationships between personality disorders, social disturbances, and physical disability following traumatic brain injury. J Head Trauma Rehabil 2:57, 1987.
12. Rappaport, M, et al: Head injury outcome up to ten years later. Arch Phys Med Rehabil 70:885, 1989.
13. Holland, AL: When is aphasia aphasia? The problem of closed head injury. In Brookshire, RH (ed): Clinical Aphasiology Conference Proceedings, BRK Publishers, Minneapolis, 1982, p 345.
14. Adamovich, BB, and Henderson, JA: Cognitive Rehabilitation of Closed Head Injured Patients. College-Hill Press, San Diego, 1985.

15. Goodglass, H, and Kaplan, E: The assessment of cognitive deficits in the brain injured patient. In Gazzaniga, MS (ed): Handbook of Behavioral Neurobiology Neuropsychology. Plenum, New York, 1979.
16. Groher, ME: Language and memory disorders following closed head trauma. J Speech Hear Res 20:212, 1977.
17. Filley, CM, et al: Neurobehavioral outcome following closed head injury in childhood and adolescence. Arch Neurol 44:194, 1987.
18. Sarno, MT, Buonaguo, A, and Levita, E: Characteristics of verbal impairment in closed head injury patients. Arch Phys Med Rehabil 67:400, 1986.
19. Malec, JF, et al: Outcome evaluation and prediction in a comprehensive-integrated post-acute outpatient brain injury rehabilitation programme. Brain Inj 7:15, 1993.
20. Hagen, C: Language disorders in head trauma. In Holland, AL (ed): Language Disorders in Adults. College-Hill Press, San Diego, 1984.
21. Pilgatano, GP, Rouche, JR, and Fordyce, DJ: Non aphasic language disturbances after closed head injury. Language Sciences 1:217, 1985.
22. Hartley, LL: Cognitive-Communicative Abilities following Brain Injury: A Functional Approach. Singular Publishing, San Diego, 1995.
23. Freund, J, et al: Cognitive-Communication Disorders following Traumatic Brain Injury: A Practical Guide. Communication Skill Builders, Tucson, 1994.
24. Jennett, B, and Bond, M: Assessment outcome after severe brain damage: Practical scale. Lancet 1:480, 1975.
25. Hagen, C, and Malkmus, D: Intervention strategies for language disorders secondary to head trauma. American Speech-Language-Hearing Association Convention Short Course. Atlanta, 1989.
26. Giles, GM, and Clark-Wilson, J: Brain Injury Rehabilitation: A Neurofunctional Approach. Chapman and Hall, London, 1993.
27. Ansell, BJ, and Keenan, JE: The Western Neuro Sensory Stimulation Profile: A tool for assessing slow-to-recover head injured patients. Arch Phys Med Rehabil 70:104, 1989.
28. Ansell, BJ, Keenan, JE, and de la Rocha, O: The Western Neuro Sensory Stimulation Profile. Western Neuro Care Center, Tustin, Calif, 1989.
29. Porch, B: Porch Index of Communicative Ability: Administration, Scoring and Interpretation, ed 2. Consulting Psychologists Press, Palo Alto, Calif, 1973.
30. Rappaport, M, Dougherty, AM, and Kelting, DM: Evaluation of coma and vegetative states. Arch Phys Med Rehabil 73:628, 1992.
31. Rappaport, M, et al: Disability rating scale for severe head trauma: Coma to community. Arch Phys Med Rehabil 63:118, 1982.
32. Thomsen, IV: Evaluation and outcome of aphasia in patients with verified focal lesions. Folia Phoniatr 28:362, 1976.
33. Holland, AL: Communicative Abilities in Daily Living. University Park Press, Baltimore, 1980.
34. Kertesz, A: Western Aphasia Battery. Grune and Stratton, New York, 1982.
35. Goodglass, H, and Kaplan, E: The Assessment of Aphasia and Related Disorders. Lea and Febiger, Philadelphia, 1972.
36. Helm-Estabrooks, N, et al: Boston Assessment of Severe Aphasia. San Antonio Special Press, 1989.
37. Helm-Estabrooks, N: Aphasia Diagnostic Profiles. Riverside, Chicago, 1992.
38. Groher, ME, and Ochipa, C: The standardized communication assessment of individuals with traumatic brain injury. Seminars in Speech and Language 13:252, 1992.
39. Hartley, LL: Assessment of functional communication. In Tupper, DE, and Cicerone, KD (eds): The Neuropsychology of Everyday Life, vol 1. Kluwer Academic, Boston, 1990, p 125.
40. Helm-Estabrooks, N, and Hotz, G: The Brief Test of Head Injury. Riverside, Chicago, 1991.
41. Barry, P, et al: Rehabilitation inpatient screening of early cognitive recovery. Arch Phys Med Rehabil 70:902, 1989.
42. Baddeley, A, Emslie, H, and Smith, IN: The Speed and Capacity of Language-Processing Test. Thames Valley Test Company, Suffolk, 1992.
43. Adamovich, B, and Henderson, J: Scales of Cognitive Ability for Traumatic Brain Injury. Riverside, Chicago, 1992.
44. McGann, W, and Werven, G: Social competence and head injury: A new emphasis. Brain Inj 9:93, 1995.
45. Prutting, C, and Kirchner, D: Applied pragmatics. In Gallagher, T, and Prutting, C (eds): Pragmatic Assessment and Intervention Issues in Language. College-Hill Press, San Diego, 1983, p 29.
46. Milton, SB, Prutting, CA, and Binder, GM: Appraisal of communication competence in head injured adults. In Brookshire, RW (ed): Clinical Aphasiology, vol 14. BRK Publishers, Minneapolis, 1984, p 114.
47. Ehrlich, J, and Sipes, AL: Group treatment of communication skills for head trauma patients. Cognitive Rehabilitation 3:32, 1985.
48. Bolton, SO, and Dashiell, SE: Interaction Checklist for Augmentative Communication. INCH Associates, Huntington Beach, Calif, 1984.
49. Penn, C: The profile of communicative appropriateness: A clinical tool for the assessment of pragmatics. S Afr J Commun Disord 32:18, 1985.
50. Kennedy, MR, and DeRuyter, F: Cognitive and language bases for communication disorders. In Beukelman, DR, and Yorkston, KM (eds): Communication Disorders following Traumatic Brain Injury. Pro-Ed, Austin, 1991, p 123.
51. Burns, M, Halper, AS, and Mogil, SI: Clinical Management of Right Hemisphere Dysfunction. Aspen, Rockville, Md, 1985.
52. Mentis, M, and Prutting, CA: Analysis of topic as illustrated in a head-injured and a normal adult. J Speech Hear Res 14:583, 1991.
53. Hartley, LL, and Jensen, P: Narrative and procedural discourse after closed head injury. Brain Inj 5:267, 1991.
54. McDonald, S: Pragmatic language loss following closed-head injury: Inability to meet the informational needs of the listener. Brain Lang 30:88, 1993.
55. McDonald, S, and Pearce, S: The dice game: A new test of pragmatic language skills after closed-head injury. Brain Inj 9:255, 1995.
56. Flavell, JH: The development of role-taking and communication skills in children. Robert E. Krieger, New York, 1987.
57. McDonald, S: Communication disorders following closed head injury: New approaches to assessment and rehabilitation. Brain Inj 6:283, 1992.
58. Flannagan, S, McDonald, S, and Togher, L: Evaluating social skills following traumatic brain injury: The BRISS as a clinical tool. Brain Inj 9:321, 1995.
59. Brookshire, RH, and Nicholas, LE: Discourse Comprehension Test. Communication Skill Builders, Tuscon, 1993.
60. Winstein, CJ: Neurogenic dysphagia: Frequency, progression, and outcome in adults following head injury. Phys Ther 63:1992, 1983.
61. Buchholtz, DW: Neurogenic causes of dysphagia. Dysphagia 1:152, 1987.
62. Robbins, JA, and Levine, RL: Swallowing after unilateral stroke of the cerebral cortex: Preliminary experience. Dysphagia 3:11, 1988.
63. Bishop, M, Weymuller, EZ, and Fink, BR: Laryngeal effects of prolonged intubation. Anesth Analg 63:335, 1984.
64. Nash, M: Swallowing problems in the tracheotomized patient. Otolaryngol Clin North Am 21:701, 1988.
65. Sasaki, CT, et al: The effect of tracheostomy on the laryngeal closure reflex. Laryngoscope 87:1428, 1977.
66. Kazandijian, MS, and Dikeman, KJ: Communication and Swallowing Management of Tracheostomized and Ventilator-Dependent Adults. Singular Publishing, San Diego, 1995.

67. Buchholtz, DW, et al: Benzodiazepine-induced pharyngeal dysphagia: Report of two probable cases. Dysphagia Research Society, McClean, Va, 1995.

68. Langmore, SE, Schatz, K, and Olsen, N: Fiberoptic endoscopic examination of swallowing safety: A new procedure. Dysphagia 1:216, 1988.

69. Thompson-Henry, S, and Braddock, B: The modified Evan's blue dye procedure in the tracheotomized patient: Five case reports. Dysphagia 10:172, 1995.

70. McKaig, TN, and Thibadeau, JA: Computer assisted cervical level auscultation: The next step. Dysphagia (in press).

71. Takahashi, K, Groher, M, and Michi, K: Methodology for detecting swallowing sounds. Dysphagia 9:54, 1994.

CHAPTER 12

A Holistic Approach to Family Assessment after Brain Injury

ANGELLE M. SANDER, PHD,
and JEFFREY S. KREUTZER, PHD

Brain injury is a catastrophic event that substantially affects the emotional well-being of the person with the injury and the entire family. Family roles, communication, and relationships are inevitably disrupted. The injury can have a devastating effect on financial security and hope for the future. Typically, family members have had no prior experience that prepares them to cope with the life-altering consequences of injury to a loved one.

Recent emphasis on family involvement in rehabilitation has made working with families an increasingly important role for all members of the treatment team.[1,2] Yet, many professionals feel they lack the time and specialized training to intervene effectively. To promote family adjustment, professionals must understand an overwhelming complexity of factors, including family dynamics, role expectations, communication styles, preinjury stresses and adjustment, coping strategies, and plans for the future.

This chapter focuses on the assessment of family reactions to traumatic brain injury. First, typical postinjury changes, including common emotional reactions, role changes, coping strategies, and family needs, are described. Second, important areas for assessment are discussed, with evaluation strategies and measures recommended for each. The chapter concludes with a discussion of special issues and challenges, including working with a culturally diverse population and evaluating noninjury stresses. Emphasis is placed on providing practical guidelines, with case studies for illustration.

☐ COMMON EMOTIONAL REACTIONS OF FAMILY MEMBERS

To best understand the impact of brain injury on families, professionals should consider the reactions of each member. Consider the following case scenario:

Case 1 ■ Brian Jones, an accountant, sustained a severe brain injury 3 months ago. Now unemployed, he stays at home doing housework and caring for his children, age 3 and 5. Mrs. Jones, who returned to full-time work, complains that her husband is childish and has difficulty controlling his anger. Brian bursts into tears when his wife describes how the children have come to fear and dislike him. Their oldest child is having nightmares and trouble in preschool. Their younger child begs to get into bed with her and has been sleeping in the couple's bed nearly every night. Mrs. Jones states, "I'm going crazy and can't take this anymore. I have to take sleeping pills to get a decent night's rest. I'm going through this by myself, and I worry all the time about what he's doing to the kids. His family won't help. They just criticize me."

This case scenario illustrates a variety of emotions commonly experienced by family members. Most common are depression, guilt, anxiety, and anger.[3-6] Most people experience a combination of emotions, which vary over time. Emotions also vary depending on each person's relationship to the injured person. Spouses, parents, children, and extended family are affected differently. For example, the literature suggests that spouses experience more emotional distress than parents.[7-11] Unfortunately, there is relatively little research on the reactions of children, and most knowledge has been derived through clinical experience. The following section describes the most common emotional reactions of family members.

Depression

Researchers have demonstrated that depression is a common and long-term consequence of traumatic brain injury, beginning as early as 3 months after injury and persisting for up to 7 years.[11-16] Virtually all family members grieve in some way for injury-related losses. Family members may grieve for a lifetime over the loss of a friend, companion, protector, and advisor. Each family member has plans and expectations for the future, which are often disrupted by the injury, perhaps leaving a sense of pessimism or futility. Frustration, despair, and the sense of isolation are increased when the injured person "looks the same to everyone else."

Because of their better developed verbal skills, adults are more likely than children to discuss their feelings of depression. In contrast, children are prone to regression and more likely to convey feelings indirectly. Common manifestations are temper tantrums, interpersonal problems, withdrawal, nightmares, bed-wetting, clinging, and academic problems.

Following are common expressions by family members that may indicate underlying depression:

- "I miss my husband, and I'm married to a stranger."
- "Our lives are a mess, and there's no reason to believe that the future's going to be any better. Everything we worked for so hard is gone."
- "My parents don't care about me anymore. They've been spending all their time with my brother since he got hurt."

Guilt

Guilt is a common reaction among family members.[3,8,17,18] Parents tend to believe that they could have or should have done something to prevent the injury. Survivor's guilt refers to situations in which family members express a desire to trade places with the injured person. Parents and spouses sometimes take personal responsibility for the patient's neurobehavioral problems. Others feel that no matter how much they do, they should always do more. Children are more likely to blame themselves for their injured parent's emotional distress.

Extended family members often feel ambivalent when asked by immediate family members to assist in the patient's care. On the one hand, relatives are upset about the patient's injury and want to offer help. On the other hand, they are concerned about the adverse impact of long-term demands on their work schedules and personal lives. Immediate family members often express guilt about burdening the extended family with responsibilities for the patient's care.

Following are examples of expressions of guilt:

- "It was my fault. I should have driven that night. It should have been me."
- "We're so focused on him and his rehabilitation, I feel like we're neglecting the children."
- "If I was more attentive, maybe he wouldn't be so angry and upset."
- "My daddy yells at me all the time. I wish I could do something right."

Anxiety

Anxiety is a common reaction to the chaotic lifestyle and uncertainties that inevitably follow brain injury.[11,13,14,19] Problems with emotional lability and temper, which are common neurobehavioral sequelae, can create an atmosphere of sustained, heightened anxiety. Adult family members worry about caring for their relative and meeting financial obligations. Parents worry about their children's welfare. Meeting children's needs for emotional support and a secure, predictable home environment with two good role models is often a major concern. Children are especially prone to fears of abandonment. Aging parents worry about alternatives for their injured children in case of their own death or serious illness.

Difficulty in meeting financial obligations is a common source of anxiety. Loss of a breadwinner and high costs of medical treatment pose serious threats to financial integrity. Family members may be faced with the loss of their home or vehicle. The problem is especially troubling for those who formerly prided themselves on having excellent credit and more than adequate financial reserves.

The following expressions suggest underlying anxiety:

- "Our entire savings are gone. If something doesn't change soon, I don't know how long we can continue to put food on the table."
- "Every day when I go to work, I wonder if Tommy and the kids will be OK when I get home."
- "There's no point in planning for the future because we're not sure what's going to happen from one day to the next."

Anger

Anger has been reported as a common consequence of injury related frustrations.[4,5,20,21] Depression may be expressed as anger. In fact, depression has been described as anger turned inward. Poor communication, lack of information and understanding regarding injury sequelae, and maladaptive coping strategies also contribute to feelings of anger. A spouse gets angry at the injured mate, who may be irritable, impatient, inconsiderate, and ungrateful for care.[3] Anger toward the patient is exacerbated when family members believe that their relative caused the injury (e.g., by driving drunk or speeding) or is failing to comply with the treatment plan. Extended family members may criticize immediate family members for not doing enough in some cases, and for being overprotective in other cases. Conversely, caregiving family members become angry at extended family members who criticize yet fail to offer help or to give help when requested. Children are angered when attention is diverted from their needs to the injured person. Hospital or medical staff members may be victims of anger when frustrated family members offer criticism for not doing more. More recently, family members have expressed anger at insurance companies that are unwilling to fund requested rehabilitation services.

Common expressions of anger include:

- "No matter what I do, it's never good enough for him."
- "Dad ignores me since Mom got hurt. I suppose I should get a head injury to get more attention."
- "His mother drives me crazy. She comes over here, stands over my shoulder, and won't lift a finger to help."

Prolonged Emotional Distress

The effects of brain injury may persist for a lifetime. Clinicians must consider each family member's ability to cope with the prolonged effects of injury in the face of diminishing internal and external resources. Over the long term, physical and mental exhaustion can reduce coping ability, diminish hope, and exacerbate emotional distress. Ultimately, prolonged emotional distress negatively affects many aspects of family functioning, especially relationships and roles.[14,22] Social isolation is especially common.[23,24]

Investigators have documented the long-term strain on coping and emotional well-being.[7,11,15,16,25] Panting and Merry[7] were among the first to comment on family members' increasing use of tranquilizers and sleep medications within the first 6 months postinjury. More recently, Hall et al.[25] found signs of increased alcohol dependence and increased use of mental health services among family members between hospital discharge and 2 years postinjury.

☐ ROLE CHANGES

In many ways, stress after brain injury results from the redistribution of responsibilities. Other family members, often with less ability and experience, assume the injured person's responsibilities. The level of stress experienced by family members is related to at least four factors: (1) amount of responsibility to be assumed, (2) their willingness and competence to assume responsibilities, (3) the length of time the injured person is unavailable, and (4) the availability of extended family and friends to provide assistance.

Common Family Role Changes

Role changes often follow serious brain injuries and influence every immediate family member. Though individual differences must be recognized, observation reveals commonalities that depend on the age of the injured person and the family composition. For injured married adults, the typical case scenario is that of the family breadwinner who is unable to return to work after injury. The uninjured spouse, who may or may not have worked prior to the injury, often assumes the role of primary breadwinner. When able, the injured spouse takes over household responsibilities, including child care. However, the injured spouse often has difficulty assuming housekeeping and parenting duties because of cognitive and emotional deficits. The result is often that the working spouse is overwhelmed and feels uncomfortable relying on the injured mate to share in responsibilities. Children may attempt to help by assuming responsibilities and roles formerly held by either parent, including caregiving of other children and acting as confidant to the uninjured parent. In most cases, children are ill equipped to assume such roles. "Parental child" refers to a child who "grows up quickly" by taking on responsibilities inappropriate for the child's age.

In many cases, injured people are unmarried, or their marriage may end in divorce after the injury. In such cases, parents often return to their former role as primary caregivers. Adult siblings and extended family may also step in to help. Years of experience in the caregiving role can give parents an advantage, facilitating adaptation soon after injury. In comparison to spouses of injured patients, parents may feel more comfortable with the prospect of patients' long-term dependence. Parents may also have an uninjured partner with whom they can share caregiving responsibilities. However, caring for an injured adult child can be stressful for several reasons. First, the many demands of caregiving may disrupt parents' plans for retirement and relaxation during their later years. Second, parents worry about their inability to provide long-term care and realize that age may bring them illness or disability. Third, divorced parents may quarrel over the adult child's "best interests." Fourth, injury may trigger a reenactment of conflicts about independence, authority, maturity, and competence that emerged during adolescence.

Some might suggest that families with an injured nonadult child are least disrupted by role changes because parents are accustomed to caregiving responsibilities and to children's dependence. However, role changes are often necessary because parental responsibilities are substantially increased by the child's injury. In two-parent households, spouses may negotiate reassignment of responsibilities. One or both parents may be forced to reduce work hours or to resign. Options are more limited in single-parent households, and reliance on extended family and friends is often necessary. Role strain is often increased as the injured child develops and impairments become more evident. Parents and siblings often take on responsibilities that would normally be assumed by the child as he or she matures. Emancipation and independence are often delayed, and parents maintain their job as supervisor, advisor, and provider for more years than originally anticipated.

Family members face unique challenges to their adjustment when the injured person is elderly. When the injured elderly person is married, the spouse may also be ill or otherwise unable to take on caregiving responsibilities. Here, the availability of adult children and ex- tended family may be critical to avoid the costs of home health or nursing home care. Caring for an elderly injured parent may be difficult for several reasons. The caregiving relationship requires a role reversal, with the child serving as the parent's "parent." Unable to care for themselves and highly dependent on their children, injured parents often feel uncomfortable. Feelings of guilt about being a "burden" are common. In turn, adult children feel uncomfortable in a supervisory role. For example, to maintain health and safety, children may find themselves in the uncomfortable position of limiting their parents' activities, such as cooking or driving. Role strain may result when children find themselves torn between responsibilities to spouse and children and obligations to their injured parent. Children who find themselves unable to care for a parent inevitably experience tremendous guilt if nursing home placement is chosen as the best overall option.

◻ COPING

For most family members, receiving bad news about their relative causes considerable emotional distress. *Coping* refers to efforts to manage the stressful situation and the resulting emotional distress.[26] Family members use widely varying coping strategies. Strategies that are successful for one family member may lead to greater distress for another. Although clinicians have a tendency to label coping strategies as good or bad, these judgments are often affected by personal prejudices, values, and preferences. Recognizing and understanding family members' unique use of coping strategies can help clinicians support family members and promote their positive involvement in rehabilitation.

Researchers have identified coping strategies family members report as helpful.[9,27,28] They include talking to friends, participating in support groups, engaging in prayer or meditation, reserving time for relaxation, and maintaining a positive outlook. Living "one day at a time" helps some family members avoid anxieties about the future. Other family members attempt to identify and focus on positive aspects of their situation. Active participation in the patient's rehabilitation, support groups, and rehabilitation advocacy efforts often help family members gain a sense of control and develop a more positive view of their life situations. Identifying and utilizing community resources for respite is also helpful.

Although family members try to cope as best they can, several common strategies are more likely to have a long-term negative impact. Denial is a common response to negative events, particularly during the first few months after injury.[3,6,17] Family members find it easier to view the injury as "only temporary" rather than face the pain associated with adverse long-term changes that destroy their hopes and dreams. Although helpful in the short term, prolonged denial is likely to be damaging and to increase the probability of mental health problems, including depression and anxiety.[29]

Denial frequently contributes to conflict between family members and rehabilitation staff, which limits the effectiveness of rehabilitation and families' planning for the future. Denial may be manifested in refusal to plan for long-term financial or health care needs. In other situations, family members may refuse to participate in treatment or fail to comply with recommendations. For example, they may refuse to seek disability benefits or purchase a wheelchair, despite repeated recommendations from the treatment team. At times, denial can be manifested by family members' scapegoating of staff for injury related problems. Repeatedly overemphasizing preexisting problems in an effort to explain injury related changes may also indicate denial. Particularly in the later stages of injury, denial may lead to "doctor shopping."[17] As a coping strategy, family members often seek opinions about the patient that are consistent with their own. Family members may reject the opinions of professionals who offer negative but realistic prognostic information in favor of those who promise that their treatment can restore lost abilities. Families should be encouraged to ask questions regarding treatment and to seek second opinions. However, repeated rejection of negative prognostic information, expressions of doubt about staff members' expertise and motivation, and playing staff members against each other are indications that family members are having difficulty in coping.

Avoidance may occur when family members recognize the adverse consequences of injury. They may sense the patient's pain, fully recognize the consequences of the injury, and fear that life will never be the same and thus avoid hospital visits, caregiving responsibilities, and participation in the rehabilitation program. The following case scenario illustrates avoidance:

> Case 2 ■ Derek, a 14-year-old only child, sustained a severe brain injury, resulting in physical and cognitive impairment, including contracture of the extremities and inability to walk. Derek's mother visited the hospital daily. In contrast, his father visited twice during the initial week in the hospital and then did not visit again. Derek's mother explained that her husband loved Derek but had been working more hours than usual since the injury. He usually left early in the morning and didn't come home until after she was asleep. Derek's mother also reported that her son and husband had been extremely close before the injury, and she was worried that her husband was having difficulty with coping.

Infantilization is a coping strategy used most often by parents of injured children. To protect against a second injury and possibly relieve guilt arising from the first, family members may restrict patients well beyond professionals' recommendations. Adolescent patients may complain that their parents refuse to let them play sports any more. Seven-year-olds may complain that they are no longer allowed to ride their bicycles. Injured adults can be infantilized by parents and spouses. For example, injured persons may complain that their spouses do not let them drive or stay home alone, even when medical restrictions have been lifted.

In summary, each family member is likely to use a combination of effective and ineffective coping strategies. Clinicians are encouraged to identify and monitor the effectiveness of each strategy and help family members rely more on effective coping strategies.

❑ FAMILY NEEDS RESEARCH

Early research investigating family members' needs after brain injury indicated that receiving a kind, clear explanation of the patient's medical condition and discussing realistic expectations for recovery were most often rated as important. Mauss-Clum and Ryan[9] noted that family members want realistic prognostic information but have a negative reaction to pessimism from health care professionals. They often have a negative reaction to statements such as "He'll never be able to hold a job" or "She'll never be able to live by herself." Family members reportedly respond best to prognostic information that is given with a hopeful, caring attitude and reassurance that optimal care is being provided. Also identified as important by Mauss-Clum and Ryan[9] were needs for emotional support, financial counseling, and information on community resources. The importance of needs for information, truthfulness, and reassurance from medical professionals has been confirmed by other researchers.[30-32]

To understand family members' needs after brain injury, Kreutzer et al.[33] developed the Family Needs Questionnaire (FNQ), a 40-item questionnaire that requests two separate ratings of injury related needs. First, needs are rated based on perceived importance (not important; somewhat important; important; very important). Afterward, family members rate the extent to which each need has been met (not met; partly met; met). Questionnaire items were based on interviews with family members, a review of literature relevant to family adjustment and neurological disability, and a review of existing needs questionnaires. The FNQ contains six factor analytically derived scales.[34] A description of scale content is provided in Table 12–1.

In a series of studies, the FNQ was used to identify needs most often perceived as important and unmet.[35–37] Receiving medical information about patients' conditions was most often identified as important. Family members rated personal needs (e.g., social and emotional support, help with responsibilities) as relatively less important. Of the needs rated as important, those relating to emotional support and caregiving were most often described as unmet. In contrast, needs for medical information and support from professional staff were most frequently reported as met.

Most studies have focused on needs soon after injury. Relatively little is known about the postacute period and changes in needs over time. Using the FNQ, Witol et al.[37] examined family needs in a longitudinal investigation at 1 and 2 years postinjury. At both time intervals, researchers examined the extent to which needs identified as important were judged as being met. Investigation revealed that health information and professional support needs were most often rated as met. Instrumental and emotional support needs were most frequently rated as unmet. Over time, family members perceived an increase in unmet needs regarding involvement with care and emotional sup-

port. At both time intervals, a majority of family members reported that none of their needs for instrumental support were met. Examination of the data suggests that creating more opportunities for respite from responsibilities and social support should be considered a priority.

☐ ASSESSMENT

Family members have different perceptions of how their lives have been and will be affected by the patient's injury. Differing perceptions, personalities, and coping styles contribute to emotional differences among family members. This section describes three techniques that provide important information about the adjustment of individual family members and the family as a whole: (1) interviews, (2) observation, and (3) quantitative assessment. Then, major assessment content areas, including emotional status, family systems functioning, coping, social support systems, and family needs, are described.

Assessment Techniques

INTERVIEWS

Perhaps the most common and flexible method of collecting information about patients and families, interviews vary in their level of structure. Some questions are commonly asked of all family members to allow for comparison of re-

---

TABLE 12–1. Description of Scales from the Family Needs Questionnaire

Factor	Description
Health information	Needs for information about the patient's medical care, physical condition, cognitive status, and psychosocial functioning
Emotional support	Needs for receiving understanding, reassurance, and nurturance from family, friends, and others in the community
Instrumental support	Needs for respite and practical assistance in meeting responsibilities; opportunities to fulfill personal, physical, and social needs
Professional support	Needs for long-term access to training and to information on how to help manage the patient's difficulties
Community support network	Needs for members of the patient's and family members' peer groups, including teachers and employers, to understand the injury and related difficulties, and to be supportive
Involvement with care	Needs to be integrated into the patient's treatment process; needs for opinions to be solicited and to be informed of rehabilitation/treatment progress

Source: Reprinted from Witol, AD, Sander, AM, and Kreutzer, JS: A longitudinal analysis of family needs following traumatic brain injury. NeuroRehabilitation 7:175, 1996, with permission.

sponses. However, clinicians typically tailor other questions to elicit information relevant to the unique issues presented by each family member. A list of important questions frequently asked during family intake sessions is shown in Table 12–2.

Interview questions are usually formatted in two ways. Open-ended questions—for example, "How do you feel about your son?" or "What do you miss about the way things were before the injury?"—invite elaboration and discussion. They develop rapport by inviting input. When confronted with strict time limits, evasiveness, or tangential responding, open-ended questions are contraindicated. Closed-ended questions are useful for soliciting specific information and developing discussion with introverted family members: "How long have you been married?" or "Have you noticed feelings of depression since the injury?"

Normalizing is a technique used to help family members feel more comfortable about answering questions. Consider the following example. A 38-year-old truck driver and his wife

were interviewed by a social worker 8 days after their son's hospitalization for severe brain injury. The social worker explained, "Even the toughest people have a terrible time when someone they love so much is hurt so badly. How have you been doing?" Normalizing helps the distraught family understand that their feelings are not unusual and may be expected, given the nature of the situation.

OBSERVATION

Careful observation provides important clues about thoughts and feelings, especially when family members find themselves confused, conflicted, or uncomfortable about their thoughts and feelings. Examples of key areas for observation include:

- Degree of eye contact reflects degree of warmth, honesty, comfort, and communication within the family
- Affect as reflected in tone of voice, facial expression, posture, and gestures
- Speech content (e.g., critical, reassuring, positive, pessimistic)
- Congruence of affect and speech content; incongruence may indicate hidden or conflicting feelings
- Seating arrangements and proximity of family members as reflections of relationship quality and the nature of alliances between family members
- Level of dominance or passivity during discussions because dominance may indicate a leadership position, self-centeredness, or isolation, whereas passivity may indicate hopelessness, pessimism, or a tendency for submissiveness

The clinician's office is an unusual environment for family members, and most people are likely to be on their best behavior. However, in time, many clinicians have an opportunity to observe enactment, spontaneous behavioral patterns that are normally displayed only in the home setting. Consider the following case example:

Case 3 ■ Mr. White, a 36-year-old man who sustained a severe brain injury 8 months ago, arrives for a family counseling session with his wife and 10-year-old son. Mother and son rush to get the two comfortable cushions on the love seat, and she sits with her arm around him. Mr. White begins the discussion by launching into a lengthy tirade about his insensitive wife and lazy son. During his tirade, he maintains eye contact with the counselor and refers to other family members in the third person. Each time his wife tries to explain herself, he interrupts her and scowls. Fi-

---

TABLE 12–2. Frequently Asked Intake Questions

1. How many people live in the home? Describe each person by age, occupation, and relationship to the patient.
2. Who are the extended family, and are they available for help?
3. Has the living situation changed since the injury in terms of where the patient lives and who is in the household?
4. Do family members feel comfortable leaving the patient alone? How much time does each family member spend with the patient, and what activities are involved?
5. If the patient is married, for how long? How would you describe the quality of the marriage (e.g., warmth, intimacy) both before and after injury? How well did all family members get along before the injury?
6. How have family members' responsibilities changed since the injury?
7. Were there any major stresses, including physical or mental health problems, before the injury?
8. What are the postinjury sources of stress, including stresses unrelated to the injury? Has anyone in the family sought help for physical or mental health problems?
9. Were family finances stable before the injury? What is the family's current financial status? Are finances a source of stress?
10. What community resources are available, including transportation, rehabilitation services, churches, and community organizations?

nally, with tears in his eyes, he remarks, "I'm just fine, I don't care if anyone likes me."

After a series of counseling sessions, everyone realized that Mr. White cared very deeply about family members' feelings toward him. He described feeling like a rejected outsider, his many years as a provider and supportive father forgotten after the injury. Mrs. White explained that her husband now behaves like a child. Their 10-year-old son had matured since the injury and taken on many of his father's responsibilities. Now, he behaved more maturely than his father. Mrs. White was eloquent in describing her loneliness and remarked, "I'm married but I don't have a husband."

QUANTITATIVE ASSESSMENT APPROACHES

Some would argue that conclusions derived from interviews and observations are tainted with subjectivity. Because of differences in training, experience, philosophical orientation, and styles, different clinicians may reach different conclusions about the same family members. Tests, questionnaires, and inventories are more structured and therefore theoretically less susceptible to clinicians' biases. Many quantitative instruments have instruction manuals for administration, scoring, and interpretation of results. Data for healthy people and other patient groups are often available for comparison. Cutoff scores may allow discrimination between healthy and unhealthy characteristics. In many cases, reliability and validity information is provided. A list of quantitative instruments that may be used to assess various aspects of family functioning is shown in Table 12–3. It is not meant to be exhaustive but rather to provide a sampling of the most widely used instruments.

The limitations of quantitative instruments should be acknowledged. Family members with limited academic skills may require help to read and interpret questions. The structured format of many instruments inherently limits flexibility and the opportunity for elaboration and explanation necessary to understand unique situations. Furthermore, caution must be exercised with the many tools not specifically developed for brain injury populations.

In summary, interview, observation, and quantitative methods offer different types of information. Each method has advantages and disadvantages. A triadic approach is most often used and most likely to offer optimal information. Clinical practice often requires a synthesis of information from different sources, including available records.

Assessment Content Areas

A thorough assessment necessitates careful collection of information in a variety of areas. Clinicians should determine how the family was functioning before the injury and how functioning has changed. Healthy and unhealthy coping and problem-solving styles before and after the injury should be identified. Many clinicians feel pressured to "figure out the family" during the course of a single assessment. Yet, the most accurate understanding is achieved when rapport has been established and information is synthesized from a variety of sources over time.

Important target areas for assessment, along with descriptions of selected quantitative instruments for each, follow:

EMOTIONAL STATUS OF EACH FAMILY MEMBER

Monitoring the emotional distress of individual family members is an important step toward formulating effective interventions. Each family member has a unique perception of the injury and a unique reaction, which may change over time. Sometimes one or two family members become the "symptom bearers," openly and repeatedly voicing distress. Here, other family members may assume a stoic attitude, provide support, and take responsibility for managing the family's affairs. Despite appearances, even the strongest family member is likely to experience distress.

Screening family members for emotional distress should include inquiry regarding mood, personality changes, sleep and appetite patterns, energy levels, interest in formerly enjoyed activities, hope for the future, levels of social interaction, and perceived sources of stress. Interviews and discussions with family members often provide a convenient opportunity to elicit information. With overwhelming responsibilities and hectic schedules, some family members may be unavailable for face-to-face discussions. As an alternative, questionnaires designed to detect depression, anxiety, and other difficulties can be mailed or sent home with visiting family members.

Among the more frequently used measures is the Brief Symptom Inventory (BSI),[38] a 53-item screening instrument that inquires about symptoms of emotional distress experienced during the past month. Items are rated on a scale ranging from 0 ("not at all") to 4 ("extremely"). Examples of items include "feeling no interest in things," "feelings of guilt," and "trouble falling asleep." Besides three global distress indices, the BSI yields nine subscale scores reflecting categories of emotional distress, such as de-

TABLE 12–3. Assessment Content Areas and Frequently Used Measures

Content	Measure	Psychometric Properties	Use with Family Members of Persons with Brain Injury
Perceived stress or burden	Perceived Burden Scale[12]	Developed for brain injury population; no reliability or validity information available	McKinlay et al.[12] Livingston et al.[13,14] Brooks et al.[15,16]
	NYU Head Injury Family Interview[42]	Developed specifically for brain injury population; good internal reliability; good content and construct validity	Cavallo et al.[53] Kay et al.[43] Rivara et al.[49,50]
	Caregiver Appraisal Scale[44]	Developed for dementia population; good internal reliability; moderate retest reliability; good construct and concurrent validity	Not yet used
Coping strategies or style	Ways of Coping Questionnaire[51]	Acceptable reliability; good content validity; 8 scales assessing problem- and emotion-focused coping; developed with a normal population; some variance in factor structure among samples	Tarter[54] Sander et al.[29]
	COPE[55]	Good internal reliability; good construct validity; 13 scales assessing problem- and emotion-focused coping; developed with a normal population	Wade et al.[56]
	Coping Health Inventory for Parents[57]	Good internal reliability; good construct validity; 3 factors assessing different coping patterns; developed for use with family members of chronically ill children	Rivara et al.[49,50]
	Family Interview Rating Scale[49,50]	Interview developed for use with family members of children with brain injury; good interrater reliability and construct validity	Rivara et al.[49,50,58]
Family functioning	Family Assessment Device[46]	Good reliability; good construct and concurrent validity	Zarski et al.[48] Kreutzer et al.[11,39] Hall et al.[25]
	Family Environment Scale[59]	Good reliability; weak validity	Rivara et al.[49,50,58]
	Family Adaptability and Cohesion Evaluation Scales[60]	Good reliability; weak validity	Zarski et al.[48]
	Family Interview Rating Scale[49,50]	See above	See above
	Family Global Assessment Scale[61]	Developed for brain injury population; good interrater reliability; no validity information available	Rivara et al.[49,50,58]
Needs	Family Needs Questionnaire[33]	Good internal consistency; good construct validity	Kreutzer et al.[35] Serio et al.[36] Witol et al.[37] Serio et al.[34]
Social support	Social Support Questionnaire[52]	Good internal and test-retest reliability; good construct validity	Sander et al.[29]

TABLE 12–3. *Continued*

Content	Measure	Psychometric Properties	Use with Family Members of Persons with Brain Injury
Emotional distress	Symptom Checklist-90 and Brief Symptom Inventory[38]	Good internal reliability; good construct and convergent validity; normative data available	Tarter[54] Kreutzer et al.[11,39]
	General Health Questionnaire[62]	Good internal consistency and test-retest reliability; good construct and concurrent validity	Livingston et al.[13,14] Sander et al.[29]
	Beck Depression Inventory[63]	Good internal consistency; good construct and concurrent validity	Not yet used
	Leeds General Scales for anxiety and depression[64]	Good reliability and validity; normative data available	Livingston et al.[13,14]
	Minnesota Multiphasic Personality Inventory[65]	Developed for use with psychiatric patients; good internal consistency and construct validity; contains scales to assess response consistency and validity	Not yet used

pression, anxiety, somatization, and hostility. The BSI has been utilized in studies of caregivers after brain injury.[11,39] Adequate internal reliability for all nine subscales and the three global indices has been demonstrated, along with convergent and construct validity.[38] Other screening measures are listed in Table 12–3.

BURDEN

Family members' perceived "burden" is a concept originally applied to the brain injury population by researchers in Glasgow.[12–16] The concept of burden was initially conceptualized as dichotomous, including "objective" and "subjective" burden. *Objective burden* referred to family members' perceptions of impairments in the patient (e.g., "Is the patient bad-tempered?") and demands of the caregiving situation (e.g., "Have you had to change your social or leisure habits since the accident because of the patient's behavior?").[12] *Subjective burden* was defined as the amount of stress experienced by the family member as a result of injury-related changes. Subjective burden was measured by a 7-point Likert scale on which family members rate the amount of stress experienced recently. In a series of studies, researchers found high levels of subjective burden in family members, beginning as early as 3 months after injury and persisting at long-term intervals of 5 and 7 years.[13–16]

Recently, the concept of burden has been redefined as equivalent to perceived stress.[40] Family members' perceptions of stress are important to assess because they can affect reaction to the injury and overall family adjustment.[41] In measuring family members' perceived stress, clinicians need to understand the specific sources of stress as well as the overall stress level. The traditional Likert scale used to assess burden among family members after brain injury is limited in its ability to assess various sources of stress. A solution to this problem is offered by the Head Injury Family Interview (HIFI).[42] The interview contains a 43-item problem checklist. Using a 7-point Likert scale, family members rate the extent to which each problem affects the daily functioning of the patient (e.g., "mood swings," "forgetful"). For each item, family members also rate the level of stress or burden they experience as a result of the problem. Responses allow clinicians to determine the primary sources of stress and enhance treatment planning. Factor analysis has supported division of items into three scales: Affective/Behavioral, Cognitive, and Physical/Dependency.[43] Evidence has been provided to support internal consistency.[43] The HIFI also contains structured interviews to assess the impact of the injury on individual family members, including specialized interviews for spouses, parents, adult siblings, siblings living at home, adult children, and children at home.

Multidimensional measures of burden developed for use with caregivers of dementia patients can be adopted for use with caregivers of people with brain injury. One such measure is the Caregiver Appraisal Scale.[44] The questionnaire is predicated on the belief that not all aspects of the caregiving situation are negative or a burden. Questions assess positive aspects of caregiving (e.g., " _____ shows real appreciation for what you do for him/her"), as well as negative aspects ("Your social life has suffered because you are caring for _____").

FAMILY SYSTEM FUNCTIONING

Research indicates that many families face a long period of social isolation after the patient's injury.[23,24] Lacking outside resources and facing many stresses, family members' relationships with one another become paramount. Relationships can serve as a source of support or a source of conflict. The behavior of family members toward one another and their ability to effectively solve problems together are critical determinants of postinjury adjustment.

Communication

Communication is perhaps the most important aspect of family behavior. Many people avoid expressing negative feelings after the injury because they fear anger, resentment, being misunderstood, and alienation from other family members. A common example involves a husband who is irritable and frequently loses his temper with family members. His wife and children avoid him and fear that honest feedback will only exacerbate his anger. A man who criticizes his injured wife's behavior may fear accusations of disloyalty and insensitivity.

Failure to honestly express feelings and provide feedback contributes to confusion and misperceptions. Even when trying to avoid direct expression, family members inevitably communicate indirectly through gestures, facial expressions, and silence. Unfortunately, indirect communication contributes to negative feelings and to family dysfunction. For example, a husband who, when his injured wife describes how hard it is to get up in the morning and care for the children, shakes his head and frowns is likely communicating frustration. However, his wife may perceive that he is angry or does not love her.

To better understand communication patterns, clinicians should consider the following questions during interviews, observations, and discussions:

- To what extent are feelings, perceptions, and beliefs communicated directly and indirectly?

- What are the individual expression styles and listening skills of each family member?

- Does the manner of speaking engage the listener or result in defensiveness? Are feelings expressed in an accusatory way?

- Do family members seem to understand one another? To what extent are paraphrase and repetition used to evaluate understanding?

- Are there topics or feelings that family members choose to avoid or focus on?

- How do family members recognize one another's feelings, especially when feelings are not expressed directly? For example, "how do you know when your husband is angry?"

Role playing may also be used to obtain a realistic picture of family members' interaction patterns.

Roles

Family members' roles are typically defined in terms of relationships and responsibilities. Society has expectations for familial roles, especially those relating to parental and spousal obligations. Family members also have responsibilities relating to housekeeping, financial management, child rearing, home maintenance, and earning income. Family members also develop roles relating to their personality style (e.g., comforter, joker).

Inevitably, brain injury necessitates role changes. Understanding family reactions necessitates understanding family members' perception of their own roles and those of other members. Soon after injury, family members may be available and willing to assume new roles temporarily. However, family members may express reluctance to assume new roles for the long term. Inquiries should be made regarding comfort levels and feelings of competence in new roles. Assessment of "role strain," which results from one person assuming too many responsibilities, is also important. The stresses associated with role changes may result in the scapegoating of the injured person. The person with the injury may be targeted for all blame, including preexisting problems. The scapegoat role is unhealthy for the patient and the entire family for several reasons. Scapegoating contributes to feelings of depression and worthlessness, which can promote suicidal ideation. Also, family members may not solve their problems because they have overlooked the real cause.

Quality of Family Relationships

Family relationships may be characterized in a variety of ways. Some clinicians focus on relationships and interactions; others focus on family activities. How much time family members spend together and the nature of their activities are important indicators of relationship quality. After a patient's brain injury, some family members report an increase in time spent together, but the quality of time is typically reduced substantially. Activities are often focused on household and injury related responsibilities, including medical care arrangements, rehabilitation, transportation, and insurance forms. When questioning family members, clinicians should identify how much time is spent together, the nature of activities, and the extent to which activities are perceived as "quality time." Perceptions of preinjury and postinjury interactions should be identified, along with expectations for the future. Consider the case of the Brown family:

Case 4 ■ Mrs. Brown resigned from her job to stay at home after having the couple's second child. Soon after her husband's injury, she began working full-time. Out of necessity, Mrs. Brown took over her husband's responsibilities for managing finances and arranging for home maintenance. In addition to being their children's primary caregiver, she has been monitoring her unemployed husband's daily activities by calling him at home throughout the day. Exhausted, she falls asleep nightly "minutes" after putting the oldest child to bed. On the weekends, she does paperwork, cleans house, and transports the children to friends' home and activities. Preinjury, the couple dined out regularly and talked for a while every evening before retiring to bed. Now, the only chance they have to "talk things over" is when she's driving him to medical and rehabilitation appointments.

A healthy family system combines encouragement of individuation and independence with emotional closeness and support. The stresses associated with brain injury often lead families to engage in unhealthy patterns of interaction. In some cases, the unhealthy interactions preexisted and are exacerbated by the injury. In other cases, previously healthy families develop unhealthy patterns. One type of unhealthy pattern is *enmeshment,* a term describing lack of clear boundaries between family members.[45] Enmeshed families overemphasize family unity and togetherness at the expense of individual identity and external social relationships. Although spending time together is important, sole reliance on each other for support and socialization may lead to social isolation and to emotional distress. Overprotectiveness, a common reaction for parents of injured children, is a primary contributor to enmeshment.

In contrast to enmeshment, *disengagement* refers to emotional distance between family members, with individual members perceiving a lack of warmth, acceptance, and support.[45] Families characterized by preinjury disengagement often have the greatest difficulty with postinjury adjustment. However, even family members who were previously close often become emotionally estranged after injury. Frustration, feelings of personal ineffectiveness, and misunderstanding the patient's behavioral problems contribute to disengagement.

Family therapists often use the term *alliance* to describe a strong bond between individuals.[45] In healthy families, alliances develop between people of equal status, such as siblings or parents. For example, parents consult in deciding on disciplinary strategies, financial planning, and assignment of household responsibilities. Effective intervention requires a thorough understanding of alliances and how they have been affected by injury. Unhealthy alliances are common after brain injury, arising from changed feelings and disrupted roles. For example, the wife of an injured man may begin turning to her adolescent son for the advice and emotional support her husband formerly provided.

Quantitative Assessment of Family Functioning

Among the most useful quantitative tools is the 60-item self-report Family Assessment Device (FAD),[46] which provides information relevant to communication, roles, and quality of relationships. Normative data and cutoff scores for dysfunction are available,[47] and investigators have used the questionnaire to characterize families after brain injury.[11,39,48] The six scales with representative items are:

■ Problem solving. "We resolve most everyday problems around the house."

■ Roles. "Each of us has particular duties or responsibilities."

■ Communication. "When someone is upset the others know why."

■ Affective responsiveness. "We are reluctant to show our affection for each other."

■ Affective involvement. "You only get the interest of others when something is important to them."

■ Behavior control. "You can easily get away with breaking the rules."

Each item is rated on a Likert scale ranging from "strongly agree" to "strongly disagree." A General Functioning Scale score can also be calculated to reflect the family's overall well-being. Other useful assessment tools are listed in

Table 12–3. Examining responses to individual items and comparing responses between members of the same family can often prove helpful.

COPING STRATEGIES

Virtually every person experiences stressful life events, and the development of coping strategies is a natural result. Coping styles emerge early in life, change over time, and relate to age, intellectual ability, experience, and genetic predisposition. As a unit, families also develop coping strategies. Characteristic strategies evolve over time and relate to experience, sources of stress, the age of individual family members, their position in the life cycle, and the nature of interrelationships between family members.

Research has shown that preinjury family coping is a strong predictor of family functioning after injury in children.[49,50] Preinjury coping styles may be ineffective, or their effectiveness may diminish over time with changing sources and levels of stress. Brain injury is a catastrophic event, and few family members have the experience or emotional stamina to cope effectively in the long term. Assessment of coping should include delineation of available resources and coping strategies. Important questions to ask include:

- What are the coping strategies used by individual family members and by the family as a whole?
- Does one person take control in stressful situations, or are problems solved through group discussion?
- Do family members ignore problems and hope for spontaneous resolution?
- Are individual members' coping strategies similar, complementary, or disparate?
- Do family members, in trying to impose their strategies on others, increase conflict?

The following case scenario illustrates the confusion that can occur when family members all attempt to impose their own coping strategies.

Case 5 ■ Joey, a 17-year-old, was discharged to his home after inpatient rehabilitation for a moderate brain injury. Returning to school on a part-time basis, Joey experienced frustration related to memory and concentration difficulties, along with persistent fatigue. Joey also felt that his friends treated him differently and did not include him in as many activities. When he complained to his family, Joey got conflicting advice. His mother responded, "If you simply have faith and trust in the Lord, everything will turn out for the best." His father advised him to be more assertive with his friends and to work in the yard as a way to relieve stress. Joey's younger brother invited him to hang out with him and his friends, and his older sister referred him to her therapist for counseling. Overwhelmed and confused, Joey withdrew from family members and became depressed.

Individual family members should be encouraged to develop coping strategies that are effective and comfortable. They should be helped to identify effective coping strategies for different situations. Some family members have difficulty identifying or analyzing the effectiveness of coping strategies. Here the therapist can act as a facilitator, prompting with questions like "What did you do when you lost your job?" or "Did talking to people in the support group help you to figure things out or feel better?" or "How did things work out when you tried not thinking about the problem?"

The Ways of Coping Questionnaire (WOCQ)[51] is a 66-item questionnaire used to identify most frequently used coping strategies. The WOCQ was developed based on Lazarus and Folkman's[26] theory that individuals use two basic types of strategies to cope with stressful events: problem focused and emotion focused. Problem-focused coping includes behaviors aimed at altering stressful situations (e.g., planning the next step, seeking information about the problem). In contrast, emotion-focused coping includes behaviors aimed at managing emotional distress (e.g., pretending that nothing has happened, focusing on the positive aspects).

To complete the WOCQ, respondents are first asked to describe a specific, recent stressful situation. Respondents can be asked to specify an injury-related situation. Each strategy is then rated on a scale of 0 (does not apply or not used) to 4 (used a great deal). The instrument has adequate internal reliability and construct validity.[51] Factor analysis supports organizing items into eight coping scales:

- Confrontive coping. "I stood my ground and fought for what I wanted."
- Distancing. "I went on as if nothing had happened."
- Self-controlling. "I kept others from knowing how bad things were."
- Seeking social support. "I talked to someone about how I was feeling."
- Accepting responsibility. "I criticized or lectured myself."
- Escape avoidance. "I hoped a miracle would happen."
- Planful problem solving. "I made a plan of action and followed it."
- Positive reappraisal. "I found new faith."

Descriptions of each scale and their loading on problem-focused or emotion-focused coping factors are shown in Table 12–4.

AVAILABILITY OF SUPPORT SYSTEMS

Support systems are an important determinant of postinjury family adjustment that provide opportunities for respite, assistance, companionship, feedback, and guidance. Caregiving family members with little support are less effective partners in the rehabilitation process. Negative perceptions about the quality of support lead to increased stress, depression, and anxiety.[29]

Parents and extended family members typically become the primary source of support over time. Friends are frequent visitors while the patient is hospitalized, but their availability and interest often diminish over time. Church members, acquaintances from social and community service groups, and former coworkers may also provide support. Distant relatives or friends may be willing to come to town and offer help on a short-term basis.

Interviews provide an important opportunity to elicit information about sources of support and feelings toward utilizing resources. Limited creativity or knowledge may lead family members to overlook viable options. Moreover, feelings about asking for help are influenced by others' reactions to past requests. A history of positive responses leads to optimism about seeking help, whereas negative reactions lead to pessimism. Guilt about relying on others or concerns about appearing inadequate may also lead to reluctance to request help.

Professionals who desire a more comprehensive assessment method are encouraged to consider the Social Support Questionnaire (SSQ).[52] With demonstrated internal reliability, the self-administered 27-item SSQ quantifies levels of social support available to individuals and levels of satisfaction with support. For each item, respondents list up to nine people on whom they could rely in a specific circumstance (e.g., "Who do you feel would help you if you were married and had just separated from your spouse?"). The number of people listed for each item can be averaged across the 27 items to provide a mean support score. To indicate satisfaction, subjects also rate each item on a scale ranging from 1 (very dissatisfied) to 6 (very satisfied). The mean score for the 27 items is used to indicate overall satisfaction.

FAMILY NEEDS

Understanding family members' needs is a first step toward developing effective intervention. Each family member usually has clear ideas about her or his most important needs and the

---

TABLE 12–4. Descriptions of Coping Scales from the Ways of Coping Questionnaire

Coping Scale	Description
Confrontive Coping*	Describes aggressive efforts to alter the situation and suggests some degrees of hostility and risk-taking.
Distancing	Describes cognitive efforts to detach oneself and to minimize the significance of the situation.
Self-Controlling	Describes efforts to regulate one's efforts and actions.
Seeking Social Support†	Describes efforts to seek informational support, tangible support, and emotional support.
Accepting Responsibility	Acknowledges one's own role in the problem with a concomitant theme of trying to put things right.
Escape-Avoidance	Describes wishful thinking and behavioral efforts to escape or avoid the problem. Items on this scale contrast with those on the Distancing scale, which suggest detachment.
Planful Problem-Solving*	Describes deliberate problem-focused efforts to alter the situation, coupled with an analytic approach to solving the problem.
Positive Reappraisal	Describes efforts to create positive meaning by focusing on personal growth; also has a religious dimension.

*Denotes that the items on this scale represent problem-focused coping strategies. All other scales represent emotion-focused coping strategies.
†Consists of both problem- and emotion-focused items.

extent to which these needs have been met. In most cases, a large number of unmet, important needs are identified. Family members may disagree on the importance of needs and their priority for intervention. A discussion with family members may suffice to establish important priorities. Sometimes there is substantial disagreement about needs, or some family members are unable to attend discussions. Here, the Family Needs Questionnaire (FNQ),[33] discussed earlier, may prove useful in soliciting input from all family members and synthesizing opinions. The comprehensive questionnaire can help to identify needs not expressed during interview.

□ SPECIAL ISSUES AND CHALLENGES

Often clinicians are asked to intervene with families at times of crisis. Naturally, attention is focused on immediate issues, including injury sequelae, needs, and sources of stress. Urgency often leads professionals to overlook a variety of factors and issues that can undermine the effectiveness of intervention.

Cultural, Ethnic, and Personal Differences

Clinicians may be unaware of their own biases and personal philosophies. They also may fail to understand the biases and philosophies of family members. For example, family members may believe that "every man should work," "a woman's place is in the home," or "no man should be asked to do housework." Such beliefs can be an obstacle to clinicians' efforts to promote renegotiation of responsibilities after injury. Clinicians should also be aware of cultural differences in family structure and interactions. For example, in many Asian cultures, elderly persons are considered the bearers of wisdom and are to be treated with deference at all times. Adult children may react negatively to clinicians' effort to have them take a supervisory role with an injured parent. Cultural traditions may also serve a beneficial role during the recovery process. For example, many cultures promote close long-term relationships between extended family members. Such relationships are likely to facilitate sharing and reassignment of responsibilities.

To be most effective, clinicians should base questions and feedback on the family's frame of reference. Clinicians should avoid asserting their own values and philosophies. Families are more likely to freely offer honest information when questioned by a clinician they perceive as nonjudgmental.

Overlooking the Patient's Point of View

Citing concerns about poor self-awareness, some clinicians undervalue patients' opinions and perceptions. Patients' perceptions are likely to be overlooked when the patient is severely impaired or placed in the scapegoat role and blamed for all the family's problems. Some clinicians may give credibility to the opinions of only one family member. Deciding who is right and wrong is a challenging and complex exercise. Nevertheless, to establish accurate conclusions, the opinions and perceptions of all involved should be solicited, compared, and carefully considered. To foster cooperation and gain complete information, every effort should be made to convey respect and appreciation for everyone's involvement.

Sources of Stress Not Related to Injury

Clinicians tend to focus on the brain injury as the primary or sole source of stress. Yet, many times family members experience stresses unrelated to the injury that far outweigh injury-related factors. Preinjury sources of stress can include pending bankruptcy or divorce and medical or emotional problems, including alcoholism and depression. Even after injury, families continue to encounter normal life problems that are independent of the injury, including unemployment, illness, or death of a loved one. During the assessment process, family members may have difficulty identifying preinjury sources of stress. They may have had sufficient coping resources, but the injury has taken them beyond the threshold of tolerance. Clinicians should carefully monitor the full spectrum of sources of stress, including those related to the brain injury and others.

□ SUMMARY AND CONCLUSIONS

Family members experience a vast array of reactions to brain injury. Their reactions are based on preinjury experiences and philosophies, individual coping styles, family dynamics, the injury consequences, and the availability of resources. Understanding family reactions requires a comprehensive assessment based on interviews, observation, records review, and quantitative measures. Considering normal changes in the life cycle, the variability of injury recovery patterns, and changing sources of stress, repeated assessments would be most beneficial in developing efficacious long-term treatment plans. Respecting cultural values, avoiding judgment, and showing respect for all family members will elicit the most valid and comprehensive conceptualization.

REFERENCES

1. Rosenthal, M, and Young, T: Effective family intervention after traumatic brain injury. J Head Trauma Rehabil 3:42, 1988.
2. Commission on Accreditation of Rehabilitation Facilities. 1996 Standards for Medical Rehabilitation. Author, Tucson, 1996.
3. Lezak, MD: Living with the characterologically altered brain injured patient. J Clin Psychiatry 39:111, 1978.
4. Lezak, MD: Psychological implications of traumatic brain damage for the patient's family. Rehabilitation Psychology 31:241, 1986.
5. Lezak, MD: Brain damage is a family affair. J Clin Exp Neuropsychol 10:111, 1987.
6. Brooks, DN: The head-injured family. J Clin Exp Neuropsychol 13:155, 1991.
7. Panting, A, and Merry, PH: The long term rehabilitation of severe head injuries with particular reference to the need for social and medical support for the patient's family. Rehabilitation (Stuttg) 38:33, 1972.
8. Thomsen, IV: The patient with severe head injury and his family. Scand J Rehabil Med 6:180, 1974.
9. Mauss-Clum, N, and Ryan, M: Brain injury and the family. Neurosurgical Nursing 13:165, 1981.
10. Allen, K, et al: Family burden following traumatic brain injury. Rehabilitation Psychology 39:29, 1994.
11. Kreutzer, J, Gervasio, A, and Camplair, P: Primary caregiver's psychological status and family functioning after traumatic brain injury. Brain Inj 8:197, 1994.
12. McKinlay, WW, Brooks, DN, and Bond, MR: The short term outcome of severe blunt head injury as reported by the relatives of the injured person. J Neurol Neurosurg Psychiatry 44:527, 1981.
13. Livingston, MG, Brooks, DN, and Bond, MR: Three months after severe head injury: Psychiatric and social impact on relatives. J Neurol Neurosurg Psychiatry 48:870, 1985.
14. Livingston, MG, Brooks, DN, and Bond, MR: Patient outcome in the year following severe head injury and relatives' psychiatric and social functioning. J Neurol Neurosurg Psychiatry 48:876, 1985.
15. Brooks, N, et al: The five year outcome of severe blunt head injury: A relative's view. J Neurol Neurosurg Psychiatry 49:764, 1986.
16. Brooks, N, et al: The effects of severe head injury on patient and relative within seven years of injury. J Head Trauma Rehabil 2:1, 1987.
17. Romano, MD: Family response to traumatic brain injury. Scand J Rehabil Med 6:1, 1974.
18. Zeigler, EA: Spouses of persons who are brain injured: Overlooked victims. Journal of Rehabilitation 1:50, 1987.
19. Oddy, M: Head injury and social adjustment. In Brooks, N, (ed): Closed Head Injury: Psychological, Social, and Family Consequences. Oxford University Press, Oxford, 1984, p 108.
20. Stern, JM, Sazbon, L, and Becker, E: Severe behavioral disturbance in families of patients with prolonged coma. Brain Inj 2:259, 1988.
21. DePompei, R, Zarski, JJ, and Hall, DE: Cognitive communication impairments: A family-focused viewpoint. J Head Trauma Rehabil 3:13, 1988.
22. Peters, LC, et al: Psychosocial sequelae of closed head injury: Effects on the marital relationship. Brain Inj 4:39, 1990.
23. Kozloff, R: Networks of social support and the outcome from severe head injury. J Head Trauma Rehabil 2:14, 1987.
24. Jacobs, HE: The Los Angeles Head Injury survey: Procedures and initial findings. Arch Phys Med Rehabil 69:425, 1988.
25. Hall, KH, et al: Family stressors in traumatic brain injury: A two year follow-up. Arch Phys Med Rehabil 75:876, 1994.
26. Lazarus, RS, and Folkman, S: Stress, Appraisal, and Coping. Springer, New York, 1984.
27. Willer, BS, et al: Problems and coping strategies of individuals with traumatic brain injury and their spouses. Arch Phys Med Rehabil 72:460, 1991.
28. Kosciulek, JF: Dimensions of family coping with head injury. Rehabilitation Counseling Bulletin 37:244, 1994.
29. Sander, AM, et al: Predictors of psychological health in caregivers of patients with closed head injury. Brain Inj 11:235, 1997.
30. Mathis, M: Personal needs of family members of critically ill patients with and without brain injury. Neurosurgical Nursing 16:36, 1984.
31. Campbell, C: Needs of relatives and helpfulness of support groups in severe head injury. Rehabilitation Nursing 13:320, 1988.
32. Engli, M, and Kirsivali-Farmer, K: Needs of family members of critically ill patients with and without acute brain injury. J Neurosci Nurs 25:78, 1993.
33. Kreutzer, JS, et al: A practical guide to family intervention following adult traumatic brain injury. In Kreutzer, JS, and Wehman, P (eds): Community Integration following Traumatic Brain Injury. Paul Brookes, Baltimore, 1990, p 249.
34. Serio, CD, Kreutzer, JS, and Witol, AD: Family needs after traumatic brain injury: A factor analytic study of the Family Needs Questionnaire. Brain Inj 11:1, 1997.
35. Kreutzer, J, Devany, C, and Keck, S: Family needs following brain injury: A quantitative analysis. J Head Trauma Rehabil 9:104, 1995.
36. Serio, CD, Kreutzer, JS, and Gervasio, AH: Predicting family needs after brain injury: Implications for intervention. J Head Trauma Rehabil 10:32, 1995.
37. Witol, AD, Sander, AM, and Kreutzer, JS: A longitudinal analysis of family needs following traumatic brain injury. NeuroRehabilitation 7:175, 1996.
38. Derogatis, LR, and Spencer, PM: The Brief Symptom Inventory. Clinical Psychometric Research, Baltimore, 1982.
39. Kreutzer, J, Gervasio, A, and Camplair, P: Patient correlates of caregiver's distress and family functioning after traumatic brain injury. Brain Inj 8:211, 1994.
40. Chwalisz, K: Perceived stress and caregiver burden after brain injury: A theoretical integration. Rehabilitation Psychology 37:189, 1992.
41. Graffi, S, and Mines, P: Stress and coping in caregivers of persons with traumatic head injuries. Journal of Applied Social Sciences 13:293, 1989.
42. Kay, T, Ezrachi, O, and Cavallo, M: Head Injury Family Interview: Problem Checklist of Significant Other Interview. New York University Medical Center, Department of Rehabilitation Medicine, Research and Training Center on Head Trauma and Stroke, New York, 1988.
43. Kay, T, et al: The Head Injury Family Interview: A clinical and research tool. J Head Trauma Rehabil 10:12, 1995.
44. Lawton, MP, et al: Measuring caregiver appraisal. J Gerontol 44:61, 1989.
45. Minuchin, S: Families and Family Therapy. Harvard University Press, Cambridge, 1974.
46. Epstein, N, Bishop, D, and Baldwin, L: The McMaster Family Assessment Device. Journal of Marital and Family Therapy 9:171, 1983.
47. Miller, IW, et al: The McMaster Family Assessment Device: Reliability and validity. Journal of Family and Marital Therapy 4:345, 1985.
48. Zarski, JJ, DePompei, R, and Zook, A: Traumatic head injury: Dimensions of family responsivity. J Head Trauma Rehabil 3:31, 1988.
49. Rivara, JB, et al: Predictors of family functioning one year following traumatic brain injury in children. Arch Phys Med Rehabil 73:899, 1992.

50. Rivara, JB, et al: Predictors of family functioning and change 3 years after traumatic brain injury in children. Arch Phys Med Rehabil 77:754, 1996.
51. Folkman, S, and Lazarus, RS: Manual for the Ways of Coping Questionnaire. Consulting Psychologists Press, Palo Alto, Calif, 1988.
52. Sarason, IG, et al: Assessing social support: The Social Support Questionnaire. J Pers Soc Psychol 44:127, 1983.
53. Cavallo, MM, Kay, T, and Ezrachi, O: Problems and changes after traumatic brain injury: Differing perceptions within and between families. Brain Inj 6:327, 1992.
54. Tarter, SB: Factors affecting adjustment of parents of head trauma victims. Archives of Clinical Neuropsychology 5:15, 1990.
55. Carver, CS, Scheier, MF, and Weintraub, JK: Assessing coping strategies: A theoretically based approach. J Pers Soc Psychol 2:267, 1989.
56. Wade, SL, et al: Childhood traumatic brain injury. Initial impact on the family. Journal of Learning Disabilities 29:652, 1996.
57. McCubbin, H, et al: CHIP—Coping Health Inventory for Parents: An assessment of parental coping patterns in the care of the chronically ill child. In McCubbin, H (ed): Family Stress, Coping, and Social Support. Springer, New York, 1979.
58. Rivara, JB, et al: Family functioning and children's academic performance and behavior problems in the year following traumatic brain injury. Arch Phys Med Rehabil 75:369, 1994.
59. Moos, R: Family Environment Scale (Form R). Consulting Psychologists Press, Palo Alto, Calif, 1974.
60. Olson, D, and Portner, J: Family adaptability and cohesion scales. In Filsinger, E (ed): Marriage and Family Assessment. Sage, Beverly Hills, Calif, 1983.
61. Mrazek, D: Family Global Assessment Scale (FGAS): Initial reliability and validity. In: Proceedings from the Thirty-Second Annual Meeting of the American Academy of Child Psychiatry. San Antonio, 1985.
62. Goldberg, DP: The Detection of Psychiatric Illness by Questionnaire. Oxford University Press, London, 1972.
63. Beck, AT, and Steer, RA: Beck Depression Inventory Manual. Psychological Corporation, New York, 1987.
64. Snaith, RP, Bridge, GWK, and Hamilton, M: The Leeds Scales for the self-assessment of anxiety and depression Journal of Psychiatry 128:156, 1976.
65. Hathaway, SR, and McKinley, JC: The Minnesota Multiphasic Personality Manual (Revised). Psychological Corporation, New York, 1951.

Treatment Approaches

MITCHELL ROSENTHAL, PHD

CHAPTER 13

Strategies to Enhance Mobility in Traumatic Brain Injured Patients

SARAH BLANTON, MPT,
LISA PORTER, MOT, OTR,
DONNA SMITH, PT,
and STEVEN L. WOLF, PHD, PT, FAPTA

This chapter reviews issues of mobility impairment among brain injured patients and avenues in which to treat these impairments. How professionals approach the problem of improving the motoric capability of this patient population largely depends on the patient's environment or facility placement. Dynamically changing health care systems dictate the need to address the circumstances under which the brain injured patient can be treated. By identifying the environment with a primary intent of promoting mobility, we can better establish the most effective strategies for treatment. The settings addressed here include acute inpatient rehabilitation, day treatment programs (outpatient rehabilitation), and community settings. Variables to consider when developing therapeutic approaches for these patients include the availability and need for interdisciplinary collaboration, appropriateness of goals, timing and degree of family involvement, and the resulting management and treatment under each of these circumstances. This chapter is divided into six sections: outcomes, goals and treatment, therapeutic environment, treatment efficacy, treatment considerations, and case studies.

The first step for the therapist in the assessment process is to determine the most appropriate goals. This process must take into account the premorbid history of the patient, the nature of the injury, any additional complications, and family involvement. Unfortunately, an additional factor often plays an important role in goal setting: insurance coverage. Length of stay—and thus realistic goals—is dictated by past decisions patients have made regarding health care coverage, long before the catastrophic injury has become a fact of life. The rehabilitation provider is forced to set the length of stay according to each patient's situation, including the extent of coverage. Consequently, goals must revolve around a functional level that is too often the bare minimum to get the patient home or to a less expensive facility. To accomplish these goals, family involvement and education are key factors, making the caregiver a vital member of the rehabilitation team.

To obtain these goals, a therapeutic environment is essential. This environment starts with the patient by considering positioning in the bed or chair, layout of the room, and scheduling of the therapeutic day. The general setting of the treatment environment includes the importance of the team approach. Therapists, physicians, and nurses must converge as a unit when dealing with this patient population. Often classes and groups are appropriate; at other times, a patient's limitations demand cotreatment by therapists for a more effective approach. Regardless of the choice, communication is the foundation for the most beneficial treatment.

With the therapeutic environment established, the treatment itself must be determined. Behavior and cognition issues, unique to this patient population, necessitate special strategies to accomplish any goals. Knowing the various Rancho levels of brain injury[1] and the best treatment approaches to most effectively handle each type of patient greatly increases the chances for successful outcomes. Determining the efficacy of different treatments, while understanding the theoretical basis behind the various "therapeutic tools," is becoming a greater professional obligation in light of the modern health care environment. Specific treatment approaches, such as Brunnstrom or Bobath techniques, are not explained in detail here; instead, references for further information are provided.

In summary, this chapter attempts to identify goals to improve mobility in the treatment of the brain injured individual, develop the therapeutic environment, and address treatment considerations and efficacy. Case histories are presented in a problem-solving format at the end of the chapter.

□ RECOVERY AND OUTCOMES

Early intervention is critical to maximize a person's recovery from a traumatic brain injury (TBI). Functional outcomes for the brain injury survivor can be improved through early onset of rehabilitation in the acute recovery stages.[2] Rehabilitation for a sufficiently stabilized patient, therefore, may begin in the intensive care unit (ICU). In some hospitals, a specialist consult is an automatic order for brain injury patients upon admission. The consult typically includes evaluations by physical and occupational therapists, speech-language pathologists, and a physiatrist.

Following a serious brain injury, most recovery seems to occur within the first 6 months, making revision of treatment plans and goals critical to ensure that rehabilitation time is efficiently used. For the purpose of this chapter, we define *outcome* as a measurable functional level directly related to spontaneous recovery and therapeutic intervention. Factors that influence recovery outcomes include age, site and size of the brain lesion, extent of diffuse injury, premorbid skills, behavior and intelligence, genetic inheritance, neural plasticity, nutritional history, environment, postmorbid emergency care, family involvement, rehabilitation and medical management, and available resources and support services.[3]

As with other central nervous system injuries, specific outcomes are difficult to predict. Among studies designed to discover methods for better predicting outcomes in the brain injury population, Swaine and Sullivan[4] documented detailed recovery profiles of motor function in TBI survivors. Their results suggest that a data base on the TBI recovery process could serve as a basis from which therapists could measure the effectiveness of treatment interventions and provide a framework for describing motor recovery.

□ DETERMINING GOALS AND THE COURSE OF MANAGEMENT

Following evaluation, the clinician targets the primary problems, based on the level of functioning. Of course, medical stability is the driving factor that sets the course for therapeutic intervention. Functional categories can be described as low, intermediate, and advanced levels. Furthermore, each category may be assigned to levels of the Rancho Los Amigos Cognitive Scale[1]: low = I–III, intermediate = IV–VI, and advanced = VII–VIII. These levels are elaborated in Table 13–1.

A wide array of impairments and potential complications may overwhelm therapists as they form a treatment plan. The therapist must use the identified problem areas and strengths of the patient to establish a functional baseline to guide treatment approaches toward attainable goals, much as would be done for patients with other diagnoses. This strategy is effectively achieved with an ongoing collaboration among all rehabilitation team members, including the physiatrist, speech pathologist, occupational and physical therapists, neuropsychologist, dietitian, therapeutic recreation specialist, respiratory therapist, nurse, case manager, family or caregiver, and the patient. Not all health care settings have access to each of these professionals, and family support systems may vary considerably. Regardless of the setting, a concentrated effort across disciplines must be maintained to provide continuity and allow a transfer of skills.

Traditional techniques and skills may be less effective than previously thought, or they may be too time-consuming to implement consistently. For example, cryotherapy to reduce spasticity in a lower extremity prior to gait training may not yield sufficient results to warrant continuation or simply may not be an option because of limited treatment time. Thus, constant monitoring and revision of the patient's functional status, response to treatment, progress, and goals are necessary to assure treatment efficiency. In addition, overemphasis on one specific intervention may hinder selec-

> **TABLE 13–1. Rancho Los Amigos Levels of Cognitive Function Scale**
>
> **I. No Response:** *Unresponsive to any stimulus.*
>
> **II. Generalized Response:** *Limited, inconsistent, nonpurposeful responses, often to pain only.*
>
> **III. Localized Response:** *Purposeful responses; may follow simple commands; may focus on presented object.*
>
> **IV. Confused, Agitated:** *Heightened state of activity; confusion, disorientation; aggressive behavior; unable to do self-care; unaware of present events; agitation appears related to internal confusion.*
>
> **V. Confused, Inappropriate:** *Nonagitated; appears alert; responds to commands; distractable; does not concentrate on task; agitated responses to external stimuli; verbally inappropriate; does not learn new information.*
>
> **VI. Confused, Appropriate:** *Goal directed behavior, needs cuing, can relearn old skills as activities of daily living (ADLs); serious memory problems; some awareness of self and others.*
>
> **VII. Automatic, Appropriate:** *Appears appropriate, oriented; frequently robot-like in daily routine; minimal or absent confusion; shallow recall; increased awareness of self, interaction in environment; lacks insight into condition; decreased judgment and problem-solving; lacks realistic planning for future.*
>
> **VIII. Purposeful, Appropriate:** *Alert, oriented; recalls and integrates past events; learns new activities and can continue without supervision; independent in home and living skills; capable of driving; defects in stress tolerance, judgment, abstract reasoning persist; many function at reduced levels in society.*
>
> **Source:** Prepared by Professional Staff Association, Rancho Los Amigos Hospital, Inc., Downey, California, 1979.

many difficult decisions. What is the best way to evaluate the patient? How much focus should be placed on assessing functional ability versus the underlying problems causing the dysfunction? How should the problems be prioritized?[5] To begin effectively assessing a patient, the clinician needs a framework to logically organize the evaluation and treatment. Shumway-Cook and Woollacott[5] suggest a "model of disablement" as a framework for structuring the effects of disease in the individual. They suggest a hierarchical system for categorizing patient problems that can be used as a framework for organizing and interpreting assessment data and for developing a comprehensive plan for treatment. Figure 13–1 illustrates one example of a model of disablement, developed by Schenkman and Butler.[6] Problems are categorized according to three levels of analysis: pathology, impairments, and functional limitations. *Pathology* refers to description of the injury process or disease at an organ level (e.g., brain injury). *Impairments* refer to problems within specific organs or systems that limit the patient's ability to function normally (e.g., cognition, decreased range of motion). Impairments are further divided into those that are a direct effect of the pathophysiology (e.g., weakness, spasticity), those that are an indirect effect (e.g., loss of joint mobility), and those that are a composite of both direct and indirect impairments. *Disability* refers to functional restrictions, such as problems with gait or activities of daily living (ADLs).

With this model of disablement, the clinician can identify and document the effects of the patient's brain injury in terms of impairment and disability, thereby allowing a clearer picture of the problems. Treatment can then focus on the most appropriate issues with knowledge of which impairments are primary or secondary to the pathology, if those impairments can be changed, and, if so, how they can be altered to improve function.

tion of creative alternatives that may better serve an individual patient's needs.

If outcomes are overestimated, then the treatment plan may appear to have failed; therefore, clinicians must keep a realistic perspective that is guided by the assessment. Less experienced clinicians may need to consult therapists who have experience with brain injury rehabilitation so that functional prognosis is reasonable.

Assessment

MODEL OF DISABLEMENT

Undertaking the analysis of movement dysfunction in the individual with TBI involves

TASK-ORIENTED ASSESSMENT

To specifically approach functional assessment, Shumway-Cook and Woollacott[5] present a task-oriented assessment that evaluates motor behavior at three levels: objective measurements of functional skills, a description of the strategies used to accomplish functional skills, and quantification of the underlying sensory, motor, and cognitive impairments that constrain performance.

The clinician can choose from a long list of tests to obtain information about the patient at different levels. This idea is represented in Figure 13–2 and is modified from the work of Shumway-Cook and Woollacott,[5] which uses a

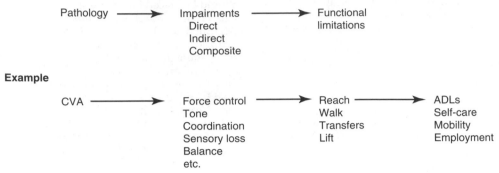

FIGURE 13–1. Model of disablement, developed by Margaret Schenkman,[6] illustrates a hierarchical system for categorizing patient problems. Problems are categorized according to three levels of analysis: pathology, impairments, and functional limitations. (Adapted from Shumway-Cook, A, and Woollacott, M: A conceptual framework for clinical practice. In Motor Control: Theory and Practical Applications. Williams & Wilkins, Baltimore, 1995, p 103, with permission.)

task-oriented model to show three levels of testing, their interrelationships, and the types of tests that could be used within each of the levels.

Performance-based functional measures are used to determine the patient's level of independence in daily life activities and are the foundation to develop functional goals during rehabilitation. These measures are the basis by which therapy is justified to the patient, the patient's family, and third-party insurers. One of the most widely used in inpatient rehabilitation is the Functional Independence Measure[7] (FIM). This test includes ADLs, such as bathing, dressing, toileting, feeding, and continence, as well as cognition and mobility. Other ADL tests are the Katz Index[8] and the Barthel Index.[9] Instrumental Activities of Daily Living (IADL) is an assessment tool that takes ADLs a step further and assesses how the individual interacts with the environment. These tests include the Scale for Instrumental Activities of Daily Living (SIADL)[10] and may measure traveling capability, telephone usage, meal preparation, housework, and handling money.

Some functional assessment measures are specific to a particular task to provide the clinician with a more detailed picture of an individual's abilities that will be directly involved in movement retraining. For example, balance can be specifically evaluated by the Tinetti Test of Balance and Mobility[11] or the Ataxia Test Battery.[12]

Strategy assessment is the second level of motor control in the task-oriented evaluation model. Shumway-Cook and Woollacott[5] define *strategy* as "not limited to the evaluation of the movement pattern used to accomplish a task, but includes how the person organizes sensory and perceptual information necessary to performing a task and how this changes under various conditions." Strategy is the most important determinant of level of performance. For example, a poor or inefficient strategy may accomplish an easy task but fail to meet the demands of a more complex task. If a patient is using circumduction to achieve adequate swing through in gait, this strategy may accomplish the task of walking on level surfaces. For ambulating on a more demanding steep incline, however, this strategy is insufficient to achieve the goal of clearing the foot in swing phase, and the patient's performance in the task is poor.

The third level of assessment in the task-oriented model is impairment assessment. This level identifies impairments that might affect functional movement skills. These tests include evaluations of strength, range of motion, coordination, muscle tone, reflexes, sensation, and cognition.

Thus, when using this task-oriented approach, the clinician attempts to evaluate (1) the patient's performance of the functional task; (2) the strategies used to perform the tasks and the adaptability of these strategies to changing tasks; (3) the motor, sensory, and cognitive impairments that limit the performance of the task; (4) changes in impairments affected through intervention; and (5) changes in performance through intervention, despite the impairments.

Establishing Therapeutic Goals

Function refers to a deliberate action or activity needed for self-care and mobility. On initiating a therapy service, the clinician evaluates the TBI

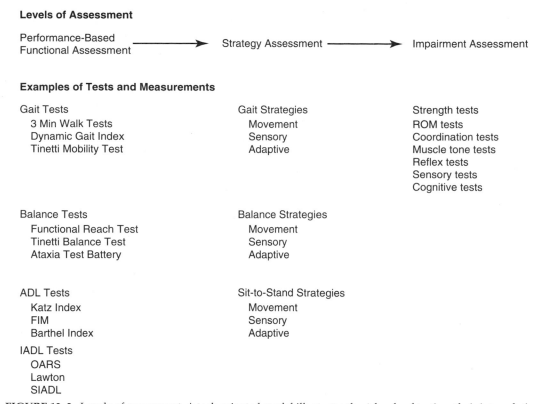

FIGURE 13–2. Levels of assessment. A task-oriented model illustrates three levels of testing, their interrelationships, and the types of tests that could be used within each of the levels. (Adapted from Shumway-Cook, A, and Woollacott, M: A conceptual framework for clinical practice. In Motor Control: Theory and Practical Applications. Williams & Wilkins, Baltimore, 1995, p 108, with permission.)

patient and then establishes a set of relevant functional goals. Timmons et al.[13] have assessed functional change in a group of survivors of severe brain injury to identify variables that affect progress. Results indicated that patients rated as level II on the Ranchos Los Amigos Levels of Cognitive Function Scale (RLCOFS; see Table 13–1) demonstrated fewer functional gains than those rated level III at admission.

The goals should describe an objective level of physical abilities that mark a progression toward independence and safety in mobility and self-care activities. When designing a treatment plan to focus on recovery of motor integrity, one must consider more than the physical disabilities and medical complications. Cognitive, emotional, behavioral, communicative, and family issues must also be assessed because they play an integral role in the patient's ability to tolerate and benefit from therapy. Another consideration in establishing therapeutic goals is the challenge to provide therapeutic services under significant financial and staffing constraints. The rehabilitation team must find a way to match their values and treatment priorities with those of the third-party payer. Frequently, health care providers have to justify that their chosen treatment modalities will lead to an outcome in a cost-effective manner.[14] Often, the family, patient, funding source, and rehabilitation facility must establish a regular dialogue to identify a small set of prioritized goals that are the most important for the patient's transition back home.[15]

In the early stages of recovery, goals focus on areas such as sensory stimulation, basic self-care activities, bed mobility, sitting tolerance, assisted transfers, pregait, and prevention of secondary complications. *Sensory stimulation,* discussed later in the chapter, might be addressed with goals that focus on eliciting visual tracking of family photographs and head turning toward a familiar sound, such as the patient's favorite song or a familiar voice. *Bed mobility* skills include rolling side to side, scooting, and transitioning between lying down and sitting up in bed. Increased independence in these purposeful activities enables patients to reposition themselves, assist in dressing and hygiene, perform exercises, and develop strength and motor control for more difficult mobility tasks. *Self-care* activities, including bathing, dental hygiene, feeding, grooming, and dressing, should be promptly incorporated into the treatment program. Each task, broken into components, may yield motoric success, such as raising hand to mouth while grasping a toothbrush. A patient's *sitting tolerance* is affected by head control, strength (especially of the trunk), endurance, range of motion, balance, and the autonomic nervous system's ability to regulate vital functions such as heart rate, blood pressure, and respiration. For a low-level treatment in a cotreatment session, the occupational and physical therapists might assist the patient in sitting on the edge of the bed, reaching for clothing, and participating in dressing. *Transferring* is a multi-task activity that mobilizes the patient to and from bed, a wheelchair, the toilet, an exercise mat, a car, a pool, and the floor. Assistive devices such as sliding boards, handrails, armrests, and trapezes enhance independence and safety. In planning for discharge from the inpatient setting, for example, the patient's caregiver may require a second helper to transfer the patient without assistive equipment but might be independent when using a sliding board. *Pregait* activities prepare the patient for gait training. The therapist facilitates neuromuscular activity, motor control, weight shifting, and balance reactions. Assistive equipment may include parallel bars, a standing table or frame, electrical stimulation units, and orthotics. As the patient's ambulatory status progresses, therapists must identify equipment needs based on safety issues, gait efficiency, the patient's endurance level, and special circumstances such as orthopedic restrictions (e.g., weight-bearing status, range of motion), visual disturbances, and cognitive deficits. For instance, a patient's gait stability may potentially improve with a cane; however, cognitive deficits, such as poor thought sequencing or limited attention span, may preclude effective use of the cane. In addition, orthotics provide stability and protection to weakened joints. Prefabricated braces may suffice, although customized equipment is often indicated because of abnormal range of motion, wearing comfort, skin integrity, abnormal tone, and substantial muscle weakness.

The degree of cognitive and motoric return dictates goal setting for gait progression, endurance, higher level balance, and safe mobility in the home and community. Considering that the leading cause of death and disability for children and adults under the age of 45 is traumatic brain injury,[16] the rehabilitation team should focus efforts toward the patient's community reentry and employability; however, third-party payers may not agree with this assumption.

In addition, shorter lengths of stay are prompting changes in how goals are established at various levels of recovery. With shortened rehabilitation stays more common because of insurance policy limitations, particularly among managed care organizations, clinicians must often downgrade initial goals to accommodate realistic treatment time. For example, achievement of independence in transfers may not be an appropriate goal for a patient in the inpatient rehabilitation setting. Rather, the goal may be a minimally assisted transfer from the wheelchair to the commode that adequately prepares the patient and caregiver for discharge to the home setting, at which time the patient may receive outpatient therapy or home health therapy services. Factors that influence the transition between therapy settings include (1) clinicians' understanding of the various levels of treatment settings and how to facilitate a smooth, timely transition along the rehabilitation continuum; (2) the patient's medical stability; and (3) the caregiver's preparedness, willingness, and ability to care for the patient. The patient's return to home allows the patient, family, and therapists to further identify functional mobility goals relative to the patient's living environment.

Prevention of Secondary Complications

Each treatment team member is responsible for carefully monitoring patients during therapy. Secondary complications may arise and subsequently slow motoric performance and impede functional progress. Complications may occur concomitantly with the brain injury or anywhere along the continuum of care, including during emergency treatment and during prolonged bedrest and inactivity. Clinicians must address these potential complications proactively to prevent compromising the patient's progress towards medical stability and functional gains, avoid the loss of valuable rehabilitation time, and conserve financial resources.

Monitoring of skin integrity should begin immediately and requires team involvement and patient and family education. Loss of sensation, poor mobility, and impaired cognition and communication inhibit the patient's ability to recognize and respond to prolonged pressure and discomfort. Frequently scheduled changes in bed and wheelchair positioning are crucial to allow adequate circulation and weight distribution. A change in position (e.g., from left to right supported sidelying and angle of recline in wheelchair) every 2 hours is usually sufficient, but this time frame must be adjusted on an individual basis considering skin, circulatory, and respiratory integrity and bony prominences. Careful selection and execution of transfers can avoid skin shearing, frictional forces, bruising, and abrasions. Splints and braces also require consistent attention to possible sites of pressure and rubbing.

In the ICU, an intracranial pressure (ICP) monitor allows the therapist to discern how specific treatment techniques affect the ICP. An increase in intracranial pressure may be indicated by increased lethargy, a decrease in motor performance, nausea and vomiting, visual losses, and seizures. This situation may cause further brain damage and is potentially life-threatening; therefore, the physician should be notified of the symptoms so that the proper measures can be taken if excessive ICP is, in fact, present. The therapist may recommend that the physician provide specific guidelines for when to hold therapy.

Medical management typically includes seizure prophylaxis. Seizures may be preceded by an aura in which the patient experiences specific sensations. The patient may appear to be in a trancelike state with a temporary disruption of the current activity; this behavior may indicate a petit mal seizure. Phenytoin (Dilantin), phenobarbital, and carbamazepine (Tegretol) are commonly used anticonvulsant medications. Therapists should be attuned to recognizing preictal and seizure activity and the possible side effects, including lethargy and ataxia, of prophylactic medications.

Joint contractures are a threat to functional progress and personal hygiene. If movement of the joints is not preserved, additional complications may result. For example, the patient will have difficulty standing with fixed ankle plantarflexion and increased tone of the finger flexors may lead to a locked fist, making hygiene difficult. Passive and active range of motion throughout the body including the neck and trunk, positioning, weight bearing, and serial casting are approaches to preserve and restore normal range of motion. Serial casting is often indicated when functional positioning of a joint cannot be achieved after immobility or severe spasticity. A series of casts can be applied to progressively increase joint range of motion and thus prevent deformity. Built-in footplates are used to allow weight bearing and gait training as well as to effectively stabilize the foot and toes for enhanced tone inhibition. Once the desired or maximal joint range of motion is achieved, the final cast may be converted to a splint of anterior and posterior halves. Physician intervention may include nerve blocks or oral antispasticity medications.

Heterotopic ossification is yet another complication that can inhibit rehabilitation of the TBI patient (see Chapter 4). Its onset is insidious and treatment is difficult; thus, prevention is of great importance. Therapists should avoid forceful range of motion to prevent physical trauma. Poor transfer techniques and falls may also lead to joint trauma. Range of motion exercises, especially active motion if the patient is able to assist, proper joint positioning, including use of splints, and progressive stretching are approaches to prevent heterotopic ossification.

Due to the nature of the trauma, TBI survivors often incur multiple musculoskeletal injuries including fractures. Some researchers have demonstrated that early stabilization of fractures reduces morbidity and mortality of multitrauma survivors, who may otherwise succumb to acute respiratory distress syndrome or late sepsis.[17] Early fracture management has become more common for patients with coexisting brain and musculoskeletal injuries. Fracture stabilization increases the patient's ability to participate in therapeutic activities, such as gait training; however, stabilization may have to be delayed because of patient agitation or risk of medical instability.

Stages of Management

As stated earlier, three functional stages can be assigned to specific levels of the Rancho Los Amigos Levels of Cognitive Function Scale. Messa[18] identifies these stages with treatment goals and interventions that, often, most appropriately address the patient's needs at various levels of recovery.

STAGE I: LOW-LEVEL MANAGEMENT

For the patient in the low-functioning category of cognitive levels I to III (Table 13–2),[19] treatment is limited by a severely impaired cognitive profile. Patient responsiveness to stimuli ranges from unresponsive to a localized response. Treatment areas emphasized at this level are sensory stimulation, cognitive arousal, basic communication, and prevention and management of specific physical impairments. Treatment focuses more on the physical impairments than on retraining for functional activities because of the patient's lack of or minimal response to meaningful tasks.

Prolonged bedrest and impaired ability to actively move body parts lead to rapid deconditioning. Patient mobilization, even for those requiring ventilators, may be accomplished through supportive sitting on the edge of the bed or in a wheelchair or recliner that offers good positioning. Time spent out of bed should

TABLE 13–2. Early Management for Patients with Rancho Levels I to III

Treatment Category	Goals	Treatment
Sensory stimulation	Arouse the senses and elicit movement.	Multisensory stimulation (e.g., smelling favorite foods, hearing familiar music, touching familiar objects and various textures). Avoid sensory overload.
Cognitive	Cognitive awareness/orientation	Identify what you are doing. Tell who, what, when, where.
Normalize tone	Increase muscle tone. Decrease dominate flexor/extensor tone. Activate righting and equilibrium reactions.	Rotation of trunk, limbs; rolling; upright position. Neuromusculature facilitation. Weight bearing. Vestibular stimuli: rapid and intermittent or slow and rhythmical. Position in neutral alignment.
Functional range of motion	Maintain range. Prevent contractures.	Ranging in proprioceptive neuromuscular facilitation patterns and straight planes. Rolling, sitting, splinting, serial casting, positioning devices. Tilt table.
Functional mobility	Improve bed mobility. Increase control and righting reactions of head and trunk.	Sitting. Rhythmic initiation. Orientation to midline. Elicit balance reactions.
Stability	Facilitate cocontraction and trunk control.	Joint compression through head and shoulders. Weight bearing. Tilt table.
Endurance	Gradually increase treatment tolerance and level of participation in therapies.	Frequent sitting.
Prefeeding	Normalize tone; develop head control; desensitize; removal of nasogastric tube.	Upright sitting; anterior pelvic tilt; neck cocontraction; oral stimulation.
Family education	Early family involvement and support.	Interview family to learn patient's premorbid interests; instruct in positioning, simple ROM, and sensory stimulation. Involve in goal setting.
Respiratory	Prevent respiratory complications. Treat current problems.	Frequent position changes; early sitting; trunk mobility.
Skin care	Prevent skin breakdown.	Frequent position changes; positioning; cushions; close monitoring; careful transfers.

Source: Modified with the permission of Sally Saadeh, PT, CCM, unpublished material, 1993.

gradually be increased as tolerated by the patient. The capacity to sit for longer periods enables the individual to engage in more complex tasks, such as early feeding and balance activities. Placing instructions and/or pictures in the patient's room may help other staff members monitor and adjust the patient for a proper sitting position or posture and cue them to the patient's endurance level.

Neuromuscular facilitation, weight-bearing positions (e.g., tilt table), range of motion exercises, vestibular stimulation, and joint positioning devices are examples of treatment tools and techniques that may enhance motoric return, tone management, body awareness, proximal stability, and basic mobility (e.g., rolling in bed).

The development of physical and cognitive abilities, such as an increased response to the environment, equilibrium and balance reactions, and head and trunk control, are stepping stones to achieve functional mobility. The therapist must connect these physical abilities to the performance of specific mobility skills so that the patient, family, and third-party payer can understand the treatment rationale.

STAGE II: INTERMEDIATE MANAGEMENT

At this stage of recovery, patients function at cognitive levels of IV to VI (Table 13–3).[19] Responsiveness ranges from confused and agitated to confused and appropriate. Physical performance and functional skills are emphasized more, partly because of the patient's increased state of arousal and ability to tolerate more complicated physical tasks. The patient can partici-pate actively in neuromuscular reeducation and mobility training that may include activities such as strengthening exercises, wheelchair propulsion, gait training with an assistive device, active-assisted transfers, and neurodevel-opmental positions (e.g., quadruped, kneeling). Neurodevelopmental sequencing is most effec-tive if implemented with functional considera-tions rather than the traditional assumption of an absolutely normal progression. For instance, the

---

TABLE 13–3. Intermediate Management for Patients with Rancho Levels of IV through VI

Treatment Category	Goals	Treatment
Sensory stimulation	Facilitate appropriate responses to stimuli. Enhance cognitive devel-opment.	Identify and eliminate stimuli that cause agitation. Provide calm stimuli if agitated, rapid stimuli if lethargic. Minimize excessive environmental stimuli.
Cognitive	Increase appropriate and self-initi-ated behavior.	Frequent orientation to person, place, and time. Provide struc-ture, consistency in behavior management. Avoid overex-plaining tasks. Provide opportu-nities for success.
Normalize tone	Break up patterned responses. In-crease righting and equilibrium reactions.	Neuromuscular facilitation. Weight bearing. Inhibitory posi-tioning.
Functional range of motion	Prevent contractures and maintain range of motion. Monitor for in-flammation and heterotopic ossi-fication.	Splinting. Serial casting. Passive and active range of motion. Heat application. Stretching and strengthening exercises.
Functional mobility	Enhance automatic activities. In-crease emphasis on skills training. Further assess need for assistive devices.	Developmental sequences. Seg-mental trunk activities. Transfer and gait training. Self-propul-sion in wheelchair.
Stability	Midline stability. Cocontraction and weightshifting in upright posi-tion. Enhance balance reactions in sitting and standing.	Weight bearing and shifting activi-ties. Facilitate postural control against gravity.
Endurance	Increase toleration of activities.	Increase time out of bed. Use of arm and leg ergometers.
Prefeeding	Improve posture and oral control.	Elongation of neck extensors. Posi-tioning to normalize tone. Touch or ice to lips. Mobilization of jaw as needed.
Family education	Encourage appropriate family in-volvement with implementing treatment plan.	Teach family members how to safely and therapeutically assist with bed mobility, dressing and self-care, transfers and walking as appropriate.
Respiration	Increase respiratory capacity.	Trunk mobility. Strengthen respi-ratory muscles. Breathing exer-cises.
Skin care	Prevent skin breakdown.	Position changes. Care with trans-fers and use of splints and braces.

Source: Modified with permission from Sally Saadeh, PT, CCM, unpublished material, 1993.

significance of transitioning from the quadruped to half-kneeling position is evident in teaching a patient how to arise from the floor after playing with grandchildren, doing exercises, or falling. Another benefit to maintaining these positions is the transfer of balance and strength training to standing and walking performance. Tailoring the treatment plan to include the patient's premorbid interests and hobbies may elicit cooperation and motivation that ultimately improve functional outcomes.

STAGE III: ADVANCED MANAGEMENT

Those patients functioning at a higher cognitive level are classified on the Rancho scale as VII to VIII (Table 13–4). Their response levels range from automatic and appropriate behavior to purposeful and appropriate. These patients demonstrate increased self-awareness and apply themselves to their environment with a heightened sense of meaning and understanding. Functional tasks should be the primary emphasis at this stage. Complex cognitive and physical activities can be integrated with treatment goals that direct the patient toward independence and safety for ADLs, community mobility, work or school reentry, and a home exercise program.

The quality of movement in performing functional tasks may be fine-tuned at this point, providing that the third-party payer supports continued therapy for this purpose. Enhanced movement quality may decrease gait deviations that could lead to future orthopedic problems, the risk of falls, overuse syndromes, the

---

TABLE 13–4. Advanced Management for Patients with Rancho Levels of VII and VIII

Treatment Category	Goals	Treatment
Sensory stimulation	Develop strategies to cope with abnormal responses to environmental stimuli.	Increase complexity of stimulation.
Cognitive	Encourage self-initiated activities and responsibility, including home and community-based skills.	Increase complexity of directions. Increase complexity of activities of daily living training. Activities that require initiation, prolonged attention, concentration, and sequencing.
Normalize tone	Increase isolated movement. Improve speed, timing, and coordination of functional movement.	Higher-level developmental sequences. Frenkel's exercises. Neuromuscular facilitation with functional integration.
Functional range of motion	Maintain range of motion. Increase function within ROM limitations. Independence with stretching exercises.	Teach functional self-stretching activities.
Functional mobility	Independence in motor skills related to activities of daily living, mobility, and work.	Advanced wheelchair and gait mobility. Perceptual motor training. Community barrier training. Higher-level balance training.
Stability	Emphasize postural symmetry. Muscular strength to allow heightened functional level.	Rhythmic stabilization. Closed-chain activities and strengthening exercises.
Endurance	Increase tolerance of community mobility and return to school or work as appropriate.	Arm ergometer. Bicycle and treadmill. Aerobic conditioning activities. Work-specific activities. Community outings.
Family education	Compliance with treatment recommendations upon discharge.	Review home exercise program and safety considerations. Home visits.
Skin care	Patient independence with self-monitoring.	Review areas of concern and reasons for monitoring.

Source: Modified with permission from Sally Saadeh, PT, CCM, unpublished material, 1993.

need for orthotic and assistive devices, and patient discomfort and hesitancy to perform physical activities.

Choosing a Treatment Strategy

One of the challenging aspects of developing an effective treatment plan with the brain injured individual is choosing an activity that fits the skill and cognitive level of the patient. In a study by Mills,[20] specific physical therapy treatments tolerated by traumatically brain injured patients in an acute rehabilitation hospital were documented as they related to the patient's cognitive ability. Twenty-one patients were evaluated and treated from admission to discharge, with each receiving intensive physical, occupational, and speech therapy. Table 13–5 describes the various categories of physical therapy treatments. From initial evaluation to discharge, participation in therapy and cognitive status, evaluated by the Rancho Los Amigos cognitive levels, were rated every 2 weeks. The treatment by the physical therapist was considered to be tolerated by the patient if no agitation was noticed or if the patient participated in the activity more than 5 minutes. At each cognitive level, the percentage of patients tolerating a treatment was calculated. As ex-

pected, the patients at Rancho levels III and IV tolerated significantly fewer types of treatments in physical therapy than cognitive levels V through VIII. At levels III and IV, the most frequently tolerated activities included the tilt table and assisted ambulation. At level 5, wheelchair propulsion and ambulation were tolerated the most frequently and for levels 6 and 7, mat exercises and ambulation were best tolerated. The lower-level patients, limited by poor attention span and difficulty following commands, were unable to participate in traditional treatment programs. Consequently, activities tolerated best were geared to function and preventing deconditioning or secondary impairments. More complicated sessions could occur once the patient was able to attend to the environment and participate well if the environment was structured, controlled, and quiet. At levels VI through VII, patients could attend to activities requiring more selective attention, cooperation, sequencing, and motivation. This study supports the concept that the types of treatments tolerated by people with TBI during their acute rehabilitation stage of recovery appeared to be related to their cognitive abilities. Intuitively, identifying a patient's cognitive abilities in therapy can help in the effort to shape motoric performance. Thus, by understanding the cognitive limitations as well as the

---

TABLE 13–5. Categories of Physical Therapy Treatments

Activity	Definition
Mat activities:	*exercises for isolated movements with or without weights and mat Bobath exercises for extremities.*
Range of motion:	*passive or active range of motion of any involved joints.*
Tilt table:	*the patient tolerates being strapped on the tilt table and raised to physiological tolerance.*
Propelling wheelchair:	*the patient follows instructions on how to propel a wheelchair or participates in propelling a wheelchair for exercise.*
Ambulation:	*encompasses walking the patient. The patient may require assistance.*
Gait:	*all types of gait training with the patient.*
Stair climbing:	*all types of stair-climbing activities.*
Developmental activities:	*developmental mat activities such as rolling, rising to prone on elbows, side sitting, quadruped, kneeling, half kneeling, and standing. The patients may weight shift in these positions or participate in rhythmic stabilization activities.*
Advanced ambulation activities:	*activities such as walking backward, walking a straight line, balancing on one foot, walking on heels or toes, jogging, running, hopping, skipping, and jumping.*
Throwing a ball:	*playing catch with either a soft, round ball or football.*
Lower extremity isokinetic machine:	*exercising the patient on the Kinetron.**

*Cybex Isokinetic System, Cybex, Division of Lumex, Inc., NY.
Source: Modified from Mills, V: Physical therapy and cognitive impairment in traumatically head injured patients: A clinical report. Neurology Report 13:51, 1989.

physical limitations, the clinician can achieve greater results with each patient.

□ THERAPEUTIC ENVIRONMENT

The therapeutic environment involves all aspects of the patient's surroundings. Physical environment is only one small part of the whole picture. Patients have different levels of tolerance for stimulation, for understanding demands placed on them, or for understanding goals set by their family or therapist. A patient's relationship with the therapist, family involvement, and types of treatment or rehabilitation settings are integral parts of each patient's therapeutic environment.

The treatment environment is an important consideration for any patient population but especially for the brain injury population. Because of advances in medical technology, patients are beginning the rehabilitation process at an earlier stage.[18] As noted later, for patients at lower classification levels, the physical and environmental conditions play a major role in rehabilitation and must be considered during treatment.

Patient Involvement with the Environment

At a Rancho level II or III (see Table 13–1), a patient has little or no interaction with the environment. For example, a patient may have only a generalized response to pain or auditory stimulation. A patient at this level probably has a low tolerance for treatment.[18] For this reason, treatment sessions should not exceed 15 minutes. The environment should be structured to maximize involvement, the patient should have a schedule of up times to be positioned in the wheelchair, and the room should be set up to encourage interaction, with the capacity to decrease stimulation as necessary. Maximizing involvement does not mean overstimulating the patient. Routine activities, such as bathing, feeding, and dispersing medications, can cause overstimulation and should be considered in outlining the patient's day. Environment is important not only to physical and occupational therapists but also to the entire treatment team plan.

At levels IV through VI, the patient's environment must still be an integral part of the treatment plan. Often a patient at a higher level physically has attentional or behavioral deficits. The family and team should be made aware of the goals and treatment approaches used by speech and occupational therapy to address cognitive and behavioral goals. Focusing on mobility and goals may be difficult for patients who have attention or behavioral deficits. This issue must be addressed by the family and the team before specific goals in strengthening or facilitation can be met. Examples include 10- to 15-minute treatment sessions, simple one-step commands, and a room without distractions. Televisions and radios should be turned off and visitors asked to leave during therapy sessions.

Social Environment

Treatment environment includes not only the physical setting but also the social and emotional environment. This environment can include the therapeutic relationship and the motivation level that patients feel to participate in therapies to reach their optimal level of function. Patients may also feel more motivated to participate in therapies if they are involved in goal setting. Any activity is more motivating if it is interesting and individualized to the person asked to perform the task. Collaboration between patient and therapist can increase patients' participation and their understanding of certain tasks. This approach can be especially important with a patient who has behavioral issues, is refusing therapies, or is unmotivated to take part in treatment sessions.

Behavior and cognition are important for the patient with mobility problems. To learn new information, a patient must retain what the therapist is trying to teach. For instance, a patient whose goal is to move independently from supine to sitting may demonstrate the task perfectly while on the mat. The therapist may be giving verbal, tactile, or visual cues and thus providing feedback to the patient during the task. The same patient may be unable to come from supine to sit in bed without assistance. In this case, the patient has been unable to generalize from one context to the next, which may be attributed to behavioral or cognitive deficits that must be addressed before or in conjunction with mobility training.[21] Patients who cannot generalize a task from the treatment setting to their own environment must take steps toward the goal. For example, increasing attention must be addressed prior to continued mobility training.

Higher-level patients must be motivated to participate in therapies and also to learn. The therapist must make the rehabilitation setting a positive and nonstressful environment. The therapist can use the environment to address cognition by adjusting the demands placed on the patient. Early in the recovery stage, patients may be overwhelmed by a crowded gym and need to be treated in a quiet area. This quiet environment may be especially important for new activities. As the level of attention increases, patients may tolerate a higher level of stimuli until they can work in an environment more similar to a home or community setting.[21] A patient functioning at low levels, both physically and cognitively, needs decreased stimulation, simple one-step commands, and repetition. Treatment at this level may include sitting balance or mat exercises. Higher-level patients may benefit by increasing both physical and cognitive challenges, for example, community mobility and map reading.

Transportation Equipment

The wheelchair, commercial vehicle, or bed can be an integral part of a patient's environment. Many patients spend most of their day in a wheelchair; therefore, early in the treatment process, positioning should be a primary goal with low-level patients. Proper positioning in both the bed and the wheelchair can diminish undesirable postures in the spastic or hypotonic patient. It may involve reflex inhibiting postures, upper extremity positioning, attention to skin integrity, use of casts or splints, and turning schedules in bed. Contractures can be more effectively prevented through a good positioning or seating program than strictly through range of motion exercises.[22]

Proper positioning inhibits undesirable tonic reflex influences and provides prolonged muscle stretch, which passive range of motion does not accomplish.[23] A good seating system also focuses on trunk stability, which, in turn, promotes good function of the extremities. Figure 13–3 illustrates proper positioning in a wheelchair with a patient who exhibits increased tone and spasticity and impaired trunk control and balance. This system promotes the patient's interaction with the environment and provides her with stability for functional activities.

When designing a seating system, the clinician should consider the changing needs of a TBI patient. Adjustable back angles accommodate hamstring length and decreased sitting balance. Adjustable seat height increases the potential for independent propulsion of the wheelchair. Seat widths should match premorbid weight, as weight gain is common after discharge to the home setting.[24] Headrests can be customized to accommodate different levels of head control as well as upper extremity supports to increase functional use and decrease deformities.

Durability should be considered for increased activity level by younger patients, agitated patients, ataxic patients, or those patients

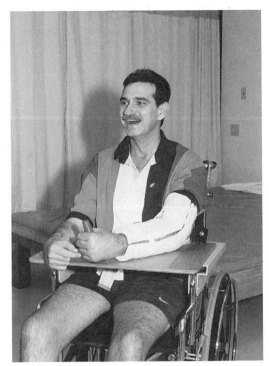

FIGURE 13–3. Proper positioning in the wheelchair can improve a patient's interaction with his environment, decrease undesirable positioning, and improve trunk stability to facilitate upper extremity function. (Photo courtesy of Rob Stanborough, SPT.)

with poor safety awareness. Seating equipment should control midline positioning to optimize proximal stabilization and distal function for either manual or power chairs.

The Environmental Surround

Sensory stimulation may include any of the five senses addressed in specific treatment sessions and/or the environmental state developed in the room. Stimulation provided by therapists and family is a significant component of the rehabilitation process for the low-level TBI patient. However, precautions are necessary because the patient may have adverse responses. Sensory bombardment may lead to increased reflex responses rather than the desired motor outcomes.[23] The treatment team should be aware of the importance of keeping sensory stimulation at a therapeutic level.

Brain injury patients, especially in the early stages of recovery, need scheduled rest periods to prevent overstimulation and fatigue. Their ability to participate in therapy can decline when they are overstimulated and become increasingly confused or agitated. This situation can also lead to increased reflex responses or avoidance reactions, which interfere with motor performance.

Families often overstimulate patients unintentionally in an attempt to speed spontaneous recovery. The treatment team must educate families on the need for down time, methods to decrease stimulation, and the importance of appropriate family involvement. The family can play a significant role in providing sensory stimulation to a comatose patient. This contribution enables the family to have some involvement in the patient's rehabilitation and gives them an opportunity to detect subtle changes in progress. Family can also give feedback about a patient's likes and dislikes. Having familiar items, pictures of family or friends, and favorite music or scents can often increase patient response to the environment.[19]

Treatment Settings

Brain injury patients may be placed in different settings. Finding the setting most appropriate for the level of care the particular patient needs and the resources approved by the insurance company is critical.

INPATIENT REHABILITATION

Acute rehabilitation consists of an inpatient stay, most often immediately following medical stabilization in an acute care hospital. This phase of rehabilitation generally involves an interdisciplinary team and focuses on physical rehabilitation, with beginning cognitive and behavioral treatment. Although patients may not reach a level of independent mobility at this stage, a goal of acute rehabilitation should allow patients to reach their highest possible level of mobility. The family must also become comfortable with assisting patients with transfers and ambulation. *Subacute rehabilitation* follows the acute phase for a patient who is not at a level to benefit adequately from intensive rehabilitation or has a decreased level of progress or participation. These patients may lack the physical or cognitive abilities to advance to the next level of treatment. The acute rehabilitation center may be a temporary step to allow the patient time to increase endurance, participation, or cognition or to control behavior. Mobility goals at this level may range from increased bed mobility and maintaining range of motion to assistance with transfers or ambulation.

OUTPATIENT REHABILITATION

Because of the high costs of inpatient rehabilitation, outpatient settings are becoming a more popular option for the patient with brain injury.[25] *Comprehensive day treatment programs* are intensive rehabilitation programs that continue with a team focus. Patients live at home and attend therapy during regular work hours. This type of program benefits patients who have the support system to live at home but requires continued interdisciplinary treatment to return to their most independent level. Often patients in a day treatment program are at a higher physical level and may require an increased endurance or strengthening program to reach an independent level. Safety judgment may also be a major issue at this level that has to be addressed before a patient can become independent. *Residential or community reentry programs* are often a final step in the rehabilitation process. These programs emphasize return to work, school, or independent living. Focus areas include higher-level balance, community mobility, route training and other higher-level self-care skills, and cognitive remediation.

Treatment settings are adapting to current changes in the health care system. Often, examining alternative or creative treatment ideas to find what is most efficient for the patient, family, therapist, and the third-party payer is a necessary precursor to treatment.

Nature of Treatment

Because of the need to cut costs and increase productivity, *group treatments* are used more widely in rehabilitation settings. However, groups are often not appropriate for brain injured patients because there is a need to decrease stimulation and distraction. At later stages in recovery, patients may be placed in gait training or balance groups. Community outings can also be a beneficial method of grouping patients to reach functional and efficient mobility goals.

One-to-one treatment is the traditional model of intensive rehabilitation. Many brain injury patients require this individual treatment because of low cognitive or physical levels. This form of treatment may be necessary to address lower extremity facilitation or intensive transfer or gait training. *Cotreatment* can combine occupational and physical therapies for a patient who is physically at a low level. Speech and occupational therapy may be necessary for a patient who requires cognitive remediation for working on basic self-care, dysphagia, or adaptive equipment for feeding.

Family Involvement

Early family involvement is essential to a successful rehabilitation process. Family education and active participation in the treatment plan, including goal setting, are vital to achieving optimal outcomes. Decreased length of stay in the inpatient setting requires that families receive training in multiple aspects of treatment. In addition, the patient and staff may be served quite well if familiar family members assist in the provision of consistent therapeutic care. Often, family members or caregivers are uncomfortable in interactions with the brain injured patient. The treatment team must assist them by providing education and resources about brain injury and the recovery process; this information must be given at a level that the family can understand. Communicating the information through jargon and unfamiliar medical language only further frustrates and confuses the family.

Prolonged family involvement from an early stage can increase understanding of the special needs of a person with a brain injury. If families are given the opportunity to feel comfortable and confident with patient care, including transfers and ambulation, then mobility training will be more therapeutic, even for patients who are functioning at a lower physical level. Simple tasks, such as assisting the patient with grooming or skin care, may help the caregiver feel useful and also comfort the patient. The family can actively participate in balance and gait training even before learning to assist with these activities independent of the therapist. Also, family members can provide assistance when other staff members are not available to help. Figure 13–4 illustrates this patient's husband assisting with ambulation. Because an extra pair of hands was available to assist with equipment and tubing, more difficult and complex treatments were possible with this patient. By assisting in patient care, the caregiver may become more comfortable with the patient and feel competent to take over the patient's care upon discharge from the rehabilitation setting.

There are situations that are less conducive to family involvement. For instance, the patient might become more distracted or agitated if a family member is present or assisting during a specific mobility training task and thus compromise the patient's performance. As a result of ongoing family education, the family becomes an active part of the rehabilitation plan. This adherence increases the likelihood that skills, exercises, and compensatory strategies will be generalized into the home setting.

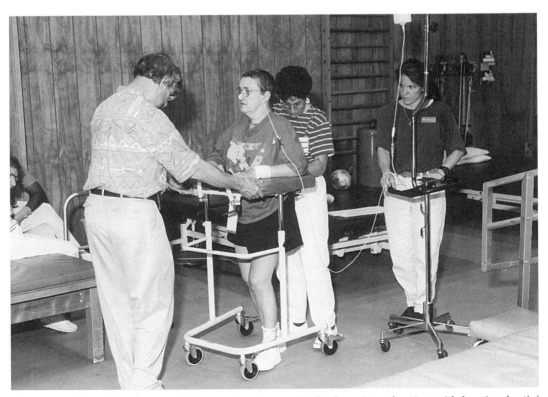

FIGURE 13–4. Family involvement during treatment can assist the therapist and patient with functional activities, as well as encourage the caregiver to be more comfortable and confident in patient care. (Photo courtesy of Rob Stanborough, SPT.)

□ EFFICACY OF TREATMENT

Treatment of the brain injured individual can be a very complex and difficult task with special challenges to the rehabilitation therapist. The clinician must evaluate not only a patient's physical status but also the patient's cognitive and social status. Once the evaluation is complete, the problems limiting the patient's function identified, and the functional goals established, the clinician and patient undergo the long, hard journey of rehabilitation, including the provision of specific therapeutic approaches.

Historical Background of Therapeutic Approaches

As rehabilitation therapies have evolved, the "tools" to treat neurologically impaired patients have become more numerous. Various treatment approaches have emerged over the decades, leaving the clinician to sift through an ever increasing library of information in an effort to decide on the most appropriate treatment for the patient. As stated earlier, the purpose of this chapter is not to inundate the reader with detailed descriptions of the various theoretical frameworks that accompany the myriad of treatment strategies today. However, a brief summary of the evolution of several neurophysiological approaches can give the clinician the theoretical background to develop appropriate intervention strategies.

Much literature lately has discussed the effect of changing scientific theories on the treatment of patients with movement disorders. Gordon[26] points out that "practical needs determine the validity of the theoretical model. A theoretical model is not simply right or wrong. It is valid only insofar as it is useful."

The historical background behind the evolution of therapeutic approaches sheds light on how our current methodology has evolved. For example, before 1950 the primary concern of therapists was the treatment of patients with poliomyelitis. The most prevalent treatment approach was muscle reeducation, with a focus on isolated, weakened muscles.[27] This technique was effective for treating focal paralysis or a lower motor neuron disease. However, with the advent of the Salk vaccine, poliomyelitis became less of a problem, and attention was turned to other neurological disorders, such as strokes and brain injuries.[26] When the central nervous system (CNS) became the focus of treatment, many treatment approaches evolved. The development of what is now referred to as the "traditional neurofacilitation approaches"

in the late 1950s and early 1960s brought about a dramatic shift in the treatment of movement disorders to an emphasis on retraining motor control through techniques designed to inhibit or facilitate specific movement patterns. The following list identifies common assumptions underlying neurotherapeutic approaches[26]:

1. "The brain controls movement, not muscles." This approach is adapted from the views of John Hughlings Jackson, a famous nineteenth-century neurologist. The focus should not be on specific muscle groups but on entire movement patterns.

2. "Movement patterns can be altered or facilitated by applying specific patterns of sensory stimulation, especially through proprioceptive pathways." This approach stems from work done by Sir Charles Sherrington (early 1900s) and Rudolf Magnus (1920s) on the function of different reflexes within various part of the nervous system that affect movement.

3. "The CNS is hierarchically organized." This approach evolved from the work of Sherrington, Magnus, and Jackson during the early to middle twentieth century. This assumption is central to determining the effects of lesions in the CNS. If the higher centers (e.g., cerebral cortex) are damaged, the lower centers are released from that higher control, and more primitive and automatic behaviors result. For example, spasticity is regarded as resulting from lack of inhibitory control from the higher centers.

4. "Recovery from brain damage follows a predictable sequence that mimics the normal development of movement during infancy." Reflex hierarchies of motor control are used to explain behaviors seen in infants. Maturation and development of the CNS is then equated with recovery of the CNS after brain damage. Thus, the developmental sequence is applied to the progression of therapeutic exercises.

The neurotherapeutic approaches include[5,28]:

Bobath (neurodevelopmental treatment [NDT])[29–31] emphasizes the importance of posture and proximal control in movement behavior as precursors for inhibition of abnormal movement patterns and facilitation of normal movement. It was developed by Karl and Berta Bobath.

Proprioceptive neuromuscular facilitation[13] (PNF) uses facilitation of normal patterns of movement to strengthen weak musculature and benefit functional training. Emphasis is placed on the role of the muscle spindle and spinal reflex mechanisms. It was developed by Kabat and Knott and expanded by Voss.

Brunnstrom[33] uses the premise that movement returns in stages, dictated by synergistic patterns. The clinician does not inhibit spastic synergy patterns (as in the Bobath technique) but rather attempts to train the patient to modify them. It was developed by Signe Brunnstrom.

Motor Control Perspective

Many neurotherapeutic approaches presume that neurophysiological basis underlies the motor behavior observed with brain damage. Currently, one primary concern with this premise is that the clinician will take a very limited viewpoint, neglecting the whole picture that involves behavioral sciences, biomechanics, and muscle biology.[26] Successful treatment of the brain injured patient demands a holistic approach to the entire individual that takes into account the many varied sources of motor behavior in this patient population.

"There is a constant tension in therapy between the desire to achieve true restitution of normal movement patterns and the practical need to train patients to carry out essential functions in their daily lives."[26] Out of this frustration, recent advances have been made in the development of the "motor control perspective," an approach that stresses specific training of motor control in everyday activities. The major assumptions that govern this new model are that a learning process is involved in the retraining of motor tasks and that this process includes practice, feedback, and understanding of the goal; motor control requires anticipatory and ongoing feedback, and postural adjustments and focal limb movements are interrelated; for a specific motor task to be performed, the task must not only be practiced but also practiced in various environmental contexts; and sensory input related to the motor task helps to modulate action.[34]

The congruency of traditional facilitation techniques with the recent advances in our understanding of the neural basis of movement is controversial. For example, one controversy revolves around the appropriateness of strength training in the spastic patient. According to Bobath, spasticity causes loss of reciprocal movement ability, increased cocontraction with movement attempts, and disturbed postural equilibrium reactions.[35] The increased effort associated with strength training would therefore increase spasticity and worsen all these associated problems. Furthermore, patients with spasticity do not pri-

marily suffer from weakness. Current research has served to refute rather than support this stance.[36–44] Limitations in movement associated with spasticity seem to stem more from inadequate recruitment of agonist motor neurons, not increased activity of the antagonist muscle.[45,46] Although many of the potential mechanisms involving spasticity are neurological, the role of mechanical factors (e.g., soft tissue tightness) must also be taken into account.[46,47] Thus, the clinician must maintain up-to-date information from current scientific and clinical research to best treat any patient population.

The appropriateness of the role of traditional facilitation techniques in current rehabilitation practice is far too broad of a topic to be taken on here, but the reader may consult excellent references by Carr and Sheperd[48] and Shumway-Cook and Woollacott.[5]

When trying to determine the most effective treatment plan for the brain injured patient the clinician must realize that each patient is different. Each patient obviously exhibits different motoric problems and responds to some approaches better than others, often with day-to-day variation. The proficiency of skills developed by each therapist is also a factor. A treatment may be more effective simply because the therapist is better trained. However, the clinician has the responsibility to fully evaluate the effectiveness of the treatment, modify as necessary, and keep up to date on the latest information available regarding treatment approaches. Balancing the traditional and contemporary models of motor control and motor learning can be difficult. Most important, no matter which neurorehabilitation approach is taken, in light of the current changes in health care today, practical application must be emphasized. There is less time to continue with the practice of reducing the actions of patients into a separate set of movements outside the context of the functional task.[28] Repetition and mastery of specific movement patterns is no longer considered essential to begin the introduction of these essential tasks. Little time exists to address all the functional goals that may have been set in the days of 3- to 4-month rehabilitation stays, much less address them in such a roundabout manner. Clinicians are called on to streamline and choose the most effective and efficient method to achieve their patients' goals.

Despite the many years of research and theory about brain injury and its subsequent functional impairments, there still remains a lack of scientific evidence to describe neural recovery and its facilitation by clinical intervention. Treatment approaches to motoric abnormalities resulting from brain trauma have proven to be effective primarily by clinical observations and must have enough flexibility to address the wide variety of symptoms and responses. Consequently, therapists must consider the mechanisms of the recovery process and the multitude of treatment options while simultaneously pursuing the most cost-effective approach.

□ TREATMENT CONSIDERATIONS

Strategies

Once the clinician has assessed the patient's performance, an important decision involves the type of strategy to teach the patient. Should the focus be recovery of normal strategies or compensatory strategies?[5] Clinical experience is valuable in making these choices. The best guideline seems to be time, emphasizing recovery of normal function in the acute stage and shifting the emphasis to compensatory strategies in the chronic patient. Obviously, the nature of the impairment itself helps to determine the strategy to teach, based on the permanence of the limitation. In the case of the brain injured individual, however, this factor is often conjecture. Once again, time is the best guideline.

Examination of Deficits

Although there are often neurophysiological explanations for movement disorders, alternative ways of explaining deficits should be considered in developing treatment strategies.[26] For example, observing deficits from a biomechanical level is vital in choosing a treatment for a spasticity related deficit. Is the gait disorder a result of the hyperactive stretch reflex in the calf or the abnormal stiffness of the passive tissues (a contracture) in the ankle joint? Is the deficit in upper extremity coordination caused by the release of abnormal synergies that prevent the normal movement pattern (per the Brunnstrom model), or are these synergies really a learned pattern of movement to compensate for weakness still present in the arm? The individual uses any strategy that facilitates the best mechanical advantage of the weakened limb. Could the phenomenon of "learned nonuse" described by Taub[49] be another explanation for limited recovery of a limb? This phenomenon refers to a patient's unwillingness to use an impaired [upper] extremity when the nonimpaired extremity is available. Thus, the nonuse of the limb is not totally a result of a neural deficit but rather because the individual learns to use the intact limb to compensate for the deficits in the affected limb. Consequently, the clinician must use analytical skills to evaluate the patient's movement disorders from not only a neurological but also a biomechanical and functional level.

Motor Learning Principles

Rehabilitation for brain injured patients must aim toward minimizing limitations to achieve the highest possible level of independence in function. To achieve this progress, efficient movement patterns must be relearned. Thus, principles and strategies of motor learning need to be incorporated into the therapist's treatment plan. Riolo-Quinn[21] addresses the areas of learning versus performance, task selection, feedback, practice schedules, and environmental effects in discussing motor learning. Learning must be distinguished from performance. Performance of a task may occur spontaneously, but for the patient to have learned the task, there must be consistency and carryover. To achieve learning, the patient needs to take an active role, and a problem-solving approach to task completion should be incorporated into treatment sessions.

In task selection, the patient's abilities must be kept in mind; too simple an activity leads to boredom, and too difficult a task causes frustration and possibly agitation. Balancing task complexity is essential for effective motor learning, and it must be done on a one-to-one basis, with ongoing evaluation of the patient's abilities.

Appropriate feedback is needed for the patient to modify actions to complete a task. Depending on the limitations of the individual, the therapist must determine the most effective sensory modality. For example, visual cues may not be useful to a patient with hemianopsia, and verbal cues may not be helpful to a patient with aphasia. Once the mode of feedback is determined, the therapist must monitor the amount and intensity of feedback to produce the best learning results. Initially, when learning a task, the individual requires more information to correctly learn the movement patterns. As the activity is learned, feedback requirements lessen, and the individual learns through trial and error. Finally, the activity has progressed to an automatic phase, where few cognitive demands are required and little intervention from the therapist is needed.

Timing of feedback is important as well. Giving feedback as close to the completion of movement as possible allows the individual to remember the task and the feeling of movement. Obviously, shorter delays are better in brain injured patients with limited attention spans and memories. In addition, emphasis should be placed on giving input for one factor at a time. Trying to correct too many issues at once only overwhelms and frustrates the individual.

Once the task has been learned, the patient must be able to practice it in different situations. A patient may learn ambulation with a narrow-base quad cane in the physical therapy gym but may not be able to ambulate at home on carpet or grass. Further practice sessions are needed to apply the knowledge and motor skills learned. If a patient is having trouble with components of a gait, the therapist may retreat and practice only that part of the gait cycle that was difficult. However, for appropriate transfer of learning, that part of gait must be put into the whole pattern of movement promptly.

☐ CASE STUDIES

These three case studies represent realistic patient situations. Each is a case history followed by a series of questions. This format is designed to encourage problem solving and stimulate discussion so that the reader has an opportunity to actively apply the information in this chapter.

Case 1 ■ Michael is a 20-year-old who suffered a brain injury in a motor vehicle accident in which he was an unrestrained driver. He also sustained multiple facial fractures and a pulmonary contusion. During his acute care hospital course, he developed a *Staphylococcus aureus* infection of his eyes and a *Pseudomonas* infection in his sputum. The Glasgow Coma Scale rating in the emergency room was 5. Upon admission to inpatient rehabilitation, Michael was unresponsive to verbal stimuli but responsive to painful stimuli and assigned a cognitive functioning level of III on the Rancho Los Amigos Scale. Stage 1 decubitus ulcers were present on his heels bilaterally, back, and buttocks. He received nourishment through a nasogastric tube and had a tracheostomy and a condom catheter. Michael had no voluntary movement of his extremities; there was significant hypertonicity throughout all four extremities and neck, with hypotonicity of the trunk and decorticate posturing. Passive range of motion was less than normal throughout his neck and all four extremities. Michael was dependent in bed mobility, sitting balance, transfers, and all self-care.

Michael's mother reported the family's goals for Michael were that he be able to walk, talk, dress himself, and function as closely to his normal lifestyle as possible, while he continued with outpatient therapy to make a full recovery. On discharge, she preferred that Michael be sent home, with the understanding that she would need assistance while she and her husband were at work. Michael's length of stay was 6 weeks, at which time he was discharged home to receive home health therapy services.

1. What initial goals and treatment approaches would you establish? Consider Michael's Rancho level upon admission, his strengths, the basic skills that will help him develop increased mobility, and ways to prevent secondary complications.

2. How would you justify each goal, approach, and expected functional outcome, therapeutically and financially? Assess the specific needs of Michael and his family. Establish functional goals that, if met, will prepare him and his family for discharge. Carefully select treatment approaches that address the goals. In general, keeping abreast of clinical research and treatment techniques helps therapists choose effective treatment approaches.

3. What are secondary complications, and how might you prevent them? Multiple fractures, a compromised respiratory system, skin sores, and hypertonicity are all complications and may lead to other complications.

4. How would you involve the family in Michael's treatment plan? Michael's family can help establish a comforting and familiar environment. They need to learn to assist with bed and wheelchair positioning, self-care activities, transfers, exercises, and mobility skills.

5. What treatment constraints and issues might affect your treatment plan? Constraints and issues, not specific to Michael's case, might include a shorter than desirable length of stay, limited resources, small staff and large caseloads, decreased time for one-to-one treatment, and lack of insurance coverage for outpatient coverage.

6. How might these constraints impact functional recovery? Michael's outpatient services are limited by his health insurance plan. A delay or suspension from therapy may mean that patients will not realize an optimal functional level. In addition, other complications, such as contractures, could develop (and did occur in Michael's situation). Because of work schedules and care for their other child, it was difficult for the family to consistently stretch and assist with range of motion exercises. Under similar circumstances, other patients often do not get the opportunity to improve mobility skills and cognitive strategies that would enhance community reentry and employability, or even would simply allow them more independence in their home setting and self-care.

7. How might the treatment team creatively deal with these constraints and treatment issues? Appropriate alternatives might include cotreatment, group settings that are suitable for Michael's cognitive and physical level, and consistent family involvement.

Case 2 ■ Ralph is a 44-year-old who sustained a traumatic brain injury as an unrestrained passenger in a motor vehicle accident. He was unresponsive at the scene of the accident. He was taken to an acute care hospital where a computed tomographic scan revealed cerebral edema, left thalamic bleed, and an intraventricular bleed. He was transferred to another acute care hospital, where he underwent a left ventriculostomy. He also suffered a left tibia fracture that was repaired by open reduction internal fixation, a left ulna fracture that was casted, and a left clavicle fracture. Thirteen days later, the patient went into respiratory failure that required a tracheostomy. He was placed on 28 percent oxygen. A G-tube was also placed at this time for nutritional needs and provision of medication.

Ralph was transferred to a rehabilitation center approximately 4 weeks postinjury. He was at a Rancho level II. He was making generalized responses to auditory stimuli but was unresponsive to both visual and tactile stimuli. He was unable to follow commands and dependent in all self-care, communication, and mobility. He continued to receive all nutrition through the G-tube and still required the tracheostomy with room air. Ralph displayed flexor spasticity in both upper extremities, primarily in the biceps and pectoralis muscles. Extensor spasticity was present bilaterally in his gastrocnemius muscles, and he was non-weight-bearing on his left upper and lower extremity. Head and trunk control were poor, requiring maximum assist of two people to maintain his balance, and no volitional movement was noted. At this time in his rehabilitation stay, he was receiving physical, occupational, and speech therapy.

Ralph's initial treatment plan consisted of (1) increasing sitting tolerance and endurance with increased time in wheelchair; (2) passive range of motion to all extremities; (3) coma stimulation; (4) family education; (5) cotreatment from physical therapy (PT) and occupational therapy (OT) to facilitate sitting balance, trunk and head control, and interaction with the environment; (6) casting of the right ankle for a contracture and to inhibit spasticity; (7) plugging of the tracheostomy tube; and (8) neurostimulants.

One month after admission to rehabilitation, Ralph's tracheostomy tube was removed. He was oriented to person and place, began following one-step commands, and was able to express 75 percent of basic needs. He had also begun therapeutic feeds. He was maximum assist in grooming and dependent in toileting and dressing. His sliding board transfers and wheelchair mobility were dependent. Bed mobility was maximum assist. Ralph was especially limited by upper extremity passive range of motion and decreased motor control.

Ralph's treatment plan at this time consisted of (1) evaluation of further cognitive areas, (2)

therapeutic feeds in a group setting, (3) tilt table, (4) casting following nerve blocks for the upper extremities, (5) continued PT-OT cotreatments to facilitate balance and trunk and head control, (6) wheelchair mobility, and (7) ADL training.

Initially, Ralph was unable to tolerate the medical neurostimulant treatment; however, after 6 weeks in rehabilitation, he was tolerating a course of methylphenidate (Ritalin) quite well. He progressed to weight-bearing as tolerated on his lower extremity. He became independent in bed mobility, minimum to moderate assist with stand-pivot transfers, and minimum assist with wheelchair mobility with his right lower extremity. He began gait training, ambulating with a platform rolling walker with minimum to moderate assist for 100 feet. He was moderate assist in upper extremity dressing and donning pants and required maximum assist for shoes and socks because of upper extremity range of motion limitations. He had improved to a transitional II diet, and the G-tube was removed. He had severely decreased memory and confabulated. Ralph's treatment plan then consisted of memory notebook, gait training, transfer training, continued nerve blocks and casting for the left upper extremity, continued ADL training, and community reentry.

Ralph continued to make progress and left inpatient rehabilitation approximately 13 weeks after his accident. He was discharged to a residential facility that offers continued PT, OT, cognitive remediation, and vocational rehabilitation. He left using the memory book with moderate verbal cues but continued to have difficulty with orientation to time and thought organization. He was ambulating 200 feet with supervision, using a narrow-base quad cane, performing stand-pivot transfers from bed to wheelchair with contact guard assist, doing wheelchair propulsion with supervision for safety, and requiring minimum assist with stairs using one rail. He was on a mechanical soft diet.

1. What are Ralph's impairments? What are his functional limitations? Some examples of impairments include decreased balance, increased tone, decreased range of motion, and weakness. Examples of functional limitations are dependent bed mobility, dependent transfers and ADLs, and poor trunk control and balance.
2. What tests could be used to assess Ralph's impairments throughout his stay at the rehabilitation center? Tests include FIM, Katz Index, Barthel Index, and goniometry for range of motion.
3. Are there sources of movement disorder other than those of neurological origin that limit Ralph's function? Yes. Multiple fractures, decreased range of motion, impaired cognition, and learned nonuse.

4. What are the benefits of using the tilt table with Ralph? When during his rehabilitation stay would this treatment be most appropriate? Benefits of the tilt table include weight bearing through lower extremities, range of motion increases in the lower extremities, sensory stimulation, prevention of respiratory complications, facilitation of muscle tone, and facilitation of interaction with the environment. This treatment would be most beneficial in the early stages of his rehabilitation, when Ralph cannot actively participate as well.

5. How might the therapist facilitate Ralph's performance of his transfers and his learning of this motoric skill? Ralph should take as active a role as possible, and the therapist should facilitate a problem-solving approach in the instruction. Once Ralph learns the skill in the gym, he should practice transfers in different environments and settings to facilitate carryover.

6. What Rancho level would describe Ralph when he was discharged from inpatient rehabilitation? Rancho level VI.

Case 3 ■ Jennifer, a 16-year-old, sustained a traumatic brain injury in a motor vehicle accident. Jennifer was admitted to an acute care hospital, where she spent 6 weeks. On admission to a rehabilitation center, 6 weeks postinjury, her Rancho level was III. She was responding to auditory, tactile, and visual stimuli with inconsistent ability to follow one-step commands. Jennifer, right hand dominant, had right hemiparesis with fair strength throughout the left side.

Upon admission, Jennifer was dependent with all self-care, communication, and mobility. At that time Jennifer received speech, occupational, and physical therapies. She had poor head and trunk control, with maximal assist to maintain sitting balance. She demonstrated inconsistent movement throughout both left extremities, with decreased tone in the right upper extremity and lower extremity with the exception of increased tone in the left and right ankle. Jennifer's mother was present during all therapy sessions. She observed treatment and was trained in range of motion exercises and coma stimulation.

Jennifer's initial treatment plan consisted of (1) increasing sitting tolerance and endurance with increased up time in the wheelchair, (2) passive range of motion to all four extremities, (3) coma stimulation, and (4) cotreating from physical and occupational therapies to facilitate sitting balance, trunk and head control, and interaction with environment.

One month following admission to the rehabilitation center, Jennifer was responding appropriately to all verbal commands. She was participating in ADLs with maximal assistance and following one-step contextual commands. She was ambulating in the parallel bars with moderate assist and required moderate assist for a stand-pivot transfer. Jennifer needed supervision and verbal cuing to push her wheelchair 100 feet.

Jennifer's treatment plan at this time consisted of (1) assessing her assistive device needs by physical therapy with continued gait training, (2) facilitating left upper and lower extremity activity by occupational and physical therapies, and (3) continued ADL training by occupational therapy for increased independence in self-care skills.

At this time, Jennifer's insurance company began requesting detailed reports of her progress in order to continue funding Jennifer's stay at the rehabilitation center. The case manager projected a 2-week stay based on the number of rehabilitation days available in Jennifer's insurance policy. The treatment team recommended a 6-week stay, and the insurance company wanted to see more progress from Jennifer, with weekly evaluation prior to recertification.

Jennifer continued to show improvement in all therapies. She required minimal assistance with bed mobility and minimal to moderate assistance with stand-pivot transfers. Jennifer required minimal assist for basic self-care and for stand-pivot transfers to a transfer tub bench. At this point, Jennifer's mother was trained in functional transfers and ADL training. She was able to assist Jennifer with her self-care routine and mobility.

Jennifer was discharged from the rehabilitation center almost 10 weeks after admission. Jennifer ambulated 200 feet with a straight cane with contact guard assist. She was able to ambulate up and down stairs with two rails with contact guard assist and required supervision and increased time for basic self-care. Jennifer's mother was comfortable in assisting her with ambulation and self-care in a therapeutic manner.

1. At what point should Jennifer's family have become involved in her treatment? This question has a different answer for each family. Some families are more accessible than others, some patients are more attentive or productive with family members present, and other patients need to work one-to-one to reach goals.

2. Name three environmental factors that would be important issues in the beginning of Jennifer's stay in the rehabilitation center. Many environmental factors are issues in the early stages of a patient's rehabilitation stay. Some important factors to remember are positioning, quiet time, and family involvement.

3. Would Jennifer have been appropriate for group treatment during the first few weeks of her stay at the rehabilitation center? Why or

why not? Jennifer would not have been appropriate for group treatment upon her admission to the rehabilitation center because of her low physical and cognitive levels.

4. What type of post acute rehabilitation setting would be most appropriate for Jennifer and her family? Jennifer's supportive family and her age made her an appropriate admission to an outpatient rehabilitation setting. This decision is made by the family with recommendations from the treatment team.

□ SUMMARY

The management of mobility problems among patients with brain injury continues to be a challenging endeavor. This challenge is augmented by an emerging need to define treatment plans in terms of length of stay, level of recovery, and the environment in which care is offered. These factors have necessitated creative intervention plans and a renewed emphasis toward functional restitution, often at the expense of comprehensive resolution of primary impairments. Management of patient problems and goal setting, more than ever before, requires collaboration among team members in each environment not only to set priorities but also to achieve goals in a cost-effective manner.

Treatment to improve mobility, in the context of constrained lengths of stay, has required clinicians to rethink the emphasis that should be placed on neuromuscular retraining approaches. More attention should be paid to integrating movement patterns as they relate specifically to functionally meaningful goals. Finally, the importance of generating quantitative outcomes that justify the intensity and duration of treatment cannot be overstated.

REFERENCES

1. Hagen, C, Malkmus, D, and Durham, P: Levels of cognitive functions. In Rehabilitation of the Head Injured Adult: Comprehensive Physical Management. Professional Staff Association, Rancho Los Amigos Hospital, Downey, Calif, 1979.
2. Mills, V: Traumatic Head Injury. In O'Sullivan, S, and Schmits, T (eds): Physical Rehabilitation: Assessment and Treatment. FA Davis, Philadelphia, 1988.
3. Cowen, T, et al: Influence of early variable in traumatic brain injury and functional independence measure scores and rehabilitation length of stay and charges. Arch Phys Med Rehabil 76:797, 1995.
4. Swaine, B, and Sullivan, J: Longitudinal profile of early motor recovery following severe traumatic brain injury. Brain Inj 10:5, 1996.
5. Shumway-Cook, A, and Woollacott, M: A conceptual framework for clinical practice. In Butler, J (ed): Motor Control: Theory and Practical Applications. Williams & Wilkins, Baltimore, 1995.
6. Schenkman, M, and Butler, RB: A model for multisystem evaluation, interpretation, and treatment of individuals with neurologic dysfunction. Phys Ther 69:538, 1989.
7. Keith, RA, et al: The functional independence measure: A new tool for rehabilitation. In Eisentberg, MG, and Grzesiak, RC (eds): Advances in Clinical Rehabilitation, vol 1. Springer Verlag, New York, 1987.
8. Katz, S, et al: Progress in development of the index of ADL. Gerontologist 20, 1970.
9. Mahoney, RI, and Barthel, DW: Functional evaluation: The Barthel Index. Md State Med J 14:61, 1965.
10. Lawton, MP: The functional assessment of elderly people. J Am Geriatr Soc 19:465, 1971.
11. Welford, AT: Motor skills and aging. In Mortimer, J, Pirozzolo, FJ, and Maletta, G, (eds): The Aging Motor System. Praeger, New York, 1982, p 152.
12. Fregly, AR, and Graybeil, A: An ataxia test battery not requiring rails. Aerospace Medicine 34:277, 1968.
13. Timmons, M, Gasquoine, L, and Scibak, J: Functional changes with rehabilitation of very severe traumatic brain injury survivors. J Head Trauma Rehabil 2:3, 1987.
14. Banja, J: Outcomes and values. J Head Trauma Rehabil 9:2, 1994.
15. Nicolaysen, L, et al: Managed care: Keying in to the challenges. Team Rehab Report 6:11, 1995.
16. Phillips, N: Personal communication, May 1996.
17. Powell, J, and Chapman, P: The impact of early orthopedic management in patients with traumatic brain injury. J Head Trauma Rehabil 9:1, 1994.
18. Messa, J: Overview of physical therapy management of patients with traumatic brain injury. Neurology Report 14:1, 1990.
19. Saadeh, S: Unpublished material, 1993.
20. Mills, V: Physical therapy and cognitive impairment in traumatically head injured patients: A clinical report. Neurology Report 13:51, 1989.
21. Riolo-Quinn, L: Motor learning considerations in treating brain injured patients. Neurology Report 14:12, 1990.
22. Roush, J, and Emory, N: Positioning the coma-emergent patient through the use of orthotics and wheelchair seating systems. Neurology Report 14, 1990.
23. Rinehart, M: Strategies for improving motor performance. In Rosenthal, M, et al (eds): Rehabilitation of the Adult and Child with Traumatic Brain Injury. FA Davis, Philadelphia, 1990.
24. Beckwith, D: Personal communication, May 1996.
25. Burke, D: Models of brain injury rehabilitation. Brain Inj 9:7, 1995.
26. Gordon, J: Assumptions underlying physical therapy interventions. In Quinlin, MM, and Bloom, R (eds): Movement Science: Foundations for Physical Therapy in Rehabilitation. Aspen, Rockville, Md, 1987.
27. Pinkston, D (ed): Analysis of traditional regimens of therapeutic exercise. Am J Phys Med 46:713, 1967.
28. Majsak, M: Consolidating principles of motor learning with neurologic treatment techniques in a professional physical therapist program. Neurology Report 20:19, 1996.
29. Bobath, B, and Bobath, K: Motor Development in Different Types of Cerebral Palsy. Heinemann, London, 1976.
30. Bobath, K, and Bobath, B: The neurodevelopmental treatment. In Scrutton, D (ed): Management of motor disorders of cerebral palsy. Heinemann, London, 1984.
31. Mayston, M: The Bobath concept: Evolution and application. In Forssberg, H, and Hirschfeld, H (eds): Movement Disorders in Children. Karger, Basel, 1992.
32. Voss, D, Ionta, M, and Myers, B: Proprioceptive Neuromuscular Facilitation: Patterns and techniques, ed 3. Harper & Row, New York, 1985.
33. Brunnstrom, S: Movement Therapy in Hemiplegia. Harper & Row, New York, 1985.
34. Carr, JH, and Sheperd, RB: A Motor Relearning Programme for Stroke. Heinemann, London, 1982.
35. Bobath, B: Adult Hemiplegia: Evaluation and Treatment, ed 2. Heinemann, London, 1978.
36. Light, KE, et al: Does heavy resistive exercise promote muscular cocontraction and loss of reciprocal movement in brain injured subjects. Society for Neuroscience Abstracts 20:2, 1994.

37. Light, KE: Is strength training contraindicated for motor coordination post CNS lesion? Presented at the Conference on Strength Training: Issues in Addressing Fundamental Impairments in Neurological Patients, Philadelphia, September 1994.

38. Giuliani, CA, Light, KE, and Purser, JL: The effects of an isokinetic exercise program on the performance of sit-to-stand in patients with hemiparesis. Presented at Combined Sections Meeting of the American Physical Therapy Association, San Francisco, February 1992.

39. Rose, DK, Giuliani, CA, and Light, KE: The immediate effects of isokinetic exercise on temporal distance characteristics of self-selected and fast hemiplegic gait. Presented at Combined Sections Meeting of the American Physical Therapy Association, San Francisco, February, 1992.

40. Hall, CD, and Light, KE: Heavy resistive exercise effect on reciprocal movement coordination of closed head injury subjects with spasticity. Presented at Combined Sections Meeting of the American Physical Therapy Association, Orlando, 1992.

41. Light, KE, and Giuliani, CA: The effect of isokinetic exercise effort on coordinated movement control of spastic hemiparetic subjects. Foundation for Physical Therapy, Alexandria, Va, 1992, unpublished data.

42. Knuttson, E, and Martensson, A: Dynamic motor capacity in spastic paresis and its relation to prime mover dysfunction, spastic reflexes and antagonist coactivation. Scand J Rehabil Med 12:93, 1980.

43. Fenichel, GM, and Daroff, RB: Hemiplegic atrophy: Histological and etiological considerations. Neurology 14: 883, 1964.

44. Harris, FA: Muscle stretch receptor hypersensitization in spasticity: Inaproprioception, part III. Am J Phys Med 57:16, 1978.

45. Sahrman, SA, and Norton, BJ: The relationship of voluntary movement to spasticity in the upper motor neuron syndrome. Ann Neurol 2:460, 1977.

46. Gowland, C, et al: Agonist and antagonist activity during voluntary upper limb movement in patients with stroke. Phys Ther 72:624, 1992.

47. Wolf, S, et al: Overcoming limitations in elbow movement in the presence of antagonist hyperactivity. Phys Ther 74:826, 1994.

48. Carr, JH, and Sheperd, RB (eds): Movement Science: Foundations for Physical Therapy in Rehabilitation. Aspen, Rockville, Md, 1987.

49. Taub, E: Somatosensory deafferentation research with monkeys: Implications for rehabilitation medicine. In Ince, LP (ed): Behavioral Psychology in Rehabilitation Medicine: Clinical Implications. Williams & Wilkins, Baltimore, 1980.

Activities of Daily Living

ROBIN McNENY, OTR

The developmental mastery of activities of daily living (ADLs) occurs during childhood and adolescence. Independence in ADLs is a function of adulthood. A brain injury can significantly affect an individual's ability to pursue routine activities and may necessitate dependence on others for completion of some or all ADLs. Performance of ADLs is vital to independent living in the home, workplace, and community and constitutes a primary focus of rehabilitation. When ADL performance is impaired in even minor ways, survivors of brain injury may require the assistance of a helper. Often this assistance comes from the survivor's social support network, which may need to alter established roles or assume new responsibilities to provide care for the person with the brain injury. Changes in roles and responsibilities among the members of the social support network may increase their sense of stress. The burden on caregivers of persons with brain injury has been well documented by Oddy et al.[1]

Retraining in ADLs is most often considered the domain of the occupational therapist. However, the subskills required for ADL performance, known as *performance components,* and the integrated nature of ADLs demand involvement from the entire rehabilitation team in the retraining effort. Occupational therapists guide the team's ADL retraining efforts by utilizing theoretically grounded and systematically applied techniques to improve function. Occupational therapists seek to understand thoroughly the individual's preinjury constellation of life tasks, interests, habits, and routines before initiating treatment. Clinicians throughout the rehabilitative continuum are wise to allow the pa-

tient's and family's goals for treatment guide the planning and implementation of intervention.[2]

The most severely injured people begin work on ADLs at the inpatient level. ADL retraining continues throughout the continuum of care. Termination of retraining usually follows a determination that maximum ADL function has been achieved; on occasion, the patient and family request cessation of treatment.

☐ EFFECTS OF BRAIN INJURY ON ACTIVITIES OF DAILY LIVING

ADLs are complex, multifaceted tasks that require integration of many areas of cerebral function.[3] Even a mild brain injury may impair performance of daily living skills.[4]

The sequelae of moderate to severe brain injury may include motor and sensory impairment,[5] visual or visual-perceptual dysfunction,[6] cognitive deficits,[3,7] language deficits,[8] and behavioral problems.[9] Concomitant medical issues also affect the performance of ADLs. Spinal cord injury as a dual diagnosis with TBI significantly complicates the performance and retraining of ADL function.[10,11] Orthopedic injuries can limit weight bearing and cause pain on movement during ADLs. Amputation, peripheral nerve injuries, and multisystem trauma can limit mobility and necessitate learning compensatory strategies. The treatment team relates these medical complications to the patient's ability to perform ADLs as they perform evaluations and plan treatment.

☐ ASSESSMENT AND DEFINITION OF FUNCTIONAL LEVEL

Discipline-Specific Evaluation

The rehabilitation of ADLs begins with an assessment of the patient's level of preinjury and postinjury performance in functional tasks. Critical to effective, relevant treatment planning is an assessment of the patient's lifestyle history. Data obtained from this history form the basis for goal setting and treatment decisions.

An occupational history interview and an interest checklist as described by Matsutsuyu[12] to explore the patient's support system, preinjury life tasks, interests, habits, and routines provide an appropriate starting point for evaluation. A comprehensive treatment plan for remediation of ADL deficits centered on patient and family needs is developed from the occupational history data.[13]

A variety of tools[3,14–17] are available for ADL assessment (Table 14–1). The majority of these assessments[3,14,16,17] were developed by occupational therapists to quantify performance in ADLs. In addition to the numerical rating, the evaluator provides qualitative comments on the patient's performance.

Comments from a skilled evaluator are very important to the process. Behavioral observations often capture the intricacies and nuances of ADL performance that elude a numerical scale. Qualitative data frequently highlight the problematic performance component. The assessment of motor and process skills (AMPS)[17] developed by Fisher and Arnadottir's OT-ADL Neurobehavioral Evaluation[3] were designed by occupational therapists to factor problems with performance components into the evaluative process.

Interdisciplinary Assessment

Interdisciplinary assessment and documentation of ADL performance are utilized frequently for patient assessment, program evaluation, and research. The numerous scales devised to document ADL function include the Disability Rating Scale (DRS),[18] Rancho Levels of Cognitive Function,[19] Level of Rehabilitation Scale (LORS),[20] Patient Evaluation Conference System (PECS),[21] the Barthel Index,[22] and the Functional Independence Measure (FIM).[23] Law and Letts[24] and Fisher[25] counsel professionals to study available functional assessments carefully prior to selecting an interdisciplinary assessment to ensure that the instrument is appropriate for persons with brain injury, accurately measures ADLs in the manner the team desires, and matches the team's philosophy regarding ADL function. For example, some teams may philosophically oppose the notion that a patient is not independent if he must utilize a device to complete an ADL and therefore reject a scale that penalizes a patient for adaptive device use.

Correct application of an interdisciplinary assessment enhances the reliability of results; therefore, training in use of an assessment is strongly recommended. Programs using the FIM may obtain certification for staff through Uniform Data Systems.* Other training methods include in-serving training, mock patient assessment, and handouts for self-study.

Clearer communication among professionals may be facilitated by the use of functional scales at the team level. Clinical discussions, professional presentations, and research that utilize familiar functional scales are easier to appreciate and apply. As a specialty, rehabilitation medicine continues to strive toward more uniform assessment and a common baseline for describing functional performance and outcome.

Elements Critical to Effective Assessment

The goal of ADL assessment is to collect information about a patient's skills in self-care and instrumental ADLs. The clinician should consider four factors during ADL assessment.

CONTEXT

A person often links the performance of ADL tasks to a place, time of day, or instruments. Even without a brain injury, a change in context can slow down or interfere with a person's pattern of performance in ADL tasks. ADL performance is optimal when the context is familiar. Home is contextually familiar and, therefore,

---

TABLE 14–1. Measures of Performance of Activities of Daily Living
Klein-Bell Scale
Kenny Self-Care Evaluation
Kohlman Evaluation of Living Skills
Arnadottir OT-ADL Neurobehavioral Evaluation (A-ONE)
Scorable Self-Care Scale
Assessment of Motor and Process Skills
Functional Task Analysis

---

*Uniform Data System for Medical Rehabilitation, UB Foundation Activities Inc., Buffalo, NY.

the ideal environment for ADL assessment. Hospitalization, however, removes the person with a brain injury from this familiar environment, thus disrupting context. Therapists use simulation in these settings to assess ADLs.

Brown et al.[26] studied evaluative simulation of ADLs in a community-based program for adults with severe mental illness. The study concluded that clinical judgment of independence based on simulated tasks was not always accurate. Although the authors recognized the potential limitations in generalization of their findings to other populations, their advice to clinicians to use caution when making judgments on functional performance outside the patient's familiar context seems appropriate. To improve the accuracy of simulated assessment, clinicians take steps to normalize the setting as much as possible. They may utilize the patient's personal items in the activity. Time of day for task performance can be manipulated in the clinical setting to match the patient's habits preinjury. Well-established routines from home can be instituted in the hospital or subacute setting.

Consider the following case illustration:

Case 1 ■ Mr. H, age 73, sustained a severe brain injury in a motor vehicle accident and presented with disorientation, ideation apraxia, decreased balance, lower extremity weakness, and cognitive deficits. The occupational therapist's (OT) initial attempts to assess Mr. H's grooming met with failure. Mr. H refused to do his morning grooming while sitting in a wheelchair, but his balance was inadequate to permit him to stand with the assist of only one person. The physical therapist (PT) joined the evaluative session and assisted Mr. H in standing. Once upright, the patient willingly engaged in the grooming assessment. Deficits in balance, praxis, and sequencing necessitated assist from the OT and PT. The coevaluation clearly enhanced the context of the grooming task for the patient.

Context is important for analyzing ADL assessment findings. If contextual familiarity is noted to improve performance, then treatment should incorporate this principle. If contextual unfamiliarity is clearly a factor in the patient's performance, therapists are obliged to qualify assessment findings with comments about context.

RELEVANCE

Administration of ADL assessments on tasks for which the patient has no responsibility or interest is pointless and irresponsible. Yet, without a carefully conducted and thoroughly reviewed evaluation of the patient's preinjury life roles and responsibilities, clinicians risk inadvertently conducting irrelevant assessments.

Only relevant ADLs should be evaluated. If a patient's money management routine involves control of checking and savings accounts, then higher-level money management evaluation is appropriate. Obviously, patients who use only cash do not require a banking assessment. The cooking evaluation for a patient who performs "survival cooking" (e.g., microwave dinners and sandwiches) should consist of simple meal preparation. Judicious cost management in health care requires clinicians to prudently regard the relevance of an assessment before its administration.

PROCESS AND PERFORMANCE

An appraisal of the process used to complete an ADL task, as well as the level of performance during the task, is critical to an analysis of the findings. Sbordone[27] encourages clinicians to assess the process of task completion, not just task performance. Qualitative information may include the frequency and types of errors made, the apparent plan developed by the patient for completion of the task, the strategy employed during task completion, and the ability to adapt an approach if an obstacle arises. The patient's verbalizations as the task proceeds provide interesting insights. Law[28] suggests that clinicians question patients about their perception of their performance during task completion. The combined findings of the process and performance assessment assist with treatment planning by highlighting both impaired and preserved performance components.

INDIVIDUALIZED ANALYSIS

There is no single standard or norm for ADL performance. Each person possesses a unique pattern of performance for ADL tasks. An individual's preinjury ADL function provides a baseline. The patient and social support network serve as resources regarding preinjury performance.

Clinicians individually compare the patient's postinjury performance with the preinjury baseline. It is not uncommon to discover that impairments in ADL noted during evaluation were troublesome to the patient prior to the injury. Indeed, many adults have difficulty making change, do not know how to use a phonebook, and eat with their elbows on the table. Careful comparison of the patient's current performance with preinjury patterns helps therapists avoid faulty judgments and wasted treatment.

Consider this example:

Case 2 ■ Mrs. R is an 87-year-old widow, mother of eight, who fell, struck her head, and presented with mild cognitive problems. Her motor skills appear intact. She has completed a cooking evaluation, during which she made an apple pie. Her occupational therapist questioned the process Mrs. R used to make the pie. Mrs. R pared the apples in the palm of her hand, refusing to use the cutting board offered by the therapist. She used a dishtowel to remove the pieplate from the oven instead of the potholders laid out next to the stove. The therapist expressed concern about the patient's kitchen safety based on the assessment. When the evaluation results were discussed with the family, they reported that Mrs. R has used these same methods when making pies for decades. By comparing preinjury and postinjury performance patterns, the OT determined Mrs. R's performance in cooking is at a supervision level. Clearly, the individual patient provides the best benchmark for ADL evaluations.

❏ CONSIDERATIONS IN RETRAINING ACTIVITIES OF DAILY LIVING PERFORMANCE

Remedial and adaptive approaches are employed in the retraining of ADLs.[29] The remedial approach focuses on component-specific deficits; intervention is designed to improve component skills. Drills, exercises, and tabletop activities are used in remedial therapy. The remedial approach is based heavily on the presumption of neural plasticity.

The adaptive approach concentrates on occupational behaviors, or ADLs, performed under the expert guidance of a clinician. The therapist provides feedback or correction during task performance. Residual skills are utilized to compensate for those skills impaired by the brain injury.[30]

Neistadt[29] advocates consideration of the neurobiology of learning in designing treatments for ADL impairment. The ability to process information and learn are important factors in the treatment planning process. Clinicians favoring this approach design intervention that engages the patient's optimal mode of learning. Neistadt[29] describes three types of learning:

■ Associational learning: The learner develops a mental connection between two ADLs, such as standing at the sink and shaving. Without this association, learning is difficult; therapy can become arduous and discouraging for patient and staff.

■ Representational learning: The learner internalizes images and symbols related to an activity, thus decreasing the need for a stimulus or cue. For example, a patient learning to use a credit card to make long-distance telephone calls gradually relies less on the instructions on the back of the card during the dialing process.

■ Abstract learning: The learner masters an activity and its associated behaviors independent of an event or context. When faced with an atypical situation, the patient engages in problem solving to complete the task.

Brain injury impairs the ability to generalize techniques and behaviors to a variety of situations. Toglia[31] has worked extensively on refining the concept of learning and information processing related to functional retraining. Using her multicontextual treatment approach in ADL retraining, the clinician designs practice of specific strategies in a variety of settings where movement requirements and task demands vary. The clinician gauges the patient's transfer of learning based on learning criteria established for the task at hand during task completion and subsequently facilitates learning by altering tasks.

Theory-based grading and saturational cuing are appropriate approaches for ADL retraining. When theory-based grading is applied to ADL retraining, the clinician gradually increases the instructions, complexity, and task-related information to stimulate higher-level performance. Saturational cuing as applied by Neistadt[32] involves a steady decrease in the specificity of cues given during task performance. As performance improves, the clinician reduces the content of the instructions to the patient. Cues become vaguer and less instructive. The patient increasingly relies on internal organization and conceptualization of the task. It is important that clinicians understand these theory-based approaches to retraining in order to provide effective services to patients.

❏ TREATMENT FOR DEFICITS IN ACTIVITIES OF DAILY LIVING

Feeding

Feeding is an intricate task involving the physical ability to manipulate utensils and food; the cognitive ability to sequence, attend to, and make judgments about the task; and the perceptual skills to permit correct identification and use of food and utensils. Successful feeding includes behavioral awareness and control, as well as the ability to conform to societal rules associated with dining. Impairment of feeding performance is common in moderate to severe brain injury.

Physical components of self-feeding include oral-motor function, balance, trunk and head control, and upper extremity movement. Dysphagia and oral musculature weakness indicate the need for involvement of a speech-language pathologist for evaluation, prescription of appropriate food consistency, and oral-motor therapy.[33,34] Use of supplemental feeding, whether by mouth or through a gastrostomy, may be indicated for patients who cannot sufficiently meet their calorie needs through self-feeding.[35]

Balance, trunk stability, and head control are prerequisites to self-feeding. Resistance to self-feeding may stem from the patient's need to support impaired balance through her or his arms. Poor head control increases the risk of aspiration and contributes to decreased neatness. Proper wheelchair positioning or head support devices can be helpful.

Motor and sensory impairments often interfere with feeding skill. Therapeutic intervention offered by physical and occupational therapy addresses these specific component deficits.

Cognitive deficits frequently underlie feeding impairments. Basic cognitive retraining techniques are often incorporated into feeding sessions. A predictable place and time for meals, coupled with consistent feedback and direction from staff, are needed. Reorientation to time, place, and the activity at hand can become a part of mealtime conversation.

Self-feeding training is by nature repetitive, which benefits patients with confusion or poor organization. Habituation of a behavior may be aided by consistent, frequent practice.[36] Staff and family collaboratively reinforce specific feeding skills and thus enhance carryover.

Comorbidities such as blindness, hemianopsia, hemi-inattention, apraxia, agnosia, spatial disturbances, or other visual-perceptual-motor problems can interfere with self-feeding skills. Compensatory retraining benefits feeding performance when perception is impaired. Erroneous assumptions may develop among staff and family regarding the patient's feeding skills unless the perceptual impairments affecting feeding ability are explained. Spillage caused by apraxia, failure to eat half a tray on account of hemianopsia, and an inability to follow instructions are at times viewed as volitional and deliberate misbehavior. Clarification of the etiology of such behaviors is helpful for staff and family.

Management of behavior issues associated with feeding should begin as soon as problems are noted. Patients with agitation benefit from eating in a quiet, distraction-free environment.

Lethargic patients need close supervision to ensure continued self-feeding and adequate intake. Initiation problems make starting to feed difficult; assistance is needed to begin self-feeding or to restart feeding if an interruption occurs. Impaired mental flexibility and perseveration are manifested in the patient's inability to shift from eating to drinking. The patient may drink liquids too quickly, overfill the mouth with food, or be unable to stop stirring cereal after adding sugar.

Brain injury programs, particularly at the inpatient level, benefit from an interdisciplinary approach to retraining feeding skills. Team members most commonly involved are the patient, family, occupational therapist, speech-language pathologist, nurse, and physician. Consultations from the dietitian regarding food consistency and choice, as well as from the neuropsychologist on behavioral issues, are valuable.

A therapeutic feeding program should be scheduled for every meal to provide consistency and reinforce newly learned skills. All patients with impairments in feeding skills should be included in the feeding program. Disciplines involved with the feeding program stagger coverage of meals. Communication among the disciplines who are providing the feeding program about diet restrictions, swallowing guidelines, and self-feeding techniques, including the use of adaptive devices, is essential to the program's success. Progress on self-feeding is monitored through medical record documentation and team conferences.

Prior to goal setting for feeding, clinicians determine baseline feeding skill, including the behavioral, cognitive, and motor performance components. During assessment, staff must consider that acceptable mealtime behavior varies from family to family. For some families, any means to get food down is permissible. For others, distinctive customs are associated with dining. Team members are urged to identify these behaviors, respect them during assessment, and incorporate them into feeding training.

Dressing

Difficulties with dressing may occur as a result of deficits in motor, cognitive, perceptual, or behavioral function. Readiness for dressing instruction must exist prior to the onset of retraining. Severely agitated or confused patients, underaroused patients, and patients with multiple medical issues benefit minimally from dressing training. Signs of readiness include a minimal ability to attend to task, the ability to engage in required motor behaviors, and stamina sufficient for the dressing task.

Cotreatment between occupational and physical therapy for the patient with severe physical impairments allows some patients earlier participation in dressing training. The involvement of two or more staff members permits patients with moderate to severe motor problems to work on dressing at a time when one therapist could not manage the patient alone. For example, while the occupational therapist instructs and assists with the task of dressing, the physical therapist facilitates the motor components of dressing, such as maintenance of sitting balance. Compensatory techniques and adaptive devices are employed as needed. However, brain injury patients with memory problems may experience limited benefit from devices; the patient simply forgets to use them.

Warren[37] and Baum and Hall[38] have demonstrated the relationship between perceptual dysfunction and dressing. Patients with apraxia or other perceptual disorders have trouble orienting clothing to the body and applying garments to the extremities. Right-left confusion or problems with spatial relations impair the patient's ability to follow verbal instructions. During treatment, therapists physically guide the patient with perceptual problems through the dressing task; this approach addresses perceptual skills while teaching compensatory techniques. Limiting verbal instructions benefits patients who need to feel and see the task but are confused when they hear what they are to do.

Patients may have limited awareness of safety and functional limitations associated with dressing. Many brain injury patients do not realize they are unable to dress themselves as they did prior to their injury. This lack of insight creates safety issues and hampers the clinician's ability to teach compensatory strategies. Although the patient's drive to be independent is commendable, such patients are at risk for falls if not supervised.

At a more advanced level, problems with error recognition, quality control, decision making, and self-assessment are manifested in the patient's inability to select appropriate clothing for an occasion, to judge cleanliness of clothing, or to assemble an outfit from several garments. These problems may be of concern for individuals attempting to return to work or school. Cue cards, labeling clothing, or preselected outfits can help with these problems.

Firm, consistent guidance to control behavioral issues during dressing may be required. Patients with manipulative behavior attempt to solicit unnecessary assistance from others. Behavior management programs utilized by the team and family to deal with manipulation, lack of cooperation, or recalcitrance can be applied.

Some patients require continued dressing retraining after discharge from the inpatient setting. Home-based therapy staff provide families and caregivers with written guidelines for dressing practice between visits. Videotapes of the clinician and patient doing dressing and undressing have proven beneficial for some families. Training sessions prior to discharge are vitally important to ensure family competency.

Grooming and Hygiene

Impairments in management of grooming and hygiene tasks often emerge as a lack of attention to and initiation of grooming, resulting in untidiness or offensive odor. Some patients' motor deficits cause execution difficulties in grooming and hygiene activities. Apraxia, agnosia, and visual-spatial impairment cause errors in performance, such as use of the toothbrush to groom hair or washing of the reflection in the mirror rather than the face. Clinicians develop strategies to assist patients in improving their performance despite such deficits.

Built-up, weighted, or adapted handles on grooming implements offset some strength and coordination deficits. Retraining in one-handed techniques is recommended for patients with hemiplegia.

Remediation of cognitive, perceptual, and behavioral deficits presents a greater challenge. Checklists and a consistent arrangement of grooming tools in the bathroom assist patients who have sequencing, organization, or memory deficits.[39] A set routine of grooming and hygiene tasks can be developed during therapy sessions for carryover after discharge. Patients experiencing apraxia and agnosia benefit most from consistent, repetitious instruction in grooming activities. Hand-over-hand guidance through the task with a minimum of verbal instruction is most useful.

Some patients seem uninterested in their appearance. Incorporating grooming activities into the daily routine early in rehabilitation may habituate appropriate behavior. Even patients at a low level of function can engage in structured, assisted grooming tasks. Behavior programs to reinforce compliance with grooming expectations may be necessary for some individuals.

❏ TREATING DEFICITS IN INSTRUMENTAL ACTIVITIES OF DAILY LIVING

Instrumental ADLs include the tasks necessary for care of the home and independence within the community.[40] Time management, homemaking, communication tasks, social skills, financial management, driving, and use of transportation are instrumental ADLs (IADLs). Because each IADL is not applicable to each adult, occupational therapists rely on data gathered during evaluation to determine pertinent IADLs. Once relevant IADLs are selected, analysis of evaluation findings identifies the problematic performance components.

Communication Tasks

Communication tasks include writing, using the telephone, correspondence, and transmittal of information. Writing is typically affected by physical impairments or language impairments. Speech-language pathology addresses language skills. In occupational therapy, attention is given to the mechanics of writing.[41] Weighted or adapted writing implements address problems with grip and control of the writing tool. Practice in letter formation is appropriate treatment for patients who must change dominance or who are experiencing apraxia. Techniques to overcome visual field cuts or hemi-inattention, such as anchoring or guidelines, are useful. Consistent verbal and tactile feedback seems to decrease perseveration during writing. Computer technology, such as touch screens, eye gaze systems, and alternative controls and keyboards, offers an alternate solution for patients unable to regain skill in writing.

Performance components of phone use include the ability to dial and handle the phone, directory use to locate a number, ability to convey and receive information, and phone etiquette. A number of adaptive devices for phones, including receiver holders, large dials, environmental control units, and speakers, are available commercially. Local telephone companies offer services and equipment to persons whose disabilities limit access to the telephone.

Phone directory use requires organizational, visual, and memory skills. Magnification devices aid patients with visual impairments. Patients with impaired organizational skills need progressively more complex practice and drill exercises. Writing down numbers before dialing can be recommended to patients as a compensatory strategy. Technology also exists to permit presetting of phone numbers to permit automatic dialing upon selection. A personalized, single-page directory kept by the phone eliminates the need to use the phone directory.

Conveying and receiving information over the phone is critical for independence in the home. During therapy, the clinician guides the patient through simulated or real conversations to make doctor's appointments, ask for product information, or deal with local service agencies by phone. Role playing in social skills training sessions serves to reinforce phone etiquette. Emergency use of the phone must be assessed prior to discharge into a residential environment. Cue cards or presetting the phone for local emergency services can be options for some patients. Some individuals must master use of computers, fax machines, copiers, and other communication technology for vocational or personal use. Job coaches, vocational trainers, occupational therapists, and others assist patients in the retraining and adaptation process.

Time Management

Performance components of time management include the ability to organize available time to meet vocational, educational, social, recreational, home, and family needs. The establishment of a therapy schedule during rehabilitation is a starting point for retraining time management. The rehabilitation schedule should include the 24-hour day; such comprehensive planning permits scheduling of therapeutic intervention during the early morning, evening, and night and provides continual structure for the patient early in recovery.

Patients experiencing disorientation benefit from inclusion in a reality orientation program.[42] As patients use their schedules throughout the day, staff provide reorientation. Clocks and calendars should be placed liberally throughout the inpatient facility, residential facility, and home for patient use. As patients are able, the use of a wristwatch is encouraged. Normalization of waking and bedtime in the inpatient setting is recommended; this helps the patient develop a sleep-wake cycle favorable to the home routine on discharge.

Although initially patients need structured assistance to follow the therapy schedule, responsibility for keeping an appointment schedule, arriving at appointments on time, and completing tasks in a timely fashion is gradually shifted to the patient. Schedules attached to wheelchairs, memory notebooks, and appointment books have been successful for some patients.[43]

Constructive use of leisure time poses problems for some patients. Patients who are unable to generate alternate activities may be found wandering, asleep, or idle during unscheduled time. The ease and accessibility of television may lead to its overuse. Escalation of agitation or restlessness has been noted during unstructured time.[44] The team and family need to guide the patient toward constructive activity. Intervention from a therapeutic recreation specialist to address avocational interests and leisure education is particularly beneficial for patients who have few leisure interests with which they can be successful postinjury.[45]

Social Skills

Impairments in social skills are manifested in a number of ways. Some patients are agitated and restless. Other patients are lethargic and uncommunicative. There may be a lack of inhibition or a diminished sense of social norms and customs. Egocentricity or lack of interest can interfere with marriage relationships and parenting. Some patients lack self-awareness and therefore do not recognize the impact of their verbalizations and behavior on others.[46]

Social skills retraining often includes group treatment, which allows opportunities for role play. Group members are encouraged to give feedback to one another on the effectiveness of interactions and behavior. Videotaping group members can promote self-awareness.[47]

Social skills group sessions often lead to community reintegration tasks, such as eating out, shopping, or going bowling. Before going into the community, the interdisciplinary team helps patients plan the outing and practice needed social behaviors. Behavioral expectations are carefully outlined. The staff-patient ratio during the outing must allow therapists to provide patients with immediate feedback and individualized guidance.

Family inclusion in the social skills retraining process is critical. Poor social skills trouble families, destroy friendships, and limit vocational opportunities. The behavior programs utilized to modify unacceptable behavior and foster acceptable behavior can be valuable to family and friends, who often benefit from early inclusion in the program. Team members provide instruction and model interactions with the patient to help family members learn effective approaches.[46]

Many families appreciate instruction and direction from the team and willingly employ learned techniques. Some families are less comfortable with the team's suggestions and may continue interactions or approaches that undermine rather than promote good social skills. Treatment teams need to accept the fact that sometimes family dynamics cannot be changed. Teams must always keep social expectations for patients high. Although it is easy for health care professionals to excuse inappropriate social interaction in a therapeutic environment, society at large is not as forgiving. Indeed, patients with poor social skills may be doomed to ostracism and isolation without the team's assistance in developing effective skills.

Homemaking

Homemaking includes tasks such as parenting, cooking, marketing, home cleaning and maintenance, clothing care, shopping, and yard duties. These tasks are highly complex and often require long, intensive retraining. Because the safety issues surrounding these activities are so significant, families need to understand the patient's level of performance in these tasks as well as supervision requirements.[48]

The patient's interest in particular homemaking tasks, as well as physical and cognitive capability, usually dictates the starting point for retraining.[32] Therapy should begin at a point where the patient will be successful and then graded into more challenging tasks. Throughout retraining, the clinician notes points of breakdown in performance; remedial activities are subsequently designed to address these areas of deficit.

Adaptive devices often prove valuable for patients with physical deficits in managing homemaking activities. Reachers, mirrors above large appliances, and adapted kitchen utensils are obtainable from mail order suppliers. Lightweight, one-handed kitchen appliances and vacuum cleaners are increasingly used by able-bodied homemakers. After a home evaluation, architectural changes to permit wheelchair access to some areas in the home are sometimes recommended. Lowered countertops, widened doors, placement of high stools in the kitchen, and ramping are all options for home adaptation.

Cognitive and behavioral deficits can affect homemaking skills. Scheduling of routine tasks aids patients with impaired memory or mildly impaired initiation. Meticulous organization and labeling of shelves, cabinets, and closets assist with retrieval of supplies. Timers remind patients to return to a task, such as checking on brownies in the oven or moving washed laundry to the clothesdryer. Checklists in strategic locations can facilitate independent completion of specific, repetitious tasks such as washing clothes or packing a child's lunch.

Home safety arises as a concern as discharge nears. When memory, attention, quality control, and initiation are significantly impaired, the patient may not be able to manage homemaking without a helper. The team's findings as the patient engages in homemaking tasks and their recommendations based on performance provide needed information for discharge planning.

Homemaking retraining continues in day treatment and transitional living programs in which continued structure and therapy for individuals who cannot manage homemaking independently but possess potential for higher-level function is offered.[49] When patients are discharged to home, homemaking can be addressed either in home health therapy or outpatient therapy. Home-based therapy is clearly optimal for retraining home management skills.

Financial Management

Financial management includes handling cash money, banking activities, and budgeting. Determination of the patient's skills before injury focuses retraining in financial management tasks.

Therapy for financial management is a sequential process. It begins with identification and valuation of coins and bills. Matching activities and drill work are beneficial for patients at this level. At the next level, patients practice basic mathematical skills as a precursor to handling money. In some cases, language function may be too impaired to permit understanding of money concepts or communication of responses to the clinicians. Cotreatment by speech pathology and occupational therapy can be attempted with these patients.

Next, patients work on simple addition of coins. Like coins are easiest to add. Patients begin by counting by denomination amounts, such as by fives or tens. Clinicians then introduce addition of unlike coins. Performing calculations on paper assists some patients who have difficulty with mental computations. As proficiency increases, paper money is added to coins during calculation practice.

Once basic computations are mastered, change-making skills are introduced. Change-making involves more complex computation, and often patients require written and verbal assistance to relearn the task. Memory impairments and decreased attention seem to particularly affect change-making skills.

Money management skills practiced in the clinical setting may be applied during community outings. Trips to restaurants, a movie, a mall, and a grocery store provide opportunities for money management. Families are advised to incorporate money management tasks into activities while the patient is on therapeutic leave.

Banking skills and budgeting can be included in the therapy program when the patient is ready. Relearning the mechanics of banking transactions is easier than becoming independent in budgeting. Writing checks, managing the check register, engaging in banking interactions, and using the automated teller are practiced within the clinical setting and then moved into the community.

Budgeting requires the ability to look ahead and make decisions based on an assessment of the past and the plan for the future. Organizational skills, memory, anticipation, and the ability to discern needs from wants are facets of this task. Budgeting training often occurs at the postacute level. Increased structure within the task assists patients who have cognitive problems. Patients with significant cognitive deficits, however, may always need assistance with this complex area of financial management. In some cases, the patient's diminished capacity for sensible decision making may necessitate appointment of a guardian to manage finances.

☐ USE OF GROUP TREATMENT IN RETRAINING ACTIVITIES OF DAILY LIVING

Utilization of group treatment varies across disciplines within rehabilitation. Neuropsychology, recreation therapy, speech pathology, and occupational therapy frequently use group treatment to meet patient goals. Among the advantages are their appeal to the social nature of humans, opportunities for peer feedback, and their cost-effectiveness.

Groups may focus on skills acquisition, support, or education. Groups may be led by a single discipline or by different specialists on the team. Frequency and duration of group treatment vary according to the goals of the sessions. Although the inclusion of families is important in some groups, such as cooking, it is deleterious in other groups. Families need clear instruction about their role in group treatment.

Skills acquisition groups are beneficial during retraining of ADLs and the performance components necessary for ADL tasks. Cooking groups,[32,50] reality orientation groups,[42] leisure skills groups,[45] and social skills groups[47,48] are examples of skills acquisition groups. Cotreatment is frequently done in skills acquisition groups. A cooking group may include physical therapy if group members need to practice ambulation skills while in the kitchen. Neuropsychology may become part of the cooking group if behavior and safety are concerns. The occupational therapist and speech pathologist may colead the social skills group. The recreational therapist may request involvement from the occupational therapist for a leisure skills group if a patient's perceptual deficits are interfering with task performance.

The format and structure of skill acquisition groups depend on the patients' needs and goals. When patients are at a lower functional level, the professionals responsible for the group play a significant role in planning and leadership. As the patients improve, they take greater responsibility for the group.

planning. Patient-centered programming seeks to meet the needs of the consumer as the team works in concert to help patients attain a maximal level of performance in their ADLs.

REFERENCES

1. Oddy, M, et al: Stresses upon the relatives of head-injured patients. Br J Psychiatry 133:507, 1978.
2. Northern, JG, et al: Involvement of adult rehabilitation patients in setting occupational therapy goals. Am J Occup Ther 49:214, 1995.
3. Arnadottir, G: The Brain and Behavior: Assessing Cortical Dysfunction through Activities of Daily Living. Mosby, St Louis, 1990.
4. Rimel, RW, et al: Moderate brain injury: Completing the clinical spectrum of brain trauma. Neurosurgery 11:344, 1982.
5. Filiatraut, J, et al: Motor function and ADL assessments: A study of 3 tests for persons with hemiplegia. Am J Occup Ther 45:806, 1991.
6. Zoltan, B, et al: Perceptual and Cognitive Dysfunction in the Adult Stroke Patient: A Manual for Evaluation and Treatment, ed 2. Slack, Thorofare, NJ, 1986.
7. Adamovich, BB, et al: Cognitive Rehabilitation of Closed Head Injured Patients: A Dynamic Approach. College-Hill Press, San Diego, 1985.
8. Groher, ME: Communication disorders in adults. In Rosenthal, M, et al (eds): Rehabilitation of the Adult and Child with Traumatic Brain Injury, ed 2. FA Davis, Philadelphia, 1990, p 148.
9. Rosenthal, M, and Bond, MR: Behavioral and psychiatric sequelae. In Rosenthal, M, et al (eds): Rehabilitation of the Adult and Child with Traumatic Brain Injury, ed 2. FA Davis, Philadelphia, 1990, p 179.
10. Davidoff, G, et al: Cognitive dysfunction and mild closed head injury in traumatic spinal cord injury. Arch Phys Med Rehabil 66:489, 1985.
11. Wilmot, CB, et al: Occult head injury: Its incidence in spinal cord injury. Arch Phys Med Rehabil 66:227, 1985.
12. Matsutsuyu, JS: Interest checklist. Am J Occup Ther 23:323, 1969.
13. Kielhofner, G, and Henry, AD: Development and investigation of the occupational performance history interview. Am J Occup Ther 42:489, 1988.
14. Kline, RM, and Bell, BJ: Klein-Bell Activities of Daily Living Scale: Manual. University of Washington, Division of Occupational Therapy, Seattle, 1979.
15. Iverson, IA: Revised Kenny Self Care Evaluation: A Numerical Measure of Independence in ADL (Publication 722). Sister Kenny Institute, Minneapolis, 1973.
16. Kohlman-Thomson, L: The Kohlman Evaluation of Living Skills, ed 3. American Occupational Therapy Association, Rockville, Md, 1992.
17. Fisher, A: The assessment of motor and process skills. In Katz, N (ed): Cognitive Rehabilitation: Models for Intervention in Occupational Therapy. Andover, Boston, 1991.
18. Rappaport, M, et al: Disability Rating Scale for severe head trauma: Coma to community. Arch Phys Med Rehabil 63:118, 1982.
19. Hagen, C, et al: Levels of cognitive functioning. In Rehabilitation of the Head Injured Adult: Comprehensive Physical Management. Professional Staff Association of Rancho Los Amigos Hospital, Downey, Calif, 1979.
20. Carey, RG, and Posavac, EJ: Rehabilitation program evaluation using a revised Level of Rehabilitation Scale. Arch Phys Med Rehabil 63:367, 1982.
21. Harvey, RF, and Jellinek, HM: Functional performance assessment: A program approach. Arch Phys Med Rehabil 62:456, 1981.
22. Mahoney, FI, and Barthel, DW: Functional evaluation: The Barthel Index. Md State Med J 44:61, 1965.
23. Keith, RA, et al: The Functional Independence Measure: A new tool for rehabilitation. In Eisenberg, MG, and Grzesiak, RC (eds): Advances in Clinical Rehabilitation, vol 1. Springer-Verlag, New York, 1987, p 6.
24. Law, M, and Letts, L: A critical review of scales of activities of daily living. Am J Occup Ther 43:522, 1989.
25. Fisher, AG: Functional assessment, Part 2: Selecting the right test, minimizing the limitations. Am J Occup Ther 46:278, 1992.
26. Brown, C, et al: Influence of instrumental activities of daily living assessment method on judgments of independence. Am J Occup Ther 50:202, 1996.
27. Sbordone, RJ: A conceptual model of neuro-psychologically-based cognitive rehabilitation. In Williams, JM, and Long, CJ (eds): The Rehabilitation of Cognitive Disabilities. Plenum, New York, 1987.
28. Law, M: Evaluating activities of daily living: Directions for the future. Am J Occup Ther 47:233, 1993.
29. Neistadt, ME: The neurobiology of learning: Implications for treatment of adults with brain injury. Am J Occup Ther 48:421, 1994.
30. Neistadt, ME: A critical analysis of occupational therapy approaches for perceptual deficits in adults with brain injury. Am J Occup Ther 44:299, 1990.
31. Toglia, J: Generalization of treatment: A multi-contextual approach to cognitive perceptual impairment in adults with brain injury. Am J Occup Ther 45:505, 1991.
32. Neistadt, ME: A meal preparation treatment protocol for adults with brain injury. Am J Occup Ther 48:431, 1994.
33. Logemann, JA: Evaluation and Treatment of Swallowing Disorders. College-Hill Press, San Diego, 1983.
34. Avery-Smith, W, and Dellarosa, DM: Approaches to treating dysphagia in patients with brain injury. Am J Occup Ther 48:235, 1994.
35. Groher, ME: Formulating feeding decisions for acute dysphagic patients. Occupational Therapy Practice 3:26, 1992.
36. Davis, ES, and Radomski, MV: Domain-specific training to reinstate habit sequences. Occupational Therapy Practice 1:79, 1989.
37. Warren, M: Relationship of constructional apraxia and body scheme disorders to dressing performance in adult CVA. Am J Occup Ther 35:431, 1981.
38. Baum, B, and Hall, KM: Relationship between constructional praxis and dressing in the head-injured adult. Am J Occup Ther 35:438, 1981.
39. Giles, GM, and Shore, M: A rapid method for teaching severely brain injured adults how to wash and dress. Arch Phys Med Rehabil 70:156, 1989.
40. Lawton, MP, and Brody, E: Assessment of older people: Self-maintaining and instrumental ADL. Gerontologist 9:179, 1969.
41. Rioux, JF, and Kagan, JR: Evaluation and treatment of adult graphomotor deficiencies. Physical Disabilities Special Interest Section Newsletter 2:1, 1988.
42. McNeny, R, and Dise, J: Reality orientation therapy. In Rosenthal, M, et al (eds): Rehabilitation of the Adult and Child with Traumatic Brain Injury, ed 2. FA Davis, Philadelphia, 1990, p 366.
43. Story, TB: Cognitive rehabilitation services in home and community settings. In Kreutzer, JS, and Wehman, PH (eds): Cognitive Rehabilitation for Persons with Traumatic Brain Injury: A Functional Approach. Paul H Brookes, Baltimore, 1991.
44. McNeny, R, and Benjamin, J: Agitation in the therapy setting: Managing the patient with brain injury. NeuroRehabilitation 5:211, 1995.
45. Berger, JP, and Regalski, AE: Therapeutic recreation. In Rosenthal, M, et al (eds): Rehabilitation of the Adult and Child with Traumatic Brain Injury, ed 2. FA Davis, Philadelphia, 1990, p 449.
46. Mateer, CA, and Williams, D: Management of psychosocial and behavior problems in cognitive rehabilitation. In Kreutzer, JS, and Wehman, PH (eds): Cognitive Rehabilitation for Persons with Traumatic Brain Injury: A Functional Approach. Paul H Brookes, Baltimore, 1991.
47. Deaton, A: Group intervention for cognitive rehabilitation: Increasing the challenges. In Kreutzer, JS, and

Wehman, PH (eds): Cognitive Rehabilitation for Persons with Traumatic Brain Injury: A Functional Approach. Paul H Brookes, Baltimore, 1991.

48. McNeny, R: Daily living skills: The foundation for community living. In Kreutzer, JS, and Wehman, P (eds): Community Integration following Traumatic Brain Injury. Paul H Brookes, Baltimore, 1990.

49. Boake, C: Transitional living centers in head injury rehabilitation. In Kreutzer, JS, and Wehman, P (eds): Community Integration following Traumatic Brain Injury. Paul H Brookes, Baltimore, 1990.

50. Phzybylak, R: Special meal preparation groups in head injury rehabilitation. OT Forum April 30, 1993, p 16.

51. Korteling, JE, and Katpein, MA: Neuropsychological driving fitness tests for brain-damaged subjects. Arch Phys Med Rehabil 77:138, 1996.

52. Galski, T, et al: Prediction of behind-the-wheel driving performance in patients with cerebral brain damage: A discriminant function analysis. Am J Occup Ther 47:391, 1993.

53. Gouvier, WD, et al: Psychometric prediction of driver performance among the disabled. Arch Phys Med Rehabil 70:745, 1993.

54. Sivak, M, et al: Driving and perceptual/cognitive skills: Behavioral consequences of brain damage. Arch Phys Med Rehabil 62:476, 1981.

Cognitive Rehabilitation

CATHERINE A. MATEER, PHD,
and SARAH RASKIN, PHD

❑ APPROACHES TO COGNITIVE REHABILITATION

Cognitive impairments are among the most common and disruptive sequelae of traumatic brain injury (TBI) and invariably are a focus of rehabilitative efforts. The goal of rehabilitation should be to improve the adaptive functioning of people in the setting in which they will be living or working. Accommodation to and for cognitive impairments is often a critical variable in the success of rehabilitation efforts. Although the nature and severity of cognitive impairments vary widely in individuals who have sustained TBI, problems with attention and concentration, with memory and new learning, and with executive functions are among the most frequent and problematic. This chapter focuses on these areas.

Problems in adaptive functioning arise in relation to cognitive impairments when there is either (1) a decrease in a given skill without an accompanying decrease in the environmental demands placed on the person or (2) an increase in environmental demands without an accompanying increase in the skills required for successful performance.[1] Consistent with this view, most rehabilitative approaches for management of cognitive impairments take one of three forms: environmental modifications, the training and implementation of compensatory skills and/or behaviors, and direct retraining in the areas of cognitive impairment.

Environmental Modifications

Environmental modifications include approaches to rehabilitation that alter factors external to the client with minimal or no expectation of underlying change in the individual's capacities. Included in this category are manipulations that decrease the demands on the individual, such as simplifying tasks, eliminating the need to do certain tasks, or allowing more time to complete activities. Other manipulations consistent with this approach include provision of external support in the form of oral or written cue systems, so that less reliance on memory is necessary, and the alteration of environmental parameters, such as reducing potential distractions. There is usually an inherent assumption that such external manipulations may need to remain in place if the improvement in functioning is to continue.

Compensatory Approaches

In contrast to approaches that focus on environmental manipulations, others have, as a primary goal, the training of compensatory behaviors or skills. Such an approach might include training the individual to independently record in and refer to a memory system or organizer. Approaches that attempt to increase self-awareness or that teach self-regulatory or metacognitive strategies could also be included here. A compensation might include a new behavior or substitute skill (such as making lists for shopping) and/or an increase in time, effort, or both (such as in studying). The injured person may also adapt to a new situation by changing self-expectations, selecting new tasks, or relaxing the criteria for success. Whether people are taught to use the compensation or develop it on their own, they are active participants in its application.

To some extent, severity of impairment is believed to affect the extent to which compensation is spontaneously adopted. Moderately impaired individuals are most likely to compensate, whereas mildly impaired individuals may be unaware of the need to compensate, and severely impaired individuals may lack the skill and insight to implement compensatory behavior without substantial training and support. It is also important to recognize that the use of a particular compensation may have a negative trade-off. Compensatory behaviors should optimize and not hinder utilization of available resources, including the residual capacity of the injured system. Implementation of compensatory behaviors should also consider the consequences for the individual and for others in the individual's environment.

Direct Interventions

Direct interventions use procedures that aim to improve or restore some underlying ability or cognitive capacity.[2] They include a myriad of approaches for improving underlying cognitive skills, such as attention, memory, planning, and problem solving. Sohlberg and Mateer[3] described what they termed a "process oriented approach" to the rehabilitation of cognitive impairments. The basic tenets of this approach include a solid understanding of the specific cognitive area involved and a detailed analysis of the nature of impairments in that area. Then, hierarchical training exercises are designed to stimulate and rebuild the impaired skills. Repetition is believed to be critical to the reautomatization of skills.

Factors Important to the Selection of a Treatment Approach

In general, patients who demonstrate little behavioral initiative or flexibility, who are environmentally dependent with apparently minimal self-regulation of behavior, or who are minimally aware of their deficits tend to respond better and more consistently to external manipulations. For these patients, environmental manipulations, behavioral strategies, and external cuing systems are often effective in decreasing maladaptive behaviors and increasing function. Patients who demonstrate greater behavioral initiative and flexibility, who initiate and direct their own behavior to some degree, and who are somewhat aware of the change in their abilities resulting from their injury are more likely to demonstrate improvements with cognitive-behavioral interventions, process-oriented cognitive training, training in the use of compensatory devices,

and training in the use of self-instructional and metacognitive strategies. It is important, therefore, to match the profile of the patient with the intervention approach.[4,5]

A comprehensive evaluation of each patient's cognitive profile is a critical first step in developing the rehabilitation plan. Although beyond the scope of this chapter, detailed cognitive, communicative, behavioral, emotional, and psychosocial evaluations should be conducted with each client. After an evaluation of the cognitive-behavioral profile of the individual and determination of the observed or anticipated real-world impact of the cognitive deficits, it is necessary to establish specific, mutually agreed upon rehabilitation goals, given the client's current and future circumstances.[6] Mutual goal setting can boost motivation and result in the patient's increased participation in the intervention. Other principles include encouraging choice in therapy, working collaboratively with clients and their families, creating a supportive environment, reinforcing clients for their efforts, asking clients to assess their progress, and providing clients with an effective and meaningful method for accomplishing tasks. The intervention plan should be constantly monitored for efficacy, in concert with the goals of treatment and with the plan for generalization.

Measurement of Generalization

The importance of generalization of treatment to daily life is ingrained in clinical practice.[7] However, an understanding of generalization and how to facilitate it is still, for the most part, lacking in the field of cognitive rehabilitation. Generalization of cognitive rehabilitation has been described by Gordon[8] in three levels: The first level is that the gains from remediation should hold true on the same materials on separate occasions. The second is that improvement on the training tasks is also observed on a similar but not identical set of tasks. The third level of generalization is that the functions gained in training are shown to transfer to functions in day-to-day living.

Sohlberg and Raskin[9] suggested a set of generalization principles or strategies that could be broadly adapted in both research and clinical practice in cognitive rehabilitation. These principles, drawn primarily from the applied behavioral literature[10] and from the cognitive psychology literature on transfer of training,[11] are (1) actively plan for and program generalization from the beginning of the treatment process, (2) identify reinforcements in the natural environment, (3) program stimuli common to both training environments and the real world, (4) use sufficient examples when conducting therapy, and (5) select a method for measuring generalization.

Perhaps the most difficult aspect of adhering to these principles is selecting the measure of generalization. Helpful in this regard is the development of a number of questionnaires that focus on everyday aspects of attention,[12] memory,[13] and executive function.[14,15] In addition to these measures, which focus on specific cognitive functions, it is also useful to incorporate measures that address broader aspects of everyday functioning and serve to structure observations related to social interaction, productive activities, and independence (e.g., the Community Integration Questionnaire[16] and the Craig Handicap Assessment and Reporting Technique[17]).

Dealing with the Emotional Consequences of Cognitive Loss

It has become increasingly evident that many individuals need assistance in dealing with the emotional consequences of acquired cognitive impairment. Because adjusting to changes in one's abilities is often difficult, fear, frustration, and feelings of loss are common emotional responses for both the brain injured individual and his or her family. The importance of providing assistance in dealing with the emotional responses to these changes in functioning cannot be underestimated. An appreciation for the organic or nonvolitional nature of the behavior is often helpful in alleviating the fears and misconceptions of family members and caregivers. Although several approaches to working with issues of adjustment are discussed in the context of specific cognitive interventions here, the reader is referred to other chapters in this book for a deeper discussion of this area.

The following sections consider assessment and intervention for three of the most common cognitive sequelae of TBI: attention, memory, and executive function disorders. The focus is on adults with TBI, although many of the rehabilitative strategies and techniques discussed have been used in children with developmental and acquired cognitive disorders. For a review of the pediatric cognitive rehabilitation literature, the reader is referred to Mateer et al.[18]

☐ APPROACHES TO MANAGING ATTENTIONAL DISORDERS

Understanding Attentional Disorders in Traumatic Brain Injury

Impairments in attention, concentration, distractibility, and "slowed thinking" are among the most commonly reported cognitive problems following TBI.[19,20] People with TBI often describe taking more time to complete tasks, having difficulty concentrating on tasks in noisy or busy environments, experiencing problems doing more than one thing at once, and forgetting what they were about to say or do. Although a comprehensive understanding of the nature of attentional problems in TBI remains to be developed, a number of possible contributors to attentional deficits have been experimentally investigated in this population.

One of the most consistent findings in individuals with a wide range of TBI severity has been slowed reaction time or slowed speed of information processing.[21–23] Several investigators have suggested that this slowness in information processing underlies most, if not all, of what is interpreted as attentional difficulties.

Despite frequent reports of oversensitivity to noise or distraction in TBI patients,[24] research regarding this aspect of attention has been mixed. Stuss et al.[25] reported that TBI subjects appeared to engage in unnecessary processing of redundant information, which might be interpreted as a kind of distractibility. Other investigators have reported generalized slowing of performance as a function of information load, but no direct correlation with degree of distraction per se.[22,26] Patients with TBI have quite consistently demonstrated difficulty on a number of measures requiring shifting of response set and inhibition of automatic responses,[27,28] as well as on tasks requiring divided attention capabilities.[25,29,30]

MEMORY DIFFICULTIES RELATED TO ATTENTION

Memory difficulties are a commonly recognized sequela of TBI. In that attention paid to information is a crucial factor in its later recall,[31,32] it has been suggested that, for a portion of the TBI population, memory may be secondarily impaired because of a disorder of attention.[33–35] Mateer et al.[13] reported results of a self-report questionnaire regarding the frequency of different kinds of forgetting failures. Subjects who had sustained TBI reported that their most frequent forgetting experiences appeared to be related to attention and prospective memory. Although beyond the scope of this chapter, a review of the experimental support for and against this notion can be found in a recent report by Schmitter-Edgecombe.[36]

The Assessment of Attention

Although a detailed discussion of the assessment of attention is not possible here, it is important to recognize that attentional capacity should be addressed from several perspectives. Observation of the individual during the evaluation can provide information about arousal levels, the ability to maintain effort over time, and distractibility. Many psychometric measures tap into different aspects of attention, and it is important to use a variety of sensitive measures to capture relevant information about the attentional system. Tests should include measurements of sustained attention or vigilance, such as continuous performance tasks; measures of working memory, such as Digit Span and mental arithmetic; measures of speeded processing, such as Digit Symbol, Paced Auditory Serial Addition Test (PASAT), and Trail Making; and measures requiring higher levels of attentional control and set shifting, such as the Stroop test.

There is increasing concern among clinicians that standardized psychometric measures of attention may not reflect the degree or nature of attention deficits in naturalistic contexts.[37] An understanding of patients' attentional abilities in the environment in which they function is necessary to allow the clinician to design a rehabilitation program that can actively facilitate the transfer of improvements in therapy to functional activities. There has been increasing interest in the use of questionnaires to investigate the degree and nature of everyday failures in cognitive ability. Ponsford and Kinsella[12] used a self-report measure of common attentional problems that conform to a hierarchical view of attention with patients with TBI. Patients' perceptions of their attentional abilities compared with others' direct observations of their functioning may provide valuable information for designing a rehabilitation program.

Specific Intervention Approaches for Individuals with Attentional Disorders

"Conventional wisdom" suggests such compensatory or environmental approaches as reducing noise or visual distraction, performing only a single task at a time, breaking down tasks into smaller steps, and reducing the impact of stress and fatigue as helpful for people who have attentional impairment. Despite limited research to support the efficacy of these interventions to guide how and when they might best be used, they certainly have some face validity. Practical suggestions for avoiding distraction, taking breaks, and reducing "cognitive overload" can help people with TBI in several respects. First, by reducing the effects of overload and fatigue, they often result in increased performance and decreased frustration. Sec-

ond, they serve as an acknowledgment to patients of their subjective experience. Recognition of people's feelings of frustration and perception of changed mental abilities often increases a sense of trust and mutual understanding between client and therapist. The suggestions assist those who are feeling overwhelmed and "victimized" by their cognitive difficulties in gaining a sense of control and self-efficacy. Use of such techniques can improve their ability to manage both the external environment and their internal emotional state.

More controversial, although actually more rigorously investigated, are the direct retraining techniques for working with individuals with attentional impairments. Many people with traumatic brain injury have been shown to benefit substantially from exercise and training of attentional skills. Indeed, some of the earliest work to demonstrate positive findings in cognitive rehabilitation involved systematic intervention focused on the attentional system,[38–42] and the literature on the rehabilitation of attention after traumatic brain injury is now substantial. (See Mateer and Mapou[43] for a review of the literature.) Table 15–1 lists studies of attention orga-

---

TABLE 15–1. Studies Demonstrating Efficacy of Attention Training

Evidence for improvement on trained tasks
Ben-Yishay, Piasetsky, and Rattock[38]
Diller, et al.[39]
Wood and Fussey[42]

Evidence for improvement on psychometric measures of attention
Ethier, Baribeau, and Braun[44]
Ethier, Braun, and Baribeau[45]
Gray and Robertson[46]
Gray et al.[47]
Sohlberg and Mateer[41]
Sturm et al.[48]

Evidence for improvement on other cognitive abilities
Mateer[33]
Mateer and Sohlberg[34]
Mateer, Sohlberg, and Youngman[49]
Niemann, Ruff, and Baser[50]
Ruff et al.[51]
Sturm and Willmes[52]

Evidence for improvement on functional tasks
Ponsford and Kinsella[53] (increased time directed to task during a clerical activity, but insignificant psychometric gains)
Sivak, Hill, and Olson[54] (improved driving performance)
Wood[55]

nized according to the level at which a significant improvement was measured—that is, on trained tasks, on independent (untrained) measures of attention, on an independent measure of another related cognitive ability, and on functional tasks.

The major premise of direct intervention approaches is that attentional abilities can be improved by exercising one or more particular aspects of attention. Treatment has usually engaged patients in a series of repetitive drills or exercises, designed to provide opportunities for practice on tasks with increasingly greater attentional demands. Repeated activation and stimulation of attentional systems are hypothesized to facilitate changes in cognitive capacity.

Although a wide variety of treatment tasks have been used in experimental studies of attention training, the *Attention Process Training*[56] and *Attention Process Training II*[57] (APT II) materials developed by Sohlberg et al. have been used in many clinical settings. The materials are hierarchically organized tasks designed to exercise sustained, selective, alternating, and divided attention. APT II, developed for individuals with higher-level attentional abilities, provides more complex and demanding tasks. In both programs, tasks make increasingly greater demands on complex attentional control and working memory. Examples of tasks are listening for descending number sequences, shifting set on a series of Stroop-like activities, alphabetizing words in sentences, detecting targets under noise conditions, and dividing attention between multiple tasks (e.g., card sorting by suit and letter; combined auditory target detection and visual cancellation). In one study,[41] multiple baseline designs revealed improvements on a complex measure of attention (i.e., the PASAT) after training, but no evidence of improvement on an unrelated visuospatial task. This latter finding argued against a generalized effect related to stimulation. Similar gains on measures of attention have been demonstrated by other researchers who used paper and pencil, auditory, or computer-based training exercises.[44-48,50]

If attention actually improves after such training, changes in other cognitive abilities dependent on attention, such as memory, would be expected, as well as in functional skills dependent on attention. In a series of studies, Mateer et al.[33,34,49] reported improved scores following attention training not only on measures of attention but also on measures of memory and learning in patients who had sustained mild and moderate to severe TBI. Similar findings of improved memory ability after attention training were reported by Niemann[58] and by Ruff et al.[51] in adults with TBI and by Sturm and Willmes[52] in patients with stroke.

A major concern about attention training exercises has been the problem of generalization. For many functions, therapy is clearly most effective when the patient practices skills in the manner and setting in which they will be used. Redevelopment of basic eating, dressing, and grooming abilities in more severely injured individuals relies heavily on repetitive practice of these abilities in as natural a context as possible. However, simply engaging an individual in a "naturalistic" activity may not be sufficient to address the specific higher-level cognitive deficits that are disrupting performance. Most naturalistic activities (e.g., cooking, money management, and driving) are multidimensional, depend on many different cognitive processes (e.g., reasoning, visuoperceptual processing, executive functions, and attention), and hence may not directly target the underlying impairments in attentional control. Attentional exercises can, however, be incorporated into natural settings and tasks as part of the generalization program.

The APT II generalization program also makes use of two attention "logs," the Attention Lapse Log and the Attention Success Log. These protocols provide an organized way of recording both breakdowns and successes in attention in naturalistic settings throughout the patient's day. They increase the patient's awareness of the situations in which attention is difficult and help in focusing treatment. Not only the nature of the lapse or the success is recorded but also how the individual responded to the lapse or failure. This program often yields insights about ways in which the individual responds emotionally and behaviorally to variations in performance. Reasons for successes and failures become more apparent, and the frequency and impact of the attentional problems may become clearer. The success log provides a focus for discussing how patients can take a more active role in managing and controlling both attentionally demanding situations and their own response to cognitive successes or failures. It can also become a focus for discussing and evaluating the effectiveness of stress management techniques. The individual can be helped to feel a greater sense of self-control over the environment. This "empowerment" phase often leads to a redefinition of self in relation to cognitive inefficiency.

Although the attentional system does appear quite vulnerable to disruption, this system also appears open to modification by targeted intervention. Indeed, among those areas of cognitive processing that have been addressed in the cognitive rehabilitation literature, perhaps the most compelling findings are those that pertain to the improvement and management of attentional impairments. A concerted and well-founded focus on these areas can often result in patients' satisfaction and in demonstrable functional improvements.[54]

☐ REMEDIATION AND MANAGEMENT OF MEMORY DISORDERS

Problems with memory and new learning are very commonly experienced following TBI. The nature and severity of memory problems vary considerably, as do approaches to management of memory impairment. Some approaches are based on techniques that help ordinary individuals remember better, and some are specifically based on what is known about the effects of brain injury. Most recently, approaches from cognitive science and learning theory have been applied to memory rehabilitation, including those that attempt to improve memory ability, provide compensatory approaches through either externally or internally focused manipulations, and maximize the likelihood of learning and remembering in individuals with memory impairments. The particular approach taken in any one case depends on the nature and severity of the deficit, the degree of insight, the goals of the patient, the environmental demands and expectations, and other factors. Before developing treatment strategies, the clinician should undertake a thorough evaluation of the client's memory functioning. There are many standardized measures of memory. Although a detailed discussion of memory assessment cannot be included here, the examination should cover all of the major divisions of memory (e.g., immediate, short term and long term, episodic and semantic, declarative and procedural) from a cognitive perspective and, most importantly, evaluate the demands on the patient in the current and projected living and/or working environment.

Externally Focused Approaches to Managing Memory Impairment

Environmental modification may decrease the need for retrieval of specific information from memory. Included in this category are environmental cues, such as large signs posted in the home that remind the person where items are located or how a machine or appliance (e.g., a computer or washing machine) is operated. These types of modifications can be used in the home, work, or school environment. Environmental modification also includes removing environmental dangers. For example, in cases of severe memory impairment, the stove may be disabled, and the patient uses only a microwave oven that cannot create a fire hazard by being left on accidentally.

Cues and checklists are a somewhat more active approach. Cues can be specific pieces of information provided by the therapist or a family member, or they can be less specific, such as an alarm watch set to go off when a task needs to be performed, a cue that requires the individual to be able to recall the task at the sound of the alarm or remember where to look up the information. Many people find it helpful to use pill boxes with alarms that remind them to take their medications.

A more sophisticated cuing system for individuals with severe memory deficits is Neuropage,[59] which uses a central computer and a paging company to page the patient automatically whenever a task needs to be completed. Patients demonstrated considerable success in carrying out tasks while wearing the pager. Obviously, this system requires the person to have the pager and to be able to respond to messages; it does not directly improve memory functioning. Increasingly sophisticated computer- and watch-based systems are also becoming available.

Strategies for Teaching Individuals with Memory Impairment

Another way of approaching rehabilitation with memory-impaired individuals is to present information in such a way as to maximize learning. Research in learning theory and cognitive neuroscience has yielded valuable new insights into the best approaches for teaching new information and training new skills in individuals with memory impairments. The "method of vanishing cues," for example, was designed to take advantage of spared priming effects in amnesic subjects.[60,61] Maximum cuing is used initially, and the amount of cuing is slowly reduced over repeated trials, similar to backward chaining techniques. For example, the individual might first be shown the word FILE, followed by FIL—, then FI—, and so forth. Glisky et al.[62,63] have used this technique in several studies in which they have shown improvement in specific functional skills (e.g., operating a computer) and maintenance of skills over time. However, despite some transfer of learning to highly similar job contexts, learning continued to be highly task-specific. In contrast, with eight memory-impaired subjects Hunkin and Parkin[64] did not find an advantage for the method of vanishing cues over rote learning (standard anticipation) in learning computer-related words and their definitions. This result might reflect differences in the subject population and points to the need for further research.

Most strategies to aid memory are based, in part, on repetition and spared procedural learning, particularly in individuals with severe amnesia. One important finding in this area is the demonstration of improved performance with "errorless learning."[65-68] In a series of studies, individuals with severe amnesia learned more quickly and accurately when they were not permitted to make incorrect guesses. Using stem-completion tasks, subjects with severe memory impairments were required to generate words that began with a particular word stem. In an errorless learning condition, the word was given and the subject told to write it down first. On subsequent trials, only correct responses were written down. In the errorful condition, subjects were allowed to generate guesses, including errors. Improved recall was seen in the errorless learning condition, presumably because individuals with amnesia have impaired explicit and episodic memory; errors are thus not recalled as errors and, by virtue of repetition, are actually primed for later recall. Errorless learning was also shown to be superior on tasks applicable to everyday life, such as recalling names or programming an electronic aid. Thus, for rehabilitation professionals, it may not be advisable to allow clients to "go ahead and guess" during the learning phase of any treatment. Instead, the correct answer should be provided, with the subject encouraged not to guess and to respond only when sure.

Another technique that has been used to aid learning is derived from studies of distributed practice. Learning is facilitated by having review occur over a longer period of time, for example, 1 hour every day for a week rather than 7 hours in 1 day. This schedule seems to allow time for memory consolidation. Landauer and Bjork[69] suggest starting with a short delay between presentation of the material and testing and then slowly increasing the delay period.

Internally Focused Approaches for Managing Memory Impairment

Some direct retraining approaches use exercises whereby an individual practices memory skills on the premise that repeated exposure and practice on memory tasks can facilitate learning. Although some authors have demon-strated improvements on specific tasks after repeated practice,[70,71] there is little evidence to suggest that this approach is helpful for memory remediation.[72]

Some memory improvements have been shown with facilitation techniques that are aimed at improving the encoding of information. Helping the person attend to the semantics or meaning of material or to organize the material to be remembered has been shown to improve recall of material in individuals without brain injury. This organization must be meaningful to the individual and is most successful if new information is integrated into material that is already familiar. Suggested techniques include elaboration (e.g., thinking about the details and relating them to information already known) and self-reference (e.g., asking learners to relate the material to themselves). Goldstein et al.[73] used computerized versions of such previously demonstrated memory training techniques in people with severe brain injuries. In the ridiculously imaged story (RIS) method, a story was presented with 20 words to be remembered, and the person was prompted to make up a story that used the list of words. In the face-name method, the person was trained to associate a person's name with a memorable physical characteristic or a memorable person he or she resembled. Although some success was reported, the study is limited by providing no data on whether these techniques could be used in daily life.

Mnemonic techniques, such as the peg words strategy[74] and method of loci, have been explored extensively in people with acquired memory disorders. Wilson[75] stresses that these techniques should not be expected to generalize but rather should be employed only in helping people learn limited amounts of domain-specific information. Reliance on the use of mnemonic strategies has been criticized for the high demand placed on encoding processes,[76] attention, planning, and vigilance, all of which may be impaired in individuals with traumatic brain injury.[77,78]

Visual imagery has been investigated in individuals with TBI[79] and used in a wide number of studies to compensate for poor verbal memory.[77,80] Wilson[71] demonstrated that people with severe memory deficits could learn to use visual imagery to learn pairs of faces and names in a series of single-subject studies and in a group study. Similarly, Twum and Parente[81] found that individuals with TBI performed better on paired associates when instructed in the use of visual imagery. Parente and DiCesare[82] trained individuals with TBI in two different mnemonic strategies. The first was to embed the list of words to be remembered in some kind of meaningful text, and the second was to use visual imagery. The subjects exhibited improved long-term storage and retrieval of a word list by using the imagery technique but not the embedding technique. Unfortunately, the authors did not provide any data indicating whether this training generalized, such that improvements were seen in recall in their daily life. Gade[83] reported that mildly amnesic subjects improved with self-generated images, moderately amnesic subjects improved when given instructions on imagery and pictures, and severe amnesics improved only minimally in any condition. In general, these studies have not shown these strategies to be useful for more than a few discrete pieces of information, and long-term retention has not been demonstrated.[76,84] Levin[85] speculates that the mental effort required to generate a visual image may reduce the cognitive resources available to the individual.

Metacognitive strategies have also been used with some success in memory-impaired individuals. These strategies use formal routines to help the person identify and structure material to be learned. Lawson and Rice[86] reported results from a single individual who had sustained a TBI in childhood. "Executive strategy training" involved identifying the problem, selecting a strategy, using the strategy, and then monitoring the outcome. These steps were first modeled by the trainer and then eventually used by the subject alone. As a result of this training, his performance improved on memory retrieval tasks.

Many academic therapies are designed to aid encoding and storage. In the PQRST (preview, question, read, state, test technique), for example, the individual is taught to first preview or skim the material. Then a series of questions are generated about the main theme and important points. The reading material is then read with a focus on finding the answers to the questions. At this point, the answers are stated. Frequent testing and probing for retention of the material are built into the technique. This procedure has been demonstrated to be effective in increasing retention of written material in a series of case studies of individuals with moderate to severe brain injury.[71]

One particularly encouraging approach to direct retraining has been prospective memory training. *Prospective memory* has been defined as the ability to remember future events or the ability to "remember to remember," as contrasted with retrospective memory, the recall of past events. Studies of prospective memory suggest its importance in people's daily lives and its susceptibility to impairment after brain dysfunction.[87,88] However, very few studies to date have

investigated the treatment of prospective memory deficits. Sohlberg et al.[89] used a within-subject operant design to evaluate the efficacy of prospective memory training in a 51-year-old brain injured man with a severe memory impairment. Training used repetitive administration of prospective memory tasks, whereby he was given actions to perform at specified future times. The length of time between task administration and task execution was gradually lengthened. Probes were taken evaluating generalization to performance on everyday prospective memory tasks and to performance on retrospective memory or recall measures. Results suggested a steady increase in the subject's prospective memory ability over time.

A follow-up study by Raskin and Sohlberg[90] used a simple within-subject operant A-B-A-B design replicated across two subjects, where A and B represented two different memory treatment conditions. The A condition represented one type of memory training termed *prospective memory training,* and the B condition represented another type of intervention termed *retrospective memory drill.* Dependent variables included performance accuracy on a test sampling prospective memory tasks in a controlled setting (PROMS[91]), the Rivermead Behavioural Memory Test,[92] a naturalistic task requiring the subject to call the examiner's office number at a specified time, and performance on a set of 10 prospective memory activities that the individual needed to carry out in daily life. Improvements were seen on all generalization measures with the prospective memory training but not with the retrospective memory training.

In a further study using the same prospective memory training procedures, Stone and Raskin[93] used electroencephalogram (EEG) measures as a measure of efficacy. Quantified EEG was recorded in a resting state prior to initiation of the training and after the completion of the training. Two subjects showed abnormal distribution of alpha activity predominating in frontal regions prior to training. Both showed a return to a more normative posterior distribution after training. Raskin[94] also measured the classic P3 response, an electrophysiological measure thought to reflect maintenance of working memory,[95] by using an auditory odd-ball paradigm, before and after prospective memory training. Two subjects with TBI showed delayed P3 before training and reduced latency after training. Interestingly, similar evoked potential changes were seen in another group of subjects with TBI before and after training of attentional skills.[96] These results suggest brain-related changes as a consequence of direct interventions and practice on specific cognitive skills.

Training Compensatory Systems for Managing Memory Impairment

Many investigations of memory rehabilitation following traumatic brain injury have involved teaching the person to compensate for the memory deficit through some external means.[73] Although prosthetic aids for memory compensation represent a valuable and essential method for managing memory impairments, these approaches focus on the symptoms of the problem rather than the cause. In addition, reliance on such techniques may actually interfere with natural recovery mechanisms[97] or may not facilitate performance for individuals with TBI.[98,99]

Prosthetic memory aids take many forms. Many individuals find helpful electronic datebooks, electronic signaling devices for keys, pill boxes with alarms, or cassette recorders for important conversations or lectures. The most widely used prosthetic aids are notebooks or organizers in which all important information is written down. The individual is trained in techniques for recording and systematically referring to the book. Memory notebook training has probably met with the most success of any memory training approach. Zenicus et al.[100] compared memory notebook use to written rehearsal, verbal rehearsal, and acronym formation to aid six individuals with TBI in learning information from a help wanted column in the newspaper. Memory notebook logging was superior to the other techniques.

Another study compared training in the use of a memory notebook to supportive therapy[101] for individuals with severe brain injury. Notebook training took place for 9 weeks in a group format. Measures of efficacy were based on experimental, questionnaire and observational measures of everyday memory failures, as well as measures of symptom distress. No significant differences were found between notebook training and supportive therapy on the laboratory-based measures or the symptom distress indicators. However, those who participated in notebook training did demonstrate significantly fewer everyday memory failures as measured by the observational technique. This technique required the subject and a significant other to complete a checklist for 7 days. One drawback may be that the subjects and others knew the type of treatment they were receiving. However, this study certainly points out the need to utilize a variety of measures of generalization to ensure that an adequate measure is included.

Sohlberg and Mateer[99] described a three-stage behavioral approach for learning to use a memory notebook. The steps involved in using the notebook in an organized fashion must be made automatic through structured training and repetition. Practice with the many different skills needed to use the book and the opportunity to use the book in both structured and naturalistic settings were essential to effective training. The sections of the notebook must coincide with the needs of the individual, and the system used must be comfortable for the person. Many commercial systems are available, and the individual can choose the most comfortable size and style. The sections we have found useful are a datebook-calendar, a list of things to do, a journal or feelings log, an events log, a telephone-address section, a things I forgot log, and a memory success log. Sections can be tailored to meet individual needs. A detailed description of the rationale and procedures for memory system training can be found in Sohlberg et al.'s manual.[103]

Another form of compensation is the implementation of organizational tools. Some people benefit from creating a specific place in the home for all important material. For example, a large calendar in the kitchen that can be used by all members of the household can reduce the frustration level of all family members. A telephone message board in the same location and a place for keys and wallets can aid in keeping track of these items.

One difficulty with many of these studies is that treatment maintenance over time has not been measured. In a series of important studies, Wilson[67,104] followed up on a group of subjects who had participated in a multimodal memory treatment program 5 to 10 years earlier. These subjects reported more use of memory aids, such as notebooks, calendars, and mnemonics, than before their injuries. In addition, performance on the Rivermead Behavioural Memory Test had improved overall; 8 subjects showed improvement, 14 showed no change, and 3 (1 of whom had had a subsequent TBI) showed deterioration in scores. In a case study of an individual with mild TBI, Crosson and Buenning[105] used a combination of strategies including feedback on performance, visual imagery, and periodic questioning to help the person improve in reading retention. Unfortunately, 9 months after training, performance had dropped because the individual had not maintained the use of the strategies.

In summary, a wide variety of approaches can be used with individuals who have memory impairments. Table 15–2 lists some of the studies that have demonstrated positive findings in memory rehabilitation. The most efficacious approaches are tailored to the specific memory profile, preserved cognitive abilities, and daily needs of the individual. Mateer and Sohlberg[34] suggested a three-pronged approach to working with individuals with memory disorders: simul-

TABLE 15–2. Studies Demonstrating Efficacy of Memory Rehabilitation Strategies

Improvement on trained tasks

Crovitz, Harvey, and Horn[80]
Goldstein et al.[73]
Grafman and Matthews[70]
Hersh and Treadgold[59]
Parente and DiCesare[82]
Twum and Parente[81]
Wilson[71]
Zenicus, Wesolowski, and Burke[100]

Improvement on psychometric measures

Crosson and Buenning[105]
Raskin and Sohlberg[90]
Sohlberg and Mateer[102]
Sohlberg et al.[89]
Wilson[67]

Improvements on functional abilities

Glisky and Schacter[63]
Lawson and Rice[86]
Raskin and Sohlberg[90]
Schmitter-Edgecombe et al.[101]
Sohlberg and Mateer[102]
Wilson[71]
Wilson[67]
Wilson and Evans[68]
Zenicus, Wesolowski, and Burke[100]

taneous attention training, prospective memory training, and training in the use of memory notebooks. Such multifaceted approaches can be individually tailored to the individual's current and future needs and abilities.

☐ MANAGEMENT OF EXECUTIVE FUNCTION DISORDERS

Individuals with frontal lobe damage and associated executive function compromise can be among the most baffling and challenging patients for rehabilitation specialists. These patients may demonstrate average or even above average intellectual abilities, seemingly adequate recall of information, and apparent knowledge when a verbal response is asked for. Yet they may demonstrate organizational, self-regulatory, and behavioral problems such that they fail to accomplish goals or complete even the simplest of tasks in the absence of cuing or structure.

Functions of the Frontal Lobe

The functions of the frontal lobe have been somewhat elusive, despite the fact that frontal lobe dysfunction can seriously impair many aspects of cognitive ability and independent functioning. The frontal lobes do not have a unitary function; rather, different regions of the frontal system are important in different aspects of cognition and behavior.[106,107] Portions of the frontal lobes play an important role in the initiation of action and behavior. Disruption of this system can result in aspontaneity or behavioral inertia.[108] Individuals with such disorders are often capable of speaking or behaving quite normally but, without substantial external cuing, fail to do so. The frontal lobes are also important in planning and organizing behavior to accomplish relevant goals and in monitoring goal directed activity.[109,110] Disruption in this system may result in behavior that seems random, disorganized, or without purpose.

The frontal lobes are also important in many aspects of attention.[111] Working memory—the capacity to hold information in a mental store during active information processing and to relate what has gone on just previously with what is going on now—appears dependent on frontal systems.[112] The ability to switch attention between tasks and the capacity for divided attention also appear, at least in part, dependent on frontal systems. In novel situations, when overlearned skills, knowledge, or responses cannot be used successfully, the frontal lobes are important in monitoring the effectiveness of behavior.[113] As a situation becomes more familiar or a pattern of response becomes more routine, there is a decreased need for frontal involvement.

Although recall of specific declarative or semantic information does not seem to depend on the frontal regions, an increasing number of mnemonic functions, such as memory for temporal order, have been ascribed to the frontal regions.[114–117] Memory for contextual information (e.g., source memory and recency memory) is also disrupted in patients with frontal involvement. Certain aspects of metamemory, such as "feelings of knowing," also appear to be frontally mediated.[118] Finally, the capacity for "remembering to remember" or prospective memory has also been related to frontal system functioning.

Evaluation of Frontal Lobe Functioning

A comprehensive discussion of the evaluation of frontal functioning is beyond the scope of this chapter. Such evaluation should include, but not be restricted to, psychometric tests shown to be sensitive to frontal involvement, behavioral observations in different settings and under conditions of varying demand, and comprehensive interviews and rating scales with family and caregivers. Determinations should be made about the individual's capacities in initiation, goal setting, planning, organizing, self-awareness of efficacy, time sense, inhibitory control, self-regulation, and cognitive and behavioral flexibility.

Rehabilitation of Impairments in Executive Function

A variety of approaches have been discussed for treatment of individuals with frontal lobe impairment. In general, they involve moving from simple structured activities with significant external cuing and support to more complex, multistep activities in which external support is gradually reduced and internal support or self-direction is required. Although articles have suggested success in using these techniques, such techniques have been experimentally evaluated in only a small number of cases and a limited number of studies.

BEHAVIOR MODIFICATION OF BEHAVIORAL DYSCONTROL

Loss of executive skills can impair a person's ability to initiate use of specific preserved abilities, monitor performance, and utilize feedback effectively to regulate behavior. Disruptive and aggressive behaviors are often a major impediment to rehabilitation. Alderman et al.[119,120] have demonstrated effective use of a particular behavior modification technique, response cost, in assisting individuals who have not responded to reinforcement or extinction techniques to gain greater inhibitory control over their behavior. In this technique, the patient is given a number of tokens, which are subsequently exchanged for tangible rewards at a later time. However, in the interim the individual is prompted to give the staff one token and state the reason for its loss whenever a target behavior (negative) is observed. The advantages of this procedure are that it facilitates directing the patient's attention to aspects of his or her behavior that are not being monitored, it enables salient feedback to be extracted from the environment, it places minimal load on memory, it facilitates procedural learning, and it increases awareness.

Alderman et al.[121] described a response cost program to reduce verbalizations in a brain injured woman who demonstrated a constant stream of verbal output. Although inhibition of speech was obtained in the institutional training environment, results did not automatically transfer to a second environment. A new program of self-monitoring training was successfully implemented to teach inhibitory control in the new environment. These results suggested that even severe disorders of behavior could come under specific control in patients with frontal compromise through use of traditional behavioral management techniques. This program was notable in that it moved from one of more externalized to more internalized behavioral control, and it demonstrated a thoughtful generalization plan as the patient moved from more controlled to less controlled settings.

BEHAVIOR MODIFICATION TO IMPROVE INITIATION AND DRIVE

The frontal lobes are essential for the effective initiation and sequencing of action programs. Disruptions of this system can be manifested in apparent lack of interest or inactivity; there may also be a significant dissociation between verbal output (e.g., what someone says they will do) and their corresponding action. Generally, it is not the case that patients with frontal lobe deficits cannot perform an action; rather, it may not occur to them to perform the action at the appropriate time or place, or they may begin an activity but fail to maintain it. Generally, such patients respond quite well to external cues or prompts to initiate activity, and their behavior can be modified through behavioral techniques, although cuing and reinforcement may need to be maintained.

Sohlberg et al.,[122] for example, demonstrated that an individual with severe frontal lobe impairment and marked initiation problems responded differentially with different types of cuing. The man with whom they worked appeared to have an adequate knowledge of and memory for what is going on in the environment, but he showed little apparent interest or involvement. During a group activity, the patient was provided with a cue, at which time he was to ask himself whether he was initiating conversation. He was also provided with some didactic training around the nature of communication and the importance of appearing involved and interested in the activity. His verbal interactions during the group session increased over a baseline period, during which no cues had been given, and following the treatment phase, during which prompts were withdrawn. Experimental control of the behavior was demonstrated by means of comparison to another measured behavior, response acknowledgments; these responses did not increase during the baseline or initial intervention stage but did increase when response acknowledgments were specifically trained and then cued by a similar prompted self-evaluation system.

REHABILITATION OF EXECUTIVE CONTROL

Executive control functions, in this context, involve the capacity to organize sequences of behavior and to carry out both familiar and novel activities. Principles of delivery, regardless of the underlying intent, would be the same. It is important to keep data on tasks presented and to build skills in a hierarchical fashion, going from more to less structured tasks and from less to more complex tasks.

Compensatory Strategies

If the patient is very acute in the rehabilitation process or is demonstrating very severe executive function disturbance, it may be profitable to initially focus on teaching task-specific routines. The assumption here is that the patient is not capable of a wide variety of different action plans in different settings because of stimulus boundedness, perseveration, severe related cognitive disorders of attention or memory, or extremely limited insight and awareness. In such individuals, it may not be reasonable to facilitate flexible, individually determined sequences, but training of particular sequences for familiar, highly repetitious functional activities may be possible.[123] Included here would be a variety of grooming and dressing procedures such as showering, taking care of one's toilet, or dressing. Other common task-specific routines that might be taught include preparation of very simple meals or going to the cafeteria for a coffee. If executive functions are severely impaired, there should probably be a limited number of steps and avoidance of potential dangers. Geyer[124] prepared a handbook for teaching such task-specific routines for just this purpose. Behavioral techniques involving shaping of behavior and reinforcement are commonly used as adjuncts to functional skills training approaches.[125] Burke et al.[126] described systematic use of checklists to guide behavior, combined with a self-instructional technique to train tasks of a similar nature.

Direct Training Approaches

Direct training approaches include a wide variety of structural exercises that provide multiple opportunities for initiating, planning, and carrying out goal-directed activities. The goal of treatment is for the patient to take on increasing responsibility for carrying out multistep plans and activities. Clinically, we have used route-finding exercises, therapy-planning exercises, and activity-planning exercises in this regard.

Although little research has been done in this area, Crepeau et al.[124] described a therapy activity designed to improve strategic time-sharing on a multistep task. The remediation technique was based on the model of executive impairment described by Shallice and Burgess[113] in their description of frontally impaired patients on the six element task. The rationale of the approach was to reduce demands on the supervisory attentional system by making routine certain specific behaviors (e.g., to record starting and ending times on a task, to shift from one activity to another after a self-directed delay). Although the authors were cautious about their findings in just three subjects, they did find an increased number of subtasks carried out (suggesting greater flexibility) and a decrease in time allocated to one subtask (suggesting improved strategy application). In addition, one subject demonstrated improved ability to monitor time passage, and one demonstrated a decrease in rule breaking.

Metacognitive Training Approaches

Insight, self-awareness, and self-regulatory capacity are thought to reflect the highest level of frontal lobe activity,[128] as many people with frontal lobe damage demonstrate limited insight into their problems and require explicit behavioral objectives in order to understand and progress in therapy. Treatment in this area presents a tremendous challenge for the rehabilitation professional.[129]

Verbal self-regulation strategies are based on the observation that it is possible to regulate one's own behavior through self-talk. Stuss et al.[130] used a verbal self-regulation approach in an individual with motor impersistence who could not maintain a simple motor movement over time. The patient did learn to alter his behavior, although he continued to need cues to initiate and maintain the self-regulation strategy.

Another kind of intervention at this level involves teaching self-instructional procedures before and during the execution of a training task. Cicerone and Wood[131] reported successful treatment with such a procedure of a patient who exhibited impaired planning ability and poor self-control 4 years after closed head injury. They used as a training task a modified version of the Tower of London. Training in the self-instructional technique involved three distinct phases: overt verbalization, overt self-guidance, and covert internalized self-monitoring. To promote generalization following the program, the client was presented with a structured interpersonal problem and asked to solve it by applying principles learned in the self-instructional training. The results supported the clinical efficacy of verbal mediation training in treating executive functions. The authors noted, however, that generalization of training occurred only after direct, extended training with real-life situations. Additional work in the use of self-instructional strategies has been carried out by Cicerone and Giacino.[132]

Von Cramon, Matthes-von Cramon, and Mai[133] described positive results in a series of patients with frontal lobe dysfunction. Their training procedure involved enabling patients to help reduce the complexity of a multistage problem by breaking it down into more manageable proportions. Problem-solving training incorporated four modules. The first was generation of goal-directed ideas, a kind of brainstorming designed to produce a variety of alternatives to a given problem. The second module was systematic and careful comparison of information provided about a problem to be solved. The third consisted of tasks requiring simultaneous analysis of information from multiple sources (such as having the patient compare catalogues from several tourist offices to find the most favorable trip to England for a family of four). The fourth module focused on improving the patient's abilities to draw inferences. Utilizing short detective stories, the authors had subjects uncover discrepancies and detect "clues" about how crimes could have been committed. The authors reported significant psychometric as well as functional gains in a group receiving this training as opposed to a group receiving more generic memory training.

As with several of the other treatment approaches discussed, the use of metacognitive strategies and self-instructional programs for patients with acquired frontal injuries is just beginning to be formally evaluated. It is encouraging, however, that positive outcomes have been reported and that there are numerous reports of success with such approaches in a variety of clinical populations, particularly children and adolescents with learning problems.[134]

The executive disorders encompass a broad range of cognitive and behavioral difficulties. Effective strategies for such patients require an appreciation for each person's cognitive profile, self-regulatory capacity, and level of awareness. Therapy usually begins by providing maximal external cuing and structure; as people develop greater behavioral initiative, flexibility, and self-regulatory capacity, they can begin to take on a greater proportion of responsibility for their function and behavior, and structure and cuing can be gradually withdrawn. Table 15–3 lists studies targeting executive control functions that have reported positive findings.

☐ SUMMARY AND CONCLUSIONS

Over the last decade, there has been increasing appreciation of the importance of cognitive abilities for everyday activities and the functional impact of cognitive impairments following TBI. Both practitioners and researchers have implemented multifaceted cognitive rehabilitation approaches, including direct training of cognitive skills through repetitive practice, well-planned environmental modifications, sophisticated behavioral and cognitive-behavioral techniques, educational approaches to increase awareness, and cognitive-behavioral approaches to alter feelings, attitudes, and behaviors. Much greater attention has been paid to the design of structured generalization approaches at home and in the workplace. No approach to cognitive impairments can afford to be office-bound or sterile, and all should incorporate techniques that reflect and affect real-life situations and demands. An ever growing cross-fertilization between the neurological, clinical, and rehabilitation sciences is leading to new procedures and approaches to working with cognitively impaired individuals. Also gratifying is an increasing recognition of the need to understand and work with individuals and their families with regard to the emotional and psychosocial impact of cognitive impairments.

TABLE 15–3. Studies Demonstrating Improvements in Executive Control and Self-Monitoring

Use of checklists and task-specific routines to guide behavior

Bergman[135]
Bergman and Kemmerer[136]
Burke et al.[126]
Craine[123]
Geyer[124]
Kirsch et al.[137]

Behavioral and cognitive-behavioral approaches

Alderman, Fry, and Youngson[121]
Alderman and Ward[120]
Sohlberg, Sprunk, and Metzelaar[122]
Wood[55]

Verbal self-regulation

Giles and Clarke-Wilson[125]
Stuss, Delgado, and Guzman[130]

Metacognitive strategies

Cicerone and Wood[131]
Cicerone and Giacino[132]
Lawson and Rice[86]
Stuss, Delgado, and Guzman[130]
Von Cramon, Matthes–von Cramon, and Mai[133]

REFERENCES

1. Backman, L, and Dixon, RA: Psychological compensation: A theoretical framework. Psychol Bull 112:259–283, 1992.
2. Meier, M, Benton, A, and Diller, L: Neuropsychological Rehabilitation. Guilford, New York, 1987.
3. Sohlberg, MM, and Mateer, CA: Introduction to Cognitive Rehabilitation: Theory and Practice. Guilford, New York, 1989.
4. Mateer, CA: Rehabilitation of individuals with frontal lobe impairment. In Leon-Carrion, J (ed): Neuropsychological Rehabilitation and Treatment of Brain Injury. St Lucie Press, Delray Beach, Fla, 1996.
5. Sohlberg, MM, Mateer, CA, and Stuss, DT: Contemporary approaches to the management of executive control dysfunction. J Head Trauma Rehabil 8(1):45–58, 1993.
6. Webb, PM, and Glueckauf, RL: The effects of direct involvement in goal setting on rehabilitation outcome for persons with traumatic brain injuries. Rehabilitation Psychology 39:179–188, 1994.
7. Raskin, S, and Gordon, W: The impact of different approaches to remediation on generalization. NeuroRehabilitation 2:38–45, 1992.
8. Gordon, W: Methodological considerations in cognitive remediation. In Meier, M, Benton, A, and Diller, L (eds): Neuropsychological Rehabilitation. Guilford, New York, 1987.
9. Sohlberg, MM, and Raskin, SA: Principles of generalization applied to attention and memory interventions. J Head Trauma Rehabil 11:65–78, 1996.
10. Stokes, TF, and Baer, DM: An implicit technology of generalization. Journal of Applied Behavioral Analysis 10:349–367, 1977.
11. Anderson, J: ACT: A simple theory of complex cognition. Am Psychol 51:355–365, 1996.
12. Ponsford, JL, and Kinsella, G: The use of a rating scale of attentional behavior. Neuropsychological Rehabilitation 1:241–257, 1991.
13. Mateer, CA, Sohlberg, MM, and Crinean, F: Perception of memory impairment in closed head injury. J Head Trauma Rehabil 2:74–84, 1987.
14. Sohlberg, MM: Manual for the Profile of Executive Control System. Association for Neuropsychological Research and Development, Puyallup, Wash, 1992.
15. Dywan, J, and Segalowitz, J: Self- and family ratings of adaptive behavior after traumatic brain injury: Psychometric scores and frontally generated ERPs. J Head Trauma Rehabil 11:79–95, 1996.
16. Willer, B, Linn, R, and Allen, K: Community integration and barriers to integration for individuals with brain injury. In Finlayson, MAJ, and Garner, S (eds): Brain Injury Rehabilitation: Clinical Considerations. Williams and Wilkins, Baltimore, 1993, pp 355–375.
17. Whiteneck, G, et al: Quantifying handicap: New measure of long-term rehabilitation outcomes. Arch Phys Med Rehabil 73:519–526, 1992.
18. Mateer, CA, Kerns, KA, and Eso, K: Management of attention and memory disorders following traumatic brain injury. Journal of Learning Disabilities 29:618–632, 1996.
19. Hinkeldey, NS, and Corrigan, JD: The structure of head injured patients' neurobehavioral complaints: A preliminary study. Brain Inj 4:115–134, 1990.
20. Lezak, MD: Neuropsychological Assessment, ed 3. Oxford University Press, New York, 1994.
21. Gronwall, D, and Wrightson, P: Delayed recovery of intellectual function after mild head injury. Lancet 2:1452, 1974.
22. Ponsford, JL, and Kinsella, G: Attentional deficits following closed head injury. J Clin Exp Neuropsychol 14:822–838, 1992.
23. Stuss, DT, et al: Traumatic brain injury: A comparison of three clinical tests, and analysis of recovery. Clinical Neuropsychologist 3:145–156, 1989.
24. Gronwall, D, and Sampson, H: The Psychological Effects of Concussion. Aukland University Press, Aukland, 1974.
25. Stuss, DT, et al: Reaction time after head injury: Fatigue, divided and focused attention, and consistency of performance. J Neurol Neurosurg Psychiatry 52:742–748, 1989.
26. Miller, E, and Cruzat, A: A note on the effects of irrelevant information on task performance after mild and severe head injury. Br J Soc Clin Psychol 20:69–70, 1980.
27. Bohnen, N, Jolles, J, and Twijnstra, A: Modification of the Stroop Colour Word Test improves differentiation between patients with mild head injury and matched controls. Clinical Neuropsychologist 6:178–188, 1992.
28. Bohnen, N, Twijnstra, A, and Jolles, J: Performance in the Stroop Colour Word Test in relationship to the persistence of symptoms following mild head injury. Acta Neurol Scand 85:116–121, 1992.
29. Stablum, F, et al: Attention and control deficits following closed head injury. Cortex 30:603–618, 1994.
30. Van Zomeren, AH, and Brouwer, WH: Head injury and concepts of attention. In Levin, HJ, Grafman, J, and Eisenberg, HM (eds): Neurobehavioral Recovery from Head Injury. Oxford University Press, New York, 1987.
31. Nissen, MJ: Neuropsychology of attention and memory. J Head Trauma Rehabil 1:13–21, 1986.
32. Russell, EW, and D'Hollosy, ME: Memory and attention. J Clin Psychol 48:530–538, 1992.
33. Mateer, CA: Systems of care for post-concussive syndrome. In Horn, LJ, and Zasler, ND (eds): Rehabilitation of Post-Concussive Disorders. Henley & Belfus, Philadelphia, 1992.
34. Mateer, CA, and Sohlberg, MM: A paradigm shift in memory rehabilitation. In Whitaker, H (ed): Neuropsychological Studies of Nonfocal Brain Injury: Dementia and Closed Head Injury. Springer-Verlag, New York, 1988.
35. Van Zomeren, AH, Brouwer, WH, and Deelman, BG: Attention Deficits: The Riddle of Selectivity, Speed and Alertness. Oxford University Press, Oxford, 1984.
36. Schmitter-Edgecombe, M: Effects of traumatic brain injury on cognitive performance: An attentional resource hypothesis in search of data. J Head Trauma Rehabil 11:17–30, 1996.
37. Kerns, KA, and Mateer, CA: Walking and chewing gum: The impact of attentional capacity on everyday activities. In Sbordone, RJ, and Long, CJ (eds): The Ecological Validity of Neuropsychological Testing. GR Press/St Lucie Press, Delray Beach, Fla, 1996.
38. Ben-Yishay, Y, Piasetsky, EB, and Rattock, J: A systematic method for ameliorating disorders in basic attention. In Meyer, MJ, Benton, AL, and Diller, L (eds): Neuropsychological Rehabilitation. Churchill Livingstone, Edinburgh, 1987.
39. Diller, L, et al: Studies of Cognition and Rehabilitation in Hemiplegia. Rehabilitation monograph no. 50. New York University Medical Center, New York, 1974.
40. Kewman, DG, et al: Stimulation and training of psychomotor skills: Teaching the brain-injured to drive. Rehabilitation Psychology 30:11–27, 1985.
41. Sohlberg, MM, and Mateer, CA: Effectiveness of an attention training program. J Clin Exp Neuropsychol 19:117–130, 1987.
42. Wood, RL, and Fussey, I: Computer-assisted cognitive retraining: A controlled study. International Disability Studies 9:149–153, 1987.
43. Mateer, CA, and Mapou, R: Understanding, evaluating and managing attention disorders following traumatic brain injury. J Head Trauma Rehabil 11:1–16, 1996.
44. Ethier, M, Baribeau, JMC, and Braun, CMJ: Computer-dispensed cognitive-perceptual training of closed head injury patients after spontaneous recovery. Study 2: Non-specified tasks. Canadian Journal of Rehabilitation 3:7–16, 1989.
45. Ethier, M, Braun, CMJ, and Baribeau, JMC: Computer-dispensed cognitive-perceptual training of closed head

injury patients after spontaneous recovery. Study 1: Speeded tasks. Canadian Journal of Rehabilitation 2:223–233, 1989.

46. Gray, JM, and Robertson, I: Remediation of attentional difficulties following brain injury: Three experimental single case studies. Brain Inj 3:163–170, 1989.

47. Gray, JM, et al: Microcomputer-based attentional retraining after brain damage: A randomized group controlled trial. Neuropsychological Rehabilitation 2:97–115, 1992.

48. Sturm, W, et al: Computer-assisted rehabilitation of attention impairments. In Stachowiak, F (ed): Developments in the Assessment and Rehabilitation of Brain-Damaged Patients. Narr: Tubingen, Germany, 1993.

49. Mateer, CA, Sohlberg, MM, and Youngman, P: The management of acquired attentional and memory disorders following mild closed head injury. In Wood R (ed): Cognitive Rehabilitation in Perspective. Taylor and Francis, London, 1990.

50. Niemann, H, Ruff, RM, and Baser, CA: Computer assisted attention training in head injured individuals: A controlled efficacy study of an outpatient program. Journal of Clinical and Consulting Psychology 58:811–817, 1990.

51. Ruff, R, et al: Neuropsychological rehabilitation: An experimental study with head-injured patients. J Head Trauma Rehabil 4:20–37, 1989.

52. Sturm, W, and Willmes, K: Efficacy of reaction time training on various attentional and cognitive functions in stroke patients. Neuropsychological Rehabilitation 1:259–280, 1991.

53. Ponsford, JL, and Kinsella, G: Evaluation of a remedial programme for attentional deficits following closed head injury. J Clin Exp Neuropsychol 10:693–708, 1988.

54. Sivak, M, Hill, CS, and Olson, P: Computerized video tasks as training techniques for driving related perceptual deficits of persons with brain damage: A pilot evaluation. International Rehabilitation Research 7:389–398, 1984.

55. Wood, RL: Rehabilitation of patients with disorders of attention. J Head Trauma Rehabil 1:45–64, 1986.

56. Sohlberg, MM, and Mateer, CA: Attention Process Training. Association for Neuropsychological Research and Development, Puyallup, Wash, 1989.

57. Sohlberg, MM, et al: Attention Process Training II: A Program to Address Attentional Deficits for Persons with Mild Cognitive Dysfunction. Association for Neuropsychological Research and Development, Puyallup, Wash, 1993.

58. Niemann, H: Retraining attention in head-injured individuals. University of Victoria, British Columbia, Dissertation.

59. Hersh, N, and Treadgold, L: NeuroPage: the rehabilitation of memory dysfunction by prosthetic memory and cueing. NeuroRehabilitation 4:187–197, 1994.

60. Glisky, EL, Schacter, DL, and Tulving, E: Computer learning by memory impaired patients: acquisition and retention of complex knowledge. Neuropsychologia 24:313–328, 1986.

61. Glisky, E, Schacter, D, and Tulving, E: Learning and retention of computer-related vocabulary in memory-impaired patients: Method of vanishing cues. J Clin Exp Neuropsychol 8:292–312, 1986.

62. Glisky, EL, and Schacter, DL: Acquisition of domain-specific knowledge in organic amnesia: Training for computer-related work. Neuropsychologia 25:893–906, 1987.

63. Glisky, E, and Schacter, D: Acquisition of domain-specific knowledge in patients with organic memory disorders. Journal of Learning Disabilities 21:333–339, 1988.

64. Hunkin, NM, and Parkin, AJ: The method of vanishing cues: An evaluation of effectiveness in teaching memory-impaired individuals. Neuropsychologia 33:1255–1279, 1995.

65. Baddeley, A: Implicit memory and errorless learning: A link between cognitive theory and neuropsychological rehabilitation? In Squire, L, and Butters, N (eds): Neu-

ropsychology of Memory, ed 2. Guilford, New York, 1992.

66. Baddeley, AD: Memory theory and memory therapy. In Wilson, BA, and Moffat, N (eds): Clinical Management of Memory Disorders, ed 2. Chapman & Hall, London, 1992.

67. Wilson, BA: Recovery and compensatory strategies in head injured memory impaired people several years after insult. J Neurol Neurosurg Psychiatry 55:177–180, 1992.

68. Wilson, BA, and Evans, JJ: Error-free learning in the rehabilitation of people with memory impairments. J Head Trauma Rehabil 11:54–64, 1996.

69. Landauer, T, and Bjork, R: Optimum rehearsal patterns and name learning. In Gruneberg, M, Morris, P, and Sykes, R (eds): Practical Aspects of Memory. Academic Press, London, 1978.

70. Grafman, J, and Matthews, C: Assessment and remediation of memory deficits in brain injured patients. In Gruneberg, M, Morris, P, and Sykes, R (eds): Practical Aspects of Memory. Academic Press, London, 1978.

71. Wilson, BA: Rehabilitation of Memory. Guilford, New York, 1987.

72. Franzen, M, and Haut, M: The psychological treatment of memory impairment: A review of empirical studies. Neuropsychol Rev 2:29–63, 1991.

73. Goldstein, G, et al: Efficacy of memory training: A technological extension and replication. Clinical Neuropsychologist 10:66–72, 1996.

74. Patten, B: The ancient art of memory. Arch Neurol 26:25–31, 1972.

75. Wilson, BA: Coping strategies for memory dysfunction. In Perecman, E (ed): Integrating Theory and Practice in Clinical Neuropsychology. Lawrence Erlbaum, Hillsdale, NJ, 1989.

76. Schacter, DL, and Glisky, EL: Memory remediation: Restoration, alleviation, and the acquisition of domain-specific knowledge. In Uzzell, B, and Gross, Y (eds): Clinical Neuropsychology of Intervention. Martinus Nijhoff, Boston, 1986.

77. Moffat, N: Strategies of memory therapy. In Wilson, B, and Moffat, N (eds): Clinical Management of Memory Problems. Aspen, Rockville, Md, 1984.

78. O'Connor, M, and Cermak, L: Rehabilitation of organic memory disorders. In Meier, M, Benton, A, and Diller, L (eds): Neuropsychological Rehabilitation. Guilford, New York, 1987.

79. Richardson, J, and Barry, C: The effects of minor closed head injury upon human memory: Further evidence on the role of mental imagery. Cognitive Neuropsychology 2:149–168, 1985.

80. Crovitz, H, Harvey, M, and Horn, R: Problems in the acquisition of imagery mnemonics: Three brain damaged cases. Cortex 15:225–234, 1979.

81. Twum, M, and Parente, R: Role of imagery and verbal labeling in the performance of paired associate tasks by persons with closed head injury. J Clin Exp Neuropsychol 16:630–639, 1994.

82. Parente, R, and DiCesare, A: Retraining memory: Theory, evaluation and applications. In Kreutzer, J, and Wehman, P (eds): Cognitive Rehabilitation for Persons with Traumatic Brain Injury: A Functional Approach. Paul Brookes, Baltimore, 1991.

83. Gade, A: Imagery as a mnemonic aid in amnesia patients: effects of amnesia subtype and severity. In Riddoch, M, and Humphreys, G (eds): Cognitive Neuropsychology and Cognitive Rehabilitation. Lawrence Erlbaum, Hillsdale, NJ, 1994.

84. Schacter, D, and Crovitz, H: Memory function after closed-head injury: A review of the quantitative research. Cortex 13:150–176, 1977.

85. Levin, H: Neuropsychological rehabilitation of head injured patients: An appraisal of recent approaches. Scand J Rehabil Med Suppl 26:14–24, 1992.

86. Lawson, M, and Rice, D: Effects of training in use of executive strategies on a verbal memory problem result-

ing from closed head injury. Journal of Clinical and Experimental Psychology 11:842–854, 1989.

87. Hannon, R, et al: Effects of brain injury and age on prospective memory self-rating and performance. Rehabilitation Psychology 40:289–298, 1995.

88. Sohlberg, MM, et al: Background and initial case studies into the effects of prospective memory training. Brain Inj 6:129–138, 1992.

89. Sohlberg, MM, et al: An investigation of the effects of prospective memory training. Brain Inj 5:139–154, 1992.

90. Raskin, S, and Sohlberg, MM: The efficacy of prospective memory training in two adults with brain injury. J Head Trauma Rehabil 11:32–51, 1996.

91. Sohlberg, MM, and Mateer, CA: Prospective Memory Screening. Association for Neuropsychological Research and Development, Puyallup, Wash, 1989.

92. Wilson, BA, Cockburn, J, and Halligan, P: The Rivermead Everyday Memory Test. Thames Valley Test Company, Flempton, Bury St Edmunds, Suffolk, 1985.

93. Stone, S, and Raskin, S: Training Prospective Memory in an Individual with Anoxic Brain Damage. International Neuropsychological Society, Chicago, 1996.

94. Raskin, S: P300 as a Measure of Brain Reorganization following Cognitive Rehabilitation. Cognitive Neuroscience Society, San Francisco, 1996.

95. Polich, J, and Kok, A: Cognitive and biological determinants of P300: An integrative review. Biol Psychol 41:103–146, 1995.

96. Baribeau, J, Ethier, M, and Braun, C: A neurophysiological assessment of selective attention before and after cognitive remediation in patients with severe closed head injury. Journal of Neurological Rehabilitation 3:71–92, 1989.

97. Stein, D, and Glasier, M: An overview of developments in research on recovery from brain injury. In Rose, F, and Johnson, D (eds): Recovery from Brain Damage. Plenum, New York, 1992.

98. Goldstein, F, et al: Facilitation of memory performance through induced semantic processing in survivors of severe closed head injury. J Clin Exp Neuropsyhol 12:286–300, 1990.

99. Shum, D, Sweeper, S, and Murray, R: Performance on verbal implicit and explicit memory tasks following traumatic brain injury. J Head Trauma Rehabil 11:43–53, 1996.

100. Zenicus, A, Wesolowski, M, and Burke, W: A comparison of four memory strategies with traumatically brain-injured clients. Brain Inj 4:33–38, 1990.

101. Schmitter-Edgecombe, M, et al: Memory rehabilitation after severe closed head injury: Notebook training versus supportive therapy. J Consult Clin Psychol 63:484–489, 1995.

102. Sohlberg, MM, and Mateer, CA: Training use of compensatory memory books: A three stage behavioral approach. J Clin Exp Neuropsychol 11:871–891, 1989.

103. Sohlberg, MM, et al: A Manual for Teaching Patients to Use Compensatory Memory Systems. Association for Neuropsychological Research and Development, Puyallup, Wash, 1994.

104. Wilson, BA: Long term prognosis of patients with severe memory disorders. Neuropsychological Rehabilitation 1:117–134, 1991.

105. Crosson, B, and Buenning, W: An individualized memory retraining program after closed-head injury: A single-case study. Journal of Clinical Neuropsychology 6:287–301, 1984.

106. Luria, AR: Higher Cortical Functions in Man. Basic Books, New York, 1980.

107. Stuss, DT, and Benson, DF: The Frontal Lobes. Raven, New York, 1986.

108. Fuster, JM: Prefrontal cortex and the bridging of temporal gaps in the perception-action cycle. Ann N Y Acad Sci 608:318–336, 1990.

109. Shallice, T: Specific impairments of planning. Philosophical Transactions of the Royal Society of London 298:199–209, 1982.

110. Shallice, T, and Burgess, PW: Higher-order cognitive impairments and frontal-lobe lesions in man. In Levin, H, Eisenberg, HM, and Benton, AL (eds): Frontal Lobe Function and Injury. Oxford University Press, Oxford, 1991.

111. Van Zomeren, AH, and Brouwer, WH: Clinical Neuropsychology of Attention. Oxford University Press, New York, 1994.

112. Goldman-Rakic, P: Specification of higher cortical function. J Head Trauma Rehabil 8:13–23, 1993.

113. Shallice, T, and Burgess, PW: Deficits in strategy application following frontal lobe damage in man. Brain 114:727–741, 1991.

114. Baddeley, AD, and Wilson, BA: Frontal amnesia and the dysexecutive syndrome. Brain Cogn 7:23–30, 1988.

115. Janowsky, JS, et al: Cognitive impairment following frontal lobe damage and its relevance to human amnesia. Behav Neurosci 103:548–560, 1989.

116. Milner, B, Petrides, M, and Smith, M: Frontal lobes and the temporal organization of memory. Human Neurobiology 4:137–142, 1985.

117. Schacter, DL: Memory, amnesia and frontal lobe dysfunction. Psychobiology 15:21–36, 1987.

118. Janowsky, JS, Shimamura, AP, and Squire, LR: Memory and metamemory: Comparisons between patients with frontal lobe lesions and amnesic patients. Psychobiology 17:3–11, 1989.

119. Alderman, N, and Burgess, PW: Integrating cognition and behaviour: A pragmatic approach to brain injury rehabilitation. In Wood, RL, and Fussey, I (eds): Cognitive Rehabilitation in Perspective. Taylor Francis, Basingstoke, 1990.

120. Alderman, N, and Ward, A: Behavioural treatment of the dysexecutive syndrome: Reduction of repetitive speech using response cost and cognitive overlearning. Neuropsychological Rehabilitation 1:65–80, 1991.

121. Alderman, N, Fry, RK, and Youngson, HA: Improvement of self-monitoring skills, reduction of behaviour disturbance and the dysexecutive syndrome: Comparison of response cost and a new programme of self-monitoring training. Neuropsychological Rehabilitation 5:193–221, 1995.

122. Sohlberg, MM, Sprunk, H, and Metzelaar, K: Efficacy of an external cuing system in an individual with severe frontal lobe damage. Cognitive Rehabilitation 4:36–40, 1988.

123. Craine, JF: The retraining of frontal lobe dysfunction. In Trexler, LE (ed): Cognitive Rehabilitation: Conceptualization and Intervention. Plenum, New York, 1982.

124. Geyer, S: Training Executive Function Skills. Good Samaritan Hospital, Puyallup, Wash, 1989.

125. Giles, GG, and Clarke-Wilson, J: The use of behavioral techniques in functional skills training after severe brain injury. Am J Occup Ther 42:658–665, 1988.

126. Burke, WH, et al: Improving executive function disorders in brain-injured clients. Brain Inj 5:25–28, 1991.

127. Crepeau, F, et al: Toward a remediation approach to improve strategic time-sharing following traumatic brain injury. Poster presented at the Baycrest Frontal Lobe Conference, Toronto, 1995.

128. Stuss, DT: Self, awareness and the frontal lobes: A neuropsychological perspective. In Goethals, GR, and Struss, J (eds): The Self: An Interdisciplinary Approach. Springer-Verlag, New York, 1991.

129. Crosson, B, Barco, PP, and Velozo, CA: Awareness and compensation in post-acute head injury rehabilitation. J Head Trauma Rehabil 23:46–54, 1989.

130. Stuss, DT, Delgado, M, and Guzman, DA: Verbal regulation in the control of motor impersistence. Journal of Neurological Rehabilitation. 1:19–24, 1987.

131. Cicerone, KD, and Wood, JC: Planning disorder after closed head injury: A case study. Arch Phy Med Rehabil 68:111–115, 1987.

132. Cicerone, KD, and Giacino, JT: Remediation of executive function deficits after traumatic brain injury. Neuropsychological Rehabilitation 2:12–22, 1992.

133. Von Cramon, DY, Matthes–Von Cramon, G, and Mai, N: Problem solving deficits in brain injured patients: A therapeutic approach. Neuropsychological Rehabilitation 1:45–64, 1991.
134. Graham, S, and Harris, KR: Addressing problems in attention, memory and executive functioning: An example from self-regulated strategy development. In Lyons, GR (ed): Attention Memory and Executive Function. Brookes, Baltimore, 1994.
135. Bergman, MM: Computer enhances self-sufficiency: Part I. Creation and implementation of a text writer for an individual with traumatic brain injury. Neuropsychology 5:17–23, 1991.
136. Bergman, MM, and Kemmerer, AG: Computer enhanced self-sufficiency: Part 2. Uses and subjective benefits of text writer for an individual with traumatic brain injury. Neuropsychology 5:25–28, 1991.
137. Kirsch, NL, et al: The microcomputer as an "orthotic" device for patients with cognitive deficits. J Head Trauma Rehabil 2:77–86, 1987.

CHAPTER 16

Psychotherapy and Psychotherapeutic Interventions in Brain Injury Rehabilitation

GEORGE P. PRIGATANO, PHD,
and YEHUDA BEN-YISHAY, PHD

Moderate to severe traumatic brain injury (TBI) produces a variety of emotional and motivational disturbances.[1] These disturbances can greatly impede long-term psychosocial adaptation and efforts at rehabilitation. Angry, depressed, agitated, and "unmotivated" TBI patients notoriously do not engage in physical therapy, occupational therapy, or speech and language therapy, let alone more extensive programs of care such as day treatment programs aimed at home independence or work reentry. At various stages after brain injury, appropriate interventions based on psychotherapeutic principles may reduce the patients' maladaptive response to disability or their resistance to engage needed rehabilitation activities. Such interventions also can reduce patients' frustration and confusion after TBI.[2] Finally, such interventions may help both family and rehabilitation staff deal with their inevitable emotional reactions to someone who has suffered a serious brain injury.[3–6]

This chapter discusses the role of formal psychotherapy in neuropsychological rehabilitation programs that foster a holistic approach. Within the context of this approach, a therapeutic milieu day treatment program is often instituted. This chapter also attempts to demonstrate how various interventions may have a psychotherapeutic effect, even when they are not part of formal psychotherapy. These interventions, which are in part based on insights about how brain injury adversely affects a person's capacity to adapt, can produce important "therapeutic breakthroughs" for some patients.

We make no claim that formal psychotherapy or psychotherapeutic intervention is always needed in brain injury rehabilitation. Much depends on the patients' premorbid psychological adjustment and how they interpret the meaning of the brain injury in their present lives.

Attempts at psychotherapy and psychotherapeutic interventions are not always helpful and may fail to achieve the desired effect. Indeed, a

This chapter emerged as a result of discussions between the two authors from May 1 through May 7, 1996, while the first author gave lectures on psychotherapy and the problem of impaired self-awareness after brain injury at the Kurt Goldstein Institute of Neuropsychological Rehabilitation, Steinach, Germany.
The authors wish to thank Shelley A. Kick, PhD, and the Neuroscience Publications Office of the Barrow Neurological Institute for their assistance in editing and preparing this manuscript

major question for this field is why these interventions sometimes are and sometimes are not helpful. Although this chapter cannot fully address this important problem, it presents empirical evidence that indirectly supports the role of psychotherapy and psychotherapeutic interventions in neuropsychologically oriented rehabilitation.

☐ "FORMAL" PSYCHOTHERAPY AND NEUROPSYCHOLOGICAL REHABILITATION

Formal psychotherapy is one of the five major components of neuropsychological rehabilitation.[2,3,7–9] The other four components are cognitive retraining and rehabilitation, protected work trials, consultation with and education of family members, and the establishment of a therapeutic milieu that incorporates these activities and permits the rehabilitation staff to deal with their personal reactions to patients.[2,10]

Psychotherapy can be defined in several ways because there are various theories about the nature of personality disorders and appropriate methods of intervention.[9,11,12] For the purpose of this chapter, it is defined as the method of helping patients establish meaning in their life in the face of (not despite) their suffering. In so doing, the process helps patients learn to behave in their own best self-interest (*not* selfish interest).[2] This generic definition has been discussed elsewhere, as have the strengths and limitations of psychotherapy after brain injury.[9] The legitimate criticism that psychotherapy for TBI patients must consider their unique neuropsychological deficits, which can and, indeed, often do affect therapeutic transactions[13] has also been addressed.[2]

Likewise, the basic assumptions underlying most formal insight-producing psychotherapeutic systems must be examined, and therapeutic techniques must be modified accordingly. This process allows practitioners to accommodate their interventions to what brain dysfunctional patients can understand and cope with at a given time.[14]

Formal psychotherapy with people who have acquired brain dysfunctions consists of individual or group therapy sessions, the express purpose of which is to discuss feelings about brain injury and the various "losses" incurred as a consequence of the injury. The sessions can also address conflicts or a patient's maladaptive responses during rehabilitation. The purpose of such discussions is to help patients clarify their emotional and motivational characteristics and how they help or impede the coping process. Psychotherapy can be distinguished from behavioral management insofar as the latter may teach individuals specific methods of coping with anxiety, depression, anger, and so on, but the former specifically deals with patients' personal reaction to what has occurred to them. Psychotherapy addresses the phenomenological concerns of the patient.

Unlike behavioral management, psychotherapy is concerned with the broader question of establishing meaning in patients' lives while dealing with their subjective feeling state. Its ultimate aims are to help people with emotional and motivational barriers that impede the process of returning to a productive lifestyle (e.g., work) and to reestablish mutually satisfying interpersonal relationships with important people in their lives. In some cases, psychotherapy also helps individuals place their uniqueness into perspective and fosters the process that Jung described as "individuation."[15] In this regard, it focuses on the problem of teaching patients "philosophical patience in the face of suffering."[15] Helping patients to construct their daily activities along the lines of "living symbols," which have traditionally proven meaningful for individuals in Western civilization, may also facilitate individuation.[2,4]

The process of psychotherapy is difficult to describe because, by its very nature, it is an individual process.[2] It can parallel various versions of what has been termed the "hero's path" in literature.[16] In the scenario of the hero's path, individuals leave the security of a certain psychological position, which is often symbolized by their home environment; that is, the hero has to leave home to face some important issue or event in life. Once people leave home (the security of a psychological position), they often confront something frightening that may even threaten their very existence. With cunning and bravery, they overcome or deal effectively with whatever threatens them. This process is analogous to facing things about the self that people wish not to consider. Once faced, however, individuals go through a transformation and emerge more mature. In the hero motif, the individual often returns home, symbolic of returning to who a person actually is, but changed or modified. This is the learning process of psychotherapy, the process by which we are constantly changed in order to face reality, the process of psychologically "growing up."

Kurt Goldstein's Insights

Kurt Goldstein[17] was concerned with the issue of how brain injured "patients might be brought to a condition where life would again be worth living" (p. 6). He recognized that for a healthy existence all of us need to make choices and to accept some restrictions in pursuit of health. He believed that the catastrophic reaction after brain injury, at its core, reflected patients' "subjective experience at being in danger of losing existence" (p. 8).

To help patients avoid the catastrophic condition and anxiety, Goldstein thought it was crucial to teach them how to make decisions (i.e., choices) that would enhance their sense of personal survival and their ability to function to maximum capacity. This concept is not far removed from Jung's notion of fostering the process of individuation. Goldstein's perspective, however, emphasizes that with the loss of the abstract attitude after brain damage, patients may need more direct guidance or teaching about what choices are actually healthy. Like other theorists, Goldstein recognized that successful therapeutic intervention required both that patients and physician (or psychotherapist) work together and that patients needed to participate actively in the process of understanding the complexity of their neuropsychological deficits and their personal reactions to those deficits.

Lost Normality and the Fear of Losing One's Existence after Brain Injury

A key concept in Goldstein's writings is that patients who cannot cope with environmental demands are thrown into a "disordered condition," and a catastrophic reaction ensues. Anxiety at such a time is a result of what patients perceive as a threat to their very existence. By restoring order, the patient "feels healthy; and one could say he is in a state of health" (p. 9). Goldstein's writings and his focus on the important of individuals' not feeling that their existence is threatened echo the existential concerns of many who have undergone the horrors of war.

Another way of approaching this same problem is to consider what it means for individuals to lose valued abilities as a result of normal aging or brain damage. In such cases, individuals may sense that their existence per se is not threatened. However, they are not the same as they were before and cannot do many of the things they once could. In this scenario, the focus is how patients can continue to derive meaning from life, given their restrictions.

Both approaches emphasize that patients' subjective sense of well-being and stability is crucial to the process of adaptation after brain injury. Psychotherapy and psychotherapeutic intervention particularly focus on helping patients gain this sense of well-being without lulling them into a false sense of security. Consequently, helping individuals relate to living symbols such as work, love, and play can be a practical, useful way of facilitating the rehabilitation process.[4]

Why Do Some Brain Dysfunctional Patients Not Benefit from Psychotherapy or Psychotherapeutic Intervention?

It has been known for some time that patients' anxiety and their catastrophic reactions may be alleviated by certain "talking therapies." Such efforts, however, are not always successful. A major problem facing the field is to reapproach the question of why some brain dysfunctional patients respond positively to either formal psychotherapy or psychotherapeutic interventions and why others do not. Clinically, at least three factors seem to contribute to this problem.

The first centers around patients' readiness to discuss important emotional and motivational issues in their lives. Patients' physical presence in a rehabilitation setting does not mean that they are ready to discuss such issues. The pressure from physicians or rehabilitation therapists, as well as financial pressures imposed by insurance carriers, may result in "psychotherapy" being done on "demand" (i.e., when the patient is seen for rehabilitation). Many patients need some time to struggle with their cognitive, motor, language, and perceptual deficits before they are in a position to talk about them in a meaningful way. The process of psychotherapy is analogous to the process of delivering a baby. Each mother-infant pair is unique, yet the laws of nature underlie the delivery process. Good physicians simply facilitate the natural sequence of events and know how to avoid catastrophes. If therapists know something about the process of psychotherapy (e.g., learning to deal with human suffering in a productive rather than a destructive manner), then they are available to help patients when they begin to deal with the natural consequences of brain injury. This natural process is often overlooked in the present managed care environment, which imposes formidable barriers to effective psychotherapy as a result.

The second reason psychotherapy may not be especially helpful centers around the actual skills of the therapist. Just because individuals are trained in some form of psychotherapy for ordinary clients does not qualify them for psychotherapeutic work with brain injured patients. Brain dysfunctional individuals have impairments at various levels of cognitive functioning that can and do affect their ability to engage in both the internal and external dialogues that are necessary for successful psychotherapeutic interactions. The therapist must be familiar with these impairments that affect the patients' ability to devote the necessary time and energy in establishing appropriate insight and a therapeutic alliance. A secondary but rarely discussed issue is therapists' capacity to tolerate how the cognitive deficits of a brain injured patient can slow the process of psychotherapy. Some therapists have difficulty in sustaining their energy to listen to such patients. Consequently, they have a difficult time entering their patients' phenomenological field to help them adjust—a process crucial to psychotherapy[18] and rehabilitation.[3]

A third factor contributing to the failure of psychotherapy is the actual extent of cognitive impairments and the premorbid personality of certain brain dysfunctional patients. Patients who have severely restricted cognitive capacities or a premorbid history of difficulty with self-control or of difficulty with demonstrating commitment to some activity or purpose find it extremely difficult to deal with the suffering associated with their brain injury. However, it is important not to assume that patients are unable to benefit from psychotherapeutic interventions because they are cognitively impaired or have a premorbid history of poor social adjustment. Rather, the therapist may judge whether a given individual has the capacity to benefit from formal psychotherapeutic dialogue. Psychotherapists who evaluate this issue carefully will make practical recommendations for the patient that avoid needless expenditures of rehabilitation dollars, a problem that is increasingly important for clinical neuropsychologists to face.[9]

Although contributory, these three factors do not completely explain why some patients respond poorly to psychotherapy. Certain patients often look like "excellent candidates" for psychotherapy but achieve little by way of formal psychotherapeutic dialogue. We continue to struggle to determine why some individuals benefit from psychotherapeutic interventions and others do not. One outcome study (discussed in more detail later) has demonstrated that the quality of the therapeutic alliance between the patient and the therapist (the therapeutic or rehabilitation team), as well as the therapeutic alliance between the patient's family and the rehabilitation team, relates to the patient's ability to maintain a productive work style. Being productive after brain injury is one of the major activities that helps patients cope with suffering and to reestablish meaning in life.

In addition to establishing a therapeutic alliance with a patient, it also is crucial to establish a therapeutic alliance with the patient's family members to achieve the best possible outcome from neuropsychologically oriented rehabilitation. The psychoanalytic tradition has emphasized total confidentiality about what is said between patient and therapist. Consequently, the patient's family members are seldom privy to information discussed in the psychotherapeutic session. Although confidentiality issues are relevant to psychotherapeutic work with both brain injured people and others, excluding key family members from the therapeutic dialogue often deprives the therapist of necessary insights about how to maintain behavioral patterns that foster good personal adjustment. This problem is especially difficult for psychotherapists who work with brain injured adults and children. We believe that incorporating key family members in the psychotherapeutic dialogue with brain dysfunctional patients often has a positive effect.

The Problem of Transference in Psychotherapy with Brain Dysfunctional Patients

Perhaps one of the major differences in doing psychotherapy with brain dysfunctional patients versus those without brain injury concerns how to handle behaviors that have traditionally been labeled under the term *transference.* In the psychoanalytic tradition, the patients' conflicts are thought to be projected onto the therapist. The therapist must therefore foster transference to help patients recognize their unconscious conflicts and to "work through the resistances to facing those conflicts." In traditional forms of psychotherapy, the therapist seldom gives advice and often does not directly answer questions, particularly as they relate to difficult interpersonal situations. For some, this style can be especially frustrating, and these patients (who have suffered brain injury or not) are discouraged with this approach. We believe that when brain injured patients ask for advice, the therapist should listen carefully to the intent of their questions and, when appropriate, provide direct answers. This stance does not mean that the therapist assumes the position of an omnipotent problem solver for patients. Rather, impaired patients need individuals who guide them in handling difficult life circumstances as they arise.

The focus of psychotherapeutic interventions with brain dysfunctional patients is to help patients find practical ways to diffuse aggression and rage and to "spell out" for them the most appropriate ways of behaving. This perspective is discussed in detail by Ben-Yishay and Lakin.[14] The phenomenon of transference can be as readily observed in brain dysfunctional patients as in other patients. We believe that it is rarely helpful to foster transference in these patients. They need help to achieve realistic insights not only about their limits but also about the limits of the therapist involved in their treatment. It is a reality-based treatment rather than a fantasy-based treatment.

☐ PSYCHOTHERAPEUTIC INTERVENTIONS THROUGHOUT THE REHABILITATION DAY

To highlight how various psychotherapeutic interventions can be applied "outside formal psychotherapy," six clinical examples are given here. The first three are from the first author's (GPP) experience. The last three are from the second author's (YBY) experience with Israeli soldiers attending a therapeutic community day program after the Yom Kippur War. In each case, the patients' personal histories were used to help them cope with the effects of their brain injury in the "here and now." The clinical neuropsychologist who appreciates the potential role of psychotherapeutic interventions after brain injury can be alert to instances when well-timed statements can contribute to the patients' adjustment process.

Learning that the Goal of Neuropsychological Rehabilitation Is Not Happiness but Independence

Case 1 ■ A middle-aged man suffered a ruptured aneurysm of the right middle cerebral artery. Before the rupture, he was diagnosed with Hodgkin's disease and was treated with radiation and chemotherapy. The patient had worked as a midlevel manager for a number of years and was in his second marriage. After the onset of his neurological difficulties, he was involved in a neuropsychological rehabilitation program aimed at helping him return to work. The biggest barrier that he experienced at that time was his depression.

The depression was partially addressed by helping him actively engage in a work trial that reinstituted a sense of competence in his life. He made considerable progress. After 6 months of

rehabilitation,[3] he, in fact, returned to work, although at a less demanding level than previously.

At this time, the patient's spouse requested a private meeting with the therapist (GPP). She stated that her husband was substantially changed by his medical difficulties and was no longer the man she had married. She had been willing to maintain her relationship with him until he could become independent, but now that he had returned to work she wanted help and support to seek a divorce. The therapist saw both the patient and his wife, who gently but directly stated that she wanted a divorce. The patient became overwhelmed and angry and threatened his spouse, stating that he would not allow her to leave him.

Over the next few weeks, the patient was seen in outpatient supportive psychotherapy (since he had completed the day treatment program). He frequently came to sessions intoxicated but denied drinking. Psychotherapy sessions consisted of pouring him coffee and discussing the realities of his life with him. At one point he asked, in effect: Who wants me? I am over 50, bald, overweight, and have bad teeth (because of his radiation treatment). The therapist responded that he had just described half the adult population. Capable of seeing the irony of his situation, the patient gave a faint laugh. He was reminded that the goal of neuropsychological rehabilitation was not necessarily happiness but the capacity to regain independence. He had achieved that goal and should not turn his back on it, given the setback of his wife's decision to divorce him.

With the benefit of the 6 months he had spent in intensive neuropsychological neurorehabilitation, the patient was able to work on this issue and again returned to a productive lifestyle. He began teaching medical transcription, lost weight, and got help with his dental problems. He eventually established a new relationship, although he never remarried. When he was seen about 2 years later, his development continued to be realistic.

Why was this patient able to turn his life around, despite this setback? He appeared to recognize that he had accomplished a lot in his life, both before and after his injury. He could recognize that the goal of rehabilitation was not necessarily happiness but the ability to be productive (and independent). His desire to be productive and his ability to comprehend this goal, in relationship with the events that occurred after his formal rehabilitation had ended, allowed him to make a good adjustment.

Learning to Show Love for a Spouse in Different Ways after Brain Injury Helps the Adjustment Process

Case 2 ■ A 63-year-old accountant suffered a right hemisphere stroke. Before his stroke, he ran his own business and provided a very good living for his wife and him. After the stroke, he cried pathologically (i.e., crying when not sad and for no apparent reason). Emotional stimuli of any type appeared to trigger the crying. During the course of a joint session with his wife, the patient emphasized that he felt useless and could no longer do anything for his wife.

The first step was to help him manage his pathological crying behaviorally. He was instructed to focus on his shoe whenever he encountered an emotional stimulus. This technique immediately neutralized his emotional reaction, and his pathological crying diminished greatly.

The patient was so relieved with the effectiveness of this minor behavioral maneuver that he became receptive to discussing how he might reinstitute a sense of meaning in his life. Although he could no longer work, provide a living, or do household chores because of his dense hemiplegia, he could still show his wife how much he cared for her. It was suggested that he buy 365 cards, in which he could write a brief loving comment. He was then to place a card under his wife's pillow every morning after she arose and went to take her shower. When she returned to make her bed, she would discover the card.

He was delighted with this simple suggestion and went out with an aide to buy the cards. Both he and his wife reported that his emotional state improved substantially after he had this simple but meaningful task to perform. This example demonstrates how psychotherapeutic interventions can greatly aid a patient's adjustment process, even though the individual can no longer work or be independent physically.

Learning That Returning to a Previous Level of Employment after Brain Injury Is Not Necessary to Derive Meaning and Satisfaction from Work

Case 3 ■ A middle-aged executive suffered a ruptured arteriovenous malformation that affected the left temporal parietal area.[19] He had alexia without agraphia and could no longer discharge his business responsibilities. Initially, he felt that he simply would take a medical retirement and stay home. With time, however, he recognized that retirement deprived him of the meaning that he had derived from work.

He enjoyed Arizona history. Consequently, an effort was made to help him to be a tour guide in a setting where he could teach others about the state's history. He could no longer read new information, but a therapist recorded information on an audiotape that he could memorize. The patient sustained this work despite the late onset of seizures. His case shows how helping patients find behavioral compensations for neuropsychological deficits not only helps them function in the real world but also helps them to reestablish a sense of meaning in their lives.

Psychotherapeutic Interventions after the Yom Kippur War

The remaining three case examples are presented in a different format[2] to illustrate how psychotherapeutic interventions can have a dramatic breakthrough effect on patients in a holistic day treatment program.[20] These interventions incorporate several principles of learning, as well as various ideas from different therapeutic systems. Each system is modified, however, to address the special needs of the brain injured soldiers. The different format gives a more comprehensive view of the patients' situations and how they were managed within the context of a neuropsychologically oriented rehabilitation program.* These case examples also show how certain interventions can provide true turning points in the rehabilitation of patients.

Case 4 ■ Reuven R. was 37 when he sustained multiple injuries during the Yom Kippur War. Shrapnel had penetrated the left frontotemporal area of his brain, and bone splinters and brain tissue had to be removed surgically. He was unconscious for 8 days. Upon recovery, he suffered right hemiplegia, dysarthria, aphasia, problems in breathing control, extreme sensitivity to heat and noise, extreme fatigability, and lability. Although his formal education had stopped after only 2 years of high school, Reuven was highly valued as the chief stock clerk of the Israel Aircraft Industries because he paid meticulous attention to his job and was reliable.

---

*As much as possible, Dr. Ben-Yishay's style of language is preserved in this portion of the chapter so that readers can share in his typical manner of telling a story.

After discharge from the hospital, Reuven returned home to live with his wife and only son (11 years old). Because of his dysarthria, injured vocal cords, breathing problems, and his constant preoccupation with his inability to control explosive outbursts of laughter and crying (when tense), he developed an elaborate repertoire of avoidance and escape behaviors, both in public and at home. Although his previous employers had offered him a range of flexible occupational options, he was unable to adapt to work life. He retreated into brooding, hypersensitivity to being "slighted," and prolonged periods of sleep. Family life became strained.

Two years after his injury, Reuven joined a special day treatment program.[21] He was a very positive, likeable, and highly motivated man who was insufficiently aware of his cognitive deficits and who was completely discouraged and overwhelmed by his inability to control his difficulties. Superimposed on his organic problems, Reuven also exhibited some hysterical features in his post-traumatic adaptation. Yet, he readily evoked empathy and sympathy in others because he radiated (somewhat naively) good will toward all members of his therapeutic community.

Immediately upon entering the therapeutic community, Reuven informed the staff that his most pressing problem was how to act like a "normal father and host" at the Bar Mitzvah party of his only son, which was to take place in 7 weeks. His deep concern was well founded. Reuven had been leading the life of a virtual recluse since his injury and had not seen most of his closest friends and many of his relatives. His desperate attempts to control his involuntary and explosive laughter having failed, he developed the habit of covering his face. When that strategy failed to help, he left the room and hid until he regained control. It was decided to tackle Reuven's problem as one of the first priorities of the therapeutic community. His "treatment" unfolded in several stages.

STAGE 1: "Objectifying" Reuven's problem. In two consecutive group sessions, the group, with Reuven present, was given a pseudoscientific explanation of the physiological mechanism of the involuntary laughter. The key points were that (1) the laughter was a matter of "scrambled messages" in the brain due to "cut" and/or "short-circuited" wires; (2) it was possible to "troubleshoot" the problem by means of "clever" training procedures; and (3) the problem was not with Reuven's personality but, rather, with the "electronics" in his brain.

STAGE 2: Modifying the hiding behavior while (through use of paradoxical intention) "liberating" Reuven from the need to control laughter and, instead, getting him to concentrate on what he wished to say to his listeners. A face mask with only two cutouts for the eyes and a handle was constructed. Reuven was instructed to cover his face whenever he "felt like laughing." However, he had to continue to participate (actively or passively) in the daily group communication exercises. His peers were instructed to act naturally and pay no attention to Reuven "hiding" behind the mask.

STAGE 3: Preparing Reuven to "come out" from his literal and figurative hiding and to invite his friends and relatives to the reception, personally, face to face. After some discussions in the group and with Reuven's final "editorial inputs," a brief script was prepared. The script explained his reasons for hiding since his injury, asserted that the hiding was over, invited the person to the party, and reassured his listener, "I will be all right and you should not feel uncomfortable if you see me laughing." Reuven practiced this invitation ritual many times during role-playing exercises with his peers by using the mask whenever he felt the need to do so. On no account was he to interrupt his speech of invitation—behind the mask or without it, laughing or not.

STAGE 4: Substituting a pair of dark sunglasses for the mask, Reuven continued to practice his person-to-person invitation ritual with his peers. This time, however, he put on sunglasses whenever he felt the need to hide. (The official cover story would be that his eyes were sensitive to bright light.)

STAGE 5: Introducing a fail-safe system. To further enforce Reuven's sense of mastery, a last-minute, cannot-fail safety procedure was added to the sunglasses. Reuven was told that if he found himself beginning to laugh, even with the glasses on, he should touch the corner of the frame of his glasses with his thumb and forefinger, mimicking the typical gesture people make when their glasses feel uncomfortable. Reuven was told that such fail-safe maneuvers could be performed as often as he needed because they appeared "natural."

STAGE 6: "Field-testing" the well-rehearsed "security" system. Armed with knowledge that he could now make a dignified appearance, Reuven visited about 20 of his friends and relatives and personally invited them to the reception. He then said, "This is enough, I am ready for the party." The party was a great success. To the surprise of his peers and therapist, Reuven removed the sunglasses about 1 hour into the party. From that point on, Reuven was cured of his problem. Reuven's ultimate rehabilitation was most successful. Ten months later, he resumed his old job and has remained fully employed since.

Case 5 ■ Matthew M. was 26 years old when he led his tank battalion into battle during the first

In many rehabilitation settings, the time and place for group programming are well established to facilitate planning and speed patient inclusion in group treatment. However, teams are advised to regularly reassess group programming to ensure that groups are suitable for their patient population. In our rapidly changing health care environment, the risk exists that patients may be thrust into inappropriate groups. Likewise, a facility's group programming may no longer meet the needs of the patients they are currently treating.

□ DRIVING

At some point during rehabilitation, patients who have previously operated a car or motorcycle need guidance from the team about resumption of driving. It is incumbent on the professionals involved to judge a patient's fitness for driving and inform the patient and his support network of their determination. Although unsafe drivers must be restricted from operating a vehicle, team members do not want to prevent individuals who are safe to resume driving from doing so.

Several studies have focused upon driving fitness assessment.[51–54] The findings of each reflected difficulty in relating the findings on psychometric measures with behind-the-wheel performance. Critical issues such as awareness and insight, as well as performance on closed-circuit versus open-road driving, were raised in these studies.

Driving is a highly complex task requiring integration of a wide range of performance components. Many discrete cognitive, perceptual, sensory, and motor skills are required for safe vehicle operation. Brain injury often causes impairments in these areas. The professionals' task is to judge a patient's readiness for driving assessment and safety in vehicle operation.

Predriving assessments are conducted prior to behind-the-wheel testing. These predriving assessments usually test perceptual and cognitive abilities judged to have predictive value for driving.[51,52] Patients who pass the predriving assessments may progress to evaluation and training with a driving simulator,* which permits patients to use the car controls and practice vehicle control. Patients engaged in simulator driving are scored on their responses, which offers quantitative feedback to the evaluator

*Driving simulators are manufactured by Doron Precision Systems, PO Box 400, Binghamton, New York, 13902. Simulators permit use of adaptive controls and offer films which create simulated driving situations in a variety of weather conditions and environs.

and the patient. The research of Galski et al.[52] indicates the potential value of combining simulator assessment with psychometric and on-the-road assessment.

Behind-the-wheel evaluations are routinely employed by driving evaluators to assess driving fitness.[51,52] Closed-circuit courses and in-traffic situations are combined. Although employees of standard driving schools may offer adequate behind-the-wheel experiences, the educated observations of a health care professional certified as a driving instructor is likely more beneficial for individuals who have experienced head injury.

When driving assessment reveals the potential for safe driving despite impaired driving skills, driving training is recommended. A combination of behind-the-wheel experiences and simulated drivers' training to teach defensive driving techniques and enhance response time is most frequently employed. When driving training is complete, retesting is done to determine driving fitness.

□ CONCLUSION

Performance of daily living skills is vital to successful, independent living for all adults. Brain injury can severely impact ADL performance and thoroughly disrupt a person's lifestyle. Recovery of ADL function is an arduous process for many survivors of brain injury. Rehabilitation professionals continually seek to refine assessment techniques and therapeutic interventions for ADL retraining. Subacute rehabilitation, day programs, transitional and assisted living, supported employment, and adult day care offer rehabilitative options for survivors who need continued therapy to regain independence. The interdisciplinary approach employed within rehabilitation settings promotes collaboration and coherence during ADL retraining. Increased integration of services offers more proficient reinforcement of newly learned strategies to promote greater reacquisition of functional skills.

Not all people with brain injury reach the point of independent living. Cognitive, behavioral, physical, and visual-perceptual deficits often combine to limit functional abilities. In such situations, families often assume responsibility for many, if not all, of the injured person's ADLs. The resulting stress within the social support network should remain foremost in the minds of rehabilitation staff as they interact with families.

In the current environment of managed care, teams seek to address ADLs quickly and efficiently. Therapists are encouraged to use innovative, creative approaches to retraining. Relevancy of therapy results from "patient-focused" few hours of the Yom Kippur War. Standing erect in his open tank, he sustained severe head wounds from shrapnel that penetrated the right frontal lobe and traveled to the left occipital region (where it is still lodged). He was evacuated by helicopter. During surgery, cerebrospinal fluid leaked from the entry site of the wound. Bone splinters were removed, and the dura mater was closed. He was unconscious for 15 days. Upon regaining consciousness, Matthew exhibited an array of bifrontal symptoms. He lacked initiation and spontaneity and had a robotlike, compliant attitude. He also had significant memory deficits and impairment of higher-level cognitive functions.

Before his injury, Matthew, a professional soldier, was a major in an armored division. When injured, Matthew had already completed 3 years of study in microbiology at a university near his camp. His objective was to obtain a doctorate in microbiology by the time he left the army.

While still on the neurosurgical service of the hospital, his fiancée (with whom he had lived for more than a year) visited him a few times. Then she left him without a word, never to return or contact him again. From the hospital, Matthew was discharged to the home of his elderly parents, where he led a sterile and robotlike existence. He uttered few words and responded in monosyllables. He showed no initiative, and his social contacts were confined to his parents and an older married sister. Two years after his injury, Matthew joined the special day treatment program.

Matthew's therapists were convinced that his fiancée's abandonment, especially the manner in which she left him, must have evoked powerful emotions in Matthew. Yet, when he was asked, "Where is your fiancée?" he replied, without a trace of emotion, with two colloquial Hebrew words: "Azva v'zehoo" (meaning "She left and that is all there is to it"). The therapists decided to "energize" and activate this severely adynamic individual, mentally as well as physically, by evoking his presumed buried emotions about the loss of his fiancée. The following procedure was adopted:

STAGE 1: The therapist undertook a painstaking effort to retrieve (by means of careful and persistent interviews) every shred of memory that could be extracted from Matthew about his fiancée's visits while he lay in the hospital. It turned out that Matthew had some fragments of verbal or visual memories (e.g., "she just sat there," "she did not smile," "her voice sounded cold," "I wanted to say come give me your hand, but I did not say anything; I just could not," "I somehow felt she does not love me anymore").

STAGE 2: The therapist told the group Matthew's "story." Having secured Matthew's permission to tell the guys what the therapist was able to dredge up from Matthew's fragmented memories, the therapist launched into a highly dramatized reconstruction of the great "betrayal of a hero" at his "most helpless" state. Most of these young, injured war veterans were moved to tears (one or two even sobbed). Witnessing his buddies' reactions, Matthew's body language registered some visible signs of emotions. Although he uttered not a single word, an embarrassed smile appeared on his face (the first smile in weeks).

STAGE 3: The betrayal was acted out by two therapists with Matthew sandwiched between them. Role playing an agreed-upon and rehearsed script, two therapists reenacted the fiancée's last visit at Matthew's bedside. Every plausible, subtle nuance of emotion that could be built around the substantially fleshed-out fragments of Matthew's recollections was explicitly verbalized by the therapists. The two "actors" in this psychodrama made a special effort to put heart and soul into their respective roles. The purpose was to move Matthew's peers and, by their reactions, to engage Matthew's own feelings. Thus, with Matthew seated between the two therapists, his peers serving as the audience, and the video camera recording the "play," one therapist (acting as Matthew) told the "fiancée" (as role-played by the second therapist) how deeply hurt he was and how angry he was with her for "walking out on me when I am down and helpless." The "fiancée" replied, in effect, "You are not the man I loved. I must leave you now because all I can feel for you is pity, and that is not a basis for a marriage." Predictably, some of Matthew's peers could not contain their emotions and jumped into the act, fiercely attacking her for her poor timing or selfishness.

This highly emotional (albeit imaginary) "dialogue" between Matthew and his fiancée did get him worked up some. He began talking at length to his peers, saying, in effect, "I don't know if I really thought those thoughts or felt such feelings, but I must have because I feel this way now."

STAGE 4: Matthew and his peers reviewed the videotaped "dialogue" with his fiancée. The therapist then asked, "So now, this intelligent, resourceful, brave, and resilient man is finished for good? Or, will he bounce back?" A series of highly charged discussions ensued.

After these dramatic sessions, Matthew came alive, so to speak. His rehabilitation then "took off." One year later, Matthew married a young teacher whom he met at a social gathering (quite a few Israeli women married war-injured veterans at the time). Shortly thereafter, Matthew was trained to perform several agricultural tests "by the numbers," following operation manuals designed to fit his special needs. Matthew is still employed by the government-owned agricultural station—and he is now a grandfather!

Case 6 ■ Aaron was 30 years old when he sustained a severe closed head injury in a parachute jump at night during a military action in the Yom Kippur War. A rotational type of acceleration-deceleration injury fractured his skull (from the left parietotemporal region to the base of his skull). He suffered from left hemiparesis, left oculomotor paresis, cognitive and perceptual deficits with extreme rigidity of thought, and agitated depression. He was unconscious for 8 days and semiconscious another 13 days.

Aaron had only 10 years of formal education, but he was self-taught (especially in military affairs) and considered to be "smart and resourceful." At the time of his injury, he was a captain in the airborne division, a career soldier, and chief instructor at the parachute school. He was famous (and, to some, infamous) for his exacting methods of parachute training and was considered to be a soldier's soldier. In his capacity as chief instructor, he trained rank-and-file soldiers, as well as high-ranking officers who wished to qualify as parachutists.

After his release from the hospital, Aaron returned home to live with his wife and 2-year-old daughter. (Some time later, a son was born.) He insisted on returning to active duty as soon as he was permitted to leave the hospital. When he proved to be inadequate on the job, he strongly objected to the suggestion that he take an extended medical leave of absence. He refused to acknowledge that he was having perceptual, cognitive, and personality problems. To prove his competence and fitness despite his hemiparesis, he parachuted into the sea to demonstrate to his superiors his preserved abilities and skills. Claiming that he had demonstrated that he was fit and competent, he steadfastly refused to be discharged from his job as chief parachute instructor.

After another brief trial at his old job, at which he was still inadequate, he was placed on "unassigned" status (i.e., earning his salary and benefits but given no assignments). Realizing that he was no longer welcome at his army base, he remained home, where he spent most of his time doing physical exercises, attempting to do woodwork, and writing a darkly brooding, rambling,

and obsessional diary and some haunting "poetry," in which he bemoaned his "great betrayal" by his former commanders and contemplated suicide as a way to punish those (including his wife) who "let him down." His marriage became very strained, largely because of his exceptionally rigid thinking and severely bruised masculine ego. Retaliating for his (mistaken) feeling that his wife no longer "respected" him (actually, she felt hurt by his sullen, accusatory, often rude behavior and yearned for her husband's preinjury "gallant" and passionate attentions), Aaron established an illicit liaison with another woman. This liaison continued until a few months after he entered the head injury day treatment program.

Soon after Aaron joined the therapeutic community, it became clear that his first priority had to be an attempt to ameliorate his problematic marital situation. At the same time, however, therapists soon realized that there was little chance of accomplishing a reconciliation by direct (one-on-one or couples) psychotherapeutic approaches. A way had to be found to break through this impasse because the success of Aaron's ultimate rehabilitation hinged on reconciling the couple fairly quickly.

After careful study of the situation, taking into account the human resources and clinical leverages available and capitalizing on the personalities, needs, and likely responses of the principal players, the therapist devised a strategy of indirect approach. This strategy was implemented in several lockstep stages as follows:

STAGE 1: Two of Aaron's peers (both of whom he greatly admired and who greatly influenced his behavior) were recruited by the therapist to serve as trained "surrogates" of Aaron and his wife in a series of carefully staged psychodramatic encounters. Aaron with "Ben" and "Dan" were invited by the therapist for a joint session. At this meeting, the therapist sought Aaron's permission to "share with them my feelings about your [Aaron's, that is] situation." Permission was granted. The therapist then launched into a detailed and dramatized description to Ben and Dan (with Aaron "listening in") of the "gallant, protective and loving" husband that Aaron was before his injury. The therapist gave detailed real-life examples, which, he admitted, were from "private conversations" with Aaron's wife. (Naturally, Aaron's wife gave the therapist permission "to use some of this information when in my judgment this might help.")

This initial briefing of his admired friends and role models had a salutary effect on Aaron. He clearly enjoyed being portrayed as the "gallant, protective, and loving" husband of yore. (Both

Ben and Dan knew about Aaron's liaison with the other woman and empathized with his attractive but greatly suffering wife.)

STAGE 2: Aaron "confronted" his wife via his surrogates in a series of staged psychodrama acts. Aaron, Ben, and Dan, with the therapist and one staff member acting as video cameraman, convened at the appointed hour. Aaron was briefed by the therapist to "tell your wife all that is in your heart. Don't mince words. Let her know what hurts you about her behavior since your injury, but don't use insulting language. Just let your feelings speak for themselves." Ben (the more astute and empathic of Aaron's two friends) was briefed (in Aaron's presence) to "tell your husband how much you miss his previous loving attentions, how hurt you have been since he has been passing you by with an angry scowl on his face. Never a nice word, never a hug." Dan was directed by the therapist to "stand behind Aaron and put into words what he secretly, in his heart, must still feel towards this beautiful woman whom he had courted so ardently and loved so passionately until the accident." Dan was told to speak out on cue from the therapist and say the words "which I will tell you." And thus, round one began in front of the camera with Ben (acting as Aaron's wife), Aaron (speaking for himself), Dan (acting as Aaron's "secret inner voice"), and the therapist (acting as director and screenwriter). Aaron restated his feelings of hurt, rage, and sense of being treated "ungratefully" and "disrespectfully" by his wife. At the end of each one of Aaron's remonstrations, Dan (his inner voice) piped in with the theme: "I wish, once again, to feel your warmth and approval." Ben (the wife) eloquently and touchingly expressed her "you don't bring me flowers any more" refrain and verbalized her yearning for the old Aaron.

STAGE 3: The videotaped session was reviewed and critiqued. With all the actors in attendance, the therapist found opportunities to further interpret and drive home different messages pertaining to Aaron's marriage and what it would take to achieve a reconciliation between Aaron and his wife.

STAGE 4: Aaron was persuaded to reverse roles and assume the identity of his wife during the role-playing exercise. Ben was asked to assume Aaron's identity and "tactfully but honestly" express Aaron's point of view, even though "I [the therapist said as an aside]know that you [Ben, that is]feel that Aaron has been mistaken about his wife letting him down, even though you feel that she is simply hurt and lonely." As before, Dan was instructed to "stand behind Ben and keep on voicing Aaron's inner feelings [on cue from the therapist]." This version, like the ones that preceded it, was a great success. Aaron (em-

ulating his idol, Ben) did an excellent job of verbalizing his wife's yearning for her "old Aaron," and the other supporting characters were likewise effective in their respective roles.

STAGE 5: The therapists met with Aaron's real wife and persuaded her to be receptive to any of her husband's "friendly overtures," should he (Aaron, that is) take the initiative to do so. While providing his wife with no details about the ongoing encounter exercises (beyond simply saying to her "I am convinced that your husband is struggling mightily to resolve his problems"), the therapist encouraged the wife to "respond in kind" to any of Aaron's friendly overtures toward her.

The therapist pointedly told the wife: "He may not say the right words. Judge him by his actions. I fully realize that after the great many hurts he inflicted on you, giving you flowers or some other gift without saying 'I am sorry for hurting you' may not be enough. . . . But, if you wish to have your husband back, you must help us guide him back toward more acceptable behavior." The wife promised to do her best to be receptive to Aaron's overtures, if Aaron made "the first move."

STAGE 6: Ben "instigated" the friendly overture. With Ben's active guidance, Aaron bought his wife some perfume and flowers for her birthday, and Aaron copied some apt phrases from a poem by which he expressed (albeit obliquely) his longing for his wife. True to her word, Aaron's wife accepted graciously her husband's gifts and refrained (at a substantial effort, no doubt) from showing overt signs that she could not simply turn off her pain (indeed, anger) "just like that." Her efforts were applauded by her peers during the spouses' weekly group session.

STAGE 7: Aaron reestablished normal relations with his wife. Shortly after these events, it became known (to those in Aaron's inner circle) that Aaron had severed his relationship with the other woman and that he now felt "much more comfortable" with his wife. (She reported in the spouses' group that Aaron was more "considerate and affectionate" now.)

The lifting of the marital siege did wonders for Aaron's morale. His rehabilitation (personal as well as vocational) could now begin. One year after entering the therapeutic community, Aaron resumed his army career with the rank of captain. With Aaron's active consent and eager cooperation, he was put in charge of a shooting range. Assisted by a smart and empathic young lieutenant and two experienced noncommissioned officers, Aaron was able to perform his duties to his satisfaction and to the satisfaction of the army.

◻ EMPIRICAL OBSERVATIONS ABOUT NEUROPSYCHOLOGICAL REHABILITATION THAT INCORPORATES PSYCHOTHERAPEUTIC INTERVENTIONS

Convergent data support the notion that rehabilitation that takes seriously the need to attend to the emotional and motivational reactions of patients with brain dysfunction may result in better outcomes. Rehabilitation outcomes can be defined in several ways. They include the patients' level of productivity and independence, the reduction of the emotional burden on family members, and the patients' need to continue psychiatric or rehabilitative services after an appropriate time has passed.

We submit that documentation of these areas helps provide evidence that neuropsychological rehabilitation has demonstrated efficacy and can be cost-efficient. To date, studies have primarily focused on the productivity of patients after rehabilitation and their ability to control negative affective reactions.

Productivity Studies

Prigatano et al.[22] reported that 50 percent of postacute young adult TBI patients who received neuropsychological rehabilitation that included psychotherapeutic interventions were working full-time or part-time or were engaged in realistic school programs at follow-up. Of the untreated TBI patients, 36 percent were similarly productive.

Several publications from the New York University Therapeutic Milieu Day Treatment Program support the notion that psychotherapeutic intervention (whether formal or specifically modified to the needs of brain injured persons) is necessary to achieve optimal outcomes from the rehabilitation process. Ben-Yishay et al.[23] reported that 63 percent of their patients attained competitive employment after completing the program (no control data are presented).

In a follow-up study from the same program,[24] factors that predicted the level of occupational success obtained by patients immediately after their rehabilitation program and their work status 6 months later were investigated. Small group therapeutic interventions, which were oriented at increasing awareness and acceptance of disability, were the most significant predictors of both initial employment status and 6-month work status. Likewise, the "supersensitivity" of specialized small group

therapeutic interventions (designed to foster awareness, malleability, and acceptance) over purely cognitive retraining methods has been demonstrated.[25]

In contrast, programs that do not actively incorporate psychotherapeutic interventions often produce outcomes comparable to the natural history of the illness[26;] that is, about a third of these patients return to a productive lifestyle with no rehabilitation or with only traditional forms of rehabilitation.

Prigatano et al.[28] replicated earlier findings and, by using a protected work trial as part of the rehabilitation program, reported a higher percentage of individuals who worked full-time after such rehabilitation efforts. Curiously, the percentage of control subjects (i.e., 36 percent) was again similar to those who were working full-time but who had not received intensive neuropsychological rehabilitation incorporating psychotherapy. These studies provide indirect evidence that such programs may, in fact, affect long-term productivity of brain dysfunction patients.

It is our impression, as it has been that of others, that 10 to 15 years after injury fewer than 10 percent of patient with severe TBI are employed. This figure contrasts with the 30 percent who are working 2 to 5 years after injury. Many of these patients continue to show a lack of insight into their disabilities and remain frustrated and confused about their problems. Consequently, they withdraw socially when they fail to maintain work. The holistic approach, which incorporates psychotherapeutic interventions as well as a variety of other activities, should result in a productive lifestyle maintained for longer periods. It should also help them maintain more stable interpersonal relationships. It is important, however, to follow these patients for several years to determine whether these goals are achieved. We predict that patients who receive treatment in such programs will maintain a level of work significantly higher than those who do not.

Accomplishments achieved through neuropsychological rehabilitation may also require maintenance and support systems to preserve patients' achievements. Therefore, it is crucial to determine what type of ongoing support will enable people to maintain the goals they achieved during rehabilitation.

Studies on Control of Negative Emotional Reactions

One of the most important contributions of neuropsychological rehabilitation is to teach patients to control negative emotional reactions.

This control can be achieved through many means, as the previous examples illustrate.

Prigatano et al.[22] demonstrated that patients who received neuropsychological rehabilitation were often described by family members (via the Katz Adjustment Scale) as being less emotionally distressed than patients who did not receive such intervention. Those undergoing rehabilitation were also often described as less negative and less verbally expansive and as showing less general psychopathology. They were also viewed as being more stable or reliable than patients who did not receive this form of treatment.

Rattok et al.[25] report data compatible with this observation. Patients with brain dysfunction who received a combination of cognitive remediation activities and small group activities aimed at improving interpersonal interaction typically showed greater control of their emotions and more involvement with others. Christensen et al.[29] also found that patients who are involved in such rehabilitation programs tend to be more socially engaged and ultimately require less financial support for their long-term care. This is an important outcome of neuropsychological rehabilitation programs that incorporate psychotherapeutic interventions.

More recently, Prigatano et al.[28] demonstrated that the working alliances between rehabilitation staff and patients and between rehabilitation staff and families relate to the patients' productivity status. A good working alliance does not mean that patients and therapists always see eye to eye about what is necessary for a patient; it is a growing sense that they are working together to help the patient become productive and independent. Furthermore, verbal agreement between the two groups about what course of action should be taken is progressive. Consequently, therapists must sometimes change their perspective, just as the patient and family must sometimes change theirs. This flexibility is the essence of a good working relationship, with both groups learning from each other. Against such a backdrop, we believe that these forms of intervention have practical payoffs for patients and their family members.

□ SUMMARY AND CONCLUSIONS

This chapter has highlighted evidence that formal psychotherapy and various types of informal psychotherapeutic interventions are important components of brain injury rehabilitation. Appreciation for their importance is growing, particularly when long-term variables such as the capacity of the patient to return to a productive lifestyle and to maintain satisfactory interpersonal relationships are considered. The most common long-term consequence of severe TBI is social isolation. Any form of intervention that helps patients to reduce their social isolation and to deal with ther emotional and motivational reactions to the perception of lost normality is an important service. Otherwise, patients remain frustrated and become increasingly isolated over the years.

Concern is growing that TBI patients are often placed into rehabilitation programs prematurely because of the financial pressures imposed by managed care. In our experience, patients placed into expensive day treatment programs within the first few months of their brain injury often seek help again 2 or 3 years after their rehabilitation has formally ended. At that time, they, their spouses, or both complain that the patient's irritability, social isolation, and paranoid ideation have increased.

It is important to assess when a patient is ready to engage a day treatment program that fosters productivity and helps cultivate the patient's acceptance of permanent disabilities without despair. When this is done, patients' adjustment can improve. Their self-esteem often improves, and their sense of meaning in life is renewed.

The measurement of any form of intervention, psychotherapeutic or not, must be based on a temporal continuum. The immediate, intermediate, and long-term effects of an intervention must be considered. In this manner, a clearer view of the role of psychotherapy and psychotherapeutic interventions in brain injury rehabilitation can be established. Such interventions are important, and failure to provide this form of assistance fragments the patients' care and ultimately frustrates both patient and family.

REFERENCES

1. Prigatano, GP: Personality disturbances associated with traumatic brain injury. J Consult Clin Psychol 60:360–368, 1992.
2. Prigatano, GP: Individuality, lesion location and psychotherapy after brain injury. In Uzzell, B, and Christensen, AL (eds): Progess in Neuropsychological Rehabilitation. Plenum Press, NY, 1994, pp 173–186.
3. Prigatano, GP, et al: Neuropsychological Rehabilitation after Brain Injury. Johns Hopkins University Press, Baltimore, 1986.
4. Prigatano, GP: Work, love, and play after brain injury. Bull Menninger Clin 53:414–443, 1989.
5. Romano, MD: Family response to traumatic head injury. Scand J Rehabil Med 6:1–4, 1974.
6. Klonoff, P, and Prigatano, GP: Reactions of family members and clinical intervention after traumatic brain injury. In Ylvisaker, M, and Gobble, EMR (eds): Community Re-Entry for Head Injured Adults. College-Hill Publications, Boston,1987, pp 381–402.
7. Prigatano, GP: Science and symbolism in neuropsychological rehabilitation after brain injury. The Tenth Annual James C Hemphill Lecture, Chicago, 1991.
8. Prigatano, GP: Disturbances of self-awareness of deficit after traumatic brain injury. In Prigatano, GP, and Schac-

ter, DL (eds): Awareness of Deficit after Brain Injury: Theoretical and Clinical Issues. Oxford University Press, New York, 1991, pp 111–126.

9. Prigatano, GP: Strengths and limitations of psychotherapy after brain injury. Advances in Medical Psychotherapy 8:23–34, 1995.

10. Prigatano, GP: Bring it up in milieu: Toward effective traumatic brain injury rehabilitation interaction. Rehabilitation Psychology 34:135–144, 1989.

11. Prigatano, GP: Disordered mind, wounded soul: The emerging role of psychotherapy in rehabilitation after brain injury. J Head Trauma Rehabil 6:1–10, 1991.

12. Hall, CS, and Lindzey, G: Theories of Personality, ed 3. John Wiley, New York, 1978.

13. Christensen, AL, and Rosenberg, NK: A critique of the role of psychotherapy in brain injury rehabilitation. J Head Trauma Rehab 6:56–61, 1991.

14. Ben-Yishay, Y, and Lakin, P: Structured group treatment for brain-injury survivors. In Ellis, DW, and Christensen, A-L (eds): Neuropsychological Treatment after Brain Injury. Kluwer, Boston, 1989, pp 271–295.

15. Jung, C: The Practice of Psychotherapy, vol. 16, Bollinger Series 2. Princeton University Press, Princeton, NJ, 1957.

16. Campbell, J: The Hero with a Thousand Faces. Princeton University Press, Princeton, NJ, 1968.

17. Goldstein, K: Notes on the development of my concepts. Journal of Individual Psychology 15:5–14, 1959.

18. Rogers, CR: Client-Centered Therapy: Its Current Practice, Implications, and Theory. Houghton Mifflin, Boston, 1965.

19. O'Brien, KP, and Prigatano, GP: Supportive psychotherapy with a patient exhibiting alexia without agraphia. J Head Trauma Rehabil 6:44–55, 1991.

20. Ben-Yishay, Y, et al: Neuropsychologic rehabilitation: Quest for a holistic approach. Semin Neurol 5:252–258, 1985.

21. Ben-Yishay, Y: Reflections on the evolution of the therapeutic milieu concept. Neuropsychological Rehabilitation 6:327–343, 1996.

22. Prigatano, GP, et al: Neuropsychological rehabilitation after closed head injury in young adults. J Neurol Neurosurg Psychiatry 47:505–513, 1984.

23. Ben-Yishay, Y, et al: Relationship between employability and vocational outcome after intensive holistic cognitive rehabilitation. J Head Trauma Rehabil 2:35–48, 1987.

24. Ezrachi, O, et al: Predicting employment in traumatic brain injury following neuropsychological rehabilitation. J Head Trauma Rehabil 6:71–84, 1991.

25. Rattok, J, et al: Outcome of different treatment mixes in a multidimensional neuropsychological rehabilitation program. Neuropsychology 6:395–415, 1992.

26. Scherzer, BP: Rehabilitation following severe head trauma: Results of a three-year program. Arch Phys Med Rehabil 67:366–374, 1986.

27. Brooks, N, et al: Return to work within the first seven years of severe head injury. Brain Inj 1:5–19, 1987.

28. Prigatano, GP, et al: Productivity after neuropsychologically oriented, milieu rehabilitation. J Head Trauma Rehabil 9:91–102, 1994.

29. Christensen, A-L, et al: Psychosocial outcome following individualized neuropsychological rehabilitation of brain damage. Acta Neurol Scand 85:32–38, 1992.

Treatment Approaches for Communication Disorders

KATHRYN M. YORKSTON, PHD,
and MARY R. T. KENNEDY, PHD

Communication dysfunction has a pervasive impact on the lives of individuals with traumatic brain injury (TBI). Early in recovery, communication is closely linked to the level of arousal. In the middle phases of recovery, confusion is manifested in communication activities. In the late phases of recovery, it is difficult to imagine many aspects of daily living that do not require some kind of communication. Because communication is so central to the rehabilitation process, intervention to minimize these deficits is critical. Although many types of communication disorders occur, the focus of this chapter is on cognitive-communication and motor speech disorders. These disorders are both common in the TBI populations and are frequently the target of intervention efforts. Communication intervention approaches are organized according to the model of chronic disease. Thus, communication interventions focusing on reduction of the impairment, functional limitation, and disability are highlighted.

□ MODEL OF CHRONIC DISEASE

The World Health Organization's model of chronic disease is a useful framework on which to organize assessment and intervention planning for a variety of communication disorders.[1-3] As revised by the Institute of Medicine and the National Center for Medical Rehabilitation Research,[4] five parameters are described: (1) *Pathophysiological* alterations occur at the cellular or physiological level; (2) *impairments* oc-

cur as loss of function (mental or physiological) of the physiology; (3) *functional limitations* are reductions in the ability to function because of an impairment; (4) *disabilities* are reductions in performance in natural environments; and (5) *societal limitations* are changes in performance that reduce or alter a person's societal roles.

The model's five parameters have been used to differentiate assessment and intervention approaches for cognitive-communication disorders and motor speech disorders, as illustrated in Table 17–1. The impairment includes cognitive processes (attention, perception, organization, reasoning and abstract thought, executive functions, awareness); memory processes and components (immediate, recent, remote, episodic, prospective, declarative, implicit); language processes (phonology, morphology, syntax, word knowledge, word retrieval, modality-specific comprehension and expression); and components of speech production (respiratory, laryngeal, velopharyngeal, and oral articulatory function). The functional limitation is reflected in a reduced ability to perform specific communicative activities (e.g., speaking, listening, reading). The disability involves reduced performance of communication activities in natural contexts. Each of these levels of deficits for cognitive-communication and motor speech disorders is described more thoroughly in this chapter.

For speech-language pathologists, assessment and intervention are typically focused in three of the five parameters of the model of chronic disease: impairment, functional limitation, and disability. A medical records review, patient and family interview and goals, standardized assessment results, informal assessment procedures, the rate of cognitive-communicative recovery in the injury, the interdisciplinary team discussion, the demands of third-party payers, and disposition plans all assist the speech-language pathologist in determining the parameter(s) that need to be targeted during intervention. Several parameters may be addressed simultaneously. For example, for a client who is highly confused, visual and auditory attention may be specifically addressed with audiotapes and printed worksheets (impairment level), while paying attention could be addressed during self-care activities in the morning (disability level).

A comprehensive communicative assessment, described in Chapter 11, provides clinicians with sufficient information to develop intervention goals and plans. However, the majority of standardized assessment tools in the field of speech-language pathology have been designed to describe deficits at the level of impairment—for example, selective attention, discrimination, short-term memory, and abstract reasoning. Such cognitive processes are believed to underlie the communication behaviors. Therapeutic goals generated from the results of these assessment tools are aimed at improving these basic cognitive processes on the assumption that communication behavior would also improve. This chapter reviews not only interventions at the level of the impairment but also those that focus on functional limitations and disability.

☐ COGNITIVE-COMMUNICATIVE DYSFUNCTION

Definitions

The American Speech-Language-Hearing Association's 1987 Subcommittee on Language and Cognition reported that *cognition* can be described as:

> specific processes which include but are not limited to attention, discrimination, sequencing, memory processes, organizational processes, comprehending, reasoning and problem solving; that use of these processes is based on knowledge (general information, rules, etc.); that use of these processes included the executive function (executions, monitoring and adjustment of behavior or response).[5] (p. 53)

Impaired cognitive and memory processes are responsible for language and nonlanguage behavioral dysfunction following TBI. The relationship between cognition and language after TBI has been described in detail in this volume

and elsewhere.[6-8] The term *cognitive communication disorder* has been used to describe the many deficits that affect communication as the result of underlying cognitive disruption. It is distinct from classical aphasia, the focal language deficit that occurs only rarely in the TBI population.

Communication is interactive behavior within an environment and includes the modalities of auditory comprehension, verbal language expression, nonverbal expression, reading, and writing. Traditionally, speech-language pathologists have viewed the primary purpose of communication to be the sharing of information.[9] However, communication has additional purposes, such as getting wants and needs met, obtaining social closeness, and expressing social and cultural etiquette.[10] Further, the communication needs of survivors of TBI change as their cognitive and behavioral status improves.[11] For example, individuals who are minimally responsive primarily express their basic wants and needs, and individuals whose behavior is appropriate but confused communicate for purposes of sharing information as well.

Treatment Issues

THE REHABILITATION TEAM

Speech-language pathologists are members of rehabilitation teams in a variety of settings, including medical settings such as acute care, acute medical rehabilitation, and subacute units and nonmedical settings such as schools and transitional living units. Because transdisciplinary and interdisciplinary team approaches encourage many rehabilitation professionals to address cognitive-communicative concerns, all team members must have a working knowledge of managing individuals with TBI.

All behaviors have the capacity to communicate.[12] The interpretation of those behaviors as a communication message is the responsibility of the communication partner. Furthermore, the appropriateness of the behavior to communicate depends on its interpretation by the communication partner(s). Because communication is interactive behavior, the burden of responsibility for a successful communication event becomes shared by both participants, the survivor of TBI and the communication partner(s). Thus, speech-language pathologists must incorporate communication partners (e.g., family, friends, rehabilitation staff) into the therapeutic process as soon after the injury as possible.

Family members are an essential part of the rehabilitation team. Throughout the management process, families provide valuable information about the injured person's prior communication

TABLE 17–1. A Conceptual Framework for Intervention Planning for Cognitive-Communicative Dysfunction and Motor Speech Disorders Following Traumatic Brain Injury

	Pathophysiology	Impairment	Functional Limitation	Disability	Societal Limitation
Definition	Interruption or interference of normal physiological and developmental processes or structures	Loss and/or abnormality of cognitive, emotional, physiological, or anatomical structure or function, including secondary losses and pain	Restriction or lack of ability to perform an action or activity as compared to preinjury performance; results from impairment	Inability or limitation in performing socially defined activities and roles within a social and physical environment as a result of internal or external factors and their interplay	Restriction attributable to social policy or barriers (structural or attitudinal) that limit fulfillment of roles or deny access to services or opportunities
Level of deficit in cognitive-communication dysfunction	Damage to brain cells in cortical and subcortical neuroanatomical structures	Components of cognitive, memory, language, and executive function systems directly and indirectly associated with trauma	Effectiveness and efficiency of cognitive-communicative performance for specific tasks	Cognitive-communication performance within its natural context	An employer's policy that mandates only full-time employment
Examples of assessment targets for cognitive-communication dysfunction	Evidence of damage using radiographic, imaging, and EEG diagnostic techniques	Selective attention, attention span, divided attention, short-term memory, word finding	Following complex instructions, explaining procedures, producing narratives, following daily schedule, planning for future events	Cognitive-communication performance observed in its natural context, e.g. "real l: e" conversations, planning and implementing actual events	Interviews with employers

Examples of approaches to intervention for cognitive-communication dysfunction	Pharmacological intervention to improve memory	Sensory stimulation for increasing alertness and attention, attention process training, verbal rehearsal practice	Training use of daily planner; internal and external compensatory strategies	Monitoring and interpretation of feedback; adjustment in use of compensatory systems; on-line flexibility in responses during conversations	Education of employers with the goal of policy change
Level of deficit in motor speech disorders	Damage to brain cells in cortical and subcortical neuroanatomical structures	Components of the speech production mechanisms of respiratory, laryngeal, velopharyngeal, and oral articulatory movements	Abnormalities of speech including reduced intelligibility, rate, and naturalness	Reduced speech performance in a physical and social context	A school policy that augmentative communication equipment may not be taken home
Examples of assessment targets for motor speech disorders	Evidence of damage using radiographic, imaging, and EEG diagnostic techniques	Determining the speaker's ability to sustain an appropriate subglottal air pressure	Speech intelligibility measurement	Interviews with communication partners	Interviews with school administrators
Examples of approaches to intervention for motor speech disorders	Early pharmacological intervention to prevent cell death and brain swelling	Exercises to increase respiratory support for speech	Training to reduce speaking rate	Teaching the speaker with dysarthria to indicate new topics	Modification of the school's policy

Source: Adapted from Disability in America: Toward a National Agenda for Prevention. Institutes of Medicine, National Academy Press, Washington, DC, 1991.

and learning style, personality, preferences, dislikes, interests, goals, and hobbies. Family responses to the catastrophic event, as well as to the injured person's recovery, can influence the eventual success of the rehabilitation process. Providing educational materials during each phase of recovery is critical.

INTERVENTION PRINCIPLES

Several intervention principles must be understood to plan intervention for cognitive-communicative dysfunction. First, clinicians should understand how to analyze and assess tasks by their component parts.[13] Task analysis provides information about components that require direct remediation in therapy by identifying the breakdown location. Second, the use of errorless repetitive practice cannot be overemphasized. The verbal memory and motor learning research literature provides evidence that retrieving the wrong answer or performing an activity incorrectly can be detrimental. Structuring activities so that performance is targeted at 100 percent results in overlearning.

Generalization effects of newly learned strategies should be facilitated as early in the rehabilitation process as possible. The client should have a basic understanding of why certain strategies are beneficial. Therapy materials should be personally relevant, and activities should take place within the natural context unless aspects of the environment are barriers to performing the activity. Facilitating awareness of disabilities by training the client in self-checking or self-quizzing behavior can ease the transition to performing the activity in a variety of settings. Additionally, a treatment plan should be structured to match the individual client's unique strengths, address weaknesses, and avoid an emphasis on what the client cannot do or communicate.

Management Approaches

Traditionally, cognitive-communicative intervention can be organized into three different approaches: process-specific approach, functional approach, and skills training. Each is discussed briefly here; extensive descriptions are provided elsewhere.[6,8,14–16]

PROCESS-SPECIFIC APPROACH

Remediation of cognitive dysfunction after TBI, which emphasizes intervention aimed at improving the underlying cognitive and memory processes (e.g., attention, figure-ground discrimination, or encoding during short-term memory), has been identified as a process-specific approach. A process-specific approach "assumes that these specific areas can be treated individually and that they can be directly retrained and remediated.... It also advocates methods to assist individuals in compensating for residual deficits, recognizing that restoration of cognitive capacity to a functional level is not always possible" (p. 22).[8]

Because cognitive impairment is believed to be the underlying cause of communicative difficulty, this approach has been widely used to address cognitive-communicative dysfunction, as well as other aspects of cognitive rehabilitation. Tasks are presented systematically, based on an assumed cognitive organizational hierarchy. Activities designed to improve attentional processes, memory, visual processing, executive functions, and problem solving are used, depending on the patient's specific impairments. For example, if a patient at level of cognitive function V (LOCF V)[17] expresses himself in a confusing manner and formulates conversations that are not coherent, the underlying cognitive impairments could be inattention to the environment and inability to inhibit verbalization of disorganized thought patterns. Tasks designed to address the attention and inhibition impairment would be used in therapy, rather than tasks that directly address the verbal output.

FUNCTIONAL APPROACH

The functional approach to cognitive-communicative intervention emphasizes useful activities in natural environments.[18–20] Addressing cognitive processes apart from their use in a functional activity is viewed as ineffective because of potential problems with generalization. Proponents of the functional approach address cognitive impairments by using everyday activities, such as verbalizing appropriate social greetings or writing down appointments in a daily planner to compensate for forgetfulness. Although it is impractical to provide therapy in natural environments for clients requiring medical care in an acute rehabilitation unit, functional activities within that environment can ease the transition into the "real world."[3,19] However, for TBI survivors who have recovered in their cognitive-communicative functioning to the point of transition back into the community, work, or school environment, addressing their communicative needs within the context of their use is critical.

Functional management based on cognitive-behavioral recovery has been applied to different phases of recovery by using the levels of cognitive functioning.[17,20] Although not new, this approach to cognitive-communicative remediation encourages the use of functional activities within the context of a patient's current environment, while using task analysis techniques to identify the cognitive requirements or components of each activity. For individuals who are just emerging from coma (generalized and localized response), a stimulation approach is warranted. For individuals who are highly confused and agitated and communicate inappropriately (confused-agitated and confused-inappropriate response), a highly structured management system is implemented. As appropriate behavior and communication emerge (confused-appropriate response), less external structure is required. As cognitive recovery continues, automatic and purposeful communication and behavior reappear, and a community-based approach to intervention is required.

SKILLS TRAINING APPROACH

Training specific skills differs from the functional approach in that it is limited to the teaching of a single skill.[3] When the goal of intervention is to teach individual skills, such as the use of a computer or note taking during lectures, then the skills training approach is warranted. The speech-language pathologist performs a task analysis of the skill and determines which component of the skill is difficult for the client. The clinician then develops strategies to facilitate improvement in or compensation for that component. The client then practices the strategy for that component and practices the entire skill with the new strategy. It cannot be assumed that the strategy learned for a specific skill will generalize to another skill. Often each skill in which the strategy is to be used must be addressed individually.

Treating the Impairment

When the component processes of cognition, memory, language, and executive function are believed to be directly amenable to intervention, the speech-language pathologist engages the TBI survivor in exercises and activities specifically designed to reduce the impairment. The tasks that are chosen are thought to demonstrate performance of the underlying processes. Intervention targeting specific impairments seeks to effect positive change in certain cognitive components. The findings of clinical research indicate that addressing some processes directly is effective, although much more efficacy research remains to be completed.[2]

For survivors functioning at Rancho levels II (generalized response) and III (localized response)[17] who are emerging from coma, cognitive-communicative intervention has two general purposes: to improve alertness and attention so as to facilitate increased communication within the environment and to increase communication of basic wants and needs.[11,20,21] Intervention at the level of impairment is exemplified by the sensory stimulation approach. Sensory stimulation, which is the systematic and direct presentation of stimuli from various input modalities (tactile, olfactory, auditory, visual, vestibular, taste), attempts to improve the consistency, rate, and quality of the client's level of alertness and responses while reducing the likelihood of sensory deprivation. Care is given to the hierarchical presentation of stimuli and to the daily recording of responses by the interdisciplinary rehabilitation team.[22,23]

As alertness and responsiveness improve and the client begins to display an array of cognitive abilities and impairments, direct intervention may be appropriate. An example of intervention designed to improve focused, selective, alternating, and divided attention is the Attention Process Training program.[8,24] The assumption of this treatment program is that these attention processes support the ability to perform tasks quickly, encode, retain, retrieve, analyze, and synthesize information from the outside environment. Using this program, the speech-language pathologist presents audiotaped tasks with and without distraction while varying the task variables. For example, to improve sustained attention, the client is at first instructed to push a buzzer each time he or she hears the number 4. The mental complexity of the activity is gradually increased by changing the requirements of the task until the client is required to push the buzzer each time he or she hears a number that is 2 less than the preceding number.

Many approaches to the remediation of memory disorders in the TBI population are designed to focus on the part of memory believed to be impaired. Encoding, retention, retrieval, and recall have all been identified as potential areas of impairment following TBI. Training in encoding strategies such as visual imagery, semantic elaboration, and mnemonics has been used frequently by clinicians to facilitate retention of new information. The notable areas of improvement after such training are usually directly related to the type of task and stimuli used in the training. For example, if story elaboration was taught, improvement was observed in story recall.[25] Memory aids, such as visual imagery, have had mixed effectiveness.[16,26,27]

Treating the Functional Limitation

The functional limitation is the behavioral manifestation of cognitive-language impairment within a category of activities. Therapeutic intervention aimed at the functional limitation level addresses cognitive-communication behavior believed to be the result of impaired cognitive and memory processes (e.g., alertness, attention, recall, executive functions).

For survivors who are minimally communicating (generalized and localized levels of response), an example of a functional limitation is the inconsistency of the yes and no response system. Eliciting yes or no verbally or with head nod or eye gaze responses by using a hierarchy of systematic cuing techniques is an example of directly addressing the limitation.[7] Therapy structured to elicit consistency in following simple verbal, single-part commands is also an example of working on the functional limitation of inability to consistently follow simple verbal commands.

As survivors of TBI recover, they progress from confused communication to automatic and purposeful communication (Rancho levels V through VIII). Depending on the individual's point of cognitive-behavioral recovery, functional limitations can include (but are not limited to) reductions in accuracy, effectiveness, and efficiency during many communication activities, such as describing (verbal or written) a narrative or procedure, social greetings, following multistage instructions, conversing about a specific topic of interest, communicating needs by using appropriate social etiquette, sharing accurate information with others (based on recall ability), using facial and gestural expression during social encounters, comprehending complex reading material, and generating and delivering written narratives, reports, and speeches.

To address these functional limitations, the speech-language pathologist creates activities that are designed to directly decrease the limitation by employing a task analysis approach to determine the "point of breakdown" in the skill. Some examples of therapy activities follow:

Producing a complete and concise narrative: training the use of the "who, what, when, where, and why" structure.

Communicating accurate information about daily routine and meetings: training the use of a daily planner or scheduler to record appointments, note taking, list making.[28,29]

Reading comprehension and recalling paragraphs: training the use of preview, question, read, study, test (PQSRT) strategy.[16]

Decision making about the use of compensatory memory strategies (writing down new information): training self-monitoring and feedback using self-questioning (Will I recall this information when I need it? no; How should I try to remember this? write it down; Did I remember this without checking my records? no; Was I able to follow through with this after checking my records? yes).

Topic selection during a "getting to know you" conversation: teaching and practicing the use of structure and topics within phases of first encounter conversations (greetings, common topics to get acquainted, "it was nice to meet you" phase).

Treating the Disabilities

Because a *disability* is defined as a functional limitation within its natural context, therapy directed at the level of disability should be structured *using* "real-life" activities and, as much as possible, *during* "real-life" activities. Disorders of pragmatics (use of language in context) and executive functions are perhaps the easiest to relate to disabilities because by definition both require the spontaneous monitoring of performance and on-line adjustments in the natural environment or activity. However, disabilities occur when any activity is performed ineffectively or inefficiently in its natural context.

Cognitive-communicative disabilities span a wide range of behaviors, depending on the interplay among the context, the activity, and the underlying cognitive, memory, and language impairments. The environmental context should be viewed on a continuum from, at one end, providing assistance to make the activity "easier" to perform to, at the other, being a barrier or hindering the performance of the activity. For example, survivors of TBI who are communicating minimally as they emerge from coma benefit from therapy in the "natural" context. However, as survivors recover cognitive and memory processing capacity, the demands of the naturally changing environment can be a barrier in which speed of processing and quick adjustments of newly learned strategies have yet to be practiced. The conversational skills of one TBI survivor with frontal lobe injury were facilitated when communicating with a single communication partner, but in a group setting, initiation was reduced. For a TBI survivor who displayed confusion and disinhibition, the group environment facilitated appropriate behavior, but face-to-face interaction with a single communication partner did not.[7]

The transition from remediating functional limitations to disabilities can be viewed on a continuum of external control to internal control. External "structure" or "control" for managing the cognitive-communication behavior may be needed initially, but the overall goal is to have clients create and use their own internal control in the natural context.[12,20] These cognitive-behavioral recovery phases are related to therapeutic stages that recovering clients go through during rehabilitation, including engagement, awareness, mastery and control, acceptance, and identity.[8] Training of a new skill or compensatory strategy may initially be performed within the constraints of the therapy setting, where the environment can be systematically controlled and variables, such as distractions, can be altered. However, generalization of the skill will not fully develop until it is being performed and practiced repeatedly in its natural context.

Individuals who are extremely limited in their cognitive-communicative performance often respond most effectively and consistently to those they know the best, such as family, friends, and nursing personnel. Because of the inability to process and retain memory of their new surroundings and physical condition, they benefit from therapy directed at the disability. For example, addressing the ability to follow simple commands could be carried out during morning self-care activities, when the activity fits within the context of the individual's daily activity routine. Furthermore, eliciting responses to structured yes-no questions that are not personally relevant is less meaningful to the individual than responses to personal questions and may not be effective. Personal items from the patient's home are likely to elicit more consistent communication responses. When family members (and friends) are communication partners, the speech-language pathologist can observe the effectiveness and efficiency of the injured person's basic communication skills and also use the interaction as an educational and training tool for family members.

Intervention addressing cognitive-communication dysfunctions as disabilities can begin within the constraints of the therapy room but at some point must move into the real-life context in which the activity occurs naturally. For survivors who are confused communicators (Rancho levels IV through VI), this means conducting therapy by using functional items and activities as they are being performed within the person's daily routine. For survivors who are transitioning back into home, school, and work, therapy tasks should be the same tasks they will need to perform in the environment. Clinicians often find themselves providing services at the workplace, in the home, or at the school. The following activities provide the clinician with some examples of how intervention should be structured[7,8,12,15,20,28,30]:

Appropriate social interaction: structuring daily routines with few to no changes; training the client and communication partners (family, hospital personnel) how to use self-monitoring checklists of performance throughout the day so that feedback is immediate; training the use of conversational scripts through videotaped role playing and repeated practice (functional limitation), prior to training in locations outside the therapy room (disability).

Telephone skills: using scripts for obtaining needed information and making emergency calls; recording of information "online" during conversations, then reviewing information later; using clarifying questions when information is not understood; location skills using the telephone directory and operator assistance.

Organization of work, home, or school day: meeting with employer (or teacher or spouse) to organize and establish job priorities for day, week, or month; reducing length of work day to accommodate for fatigue; rearranging job tasks so that most demanding activities are completed during the client's "peak" energy hours.

Communicating accurate information and completing tasks: using daily planners, memory notebooks, and logs throughout daily activities; using "things to do" checklists to compensate for forgetfulness and reduce mental energy expended trying to retain information.

Study skills: using actual readings from school assignments, training the use of techniques such as PQSRT, audiorecording the material and taking notes from the recording.

❑ DYSARTHRIA

Description and Characteristics

DEFINITIONS

Because of the diffuse and variable neuropathology associated with TBI, motor speech disorders, including types of dysarthria and apraxia of speech, are common. Dysarthria is a motor speech disorder caused by disturbances in neuromuscular control of components of the speech mechanism. Weakness, spasticity, or incoordination of the muscles caused by damage to the central or peripheral nervous system makes execution of movements during speech difficult. Although much less common than dysarthria, apraxia of speech, a disturbance in motor programming of sequential movements for volitional speech production, may also be present.

The characteristics of dysarthria depend on the locus and severity of the injury. Diffuse neural injuries often produce a mixed type of dysarthria,[31] but predominantly ataxic[32] and flaccid dysarthria[33] have also been described. Overall, dysarthria is present as a sequela to TBI in approximately one-third of the population.[34,35] However, the prevalence depends on the time postonset, with estimates of 60 percent of individuals acutely exhibiting dysarthria and 10 percent exhibiting the disorder at long-term follow-up.[36]

COURSE OF RECOVERY

Long-term studies of dysarthria associated with TBI are becoming available for both children and adults. Although dysarthria may resolve during the early and middle stages of recovery, severe motor speech deficits may persist. In the case of severe dysarthria, a strong trend emerging from the literature is the idea that important changes in speech can be obtained many years after the onset of TBI.[37–44] For example, Enderby and Crow[37] followed four individuals with head injury and severe bulbar dysfunction. They noted that few gains were made within the first 18 months, and substantial changes in function were noted as long as 48 months after onset. The implication is that long-term follow-up is necessary to exploit and extend return of motor speech function.

Treating the Impairment

At times the focus of treatment is to reduce the impairment, in other words, to develop physiological support for speech. Documentation of the effects of physiological intervention has been the major focus of treatment research in dysarthria.[45] This physiological approach is particularly relevant during a period of spontaneous recovery but may also be appropriate in the chronic phase. Early intervention can be viewed as a process of creating the physiological building blocks of speech. These blocks are the minimal physiological requirements to support intelligible speech. If they are not present (as is the case with severe dysarthria), then the therapist must work to develop the physiological components of speech.

ESTABLISHING RESPIRATORY SUPPORT FOR SPEECH

Because the respiratory system provides the energy for speech production, it is frequently the focus of physiological intervention. Failure to establish respiratory-phonatory support for speech may be an important factor in preventing the return of intelligible natural speech and necessitating the long-term use of augmentative communication approaches. The impact of respiratory impairment on the performance of speakers with dysarthria is a complex phenomenon. Perceptual indicators of respiratory inadequacy include inability to initiate phonation, abnormal loudness alterations, and abnormal patterns of the timing of inhalation and exhalation. Breath patterning abnormalities are characterized by a deviation from the normal speech breathing pattern of a quick inhalation followed by a prolonged exhalation.

If respiratory impairment is suspected, then assessment focuses on estimating the adequacy of respiratory support (the speaker's ability to sustain adequate levels of subglottal air pressure) and the pattern of respiratory movements. By measuring oral air pressure during the stop phase of the voiceless plosive sounds (such as the /p/), the clinician can estimate the amount of subglottal air pressure a speaker is using.[46,47] Clinically, the 5 for 5 rule is helpful.[48] This rule suggests that respiratory support should be adequate for speech if an individual is able to sustain 5 cm of water pressure with a bleed in the system for 5 seconds. Respiratory support for speech can also be estimated by assessing the speaker's ability to produce sustained phonation.

Respiratory movement—changes in shape of the thorax and abdomen during speech—may also be disrupted in dysarthria associated with TBI. Speakers with reduced vital capacity may routinely need to inhale more deeply prior to speaking than unimpaired individuals. Other individuals with TBI fail to inhale before speaking and may begin to speak at improper lung volume levels. Still other individuals with TBI may exhibit a strong but uncoordinated respiratory system. These speakers may attempt to compensate for phonatory, velopharyngeal, and articulatory problems by inhaling to excessively high lung volume level, which results in speech that is excessively loud.

The overall treatment goal for patients with respiratory impairments is to achieve consistent subglottal air pressure during speech. A variety of approaches can be found in the literature. Blowing techniques in which the speaker is taught to blow into a pressure sensor, which contains a leak tube allowing air to escape at a rate associated with normal phonation, has been described for individuals with severe dysarthria.[33,49] Postural adjustments and prosthetic assistance have been reported to assist individuals with severe motor impairment.[50] Although there is no "perfect" respiratory shape for dysarthria speakers, some patterns of speech breathing may be fatiguing or unnatural and can be eliminated with training.

LARYNGEAL FUNCTION

Phonatory dysfunction associated with an impairment of laryngeal function is common following TBI. This dysfunction may range from a severe impairment associated with the inability to generate a sound source or voice during speech to a mild impairment associated with a slightly abnormal voice quality. Clinical assessment of phonatory dysfunction is made largely on the basis of perceptual judgments, such as judgments of features like pitch level, pitch breaks, and harsh or breathy voice quality. Instrumental measures of laryngeal function such as air flow through the vocal folds during phonation and laryngeal resistance are also available.[51,52]

Treatment of laryngeal impairment can be viewed as a hierarchy from techniques appropriate for severe impairment to those appropriate for mild involvement. Intervention at the most severe levels focuses on establishment of voluntary phonation. Generally an attempt is made to move from reflexive activities such as laughing and coughing to more voluntary voice production.[1] Reduced vocal loudness, common in speakers with dysarthria, may be addressed by training the speaker to generate greater levels of subglottal air pressure. As in the case of loudness modification, training of respiratory and phonatory aspects of speech often go hand in hand. When voice quality disorders are associated with hyperadduction of the vocal folds, traditional voice therapy techniques designed to reduce laryngeal hyperadduction and increase airflow through the glottis may be appropriate.[53]

VELOPHARYNGEAL FUNCTION

Velopharyngeal dysfunction of speakers with dysarthria is extremely important because it distorts the production of vowel and consonant sounds, thus exaggerating the impairment of other aspects of speech production such as respiratory-phonatory function and oral articulation. The patterns of velopharyngeal dysfunction in dysarthria include abnormal timing of velar movements related to other articulatory movement, incomplete velopharyngeal contact, and inconsistency of movement.[46] Perceptual indicators of velopharyngeal impairment include hypernasality, nasal emission during the production of consonants, and a disproportionate inability to produce pressure consonants. Instrumentally, velopharyngeal function has been assessed with aerodynamic measures of oral air pressure and volume velocity of airflow across the velopharyngeal port.[54] The velopharyngeal mechanism can be directly visualized with fiberoptic equipment.

The three general categories of treatment approaches for speakers with velopharyngeal impairment are behavioral, prosthetic, and surgical intervention. Generally, behavioral approaches are considered for speakers with mild or moderate impairment, who are taught to achieve adequate velopharyngeal closure by speaking at the appropriate rate and adequately monitoring their general articulatory precision.[55] The most common prosthetic method of treating velopharyngeal dysfunction in dysarthric speakers involves fitting of a palatal lift. A lift consists of a retentive portion that covers the hard palate and fastens to the maxillary teeth by wires and a lift portion that extends along the oral surface of the soft palate. Discussion of candidacy and timing of palatal lift fitting for speakers with TBI can be found elsewhere.[56,57] Surgical procedures for velopharyngeal management are rarely reported for speakers with TBI because of the permanence of the procedure and the speaker's potential for recovery of function.[58]

ORAL ARTICULATION

Impairment in oral articulatory function is almost universal in speakers with dysarthria and TBI. The most prevalent articulatory error in dysarthria is distortion of vowels and consonants. Treatment of oral articulatory impairment has often included attempts to normalize function. For example, exercises for strengthening the oral structures have been used with speakers with muscle weakness. However, caution is warranted because weakness is not universally present in dysarthria. Other abuses of strengthening exercises include delaying of the other intervention approaches until strengthening is "finished" and increasing the strength of certain muscles so that they overwhelm the efforts of others.[51] Other treatment approaches emphasize compensation for the impairment. For example, contrastive production or intelligibility drills have been used to assist speakers to modify production to make the final speech end product sound distinctive—for example, to differentiate *pat* and *bat*.[1] These approaches do not attempt to train the speaker to change specific movement patterns. Instead, general feedback about the adequacy of the production is given, and the speaker is expected to make the modifications necessary to accomplish the changes.

Treating the Functional Limitation

Treatment of dysarthria associated with TBI may also emphasize improvement in functional communication. When dysarthria is severe, this effort may involve the use of augmentative communication approaches rather than natural speech. For speakers with moderate dysarthria, speech intelligibility may be improved by using speaking rate control techniques. For speakers with mild dysarthria, treatment may emphasize improving the naturalness of speech production.

AUGMENTATIVE COMMUNICATION

The philosophy of augmentative communication applications has changed considerably in recent years.[59] The focus of intervention has shifted from providing a single, long-term communication system for those individuals with persistent, severe dysarthria to providing a series of systems that meet short-term communication needs while continuing efforts to reestablish natural speech. Case examples of the transitions through many augmentative systems are available.[40] Long-term follow-up studies of individuals who were nonspeaking on admission to rehabilitation are also available.[60,61] These studies suggest that approximately half of these individuals become functional natural speakers during inpatient rehabilitation, often when they achieve cognitive function levels V and VI.[62]

Appropriate augmentative communication systems depend on the level of cognitive recovery.[11,60,63] During the early phase of recovery (LOCF I, II, and III), the goal of intervention is to assist the patient in responding consistently to simple commands. Thus, augmentative communication approaches may include simple yes-no signaling systems. During the middle phases of recovery (LOCF IV and V), communication of basic wants and needs may become important. Thus, simple communication boards with frequently occurring messages may be appropriate. A simple switch to call for attention or running tape recorders may also be used. During this phase, natural speech may also be supplemented with the use of an alphabet board. With this technique, speakers point to the first letter of a word on an alphabet board as the word is spoken.[64] This technique not only reduces the speaker's rate but also gives the listener the extra information about the first letter of the word. Speakers who use this technique are often able to use natural speech earlier in the course of their recovery than they would without the alphabet supplementation. During the later phases of recovery (LOCF VI, VII, and VIII), severe physical impairment may persist. If this is the case, traditional augmentative communication systems may be used to produce unique messages. Most of these individuals are able to use their fingers or hands to select letters, words, or messages.[63] Systems appropriate during the late phases of recovery range from simple typing systems to more complex devices with multiple functions, such as message encoding and synthesized speech output.

RATE CONTROL

Rate reduction is an important strategy in speech treatment with speakers following TBI. Ataxia is a frequent component of dysarthria in TBI. Sudden onset of ataxia, coupled with poor monitoring associated with reduced cognitive functioning, frequently contributes to unintelligible speech. A variety of rate control techniques are available.[1] Some of these techniques are described as rigid because they impose a slow speaking rate, often at the expense of speech naturalness. Included in the category of rigid techniques are the alphabet supplementation described earlier and pacing boards on which the speaker points to a different location on a color board as each word is spoken. These techniques are generally reserved for those speakers who cannot learn to speak more slowly by using other techniques. Computerized rhythmic pacing and delayed auditory feedback are techniques that slow speaking rate but preserve speech naturalness.

MAXIMIZING SPEECH NATURALNESS

For individuals with mild dysarthria, speech naturalness often remains a concern, even after problems with speech intelligibility have been resolved. To achieve natural-sounding speech, attention is focused on the prosodic or melodic components of speech, including stress patterning, intonation, and rhythm. Contributors to reduced naturalness of speech include monotony (an excessively even rhythmic patterning of syllables, an evenness of stress patterning, or reduction in intonation contours) and mismatches between the prosodic features and the grammar of the utterance.[65]

Treating the Disability

Comprehensibility has been defined as the extent to which a listener understands utterances produced by a dysarthric speaker in a natural communication situation.[66] The adequacy of communication can be improved by a variety of simple techniques. For example, speakers with decreased speech intelligibility may improve their adequacy of communication by introducing a new topic in writing and by signaling listeners when they are changing topics. Other techniques to improve comprehensibility involve the listener and the communication environment. Severely distorted speech is easier to understand if the room is quiet and listeners are able to watch the speaker's face. Intervention focusing on improved comprehensibility of speech is dependent on a detailed understanding of the environments in which communication is likely to occur and on well-instructed communication partners who take an active role in facilitating the communicative interaction.

□ FUTURE NEEDS

Knowledge related to the management of communication disorders associated with TBI has grown tremendously in the last 15 years. Few publications on this topic were available before 1980, but currently several entire textbooks are devoted to the problem.[3,6,8,18,67] Despite the progress, the field of management of cognitive-communication and motor speech disorders in TBI is faced with a number of challenges.

Perhaps the most serious challenges are the documentation of treatment efficacy and the development of adequate outcome measures. The model of chronic disease that is reviewed in this chapter may be useful in establishing a framework for describing outcomes.[68] Future outcome studies may need to target multiple level of deficits, including impairment, functional limitation, and disability. Better communication outcome measures would no doubt allow us to provide more effective, timely, and efficient treatment to individuals with TBI.

REFERENCES

1. Yorkston, KM, Beukelman, DR, and Bell, KR: Clinical Management of Dysarthric Speakers. ProEd, Austin, 1988.
2. Coelho, CA, DeRuyter, F, and Stein, M: Treatment efficacy: Cognitive-communication disorders resulting from traumatic brain injury. J Speech Hear Res 39:S5–S17, 1996.
3. Gillis, RJ, Pierce, JN, and McHenry, M: Traumatic brain injury rehabilitation for speech-language pathologists. Butterworth-Heinemann, Boston, 1996.
4. Disability in America: Toward a National Agenda for Prevention. Institutes of Medicine, National Academy Press, Washington, DC, 1991.
5. The role of the speech-language pathologist in the habilitation and rehabilitation of cognitively impaired individuals. ASHA 29:53–55, 1987.
6. Adamovich, BB, Henderson, JA, and Auerbach, S: Cognitive rehabilitation of closed head injured patients: A dynamic approach. ProEd, Austin, 1985.
7. Kennedy, MRT, and DeRuyter, F: Cognitive and language bases for communication disorders. In Beukelman, DR, and Yorkston, KM (eds): Communication Disorders following Traumatic Brain Injury: Management of Cognitive, Language, and Motor Impairment. ProEd, Austin, 1991.
8. Sohlberg, MM, and Mateer, CA, eds: Introduction to Cognitive Rehabilitation: Theory and Practice. Guilford, New York, 1989.
9. Davis, A: A Survey of Adult Aphasia. Prentice Hall, Englewood Cliffs, NJ, 1983.
10. Light, J: Interaction involving individuals using augmentative communication systems: State of the art and future directions for research. Augmentative and Alternative Communication 4:66–82, 1988.
11. DeRuyter, F, and Kennedy, MR: Augmentative communication following traumatic brain injury. In Beukelman, DR, and Yorkston, KM (eds): Communication Disorders following Traumatic Brain Injury: Management of Cognitive, Language, and Motor Impairments. ProEd, Austin, 1991, pp 317–365.
12. Ylvisaker, M, and Feeney, TJ: Communication and behavior: Collaboration between speech-language pathologists and behavioral psychologists. Topics in Language Disorders 15:37–54, 1994.
13. Lezak, M: Neuropsychological Assessment, ed 2. Oxford University Press, New York, 1983.
14. Bracy, O: Cognitive rehabilitation: A process approach. Cognitive Rehabilitation 4:10–17, 1986.
15. Kreutzer, JS, Gordon, WA, and Wehman, P: Cognitive remediation following traumatic brain injury. Rehabilitation Psychology 34:117–133, 1989.
16. Wilson, BA: Rehabilitation of Memory. Guilford, New York, 1987.
17. Hagen, C, Malkmus, D, and Durham, P: Levels of cognitive functions. In Rehabilitation of Head Injured Adults: Comprehensive Physical Management. Professional Staff Association of Ranchos Los Amigos Hospital, Downey, Calif, 1979.
18. Hartley, LL: Cognitive-Communicative Abilities following Brain Injury. Singular Publishing, San Diego, 1995.
19. Giles, GM, and Clark-Wilson, J: Brain Injury Rehabilitation: A Neurofunctional Approach. Chapman and Hall, London, 1993.
20. Malkmus, D, Booth, BJ, and Kodimer, C: Rehabilitation of the Head Injured Adult: Comprehensive Cognitive Management. Professional Staff Association of Ranchos Los Amigos Medical Center. Downey, Calif, 1980.
21. Whyte, J, and Glenn, MD: The care and rehabilitation of the patient in a persistent vegetative state. J Head Trauma Rehabil 1:39–54, 1986.
22. Finger, S, and Stein, DG: Brain Damage and Recovery: Research and Clinical Perspectives. Academic Press, New York, 1982.
23. Ansell, B, and Keenan, J: The Western Neuro Sensory Stimulation Profile: A tool for assessing slow-to-recover head injured patients. Arch Phys Med Rehabil 70:104–108, 1989.
24. Sohlberg, MM, and Mateer, CA: Effectiveness of an attention-training program. J Clin Exp Neuropsychol 9:117–130, 1987.
25. Malec, J, and Questad, K: Rehabilitation of memory after craniocerebral trauma. Arch Phys Med Rehabil 64:436–438, 1983.
26. Daniel, M, Webster, JS, and Scott, RR: Single-case analysis of the brain-injured patient. Behavior Therapist 4:71–75, 1986.
27. Ryan, TV, and Ruff, RM: The efficacy of structured memory retraining in a group comparison of head trauma patients. Archives of Clinical Neuropsychology 3:165–179, 1988.
28. Honsinger, MH, and Yorkston, KM: Compensation for memory and related disorders following traumatic brain injury. In Beukelman, DR, and Yorkston, KM (eds): Communication Disorders following Traumatic Brain Injury: Management of Cognitive, Language, and Motor Impairments. College-Hill Press, Boston, 1991.
29. Sohlberg, MM, and Mateer, CA: Training use of compensatory memory books: A three stage behavioral approach. J Clin Exp Neuropsychol 11:871–891, 1989.
30. Tefft, D, Briggs, D, and Stone, D: Functional Skills Profile. Professional Staff Association of Rancho Los Amigos Medical Center, Downey, Calif, 1986.
31. Yorkston, KM, and Beukelman, D: Ataxic dysarthria: Treatment sequences based on intelligibility and prosodic considerations. Journal of Speech & Hearing Disorders 46:398–404, 1981.

32. Simmons, N: Acoustic analysis of ataxic dysarthria: An approach to monitoring treatment. In Berry, W (ed): Clinical Dysarthria. ProEd, Austin, 1983.

33. Netsell, R, and Daniel, B: Dysarthria in adults: Physiologic approach to rehabilitation. Arch Phys Med Rehabil 60:502, 1979.

34. Sarno, MT, Buonaguro, A, and Levita, E: Characteristics of verbal impairment in closed head injured patients. Arch Phys Med Rehabil 67:400–405, 1986.

35. Costeff, H, Groswasser, Z, and Goldstein, R: Long-term follow-up review of 31 children with severe closed head trauma. J Neurosurg 73:684–687, 1990.

36. Yorkston, KM, et al: The relationship between speech and swallowing disorders in head-injured patients. J Head Trauma Rehabil 4(4):1–16, 1989.

37. Enderby, P, and Crow, E: Long-term recovery patterns of severe dysarthria following head injury. Br J Disord Commun 25:341–354, 1990.

38. Harris, B, and Murry, T: Dysarthria and aphagia: A case study of neuromuscular treatment. Arch Phys Med Rehabil 65:408–412, 1984.

39. Keatley, A, and Wirz, S: Is 20 years too long? Improving intelligibility in longstanding dysarthria: A single case treatment study. Eur J Disord Commun 29:183–201, 1994.

40. Light, J, Beesley, M, and Collier, B: Transition through multiple augmentative and alternative communication systems: A three-year case study of a head injury adolescent. Augmentative and Alternative Communication 4:2–14, 1988.

41. Workinger, MS, and Netsell, R: Restoration of intelligible speech 13 years post-head injury. Brain Inj 6:183–187, 1992.

42. Jordan, FM, Ozanne, AE, and Murdoch, BE: Long term speech and language disorders subsequent to closed head injury in children. Brain Inj 2:179–185, 1988.

43. Jordan, FM, and Murdoch, BE: Unexpected recovery of functional communication following a prolonged period of mutism post-head injury. Brain Inj 4:101–108, 1990.

44. Najensen, T, et al: Recovery of communicative functions after prolonged traumatic coma. Scand J Rehabil Med 10:15–21, 1978.

45. Yorkston, KM: Treatment efficacy: Dysarthria. J Speech Hear Res 39:S46–S57, 1996.

46. Netsell, R, Lotz, WK, and Barlow, SM: A speech physiology examination for individuals with dysarthria. In Yorkston, KM, and Beukelman, DR (eds): Recent Advances in Clinical Dysarthria. College-Hill Press, Boston, 1989, pp 3–33.

47. McHenry, M: Motor speech disorders. In Gillis, RJ (ed): Traumatic Brain Injury: Rehabilitation for Speech-Language Pathologists. Butterworth-Heinemann, Boston, 1996, pp 223–254.

48. Netsell, R, and Hixon, T: A noninvasive method for clinically estimating subglottal air pressure. J Speech Hear Disord 43:326–330, 1978.

49. Hixon, T, Hawley, J, and Wilson, J: An around-the-house device for the clinical determination of respiratory driving pressure. J Speech Hear Disord 47:413, 1982.

50. Rosenbek, JC, and LaPointe, LL: The dysarthrias: Description, diagnosis, and treatment. In Johns, D (ed): Clinical Management of Neurogenic Communication Disorders. Little, Brown, Boston, 1985, pp 97–152.

51. Netsell, R: Physiological studies of dysarthria and their relevance to treatment. Seminars in Language 5:279–292, 1984.

52. Smitheran, J, and Hixon, T: A clinical method for estimating laryngeal airway resistance during vowel production. J Speech Hear Disord 46:138–146, 1981.

53. Prator, RJ, and Swift, R: Manual of Voice Therapy. Little, Brown, Boston, 1984.

54. Warren, DW: Aerodynamic measurement of speech. In Cooper, J (ed): Assessment of Speech and Voice Production: Research and Clinical Applications. National Institute of Deafness and Other Communication Disorders, Bethesda, Md, 1992, pp 103–111.

55. Liss, JM, Kuehn, DP, and Hinkle, KP: Direct training of velopharyngeal musculature. Journal of Medical Speech-Language Pathology. 2:243–251, 1994.

56. Yorkston, KM, and Beukelman, DR: Motor speech disorders. In Beukelman, DR, and Yorkston, KM (eds): Communication Disorders following Traumatic Brain Injury: Management of Cognitive, Language, and Motor Impairment. College-Hill Press, Boston, 1991.

57. Yorkston, KM, et al: The effects of palatal lift fitting on the perceived articulatory adequacy of dysarthric speakers. In Yorkston, KM, and Beukelman, DR (eds): Recent Advances in Clinical Dysarthria. College-Hill Press, Boston, 1989, pp 85–98.

58. Dworkin, JR, and Johns, DF: Management of velopharyngeal incompetence in dysarthria: A historical review. Clin Otolaryngol 5:61, 1980.

59. Beukelman, DR, and Mirenda, P: Augmentative and alternative communication: Management of severe communication disorders in children and adults. Paul H Brookes, Baltimore, 1992.

60. Ladtkow, MC, and Culp, D: Augmentative communication with the traumatic brain-injured population. In Yorkston, KM (ed): Augmentative Communication in the Medical Setting. Communication Skill Builders, Tucson, 1992.

61. Dongilli, JP, Hakel, M, and Beukelman, D: Recovery of functional speech following traumatic brain injury. J Head Trauma Rehabil 7:91–101, 1992.

62. Hagen, C: Language disorders in head trauma. In Holland, A (ed): Language Disorders in Adults: Recent Advances. ProEd, Austin, 1984.

63. DeRuyter, F, and Lafontaine, LM: The nonspeaking brain injured: A clinical and demographic database report. Augmentative and Alternative Communication 3:18–25, 1987.

64. Beukelman, DR, and Yorkston, KM: A communication system for the severely dysarthric speaker with an intact language system. J Speech Hear Disord 42:265–270, 1977.

65. Bellaire, K, Yorkston, KM, and Beukelman, DR: Modification of breath patterning to increase naturalness of a mildly dysarthric speaker. J Commun Disord 19:271–280, 1986.

66. Yorkston, KM, Strand, EA, and Kennedy, MRT: Comprehensibility of dysarthric speech: Implications for assessment and treatment planning. American Journal of Speech-Language Pathology 5:55–66, 1996.

67. Beukelman, DR, and Yorkston, KM, eds: Communication disorders following traumatic brain injury: Management of cognitive, language, and motor impairments. ProEd, Austin, 1991.

68. Beukelman, DR, Mathy, P, and Yorkston, KM: Outcomes measurements of motor speech disorders. In Fratelli, C (ed): Measuring Outcomes in Speech Language Pathology. Thieme, New York, 1998, pp 334–353.

CHAPTER 18

Behavior Analysis and Brain Injury Rehabilitation

HARVEY E. JACOBS, PHD

❏ CYCLES OF BEHAVIORAL INTERVENTION

The value of behavioral intervention following traumatic brain injury has been acknowledged for at least 15 years.[1,2] Early work by Eames and Wood,[3,4] among others, reported the reduction of aggression and other aberrant patterns of behavior with the aid of token economies, time out, single-subject evaluation methodology, and other commonly acknowledged behavioral procedures. By the mid-1980s, the concept of neurobehavioral intervention was well accepted within the care continuum of brain injury services.[5]

Use of this methodology has not been without controversy, however, and its introduction within brain injury rehabilitation has followed patterns similar to its introduction among other people and populations.[6] Initial referrals were characteristically for situations involving aggression, self-injury, or refractory conditions that had not responded to other forms of intervention—the last chance scenario. Behavioral intervention became validated as a means to help clients return to their previous treatment or to allow maintenance in less restrictive and less costly environments.

Subsequently, behavioral techniques were regarded for their ability to motivate client participation in other treatments through token economies[7] and other incentive programs. At this point, behavioral intervention was recognized for basic contingency management systems—the management of consequences to mediate behav-

ior. Over time, more profound aspects of formal behavioral intervention, especially those involving stimulus control and teaching, began taking root and contributing to overall treatment and outcomes.

❏ WHAT IS BEHAVIORAL?

What constitutes proper behavioral intervention is important. Many people outside the field have often considered any event that is *assumed* to change behavior as *behavioral*. Medications, surgeries, token economies, verbal mediation, education, coercion, restraint, torture, laws, access to sexual activity, counseling, food and water deprivation, motivational speakers, shelter, pay raises, downsizing, and so on have at one time or another all been noted to effect behavior, although not always according to the goals and values of the individual.

Obviously, only a few such interventions are acceptable in rehabilitation programming, but, rightly or wrongly, each has at some time been cited as a form of behavior modification within some social institution (e.g., schools, hospitals, prisons). Concern over actual or possible repercussions of the uncontrolled application of such interventions has also spawned decades-long concern and debate.[8,9] A specific intervention or event by itself does not constitute proper behavioral intervention, and there are specific guidelines for the context, focus, and manner in which a behavioral procedure is developed, applied, and evaluated.

☐ WHAT IS BEHAVIOR?

Behavior can be defined in many ways.[9] Sometimes it is defined according to topic or specific action. For example, instrumental skills may be considered behavior and different from other human activity, such as thinking or language. Interventions directed toward the former are subsequently considered *behavioral* in nature. Other times, *behavior* may be defined relative to its adverse effect on others (e.g., hitting or yelling) or negative judgment by others. Hence, unsanctioned actions involving violence, aggression, or noncompliance may be appropriated for *behavioral* intervention, whereas other actions, such as getting dressed, reading a book, or successfully following a treatment protocol, come under the purview of some other form of intervention.

Human activity has also been appropriated to behavioral or nonbehavioral categories according to the variables identified as effecting such action. Action that appears amenable to change through environmental manipulation (i.e., antecedents and consequences) is often considered behavior, whereas action that does not appear to have such immediate correspondence is often attributed to other causes. This division presents two problems. First, manipulation of environmental variables alone is insufficient for proper behavioral intervention. Second, few forms of human action are under single sources of control.

People are complex beings, and full understanding of the causes, attributions, actions, and relations of the human condition are beyond the scope of this chapter. However, we rarely have access to these complex relations. What we usually observe and experience are the products of such interactions by others—behavior. Thus, we do not directly observe memory but a person's performance on various tasks and tests. To say that someone loves another person is not based on a direct measure of love but on observation and interpretation of actions relative to given circumstances over time. We may measure thinking by virtue of a person's verbal reports (e.g., "Not right now, I'm thinking about an answer to this problem"), by observing their actions in a given test or situation, or through other indices that are attributed to ongoing processes. We may even attempt to measure elements of these processes while they are in progress through self-reports, neuroimaging, or other technologies. However, at this stage of scientific and technological development, we still have to correlate data from these processes with the action of the individual (e.g., there was increased activity in the left temporal lobe when the individual was talking; conversely, simply observing increased activity in the left temporal lobe would not necessarily mean that the individual was talking).

Defining all observable actions by another person as behavior does not relegate the cause of all actions to stimulus-response or other so-called behavioral paradigms. We are solely defining a product of the complex interactions among many salient factors at a given place and time. The procedures and techniques that we use are as diverse as the challenges we address.

☐ WHAT IS APPLIED BEHAVIOR ANALYSIS?

Behavior analysis incorporates specific dimensions of design, implementation, and evaluation into responsible programming. A classic article by Baer, et al.[10] noted that behavior analysis involves procedures that are applied, behavioral, analytic, technological, involve conceptual systems, are effective, and promote generality. These seven guidelines still provide a means of exploring this field and its application to brain injury rehabilitation programming, although some of the original language is dated.

Applied

> The label *applied* is not determined by the research procedures used but by the interest which society shows in the problems being studied.

Applied intervention focuses on practical presenting issues that are considered important by the prevailing community, the client, and his or her circle of support. It contrasts with basic research, in which findings that advance a body of knowledge may or may not have an immediate social effect. Basic research is obviously important, but it is conducted for other reasons. This guideline delineates between these different types of investigation.

Applied research also requires social validity. Simply incorporating full or partial research protocols into a treatment application does not constitute adequate validity for any procedure. Thus, the use of a single-subject design to evaluate treatment does not constitute an applied behavioral intervention if other subsequently noted criteria for behavior analysis are not included.

Behavioral

> Applied research is eminently pragmatic; it asks how it is possible to get an individual to do something effectively. Thus it usually

studies what subjects can be brought to do rather than what they can be brought to say; unless, of course, a verbal response is the behavior of interest.

Behavior analysis focuses on actual outcomes rather than correlates of outcomes. From its early roots, its practitioners have noted the inconsistent relationship between what people say and what people do.[11] They may report they are calm when other people see them as agitated because of their pacing, clenched fists, red face, and shouting. They may master a new skill as assessed by a paper-and-pencil test yet not be able to successfully employ the skill at work. They may report that they are paying attention when in fact they are looking at other activities and then cannot repeat the task they were just shown.

Accordingly, behavior analysis focuses on the actual behavior of interest within its prevailing environment for primary measurement, intervention, and evaluation. Standardized tests, surveys, checklists, and other correlational measures may serve as supplemental indices, help to further document and explain the main ef-

fect, or relate current results to others within a given population, but they are insufficient as primary indices.

Clear behavioral definitions require (1) precise specification of the topography (form) of the behavior and (2) specification of the environment or stimulus situation where the behavior is expected to occur. This specificity is key to program definition, measurement resolution, and treatment success. Thus, identifying a problem of poor memory provides little direction for intervention or articulate measurement; conversely, noting that a person is unable to independently take medication at school according to a prescribed daily schedule offers better definition for both measurement and intervention. Table 18–1 provides examples of prospective behavioral definitions.

Preferably, behaviors of interest are measured through direct observation, and techniques involving incidence, frequency, and interval measurement have been established for this purpose.[12–14] However, direct observation is not always possible, and it can sometimes confound results, such as having an observer accompany someone who is practicing independent com-

---

TABLE 18–1. Examples of Acceptable and Unacceptable Behavioral Definitions

Acceptable Definition	Unacceptable Definition
Stop throwing personal belongings out of the bedroom when angry and instead ask a house staff member in a calm voice if he can go outside for a 5-min walk to cool down.	Stop throwing things.
Eat lunch with other clients at the table within a 30-min period. During the meal, she will use a fork, spoon, and knife to pick up food items, as appropriate to the food being eaten. The client will chew food with her mouth closed, taking a bite no bigger than the size of the utensil at a time, chew, and swallow the food before taking another bite. The client will take food from her own tray only.	Eat lunch appropriately.
In the presence of members of the opposite sex, the client will not touch the other person and will remain at an appropriate social distance (i.e., at least 18 inches when standing and not bodily touching the person when sitting next to them). The client may talk on impersonal issues, recent accomplishments, joint interests of the other person, and similar topics, but may not talk about anything of a sexual nature. The client must remain in the presence of a staff member whenever with a member of the other sex.	Quit coming on to members of the opposite sex.
The goal of the program is for the client to walk 100 ft in the therapy room without any assistive devices or the assistance of another person.	Independent ambulation.

Source: Jacobs, HE: Behavior Analysis Guidelines and Brain Injury Rehabilitation: People, Principles and Programs. Aspen, Gaithersburg, Md, 1993, p 27, with permission.

munity transportation skills. Here, we may have to rely on products of the behavior as another means of measurement. For example, we might ask clients to bring back evidence of a journey, such as a bus transfer or a napkin from the restaurant where they ate. Ultimately, functionally related measures allow greater management of intervention and greater likelihood of success.

Analytic

> The analysis of a behavior, as the term is used here, requires a believable demonstration of the events that can be responsible for the occurrence or non-occurrence of that behavior.

Because behavior analysis recognizes the variability of people and intervention effect across people, it requires documentation of effect for each treatment application. Simply speaking, what may work for one person or the past 100 people may not work for the next person. Obviously, as the number of successful replications increase, the degree of documentation required may be reduced. However, it is still important to monitor individual performance to ensure that each outcome is having its intended effect.

Behavior analysis emphasizes the assessment of functional relations[15]: demonstration that a given variable (intervention) effects a change in another variable (behavior). Correlations—relations in which two events, such as treatment and outcome occur together—are insufficient for a behavior analysis. Ideally, a functional analysis documents targeted behavior change each time an intervention occurs. For example, whenever a specific medication was at a given blood level concentration, the person was able to sleep all night, but when the medication concentration fell below the given blood level, the person did not sleep. Or, after teaching each client a specific community transportation skill, each client was able to successfully access public transportation.

Single-subject designs remain the most common evaluation methodology in behavior analysis.[13,16] These designs are sensitive to individual variation, and different designs are available for different clinical conditions. A-B, reversal, additive, and multielement designs can be used to assess *present-state effects*, changes that remain only as long as the intervention is present. Multiple baseline designs are frequently used to evaluate *learning effects*, changes in behavior that remain after termination of intervention.[17]

Single-subject designs also have their vulnerabilities. Their purposely high levels of sensitivity make them vulnerable to unexpected changes in the environment, such as personnel, protocols, or other ongoing treatment. Dependent (behavior) and independent (treatment) variables must also be carefully defined, or the data are ambiguous at best, if the treatment effect is obscured by error variance. These challenges are best addressed through proper program design and careful management of the treatment setting during intervention. Critics of single-subject designs contend that generality of effect cannot be determined from an individual case study. Behavior analysts agree but note that the purpose of evaluation at a given time is the individual client at hand. Successive replications across additional individuals help to assess generalization.

Technological

> "Technological" here means simply that the techniques making up a particular behavioral application are completely identified and described. In this sense, "play therapy" is not a technological description, nor is "social reinforcement." For purposes of application, all salient ingredients of play therapy must be described as a set of contingencies between child response, therapist response, and play materials before a statement of technique has been approached. Similarly, all the ingredients of social reinforcement must be specified (stimuli, contingency, and schedule) to qualify as a technological procedure.

Interventions must be just as carefully defined as target behaviors. For example, a physician does not simply prescribe antiseizure medication but selects a specific type, at a specific dosage, at specific intervals, and perhaps under specific conditions (e.g., with or without food). However, we frequently do not rigorously define other types of intervention. Thus, two staff following the same procedure to cue the client through a morning dressing routine may implement very different programs. One may begin with a verbal prompt to get dressed and then verbally prompt the client to the next article of clothing after he or she has donned the previous piece without attending to other details of the client's behavior. The other staff member may break down the cuing regimen into smaller steps and use a greater variety of cuing procedures. This second staff member may also be more sociable to the client as he or she dresses (a form of social reinforcement). Hence, even a simple procedure can become two different programs by two different staff members.

Staff sometimes object to such specificity if it locks them into a regimented approach with no room for variation. Conversely, they may find provided specification too broad relative to the intricacies of the task at hand. Properly described interventions minimize these problems, and procedures that do not prove effective are modified. Data are consistently reviewed and programs adjusted as required to optimize effect. With time, properly trained staff become more articulate in defining interventions. Greater transfer of successful effect across staff, clients, and settings can also result because the variables that effect change are better understood and communicated.

Conceptual Systems

The field of applied behavior analysis will probably advance best if the published descriptions of its procedures are not only precisely technological, but also strive for relevance to principle. To describe exactly how a preschool teacher will attend to jungle-gym climbing in a child frightened of heights is good technological description; but further to call it a social reinforcement procedure relates it to basic concepts of behavioral development.

The conceptual systems of behavior analysis develop from its basic procedural building blocks. Most behavioral concepts focus on stimulus situation, topography of action, and probability of effect. A program is not judged by its intended effect but by its actual effect. Thus, an event can be considered a reinforcer only if it follows the occurrence of an identified behavior *and* increases the future probability of that response. We may subsequently consider some form of reinforcement procedure when considering a means to increase the occurrence of already established skills. A stimulus is a discriminative stimulus only if a person responds in a characteristic manner in its presence and not in its absence. Discrete behaviors that share one or more properties belong to the same class or operant by the fact that they all *operate* on the environment in a similar manner. Thus, after teaching someone a new skill, we may try to teach that person the class of behaviors, or *concept*, so that they will be equally adept in responding to a variety of like situations (i.e., generalization).

Effective

If the application of behavioral techniques does not produce large enough effects for practical value, then the application has failed.

The efficacy of any behavior analysis is determined by its practical value to the people who are directly involved in the intervention. Statistically significant effects that do not produce practical change for the consumer are simply ineffective. Within the pragmatic focus of applied intervention, they have failed to appreciably improve a person's quality of life.

This emphasis fits well with most requirements for successful rehabilitation programming. This standard directly addresses the role of client-consumer determination. Successful outcomes have to account for consumer goals and values during program design and application. Effect must also occur in situations and environments that are relevant to the consumer. Hence, treatment that is effective within a rehabilitation program but fails to sustain effect at the client's destination is not considered successful. Deciding what constitutes a practically significant effect obviously injects some level of subjectivity into any evaluation, which is why client input is so critical during all phases of programming.

Generality

A behavioral change may be said to have generality if it proves durable over time, if it appears in a wide variety of possible environments, or if it spreads to a wide variety of related behaviors.

Behavior analysis recognizes several forms of generalization. First, generalization can be considered to occur if an effect developed in one situation or environment spreads to others. It may occur as a result of direct intervention with the same procedure in new environments, such as teaching the client the skill in successive settings, or independent of direct intervention, such as learning paradigms in which an individual learns a skill in one setting and can then apply it in other settings. Second, techniques developed for one goal or behavior may be considered to have generalized if they then prove effective with other behaviors. Finally, we may conclude the generality of the technique across a group or population when the same intervention, or class of intervention, results in similar effects upon multiple replications. However, true to behavioral principles, procedural efficacy must be documented for each application.

These seven elements constitute accepted practices of behavior analysis and may be useful in considering behavioral intervention in brain injury rehabilitation. Ideally, each behavioral intervention incorporates all seven elements. Individual elements from this approach may also be combined with effective procedures from other orientations to provide successful and comprehensive services.[18]

□ TOPICAL *BEHAVIORAL* APPLICATIONS IN BRAIN INJURY REHABILITATION

The following section summarizes selected literature according to characteristic clinical topic areas. It should not be surprising to find similarity between some of the noted behavioral interventions and cognitive strategies; similar interventions are always open to different interpretations of the mechanism of effect. Most of the studies integrate several different procedures into a packaged intervention. Description of the individual elements are found elsewhere in the literature.[16,17,19]

Aggression and Agitation

Most early behavioral applications in brain injury rehabilitation focused on reduction of aberrant behavior and demonstrated how selected procedures could benefit many individuals who were refractory to other forms of intervention.[3,4] This early work was important for many reasons. First, it contributed to a then growing body of evidence that people can learn following brain injury.[20] Second, it focused on functional (and obvious) changes in behavior. Third, treatment was tailored to each individual and evaluated accordingly. Fourth, although most of the work focused on amelioration of aggressive behavior, it was implicit that successful outcome allowed a person to move to a less restrictive environment. Fifth, data frequently reported successful maintenance and generalization of treatment effect. Sixth, true to historical form, the ability to manage previously uncontrollable situations ushered behavioral intervention into other areas of brain injury rehabilitation programming.

Over the past 15 years, the concept of neurobehavioral rehabilitation has become synonymous with management of aberrant and aggressive behavior. However, not all neurobehavioral programs follow the same focus, design, or treatment philosophy. There are few standards for neurobehavioral rehabilitation, and treatment techniques vary across programs. Programs may exist in rural or urban communities, within existing brain injury rehabilitation programs, as locked units in psychiatric hospitals, or in state institutions. Many programs take on the character of their location. Not surprisingly, outcomes across programs range from basic containment

of uncontrollable individuals to positive and prospective programming that generalizes to normative, less restrictive, and long-term living environments. More work is needed to properly define what *neurobehavioral intervention* actually means.

Techniques for managing aggressive and agitated behavior have also expanded over time. Different forms of agitation have different loci of origin and require different forms of management. For example, early stages of agitation associated with Rancho Level IV[21] are now commonly managed by minimizing patient restraint while assuring safety through environmental management[22] rather than the physical and chemical restraints previously used.

Medications such as haloperidol are used less, in part because of concerns about paradoxical and possibly harmful effects.[23,24] Containment, restraint, and other forms of active suppression are more frequently considered as final alternatives rather than treatments of choice[25] because of their own iatrogenic effects. Too often, improper use of these procedures causes their own aggressive retort and results in overall suppressive rather than rehabilitative programming. Self-fulfilling prophecies can result, in which a client is assumed dangerous and is treated accordingly, which increases the danger of the client.

Intensive and active forms of containment may occasionally be warranted but as the exception rather than the rule. These procedures inevitably fail without properly trained staff who can fairly and consistently apply the intervention, coupled with facilitative programming to teach prosocial interaction.[17,27,41]

Jacobs et al.[28] unsuccessfully attempted a series of less restrictive procedures before implementing contingent restraint to address aggression in an adolescent male who was refusing food, medication, and basic care. Subsequently, contingent restraint worked quickly to decelerate aggression and allowed the implementation of facilitative programming to teach eating, self-care, and group interaction skills. The client's aggression was also affected by a variety of factors and situations. Although contingent restraint appeared to counteract any opportunities of avoidance or escape that aggression provided from most daily care activities, this procedure was not effective during showering or in small therapy rooms. Here an in vivo desensitization procedure worked best, demonstrating again the importance of assessing treatment efficacy with each intervention, in each situation, and with each presentation of behavior.

Delineating how components of organic or environmental factors can contribute to unsanctioned behavior is critical for successful programming. Treadwell and Page[29] and Pace et al.[30] have used functional analysis procedures to isolate the relative effects of environmental factors on behavior. Targeted behaviors are first recorded across a variety of stimulus conditions via single-subject methodology to identify which situations are more and less likely to evoke the unsanctioned response. For example, one person may demonstrate greater agitation under demand conditions but be cooperative in distracting environments with lower task demands; another person may decompensate in situations with high stimulus loads but not when receiving profuse attention. Each client's environment and treatment program are subsequently modified to create settings that optimize individual abilities. The resulting behavior change can be dramatic, and in some cases chronic and severe behavior dysfunction has been successfully addressed within weeks.

Procedures involving situational time-out, observational time-out, or cool down[31] have reduced or prevented aggression by preempting such episodes. These techniques help the client leave the setting until the situation passes or until he or she is able to return with a better management strategy. Although staff may first have to initiate each episode, some clients learn the cues to independently initiate successful action. This ultimate transition from therapist-directed intervention to client self-control represents one of the highest values in behavior analysis: helping people gain greater understanding and control of their own environment, goals, and personal affairs.

Haley[32] reported an early model of consumer involvement with a nursing home resident who persistently yelled and screamed. After spending considerable staff time to develop different interventions, the resident was asked for her input. Whereas staff were concerned about the resident's yelling and screaming, the resident was concerned that staff were not fairly distributing her cigarettes. A behavioral contract was established between the parties that clearly specified their rights and responsibilities. Problem behaviors quickly vanished, and within 1 week the resident was discharged to a rehabilitation program and then home.

Uomoto and Brockway[33] established successful home-based anger management training in which patients were taught to implement a self-talk method to decrease escalating tension prior to anger and a brief time-out when they became aware of increased anger. Family members learned how to monitor this behavior and to identify the antecedents of an outburst. They were also taught how to modify their communication style to reduce patient irritability, when to verbally cue the patient to use self-control methods, and how to increase overall family cohesion.

Natural Setting Behavior Management[34] addressed a variety of in-home and community challenges, including aggression, self-injury, noncompliance, and disinhibition. Clients and their families were first assessed by a mobile treatment team, who provided training on how to address presenting problems. This training included education about brain injury and basic behavior management strategies. Trained family units were able to sustain programming and maintain treatment outcomes. Interestingly, most improvements occurred during the education component as family members learned that problems could be addressed with procedures that were within their abilities. They had previously assumed that the presenting behaviors were *organic* and something they would have to live with.

Feeney and Ylvisaker[35] focused on consumer involvement and antecedent intervention to help aggressive high school students succeed in the classroom. The program included concrete task organizers to help each student compensate for cognitive impairments, daily routines to maintain behavioral self-regulation, student involvement in program development, and programming for frequent success as a means of maintaining momentum to the task.[36] Aggression decreased and compliance increased as long as the training conditions were maintained. The study recognized that the aggression was a response to other variables (e.g., student inability to succeed academically) and emphasized the use of antecedents over consequences to mediate these challenges.

Compliance

Compliance training remains a frequent source of referral for behavioral intervention. Requests usually involve development of motivation systems to increase patient participation, client-program interfaces to maximize therapeutic gains, and procedures to moderate disruptive behaviors that interfere with treatment efficacy. Properly constructed reinforcement systems can increase participation over a wide range of tasks *when the requisite skills are already in the client's repertoire.* Otherwise, skill development protocols are first required.

When developing compliance programs, most people overlook powerful and readily available reinforcers—frequent verbal feedback and social approval. Access to preferred activities or specific goods, point systems, check systems, and token economies can also be useful in postacute settings.[22,37] Properly designed token economies not only deliver reinforcement but also specify program goals and expectations from both clients and staff. These systems are generally not useful during early phases of recovery, however; many people cannot remember what the tokens signify, or they lose them. The use of naturalistic contingencies, in which one activity sets the occasion for the next, may be more effective in such situations.[38] Hence, scheduling breakfast to occur after morning self-care may relinquish the need for points and establish a morning routine.

Silver et al.[39] added a monetary reinforcement system to the daily self-care regimen of a 12-year-old with anoxic brain injury to reduce the level of staff assistance required for daily dressing, toileting, and undressing. The steps in the child's daily protocol had already been established, and intervention consisted of paying the client a penny for each successfully completed step. Pennies were empirically selected as a potential reinforcer because of their previously observed effect and not because of assumed value. Treatment gains were maintained at home 6 months later.

Although amotivation is often considered a key factor in noncompliance, lack of salient information can also substantially contribute to such problems. Established directions may seem clear to those designing a program but not to someone with a wide range of postinjury challenges. Zencius et al.[40] documented how simple, common, and *client-relevant* antecedents (cues) such as written instructions, maps, and strategically placed signs rapidly reduced noncompliance. These findings seem obvious but are not always followed.

Burke and Wesolowski[41] used a multicomponent program to reduce memory failure, increase worksite attendance, and reduce assaultive behavior. A careful analysis indicated that these behaviors were interrelated. Failure to remember a task usually produced increased staff attention and prompting, both of which can be powerful social reinforcers. Once off task, the client sometimes became disoriented and disruptive, which resulted in containment by male staff, which physically agitated the client and often resulted in his subsequent removal from treatment. The client would subsequently miss work and receive significant attention by female nursing staff, who treated his wounds. The client's environment was rearranged with cues and mnemonics that he could use to participate in daily tasks. A token economy was established to promote attendance and work participation, and he was taught to use relaxation techniques when he started to become tense. Finally, time to interact with female staff was made available each day he participated in his program. Within 2 months, disruptive episodes

ceased; the client consistently used his memory aids and was regularly participating at work.

Zhou et al.[43] modified the Trivial Pursuit game to increase knowledge and awareness about brain injury residuals. The participants previously refused to participate in other forms of knowledge and awareness training and had trouble staying on task. Eighteen questions were developed for each of six content areas: behavior, emotion, cognition, communication, physical, and sensory. Players advanced on the game board by answering the questions correctly and earned small amounts of money for their progress. All participants completed the training and gained substantial topical knowledge.

Slifer et al.[44,45] documented how operant conditioning techniques could reduce noncompliance and engender treatment gains when other forms of training were not successful for children who were still in post-traumatic amnesia. Once each child's amnesia had cleared, they were able to achieve greater gains through verbally mediated procedures than through operant conditioning. The authors suggested that these different techniques of learning might be associated with different neurological processes that unfold during recovery from brain injury, making each teaching technique more relevant at different times.

Skills Training

Behavioral strategies have been successfully incorporated into a variety of skills training programs. Task analyses can promote the careful definition of target behaviors and their aggregate into more complex skills. Emphasis on behavioral and environmental relationships helps to identify the precise stimulus conditions in which skills are expected to occur. Reliance on empirical outcomes to direct program design engenders adaptation of training strategies until targeted goals are achieved. Training is not complete at the end of a curriculum but rather when the client is capable of the specified goals. Most training protocols consist of a variety of integrated procedures.

HOME AND COMMUNITY SKILLS

Giles et al.[46,47] taught severely impaired and chronically dependent individuals to independently wash and dress. Intervention was adapted to each client's morning routine and involved breaking down complex tasks to simpler elements, establishing chains of behavior, teaching clients to follow the skill sequences, and reinforcing completed steps of the task.

O'Reilly et al.[48] modified in-home checklists to promote home accident prevention. Existing checklists identified potential home hazards but did not specify what clients were to do in each situation. Each client's accident prevention skills were first assessed, and task analyses of requisite skills were developed and incorporated into existing checklists. Training was then provided, as necessary, to assure skill proficiency. The revised checklists alone were sufficient to sustain the accident prevention skills as measured throughout treatment and at 1 month follow-up.

Godfrey and Knight[49] used functional skills training to assist a 33-year-old man who had failed to return to the community after intensive memory training. That training improved his concentration and reduced his aggression in group therapy sessions but not on his home unit. Skills training first focused on self-medication and participation in a community-based sheltered workshop. Skills were dissected via task analyses and trained sequentially through verbal prompting and social reinforcement, with supports faded as skills improved. The client was subsequently taught to live in a community-based lodge and use public transportation. Twelve-month follow-up indicated stable community placement. The client clearly spent much more time in functional skills training than in the memory training program, and it could be debated whether equivalent memory skills training would have produced similar outcomes. The functional skills training, however, focused directly on requisite skills for community habitation, whereas the memory skills program addressed more global concepts.

SOCIAL AND PROBLEM-SOLVING SKILLS

A variety of techniques have been reported to facilitate social skills in home, group, and community settings. In some cases, the use of consequences to reduce aberrant behavior has been sufficient. Burke and Lewis[50] implemented a point system for a 21-year-old postanoxic male who shouted, interrupted others, and engaged in nonsensical talk. Points, which could be exchanged for a variety of reinforcers, were awarded for the absence of such behaviors during mealtimes. Results indicated a substantial reduction in all three behaviors in residential and community settings even after treatment had been terminated. Unfortunately, the authors do not indicate what prosocial behaviors replaced the behaviors that were reduced by this procedure.

Turner et al.[51] reduced dysfunctional verbal and physical social behaviors with a changing criteria design in which progressively more time had to elapse with no unsanctioned behavior for the client to receive tokens. Initial periods free of dysfunctional social behaviors were relatively short to give the client a chance to succeed in the task. Over 15 weeks, required intervals of no dysfunctional behavior were gradually lengthened until the behavior was no longer considered a problem.

Gajar et al.[52] used feedback to teach conversational skills to young adults with head injury and evaluated effect according to norm-referenced criteria—another demonstration of the importance of the consumer and the community when determining effect. Notable speaking skill deficits included confabulation, preservative responding, inability to stay on topic, excessive self-disclosures, interruptions, and inappropriate laughter. Baseline assessment noted that the two participants were at least 1 standard deviation below their peers on these measures. During training, the clients were first asked to talk about selected topics while observers in another room flashed a green light when their conversation was on topic and a red light when their conversation was off topic. In a subsequent self-monitoring condition, each participant was trained to flash either the green light or the red light, based on the appropriateness or inappropriateness of the conversation.

Figure 18–1 presents results of this ABC additive design with reversal[12,13,18] for one of the two participants in the study (the other participant demonstrated similar results). As noted, conversational skills improved to levels equivalent to the peer comparison group during the therapist feedback intervention and during the self-monitoring condition but deteriorated below normed skill levels when baseline conditions were reinstated. Skills returned within normed levels with reimplementation of treatment. These same procedures were subsequently used to teach heterosexual conversational skills to head injured youth.[53]

Demonstrating the importance of individualized assessment and treatment, Zencius et al.[54] used various techniques across clients to manage hypersexual disorders. Verbal feedback regarding appropriate and inappropriate social interaction was sufficient to redirect a female client who was promiscuous with males. Exhibitionism by a male client was first addressed through a detailed interview about the client's urges, feelings, and fantasies before and during acts of exhibitionism. The client was also provided with a self-monitoring notebook to record his urges when he had the desire to expose himself. He could then masturbate in a secluded area to fantasies of situations presented to him in a dating skills training

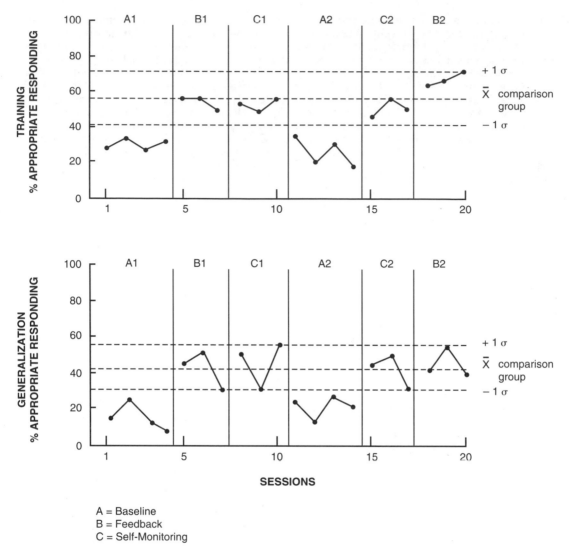

A = Baseline
B = Feedback
C = Self-Monitoring

FIGURE 18–1. Percentage of appropriate conversational behaviors produced by client 2 during baseline, treatment, and generalization sessions. (From Gajar, A, et al: Effects of feedback and self monitoring on head trauma youths' conversation skills. J Appl Behav Anal 17(3):353, 1984, p 357, with permission.)

class. These combined procedures reduced exhibitionism from two episodes during the first week of his admission to two total episodes over 15 subsequent weeks of treatment and 4 weeks of follow-up data. Finally, inappropriate touching and hand kissing by a male client was reduced 300 percent through redirection and stimulus specificity. The client was allowed to give back rubs during a scheduled relaxation class but not at other times.

Two groups of investigators[55,56] used a composite program to teach community problem-solving skills involving community awareness and transportation; medication, alcohol, and drugs; stating one's rights; and emergencies, injuries, and safety. In both studies, the trainer first modeled effective skills in selected community situations and then presented a cue card listing criterion components for solving problems. Participants then used the criteria to formulate their own solutions with feedback, prompting, and coaching by the trainer. Later, the criterion cue cards were dropped from training, and participants had to formulate their solutions. Participants quickly grasped the training and demonstrated from 55 to 200 percent improvement over baseline scores compared to no improvement for a contrast group that participated in pretest and post-test assessment but no training.

Other Clinical Challenges

Shutty et al.[57] adapted a multicomponent air sickness management program used with student pilots to help a postconcussional patient overcome benign positional vertigo (BPV). The program consisted of education about BPV, self-monitoring of physical activity and frequency of dizzy spells, biofeedback-assisted relaxation training, stress management and counseling, gaze fixation as a means to prevent dizziness, desensitization to increasingly severe degrees of vestibular disruption, and generalization training in daily routines and real-life situations. The client was subsequently able to return to community activities such as driving a car, and treatment effects were sustained 2 months later.

Silver and Stelly-Seitz[58] addressed adipsia in a child with a gunshot-induced hypothalamic injury who had received a gastrostomy tube. A multicomponent program was established in which social approval and preferred foods were first provided during each meal following any sip of liquid. Social interaction was also removed for 30 seconds each time the child refused the liquid. Shaping procedures subsequently made access to preferred food contingent on progressively larger sips of water. Once preliminary effect was established by one staff member, other staff and the child's mother were also trained in the technique. Within 17 days, oral consumption of liquid increased to the point where there was no clinical evidence of dehydration. Ten days later, the gastrostomy tube was removed, and the child returned home, where normal patterns of drinking gradually returned over time.

Papworth[59] adapted nocturnal enuresis programs commonly used with children[60] for a 42-year-old man with severe brain injury. The program involved bladder training to void on schedule, regular awakenings throughout the night to reduce the likelihood of in-bed accidents, a positive practice component in which the client was responsible for cleaning up after an accident, and reinforcement for a dry bed throughout the night. Complete remission of nocturnal enuresis was reported after 4 weeks of training and sustained 6 months later.

Lane et al.[61] combined stimulus control, a token economy, and brief time-out to reduce trash hoarding. Previous interventions including counseling, fines, a separate token economy system, differential reinforcement of incompatible behavior, overcorrection, and time-out had all been ineffective. The present program was conducted in two phases. First, the client was given baseball cards throughout the day when he did not hoard trash in his clothing. Within a week, the cards were established as conditioned reinforcers that could also be exchanged for hats, posters, and other items. Next, the stimulus conditions were established for picking up trash, namely, when wearing an apron and gloves and cleaning up in the dining room after meals. The client earned baseball cards when he collected trash at these times and disposed of it properly. He was verbally reprimanded when he picked up trash at other times and escorted to a brief time-out of 10 to 15 seconds. Trash hoarding was eliminated within 15 days, and the effect was sustained 1 year later.

Jacobs et al.[18] combined behavioral techniques and other approaches within a variety of multidisciplinary treatment settings. A changing criterion design with feedback for performance was used to increase standing balance for one client as a prelude to walking. Previous attempts had been unsuccessful because they were too ambitious. By evaluating baseline abilities and developing incremental tasks, the client and his therapist were able to establish the intervention and accomplish the overall goal, literally, one step at a time.

A changing criterion design and shaping procedure was used to help a postanoxic and amnesic female who was unable to swallow any texture of food or liquid and who was scheduled for nursing home placement. Scattered clinical evidence indicated the possibility that she could still swallow, but previous interventions were unsuccessful. The act of swallowing was broken down into a series of steps, and a backward chaining procedure was established. At first 1 cc of grape juice was squirted to the faucial pillars at the rear of her mouth, and the client was encouraged to swallow. Three weeks later, the amount was increased to 3 cc, as she successfully mastered the first step. The juice was then administered via a cup, so she had to move the liquid with her tongue from the front to the back of her mouth before swallowing, and the volume was gradually increased according to her progress. Soon the client began eating solid food off meal trays that were provided throughout treatment. Within 1 month, the client was eating regular meals and eventually returned home.

Staff Management

Several studies have evaluated the effects of managing staff behavior as a means of increasing client gains. Mozzoni and Bailey[62] first assessed the teaching techniques of staff working with inpatients who were not making expected progress. Therapist skills were first rated by a checklist that focused on 14 teaching techniques. Therapists were then provided with specific feedback and brief training to incorporate suggested teaching skills into daily practice. These changes produced dramatic improvement in each patient's therapeutic progress and goal attainment, yet required only 1 hour of time to teach each therapist the necessary teaching skills.

Pace and Colbert[63] incorporated principles of behavior analysis into the organization of a home and community rehabilitation program. Specific treatment goals that were required for the client to complete medical rehabilitation and live at home were first established between the client, his family, and the treatment team, and the insurance company. Individual therapists then assumed particular goals for their treatment, followed prescribed protocols, and reported their progress each session through objective data that were reviewed by the case coordinator, which allowed procedures to be modified as needed during the course of treatment. The length of individual therapies was based on client goals and progress and ended as specific goals were attained. As a result, over the course of in-home treatment, therapy costs were reduced from more than $1700 per week at the start of treatment to $550 per week at the end of treatment, when all goals had been achieved. The authors credit the implicit functional definitions, data management, and evaluation techniques of behavior analysis as the key to successful operation of the program.

·

☐ MEDICATION AND BEHAVIOR CHANGE

There is no doubt that medications change behavior. For too long, however, too many people have been divided about whether to use medication or behavior modification. Both approaches have their uses, either alone or in combination. For example, changes in physiological status, such as reduction of seizures or stabilization of metabolic imbalances, can open new opportunities to return to work or driving. Improvement in arousal or attention may enhance responsiveness to other forms of rehabilitation treatment. Conversely, a self-medication skills training program may help to ensure medication compliance and the intended chemotherapeutic effect.[49] Direct observation and single-subject evaluation protocols can be used to empirically document medication effects.[17,64,65]

A clinical body of knowledge about medication effects following brain injury is beginning to accumulate, although many findings remain contradictory, and individual differences across patients remain prominent. Still, promising effects that can facilitate overall programmatic gains have been reported in areas such as arousal and attention,[65–67] learning,[64,68] selected affective and psychotic disorders,[69] and aggression and agitation.[70–74] (Interested readers are referred to comprehensive reviews of the literature[24,75] and Chapter 30 for additional information.)

However, medication is no panacea, and the promise of rapid case management or the quick fix through chemistry offers its own problems. First, knowledge about drug effects and interactions remains very limited, and there is even less understanding about the number, type, and operation of the brain's neurotransmitters.[24,76,77]

Second, like any form of intervention, there are often discrepancies between intended effect and actual outcomes. In addition to differential effects across people, many commonly used medications were initially developed for individuals with other forms of impairment (e.g., psychiatric), who may respond to them differently than people with neurological impairment.[78] Beneficial effects may also be moderated by side effects in other areas of functional performance, such as the use of phenytoin to control seizures with possible adverse effects on memory and learning[79] or the use of haloperidol and other psychotrophics to mediate aggression, which may inhibit motor learning,[23] arousal, and attention.[80] Another concern is that too many prescribers have inadequate training to implement and sustain successful psychopharmacological treatment,[24] and it is not unusual to find a refractory client on high doses of a medication who actually improves when the drug is eliminated.

Third, medication is too frequently used for its suppressive effects, as a means of reducing some undesirable behavior, without concurrent goals of skills facilitation. This approach may be warranted in selected situations if the safety of the individual or others is imminently at risk, *and no other treatment alternatives are available.* However, in such situations the client should be quickly transitioned to a setting that can productively manage the presenting challenge and promote positive and prospective programming, in which medication may continue to play an important role.

Other problems occur when medication is used singularly for behavioral control, especially in institutional settings, because it is administratively considered as a cheaper but equally effective treatment or effective within the contractual obligation of the funding source. *Caveat emptor* remains a clearly unconscionable clinical strategy, especially among vulnerable patients.

☐ LIMITATIONS OF BEHAVIOR ANALYSIS

As the previous studies note, behavior analysis can offer useful options to address a wide variety of challenges after brain injury. Nevertheless, it is only one approach and cannot independently address the myriad of medical, neurological, social, financial, and political sequelae that follow catastrophic injury. No discipline or individual orientation is capable of making such a claim. Intervention generally works best when effective procedures are combined for the functional benefit of the client rather than according to dubious disciplinary distinctions (e.g., cognitive vs. behavioral or behavioral vs. psychopharmacology).

Perhaps the biggest obstacle to the proper use of behavior analysis in brain injury rehabilitation programming is the lack of skilled and experienced practitioners.[17,27] Too often, those who are responsible for behavioral intervention within a brain injury program do not have formal training in behavior analysis, and interventions are not unusual that would be considered inappropriate, unethical, or illegal if they were applied to people with developmental disabilities, psychiatric impairment, or challenges of learning. It is similarly not surprising when such procedures have an iatrogenic effect and promulgate the problem they were designed to address.

Similarly, many currently trained behavior analysts developed their skills with clients in other settings and with other forms of impairment. Too often, such inexperienced practitioners may emphasize consequences of behavior over antecedents and skills development. They may also neglect to acknowledge the practical changes in learning and perception that may follow neurological impairment. Catastrophic brain injury changes the way a person senses, perceives, learns, and interacts with the world. Frequently, presenting challenges are a function of *can't do* over *won't do*. Successful programming requires sensitive and practical interfaces between environmental demands and individual ability.

☐ SUMMARY

Behavioral intervention involves much more than suppressing aberrant behavior and applying positive reinforcement. Individual elements of behavior analysis can be combined into comprehensive behavioral programs that address a variety of challenges and opportunities that may occur following brain injury. These techniques of assessment, intervention, and evaluation can also be used as individual components within comprehensive treatment that is conducted by multiple disciplines.[18]

Some of the studies presented in this chapter used techniques comparable to cognitive rehabilitation strategies, which should not be surprising because both disciplines focus on similar challenges: helping people who experience disability following neurological impairment improve their skills and reduce their handicaps. In many cases, the mode of treatment may be equivalent, but the explanation may differ with theoretical orientation. If clinical intervention is focused on outcome, then the most effective techniques for the individual client will be used, regardless of theoretical orientation.

Many people question who should use this technology. The field of behavior analysis was established and has developed with an eye toward consumer empowerment. Thus, as practical, behavior analysts seek to make programs and techniques available to people in the situations where specific needs are being addressed; school-based interventions can be developed and managed by students and teachers, family training by children and parents, and rehabilitation interventions by clients and therapists.

REFERENCES

1. Wood, MM: Behavioural methods in rehabilitation. In Dinning, TAR, and Connelley, JJ (eds): Head Injuries: An Integrated Approach. Metheun, New York, 1981, p 66.
2. Wood, RL, and Eames, PG: Behaviour modification in the rehabilitation of brain injury. In Davey, G (ed): Applications of Conditioning Theory. Metheun, London, 1981, p 81.
3. Eames, P, and Wood, R: Rehabilitation after severe brain injury: A special unit approach to behavior disorders. International Rehabilitation Medicine 7:130, 1985.
4. Eames, P, and Wood, R: Rehabilitation after severe brain injury: A follow up study of a behavior modification approach. J Neurol Neurosurg Psychiatry 48:613, 1985.
5. Wood, RL: Brain Injury Rehabilitation: A Neurobehavioral Approach. Croom Helm, Wolfeboro, NH, 1987.
6. Martin, R: Legal Challenges to Behavior Modification: Trends in Schools, Corrections and Mental Health. Research Press, Champaign, Ill, 1975.
7. Ayllon T, and Azrin, NH: The Token Economy: A Motivational System for Therapy and Rehabilitation. Appleton-Century-Crofts, New York, 1968.
8. Skinner, BF: Beyond Freedom and Dignity. Alfred A Knopf, New York, 1974.
9. Skinner, BF: About Behaviorism. Alfred A Knopf, New York, 1974.
10. Baer, DM, Wolf, MM, and Risley, TR: Some current dimensions of applied behavior analysis. J Appl Behav Anal 1:91, 1968.
11. Skinner, BF: Verbal Behavior. Appleton-Century-Crofts, New York, 1957.
12. Bailey, JS, and Bostow, DE: A Handbook of Research Methods in Applied Behavior Analysis. Author, Tallahassee, Fla, 1980.
13. Hersen, M, and Barlow, DH: Single Case Experimental Designs: Strategies for Studying Behavior Change. Pergamon, Elmsford, NY, 1976.

14. Hersen, M, and Bellack, AS: Behavioral Assessment: A Practical Handbook, ed 2. Pergamon, Elmsford, NY, 1976.
15. Skinner, BF: Science and Human Behavior. Free Press, New York, 1953.
16. Kazdin, AE: Behavior Modification in Applied Settings, ed 4. Brooks Cole, Calif, 1989.
17. Jacobs, HE: Behavior Analysis Guidelines and Brain Injury Rehabilitation: People, Principles and Programs. Aspen, Gaithersburg, Md, 1993.
18. Jacobs, HE, et al: Single subject evaluation designs in rehabilitation: Case studies on inpatient units. J Head Trauma Rehabil 11(1):86, 1996.
19. Martin G, and Pear, J: Behavior Modification: What It Is and How to Do It. Prentice Hall, Englewood Cliffs, NJ, 1983.
20. Ben-Yishay, Y, et al: Relationship between initial competence and ability to profit from cues in brain-damaged individuals. J Abnorm Psychol 75:248, 1970.
21. Hagen, C, Malkmus, D, and Durham, P: Levels of cognitive functioning. Head Trauma Rehabilitation Seminar, Rancho Los Amigos Hospital, Los Angeles, Calif, 1977.
22. Tate, RL: Behavior management techniques for organic psychosocial deficit incurred by severe head injury. Scand J Rehabil Med 19:19, 1987.
23. Feeney, D, Gonzalez A, and Law, W: Amphetamine, haloperidol and experience interact to affect rate of recovery after motor cortex injury. Science 27:855, 1982.
24. Cope, DN: Psychopharmacologic aspects of traumatic brain injury. In Cope, DN, and Zassler, N (eds): Medical Rehabilitation of Traumatic Brain Injury. Hanley and Belfus, Philadelphia, 1996, p 573.
25. Gregory, HH, and Bonfiglio, RP: Limiting restraint use for behavior control: The brain injury rehabilitation unit as a model. Md Med J 44:279, 1995.
26. Pace, GM, and Nau, PA: Behavior analysis in brain injury rehabilitation: Training staff to develop, implement, and evaluate behavior change programs. In Durgin, CJ, Schmidt, ND, and Fryer, LJ (eds): Staff Development and Clinical Intervention in Brain Injury Rehabilitation. Aspen, Gaithersburg, Md, 1993.
27. Jacobs, HE: Yes, behavior analysis can help, but do you know how to harness it? Brain Inj 4:339, 1988.
28. Jacobs, HE, et al: Behavior management of aggressive sequelae in Reyes' syndrome. Arch Phys Med Rehabil 67:558, 1986.
29. Treadwell, K, and Page, TJ: Functional analysis: Identifying the environmental determinants of severe behavior disorders. J Head Trauma Rehabil 11(1):62, 1996.
30. Pace, GM, Ivancic, MT, and Jefferson, G: Stimulus fading as treatment for obscenity in a brain-injured adult. J Appl Behav Anal 27:301, 1994.
31. Crane AA, and Joyce, BG: Cool down: A procedure for decreasing aggression in adults with traumatic head injury. Behav Res Treat 6:65, 1991.
32. Haley, WE: Behavioral management of the brain damaged patient: A case study. Rehabilitation Nursing 26:26, 1983.
33. Uomoto, JM, and Brockway, JA: Anger management training for brain injured patients and their family members. Arch Phys Med Rehabil 73:674, 1992.
34. Carnevale, GJ: Natural setting behavior management for individuals with traumatic brain injury: Results of a three year caregiver training program. J Head Trauma Rehabil 11(1):27, 1996.
35. Feeney, TJ, and Ylvisaker, M: Choice and routine: Antecedent behavioral interventions for adolescents with severe traumatic brain injury. J Head Trauma Rehabil 10:67, 1995.
36. Mace, FC, et al: Behavioral momentum in the treatment of noncompliance. J Appl Behav Anal 21:123, 1988.
37. Zencius, A, Wesolowski, MD, and Burke, WH: Comparing motivational systems with two noncompliant head injured adolescents. Brain Inj 3:67, 1989.
38. Premack, D: Reinforcement theory. Neb Symp Motiv 123, 1965.
39. Silver, BV, Boake, C, and Cavazos, D: Improving functional skills using behavioral procedures in a child with anoxic brain injury. Arch Phys Med Rehabil 75:742, 1994.
40. Zencius, AH, et al: Antecedent control in the treatment of brain injured clients. Brain Inj 3:199, 1989.
41. Burke, WH, and Wesolowski, MD: Applied behavior analysis in head injury rehabilitation. Rehabilitation Nursing 13:186, 1988.
42. Winett, RA, and Winkler, RC: Current behavior modification in the classroom: Be still, be quiet, be docile. J Appl Behav Anal 5:499, 1972.
43. Zhou J, et al: The utilization of a game format to increase knowledge of residuals among people with acquired brain injury. J Head Trauma Rehabil 11(1):51, 1996.
44. Slifer, KJ, Cataldo, MD, and Kurtz PF: Behavioral training during acute brain trauma rehabilitation: An empirical case study. Brain Inj 9:585, 1996.
45. Slifer, KJ, et al: Operant conditioning for behavior management during posttraumatic amnesia in children and adolescents with brain injury. J Head Trauma Rehabil 11(1):39, 1996.
46. Giles, GM, and Clark-Wilsho, J: The use of behavioral techniques in functional skills training after severe burn injury. Am J Occup Ther 42:658, 1988.
47. Giles, GM, and Shore, M: A rapid method for teaching severely brain injured adults how to wash and dress. Arch Phys Med Rehabil 70:156, 1989.
48. O'Reilly, MF, Gren, G, and Braunling-McMorrow, D: Self administered written prompts to teach home accident prevention skills to adults with brain injuries. J Appl Behav Anal 23:431, 1990.
49. Godfrey, HDP, and Knight, RG: Memory training and behavioral rehabilitation of a severely head injured adult. Arch Phys Med Rehabil 69:458, 1988.
50. Burke, WH, and Lewis, FD: Management of maladaptive social behavior of a brain injured adult. Int J Rehabil Res 9:335, 1986.
51. Turner, JM, Greene, G, and Braunling-McMorrow, D: Differential reinforcement of low rates of responding (DRL) to reduce dysfunctional social behaviors of a head injured man. Behav Res Ther 5:15, 1990.
52. Gajar, A, et al: Effects of feedback and self monitoring on head trauma youths' conversation skills. J Appl Behav Anal 17:353, 1984.
53. Schloss, PJ, et al: Influence of self-monitoring on heterosexual conversational behaviors of head trauma youth. Applied Research in Mental Retardation 6:269, 1985.
54. Zencius, A, et al: Managing hypersexual disorders in brain injured clients. Brain Inj 4:175, 1990.
55. Foxx, RM, et al: Teaching a problem solving strategy to closed head injured adults. Behav Res Ther 3:193, 1988.
56. Foxx, RM, Martell, RC, and Marchand-Martella, NE: The acquisition, maintenance, and generalization of problem-solving skills by closed head injured adults. Behavior Therapy 20:61, 1989.
57. Shutty, MS, et al: Behavior treatment of dizziness secondary to benign positional vertigo following head trauma. Arch Phys Med Rehabil 72:473, 1991.
58. Silver, BV, and Stelly-Seitz, C: Behavioral treatment for adipsia in a child with hypothalamic injury. Dev Med Child Neurol 34:539, 1992.
59. Papworth, MA: The behavioral treatment of nocturnal enuresis in a severely brain damaged client. J Behav Ther Exp Psychiatry 20:265, 1989.
60. Doleys, M: Behavioral treatments for nocturnal enuresis in children: A review of the recent literature. Psychol Bull 84:30, 1977.
61. Lane, IM, Wesolowski, MD, and Burke, WH: Teaching socially appropriate behavior to eliminate hoarding in a brain injured client. J Behav Ther Exp Psychiatry 20:79, 189.
62. Mozzoni, MP, and Bailey, JS: Improving training methods in brain injury rehabilitation. J Head Trauma Rehabil 11(1):1, 1996.

63. Pace, GM, and Colbert, B: Role of behavior analysis in home and community based neurological rehabilitation. J Head Trauma Rehabil 11(1):18, 1996.

64. Evans, RW, Gualtieri, CT, and Patterson, D: Treatment of chronic closed head injury with psychostimulant drugs: A controlled case study and an appropriate evaluation procedure. J Nerv Ment Dis 175:106, 1987.

65. Glenn, MB: CNS stimulants: Applications for traumatic brain injury. J Head Trauma Rehabil 1(1):74, 1986.

66. Whyte, J: Toward rational psychopharmacological treatment: Integrating research and clinical practice. J Head Trauma Rehabil 9(3):91, 1994.

67. Whyte, J: Neurologic disorders of attention and arousal: Assessment and treatment. Arch Phys Med Rehabil 73:1094, 1992.

68. Evans, RW, and Gualtieri, CT: Psychostimulant pharmacology in traumatic brain injury. J Head Trauma Rehabil 2(4):264, 1987.

69. Silver, JM, and Yudofsky, SC: Psychopharmacological approaches to the patient with affective and psychotic features. J Head Trauma Rehabil 9(3):61, 1994.

70. Barratt, ES: The use of anticonvulsants in aggression and violence. J Head Trauma Rehabil 29:75, 1993.

71. Glenn, MB, et al: Lithium carbonate for aggressive behavior or affective instability in ten brain-injured patients. Am J Phys Med Rehabil 68:221, 1989.

72. Mooney, GF, and Haas, LJ: Effect of methylphenidate on brain injury-related anger. Arch Phys Med Rehabil 74:153, 1993.

73. Mysiw, WJ, and Jackson, RD: Tricyclic antidepressant therapy after traumatic brain injury. J Head Trauma Rehabil 2(1):34, 1987.

74. Yudofsky, S, Williams, D, and Gorman, J: Propranolol in the treatment of rage and violent behavior in patients with chronic brain syndromes. Am J Psychiatry 138:218, 1981.

75. Whyte, J, and Cope, DN (eds): Psychopharmacology. J Head Trauma Rehabil 9(3), 1994.

76. Cope, DN: An integration of psychopharmacological and rehabilitation approaches to traumatic brain injury rehabilitation. J Head Trauma Rehabil 9(3):1, 1994.

77. Kolata, GB: New drugs and the brain. Science 205:774, 1979.

78. Helms, PS: Efficacy of antipsychotics in the treatment of the behavioral complications of dementia: A review of the literature. J Am Geriatr Soc 33:206, 1987.

79. Reynolds, EH: Anticonvulsants and mental symptoms. In Sandler, M (ed): Psychopharmacology of Anticonvulsants. Oxford University Press, Oxford, 1982.

80. O'Shanick, GJ: Clinical aspects of psychopharmacologic treatment in head-injured patients. J Head Trauma Rehabil 2(4):59, 1987.

Community Integration and Quality of Life of Individuals with Traumatic Brain Injury

WAYNE A. GORDON, PHD,
MARY R. HIBBARD, PHD,
MARGARET BROWN, PHD,
STEVEN FLANAGAN, MD,
and MAUREEN CAMPBELL KORVES

The primary purpose of this chapter is to expand our understanding of who the people are who have experienced traumatic brain injury (TBI) and live in the community. What characterizes them, and what is life like for them? Previous studies of individuals with TBI living in the community largely focused only on subsets of the population of people with TBI living "at home." Because of sampling and other methodological biases, the picture that emerged from this literature is of questionable validity and breadth. The newly emerging data from a large, community-based study of individuals with TBI—the Research and Training Center (RTC) on the Community Integration of Individuals with TBI at the Mount Sinai Medical Center in New York City—presented in this chapter provide a substantial contribution to the current knowledge base. A secondary goal of this chapter is to discuss several societal "forces" that either threaten the quality of community living of individuals with TBI or offer promise. Thus, the continuum of services needed by individuals with TBI, public policy affecting such services, and managed care are reviewed in this chapter's final sections.

The preparation of this manuscript and the research reported herein was supported by Grant No. H133B30038 to the Research and Training Center (RTC) on Community Integration of Individuals with Traumatic Brain Injuries, Department of Rehabilitation Medicine, The Mount Sinai Medical Center, New York, NY, from the National Institute on Disability and Rehabilitation Research, United States Department of Education. The authors wish to acknowledge the important contributions of current and past RTC staff members to the research described herein: Jennifer Bogdany, Joyce Echo, Deborah Fedor, Rachelle Kalinsky, Karen Kepler, Naomi Tyler Lloyd, Pam Merritt, John O'Neill, Nina Patti, William Schalk, Michael Sheerer, Ralph William Shields, Suzan Uysal, and David Vandergoot.

□ PREVIOUS STUDIES OF INDIVIDUALS WITH TRAUMATIC BRAIN INJURY LIVING IN THE COMMUNITY

The extensive literature[1-14] on long-term outcomes of individuals with TBI living in the community suggests that, after TBI, most people experience significant barriers to successful community reentry (Table 19–1). The wide range of cognitive, physical, psychosocial, behavioral, and vocational challenges that persist through many years of community living negatively affect quality of life not only of people with TBI but also of their spouses, other family members, and caretakers.

Taken as a whole, this literature presents a fairly pessimistic view of life after brain injury. However, these consistently negative findings may partially be caused by factors other than TBI:

■ *Restrictive sampling.* Researchers have primarily sampled directly from rosters of previously hospitalized individuals, resulting in studies of people primarily with moderate to severe TBI, the majority of whom are male. Typically ignored has been the larger and more representative group of individuals— both male and female—experiencing the full range of brain injury severity, including so-called mild brain injury.

■ *Framework for comparison.* The strength of the negative results also may be partly attributable to the particular frame of reference chosen for defining *difficulty*. In most cases, it has been a comparison of the preinjury to the postinjury status of the individual with TBI. None of the studies compare individuals with TBI to similar groups of people with other disabilities or without a disability. The latter framework for comparison may provide broader insights about TBI than findings relying on an informant's judging how things are "better" or "worse" since the TBI.

■ *Deficit focus.* The negative results are also not surprising, given that all studies are largely deficit- or impairment-driven; that is, they focus only on what individuals with TBI *cannot* do, with minimal attempts to explore domains of successful reintegration. As summarized in Table 19–1, long-term outcomes are largely conceived in terms of impairments or barriers for the individual and the negative impact on family members and other caregivers.

■ *Data source.* The evaluation of quality of life of individuals with TBI is routinely based on data obtained not from the person with TBI per se but instead from other sources: neuropsychological evaluations or reports of relatives. Individuals living with the brain injury were rarely asked about their own lives, their feelings of satisfaction and accomplishment, or the unique challenges and problems they experience in day-to-day living.

□ A COMMUNITY-BASED STUDY OF INDIVIDUALS WITH TRAUMATIC BRAIN INJURY: WHO ARE THEY AND HOW DO THEY FARE IN LIFE?

Since 1993, the Research and Training Center (RTC) on Community Integration of Individuals with TBI at the Mount Sinai Medical Center in New York City has taken a different approach to researching outcome after TBI. Most striking in the RTC's five-year program of research (completed in 1998) is its incorporation of people with TBI—both as staff and as volunteers—to help shape and carry out every aspect of the program. The Quality of Life (QOL) Study is a major component of this research program. In this study, two areas of question were given primacy:

■ What are the characteristics of individuals who have experienced a TBI and live in the community?

■ What is the subjective QOL of people with TBI living in the community, and what variables predict good QOL?

The Quality of Life Study Sample

In designing the QOL Study, six principles governed the selection of the study sample:

1. The focus of the study was the individual with TBI rather than a broader view of the family unit affected by a member with TBI.

2. The source of information was solely the individual with TBI; other informants, clearly, provide complementary views of life after TBI, but we chose to limit the study to the view provided by the person at the center of the TBI experience.

3. "Community living" was conceptualized as encompassing only individuals living in noninstitutional settings.

4. The framework for comparison was that the sample of people with TBI was to be compared to samples of people who are similar but without a disability.

5. Because one goal of the study was to document the characteristics of the population of community-based individuals with TBI,

TABLE 19–1. Long-Term Outcome Studies in Individuals with Traumatic Brain Injury: 1970 to Present

Author(s)	Sample Size and Severity of TBI	Gender	Mean Duration between Onset and Follow-up	Informant or Source(s)	Core Findings
Thomsen, 1974	50 severe TBI (23/50 w/aphasia)	74% male, 26% female	12–70 mo	Patient & relatives	▪ Patients report few changes except lack of contact with people and loneliness ▪ Relatives report irritability, hot temper, aspontaneity, restlessness, emotional regression, emotional lability, and stubbornness
Rosenbaum & Najenson, 1976	10 severe TBI, 9 paraplegia, 14 nondisabled	100% male	1 yr	Wives	▪ Wives of Ss with TBI had greater stress and more role reversal than other wives ▪ Wives of Ss with TBI were more isolated and lonely ▪ TBI resulted in reduction in sexual relationships ▪ Ss with TBI were more self-oriented and childlike

Levin, et al, 1979	27 severe TBI	Unspecified	3 yr	Patient & relatives Cognitive testing	▪ Recovery patterns were heterogeneous on Glascow Outcome Scale (GOS)
					  □ 10 made good recovery
					  □ 12 remained moderately disabled
					  □ 5 remained severely disabled
					▪ Intellectual and social (i.e., work) adjustment related to overall outcome (GOS)
					▪ Mild anxiety and depression noted in persons with good recovery (GOS)
					▪ Psychiatric disorders requiring hospitalization noted in moderately to severely disabled (GOS) individuals

Weddell, Oddy & Jenkins, 1980	44 severe TBI	70% male, 30% female	2 yr	Patient & relatives	▪ Increased irritability noted ▪ 11/44 returned to work in reduced capacity ▪ Fewer interests, fewer friends, and more anxiety noted
McKinlay, et al, 1981	55 severe TBI	84% male, 16% female	3, 6 & 12 mo	Relatives	▪ Emotional disturbances (bad temper, mood swings), poor memory, and physical complaints persisted ▪ Stress for relatives increased as duration postinjury increased
Thomsen, 1984	40 severe TBI	70% male, 30% female	2–5 yr & 10–15 yr	Patient & relatives	▪ Permanent personality changes in two-thirds of sample ▪ Irritability and social isolation are major handicaps
Oddy, et al, 1985	42 severe TBI	74% male, 26% female	2 & 7 yr	Relatives & patient Cognitive testing	▪ At 2 yr, 71% of patients had some personality changes, with irritability most common ▪ At 7 yr, impatience, decreased interest, childishness, and loss of temper most common ▪ No significant changes in cognitive testing or employment over time span examined

Study	Sample	Gender	Time	Source	Findings
Brooks, et al, 1986	42 severe TBI	100% male	5 yr	Relatives	▪ Personality changes, tension, tiredness, difficulty with self-control, irritability frequently observed ▪ Changes may remain stable or worsen over time ▪ Stress on relatives proportional to magnitude of behavioral personality changes
Klonoff, Snow & Costa, 1986	78 TBI □ 60% mild □ 10% moderate □ 30% severe	82% male, 18% female	2–4 yr	Patient	▪ 14% decline in proficiency with household chores ▪ 39% unable to maintain full-time employment ▪ Physical complaints reported by 57% (i.e., limb weakness, reduced strength/power, stiffness, pain) ▪ Psychological complaints reported: memory (60%), irritability (53%), concentration (24%) ▪ Psychosocial functioning, work, and recreation impaired ▪ Residual impairments in most domains of quality of life
Brooks, et al, 1987	134 severe TBI	Unspecified	2–7 yr	Relatives Cognitive testing	▪ Preinjury, 86% working; postinjury, 29% working ▪ Younger, less severe TBI and high prevocational level predictive of return to work post-TBI
Jacobs, 1988	142 severe TBI	72% male, 28% female	1–6 yr	Relatives	▪ Wide range of skill deficits ▪ Patients functioning independently across 75% of skills ▪ Majority of survivors did not live on own, work, or attend school; were dependent on others for skills, finance, and services outside the home ▪ Significant burden on families
Lezak & O'Brien, 1988, 1990	39 moderate to severe TBI	100% male	Serial reevaluations, 6 mo to 5 yr	Observer ratings	▪ Impairments noted most frequently in social adjustment, i.e., work/school, social contact, driving, and appropriate social interactions ▪ Persistent social dislocation and social withdrawal ▪ Depression, anxiety, and relationship difficulties increase 6–12 mo post-TBI ▪ 40% of sample had difficulty with control of anger at 5 yr post-TBI
Thomsen, 1989	40 severe TBI	70% male, 30% female	2–5 yr 10–15 yr	Relatives & patient	▪ Younger, onset of TBI = higher risk of late behavioral and emotional sequelae ▪ Changes in personality, emotion, social problems observed ▪ Behavioral crisis in families occurs at differing times for married and single patients

highly varied recruitment methods and sources were used, such as independent living centers, newspaper ads, and articles in publications of the Brain Injury Association of New York State.

6. Individuals had to be self-identified as having a TBI (or other disability) or as being nondisabled.

Based upon these principles, at completion the study sample will include 400 individuals with TBI, 300 without a disability, 100 whose brain injuries were nontraumatic, 100 with spinal cord injury, and 100 with HIV. All participants are between the ages of 18 and 65. Participants with disabilities had to be at least 1 year post-onset or 1 year post diagnosis. Only data from the TBI sample (the TBI group) and the sample of individuals without a disability (the nondisabled group) are presented here.

Because the QOL Study has not yet been completed, the results reported in this chapter are based on data collected from 298 individuals with TBI and a comparison group of 127 individuals without a disability. These data should be interpreted with some caution because the nondisabled group is considerably smaller than the TBI group, and it is not well matched* in terms of gender and education (Table 19–2). Because the current data represent 75 percent of the complete TBI sample and only 40 percent of the complete nondisabled sample, only the most robust findings—that is, those with sufficient power—are presented.

The Study Interview

The interview was designed to provide a structured exploration of "community life after TBI," which was refocused as a study of determinants of the individual's subjective QOL.[15,16] Three sets of variables were judged to be predictors of subjective QOL and were used as the basics for designing the clinical interview used in the QOL study:

1. Community integration variables focus on social and role activities of the individual:
□ *Vocational and economic role activities.* Higher levels of integration into the community require that an individual have a meaningful and culturally appropriate vocational or economic role to play—that is,

working as a student, volunteer, or homemaker or in a paid job.
□ *Integration into social networks.* Community integration also has a social component. Thus, as an individual is more broadly integrated into social networks, he or she is better integrated into the community.
□ *Participation in community- and home-based activities.* The community-integrated individual engages in a variety of activities inside and outside the home that define daily life for active community members, such as grocery shopping, church going, and eating out.

2. The second set of QOL variables describes the individual's intrapersonal functioning, primarily variables assessing health, needs, cognition, and emotional well-being.

3. The third set of variables refers to the resources to which the individual has access: social, economic, and societal resources that enable or disable the individual in living life to the fullest, such as access to needed services, household income, and the size and nature of social networks on which the individual can draw.

Using this broad definition of quality of life determinants, a standard interview was developed, based on adaptation of existing instruments, many of which are described in the discussion of results. The clinical interview was conducted by phone or in person, and each interview took 2 to 4 hours.

Results

WHAT ARE THE CHARACTERISTICS OF THIS GROUP OF INDIVIDUALS WITH TRAUMATIC BRAIN INJURY LIVING IN THE COMMUNITY?

The 298 individuals in the TBI group (Table 19–2) are, on average, 37 years old and 9 years postinjury (range: 1 to 44 years). The group covers a wide range of severity of injury: 24 percent sustained a loss of consciousness (LOC) of less than 20 minutes, 13 percent an LOC between 20 minutes and 1 day, 14 percent between 1 and 7 days, 11 percent between 1 and 2 weeks, and 38 percent 3 weeks or more. The majority of people in the TBI group are male, white, and high school graduates or higher. The nondisabled group (*n* = 127) is similar in age and ethnicity; however, fewer are male, and more have completed at least high school.

The characteristics of the sample of individuals with TBI described in this chapter, which

---

*The nondisabled group is being selectively recruited to remedy this problem; the goal is to match it to the TBI group on diverse demographic characteristics.

TABLE 19–2. Demographic Characteristics of the Two Samples in the Quality of Life Study

Demographic Variables	Traumatic Brain Injury (n = 298)	Nondisabled Group (n = 127)
Age	37.2 (9.9)	34.8 (12.6)
Gender		
% Male	61.7	26.8
% Female	38.3	73.2
Race		
% White	69.5	55.9
% Black	13.1	21.3
% Hispanic	9.1	11.0
% Other	8.3	11.8
Education		
% >High school	11.8	3.2
% High school	22.9	11.9
% Some college	30.0	39.7
% College	12.8	23.8
% Postgraduate	22.5	21.4

was drawn from diverse community-based sources, vary from those reported in previous studies. In part, these differences may be because prior samples were typically drawn solely from institutional settings. Most striking is the wider variation in terms of severity of injury in the QOL study sample. Further, males (60%) are proportionally fewer in this sample than in many studies; females may represented more in this sample because of the inclusion of many more individuals with mild TBI. The sample is also unusual in its inclusion of people studied so long after injury, up to 44 years posttrauma. In addition, the TBI group is relatively well educated. These variations from samples studied in previous research invite further study to determine the degree to which repeated sampling produces consistency of sample characteristics and to provide better estimates of the "true" population of individuals with TBI living "at home."

WHAT IS THE OVERALL QUALITY OF LIFE OF THESE INDIVIDUALS WITH TRAUMATIC BRAIN INJURY LIVING IN THE COMMUNITY?

Of the many measures of QOL in the literature, none has been systematically applied to individuals with TBI in the community. The 263-item Bigelow Quality of Life Questionnaire (BQOL)[17] was therefore incorporated into the study interview. The 13 BQOL scales are psychological distress (e.g., anxiety, depression, somatic disturbance), psychological well-being (e.g., optimism, contentment), interpersonal interaction (e.g., satisfaction of affiliation needs), spouse role, basic need satisfaction, indepen-

dence, social support, work at home (i.e., performance of household tasks), employability, work on the job (e.g., ability to accept supervision, quality of work, motivation), use of leisure time, negative consequences of alcohol use, and negative consequences of drug use.

Differences between the TBI and nondisabled groups were found on seven BQOL scales: psychological distress, basic need satisfaction, independence, social support, work at home, employability, and use of leisure time (Table 19–3). In each instance, the direction of difference favored the nondisabled group. No differences were found between the two groups on the remaining six scales. Although some of these findings might appear contradictory, when the items comprising each scale are examined, a more coherent picture emerges. For example, although those in the TBI group are relatively more anxious and depressed (i.e., scoring lower on the psychological stress scale) than those in the nondisabled group, the degree of their upset was not sufficient to negate the feelings of general contentment tapped in the psychological well-being scale. Similarly, although people with TBI experience less social support (i.e., scoring lower on the social support scale), they find their relationships with their friends, family, and spouse satisfying (i.e., no difference in scores on the interpersonal interactions scale). The data also suggest that those individuals with TBI who work fare as well as workers in the nondisabled group (i.e., no difference in scores on the work on the job scale) but that unemployed people with TBI report being worse off than their nondisabled counterparts (i.e., the former scoring lower on the employability scale).

TABLE 19–3. Means (Standard Deviation) of Bigelow Quality of Life Questionnaire Scores in Groups in Quality of Life Study

	Traumatic Brain Injury Group	Nondisabled Group
Psychological Distress	71.9 (18.2)	82.0 (13.1)[‡]
Psychological Well-being	40.6 (19.2)	44.1 (15.9)
Basic Need Satisfaction	88.9 (23.8)	94.7 (23.1)[*]
Independence and Assertiveness	54.8 (11.3)	59.9 (8.5)[‡]
Interpersonal Interaction	43.8 (13.4)	42.0 (11.8)
Spouse Role	57.8 (20.0)	60.8 (17.5)
Social Support	59.8 (20.2)	66.7 (17.0)[†]
Work at Home	49.2 (22.9)	58.7 (19.2)[‡]
Employability	47.8 (11.1)	53.5 (8.7)[‡]
Work on the Job	60.4 (10.6)	58.1 (12.3)
Meaningful Use of Leisure Time	35.6 (15.4)	40.4 (12.5)[†]
Negative Consequences of Alcohol	51.7 (6.8)	52.9 (4.3)
Negative Consequences of Drugs	10.4 (.7)	7.1 (.8)

[*]$p < .01$.
[†]$p < .001$.
[‡]$p < .0001$.

HOW WELL INTEGRATED INTO THE COMMUNITY ARE INDIVIDUALS WITH TRAUMATIC BRAIN INJURY?

The Community Integration Questionnaire (CIQ)[18] consists of 15 items, which produce a total score reflecting three subscales: the individual's degree of integration within the home, in social networks, and into productive activities. The TBI group had a lower CIQ total score than the nondisabled group (16.1 vs. 19.5) and lower scores on each of the three CIQ subscales (Table 19–4).

The TBI group's overall CIQ mean is equivalent to a sample of individuals with TBI assessed by Willer et al.[18] and slightly higher than means reported for community-based samples by Corrigan and Deming.[19] What might account for these latter differences? The lower-scoring sample included more recently injured people, who on average were only 3 months postinjury and thus had less time to resume community activities. Of interest is the finding that Corrigan and Deming's sample scored lower than the current sample primarily on the productive activities scale, suggesting that participation in vocational activities may be positively associated with time since injury.

WHAT ARE THE NEEDS OF INDIVIDUALS WITH TRAUMATIC BRAIN INJURY LIVING IN THE COMMUNITY?

In a study of quality of life, Flanagan[20] factor-analyzed 15 categories of needs critical to the concept of QOL. His categories were adapted for incorporation into the study interview: material well-being and financial security; health and personal safety; relations with a spouse or significant other; having and raising children; relations with parents, siblings, and other relatives; relations with friends; activities related to helping or encouraging others; activities relating to local and national governments; intellectual development; personal understanding and

TABLE 19–4. Means (Standard Deviation) of Community Integration Questionnaire Scores in Quality of Life Groups

	Traumatic Brain Injury Group	Nondisabled Group
Total Score	16.1 (4.6)	19.5 (3.6)
Subscale Scores		
Social Integration	6.8 (1.9)	7.5 (1.7)
Home Integration	5.2 (3.5)	6.9 (3.1)
Productive Activity	4.0 (1.5)	5.1 (1.0)

planning; occupational role; creativity and personal expression; socializing; passive and observational recreational activities; and active and participatory recreational activities. Each interviewee was asked to rate both the importance of each need area and the degree to which the need was currently being met, on a 3-point scale (well met, somewhat met, or not well met).

Interestingly, the number of needs rated by individuals with TBI as important was similar to that of the nondisabled group (12.3 vs. 12.8). However, fewer "important" needs were seen as "well met" within the TBI group (Table 19–5). For the TBI group, only one important need (passive recreation) was rated well met by more than 50 percent of the sample. In contrast, in the nondisabled group, four important needs (close friends, relationships with family, health, passive recreation) were well met in a majority of the sample. Similar results were found when unmet needs were examined. Three needs (work, close relationships with spouse or significant others, raising children) were "not well met" in the TBI Group, and only one need (raising children) was not well met in the nondisabled group.

WHAT ARE THE SERVICE UTILIZATION PATTERNS OF INDIVIDUALS WITH TRAUMATIC BRAIN INJURY LIVING IN THE COMMUNITY?

Typically, cognitive, physical, and behavioral sequelae of TBI endure over the life span. It is no surprise, then, that despite the length of time since their injuries, many individuals in the TBI group were still utilizing a variety of services (Table 19–6). Counseling and other psychological services were among those most frequently used many years post-TBI. No significant correlation was found between service utilization and either the duration of unconsciousness—an indicator of severity of injury—or time since injury. This finding suggests the need for services that are focused on coping

TABLE 19–5. Percentage of Needs Rated "Important" That Are "Well Met," "Somewhat Met," or "Not Well Met" in Quality of Life Study Groups

	Well Met	Somewhat Met	Not Met
Nondisabled Group	44.6%	45%	10.3%
TBI Group	36.4%	43.4%	20.2%

TABLE 19–6. Percentage of Traumatic Brain Injury Group ($n = 298$) Using a Variety of Community Services

Service	Percent
Individual counseling	40.9
Support group	26.4
Physical therapy	19.0
Case manager	18.4
Head injury association	17.2
Vocational rehabilitation	15.9
Group counseling	13.6
Cognitive rehabilitation	13.3
Companion	13.2
Psychological testing	10.9
Occupational therapy	9.2
Nurse	9.5
Twelve-step program	9.1
Therapeutic recreation	7.8
Speech	7.4

with the effects of TBI as an *ongoing* process for individuals with TBI, regardless of the severity of their injury.

IS SUBSTANCE ABUSE A PROBLEM FOR INDIVIDUALS WITH TRAUMATIC BRAIN INJURY LIVING IN THE COMMUNITY?

Previous research[21] suggests that, both before and after injury, alcohol and substance abuse problems are common in individuals with TBI. However, the findings that emerged from the QOL study only partially corroborate these findings. More specifically, although the number of individuals who *ever* had a drink is similar in the nondisabled (95.3%) and TBI (92.2%) groups, fewer individuals in the TBI group (44.6%) than in the nondisabled group (61.3%) had a drink "in the last month" ($p < .002$). These findings suggest that education regarding the negative effects of alcohol following TBI is effective, at least with some members of the TBI group. When asked if they had difficulty controlling drinking or if they had behavioral, health, or marital problems as a result of the drinking, the groups were similar. A larger proportion ($p < .05$) of those in the TBI group than in the nondisabled group (10.74% vs. 1.3%) acknowledged that they had emotional difficulties as a result of drinking. More than 9 percent of those in the TBI sample and 4 percent of those in the nondisabled group acknowledge participating in a 12-step program.

When drug use was examined, the pattern was somewhat different. More specifically, although 51 percent of those with TBI versus 35 percent of the nondisabled group ($p < .003$) acknowledge use of street drugs, few in either group acknowledge difficulties in controlling their drug use (3.3% in the TBI group vs. 1.3% in the nondisabled group). Despite the fact that few people in the study admit to having difficulties controlling the use of drugs per se, several types of specific problems *were* attributed to drug use: behavioral (TBI = 4.27%; nondisabled = 2.5%; n.s.), and marital (TBI = 11.8%; nondisabled = 7.4%; n.s.) problems. These data suggest that admitting specific problems attributable to drug use was easier than admitting to having a general problem with drugs, and these difficulties were equally common in individuals in the TBI and nondisabled groups.

IS DEPRESSION A PROBLEM FOR INDIVIDUALS WITH TRAUMATIC BRAIN INJURY LIVING IN THE COMMUNITY?

In the QOL study, assessment of mood included the Beck Depression Inventory (BDI).[22] Although the majority of the TBI group (75%) and the nondisabled group (96%) were *not* depressed, significantly more individuals with TBI were depressed (Table 19–7). More specifically, 25 percent of those with TBI reported moderate to severe depression (BDI >16), compared with only 4 percent of those in the nondisabled group. Thus, the proportion of those in the TBI sample who were depressed was 8 times greater than in the nondisabled group (Chi-square = 25.96; df = 3; p <.001). Further, on average, the TBI group had higher total BDI scores (p <.001) and endorsed a greater number of somatic (p <.0001) and nonsomatic items (p <.0001) than did individuals without a disability.

The results on depression from the QOL Study need to be interpreted carefully.[23] Research on poststroke depression with measures other than the BDI suggests that somatic items (e.g., feeling tired, having difficulty concentrating) are not depression-sensitive in individuals with acquired brain pathology (i.e., stroke) because they usually represent physical or cognitive sequelae of the brain injury rather than indicators of mood.[24] Until appropriate studies have been done, clinicians should give credence to nonsomatic, intrapsychic symptoms as more sensitive indicators of mood and question "evidence" of depression based primarily on somatic complaints. Such a study is being carried out within the RTC's research program.[25]

Discussion

How do the study's results advance our knowledge of the quality of life of people with TBI who are living in the community? A basic premise of this body of research has been that a less pessimistic picture of community living for people with TBI might emerge from broader-based samples, by asking individuals with TBI directly about their experiences and perceptions, and by focusing on a broad range of variables, both assets and challenges. Do these preliminary results support this stance?

Certainly, the results do not paint a rosy picture of the group studied. For example, the majority of individuals with TBI in our sample continue to experience a broad range of symptoms and difficulties that persist long after injury, up to 44 years. Considering that the average length of time since injury for the group was 9 years, it is likely that the symptoms reported are chronic and the permanent residuals of TBI. Furthermore, the individuals with TBI had more unmet needs and were more depressed than the comparison group.

Nevertheless, many of the QOL measures point to positive outcomes for individuals with TBI. For example, more individuals with TBI than in the nondisabled group avoid alcohol altogether. This group is in this way living a more healthful life, as alcohol clearly (from our results and others') creates more problems for people who have had a brain injury than for those who have not. Second, while the total scores on QOL and community integration measures were typically lower for people with TBI than for the nondisabled comparison group, many of the subscales for these measures were equivalent across groups (e.g., six scales of the Bigelow[17] QOL Questionnaire: psychological well-being, interpersonal interaction, spouse role, work on the job, and negative consequences of alcohol and of drugs).

TABLE 19–7. Beck Depression Inventory: Mean Total Score and Somatic and Nonsomatic Item Scores (Standard Deviation) in the Quality of Life Study Groups

Score	Traumatic Brain Injury Group	Nondisabled Group
Total Score	11.3 (8.8)	4.4 (4.8)
Somatic Items	4.0 (3.3)	1.6 (2.1)
Nonsomatic Items	7.4 (6.6)	3.0 (3.5)

The major challenge in this research is to enlarge our understanding of those factors that aid successful integration into the community after TBI and those factors that constitute the strongest barriers. We will continue to look within this data base to better answer our questions about who does well, in what ways, and how.[15,23,25–28]

□ INDIVIDUALS WITH TRAUMATIC BRAIN INJURY IN THE COMMUNITY: SERVICE DELIVERY AND PUBLIC POLICY CHALLENGES

To this point in the discussion, the perspective taken has been that of individuals with TBI. The focus in this section now shifts to the society in which the individuals with TBI lives: What is society's perspective of TBI? What does the individual with TBI need, including medical care and long-term services, from his or her societal context to maximize community living? How are people with TBI faring in getting those needs met that can be met only with the input of societally based resources?

From society's perspective, the key concern about life after TBI is economic. A recent study, in fact, estimates that medical costs associated with new cases of TBI emerging *in any given year* exceeds $8 billion over the course of the first 4 years following injury, a figure that does *not* cover indirect costs to society, such as lost earnings.[29] Within the societal viewpoint, fuller community integration is synonymous with less institutionalization, as institutionalization is clearly the most expensive "outcome" of TBI. Benefits are thus measured in terms of decreased fiscal demands on government. Medicaid in New York State, for example, is currently paying more than $50 million per year for the continued *out-of-state* placement (i.e., institutionalization) of individuals with TBI.[30] Returning these individuals to residences in their own communities (primarily through implementation of a Medicaid waiver program) will reduce overall expenditures and keep revenues within the state.

How have individuals with TBI fared in getting their needs met through organized societal efforts such as medical services, community-based services, and residential programs? Only in recent years are we beginning to see improvements that would have seemed unlikely in previous editions of this book. Thus, although individuals with TBI have been described as sometimes being "unaware,"[31] this term can just as easily be applied to rehabilitation service providers, insurance companies, and government officials in years past in describing their understanding of the impairments and service needs of individuals with TBI. Many of these wielders of power in the lives of people with TBI had been (and some continue to be) ignorant of the diverse physical, cognitive, and behavioral impairments that require treatment and, as a result, were unaware of the complex continuum of inpatient, outpatient, and community-based services needed by individuals with TBI. The result was inflexible treatment planning and inadequate mechanisms for paying for services, which left individuals with TBI and their families in the lurch. Thus, while medical science was making significant advances in learning to reduce morbidity and mortality following TBI, similar gains were not being made, until very recently, within the service system as a whole.

Stroke rehabilitation was the original treatment model for brain injury rehabilitation. Over the past two decades, a slow but steady increase in the diversity and quality of services for individuals with TBI has been matched by an increased willingness by public and private insurers to pay for the long-term services needed by individuals with TBI. These changes have been, in large part, caused by intense advocacy efforts by the Brain Injury Association, the creative thinking of many in the field, and some critical paradigm shifts in public policy.

The Brain Injury Association (BIA) was instrumental in increasing awareness of TBI and actions directed toward TBI at the federal level, as evidenced in:

■ The signing in 1985 of a cooperative agreement between the BIA (formerly the National Head Injury Foundation) and the Office of Special Education Programs, the Rehabilitation Services Administration (RSA), the National Institute of Handicapped Research (NIHR), the Council of State Administrators of Vocational Rehabilitation, and the National Association of State Directors of Special Education.

■ The increased willingness of the Social Security Administration to consider individuals with brain injury as eligible for Social Security disability insurance benefits.

■ The funding by the National Institute on Disability and Rehabilitation Research (formerly the NIHR) not only of research and training centers in the area of TBI but also of TBI model systems of care.

■ The funding by RSA of six regional TBI comprehensive rehabilitation and prevention centers.

■ The inclusion of TBI as a disability that is eligible for special education services under the Individuals with Disabilities Education Act (IDEA).

- The passage by Congress in 1996 of the TBI Act.

Service delivery has also benefited from our growing knowledge of the dynamics of recovery of cognitive function following TBI and by the development of interventions that enhance recovery. Prior to the late 1960s, although the dynamics of motor recovery were somewhat understood and rehabilitation treatments were available for some physical impairments, little was known about cognitive impairments and their potential for recovery or treatment. In the late 1960s and early 1970s, Leonard Diller, Yehuda Ben-Yishay, Joseph Weinberg, and their colleagues at the Rusk Institute in New York began to examine the learning styles of individuals with brain injury. They demonstrated that, following brain injury, individuals could benefit from interventions aimed at improved performance of cognitive tasks that they had failed prior to training.[32] This research led to the development of cognitive remediation as a rehabilitation therapy and to Ben-Yishay's comprehensive day treatment program for individuals with TBI.[33] Another key innovation in the rehabilitation of individuals with TBI was the demonstration by Paul Wehman[34] and his colleagues that supported employment was effective in improving the vocational outcomes of people with TBI.

The ability of individuals with TBI to obtain needed services has also been improved through shifts in public policy. For example, states such as Florida, Massachusetts, Minnesota, Missouri, and New York have developed statewide approaches to service delivery and service coordination for people with TBI.[35] In other states, when it became apparent that Medicaid was to become the primary payer of services for TBI and that, as originally structured, Medicaid would not pay for many of the services needed by people with TBI, waivers were developed to give states flexibility in the use of Medicaid dollars.[36] Approved Medicaid waivers that allow for the purchase of services not ordinarily covered now exist in 15 states: Colorado, Connecticut, Iowa, Kansas, Louisiana, Minnesota, New Hampshire, New Jersey, New York, North Dakota, South Carolina, Vermont, Washington, Wisconsin, and Utah. Although the waivers in these states differ, the impact is the same: Each provides payment for many of the "nontraditional" services required by individuals with TBI and thereby promotes decreased institutionalization and better quality of life.

In 1992, New York State changed the regulations under which rehabilitation programs operated to encourage more flexible yet cost-effective service delivery for individuals with TBI.[29] This change permitted individuals in coma to be admitted to acute rehabilitation programs. If these individuals began to make progress, they could remain in acute facilities for the duration of their inpatient rehabilitation stay (calculated to be about 85 days); if they did not make progress, they could be transferred to a skilled nursing facility. The state gave the nursing home a financial incentive (an increased level of reimbursement) to admit these individuals and develop needed programming. Of interest was the provision that, if these individuals began to make progress in the nursing home and could benefit from more intensive inpatient rehabilitation services, they could be transferred back to the acute inpatient facility. This innovation created flexibility in the continuum of care, which took into account the person's cognitive status and the extent to which he or she could benefit from intensive inpatient services at any given point in time. In addition, because individuals in coma could be admitted to acute rehabilitation programs in the state, the need decreased to send people to out-of-state facilities. This change, in turn, reduced both the stress on families and the potential for abuse.[37,38]

Important changes have also occurred in the ways in which issues of living with a brain injury are being conceptualized. For example, Jacobs et al.[29,40] make the observation that a "lifelong" perspective is needed to conceptualize the service needs of individuals with TBI. Condeluci[41] has advocated that a *medical* service delivery model is inappropriate for individuals with TBI. Instead, he urges an "interdependence" paradigm. Rather than focus on deficits, this model seeks to create supports for and empower consumers. A similar shift away from the medical model toward one that is more person centered has been called the "Whatever It Takes" approach to the delivery of community-based services.[42]

In a previous edition of this book, Cervelli[43] discussed the concept of a "continuum" of care for individuals with TBI. This continuum is meant to incorporate the needs of individuals with TBI into a single service system with all the necessary components, including acute medical and rehabilitation services, comprehensive outpatient and day treatment programs, transitional living programs, and supported housing. What is clear at present is that no single provider or institution can deliver the full range of services needed. Instead, regional alliances must be developed to create a network of service providers who hold a common vision. This, too, is a change in thinking that reflects the desire to increase access to services for the broadest group of people with TBI.

□ INDIVIDUALS WITH TRAUMATIC BRAIN INJURY: THE CHALLENGE OF MANAGED CARE

What is the expectable impact of managed care on the gains that have been made in increasing access to services by individuals with TBI? Managed care is designed to reduce health care costs by reducing visits to medical specialists, shortening the length of inpatient hospital stays, and limiting the diversity and intensity of outpatient services. In New York State, for example, the basic managed care contract pays for only 60 consecutive days of outpatient rehabilitation per diagnosis over the lifetime of the insured. Thus, although the managed care approach will certainly save money by reducing services (but presumably not benefits) for those in good health, for individuals with TBI, managed care threatens to limit the individual's access to services and, thereby, recovery of function. This, in turn, threatens to restrict community integration and quality of life, while increasing the likelihood of secondary disabilities and long-term institutionalization.

The causes of problems individuals with TBI face under managed care fall into two categories:

1. Caps on services mean that the *number* of services that the managed care company will pay for will often be inadequate to meet needs. Thus, in seeking to cut costs, managed care companies restrict access to services, without allowing sufficiently for variations in needs for services across individuals and across situations. Similarly, services under managed care often cannot be continued over a long enough period. Even under managed care systems with relatively liberal benefits, those who coordinate services are often insensitive to the lengthy periods of intensive services that typically are needed to attain desired outcomes following TBI. Too frequently ignored is the fact that the person receiving the service has experienced a brain injury, and thus his or her rate of learning has been significantly slowed.

2. The *mix or nature* of services is inappropriate because the coordinator or controller of allowable services—who is employed by the insurance carrier—is neither the rehabilitation team nor any other entity that places the individual with TBI at the center. This immediately sets up an adversarial relationship, with the person with the brain injury and his

or her family caught in the middle. Consequently, all too often, the real needs of the individual with TBI are lost in the name of "cost containment."

In the managed care milieu, the costs of care are often shifted from inpatient to outpatient services. In many instances, the burden of care is thus shifted onto the family, which becomes the untrained provider of needed services. The costs, in many such cases, are also shifted to the individual with TBI, to the extent that he or she achieves lesser outcomes because of truncated services under managed care. In some cases, the costs shift further, as either society or the family has to assume the financial responsibility for maintaining the individual with TBI in an institution because managed care falls far short of allowing the individual with TBI to function adequately in the community.

In terms of these threats to access to services and the shift of costs onto families and society, what responses will help? In raising our voices and seeking solutions to these problems revolving around managed care, we suggest, first, that more outcome research is needed to better bolster the assertion that specific services do matter and do lead to functional, real-life gains. Whether services are funded by managed care companies, families, or society, we need more than anecdotal data to make decisions about the best use of scarce resources.

Second, "sense" all too often has been missing under managed care, in terms of it being *sens*itive to and *sens*ible about the challenges of TBI (and other chronic conditions). TBI cannot be treated like an outbreak of the flu. Basic managed care contractors are not prepared to confront the complexities of catastrophic disability. To provide a rational basis for cost-effective service delivery, managed care companies should be urged to contract services for people with severe disabilities with providers that demonstrate "expertise." In this way, costs can be controlled through the necessary input of those with appropriate know-how.

Third, the goal for any individual who has experienced a TBI is not solely medical. It focuses more broadly on recovering function and reconstructing a life after TBI. Here, fiscal bottom-line thinking should not be given primacy (a voice, yes, but not primacy). When the aim is to reconstruct a life, all involved may benefit by exploring alternative ways to respond sensibly and sensitively to the long-term, complex needs of individuals with TBI. We would argue that, even within a managed care context, the hopes and aspirations of the person with TBI need to become the center and the driving force of service delivery. In this approach, a "case" is not "managed"; rather, a broker of services advocates on behalf of the brain injured person to ensure that he or she gets what is needed to reconstruct a life.

Exploring ways to encourage person-centered planning, researchers at the RTC on the Community Integration of Individuals with Traumatic Brain Injury have adapted personal futures planning[44,45] (PFP) to fit the needs of individuals with TBI. PFP has been widely used in the developmental disability community but has not been systematically used with individuals with TBI. Pilot testing of this adapted PFP[46] in New York State with individuals with moderate to severe TBI, both living in the community and trying to return to community living, has resulted in life plans that are both useful and inexpensive. Consequently, the New York State Department of Health (DOH) is supporting the training of DOH personnel across the state to use this method for planning service delivery—with the person with TBI at the center of the process and with the person's vision of a positive future as the driving force.

Without a realistic view of TBI and other chronic disabling conditions, managed care is likely to limit community options and outcomes for individuals with TBI, inadvertently driving up the economic costs of injury and potentially increasing the rates of reinstitutionalization.

□ CONCLUSION

The concepts of community integration and quality of life following TBI are complex. Criteria have not yet been generated that distinguish between those who "successfully" versus "unsuccessfully" integrate themselves into the community. Clearly, the quality of life of individuals with TBI tells many stories—some negative, some positive. On the one hand, results from the QOL Study tell an upsetting story—for some individuals in the sample. That story is one of depression, limited vocational outcomes, and other signs of a reduced quality of life. On a positive note, many of the people included in this study *have* returned to work or school, *do* participate in the community life, are *not* depressed, and remain free from alcohol and drugs. Nevertheless, they still confront many barriers to community living every day of their lives, including a variety of chronic physical, cognitive, and social challenges and unmet needs. These individuals are living their lives, successfully walking the sometimes conflicting paths of "who they were," "who they are," and "who they want to be."

In considering the research results reviewed and the discussion of external forces that threaten and/or hold promise for improving the lives of people who have experienced a TBI, we are reminded that brain injury does not destroy a person's individuality or his or her hopes and aspirations. People with TBI have dreams and goals, and like all of us are entitled to be supported in their quest toward a positive future. Rehabilitation and community integration are about facilitating the unfolding of each person's story so that it may better correspond to his or her hopes.

REFERENCES

1. Thomsen, I: The patient with severe head injury and his family. Scand J Rehab Med 6:180, 1974.
2. Rosenbaum, M, and Najenson, T: Changes in life patterns and symptoms of low mood as reported by wives of severely brain-injured soldiers. J Consult Clin Psychol 44:881, 1976.
3. Levin, H, et al: Long-term neuropsychological outcome of closed head injury. J Neurosurg 50:412, 1979.
4. Weddell, R, Oddy, M, and Jenkins, D: Social adjustment after rehabilitation: A two year follow-up of patients with severe head injury. Psychol Med 10:357, 1980.
5. McKinlay, W, et al: The short-term outcome of severe blunt head injury as reported by relatives of the injured persons. J Neurol Neurosurg Psychiatry 44:527, 1981.
6. Thomsen, I: Late outcome of very severe blunt head trauma: A 10-15 year second follow-up. J Neurol Neurosurg Psychiatry 47:260, 1984.
7. Oddy, M, et al: Social adjustment after closed head injury: A further follow-up seven years after injury. J Neurol Neurosurg Psychiatry 48:564, 1985.
8. Brooks, N, et al: The five year outcome of severe blunt head injury: A relative's view. J Neurol Neurosurg Psychiatry 49:764, 1986.
9. Klonoff, P, et al: Quality of life in patients 2 to 4 years after closed head injury. Neurosurgery 19:735, 1986.
10. Brooks, N, et al: Return to work within the first seven years of severe head injury. Brain Inj 1:5, 1987.
11. Jacobs, H: The Los Angeles head injury survey: Procedures and initial findings. Arch Phys Med Rehabil 69:425, 1988.
12. Lezak, M, and O'Brien, KP: Longitudinal study of emotional, social, and physical changes after traumatic brain injury. Journal of Learning Disabilities 21:456, 1988.
13. Lezak, M, and O'Brien, KP: Chronic emotional, social, and physical changes after traumatic brain injury. In Bigler, ED (ed): Traumatic Brain Injury: Mechanisms of Damage, Assessment, Intervention, and Outcome. Pro-Ed, Austin, 1990, p 365.
14. Thomsen, I: Do young patients have worse outcomes after severe blunt head trauma? Brain Inj 3:157, 1989.
15. Brown, M, and Vandergoot, D: Quality of life of individuals with traumatic brain injury: Comparison with others living in the community. J Head Trauma Rehabil 13:1, 1998.
16. Brown, M, and Gordon, WA: Quality of life as a construct in health and disability research. Mt Sinai J Med (in press).
17. Bigelow, DA, Gareau, MJ, and Young, DJ: A quality of life interview. Psychosocial Rehabilitation Journal 14:94, 1992.
18. Willer, B, et al: Assessment of community integration following rehabilitation for traumatic brain injury. J Head Trauma Rehabil 8:75, 1993.
19. Corrigan, J, and Deming, R: Psychometric characteristics of the Community Integration Questionnaire: Replication and extension. J Head Trauma Rehabil 10:41, 1995.
20. Flanagan, JC: A research approach to improving our quality of life. Am Psychol 33:138, 1978.

21. Corrigan, J: Substance abuse as a mediating factor in outcome from TBI. Arch Phys Med Rehabil 76:302, 1995.
22. Beck, A: Beck Depression Inventory: Manual. Psychological Corporation, San Antonio, 1987.
23. Hibbard, MR, et al: Axis I psychopathology in individuals with traumatic brain injury. Head Trauma Rehabil 13:24, 1998.
24. Stein, PN, et al: The discriminative properties of somatic and non-somatic symptoms for post-stroke depression. Journal of Clinical Neuropsychology 10:142, 1996.
25. Sliwinski, M, Gordon, WA, and Bogdany, J: The Beck Depression Inventory: Is it a suitable measure of depression for individuals with traumatic brain injury? J Head Trauma Rehabil 13:40, 1998.
26. O'Neill, J, et al: The impact of employment on quality of life and community integration after traumatic brain injury. J Head Trauma Rehabil (in press).
27. Gordon, WA, et al: The enigma of hidden TBI. J Head Trauma Rehabil (in press).
28. Hibbard, MR, et al: Undiagnosed health issues in individuals with traumatic brain injury living in the community. J Head Trauma Rehabil 13:47, 1998.
29. Brooks, CA, et al: Cost of medical care for a population-based sample of persons surviving traumatic brain injury. J Head Trauma Rehabil 10(4):1, 1995.
30. Milliren, JR, and Gordon, WA: The development of an integrated rehabilitation system for persons with traumatic brain injury: The evolution of public policy in New York. J Head Trauma Rehabil 9:27, 1994.
31. Hackler, E, and Tobis, JS: Reintegration into the community. In Rosenthal, M, et al (eds): Rehabilitation of the Head Injured Adult. Philadelphia: FA Davis, 1983, p 421.
32. Diller, L, and Gordon, WA: Rehabilitation and clinical neuropsychology. In Filskov, S, and Boll, T (eds): Handbook of Clinical Neuropsychology. John Wiley, New York, 1981, p 702.
33. Ben-Yishay, Y, and Prigatano, G: Cognitive remediation. In Rosenthal, M, et al (eds): Rehabilitation of the Adult and Child with Traumatic Brain Injury. Philadelphia: FA Davis, 1990, p 393.
34. Wehman, P, et al: Return to work for persons with traumatic brain injury: A supported employment approach. Arch Phys Med Rehabil 71:147, 1990.
35. Digre, PG, et al: Selected states' public policy responses to traumatic brain injury. J Head Trauma Rehabil 9:12, 1994.
36. Rosen, B, and Reynolds, WE: The impact of public policy on persons with traumatic brain injury: The evolution of public policy in New York. J Head Trauma Rehabil 9:1, 1994.
37. Kerr, P: Center of head injury accused of earning millions for neglect. The New York Times, March 16, 1992, p 1.
38. House Committee on Government Operations: Fraud and Abuse in the Head Injury Rehabilitation Industry. House Report 102-1059. Government Printing Office, Washington, DC, 1992.
39. Jacobs, HE (ed): Lifelong living. J Head Trauma Rehabil 5(1):1, 1990.
40. Jacobs, HE, Blatnick, M, and Sandhorst, JV: What is lifelong living, and how does it relate to quality of life? J Head Trauma Rehabil 5:1, 1990.
41. Condeluci, A: Brain injury rehabilitation: The need to bridge paradigms. Brain Inj 5:543, 1992.
42. Willer, B, and Corrigan, J: A model for community based services: The Whatever It Takes Model. Brain Inj 7:647, 1994.
43. Cervelli, L: Re-entry into the community and systems of posthospital care. In Rosenthal, M, et al (eds): Rehabilitation of the Adult and Child with Traumatic Brain Injury. Philadelphia: FA Davis, 1990, p 463.
44. O'Brien, J, and Mount, B: Telling new stories: The search for capacity among people with severe handicaps. In Meyer, LH, Peck, CA, and Brown, L (eds): Critical Issues in the Lives of People with Severe Disabilities. Paul Brooks, Baltimore, 1991, p 89.
45. Mount, B: The benefits and limitations of personal futures planning. In Bradley, VJ, Ashbaugh, JW, and Blaney, BC (eds): Creating Individual Supports for People with Developmental Disabilities. Paul Brooks, Baltimore, 1994, p 97.
46. Mount, B, et al: Moving on: A Personal Futures Planning Workbook for Individuals with Traumatic Brain Injury. The Mount Sinai Medical Center, RTC on Community Integration of Individuals with TBI, New York, 1997.

Vocational Rehabilitation for Individuals with Traumatic Brain Injury

PAUL WEHMAN, PHD,
MICHAEL WEST, PHD,
ANGELA JOHNSON, MAED,
and DAVID X. CIFU, MD

In recent years, the education, rehabilitation, and treatment of people who have experienced traumatic brain injuries (TBI) have been emphasized. As a result of advances in emergency evacuation procedures, neurosurgical and rehabilitation techniques, psychopharmacological methods and interventions, and the use of motorcycle and bicycle helmets and other safety devices, more of these individuals are surviving motor vehicle crashes and other accidents.[1] Individuals with severe TBI are usually quite disabled and require special vocational help and other community support services to reenter the competitive work force.

Annually, close to 500,000 people sustain a brain injury of sufficient degree to require treatment, with approximately 50,000 sustaining an injury resulting in severe, chronic, debilitating impairments.[2] Survivors of severe brain injury typically exhibit cognitive, physical, and/or psychosocial impairments that inhibit employment and other activities of daily living and adversely affect their quality of life.[3]

Because a significant proportion of TBI survivors are young adults who are just beginning their careers, brain injury frequently results in long-term economic hardship on victims, their families, and society. At every level, the costs of TBI are staggering. An estimate for people injured in 1985 yields a societal cost of $37.8 billion, or $115,300 per person, including both survivors and fatalities.[4] For those who survive their injuries, lifelong costs for lost productivity and wages, ongoing income and health maintenance, long-term care, and other needs averaged $71,000 per person injured in 1985.

Let's examine the case of Nick, who was an insurance sales executive and recently graduated from a masters in business administration program. Nick was hit at a crosswalk by a drunk hit-and-run driver and suffered massive injuries to his head and chest. Nick was taken to the nearest hospital trauma center. Within days he stabilized but remained unconscious for several months. Slowly Nick woke up and over six months began to recover, although at this point he has severe headaches and needs extensive physical therapy. Intellectually and psychologically, he has significant problems. He has memory difficulties, his planning and organizing skills are jumbled, and he becomes angry and frustrated for no apparent reason. Most of his preinjury friends are gone or see him only for short visits, and Nick is confused about his future. What is Nick's outlook for getting and holding a job and maintaining his career?

A significant proportion of the costs of TBI can be linked to low rates of postinjury employment.

Estimates of those who will enter or reenter the competitive work force following injury have been very low, often below 30 percent.[5-7] Moreover, "employment" of brain injury survivors is often determined by the percentage of those who find work after their injury. Research indicates that individuals who return to work do so in less demanding or menial positions, in sheltered employment or volunteer work, or for only short periods.[8] Individuals who return to work frequently require assistance from coworkers to perform their duties.[9] These findings underscore the difficulties individuals with TBI experience in attempting to return to productive lives. This chapter presents an overview of the importance of choice in vocational planning, a description of different vocational rehabilitation models, and an overview of training and employment issues.

◻ INDIVIDUAL CHOICE

Historically, individuals with TBI have often been given a choice regarding the vocational services that were available to them. An individual either met the eligibility criteria for vocational rehabilitation services or was referred for extended evaluation, training, or work adjustment to "get ready" to go to work. Individuals with severe TBI have often been seen as "too disabled" to benefit from rehabilitation and receive little or no help or support from the state vocational rehabilitation program.

Fortunately, as people with TBI have demonstrated work potential and as services for consumers with severe disabilities have emerged (e.g., assistive technology and supported employment), access to vocational rehabilitation (VR) services has improved. One of the mandates of the Rehabilitation Act Amendments of 1992 (P.L. 102-569), the funding authority for the VR program, is that rehabilitation goals and services should be guided by the choices of the consumer. Our clinical observations from nearly a decade of service to members of this population suggest that opportunities to make career choices and job changes can have a significant impact on a person's degree of job satisfaction and job retention.

Choosing a Career

Identified career preferences provide broad parameters that can guide the employment specialist's job development activities. However, the specific characteristics of each potential job opening and work environment (e.g., salaries, benefits, and degree of integration and interaction) vary and affect the desirability of the specific job to the consumer. For example, an individual may prefer the higher wages of one job over the "nine to five" hours of another. Similarly, an individual may choose the social atmosphere of one job over the geographical location of another. An indication of the job characteristics that are valued by an individual can be identified during the consumer assessment process by (1) interviewing the consumer and family members, (2) observing the consumer in different environments, (3) reviewing records and evaluations that document previous experiences, (4) repeatedly visiting and communicating with the consumer and/or family in familiar surroundings, (5) conducting community-based situational assessment work experiences, and (6) arranging on-site visits at different businesses in the community.

Selecting a Counselor

In areas that have multiple providers of employment services, funding and referral agencies can give an individual and, if desired or needed, his or her family the opportunity to express a preference for a particular employment counselor. This preference may be based on prior experiences, good and bad track records with job placements and retention, geographical proximity, or level of comfort with agencies or staff within agencies.

Usually a human service program assigns an employment counselor or specialist to assist a consumer according to availability and caseloads. Typically, an individual does not know the employment specialists well enough to select one over another at the time of referral. As the consumer and employment specialist work together more closely during job development, consumer assessment, and job site training, provisions should be made to accommodate an individual's request for a different counselor. For example, the individual may find that it is difficult working with a certain counselor because of conflicting values or ideas regarding employment. It is important to listen to what the individual with a disability is saying and to pay attention to a change in behavior at the job site that may signal a problem with the current training arrangements. Perhaps increasing the involvement of family, friends, and coworkers in job development and training or another change can alleviate the problem without a change of counselors.

Participation in Decisions on Training Methods

Individuals with TBI can and should be involved in selecting training methods, adaptive devices, or compensatory strategies. They may suggest options that would be more effective, more comfortable to use, or less stigmatizing or have preference concerning the level of help being provided at the job site. Some individuals with TBI feel that the employment counselor is checking up too often, embarrassing them in front of coworkers, or otherwise making it more difficult to blend into the workplace culture. They may feel that picture prompts are too juvenile, or call attention to their inability to read or follow instructions.

Deciding to Keep a Job

This choice is most problematic for many human service agencies to accept and implement. Because of financial and personnel commitments or relationships with employers, placement agencies and counselors frequently attempt to maintain placements as long as possible, regardless of the level of satisfaction or vocational aspirations of the service recipient. However, in terms of consumer empowerment, human service provider agencies have two major tasks. The first is to acknowledge that long-range vocational success begins with consumer-directed placement in positions which they choose. Frequently, agencies target positions into which the greatest number of potential clients can"fit," rather than attempting to match the abilities and interests of individuals with motivating, challenging jobs. Second, human service agencies need to develop more positive attitudes regarding job separations. Job separations should be viewed not as failures on anyone's part but as a stage of growth in the development of work preferences and capacity; that is, the consumer has learned more about preferred work situations and has established a competitive employment baseline (e.g., 1 wk, 1 mo, or 6 mo) on which to improve during the next attempt.

These areas of choice are an important foundation for understanding the value of the different models and processes of vocational rehabilitation that are described later in the chapter. First, however, is a case study in choice for a young man with a TBI, in his own words, who received services from our supported employment program.*

Case 1 ▪ Let me begin by telling you how I discovered supported employment. A friend of mine asked me to go with her to an appointment at a supported employment program because she was nervous. I had heard about supported employment from another friend who was using it, but I really did not know much about it. Anyway, I agreed to accompany my friend. During the meeting, I thought this sounded like an interesting idea. So, soon afterwards, I went to see my [VR] counselor, requested supported employment, and that is when things began.

I knew which service provider I wanted, the same one my friend had chosen. During the first meeting, we completed some paperwork. Then I was given the option to either have an employment specialist assigned or to interview and select who was going to work for me. I decided to interview and met with four candidates. I chose someone who I felt had a genuine interest and desire to assist me.

In order to look for jobs, the employment specialist needed to know my expectations. She came to my home and we had discussions about where I would like to work and my strengths. I was very interested in a job that would allow me to transport myself to work. I did not want to be dependent upon an unreliable specialized transportation system. Next, we discussed how I wanted to be involved in "finding a job." I decided to contact businesses near my home. Also, my wife, the employment specialist, and I brainstormed a list of businesses to contact. We also scheduled to meet and review the classified ads and progress to date.

Eventually, the employment specialist discovered an opportunity at a restaurant. The employer wanted someone to clean the dining area prior to opening. Over the years, I had cleaned house and enjoyed this type of work, so I decided to check it out. The employment specialist arranged for an interview. During the interview, I emphasized to the employer that although I had no paid work experience that I would be a dependable and hard worker. I got the job. The employer let me establish my work schedule, and we negotiated a starting rate of pay.

The employment specialist went to work with me and provided recommendations on how to do the job in the most efficient manner. For example, while learning to vacuum, we experimented with several different routes or patterns to follow until a best way was agreed upon. I also needed some modifications to the vacuum, because the cord constantly got entangled in the wheels of my chair. The employment specialist encouraged me to contact my counselor [for the authorization of funds for equipment modification], which I did. Then I turned it back over to the employment specialist. It took longer than I expected, but finally the vacuum was modified. The changes allowed me to work much faster.

Today the employment specialist visits the job site on occasion to see how things are going. My

*This case study is adapted from a case study for Customer Initiated Supported Employment . . . Partnerships for Success, developed by the Virginia Commonwealth University Rehabilitation Research and Training Center on Supported Employment.

supervisor, at my request, uses an evaluation that I designed to provide me with feedback on certain aspects of my job performance. The feedback is helpful and I have remained open to new ideas on how to do the best job. My success has been in part because of my dependability, hard work, and good interpersonal skills. I have come a long way—a year ago unemployed and look where I am today!

☐ MODELS AND PROCESSES OF VOCATIONAL REHABILITATION

There are several different approaches to the vocational rehabilitation of people with TBI. Clearly, a community-based orientation seems to be the most effective because this is where people with TBI live and function. However, different models exist and are being used.

Supported Employment

WHAT IS SUPPORTED EMPLOYMENT?

Supported employment evolved from federally funded research and demonstration projects, particularly in Virginia, Oregon, and Illinois, in the late 1970s and early 1980s. These demonstrations showed that people with severe cognitive, physical, and behavioral impairments, typically in sheltered employment or deemed inappropriate for state VR services, could work competitively if given the opportunity and necessary supports.[10] Those supports typically included intensive training and adaptation after placement into a job (often referred to as "place, then train" methodology), followed by ongoing assistance to the individual, family, employer, and coworkers. This concept of supporting individuals with disabilities in natural environments has since been extended to education, housing, recreation and leisure, family assistance, behavioral intervention, and other areas.

Supported employment became a service option within the VR service system via the Rehabilitation Act Amendments of 1986. The regulations for this Act[11] defined *supported employment* as time-limited employment services (up to 18 mo), including job placement, training, and modifications (funded by the state VR agency; and extended services, including periodic job skills reinforcement and ongoing support, funded by non-VR sources. Typically, these non-VR sources have been state mental retardation, developmental disability, or mental health funding agencies.

The supported employment regulations also defined the target population as individuals with severe disabilities for whom competitive

employment has not traditionally been an option and for whom ongoing support services are essential to perform competitive work. Those who are severely disabled because of mental retardation or psychosocial disabilities have been the primary recipients of supported employment services, although supported employment programs serve a diverse population. Amendments to the Rehabilitation Act in 1992 and subsequent regulations[12] added language that defined the target population as VR consumers "with the most severe disabilities" in an effort to ensure that programs serve those who are truly in need of intensive long-term supports.

Supported employment participants can be placed into jobs individually by a job coach or employment specialist or in small group models such as work crews, enclaves, and small businesses developed specifically for supported employees. A growing body of research shows that people in individual placement fare better than those in group options in wages, benefits, and levels of integration with coworkers.[12,13] Perhaps for this reason, group options appear to be used far less frequently than in the early years of the program.[14]

Much of the research literature on supported employment has focused on the impact of the program on participants and on society in general. Because the target population is those who have been excluded from competitive employment opportunities, participants have generally been unemployed or engaged in segregated workshops or work activity programs prior to entry. Those who enter supported employment from segregated work options have greatly increased their earnings, job satisfaction, community participation, and self-esteem.[15] Society benefits as well in that supported employment programs tend to be less costly over time than segregated programs and participants return more in income taxes and savings in other types of taxpayer-funded supports.[16,17]

SUPPORTED EMPLOYMENT FOR PERSONS WITH TRAUMATIC BRAIN INJURY

Only in recent years has supported employment been viewed as a viable alternative for individuals with brain injuries. Severe injuries typically result in long-term deficits in cognition, often with attendant impairments in health, physical capacity, mobility, social behavior, and other areas.[18–20] These problems result in very low rates of return to work and a generally low expectation of employability following severe injury.[6,7] However, the research base for this assumption generally assumes an unassisted return to work or short-term vocational interventions, such as counseling, work adjustment, and work hardening. The combination of (1) intensive training, adaptation, and accommodations provided initially and (2) ongoing support to the individual and the employer can alleviate the deleterious effects of severe injury that inhibit return to work and a productive life.[21]

Outcome studies of supported employment for people with severe brain injuries have found that individuals have greatly increased their earnings and employment participation to approximately their preinjury levels. For example, Table 20–1, from a report by Wehman et al.[22] summarizes comparisons of hourly salaries, work hours per week, and a measure of labor force participation, the monthly employment ratio (calculated by dividing months employed during a specified time period by the total months in that period). A later report[23] with an increased number of consumers and a longer time period showed that the average employment ratio increased from 13 to 67 percent; while receiving services, individuals who had been employed an average of only about 47 days in any given year were now employed about 245 days a year.

However, this last finding also points out a significant problem in assisting persons with severe brain injuries to return to work. Many such individuals experience frequent job changes because of either the problems they exhibit, their need to relearn work skills and job preferences, or frequent layoffs. This pattern has prevailed with those who are in supported employment as well; on average, one third of their supported employment service time is spent between jobs. These data, however, do not imply that the program has failed. For many, job tenure improves with second, third, and subsequent placements as they continue in the program.[21] Because the program offers long-term support, even in periods of unemployment, successful return to work in the supported employment model is not measured by retention of a single job but by steady participation in the workforce, perhaps in repeated jobs.

People with TBI represent only a small fraction of the supported employment program; in fact, estimates provided by state VR supported employment directors indicate that probably fewer than 2000 individuals with brain injuries are receiving supported employment services.[14] However, many rehabilitation centers have recently added supported employment to their array of post acute services for their patients. Most recent estimates of costs of services[24] showed an average of $10,198 for the first year of service ($6,942 median).

Natural Supports

WHAT ARE NATURAL SUPPORTS?

At some time, all members of a community—whether they are family members, friends, coworkers, or others—rely on each other for specific types of assistance. *Natural supports* is a term used to refer to the informal support networks that people develop to enhance functional performance and pleasure in their communities and workplaces. This concept has become a major component of employment services for individuals with disabilities as well. These natural supports can include coworkers, supervisors, employee assistance programs, neighbors, family members, public accommodations such as transportation services, and community service organizations.[25,26]

The 1992 Amendments to the Rehabilitation Act endorse natural supports for a VR service consumer as long as the supported functions are consistent with needs identified in the individualized written rehabilitation plan (IWRP). If ongoing transportation assistance and monitoring of health status are identified needs, family members or coworkers can be designated as support options to meet those needs and, if necessary, can be reimbursed for providing those services. Natural supports have been

---

TABLE 20–1. Employment Outcomes for Supported Employment Compared to Preinjury and Postinjury Employment Status

	Preinjury Employment	Postinjury Employment	Supported Employment
Hourly wage	$ 5.11	$ 3.45	$ 4.52
Work hours per week	34.7	27.7	29.2
Employment ratio	.839	.224	.876

Source: Adapted from data reported by Wehman, P, et al: Employment outcomes of persons following traumatic brain injury: Pre-injury, post-injury, and supported employment. Brain Inj 3:397, 1989.

proposed as a cost-effective means of achieving maximum integration at work, at home, and in the community.[27]

NATURAL SUPPORTS FOR PEOPLE WITH TRAUMATIC BRAIN INJURY

The use of natural supports to enhance the employment and independent living outcomes for people with brain injuries and their families has only recently been explored.[28,29] In vocational rehabilitation, Curl et al.[30] described a return to work program that used coworkers as trainers for individuals with severe brain injuries. Selected coworkers were trained and monitored by rehabilitation professionals and received stipends for additional mentoring responsibilities. The model proved effective in terms of employment success for approximately one third of the project's client pool.

Natural supports have particular significance for those with severe brain injuries who need supported employment services. The supported employment regulations require the VR counselor to ensure that sources of ongoing support are likely to be available before the initiation of time-limited services. In many states, people who acquire brain injuries as adults do not have ready access to extended service funding streams (e.g., mental retardation, developmental disability, or mental health agencies), particularly if the injury occurred after the age of 22. Planning for natural supports as extended service options can make supported employment available to individuals with brain injuries who might otherwise not be able to access services.[29]

The availability of natural supports at the work site can have very positive impacts on employment outcomes. West[31] conducted a prospective study of 37 individuals with severe TBI who were placed into supported employment positions. All were assessed using the Vocational Integration Index (VII), an observational tool for rating the opportunities for integration within a work setting and the extent to which an individual participates in those opportunities. Individuals who retained their employment for 6 months or longer had been rated higher than nonretainers on all eight VII subscales, with significant differences on seven subscales. Key items that discriminated between successful and unsuccessful placements included physical proximity with coworkers, common areas for lunches and breaks, opportunities for social interaction both on the job and during off-hours, regular meetings, and economic benefits such as regular merit reviews and health insurance. West[31] concluded that the social and economic aspects of a position are important but often overlooked factors in promoting return to work for this population.

Job Clubs

WHAT IS A JOB CLUB?

Job clubs originated in the 1970s through the work of Nathan Azrin and his colleagues. The job club approach combines (1) instruction and practice in job-seeking skills, such as job search and interviewing skills and (2) support and encouragement from a counselor and other members of the club.[32] The approach has standard procedures that are followed by the counselor with all participants, who track their own performance with the counselor's help.

The job club approach has been most frequently associated with people who have psychosocial disabilities such as substance abuse, depression, bipolar disorders, and anxiety disorders.[33] However, the model has also been used successfully with other groups of individuals who are experiencing difficulties in entering or reentering the work force, such as workfare participants,[34] displaced older workers,[35,36] offenders,[37] and students with and without disabilities who are entering the work force.[38,39] Job clubs are typically funded through state departments of VR, mental health, substance abuse, or employment.

JOB CLUBS AND PEOPLE WITH TRAUMATIC BRAIN INJURY

The job club approach has been utilized with persons with TBI to only a limited degree. However, the components of the model are well suited to this population. The repetition and practice of job search skills can be beneficial to those who have memory impairments or who experience excessive anxiety before job interviews. The support of a counselor and other individuals with brain injuries can provide potential job leads, comfort, and encouragement for the person with TBI who attempts to reenter the work force.

Mann and Svorai[40] describe a modification of the job club program for individuals with mild to moderate cognitive disabilities from mental retardation, brain injury, or learning disabilities, called COMPETE (computer preparation: evaluation, training, and employment). As evident from the title, the project focuses on information-age occupations and training methods and includes job modifications and support from a job club as well. During the course of this 3-year project, 17 of 27 participants achieved full-time employment in computer applications.

Vocational Rehabilitation Counseling

Vocational counseling is available from state VR programs and from private for-profit or nonprofit agencies. Although the goals and processes are similar, state VR agencies are more strictly and consistently regulated in areas of admissions, documentation of services, and service availability.

To be eligible for state VR-funded counseling services, an individual must (1) have a disability (i.e., a physical or mental impairment that constitutes or results in a substantial impediment to employment), (2) require VR services to prepare for, enter, engage in, or retain gainful employment, and (3) be able to benefit from VR services in terms of an employment outcome.

The goal of VR counseling is to assist persons with disabilities in developing accurate self-knowledge, identifying a variety of employment alternatives that are available, realistically considering and selecting an employment option, and preparing the individual to make career changes or adjustments as independently as possible.[41]

VOCATIONAL REHABILITATION COUNSELING FOR PEOPLE WITH TRAUMATIC BRAIN INJURY

The VR counselor plays a pivotal role in helping people with TBI to successfully enter or return to employment. The VR counselor is able to access services from other professionals involved in the rehabilitation team, which can directly or indirectly affect the client's ability to enter and maintain employment. At every step of the rehabilitation process, including eligibility determination, the VR counselor must consider how rehabilitation technology can help people with TBI successfully return to work. Rehabilitation technology encompasses a broad range of assistive technology devices and services (e.g., wheelchairs, watch alarms, and memory books) designed to aid individuals with disabilities in performing daily life activities.

When informing a person with TBI of available employment options, the VR counselor must inform the client of supported employment services if they are a viable option. For people with TBI who are eligible for VR, an IWRP must be written. This plan is developed by both the counselor and the client and includes a statement of the specific rehabilitation technology services needed to help the client achieve his or her intermediate rehabilitation objectives and long-term rehabilitation goals.

To effectively serve individuals with traumatic brain injuries, VR counselors should carefully evaluate (1) the job or school setting of interest to the client, (2) the nature of the deficit, (3) the severity and type of brain damage, (4) the type of job and its location, and (5) the job requirements (e.g., physical demands, complexity, interpersonal requirements, language and visual perceptual requirements, and the degree of new learning required).[42]

Because people with TBI experience a wide array of problems, such as difficulty with new learning and interacting inappropriately in social settings, many disciplines need to be involved in the rehabilitation process. The VR counselor can include persons from various professions on the rehabilitation team to provide different insights into the client and the type of assistive technology that would best benefit the client in a job setting. For example, in training a person with a TBI on how to interact in an interview, the VR counselor may rely on a speech-language pathologist to teach effective communication skills (e.g., maintaining eye contact, speaking at an optimal voice tone, focusing on the topic at hand, and asking appropriate questions).[43]

The VR counselor can establish one or more nonpaid community assessments to evaluate the client's vocational strengths, abilities, and deficits. The U.S. Department of Labor allows a community-based assessment, which includes vocational exploration, assessment, and training, to occur on a nonpaid basis within the private sector for up to 120 hours.[43] Based on these assessments and the client's job preferences and interests, the VR counselor can determine the job placement model that would be most appropriate and identify reasonable accommodations that may be needed to help the client function as independently as possible at the job site.

People with traumatic brain injuries often experience persistent symptoms well after the injury has occurred. For instance, Fraser et al.[44] studied 107 individuals across all levels of TBI severity and found that 40 percent of the individuals who returned to work reported one or more symptoms such as fatigue or irritability. In the same study, 17 percent of those with TBI had not been employed during the year postinjury because of the persistent effects of their injuries. Because the time-limited component of VR services (i.e., providing job development and training services for up to 18 mo after employment) do not address the additional problems experienced by people with TBI, supported employment services may be the best employment option. Ellerd and Moore[45] examined the effects of supported employment on the job retention rates of 24 employees with TBI at 12 and 30 months. After 12 months, 71 percent of employees with TBI were still employed, and approximately 38 percent were employed after 30 months.

Independent Living Centers

WHAT ARE INDEPENDENT LIVING CENTERS?

Independent living centers (ILCs) are facilities funded under Title VII of the Rehabilitation Act that are designed to help people with disabilities to live and function more independently and become active members in their communities, including enhanced employability. Services funded under this rehabilitation program include counseling, housing, transportation, job placement, attendant care, physical rehabilitation, prosthetics and other appliances, health maintenance, and recreation.

According to Mathews,[46] ILCs operate on the premise that people with severe disabilities are capable of exercising self-determination and participating in all aspects of society, given appropriate support services, accessible environments, and the necessary skills and information. Furthermore, persons with disabilities are given control over the choice of goals and solutions to problems.

INDEPENDENT LIVING CENTERS AND PEOPLE WITH TRAUMATIC BRAIN INJURY

Despite the usefulness of ILCs in helping persons with disabilities integrate into their communities, most people with TBI are not able to access these services. According to a study by Jones et al.,[47] some ILCs do not serve people with TBI because the staff lack the experience and expertise to work with this population. Fortunately, they also report increased requests for services for people with TBI and increased literature documenting the success rates of persons with TBI in rehabilitation programs designed to improve their independent living skills. For example, Johnston and Lewis[48] evaluated the independent living skills of people with TBI after they participated in a community reentry program. Independent living was based on improvements in the total amount of supervision or help time required. One year after discharge from the program, only 13 clients (16%) required constant supervision compared to 72.8 percent before admission to the program. Only 4 percent of persons with traumatic brain injuries were considered independent and re-

sponsible for their self-care needs upon admission to the rehabilitation program; one year after discharge, however, 46 percent of the participants were rated completely independent and responsible for their own self-care needs. The program was not a VR-funded ILC, but the findings of this study showed that these types of services can contribute to increased independent living skills for this population.

People with TBI are capable of becoming productive members of their communities, provided that they are able to access support services and skills training. The ILC can provide necessary information about the services available in the community, accessible housing, and housing assistance services or create roommate matching services.[46] People with TBI can also participate in independent living skills training, including health care, hygiene, financial management, consumer rights, and self-advocacy. ILCs can also be a great source of information for persons with TBI and their families. An increasing number of ILCs have started brain injury support groups,[46] which can expand the social network of persons with TBI and provide them with peers who can demonstrate the appropriate skills they need to learn.

◻ TRAINING AND EMPLOYMENT ISSUES

Career Planning

Helping individuals with TBI and other severe disabilities identify *what* type of work they wish to do is a critical first step in the vocational rehabilitation process. It has been well established through research and "best practices" that individuals with disabilities who are placed in jobs they do not like will ultimately fail.[21]

One factor that can make job selection and skill instruction challenging is that many people with TBI are unable to consistently express their preferences. Sometimes a client with TBI vacillates from week to week, giving the counselor inconsistent feedback about the type of work she or he would like to perform. This uncertainty should not be surprising because many youth with TBI have never held jobs. In the case of adults with TBI, the type of work performed preinjury is often not feasible postinjury.

It is essential, therefore, that the counselors give people with TBI the opportunity to try out different types of jobs. Furthermore, in any vocational instruction curriculum, teachers must look to the community labor market to see what types of jobs are available. It makes no sense to teach an individual how to repair air conditioners if there are few or no such positions in the community.

In the development of a set of materials in a vocational curriculum, it is always difficult to know which sample jobs to include and which to delete because there are thousands of different types of jobs that people with disabilities can perform well. The categories or types of jobs for the counselor to consider in helping the individual decide his or her preferences include:

1. Cleaning and laundry services
2. Clerical services
3. Grounds and greenhouse work
4. Food service
5. Warehouse, distribution, and factory work
6. Retail work

Of the many categories of possible employment, these are common across most parts of the country. More important are the different components of job identification. For example, every job should have a position title, a job and work site description, a listing of the specific tasks, and the equipment and supplies needed. To teach specific jobs, instruction is best done at a real job site, ideally under some form of fully or partially paid arrangement. However, the next best situation is to approximate as closely as possible the type of work activity that is related to this job. Furthermore, because many individuals with TBI are unsure of the type of job they ultimately want, setting up a series of work trials across four or five jobs during the course of a year can be very beneficial. Tables 20–2 and 20–3 show sample jobs that may be appropriate for individuals with severe TBI or other disabilities.

Assistive Technology

Survivors of TBI can be helped in many ways through assistive technology, such as electrical feeding devices, touch talkers, voice-activated environmental control units, vehicles with adaptive driving controls and lifts, power wheelchairs propelled by slight head movements, and computers for cognitive training.

When accessing assistive technology, individuals may require services as well as devices. An assistive technology service directly assists an individual with a disability in the selection, acquisition, or use of an assistive technology device. A few illustrations of assistive technology services are:

1. Functional assessment of an individual's environments to determine needs
2. Assistance in acquiring assistive technology through purchasing, leasing, or other methods
3. Aid in selection, design, fitting (customizing, adapting, applying), and maintaining (repairing or replacing) of devices

There are many types of assistive technology, products, and services.[49] However, individuals

---

TABLE 20–2. Cleaning and Laundry Services

SCHOOL JANITOR

Job description

The custodian is responsible for cleaning the school interior and maintaining the grounds. The employee begins the shift by vacuuming the hallways before school starts. Next, all restrooms are checked for cleanliness and paper products. The restrooms are wet mopped whenever necessary. The custodian continues by dust mopping each floor on the three-storied building. The cafeteria lobby is also cleaned daily. This involves dust mopping the floor, cleaning all tables, and emptying the trash. Occasionally, the custodian may be asked to assist with maintenance repairs, such as changing light bulbs or repairing school equipment. Throughout the spring and summer months, the employee is responsible for keeping the lawn mowed. This involves cutting the grass with a lawnmower and removing weeds with a weed eater.

Worksite description

The custodian works in a well-lit, temperature-controlled, three-story school building. The type of flooring ranges from tiled to carpeted. Depending on the time of day, background stimuli range from quiet to noisy. Supervision is minimal, and the employee usually works independently. The majority of interactions with coworkers occur during lunch and breaks. Task completion is not dependent upon other workers. There are more female than male employees, and the environment is not diverse, with the majority culture dominant. The custodian wears a uniform. Only the first floor of the building and the grounds is accessible.

TABLE 20–3. Greenhouse Attendant

Job description

The greenhouse attendant is responsible for watering plants, constructing boxes, weeding, and dumping trash and compost. All plants located outside and within the greenhouse are watered daily except for the roses. A hose is connected to the water outlet, and each plant is thoroughly drenched. After all plants are watered, the attendant checks on the box supply and, if needed, constructs boxes. If the supply is adequate, the attendant should perform plant maintenance. This involves weeding, removing dead flower blooms, and straightening the potted plants.

At the end of the shift, the attendant should inspect and clean the parking lot, as well as the surrounding property. This primarily involves trash removal and disposal. Also waste plant material is collected and dumped onto the compost pile. At times, the attendant will be interrupted during a task to assist customers. Customer service entails carrying customer merchandise and loading it in a vehicle.

Worksite description

The greenhouse attendant works outdoors and within a large greenhouse. The attendant is exposed to weather, and the greenhouse temperature is higher than the outdoors. The noise level is generally quiet in the greenhouse, including the sounds of moving and passing vehicles outdoors. Task completion is not dependent upon others. Coworker and customer interactions vary, depending on the time of day, from low to high. Employee contact varies throughout the day. Supervision is minimal. There is approximately an equal number of male and female employees, with the majority culture dominant. Employees may dress casually and wear shorts in the summer. All work areas are accessible.

---

often do not know how to obtain the information necessary to locate, choose, and utilize the appropriate product or service. Basic information such as cost, product names and descriptions, vendors, and consumer satisfaction reports must be gathered. Service information includes type and cost of service, eligibility requirements, and descriptions of available training.

The individual who uses assistive technology should be an active participant and decision maker throughout the process, particularly during selection and evaluation. Users of assistive technology should learn about available devices and try them out at school, work, home, and play before purchasing them. Training and follow-up on a device should be provided; if a particular device is not effective, the search for an appropriate one should be continued. Needs change over time; users should provide input to a vendor on the effectiveness of a device every few years. This feedback is important because vendors continually make improvements based on users' evaluations.

Case 2 ■ William, 30, suffered a traumatic brain injury as a result of a motor vehicle crash. He was in a coma for more than 3 weeks and was described as "beyond medical rehabilitation" because of the severity of his orthopedic and neurological injuries. Following extensive medical rehabilitation, he was transferred to a long-term care facility for convalescence.

William was discharged to his mother's home after several months. He was able to move about with the assistance of a walker and was able to perform basic activities of daily living. His receptive and expressive language skills were intact, and he was able to communicate his needs adequately to his family, although his speech was difficult to understand. However, William showed moderate to severe deficits in immediate and delayed recall of auditory-verbal information.

More recently, William's problems include short-term memory impairment, poor impulse control, disorientation in new surroundings, and decreased motor control because of ataxia. His speech is difficult to understand, particularly over the telephone. He is independent in activities of daily living but unable to manage on his own because of short-term memory problems and impaired decision-making ability. His mother eventually quit her job because she feared for her son's safety when he was left alone.

William is energetic, creative, and fun, and he does well socially despite impulse behavior and difficulty in recalling names. His goals are to work with a local welding firm (prior to his accident, William worked as a welder at a local shipyard) and to live in his own apartment. William's inability to function independently has resulted in social isolation and feelings of hopelessness.

William needs assistance in using the telephone, accessing emergency assistance via telephone, identifying guests before opening the door (he often lets in strangers without regard to safety), and using the stove, microwave, and other appliances safely. He also needs help in managing his finances and personal affairs (paying bills, keeping appointments, taking medications). His overriding goal is increased independence and less dependence on family members and others. William has a variety of needs, many of which were successfully met through the use of "high-tech" and "low-tech" assistive technology products and services (Table 20–4).

A few well-chosen assistive technology devices have enabled William to lead a fuller, more productive life, reduced the stress on his family, and allowed William to stay in the home independently. For William, assistive technology has made the difference between living fully in an environment of his choosing and living in isolation.

Compensatory Strategies

Compensatory strategies have been defined as the deliberate, self-initiated application of sometimes unconventional procedures to achieve desired goals.[50] They are the adjustments an individual makes to solve a problem and therefore succeed at a task. Compensatory strategies and adaptations have been extremely effective in providing success in the workplace for people with TBI. Developed as the individual encounters difficulty with issues or tasks associated with job success, compensatory strategies range from simple to complex and from expensive to free. They can be taught by counselors, family members, or rehabilitation professionals or may develop spontaneously from the individual's experiences. Because of this variability, the person with TBI should ideally be directly involved in developing compensatory strategies to increase her or his acceptance and likelihood of success.

Compensatory strategies include work environment modifications, adaptive equipment, and reorganization of necessary equipment. Self-recording checklists, picture cues, elevated tables, a magnifying glass, and adaptive reachers for high shelves are examples of individualized modifications that may enable an individual to perform a job task. Individualization is the key to effective compensatory strategies; what is effective and comfortable for one person may not be so for the next, even when their problems and the tasks to be performed are similar. Previous learning history both before and after injury provides useful strategies in developing compensatory skills. Additionally, family members or coworkers are excellent sources to provide effective ways of dealing with specific problems.

Learning the Job

The purpose of employment training is to enable the individual with a traumatic brain injury to perform a job independently, which is achieved by one-to-one instruction, development and implementation of compensatory strategies, advocacy, and ongoing case management. This section outlines effective strategies that have been successfully used during this phase of the supported employment model.

Designing a program unique to the individual's special needs is the key to success. Training techniques must be adapted to maximize strengths and preferences. Supported employment program personnel should be flexible in providing job site training assistance.

The employment specialist observes the individual to assist with structuring the work day and in developing and training compensatory strategies to facilitate independence. The specialist also solicits feedback about job performance from the supervisor. Relearning is often rapid if the individual has residual skills or knowledge from past experience.

TABLE 20–4. Assistive Technology for William

Problem	Assistive Technology Solution
Forgets to pay bills	Electronic payment for regular expenditures (e.g., rent, utilities, telephone)
Forgets to take medication	Weekly medication box with electronic timer for doses
Difficulty dialing phone numbers	Programmable phone for frequently called numbers and emergency numbers
Difficult to understand over phone	Personal computer with e-mail and fax capability Speech-synthesizing software
Forgets appointments	Personal electronic appointment calendar and reminder
Forgets to turn off appliances	Appliances with automatic cutoffs and timers
Opens door to strangers	Locate apartment with security features (e.g., video monitor, buzzer access)

If an individual is placed in a new nontechnical position, the specialist provides one-to-one skill training by using systematic instruction, while maintaining the employer's production standards until the individual completes the job independently. The employment specialist will have worked the job at least 1 full day before making the placement to create a foundation for training. In most cases, the specialist has observed the job but had limited time to perform his duties. Sometimes an employer wants a new employee to start work immediately. The specialist should try to renegotiate the start date to develop a comprehensive training schedule to analyze the tasks in the job duties prior to placement.

The major phases of job training are (1) learning a skill, (2) performing the skill, and (3) advocacy for the worker. During the learning phase, the individual studies the job and related skills needed to perform it successfully. Job-related skills include entering and exiting the building, orienting to the break area or rest room, punching in and out on the timeclock, using vending machines, and appropriately greeting coworkers. After the skill has been acquired, the specialist works on increasing the individual's speed and ensures that quality standards continue to be met.

TASK ANALYSIS

During the first days of employment, the specialist determines which tasks the individual can perform independently and which may need assistance. The employment specialist should develop a task analysis (TA) for each job task for which the individual does not possess the necessary skills to perform independently. These are the job tasks in which the specialist provides training. If the individual can perform a task independently, the specialist does not need to develop the comprehensive TA. The specialist can simply check off the task on a sequence of job duties as the individual demonstrates proficiency.

In writing a task analysis, the specialist develops a sequence of job duties. Next, the specialist either performs the tasks or observes coworkers as they perform the tasks to identify the sequential steps for completing each one. The specialist then writes down how to perform the job duties in concrete, observable steps. Once training begins, the specialist should revise the task analysis to reflect the individual's style and preference in performing each job duty.

SYSTEMATIC INSTRUCTION

Systematic instruction is used in job site training to teach job duties and related tasks in a consistent manner. Systematic instruction uses prompts, reinforcements, data collection methods, and general training techniques. Neuropsychological evaluations are reviewed to assure that the individual's cognitive strengths are used in the development of instruction strategies. For example, if deficits exist in auditory recall, the employment specialist should implement visual or tactile learning strategies.

Systematic instruction also provides a method of data collection about the individual's performance level. Using this information to monitor progress during training provides structure and minimizes confusion for both client and specialist.

Performing the Job

Once an individual has learned to perform a specific job duty correctly and independently, the employment specialist must assure that the performance is maintained at employer standards under normal working conditions. The training is based on implementing the following procedures:

1. Review the job site production standards for the job duty based on job analysis.

2. Determine the individual's current production rate.

3. If needed, design and implement a program to increase production to employer standards.

DETERMINING PRODUCTION STANDARDS

The first step in increasing the production rate is to determine the employer standard as a comparison. Ask the supervisor if there is a production standard for each job duty the individual performs. After the employer provides a production rate standard (or if no standard existed), the employment specialist verifies a rate based on the performance of coworkers in the same position by observing them for several days and computing an average of their production rates.

If the production rate is defined by the length of time needed to perform a job duty, the following steps should be completed to verify the company standard:

- Collect information on how long the worker being observed takes to perform the job duty.

- Observe a coworker performing the task.

- Time when the coworker begins the job duty and completes the task.

- Take an average production rate across several days to establish a company standard.

These data may have already been determined during the job analysis preplacement phase. In that case, the employment specialist just verifies previous data.

Determining the Individual's Current Production Rate

The second step determines the consumer's current production rate. If the production standard is defined by the length of time taken to perform the job duty (e.g., 90 minutes to shred wastepaper into a bail), the employment specialist should implement the following procedures:

- Note the time the individual begins the job duty.
- Observe the individual performing the task.
- Note the time the individual completes the task.
- Subtract the beginning time from the ending time to determine how long the individual takes to complete the task.
- Divide the company standard by the time the individual takes to complete the job to get a production rate percentage.
- Record the data.

Job duties that must be complete within a prescribed period of time, such as logging on a computer, restocking a shelf of items, or machine maintenance, may occur only once during the employee's shift. In these cases, the employment specialist records the production data over 3 consecutive days to determine if the employee performs at or near standard rates. In other instances, job duties such as visiting room-bound residents at a nursing home, photocopying printing requests, refilling orders, or pricing items may occur throughout the day. In these situations, the employment specialist records production data 2 or 3 times a day for 2 days.

Finally, if the production standard is determined by counting the number of units completed during a given time period (typing 45 wpm, collecting tolls for x cars per minute, or bagging x garments in 20 min), the employment specialist should implement the following procedures to determine the employee's production rate:

- Identify two short periods to sample and record production rate.
- Count and record the number of units completed (e.g., number of cupcakes to be iced) during the identified sample period (e.g., 10 min).

- Divide the number of units the individual completes by the company standard to determine production rate (percentage of standard).
- Record the rate on the data sheet.
- Collect and record the production rate at least twice during the day for 2 consecutive days.

If the production standard is determined by counting the number of units completed during a given period, complete the following steps to verify a company standard:

- Collect information on how long the worker being observed has worked.
- Identify two short periods during the day to observe a coworker performing the job duty.
- Count and record the number of units completed (e.g., number of keystrokes entered into computer) during the identified sample time period (e.g., per minute)
- Take an average of a coworker's production rate to verify a company standard.

Table 20–5 describes how work production can be increased for a young person with TBI.

Keeping the Job

Many individuals with severe TBI have problems with job retention. Professionals, consumers, and families have learned that having a staff person provide follow-along at the job is helpful. *Follow-along* may be defined as an ongoing assessment and monitoring of the individual's work performance. During this time, the employment specialist collects data, makes observations, and provides advocacy as needed. Additional intervention and support services are available for the duration of the individual's employment. During this phase, the employment specialist is no longer at the work site on a daily basis but continues to have contact with the individual and employer.

Formal and informal methods can be used to provide follow-along services. Informal methods include conversations with the consumer, supervisors, coworkers, and family members and unobtrusive observations on the job site. Formal methods include collection of data to assess the consumer's current work performance in areas such as task performance, production, and quality. To ensure that employment continues during follow-along, the specialist gathers data to provide ongoing assessment in the following areas:

- Dependability
- Current job performance

TABLE 20–5. Case Study: Increasing Production Rate

MA is employed as a microfilm processor for a national electronics retail company. His job duties are processing expense and merchandise checks and microfilming documents. Problems encountered and adaptations that alleviate the problems are:

- **Forgetting to reset the date stamp machine (short-term memory problems).**
  Possible solution:
  ▫ Visual cue, such as written note or checklist
- **Difficulty picking up paper clips from table tops (poor fine motor ability, right hand ataxia).**
  Possible solutions:
  ▫ Substitute large paper clips for small ones
  ▫ Put clips in a bowl
  ▫ Use a magnetized paper clip holder
- **Difficulty distinguishing work already finished from work to be done (problems with discrimination; finished work and unfinished work look similar).**
  Possible solutions:
  ▫ Plexiglas divider
  ▫ Use a yellow self-stick note on finished work
  ▫ Use a file box for work that is finished
- **Slow rate restapling work after microfilming (right hand ataxia: cannot use both hands simultaneously).**
  Possible solution:
  ▫ Electric stapler
- **Forgetting sequence of job duties throughout the day (problems with learning, short-term memory, and disorganized thinking).**
  Possible solution:
  ▫ Written checklist posted above desk

- Adherence to company policies
- Employer's perceptions of performance
- Appropriateness of compensatory strategies
- Dynamics of interpersonal job site relations
- Relations with job site personnel
- Changes in work routine or work environment
- Job satisfaction
- Factors outside work that affect job performance

During the first month of follow-along (after the employment specialist has faded from the job site), staff continues to schedule at least two visits each week. Based on the outcome of these job site visits, the specialist and program manager establish the level of follow-along to provide. The number of scheduled contacts most likely will not remain constant but will fluctuate over time, based upon job performance.

An analysis of the following information can assist in determining the appropriate level of follow-along for the individual:

- Attendance and punctuality during job site training
- Consistency of job performance and use of compensatory strategies
- Number and type of incidents that occurred during training

- Current case management needs (stability of living situation, relationships outside work, ability to monitor medication)
- Emotional stability of client, particularly if the individual is at risk for depression, anxiety attacks, or substance abuse
- Support system available in the work or home environment
- Need for contact as identified by the individual, employer, or data

Employment specialists provide intervention, either on or off the site during the follow-along phase. Areas requiring intervention become apparent during follow-along visits or through ongoing communication with the family, employer, or coworkers.

Advocacy for the Worker

Advocacy is the most important tool the employment specialist uses during job training. Advocacy facilitates rapport among coworkers, employers, parents, case managers, and the general population. It is important to be proactive as an advocate by preplanning likely scenarios and identifying concerns before they become major issues. This practice allows the employment specialist to discuss issues with the employer that may arise during job site training and follow-along. Discussions concern appropriate responses to different situations and empower the employer to make informed decisions when and if these issues arise.

Advocacy encompasses delicate issues for the individual, such as revealing the nature of the injury and her or his emotional and cognitive deficits. The employment specialist and the consumer must discuss beforehand what information is relevant and can be shared with potential or current employers. Another sensitive issue is that of employee rights. Under the Americans with Disabilities Act (PL 101-336 ADA), qualified individuals with disabilities are protected from discrimination in hiring and promotion, and employers are required to provide reasonable accommodations for handicapping conditions. VR consumers with TBI need to be informed of those rights by the employment specialist and assisted in the prescribed avenues for seeking remedy. However, when problems occur, some may choose not press the issue if it means making waves within the organization or if the individual does not consider it worthwhile to proceed. The extent to which ADA noncompliance cases are pursued should be at the discretion of the individual with the disability.

The employment specialist is often placed in the difficult situation of trying to meet the needs of both parties. The most important underlying theme during job site training is to be honest while maintaining confidentiality. Honesty with the individual and employer enhances and facilitates communication. Actively involving all parties during job site training increases the chances of a successful placement—the ultimate goal of advocacy during job site training.

□ CONCLUSION

This chapter has discussed the importance and role of vocational rehabilitation in the return to work activities by people with TBI. Choice and consumer preference are viewed as a critical cornerstone for all vocational services that are provided to people with TBI and other disabilities. Those who facilitate return to work for members of this population must attend to this philosophy and dimension of service delivery.

The models or approaches to vocational rehabilitation discussed range from the more traditional rehabilitation counselor model to consumer-oriented approaches such as supported employment and job clubs. Centers for independent living can provide complementary services for enhancing greater community independence and mobility. Key training and employment issues discussed in the chapter include career de-

velopment, behavior training, production training, and self-advocacy.

There are many challenges in the vocational rehabilitation of people with TBI. This chapter has presented some contemporary ways of managing these challenges and helping these individuals be successful. Although people with severe TBI have traditionally experienced limited access to VR services and normal workplaces, new service technologies such as supported employment and assistive technology, along with protections and mandates under the ADA, show promise for reversing these trends. The keys to successful employment for members of this population are (1) individualized services and supports that focus on the career goals and preferences of the consumer and (2) knowledge of legally mandated rights and the means for exercising them.

REFERENCES

1. Sosin, DM, Sniezek, JE, and Waxweiler, RJ: Trends in death associated with traumatic brain injury, 1979 through 1992. Success and failure. JAMA 273:1778, 1995.
2. National Head Injury Foundation: Trauma: The Silent Epidemic. National Head Injury Foundation, Framingham, Mass, 1986.
3. Webb, CR, et al: Explaining quality of life for persons with traumatic brain injuries 2 years after injury. Arch Phys Med Rehabil 76:1113, 1995.
4. Max, W, MacKenzie, EJ, and Rice, DP: Head injuries: Costs and consequences. J Head Trauma Rehabil 6:2, 1976.
5. Tennant, A, Macdermott, N, and Neary, D: The long-term outcome of head injury: Implications for service planning. Brain Inj 9:595, 1995.
6. Dawson, DR, and Chipman, M: The disablement experienced by traumatically brain-injured adults living in the community. Brain Inj 9:339, 1995.
7. Dikmen, SS, et al: Employment following traumatic head injuries. Arch Neurol 51:177, 1994.
8. McMordie, WR, Barker, SL, and Paolo, TM: Return to work (RTW) after head injury. Brain Inj 4:57, 1990.
9. Jacobs, HE: The Los Angeles Head Injury Survey: Procedures and initial findings. Arch Phys Med Rehabil 69:425, 1987.
10. Wehman, P: Competitive Employment: New Horizons for Severely Disabled Persons. Brookes, Baltimore, 1981.
11. Federal Register 52(157):30546, 1987.
12. Coker, CC, Osgood, K, and Clouse, KR: A Comparison of Job Satisfaction and Economic Benefits of Four Different Employment Models for Persons with Disabilities. University of Wisconsin–Stout, Rehabilitation Research and Training Center on Improving Community-Based Rehabilitation Programs, Menomonie, Wisc, 1995.
13. West, M: Supported employment. In Del Orto, AE, and Marinelli, RP (eds): Encyclopedia of Disability and Rehabilitation. Macmillan, New York, 1995, p 708.
14. Wehman, P, Revell, WG, and Kregel, J: Unpublished material, 1995.
15. West, M: Choice, self-determination, and VR services: Systemic barriers for consumers with severe disabilities. Journal of Vocational Rehabilitation 5:281, 1995.
16. Baer, R, et al: A study of the costs and benefits of supported employment for persons with severe physical and multiple disabilities. Journal of Rehabilitation Administration 18:46, 1995.
17. Lewis, DR, et al: Is supported employment cost-effective in Minnesota? Journal of Disability Policy Studies 3:67, 1992.

18. Vogenthaler, DR: An overview of head injury: Its consequences and rehabilitation. Brain Inj 1:113, 1987.
19. Horn, LJ, and Zasler, ND (eds): Medical Rehabilitation of Traumatic Brain Injury. Hanley & Belfus, Philadelphia, 1996.
20. Fann, JR, et al: Psychiatric disorders and functional disability in outpatients with traumatic brain injuries. Am J Psychiatry 152:1493, 1995.
21. Wehman, PH, et al: Return to work for persons with severe traumatic brain injury: A data-based approach to program development. J Head Trauma Rehabil 10:27, 1995.
22. Wehman, P, et al: Employment outcomes of persons following traumatic brain injury: Pre-injury, post-injury, and supported employment. Brain Inj 3:397, 1989.
23. Wehman, P, et al: Return to work for persons following severe traumatic brain injury: Supported employment outcomes after five years. Am J Phys Med Rehabil 72:355, 1993.
24. Wehman, P, et al: Return to work for patients with traumatic brain injury: Analysis of costs. Am J Phys Med Rehabil 73:280, 1994.
25. Albin, J, and Slovic, R: Resources for Long-Term Support in Supported Employment. University of Oregon, The Employment Network, Eugene, 1992.
26. West, MD, and Parent, WS: Community and workplace supports for individuals with severe mental illness in supported employment. Psychosocial Rehabilitation Journal 18:13, 1995.
27. Nisbet, J (ed): Natural Supports in School, at Work, and in the Community for People with Severe Disabilities. Brookes, Baltimore, 1992.
28. Racino, J, and Williams, JM: Living in the community: An examination of the philosophical and practical aspects. J Head Trauma Rehabil 9(2):35, 1994.
29. West, MD, Gibson, K, and Unger, D: Unpublished material, 1996.
30. Curl, RM, et al: Traumatic brain injury vocational rehabilitation: Preliminary findings for the coworker as trainer project. J Head Trauma Rehabil 11(1):75, 1996.
31. West, M: Aspects of the workplace and return to work for persons with brain injury in supported employment. Brain Inj 9:301, 1995.
32. Azrin, NH, and Besalel, VA: Job Club Counselor's Manual. University Park Press, Boston, 1980.
33. Ford, LH: Providing Employment Support for People with Long-Term Mental Illness. Paul H Brookes, Baltimore, 1995.
34. Stidham, HH, and Remley, TP: Job club methodology applied in a workfare setting. Journal of Employment Counseling 29:69, 1992.
35. Braddy, BA, and Gray, DO: Employment services for older job seekers: A comparison of two client-centered approaches. Gerontologist 27:565, 1987.
36. Rife, JC, and Belcher, JR: Assisting unemployed older workers to become reemployed: An experimental evaluation. Research on Social Work Practice 4:3, 1994.
37. Cellini, HR, and Lorenz, JR: Job club group training with unemployed offenders. Federal Probation 46:46, 1983.
38. Elksnin, LK, and Elksnin, N: The school counselor as job search facilitator: Increasing employment of handicapped students through job clubs. School Counselor 38:215, 1991.
39. Murphy, GC, and Athanasou, JA: School to work transition: Behavioural counseling approaches to the problem of finding jobs for unemployed adolescents. Behaviour Change 4:41, 1987.
40. Mann, WC, and Svorai, SB: A model for vocational evaluation, training, employment, and community integration for persons with cognitive impairments. Am J Occup Ther 48:446, 1994.
41. Marme, M, and Skord, K: Counseling strategies to enhance the vocational rehabilitation of persons with traumatic brain injury. Journal of Applied Rehabilitation Counseling 24:19, 1993.
42. Moore, R, and Bartlow, C: Vocational limitations and assessments of the client who is traumatically brain injured. Journal of Applied Rehabilitation Counseling 21:3, 1990.
43. Fraser, R, and Baarslag-Benson, R: Cross-disciplinary collaboration in the removal of work barriers after traumatic brain injury. Topics in Language Disorders 15:55, 1994.
44. Fraser, R, et al: Employability of head injury survivors: First year post-injury. Rehabilitation Counseling Bulletin 31:276, 1988.
45. Ellerd, D, and Moore, S: Follow-up at twelve and thirty months of persons with traumatic brain injury engaged in supported employment placements. Journal of Applied Rehabilitation Counseling 23:48, 1992.
46. Matthews, R: Independent living as a lifelong community service. J Head Trauma Rehabil 5(1):23, 1990.
47. Jones, M, et al: A survey of service by independent living centers to people with cognitive disabilities. Rehabilitation Counseling Bulletin 31:244, 1988.
48. Johnston, M, and Lewis, F: Outcomes of community reentry programmes for brain injury survivors. Part 1: Independent living and productive activities. Brain Inj 5:141, 1991.
49. Inge, K, Flippo, K, and Barcus, M: Assistive Technology. Paul Brookes, Baltimore, 1995.
50. Wehman, P, et al: Cognitive impairment and remediation: Implications for employment following traumatic brain injury J Head Trauma Rehabil 4(3):66, 1989.

Rehabilitation of the Child with Traumatic Brain Injury

ERNEST R. GRIFFITH, MD

CHAPTER 21

Specific Problems Associated with Pediatric Brain Injury

LINDA J. MICHAUD, MD,
ANN-CHRISTINE DUHAIME, MD,
and KENNETH M. JAFFE, MD

Each year approximately 200 of every 100,000 children in the United States sustain traumatic brain injury (TBI).[1] Although most (82%) of these injuries are mild, many are moderate to severe (14%) or fatal (5%); incidence of significant disability is approximately 20 percent among survivors.[2] Traumatic brain injury is the most common cause of acquired disability in pediatrics.

The majority of children with severe brain injuries also have additional injuries to other body systems, some of which independently have an impact on outcome.[3] Injuries to other body systems may result in increased disability by contributing to secondary brain injury associated with hypoxia and hypotension[4,5] or may directly increase disability independent of problems caused by the brain injury—for example, fractures. These additional injuries and their management may delay and lengthen the duration of the rehabilitation process for children and adolescents with brain injuries.

Traumatic brain injury in children is associated with both medical and surgical complications involving the nervous system and other body systems. Although some complications present during the early days following injury, others do not become evident for months. Any organ system can be affected, depending on the severity and mechanism of the injury to the brain, the nature and severity of additional in-

juries to other body systems sustained at the time of the brain injury, subsequent treatment, and complications of the injuries to the brain or other systems or of their treatment. Familiarity with the constellation of problems that can potentially complicate recovery leads to early recognition, prompt treatment, and reduced morbidity.

☐ FUNCTIONAL CONSEQUENCES OF SPECIFIC BRAIN INJURY CATEGORIES

In approaching a child who has suffered a brain injury, it is helpful to understand the anatomic structures involved, the function of those structures, and the typical course of recovery from that particular injury category. The following categories are not mutually exclusive, and a given patient may sustain more than one injury type.

Diffuse Axonal Injury

In the pediatric age group, diffuse axonal injury occurs almost exclusively as a consequence of motor vehicle trauma. Children are pedestrians or bicycle riders struck by vehicles or passengers in vehicle crashes. The terminology *diffuse axonal injury* has been used to describe different but related phenomena. It was first used to describe the pathological findings on autopsy of certain patients who had died from severe non-missile head injury and whose brains showed widespread microscopically visible tears in the nerve fibers (axons) of the brain.[6] Biomechanical analysis of the forces required to cause this injury showed that large, angular deceleration forces, such as those generated by motor vehicle injuries, were responsible.[7] Clinically, such patients were comatose immediately after the injury and remained unconscious for at least 6 hours. This type of injury was discovered to be most often responsible for prolonged or persistent coma after brain trauma.[8] Later, the radiological findings of diffuse axonal injury came to be recognized, both on computed tomography (CT) and magnetic resonance imaging (MRI), in which scattered areas of tissue tears and tiny hemorrhages could be seen. Milder forms of similar pathological changes were discovered in humans and animals whose symptoms spanned a spectrum of severities from concussion through unconsciousness lasting less than 6 hours. For this reason, the term *diffuse axonal injury* is sometimes also applied to patients in whom the typical radiological features are demonstrated but who have durations of unconsciousness less than 6 hours. However, in its most common usage, the term implies a more severe injury with particular clinical features including prolonged unconsciousness, abnormal motor signs such as extensor or flexor posturing, and autonomic dysfunction.

Children with diffuse axonal injury (DAI) recover from their injuries in a fairly stereotyped manner. Initial deep coma with posturing, sweating, intermittent hypertension, and central fever is often seen. Bruxism (tooth grinding) is common. The eyes may open, but there is no visual responsiveness. As recovery continues, posturing may be replaced gradually by purposeless flailing of the extremities, hyperventilation, and agitation. Eye opening becomes more frequent. Responsiveness to touch or voice may begin to become apparent. Finally, the ability to follow some simple commands develops; it is usually intermittent at first and then gradually becomes more consistent. Expressive speech lags behind receptive abilities in most children. Marked difficulties with attention and behavior appear as abilities return, and the child is unable to remember new information. Gradual improvement leads to the end of post-traumatic amnesia and the resumption of the ability to participate actively in rehabilitation.[9] Motor and cognitive difficulties, especially with memory, attention, and executive functions, usually persist to some degree in children with severe injuries.[10] Follow-up imaging most often shows a degree of diffuse atrophy of the brain.

Focal Parenchymal Injuries

Focal parenchymal injuries include contusions (bruising) and lacerations (tearing) of the brain. Such injuries result from impact injuries to the head (usually from falls), depressed skull fractures, and localized penetrating injuries.

Children who sustain this sort of injury without a concomitant diffuse injury often have minimal or no loss of consciousness. Surgery may be needed to repair the skull or dura and decrease the risk of infection. The consequences of the injury depend on the specific area of the brain involved. For example, children with contusions of the dominant (usually left) temporal region may show language difficulties; damage to the posterior frontal region may affect the motor cortex and result in weakness of the opposite extremities. Injury to the anterior frontal region may be associated with changes in behavior, especially if the injury affects both sides.

Children with focal deficits may recover significantly and show gratifying improvement in the months after injury. One exception may be infants, in whom focal weakness of the extremities may be less apparent early in life but may become more obvious with maturation as spasticity and differential growth occur. It is useful to anticipate these developmental changes in counseling the family to alleviate concerns of an active, progressive problem.

Epidural Hematoma

Blood clots in the epidural space occur as a result of focal impact forces and, like surface contusions and lacerations, are not associated with major diffuse brain injury. Arterial epidural hematomas result from a tear through a dural artery and usually are associated with skull fracture. In young children, whose skulls are thin, this can occur after relatively minor trauma; in older children, somewhat higher forces are involved. At the time of impact, the child may suffer a brief concussion or have no loss of consciousness, but the clinical hallmark of arterial epidural hematoma is a progressive deterioration in neurological status over minutes to hours as the clot enlarges and compresses the underlying brain. Prompt surgical evacuation leads to a good to excellent outcome.[11] Delay in clot removal can result in dangerous or fatal increases in intracranial pressure, with herniation, cerebral infarction, and significant neurological morbidity. Specific deficits in this situation may include prolonged coma, visual loss, weakness especially on the side opposite the clot, and cognitive impairment. Eventual outcome depends largely on the amount and distribution of irrecoverably injured tissue.

Epidural hematomas can also occur from tears in the dural venous sinuses. Because venous pressure is lower than that in the arteries, these clots tend to enlarge more gradually, and symptoms may be delayed in onset. Hematomas in the posterior fossa may lead to obstructive hydrocephalus. Surgical evacuation is needed if the clot enlarges or if the child is symptomatic.

Small epidural hemorrhages often accumulate under fracture sites as a result of bleeding from the fractured bone itself. The majority of these clots remain small and do not require surgical drainage. Close clinical follow-up is important, however, for occasionally these collections are associated with persistent or progressive symptoms (usually headache and vomiting) that are amenable to surgical evacuation.

Subdural Hematoma

Like diffuse axonal injury, the majority of subdural hematomas result from large, angular acceleration-deceleration forces in which the head stops but the brain continues to rotate within the skull.[12] Under these circumstances, the bridging veins, which course from the brain surface to the dural venous sinuses, are torn as they are stretched between the moving brain and the stationary dura.

Brain injury in subdural hematoma occurs for two reasons. First, the clot itself produces mass effect, compresses the brain, and causes increased intracranial pressure. Emergent surgical evacuation can reduce the contribution of the clot itself to the damage.[13] However, unlike the situation with epidural hematoma, in which the primary injury to the brain is minimal, the forces required to cause rupture of the bridging veins are significant, and therefore the associated injury to the brain itself is considerable. Therefore, patients with subdural hematomas generally have much worse outcomes than those with epidural hematomas, in spite of prompt surgical treatment of both types of clots.

Typically, patients demonstrate deficits related to increased intracranial pressure and angular deceleration, which affect the brain diffusely, as well as specific focal deficits related to damage on the side of the clot. Infants are particularly susceptible to damage from subdural hematoma and may show massive loss of brain tissue, which is associated with severe disability.[14] This happens most often in the setting of inflicted injury; infants with the shaking-impact syndrome may have deficits ranging from mild to severe. Outcome in this setting can be predicted by the level of consciousness at presentation and by the finding of diffuse hemispheric hypodensity on CT scan. Infants with bilateral diffuse hypodensity appear to have a uniformly poor outcome, and remain blind, nonverbal, and nonambulatory, even many years after injury.[15]

Gunshot Wounds

Both focal and generalized deficits result from gunshot wounds to the head. The specific focal deficits encountered depend on the particular trajectory of the missile and the resultant anatomic damage to eloquent areas of the brain. In addition, unlike low-velocity penetrating injuries in which damage is confined to the site of cerebral laceration, gunshot wounds are also associated with shock waves and widespread transmission of energy that cause damage beyond the actual bullet path. Intracranial pressure may be extremely elevated after gunshot wounds, and this, too, adds to the damage. Nonetheless, gradual recovery from initially severe injuries can occur, and the eventual outcome in children may be better than initially predicted in selected cases.[16]

◻ NEUROLOGICAL AND NEUROSURGICAL COMPLICATIONS

Infections

Late infections after civilian head trauma are uncommon. In children, meningitis caused by occult cerebrospinal fluid (CSF) leak occasionally occurs after basilar skull fracture. If meningitis occurs more than a few weeks after the acute injury, a metrizamide CT scan or radionuclide study may be necessary to identify and localize a persistent leak. Lumbar drainage is usually the initial treatment for CSF otorrhea or rhinorrhea lasting more than a few days. Refractory leaks may require direct or endoscopic surgical repair.

Another source of delayed infection is a fracture through the posterior wall of the frontal sinus, which can result in an intracranial abscess from contamination through the torn sinus mucosa. This problem presents with headache, fever, or seizures; CT scan or MRI with and without contrast helps to differentiate a resolving contusion from cerebritis or abscess formation.

Penetrating injuries can also lead to late infection. Foreign bodies such as sticks or pencils, which commonly enter the brain through the thin orbital roof in children, may be radiolucent, and small bits of contaminated material may be left behind when the object is removed. Close follow-up with serial scans is needed to check for the development of an abscess in this situation, particularly once antibiotic coverage is discontinued.

In some situations, parenchymal penetrating injuries are not recognized acutely. For example, animal bites may leave only small lacerations in the skin, and objects such as hair ornaments, sharp toys, or household items may enter the brain through the thin calvarium or skull base. In the latter situation, intermittent CSF leakage may persist if a fistula forms between the nasopharynx or sinuses and the brain. The fistula may not be clinically apparent because drainage may be intermittent and scant, and the leak often empties into the nasopharynx, where it is not noticed. Such fistulas may be a cause for recurrent meningitis years after what originally might have seemed a superficial injury. Therefore, any injury in which penetration of a sharp object to the eye, face, or mouth might include a trajectory through the skull should be investigated carefully with appropriate radiological studies to anticipate and prevent later complications.

Growing Fractures

The unusual phenomenon of growing fractures occurs when a linear skull fracture in an infant gradually enlarges rather than healing over time. Such fractures are accompanied by a tear of the dura under the fracture line and present as a pulsatile swelling at the site. Fractures that go on to enlarge occur most often from falls from more than a few feet in height or from other mechanisms such as motor vehicle collisions because these forces result in a fracture that usually appears rather widely separated acutely, often associated with an underlying contusion. The diagnosis can be made by skull radiographs. Treatment is surgical and consists of dural repair and split-thickness cranioplasty.[17]

Hydrocephalus and Extra-Axial Collections

Ventricular enlargement after diffuse brain injury is common and in most cases related primarily to atrophy. It is usually mild to moderate after diffuse axonal injury but may be marked after subdural hematoma (especially in infants) or after diffuse hypoxia or ischemia, such as after cardiac or respiratory arrest. In addition, some degree of impairment of CSF absorption may occur as a consequence of subarachnoid hemorrhage or inflammation, leading to enlargement of the CSF spaces. On CT scan or MRI, the ventricles, convexity subarachnoid spaces, or both may appear enlarged, compared with the acute studies. In most cases, this process is self-limited and stabilizes or resolves with time.

Although increases in intracranial CSF volume that are mild and asymptomatic are common after severe brain injury, occasionally the question of symptomatic ventricular hydrocephalus or extra-axial loculated CSF collections (hygromas) arises. The diagnosis may be difficult to establish on clinical grounds, because the primary injury itself often accounts for the majority of symptoms; ideally, the clinician should document a decrement in abilities that corresponds temporally to the enlargement of the ventricles or CSF space. Occasionally, an ophthalmologic exam is useful, although the absence of papilledema does not completely rule out increased pressure. Neuroimaging may not distinguish atrophy or benign ventricular enlargement from that associated with increased intracranial pressure. When the process appears to be communicating hydrocephalus (i.e., the ventricles communicate with the subarachnoid space), lumbar puncture with careful pressure measurement may be of use. A therapeutic trial of acetazolamide also may be helpful. Finally, if suspicion is reasonably high for true symptomatic hydrocephalus or hygroma, a therapeutic trial of shunting or drainage may be justified. It is important to avoid unrealistic expectations of these procedures in the setting of major brain injury.

Proteinaceous subdural fluid collections often occur after subdural hemorrhage in infants. Like CSF collections, they usually resolve with time. Occasionally, children demonstrate an enlarging head circumference, bulging fontanelle, vomiting, and other signs of increased pressure; draining or shunting the collections may result in clinical improvement. In infants with severe brain injury, large subdural collections related primarily to underlying brain atrophy may be present; surgery in this setting is unlikely to improve the long-term outcome and is usually not necessary.

Post-Traumatic Seizures

Seizures within the first hours after head injury are probably more common in children than in adults; they do not have predictive value with respect to eventual development of epilepsy.[18] The decision to treat with anticonvulsants is made on an individual basis; early treatment has been shown to decrease the risk of seizures in the first week after injury but does not decrease the risk of later development of epilepsy.[19] In general, children at high risk for recurrent seizures (those with cortical contusions or lacerations) or those in whom recurrent seizures would complicate acute management are treated with early institution of anticonvulsants. Children with low-risk injuries and stable neurological exams who have an early seizure may be managed without medication unless seizures recur. In most children with TBI with a single early seizure, anticonvulsants are discontinued after 1 week of treatment if no further seizures have occurred.

Seizures that begin later after injury usually warrant anticonvulsant therapy. Optimal duration of treatment is unknown, but in most instances anticonvulsants are administered for 3 to 6 months, then tapered, and discontinued if the child remains seizure-free. The overall risk of the development of post-traumatic epilepsy in children is less than 5 percent; as in adults, direct injury to the cortex is a relative risk factor.[18]

Auditory and Vestibular Disorders

There is a significant incidence of hearing loss following TBI in children. Zimmerman et al.[20] observed hearing losses in 48 percent of a series of 50 children with TBI. Post-traumatic hearing loss is most commonly the result of a fracture of the temporal bone and is usually unilateral. Both longitudinal and transverse fractures can result in sensorineural and conductive hearing loss, vertigo, facial paralysis, CSF leak, and meningitis.[21] The more common longitudinal fractures are more likely to result in a mild to moderate hearing loss and normal facial nerve function, whereas 50 percent of transverse fractures result in both profound hearing loss and facial nerve injury.[21] Longitudinal fractures tend to involve middle ear structures and result in conductive hearing loss; transverse fractures often affect the cochlea and cause a sensorineural deficit.[22] Prognosis for recovery is better for conductive than for sensorineural hearing impairment. Audiologic referral is indicated for children with TBI,[20] with complete otolaryngologic evaluation for those with known or suspected problems. Depending on the type and severity of hearing loss, amplification may be indicated.

Although objective vestibular disturbances occur with similar frequency in children and adults, subjective symptoms are less common in children.[23] Vartiainen et al.[23] examined 199 children with blunt head trauma and found 46 percent with spontaneous and/or positional nystagmus and 43 percent with central disturbances on electronystagmography immediately after trauma but observed only 1.5 percent with complaints of vertigo more than 6 months after injury.[23]

Visual Impairment

Visual deficits after pediatric TBI can result from crush injuries to the globe, cranial nerve (CN) involvement (II–VII), cerebellar injury, or lesions affecting the visual pathway or cortex. Orbital fractures may result in extraocular muscle entrapment.

Optic nerve injuries can be associated with TBI and include laceration or avulsion, usually from a direct penetrating orbital injury and occasionally from fracture fragments associated with blunt orbital trauma; blunt trauma can thrombose, compress, or tear the vascular supply to the optic nerve.[24] Traumatic optic neuropathy, usually characterized by swelling of the optic disk and central retinal vein occlusion, may result in permanent visual loss unless the optic nerve sheath is decompressed or high-dose steroids given.[24]

Diplopia resulting from CN involvement (III, IV, VI) after TBI in children frequently resolves without surgical intervention. Functional improvement usually results from alternate eye patching under the guidance of an ophthalmologist. Preschoolers are at risk for permanent suppression of vision in the weaker eye when ophthalmoplegia occurs; it is potentially preventable by appropriate early patching.[25]

Loss of either the afferent or efferent limb of the corneal reflex arc (CN V or VII) or incomplete eye closure caused by facial nerve (CN VII) palsy can be associated with corneal abrasions. Appropriate lubrication must be provided for prevention.

Visual field defects may occur, the nature of which are determined by the site of damage along the optic pathway. Optic nerve damage may cause visual impairment of the affected eye. Chiasmatic lesions usually affect vision bilaterally. Involvement of the optic tract, radiations, or cerebral cortex may produce cuts in visual fields opposite the side affected. Damage to visual association areas may lead to visual perceptual deficits. Cortical visual impairment (CVI) in children may differ in prognosis from cortical blindness in adults, and clinicians should maintain optimism about the potential for some recovery of vision.[26] Visual evoked potentials are not usually helpful in predicting outcome.[26]

Ophthalmologic findings may be strongly associated with specific mechanisms of TBI. Although retinal hemorrhages can occur under a variety of circumstances, they are highly associated with inflicted injuries in very young children.[27]

In view of the high frequency of visual impairment after pediatric TBI, a high index of suspicion should be maintained and ophthalmologic assessment obtained when problems are suspected. Evaluation of visual function may require the participation of a multidisciplinary team and special testing techniques.[26]

Spinal Cord Injury

Acute mechanical high-force events may result in spinal cord injury (SCI) with TBI. The early diagnosis of SCI in a comatose child can be easily missed, and radiological evaluation of the cervical spine should be routine when indicated by the mechanism of injury. The diagnosis should be suspected if there is flaccid paraparesis or paraplegia, a differential response to pain in the upper versus the lower extremities, or abnormal anal sphincter tone.

Cervical spine injuries in children more commonly affect the soft tissues than the vertebrae. For this reason, they may remain undetected in children with normal plain spinal x-rays who have a decreased level of consciousness or other conditions precluding a full physical examination. This situation is known as SCIWORA, or spinal cord injury without radiographic abnormality.[28] Children with ligamentous injuries may have spinal instability, predisposing them to increased injury on movement. Therefore, plain films alone are insufficient in children for "clearing" the spine. Injury must be ruled out by clinical examination (absence of pain on full active or passive range of motion of the neck, absence of neurological signs or symptoms referable to possible neck injury) or by a normal MRI scan done with particular attention to possible ligamentous injuries.[29,30]

Peripheral Nerve Injury

Peripheral nerve injury must be considered when flaccid paralysis or weakness or a differential response to pain is observed in the distribution of the brachial or lumbosacral plexus or other peripheral nerves. Fractures of the clavicle and pelvis should increase suspicion of brachial and lumbosacral plexus injuries, respectively. Fractures of long bones may be associated with direct injury to other peripheral nerves, in particular, the peroneal and radial

nerves. Peripheral nerve injuries may also be caused by compartment syndromes. The diagnosis of peripheral nerve injury can be confirmed by electromyography and nerve conduction studies.

☐ MEDICAL AND SURGICAL PROBLEMS

Traumatic brain injury in children is associated with both medical and surgical complications and with concurrent injuries to other body systems. Many of them present at or near the time of injury, whereas others do not become evident until later. Delayed diagnosis of additional injury in multiple trauma is especially likely with greater severity of TBI, and ongoing evaluation is indicated to identify and manage initially unrecognized injuries.[31] Early detection and management of the complications of TBI and associated injuries are essential skills in pediatric rehabilitation.

Nutrition and Feeding Problems

Nutritional management is an essential and challenging aspect of the care of children with TBI. The nutritional needs of injured children have not been well studied, and provision of nutritional support is generally based on studies of animals and adult trauma patients.[32] Children have higher metabolic rates, smaller nutrient stores, and greater nutrient requirements per kilogram than adults.[32] Phillips et al.[33] have demonstrated increased mean measured energy expenditures (to 130%) over Harris-Benedict predicted values in children and adolescents with severe TBI during the first 2 weeks after injury. Mean nitrogen excretion values in that study were observed to be less than those in adults with severe TBI. The frequently elevated core temperature in children with severe TBI is also associated with an increase in whole body energy expenditure, with expenditure increasing by a mean of 7.4 percent per degree centigrade in a study by Matthews et al.[34] This high rate of energy expenditure contributes to the increase in nutritional demands in the child with TBI.[34] Accurate estimation of the caloric needs of the child with TBI is essential to avoid both inadequate and excessive intake. Underestimation has adverse effects on wound healing, immunocompetence, and organ functions, and overestimation can cause complications of hyperglycemia, liver abnormalities, and respiratory distress.[32]

Children in coma after severe TBI require administration of nutrients via the enteral or parenteral routes.[32] When possible, enteral feeding is preferable because of greater metabolic efficiency, lower cost, and greater safety.[35] Even in the absence of gastrointestinal tract injury, gastric ileus may occur in children with trauma; because the small bowel usually maintains normal motility and absorption, it may be preferable to feed into the small bowel.[32] Oral motor impairment and/or dysphagia may persist in children recovering from TBI, and prolonged enteral feeding may be indicated. Feeding through nasogastric tubes may contribute to patient discomfort and disrupt function of the lower esophageal sphincter, promoting gastroesophageal reflux; prolonged use may lead to erosion of the nares.[35] For those children requiring prolonged enteral feeding, gastrostomy or gastrojejunostomy tube placement may be indicated. Percutaneous placement of these tubes has been demonstrated to be safe and applicable to children of all ages.[36,37] Enteral feedings are usually initially administered by continuous infusion.[35] Continuous tube feedings can generally be advanced to bolus feedings, which allow greater approximation to normal physiological function, longer periods of time during which the child can participate in therapies without the additional encumbrance of the feeding tube, and increased ease for caregivers.

Children with severe TBI and prolonged acute hospital courses may have significant weight loss and be at risk for refeeding syndrome during rehabilitation. *Refeeding syndrome* may be defined as "the occurrence of severe fluid and electrolyte shifts (especially, but not exclusively, phosphorus) and their associated complications in malnourished patients undergoing refeeding either orally, enterally, or parenterally."[38] In addition to hypophosphatemia, additional metabolic complications with refeeding syndrome may include hypokalemia, hypomagnesemia, glucose and fluid intolerance, and thiamine deficiency.[38] Recommendations for anticipating, preventing, and managing refeeding syndrome include awareness of the syndrome and recognition of patients who are at risk; appropriate monitoring and supplementation of electrolytes, including phosphorus and magnesium, before and during refeeding; gradual progression of volume and calories in patients at risk; routine administration of vitamins; and monitoring of cardiac, respiratory, neuromuscular, and hematological systems for complications of the syndrome.[38]

Later during recovery, caloric intake exceeding metabolic requirements can lead to obesity, which may be associated with hypothalamic injury. Weight should be monitored for early detection of this complication.

Respiratory Problems

Airway management is the first priority after brain injury. Endotracheal intubation in patients with severe injury is frequently indicated early, often in the field. Patients with delayed or poor neurological recovery may require tracheostomy for longer-term airway management. Major airway complications in children and adults with brain injuries and tracheostomies who were studied by Woo et al.[39] included aspiration, airway stenosis involving both the larynx and trachea, and dysphonia. Airway obstruction was observed by those authors to be a frequent complication because of the initial intubation, tracheostomy, or neurological dysfunction.[39] In the study of 50 patients with brain injuries and tracheostomies reported by Woo et al.,[39] complications related to the trachea and tracheostomy included stenosis, malacia, and granulation; laryngeal and intubation injuries included subglottic or glottic stenosis, subglottic airway collapse, and fractures of the thyroid and cricoid cartilages; and neurological injuries included vocal cord paralysis, abnormalities of supraglottic sensation, absence of the gag reflex, and cricopharyngeal spasm associated with aspiration. The majority of patients in this study (37/50) could be decannulated.[39] In view of the high incidence of airway complications, consultation by otolaryngology with consideration of direct laryngoscopy and bronchoscopy prior to decannulation is generally indicated.

Dysphonia may result from intubation, peripheral laryngeal or nerve injury, or central laryngeal movement dysfunction.[39]

Chest injury concurrent with severe TBI in children has been correlated with the level of oxygenation during the immediate period after injury and associated both with survival and with severity of disability in survivors.[3] Pneumonia may be a consequence of aspiration and is a common complication of tracheostomy.[40] Additional pulmonary complications in children with TBI include atelectasis and acute respiratory distress syndrome. Pulmonary embolus formation occurs rarely in children.

Gastrointestinal Problems

Abdominal trauma is usually not encountered as an isolated injury in children but is typically seen in the context of multiple trauma.[41] Most pediatric abdominal trauma is caused by motor vehicle, pedestrian, and bicycle injuries, with significant numbers of injuries caused by falls, sports, and child abuse.[41] These mechanisms are similar to those causing most brain injuries in children, and abdominal injuries are frequently seen concomitantly with pediatric TBI. Injuries to solid organs predominate in children with abdominal trauma, with approximately equal incidence of liver and spleen injuries; the majority of these injuries are self-limited.[41] Extensive hemorrhage, hollow viscus perforation, and other life-threatening injuries do occur, and careful evaluation and management are indicated.[41] The presence of abdominal injury concurrent with severe TBI is associated with worse TBI outcome, as measured by the Glasgow Outcome Scale.[3]

Children are at risk during the acute stage after injury for upper gastrointestinal (GI) tract bleeding for a variety of reasons, including stress ulceration, irritation from nasogastric tubes, and medications.[42] Monitoring the stool for occult blood should be a routine nursing practice. Use of antacids and histamine-2 receptor (H_2) antagonists is appropriate for children at risk of stress ulceration and likely prevents progression in those with evidence of GI bleeding.[42] Children with TBI with delayed or limited recovery of neurological function, especially in association with spasticity and gastrostomy tubes, are at increased risk for gastroesophageal reflux (GER). Medical therapy with antacids or H_2-receptor antagonists can be helpful if esophagitis is present. Omeprazole may be indicated to reduce acid secretion. Motility agents, including metoclopramide and cisapride, are commonly used in pediatrics to reduce GER. Cisapride may be preferable in children with TBI because of lesser adverse central nervous system (CNS) effects. Medications to reduce GI complications, like all medications in children with TBI, must be used with caution to minimize unnecessary exposure to agents that may have additional CNS consequences. Operative intervention may be indicated for those children with GER that is not responsive to medical therapy.

Pancreatitis has been associated with increased intracranial pressure[43] and has been observed in children with recent or remote TBI without obvious concurrent abdominal trauma.[44]

Unusual later GI complications of TBI include superior mesenteric artery (SMA) syndrome, associated with risk factors including prolonged recumbency, weight loss (loss of mesenteric and retroperitoneal fat), spasticity, and hip flexion contractures that cause increased lumbar lordosis.[45] These factors can decrease the angle formed by the SMA and aorta and lead to obstruction of the duodenum as it is crossed by the SMA.[45] The SMA syndrome usually occurs during the adolescent growth spurt, which also temporarily reduces the SMA angle.[45] Treatment should include identification and correction of precipitating factors, gastric decompression, use of left lateral or prone positioning, and, for children receiving tube feedings, placement of the tube into the jejunum (i.e., distal to the obstruction); surgical management may be indicated.[45]

Genitourinary Problems

Injury to the kidney is the most common type of genitourinary injury in children with trauma.[46] Bladder rupture is the most common major bladder injury in pediatrics; it is typically seen with multiple trauma in association with pelvic fractures.[46] Although uncommon, ureteral, urethral, testicular, and scrotal injuries may also occur in pediatric trauma.[46] Because genitourinary injury, even when severe, results in few signs and symptoms and is frequently present with more life-threatening injuries, including those to the CNS, it is likely underrecognized.[46]

Urinary tract infections are common complications of indwelling urinary catheters, which are frequently used in the early management of children with severe TBI. Urinalyses and urine cultures are therefore frequently obtained on rehabilitation admission from acute care settings, as well as during evaluation of fevers when the source is unknown.

Brain injury may cause impaired bladder control, resulting in incontinence in previously toilet-trained children because of an uninhibited detrusor or detrusor-sphincter dyssynergia. Intermittent catheterization may be indicated if dyssynergia is present and results in high postvoid residual volumes. If bladder dysfunction persists during rehabilitation, urologic assessment with renal ultrasound, a voiding cystourethrogram, and urodynamic studies should be considered to guide further management. Medications must be used with caution to minimize adverse effects in the child with TBI.

Musculoskeletal Disorders

FRACTURES

Fractures are more common and more likely after seemingly minimal trauma in children than in adults.[47] Uncomplicated long bone fractures in children usually heal quickly and with minimal sequelae following reduction and fixation by an orthopedist.[48] Fractures caused by high-energy trauma are often associated with significant concurrent injuries to other body systems,[47] including the nervous system. When there is polytrauma (injuries to other body systems), fracture healing in children is slower, less predictable, and with greater risk of complications.[47] In children, complications of fractures differ from those in adults, and methods of treatment receive different emphasis.[47] Later complications of pediatric fractures are especially associated with fractures through the growth plate. Altered growth of bone may follow these fractures and result in leg length discrepancy or progressive angular deformity.[48]

Fracture diagnosis, management, and the extent of associated disability may be complicated by the presence of the concomitant brain injury in children. Less obvious fractures and musculoskeletal injuries may be missed with multiple trauma, especially if the other injuries are severe and the child's ability to communicate is affected.[47] To determine the frequency of undetected musculoskeletal trauma in children with neurotrauma who were admitted to rehabilitation, Sobus et al.[49] obtained total body bone scans on rehabilitation admission. In that study, 16 of 60 patients from 4 months to 21 years of age with TBI (27%) had undetected fractures, and 19 (32%) had undetected areas of soft tissue injury. These undiagnosed injuries were considered to have impeded progress in rehabilitation in 12 of the patients. Heinrich et al.[50] also used whole body bone scans to study 48 severely injured patients less than 22 years old who had multiple injuries, a head injury, or both to detect undiagnosed fractures. Ten patients had previously undetected fractures, among whom 6 patients had altered treatment, consisting of cast application in all cases. Children may demonstrate deficits in mobility and age-appropriate activities of daily living following multiple trauma involving the brain and musculoskeletal system because of either or both types of injury. Individualized assessment of the child's rehabilitation needs is indicated in these complex patients with multiple trauma.

HETEROTOPIC OSSIFICATION

Ectopic bone formation may occur as a consequence of brain injury in children and adolescents. Incidence was 22.5 percent in a study by Citta-Pietrolungo et al.[51] of 111 patients with TBI, ages 6 to 21 years, who prospectively underwent routine triple-phase bone scans within 3 weeks of rehabilitation admission. Among the 25 patients with heterotopic ossification (HO) in this study, 10 remained asymptomatic, and only 3 were discharged with reduced range of motion in an affected joint. Citta-Pietrolungo et al.[51] concluded that HO is more common in children and adolescents with TBI than previously believed. They also suggested that the

beneficial effects of early therapy for HO must be demonstrated before widespread use of routine bone scans for detection can be justified.

The cause of HO after TBI in children remains unknown. Management includes passive range of motion exercises, carried to the point of joint resistance, to prevent joint ankylosis. Treatment with etidronate disodium has not been well studied in children who have not completed skeletal growth. Rachitic changes have been infrequently observed in the epiphyses with its administration; radiological changes and symptoms have been reversible following withdrawal of the drug. Surgical excision may infrequently be indicated. It should be considered after the ectopic ossification has matured if the restricted joint range of motion results in functional limitation. Mital et al.[52] have suggested that salicylate administration (60 mg/kg of body weight/day) may prevent recurrence after excisional surgery.

SCOLIOSIS

Scoliosis can occur in children with spasticity after TBI. In a series of 221 children with severe TBI, 19 (9%) developed scoliosis of greater than 30 degrees.[53] Children should be observed carefully for this complication, especially as they go through the accelerated growth of puberty.

LEG LENGTH DISCREPANCY

In addition to children with TBI who have multiple trauma with lower extremity fractures, as discussed previously, children with hemiplegia following TBI should be monitored for development of a discrepancy in leg lengths. Particularly for the child who is very young at injury, asymmetry may increase with growth as persistently decreased ground reaction and muscular forces differentially stimulate less growth on the already shorter limb. A shoe lift frequently provides adequate treatment for a milder (2–5 cm) leg length discrepancy.[54] When the magnitude of the discrepancy is greater, surgical intervention, such as an epiphysiodesis to shorten the eventual length of the unaffected limb or a lengthening procedure for the shorter limb, may be warranted.[54]

Endocrine Disorders

Disruption of the hypothalamic-pituitary area can lead to neuroendocrine dysfunction after TBI in children and adolescents. Hypothalamic-posterior pituitary disorders include the syndrome of inappropriate antidiuretic hormone secretion (SIADH) and central diabetes insipidus. Although onset is usually early and these disorders are usually transient, either may occur months after injury and warrant pharmacological intervention.

Dysregulation of thyroid, growth, and adrenocorticotropic hormones, gonadotropins, and prolactin may result from hypothalamic-anterior pituitary injury. Premature activation of the hypothalamohypophyseal axis can also result in precocious puberty,[55] although this complication is rare relative to the pituitary hormone deficiencies after pediatric TBI. Growth and sexual development should be monitored and symptoms and signs of endocrinopathy evaluated because hormonal replacement may be indicated.

Fever and Infection

Most children become pyrexial after severe TBI, probably because of elevation in the central temperature setpoint controlled by the thermoregulatory center in the anterior hypothalamus.[34] Hyperthermia may be accompanied by hypertension, hyperventilation, and decerebration with hypothalamic-midbrain dysfunction, possibly because of interruption of higher-level reflex regulation of lower brain stem mechanisms.[56]

Fever in children with brain injury is often caused by infection. In addition to intracranial infections, discussed previously, infections that complicate the recovery of children with TBI include sepsis, pneumonia, sinusitis, urinary tract infection, cellulitis, and infections caused by foreign bodies, such as intravascular catheters. Physical examination and laboratory and radiological evaluation must be performed before assuming fever in the child with TBI is of central origin. Identified infections are treated with appropriate antibiotics. Altered cell-mediated immune function is associated with pediatric TBI and likely contributes to the high rate of infection.[57,58] Anergy has been demonstrated in the majority of children with severe brain trauma on the day of injury in two recent studies.[57,58] In the study by Wilson et al.,[58] 79 percent of 14 anergic children identified by delayed-type hypersensitivity skin testing became infected, in contrast to 27 percent of nonanergic children; the average length of stay in the intensive care unit was 17 days longer and in the hospital was 31 days longer for the anergic children. Meert et al.[57] did not find the expected difference in the frequency of infection between anergic and nonanergic children, but there were only four patients in the nonanergic group.

Other potential causes of fever that should be considered in children with TBI include drug fever, deep vein thrombosis (rare in preadolescence), and heterotopic ossification.

Centrally acting antipyretics such as acetaminophen may reduce the thermoregulatory setpoint and are reasonable treatment for central fever.[34] Surface cooling does not alter the central thermoregulatory setpoint and may have an adverse effect on the child with TBI by further increasing body metabolism.[34] Propranolol may be useful when hypothalamic-midbrain dysregulation is present.[56]

Dermatologic Problems

Pressure sores, although preventable, are not uncommon in the child with TBI who remains at bed rest for an extended period. Predisposing factors include incontinence, poor nutrition, spasticity, casting, and positioning problems. Young children are predisposed to development of occipital ulcers. The site of greatest supine interface pressure changes with increasing age from the occipital to the sacral area.[59] The cornerstone of treatment remains strict pressure relief complemented by proper nutritional support, local wound care that includes debridement of necrotic tissue, and antibiotic treatment of significant wound infections.

◻ SUMMARY

Pediatric TBI is associated with medical and surgical complications involving the neurological and most other organ systems. Knowledge of the range of these complications can prevent many and lead to early recognition and appropriate management of most. Minimizing the impact of these complications is essential to achieving our primary goal of maximizing functional outcomes after TBI in children.

REFERENCES

1. Division of Injury Control, Center for Environmental Health and Injury Control, Centers for Disease Control: Childhood injuries in the United States. Am J Dis Child 144:627, 1990.
2. Kraus, JF, Rock, A, and Hemyari, P: Brain injuries among infants, children, adolescents, and young adults. Am J Dis Child 144:684, 1990.
3. Michaud, LJ, et al: Predictors of survival and severity of disability after severe brain injury in children. Neurosurgery 31:254, 1992.
4. Miller, JD, et al: Early insults to the injured brain. JAMA 240:439, 1978.
5. Walker, ML, et al: Pediatric head injury: Factors which influence outcome. In Chapman, PH (ed): Concepts in Pediatric Neurosurgery, vol 6. Karger, Basel, 1985, p 84.
6. Adams, JH, et al: Diffuse axonal injury due to nonmissile head injury in humans: An analysis of 45 cases. Ann Neurol 12:557, 1982.
7. Adams, JH, Graham, DI, and Gennarelli, TA: Head injury in man and experimental animals: Neuropathology. Acta Neurochir Suppl (Wien) 32:15, 1983.

8. Gennarelli, TA: Head injury in man and experimental animals: Clinical aspects. Acta Neurochir Suppl (Wien) 32:1, 1983.

9. Ewing-Cobbs, L, et al: The Children's Orientation and Amnesia Test: Relationship to severity of acute head injury and to recovery of memory. Neurosurgery 27:683, 1990.

10. Levin, HS, et al: Memory and intellectual ability after closed head injury in children and adolescents. Neurosurgery 11:668, 1982.

11. Schutzman, SA, et al: Epidural hematomas in children. Ann Emerg Med 22:535, 1993.

12. Gennarelli, TA, and Thibault, LE: Biomechanics of head injury. In Wilkins, RH, and Rengachary, SS (eds): Neurosurgery, vol 2. McGraw-Hill, New York, 1985, p 1531.

13. Dent, DL, et al: Prognostic factors after acute subdural hematoma. J Trauma 39:36, 1995.

14. Duhaime, AC, Bilaniuk, L, and Zimmerman, R: The "big black brain": Radiographic changes after severe inflicted head injury in infancy. J Neurotrauma 10(suppl 1):S59, 1993.

15. Duhaime, AC, et al: Long-term outcome in infants with the shaking-impact syndrome. Pediatr Neurosurg 24:292, 1996.

16. Michaud, LJ, and Duhaime, AC: Gunshot wounds to the brain in children. J Head Trauma Rehabil 10(5):25, 1995.

17. Winston, K, Beatty, RM, and Fischer, EG: Consequences of dural defects acquired in infancy. J Neurosurg 59:839, 1983.

18. Hahn, YS, et al: Factors influencing post-traumatic seizures in children. Neurosurgery 22:864, 1988.

19. Temkin, NR, et al: A randomized, double-blind study of phenytoin for the prevention of post-traumatic seizures. N Engl J Med 323:497, 1990.

20. Zimmerman, WD, et al: Peripheral hearing loss following head trauma in children. Laryngoscope 103:87, 1993.

21. Milmoe, G: Otolaryngologic injury. In Eichelberger, MR (ed): Pediatric Trauma: Prevention, Acute Care, Rehabilitation. Mosby, St Louis, 1993, p 423.

22. Healy, GB: Current concepts in otolaryngology: Hearing loss and vertigo secondary to head injury. N Engl J Med 306:1029, 1982.

23. Vartiainen, E, Karjalainen, S, and Kärjä, J: Vestibular disorders following head injury in children. Int J Pediatr Otorhinolaryngol 9:135, 1985.

24. Catalano, RA: Eye injuries and prevention. Pediatr Clin North Am 40:827, 1993.

25. Cockrell, J: Pediatric brain injury rehabilitation. In Horn, LJ, and Zasler, ND (eds): Medical Rehabilitation of Traumatic Brain Injury. Hanley & Belfus, Philadelphia, 1996, p 171.

26. Good, WV, et al: Cortical visual impairment in children. Surv Ophthalmol 38:351, 1994.

27. Duhaime, AC, et al: Head injury in very young children: Mechanisms, injury types, and ophthalmologic findings in 100 hospitalized patients younger than 2 years of age. Pediatrics 90:179, 1992.

28. Pang, D, and Pollack, IF: Spinal cord injury without radiographic abnormality in children: The SCIWORA syndrome. J Trauma 29:654, 1989.

29. Tracy, PT, Wright, RM, and Hanigan, WC: Magnetic resonance imaging of spinal injury. Spine 14:292, 1989.

30. Grabb, PA, and Pang, D: Magnetic resonance imaging in the evaluation of spinal cord injury without radiographic abnormality in children. Neurosurgery 35:406, 1994.

31. Furnival, RA, Woodward, GA, and Schunk, JE: Delayed diagnosis of injury in pediatric trauma. Pediatrics 98:56, 1996.

32. Trocki, O: Nutritional management of children with burns and trauma. In Eichelberger, MR (ed): Pediatric Trauma: Prevention, Acute Care, Rehabilitation. Mosby, St Louis, 1993, p 591.

33. Phillips, R, et al: Nutritional support and measured energy expenditure of the child and adolescent with head injury. J Neurosurg 67:846, 1987.

34. Matthews, DSF, et al: Temperature response to severe head injury and the effect on body energy expenditure and cerebral oxygen consumption. Arch Dis Child 72:507, 1995.

35. Seashore, JH: Nutritional support of children in the intensive care unit. Yale J Biol Med 57:111, 1984.

36. Towbin, RB, Ball, WS Jr, and Bissett, GS III: Percutaneous gastrostomy and percutaneous gastrojejunostomy in children: Antegrade approach. Radiology 168:473, 1988.

37. Gauderer, MWL: Percutaneous endoscopic gastrostomy: A 10-year experience with 220 children. J Pediatr Surg 26:288, 1991.

38. Solomon, SM, and Kirby, DF: The refeeding syndrome: A review. JPEN J Parenter Enteral Nutr 14:90, 1990.

39. Woo, P, Kelly, G, and Kirshner, P: Airway complications in the head injured. Laryngoscope 99:725, 1989.

40. Citta-Pietrolungo, TJ, et al: Complications of tracheostomy and decannulation in pediatric and young patients with traumatic brain injury. Arch Phys Med Rehabil 74:905, 1993.

41. Thompson, WR: Patterns of injury. In Eichelberger, MR (ed): Pediatric Trauma: Prevention, Acute Care, Rehabilitation. Mosby, St Louis, 1993, p 451.

42. Cochran, EB, et al: Prevalence of, and risk factors for, upper gastrointestinal tract bleeding in critically ill pediatric patients. Crit Care Med 20:1519, 1992.

43. Eichelberger, MR, et al: Acute pancreatitis and increased intracranial pressure. J Pediatr Surg 16:562, 1981.

44. Urban, M, Splaingard, M, and Werlin, SL: Pancreatitis associated with remote traumatic brain injury in children. Childs Nerv Syst 10:388, 1994.

45. Philip, PA: Superior mesenteric artery syndrome in a child with brain injury: Case report. Am J Phys Med Rehabil 70:280, 1991.

46. Allshouse, MJ, and Betts, JM: Genitourinary injury. In Eichelberger, MR: Pediatric Trauma: Prevention, Acute Care, Rehabilitation. Mosby-Year Book, Inc, St Louis, 1993, p 503.

47. Thomas, MD: Musculoskeletal Injury. In Eichelberger, MR (ed): Pediatric Trauma: Prevention, Acute Care, Rehabilitation. Mosby, St Louis, 1993, p 533.

48. Stempien, LM, and Glancy, GL: Special considerations in the rehabilitation of fractures in children. Physical Medicine and Rehabilitation: State of the Art Reviews 9:175, 1995.

49. Sobus, KML, Alexander, MA, and Harcke, HT: Undetected musculoskeletal trauma in children with traumatic brain injury or spinal cord injury. Arch Phys Med Rehabil 74:902, 1993.

50. Heinrich, SD, et al: Undiagnosed fractures in severely injured children and young adults: Identification with technetium imaging. J Bone Joint Surg 76A:561, 1994.

51. Citta-Pietrolungo, TJ, Alexander, MA, and Steg, NL: Early detection of heterotopic ossification in young patients with traumatic brain injury. Arch Phys Med Rehabil 73:258, 1992.

52. Mital, MA, Garber, JE, and Stinson, JT: Ectopic bone formation in children and adolescents with head injuries: Its management. J Pediatr Orthop 7:83, 1987.

53. Hoffer, MM, and Brink, J: Orthopedic management of acquired cerebrospasticity in childhood. Clin Orthop 110:244, 1975.

54. Moseley, CF: Leg-length discrepancy. In Morrissy, RT (ed): Lovell and Winter's Pediatric Orthopaedics, ed 3. JB Lippincott, Philadelphia, 1990, p 767.

55. Maxwell, M, et al: Precocious puberty following head injury: Case report. J Neurosurg 73:123, 1990.

56. Pranzatelli, MR, et al: Hypothalamic-midbrain dysregulation syndrome: Hypertension, hyperthermia, hyperventilation, and decerebration. J Child Neurol 6:115, 1991.

57. Meert, KL, et al: Alterations in immune function following head injury in children. Crit Care Med 23:822, 1995.

58. Wilson, NW, et al: Anergy in pediatric head trauma patients. Am J Dis Child 145:326, 1991.

59. Solis, I, et al: Supine interface pressure in children. Arch Phys Med Rehabil 69:524, 1988.

Traumatic Brain Injury in Children and Adolescents: Assessment and Rehabilitation

MARK YLVISAKER, PHD,
ANNA J. L. CHORAZY, MD,
TIMOTHY J. FEENEY, PHD,
and MARY LOUISE RUSSELL, MD

This chapter describes assessment and intervention approaches for selected problems associated with pediatric traumatic brain injury (TBI). In that several books would be required to deal comprehensively with all aspects of rehabilitative assessment and intervention for children with brain injury, we had difficult decisions to make about what to include and what to exclude. We considered the following questions: (1) Which issues associated with pediatric TBI tend to be the most common? (2) Which issues tend to be the most troubling for the children and their caregivers? (3) Which rehabilitation themes have a critical developmental component, necessitating attention to issues not covered in the chapters dealing with adults? (4) Which rehabilitation themes are uniquely associated with acquired versus congenital brain injury in children?

□ A LONG-TERM DEVELOPMENTAL PERSPECTIVE

Children are "a work in progress."[1] Brain injury at different developmental stages creates im-

portantly different challenges for the child and for family members and staff. For example, the rehabilitation needs of a child injured at age 3, coming from and returning to a highly structured, supportive, nurturing, routine, and relatively undemanding life, are quite different from those of a comparably injured 10-year-old. Similarly, the 10-year-old's needs differ from those of an 18-year-old, who, before the injury, was about to graduate from high school and begin vocational and social life as an independent young adult. In this obvious way, pediatric rehabilitation mandates a developmental perspective.

In addition, because children are a work in progress, brain injury has the potential not only to rob the child of knowledge and skills already acquired and create obstacles to success at the current developmental stage but also to jeopardize the child's ability to master new skills, acquire new knowledge, and successfully negotiate progressively more difficult developmental challenges over the years following the injury. To be sure, some children, including many with mild to moderate injuries, experience excellent recovery, resume their preinjury developmental careers and trajectories, and achieve success at levels unaffected by the injury. However, many children, including large numbers with severe injuries, have significant disability in the weeks and months after the injury and, in many cases, experience new and possibly growing cognitive, academic, and psychosocial difficulties in the years thereafter.

Delayed Developmental Consequences

The likelihood of delayed developmental consequences has become one of the salient themes in outcome research following frontal lobe injury in children, as well as in immature animals. Because the frontal lobes are the most common locus of damage in closed head injury,[2] it is critical that this well-documented phenomenon guide assessment and management planning for children with such injuries.

There are several possible contributors to delayed developmental consequences following pediatric TBI. From a neurological perspective, prefrontal injury has long been associated with delayed consequences in children[3-13] and in immature animals.[14,15] Because prefrontal regions of the brain and their interconnections with posterior areas mature slowly, the "executive" or self-control functions associated with these parts of the brain have a prolonged developmental course. This fact explains the common clinical observation that preschoolers with selective prefrontal injury may be very much like their uninjured peers: impulsive, egocentric, labile, episodically aggressive, "childlike," disorganized, and not given to long-range planning, deferred gratification, and dogged perseverance with difficult and frustrating tasks. However, the same child who appears adequately recovered at age 3 may have significant disability at age 6 and beyond if prefrontal regions have not recovered and matured sufficiently to support the growing self-control and planful thinking expected of schoolage children. Similarly, a third-grader with recently acquired prefrontal injury may evidence a degree of concreteness, egocentrism, inflexibility, impulsiveness, nonstrategic thinking, and need for externally imposed structure that is not unusual for third-graders. However, without ongoing development of the frontal lobes, that same child may demonstrate these characteristics to a degree that creates a substantial disability in middle school or high school.

In addition to neurological contributors to delayed consequences of TBI, preinjury and environmental factors account for many of the academic, social, and behavioral problems first identified long after the injury.[16-19] For example, Brown et al.[17] found a relatively high rate of new "psychiatric" disorders (problems that did not predate the injury) among children whose life circumstances before and after the injury were rated high on a psychosocial adversity scale. Similarly, Greenspan and MacKenzie[19] found poverty to be a better predictor of long-term outcome than severity of injury in their group of children and adolescents with TBI; that is, injury may heighten vulnerabilities present before the injury. Thus, the interaction of injury, disability, and environmental factors must be considered in designing long-term care and management.

Moreover, because of the frequency of new learning problems after TBI (associated with a high frequency of injuries to the hippocampus and to parts of the frontal lobes responsible for deliberate or strategic learning), disability after the injury may grow over time; that is, recovery of knowledge and skill acquired before the injury may enable the child to perform adequately in school for several months or even a year or two. However, inefficient new learning can have a snowball effect, as the child falls further and further behind in the curriculum. This phenomenon is far from universal but common enough that educators and others must adopt a long-term perspective in serving these students.

Increasing academic difficulties are one contributor to another possible explanation for delayed negative consequences of TBI in children—namely, increasing emotional and behavioral problems. Children with residual disability inevitably fail to meet their preinjury standards of success and are therefore vulnerable to anger, depression, withdrawal, acting out, and other psychoreactive disorders. In addition, severe TBI has a predictable negative impact on peer relations, with preinjury friendships difficult to maintain and a satisfying postinjury social life difficult to create. Resilient children and those with very strong support systems (especially family and friends) may escape the cascade of negative emotions associated with loss of ability, of success, and of friends. However, the downward emotional spiral set in motion by academic and social failure is sufficiently common and powerful in its negative impact to be considered central to rehabilitative efforts after pediatric TBI.[5,13]

Finally, poorly conceived systems of care, rehabilitative management, and education may contribute to delayed negative consequences. Included in this set of possible contributors are (1) decontextualized therapy and teaching procedures for children who require concrete contextual cues to learn efficiently and to effectively generalize their learning; (2) consequence-oriented behavior management for children who are severely disinhibited and who learn inefficiently from feedback, thus requiring positive,

TABLE 22–1. Immediate and Delayed Consequences of Traumatic Brain Injury in Adolescence

Key Developmental Issues	Common Concerns with TBI at This Stage	Common Delayed Symptoms Related to Earlier Injury
EARLY ADOLESCENCE		
Social-emotional-behavioral issues		

■ Emerging personal identity associated with short-term future goals, often involving physical accomplishments
■ Emphasis on following a rigid code of behavior and on punishment in moral thinking
■ Development of a cognitive map of social networks with primary emphasis on same-sex peers
  □ Emergence of fixed friendships, along with crowds and cliques
  □ External locus of control, with deference to the approval or disapproval of peers
	■ Social vulnerability, related to:
	  □ Separation from the clique
	  □ Socially awkward behavior (associated with frontal lobe injury)
	■ Role confusion and psychogenic problems ("I am not who I was") possibly associated with physical changes caused by the injury
	■ Likelihood of behavior problems associated with vulnerability to environmental stressors (especially with frontal lobe injury)
		■ Behavior problems associated with decreasing external control and an inability to meet the expectation for increasing behavioral self-regulation
		■ Inability to meet increasing social demands associated with puberty

Cognitive-academic issues		

■ Increase in abstract thinking and hypothetical-deductive reasoning
■ Increase in ability to use organizing schemes deliberately to process large amounts of information (e.g., for reading texts and writing essays)
	■ Increasing concerns with the academic curriculum, associated with:
	  □ Cumulative effects of new learning problems
	  □ Difficulty organizing large amounts of information
	  □ Difficulty with increasingly abstract information
		■ Increasing academic problems, associated with:
		  □ Cumulative effects of new learning problems
		  □ Difficulty organizing large amounts of information
		  □ Difficulty with increasingly abstract information

MIDDLE ADOLESCENCE		
Social-emotional-behavioral issues		
■ Increasing awareness of changes associated with puberty; increasingly heterosexual social networks ■ Increasing need to experiment and take risks ■ Increasing ability to manage environmental stressors, profit from feedback, and make flexible and autonomous decisions ■ Increasing ability to read social cues	■ Discontinuity of personal identification because of physical and cognitive changes; breakdown in social grouping associated with communication and other changes ■ Difficulty managing increasing environmental stressors; ongoing rigidity in responding; inability to profit from feedback ■ Experimentation and risk taking at dangerous levels ■ Possible "hyperegocentrism," with focus on the injury ■ Difficulty reading social cues	■ Continued rigidity and dependence on external control while peers become increasingly flexible and autonomous ■ Hypersexuality ■ Social withdrawal
Cognitive-academic-vocational issues		
■ Decreasing egocentrism, resulting in increasing ability to communicate varied thoughts and feelings competently in varied social settings ■ Emerging vocational goals and long-range goal planning	■ Difficulty with increasingly demanding curriculum ■ Possibly increasing incongruity between vocational goals and vocational potential after the injury	■ Increasing academic failure because of cumulative effect of new learning problems ■ Difficulty achieving communicative effectiveness in varied social settings requiring varied social registers ■ General difficulty with divergent thinking and flexible problem solving

TABLE 22–1. *Continued*

Key Developmental Issues	Common Concerns with TBI at This Stage	Common Delayed Symptoms Related to Earlier Injury
LATE ADOLESCENCE		

Social-emotional-behavioral issues

■ Loosening and shifting of social networks, based on vocational and social needs ■ Reduction in risk taking ■ Increasing ability to identify source of stress and adjust behavior accordingly (self-management) ■ Continued reduction in egocentrism and growth in attention to the needs of others (a life-long process) ■ Romantic relationships increasingly focused on companionship and love ■ Solidification of communication styles	■ Regression to rigid behavior, egocentric perspective, and dependence on external control; difficulty considering alternative perspectives ■ Inability to anticipate and recognize stressors and alter behavior accordingly ■ Loss of social networks; possible dependence on old social networks ■ Sexual relations persistently focused on physical aspects	■ Retention of concrete thinking and rigid responding ■ Immature social skills; continued dependence on cliques while peers move on ■ Continued dependence on same-sex peers for support; relations with opposite sex possibly characterized by hypersexuality ■ Possible perception of differences between self and others as representing a psychiatric problem

Cognitive-academic-vocational issues

■ Solidification of vocational and academic goals; organization of behavior in pursuit of these goals ■ Increasingly mature understanding of academic and vocational potential	■ Regression to rigid and concrete communication; loss of subtlety, abstractness, and flexibility in communication ■ Incongruity of previous academic/vocational goals and current abilities	■ Possible failure in college or on the job due to the elimination of the supports provided in high school

By "delayed consequences" we mean symptoms associated with an earlier injury (probably incurred at the previous developmental stage) often observed in individuals whose recovery had appeared to be generally good.

Source: From Ylvisaker, M, and Feeney, T: Traumatic brain injury in adolescence: Assessment and reintegration. Seminars in Speech and Language 16:32, 1995, with permission.

proactive, antecedent-oriented approaches to behavior management; (3) inadequate external organizational support for children who have difficulty planning and organizing behavior, thought, and language; and (4) systems of care and intervention that fail to engage executive functions in meaningful and developmentally appropriate ways, thereby contributing to learned helplessness over time.

It is quite easy to understand why the consequences of frontal lobe injury may be delayed in *young* children; furthermore, there is considerable empirical verification of this unwelcome phenomenon. In contrast, documentation and description of delayed developmental consequences of injury have only recently emerged in the literature on *adolescents* with TBI.[5,13,20] Table 22–1 outlines possible immediate and delayed consequences of TBI over three broad stages of *adolescent* development, not to suggest the inevitability of such consequences but rather to alert professionals to the possible need for preventive measures for this age group.

The point of this discussion of delayed consequences is that management of the cognitive, behavioral, psychosocial, and academic dimensions of the life of a child or adolescent with severe TBI requires a long-term focus and a dynamic understanding of new disability, interacting in often unpredictable ways with preinjury challenges, environmental vulnerabilities, and increasingly demanding developmental tasks. A proactive, long-term management system does much more than remain alert to the possible onset of delayed developmental consequences. Rather, the goal should be to prevent academic and social failure with a rich system of appropriate supports, thereby short-circuiting the downward behavioral and emotional spiral that is often the most painful and troubling consequence of TBI in children.

In the early weeks and months after the injury, the evolution of long-term needs and concerns cannot be confidently predicted. Therefore, acute rehabilitation staff have the daunting responsibility of orienting school staff and family members to possible future difficulties and possibly needed supports related to those difficulties, without losing optimism or creating self-fulfilling prophesies.[21,22] With each developmental transition—for example, from one level of schooling to another—staff must then "pass the baton" to staff at the new level so that they are alert to possible emerging difficulties for the child and equipped with an appropriate set of supports with which to ensure the child's successful transition. Although acute rehabilitation staff cannot foresee the future and dictate appropriate management procedures for every possible long-term outcome, they can and must dedicate themselves to educating, training, and supporting family members and staff at the next level of care, and they must insist that a long-term monitoring and safety net system be in place when the child leaves the rehabilitation hospital. Severe behavior problems require extraordinary effort to reverse if they are allowed to escalate in the years after injury.[6] Prevention of long-term sequelae by means of creative supports and antecedent-focused interventions is clearly preferable and often effective.[5]

◻ EXECUTIVE FUNCTIONS, COGNITION, COMMUNICATION, AND BEHAVIOR: AN INTEGRATED APPROACH TO REHABILITATION

Virtually any combination of strengths and weaknesses is possible after TBI, depending on the interaction of the individual's age, resilience, and profile of abilities before the injury with the location, nature, and severity of the injury and with postinjury treatment, support, opportunities, and emotional factors. However, despite the diversity in this population, TBI is considered a useful disability category by professionals in rehabilitative, educational, and vocational contexts, in part because of the frequency of frontal lobe (or frontolimbic) injury in closed head injury[2] and of associated executive system impairment. When frontal lobe injury dominates the outcome picture, as it often does, then problems with cognition, communication, behavior, and academic performance may have common roots in executive system dysfunction and must therefore be addressed by rehabilitation and special education professionals in an integrated manner. The premises that follow represent an outline of an approach to rehabilitation that embodies this integrated perspective.

PREMISE 1: Effective intervention integrates behavioral, social, cognitive, and communication perspectives and requires collaboration among professionals and others involved in the child's rehabilitation and education.

In an important sense, behavioral, social, communicative, cognitive, and academic problems associated with frontal lobe injury are best understood as different manifestations or components of executive system impairment.[13] For this and other reasons, it is critical for staff, family members, and others to fashion an integrated approach to intervention. Fragmentation in the delivery of services to children who are already fragmented by the injury can result in only increased fragmentation.

PREMISE 2: The most useful assessment for planning intervention occurs in natural contexts, is ongoing and collaborative, and involves testing hypotheses regarding the individual's performance and what can be done to improve it.

Behavioral psychology has a rich history of evaluating behavior in natural contexts and identifying the most effective management strategies by actively experimenting with potentially useful procedures in normal contexts.[23–25] In the section of this chapter dealing with cognitive assessment, we recommend the same approach to assessment of cognitive, communicative, and academic functioning. Contextualizing assessment addresses the ecological validity hazards that are a major theme in the literature on frontal lobe and executive system assessment and ensures practical application of findings. Collaboration increases the number and variety of observations and dramatically increases the likelihood that all members of the team agree to the resulting intervention decisions. Active testing of carefully selected hypotheses is typically required to identify the specific contributors to failure on tasks and the modifications and supports that can turn failure into success.

PREMISE 3: The most effective intervention occurs in meaningful contexts and is designed to influence routines in those contexts. The most important providers of services and supports are often everyday people in the individual's environment, including direct care staff, family members, and friends.

Behavioral psychologists have long recognized the impact of context on behavior and have sought to positively influence behavior by systematically modifying antecedents and consequences in everyday contexts of behavior.[26] More recently, cognitive scientists have experimentally verified the "domain specificity" (i.e., context dependence) of cognitive skill and have developed theories of internal cognitive representations to reflect these findings.[27] These findings challenge glib assumptions about the transfer of cognitive skill from training contexts and tasks to application contexts and tasks. In this chapter, we translate decades of research in behavioral and cognitive science into an approach to rehabilitation and special education that focuses on the child's everyday routines and the everyday individuals who interact with the child during everyday routines. This focus on social-behavioral routines as the basis for improved cognition and communication is most obviously associated with the developmental theories of Vygotsky[28] but is also consistent with other theoretical orientations.

PREMISE 4: Normal development of executive functions in children yields insights for intervention.

All aspects of cognition and executive system functioning develop simultaneously and in mutual interaction over the course of the developmental years.[29–31] Therefore, although there are hierarchies in cognitive rehabilitation based on task difficulty and required levels of support, aspects of cognition themselves (e.g., attention, perception, organization, memory, reasoning, executive functions) should *not* be serially arranged in rehabilitation (i.e., *not* first attention, then perception, and so on). As with normally developing infants, preschoolers, and older children, the best cognitive intervention after brain injury is engagement of individuals in real-life executive function routines connected with personally meaningful activities, at the child's level of ability, and with sufficient support and coaching to ensure success, gradually increasing expectations and withdrawing supports as improvement occurs.

PREMISE 5: Intervention for individuals with behavior problems focuses more on antecedents than on consequences.

Parents of infants and toddlers are well aware of the importance of antecedent control procedures relative to manipulation of consequences in managing the young child's behavior. Because prefrontal injury is often associated with impaired inhibition and relative inefficiency in profiting from feedback, antecedent control procedures are also of primary importance after TBI. These procedures include eliminating triggers for challenging behavior, ensuring that background setting events are positive before presenting stressful tasks, helping the individual generate positive behavioral momentum before

attempting difficult tasks, providing ample opportunities for choice and control, helping the individual develop positive scripts and social roles that are emotionally satisfying, and encouraging the individual to control his or her own antecedents. This perspective on behavior management is in sharp contrast to the traditional focus on consequences in programs that highlight token economies, time-out, response cost, and other contingency management procedures.

PREMISE 6: Recovery after brain injury progresses gradually and systematically from external control to internal self-control of social behavior and of covert cognitive behavior. Good rehabilitation facilitates this progression.

Just as normal child development proceeds slowly and through many stages from external to internal control of behavior and thought processes, good rehabilitation promotes the same progression. It includes a problem-solving, self-management approach to behavior and a metacognitive or strategic thinking approach to education, consistent with the child's developmental level. At the same time, internal control requires sufficient practice with skills and behaviors that they become as routine and habitual as possible, thereby not competing for limited resources in the child's working memory.

PREMISE 7. In the absence of meaningful engagement in chosen life activities, all interventions ultimately fail.

Although children as a group may be somewhat more willing than adults to engage in seemingly pointless activities simply because they are told to do so, their learning is more efficient and their engagement more intense if the activities are personally meaningful and have a purpose. There is an affective and motivational dimension to all behavior resulting, among other things, in deeper processing and more effective learning of information that is personally meaningful or important. This principle supports an active embedding of all aspects of rehabilitation in meaningful activities. Furthermore, supporting the child's need for success in chosen activities may reduce the likelihood of depression, resulting in part from a lack of meaningful engagement in chosen activities.

PREMISE 8. Professionals must quickly move beyond narrow medical and training models of intervention after TBI.

Social and academic behavior is a complex interaction between individuals, their abilities and motivation, the contexts in which they act, and the individuals with whom they interact. The traditional medical model of rehabilitation identifies the source of the disability primarily in the impairment internal to the individual and seeks to improve the individual's performance largely by remediating internal deficits with targeted retraining tasks. The training model, which is the primary tradition in developmental disabilities, similarly identifies the problem as in the learner, who is then subjected to a large number of isolated and decontextualized training tasks in a training environment with carefully managed contingencies for successful and unsuccessful performance. In other areas of cognitive and behavioral intervention that have a longer history than brain injury rehabilitation (e.g., mental retardation, learning disabilities), the combination of medical and animal trainer models has been disappointing in its long-term effectiveness in relation to functional cognitive and academic goals.[32]

A more productive model of intervention sees the professional as more like a cross between a coach,[33] a master craftsperson guiding an apprentice, and an environmental engineer. These metaphors lend themselves more readily to intervention that occurs in meaningful contexts, targets functional goals and objectives, and focuses as much on environmental supports and the behavior of others as on the individual's internal impairment.

These eight premises shape a general approach to integrated cognitive, communicative, behavioral, and academic intervention for children and adolescents with TBI, especially those with executive system impairment associated with frontal lobe injury.

Functional Assessment

Cognitive, behavioral, communication, and academic assessment can serve a variety of purposes, including diagnosing disorders, investigating characteristics of clinical populations, investigating characteristics of tests, qualifying children for special services, establishing the effectiveness of those services, and preparing for legal testimony. Here our interest is solely in assessment as it relates directly to decisions about functional intervention. With the goal of making the best decisions about supports and intervention, the most useful assessment engages a variety of staff and family members in ongoing collaborative testing of thoughtfully selected hypotheses in important contexts of the individual's life. Ongoing, collaborative, contextualized

hypothesis testing, familiar to many functional behavioral psychologists, should routinely be added to the common practice of administering standardized tests in a controlled assessment context and then using test performance to make judgments about the child's profile of abilities and about appropriate intervention (a practice familiar to many neuropsychologists, speech-language pathologists, and others).

ONGOING, CONTEXTUALIZED, COLLABORATIVE, HYPOTHESIS-TESTING ASSESSMENT

From a rehabilitation perspective, the goal of cognitive, behavioral, academic, and communication assessment is not only to identify performance strengths and weaknesses but also to explain why performance is poor in certain areas (compare "process assessment"[34]) and to identify what supports or task modifications the individual may need to perform at a higher level (compare "dynamic assessment"[35]). Following TBI, it is critical that assessment be ongoing, contextualized, collaborative, and experimental, an approach that has its roots in process assessment and dynamic assessment.

Ongoing Assessment

Following severe TBI, neurological improvement can continue for months and even years. Therefore, formal assessment completed early in this process may be an accurate description of the child's functioning for, at best, a brief period of time. Furthermore, the complexity in the profile of many students with TBI necessitates frequent adjustment and refinement of rehabilitation and education programs. Ongoing assessment contributes to this process. Finally, the frequently observed phenomenon of delayed onset of deficits mandates careful monitoring over time.

Contextualized Assessment

Studies of adults[36–38] and children[3,6,10,39,40] with frontal lobe injury have underscored the difficulty of capturing executive system impairment by using only structured, standardized tasks. Thirty years ago, the neurologist Teuber described "the curious dissociation between knowing and doing" in patients with frontal lobe injury. Since then, investigators have found that children and adults with executive system impairment can score adequately or even well on tests of intelligence, language, and academics—and even on neuropsychological tests designed to reveal the consequences of frontal lobe injury—despite potentially debilitating disability in demanding, nonroutine, real-world contexts. Kolb[15] has similarly found that animals with experimentally induced frontal lobe lesions may perform adequately on structured tasks (e.g., maze running) but fail to engage efficiently in important life-preserving tasks (e.g., foraging for food) in their natural environment.

This profound challenge to the ecological validity of standardized tests is probably related to what Lezak[41] referred to as the paradox of executive system impairment—that is, the difficulty of identifying how effectively people can identify what they need to do in the real world to achieve goals, plan how to do it, initiate behavior, monitor and evaluate performance, and choose a different course in the event of failure, when very little of this type of behavior is elicited by standardized tests. The evaluator and context of formal, standardized assessment take over most of what are referred to as the executive dimensions of tasks.

To be sure, there are tests that are better than others at capturing executive system impairment.[42–46] However, practicing clinicians and teachers should be alert to the critical need to supplement tests with real-world exploration when working with children with TBI.

Collaborative Assessment

Collaboration in assessment serves three important purposes. First, there is value in increasing the number of people available to observe the child's performance under a variety of circumstances in a variety of settings, to brainstorm about hypotheses, to test the hypotheses, and subsequently to implement intervention in a consistent manner. Specialists are often limited in the settings they can enter and must therefore rely on others' observations. If everyday people can learn to be reliable reporters of relevant behaviors, then specialists have a much broader data base from which to draw conclusions. In the case of direct care staff (e.g., nursing assistants, aides), it is most useful to request specific observations of specific behaviors under specific circumstances as part of the collaborative testing of hypotheses.

Second, compliance with intervention recommendations increases when the staff and family members responsible for implementing the intervention are actively involved in the assessment. Direct care staff, teachers, therapists, and others are notorious for ignoring or sabotaging treatment plans that are simply presented to them as finished products by behavioral psychologists, neuropsychologists, or other specialists who completed their assessments in isolation. In contrast, when relevant staff and family members share ownership of the assessment and see firsthand the effects of trial man-

agement procedures, teaching procedures, or behavioral and cognitive supports during the hypothesis-testing phase of assessment, the likelihood of compliance with the ultimate recommendations is increased, and mutually respectful relationships among staff and others are created.

Third, collaborative hypothesis testing is an ideal context within which specialists in cognition, communication, behavior, and education can integrate their diverse perspectives and also orient and train nonspecialists.

Experimental (Hypothesis-Testing) Assessment

Because successful performance on all real-world tasks is a result of a large number of cognitive and noncognitive processes and factors working in concert, failure on any task can potentially be explained by reference to a large number of breakdowns. Knowing how to help a child improve performance requires understanding why performance is weak. Furthermore, it is insufficient to know simply that performance in a given area is weak and that a deficit has been identified that could explain the weak performance. For example, a child may score badly on reading tests and also have visual perceptual deficits, but the latter may not account for the former; a child may exhibit acting out behavior and also be depressed, but the latter may not be causally related to the former.

Identifying what factors account for impaired performance and how failure can be turned into success requires active experimentation with aspects of the problematic tasks and with task modifications and supports that might improve performance. For example, if compensations for visual-perceptual problems (e.g., enlarged print, line markers) improve reading scores substantially, then a contributor to failure has been identified, and guidelines for intervention can be intelligently developed. Similarly, if experimental intervention for depression (e.g., antidepressant medication, intensive counseling, increase in life activities incompatible with depression) substantially decreases acting out behavior, then a major contributor to behavior problems has been identified, and intervention plans can be developed accordingly.

Contextualized, collaborative, hypothesis-testing assessment has its roots in process assessment[34] and dynamic assessment.[35] Within this test-oriented, hypothesis-testing approach, Denckla[42] recommended systematically pairing and comparing results on tests that vary primarily in their executive function demands as a way of evaluating executive system functioning in children with cognitive disability. For example, she recommends comparing (1) recall across five trials on the California Verbal Learning Test[47] with (2) clustering across five trials on the same test. In this way, the executive contribution to verbal learning (strategically organizing information to be learned) can be experimentally separated from the varied nonexecutive dimensions of the task.

The approach to cognitive, behavioral, communication, and educational assessment that we recommend adds to this experimental approach the important dimensions of collaborating with others and contextualizing the assessment tasks. Table 22–2 illustrates this approach. Real-world hypothesis testing has been increasingly used in varied domains, including assessment of children with behavior problems[13,48] and vocational assessment.[49] Ylvisaker and Gioia[50] present an extended discussion of contextualized, collaborative, hypothesis-testing assessment, including illustrations applicable to children with TBI.

COGNITIVE ASSESSMENT: SPECIAL CONSIDERATIONS

Depending on the purpose of testing and a variety of child-specific factors, the standard domain of intellectual and other cognitive tests used by neuropsychologists, school psychologists, and psychoeducational evaluators may be helpful in developing rehabilitation and educational programs for children with TBI. Furthermore, neuropsychological assessment of children has improved with the acquisition of pediatric norms for measures that are considered parts of a sensitive "frontal lobe battery" for adults[44] and with neuropsychological interpretations of developmental measures, particularly those sensitive to the development of executive functions.[31,51] However, studies of the consequences of frontal lobe injury in children and adults (cited earlier) raise serious questions about the validity and completeness of batteries of standardized tests.

Professionals with special expertise in cognition can contribute to the development of rehabilitation programs for children with TBI by (1) identifying specific hypotheses regarding the child's performance and what can be done to enhance it, based on history, neuropathological information, and, possibly, test data; (2) helping staff and family formulate contextualized tests of those hypotheses; and (3) helping staff and family translate the results of this hypothesis testing into appropriate intervention plans. Guidance of collaborative cognitive assessment can occur within rehabilitation hospitals and schools and also between hospital and school. For example, useful neuropsychological reports that accompany children with TBI from hospital to school are designed, in part, to guide school staff in their ongoing exploration of the child's abilities and disabilities. In contrast, reports that simply describe static levels of performance at a specific time, associate deficits with lesion sites, and postulate specific educational recommendations based on test results are often unhelpful to school staff and, therefore, ignored. This approach to cognitive assessment following TBI in children is elaborated by Ylvisaker and Gioia.[50]

BEHAVIORAL ASSESSMENT: SPECIAL CONSIDERATIONS

Behavioral psychologists who work within the tradition of applied behavior analysis are accustomed to using real[52–54] or contrived (i.e., "analogue"[55]) contexts to experimentally derive explanations of behavior by reference to that behavior's antecedents and history of consequences. More recently, many behavioral psychologists have placed this exploration within the useful framework of the child's communication ecology[56–58]; that is, a goal of behavioral assessment is to identify the communication value of behavior and the effects of the partner's communication on the child's behavior.

Behavioral psychologists with additional expertise in neuropsychology are particularly useful in serving children with TBI. For example, children with orbital-frontal injury may engage in challenging behavior not simply because of the present antecedents combined with the child's history of reinforcement but rather because of severe, neurologically based disinhibition. Similarly, children who appear lazy or unmotivated may have some degree of neurologically based lack of activation or initiation related to dorsolateral or medial prefrontal injury. Children with right frontal injury often behave in unwanted ways because of serious misperception of their social situation. Children with ventromedial prefrontal injury may fail to profit efficiently from feedback or from a carefully designed program of contingency management. Knowledge of these neuropsychological factors is critical in serving children with TBI effectively, not by giving the child an excuse for undesirable behavior but rather by appropriately focusing intervention efforts (e.g., on antecedents rather than consequences) and by helping adults understand the constraints on the child's behavior.

In the real world, of course, behavior is often a result of a confusing interaction between pre-injury characteristics and behavior patterns, neurologically based factors, and the child's environment and history since the injury. In light of this complexity, collaborative, contextualized, hypothesis testing is particularly useful in behavioral assessment.

TABLE 22–2. Illustrations of Collaborative, Contextualized, Hypothesis-Testing Assessment for Developing an Educational Program

FORM

In order to answer the question: _____,
staff (and family) will systematically collect and compare performance data gathered under the following conditions:

1. _____

versus

2. _____

Results will be evaluated by the team, leading to decisions about the educational program.

Example 1: Attention

Question: "Is John's ability to focus his attention better facilitated by removing distractions or by ensuring that the routine/activity that he is involved in is well understood and interesting?"

Experiment: Staff and family will systematically collect and compare data on attention span and quality of attending gathered under the following conditions:

1. 1:1 interaction in a quiet environment

versus

2. Highly routine story time in the classroom with many other children present and with an interesting story

versus

3. Small group instruction

Example 2: Oppositional Behavior

Question: "Does John routinely reject tasks simply because they are explicitly presented as demands?" An answer to this question will help staff know how to present tasks, including specific instructional tasks, in the most efficient manner.

Experiment: Staff and family will systematically observe and compare John's performance (especially resistive behavior) on equally interesting and equally difficult tasks in response to:

1. Instructions that are explicit—that is, introduced with words like, "John, I would like you to," "We are going to," or "Your job is to"

versus

2. Tasks that are presented without instructions; that is, the environment is organized so that John has access to activity materials and teacher support but receives no explicit instruction to do the task (e.g., the math workbook and teacher are available during math time, but John is not directly told to do his math).

Example 3: Deliberate versus Incidental Learning

Question: "Does John perform better and learn more efficiently when the task is organized (1) so that his goal is to learn or (2) so that he is pursuing his own concrete meaningful tasks and learning is a byproduct?" An answer to this question will help staff know how to design learning tasks for John.

Experiment: Staff and family will systematically observe and compare John's performance (especially learning rate) on equally demanding tasks, but with a different task orientation for John:

1. *Deliberate Learning:* The task is preceded with a statement such as "John, today we will work on," "John, let's see if you can remember," or "John, I bet you can learn this if you try hard." With these orienting words, John's goal becomes the goal of learning.

versus

2. *Incidental Learning:* John is engaged in a play activity or in a practical activity that is designed in such a way that mastering the concept or learning the information is a by-product of completing the personally meaningful activity. His goal is not to learn but rather to play, accomplish the practical task, or produce a concrete product. For example, John is asked to write a story for the class newspaper. The teacher introduces an outline format which John is to learn. However, John's goal is not to learn the format (the teacher's goal for John) but rather to produce the story.

Source: From Ylvisaker, M, et al: School reentry following severe traumatic brain injury: Guidelines for educational planning. J Head Trauma Rehabil 10(6):25, 1995, with permission.

COMMUNICATION ASSESSMENT: SPECIAL CONSIDERATIONS

Although communication deficits are common components of global disability after the most severe cases of TBI and also of generalized executive system impairment, *specific* speech and language disorders are relatively rare.[12] The most common language-related deficits after closed head injury are not effectively explored by language tests in common use, with the possible exception of word-retrieval deficits. Therefore, speech-language pathologists must not consider a language assessment complete after administering a typical battery of tests designed for children with developmental language problems. Furthermore, they must not assume that a child with TBI who scores within normal limits has the language competence needed to succeed in the classroom and social environments. Table 22–3 includes a list of language-related concerns associated primarily with frontal lobe injury, along with informal procedures for exploring skills in those areas. Dennis et al.[43,59] have recently developed a number of tasks for exploring areas of language weakness following

---

TABLE 22–3. Procedures for Exploring Commonly Occurring Cognitive-Language Deficits in Children with Traumatic Brain Injury

Area of Concern	Possible Assessment Procedures
Disorganized discourse	1. *Expressive language: speech and writing.* Does language expression deteriorate rapidly with increases in organizational demands? Use varied discourse tasks (e.g., narrative, procedural, descriptive, explanatory) up to a length and complexity expected at the child's age and grade level. Analyze the amount and organization of content (number of pieces of information and coherence of presentation) and of linguistic markers of organization (cohesion). 2. *Receptive discourse: reading.* Does reading comprehension deteriorate rapidly with increases in the amount to be read? Use reading tasks up to a length and complexity expected at the child's age and grade level. Does reading comprehension deteriorate rapidly with increases in reading rate? Is comprehension of factual information significantly better than comprehension of themes and indirect meaning? 3. *Receptive discourse: listening.* Does listening comprehension deteriorate rapidly with increases in the amount of language to be processed? Use listening tasks up to a length and complexity expected at the child's age and grade level. Compare comprehension of factual information with comprehension of themes and inferences. Explore the influence of increases in speaking rate on listening comprehension. 4. *Receptive/expressive discourse: conversation.* Explore all dimensions of conversation, ideally in social context. Prutting and Kirchner's taxonomy of components of conversation[60] is useful for this purpose.
Inefficient word retrieval	1. Consider standardized tests of word finding.[61–63] 2. Consider word fluency measures.[64] 3. Explore effects of psychosocial stress (e.g., classroom recitation) and cognitive stress (e.g., time pressure) on efficiency of word retrieval.
Linguistic inflexibility	1. Does the child have difficulty interpreting sentences with multiple meanings?[65] 2. Does the child have difficulty with topic shifts? With alternative formulations of a given thought?
Concreteness	1. Does the child have relatively severe difficulty with comprehending metaphors and figures of speech?[59] 2. Does the child have relative difficulty with abstract vocabulary? Metalinguistic reference?[43]
Inefficient verbal learning	1. Does the child learn new vocabulary at a rate commensurate with current knowledge? Teach new vocabulary, carefully documenting rate and style of learning. 2. Does the child use strategic procedures in learning verbal information?[47]
Social awkwardness	1. Does social interactive competence deteriorate with increases in social stress? Observe communicative interaction in a variety of natural settings and under a variety of circumstances.[60] Social skills inventories may be useful.

closed head injury in children, including metalinguistic awareness and indirect meaning.

ACADEMIC ASSESSMENT: SPECIAL CONSIDERATIONS

Standardized, norm-referenced tests of performance in varied academic areas are useful in identifying current levels of performance and assisting in decisions about placement and needed supports. In addition, creative educational diagnosticians can use tests to begin the process of dynamic, hypothesis-testing assessment. It is common for evaluators to administer a test in a standardized manner, followed by variation of one test factor at a time to isolate reasons for failure and the need for specific supports; for example, if a child scores poorly on a reading test, the evaluator might next give the same or a comparable task but without time constraints, with enlarged print or other visual-perceptual support, with an advance organizer to guide the reading, with fewer environmental distractors, with increased motivation for successful performance, or with another modification of the task. If performance improves substantially with one or more of the modifications, then the evaluator can recommend that classroom staff use that modification, at least on a trial basis. This systematic exploration should continue in the classroom with procedures that educators refer to as diagnostic teaching.

However, children with frontal lobe injury often score better on tests than would be expected in light of their relatively weak classroom learning and performance. Reasons for this possible discrepancy were discussed earlier. The phenomenon of relative superiority of performance on tests yields cautions about making judgments about needed supports based on test results alone. Often educational disability is not fully revealed until the child is in the classroom and exploratory teaching has begun.

Furthermore, because test results may not reveal all aspects of educationally relevant disability, educational evaluators must collaborate with classroom staff (or tutors in the case of hospitalized children) to derive an accurate description of contextualized academic performance and to systematically explore possible classroom supports. Ylvisaker et al.[66] described procedures for collaborative hypothesis testing involving formal or informal interaction between classroom staff and other specialties (e.g., school psychologist, TBI consultant), with hypotheses generated in one context possibly tested in the other. For example, because children with closed head injury commonly experience organizational impairment, a hospital- or school-based evaluator may propose experiments with varied advance organizers for organizationally demanding tasks in the classroom. Advance organizers can range from a visual (e.g., photograph) plan for the day to a diagram organizer for reading and writing tasks to simple checklists for activities of daily living. Ylvisaker et al.[67] presented an extended discussion of advance organizers for children with organizational impairment after TBI. Student performance with and without various types of advance organizers can then be used by the total education or rehabilitation team to refine the student's program and set of cognitive supports.

Finally, relatively well-recovered students (older children and adolescents) should participate in their own evaluation and educational planning process as an excellent way to begin an executive system focus in intervention and to encourage students to gain progressively greater insight into their abilities. Ylvisaker et al.[68] presented a student self-assessment questionnaire and a process for student engagement in developing educational programs for high school special education resource rooms.

Functional, Everyday, Routine-Based Intervention

Internal cognitive and linguistic processes and systems have their developmental origin in simple, everyday interaction routines between young children and their caregivers. This developmental theory, formulated and elaborated more than 50 years ago by Vygotsky,[28] has received empirical support from explorations of varied aspects of cognitive and language development. For example, Ratner and Bruner[69] traced the origin of rules of conversation to simple, prelinguistic, gamelike routines that babies enjoy with their parents. Similarly, several developmental cognitive psychologists have recently supplied evidence for the claim that internal cognitive organization and autobiographical memory are grounded in part in simple narratives about the past that parents construct conversationally with their young children.[70-74] Furthermore, contemporary approaches to facilitating development in children with congenital disability have made extensive use of this Vygotskyan theme in areas ranging from early language development[75] to later language development[76] to reading acquisition[77] to general cognitive development.[78]

Furthermore, the notion of an everyday routine provides an ideal meeting place for behavioral and cognitive approaches to rehabilitation. From a behavioral perspective, a routine is a behavior chain in which each behavior is a discriminative stimulus for the next (in specific contexts). A goal of behavioral intervention is to teach positive routines that are sufficiently flexible to support successful behavior in an ever-changing world; that is, the stimuli and responses that comprise the routine are identified as expanding *classes* of behaviors versus specific behaviors. From a cognitive perspective, a routine is a specific sequence of actions that comes to be represented internally as a knowledge structure that has potential to become increasingly general and abstract as children mature and expand their domain of experiences. General knowledge structures (e.g., an "eating out schema" that is capable of guiding behavior in a wide variety of restaurants), derived from concrete routines (e.g., eating at one's favorite McDonald's), are referred to as scripts or schemas and guide mature thinking, acting, talking, and remembering. In summary, rehabilitation understood as conversational modeling and coaching within the context of everyday routines has support within both behavioral and cognitive theoretical perspectives.

In an interesting way, Vygotskyan theory dictates intervention practices that are the opposite of the tradition in rehabilitation for cognitive, communicative, and behavioral impairment. Using World Health Organization language, traditional rehabilitation attempts to reduce the underlying neurologically based *impairment* (often with decontextualized exercises), in hopes of reducing the functional *disability* and then the social, vocational, and academic *handicap* associated with that disability. The approach that we describe can be understood as addressing the *disability* (and possibly also *handicap*) first, by creating supports for successful performance in everyday routines, with reduction in underlying *impairment* a secondary goal as the child internalizes the routines, creates more general knowledge structures, and thereby improves cognitive function and behavioral self-regulation. Cognitive supports have been referred to in the developmental cognitive psychology literature as "scaffolds,"[79] a concept that has been fruitfully applied to adult brain injury rehabilitation.[80,81] To succeed within this framework, rehabilitation clinicians must think of themselves *less* as a cross between a surgeon and animal trainer (focusing directly on eliminating the impairment) and *more* as a combination of coach, master craftsperson, and consultant.[82]

EVERYDAY EXECUTIVE SYSTEM ROUTINES

Executive functions include the self-regulatory or control functions that direct and organize all nonreflexive or nonautomatic behavior, including readily observable behavior in a social context, as well as covert cognitive and linguistic

behavior. From a practical, everyday vantage, executive functions include (1) having some sense for one's strengths and weaknesses and, on the basis of that understanding, (2) knowing what is easy and what is hard to do, thereby being able to set reasonable goals for oneself, (3) planning and organizing behavior to achieve the goals (i.e., making active use of knowledge and skill in the pursuit of goals); (4) initiating goal-directed behavior; (5) inhibiting behavior that is inappropriate or interferes with achieving goals; (6) monitoring one's behavior; (7) evaluating it in relation to goals; and (8) flexibly shifting sets, thinking strategically, and solving problems in the event of obstacles. In this broad sense, development of executive functions is critical in achieving any meaningful goals in life that require effort.

Developmental neuropsychologists have recently sought to characterize executive functions in children by administering a battery of tests to various clinical populations, including children with TBI, and deriving relatively independent components of the executive system by means of factor analysis. Using this methodology, Levin et al.[45] examined children and adolescents with TBI and proposed five factors: conceptual/productivity (e.g., word fluency), planning/execution (e.g., number of rules broken on the Tower of London task), schema (e.g., number of constraint-seeking questions on a 20-question task), cluster (e.g., use of organizational strategies in memory tasks), and inhibition (e.g., false alarm errors on a Go/No Go task). In contrast, Taylor et al.[46] proposed a three-factor analysis of executive functions in children: response speed, planning/sequencing, and response inhibition. Because these characterizations of executive functions in children are based on administration of available tests, it is not surprising that they both omit critical components of the executive system, including self-awareness (few tests require the individual to accurately predict performance), initiation (in testing situations, the examiner is responsible for initiation), and self-evaluation (those being tested are rarely responsible for evaluating their own performances). A clinically more meaningful methodology for examining executive functions is that preferred by many investigators in the field of attention deficit–hyperactivity disorder (another disability associated with executive system impairment)—namely, characterizing the disability as it manifests itself in real-world activities and then creating assessment tasks that are tested for validity against that real-world standard.

An advantage of the operational definition of executive functions proposed earlier in this section is that it naturally captures the elements critical to success on any difficult task and lends itself to implementation through everyday routines. Following Vygotsky's theories of cognitive development, supported by research with other disability populations,[83] and guided by our experience with hundreds of children with frontal lobe injury after TBI, we recommend that the focus of intervention be creative manipulation of everyday routines to incrementally facilitate development, habituation, and internalization of executive behaviors.

GENERAL EXECUTIVE SYSTEM ROUTINES: GOAL-PLAN-DO-REVIEW

Figure 22–1 illustrates a general guide for practicing executive functions in the context of everyday tasks. The routine could involve no more than a few seconds of adults' reflections out loud about the child's activity or at the other extreme could involve extensive and independent planning and reviewing on the child's part. The child's cognitive and language levels, atten-

WHAT IS MY GOAL?

WHAT IS MY PLAN? (Could be generated by the individual or collaboratively with a professional)

1

2

3

4

5

HOW WELL DO I THINK I WILL DO? (Could be a grade, rating, or any relevant measure of success)

1	2	3	4	5	6	7	8	9	10
lousy									great

HOW WELL DID I DO? (Could be a grade, rating, or any relevant measure of success)

1	2	3	4	5	6	7	8	9	10
lousy									great

WHAT WORKED FOR ME?		**WHAT DIDN'T WORK FOR ME?**
1	■ 1	
	■	
2	■ 2	
	■	
3	■ 3	
	■	
4	■ 4	
	■	
5	■ 5	

WHAT WILL I TRY NEXT TIME? (Remember: Stick with winners; discard losers; try new possibilities)

FIGURE 22–1. Structure of a general executive system routine.

tion span, motivation, and other factors influence decisions about how to implement the routine on any given occasion.

Professionals who fear that such a routine is applicable only to older and well-recovered children should be reminded that one of the most popular preschool curricula, High Scope,[84] designed for at-risk and mildly delayed Head Start children, is structured around a daily plan-do-review routine. Clearly, the routine is a very simple one for children who are highly distractible or have little language. Planning may be little more than selecting a toy or activity and having an adult briefly comment on what a great plan that is; reviewing may be little more than the adult's description of what the child did during play time, along with possible problems that arose. However, as the children's cognitive and verbal functions improve, they can become more active contributors to the process of selecting goals, making plans, and reviewing accomplishments.

In rehabilitation hospitals and schools serving children with executive system impairment, the day ideally begins with the children actively involved in making their plan for the day (e.g., placing photographs of themselves, engaged in scheduled activities, on a planning board that can later be used for reorientation throughout the day). The children's day ends with a review of the day's activities, made meaningful because a concrete product has to be generated (e.g., a letter to parents describing the day's activities, highlighting accomplishments as well as problems that arose and how they were solved). Over the course of the day, staff and family members can begin each new activity with the routine: "Ok, what are we trying to accomplish? . . . Good! So what's our plan? . . . Great! How well do you think you will do?" In our experience, children who know that their involvement in planning is part of the routine not only become engaged in planning activities but also indicate that they appreciate the respect implicit in this involvement.

More demanding elements can be incrementally added to this basic routine as the child recovers or matures. For example, it is useful to require children with weak self-awareness of strengths and weaknesses to predict how successful they will be on a task after they have formulated their plan and later compare that prediction with their actual performance. Alternatively, children may be asked to rate their performance and compare that rating with an adult's rating. Furthermore, relatively well-recovered children, grade school age and older, can be engaged in a brief "What worked? What didn't work?" discussion after completing a difficult task. In this way, strategic thinking, starting very simply and concretely, can be in-jected into daily routines. What is most critical is that everyday routines emphasize the executive dimensions of tasks and that the children's processing of the executive dimensions is deep because they find the activity personally meaningful and important.

Empirical verification of the long-term effectiveness of daily goal-plan-do-review routines, combined with everyday coaching in practical problem solving in the context of everyday problems, has been provided by long-term outcome studies—to age 27—of the High Scope preschool curriculum.[85] The High Scope approach combines a daily plan-do-review routine with intensive, contextualized coaching in strategic thinking, as well as training for parents so that the executive function routines established at school are reinforced by positive executive function routines at home. Admittedly, cross-population inferences regarding effectiveness of intervention require great caution. Indeed, in the case of severe frontal lobe injury, children may continue to require considerably more external support and direction than the high-risk children served in Head Start programs. However, these data are exceedingly welcome in their suggestion that early establishment of positive executive system routines with children and families can have a dramatic impact on functional, real-world outcomes in adolescence and young adulthood.

PROBLEM-SOLVING ROUTINES

Between 6 and 18 months of age, there is a burst of development of executive functions (corresponding to what Piaget referred to as development of means-ends relations or problem-solving behavior[86]). Simple problem-solving routines for toddlers (and older children early in recovery after brain injury) are illustrated by the interaction between a 15-month-old toddler and his father, presented in Table 22–4. The critical features of this routine are (1) the child has an important goal (e.g., make the toy work); (2) there is an obvious obstacle, making it difficult to achieve the goal without doing something special; (3) the father verbally and nonverbally encourages a variety of possible solutions; (4) the father highlights the difficulty of the task; (5) the father praises the child for his efforts and perseverance; and (6) the father confirms that there is one solution that always works.

As normally developing children mature and as injured children improve, everyday problem-solving routines can increase in complexity and expectations for the child's contribution. Complexity increases in the areas of (1) clarifying the nature of the problem, (2) gathering information relevant to solving the problem, (3) clearly articulating alternative solutions, (4) considering ad-

---

TABLE 22–4. Illustration of a Problem-Solving Routine for a Toddler

CHILD:	(Picks up a small wind-up toy.)
FATHER:	That's a funny thing. I wonder how it goes.
CHILD:	(Tries to manipulate the wind-up key but can't turn it.)
FATHER:	Boy, that's hard to do, isn't it. I wonder what else you could do.
CHILD:	(Turns the toy; hits it on the head; drops it.)
FATHER:	You tried lots of things. That's great! But it's still not working, is it? Let me show you. (Models the correct solution to the problem.)
CHILD:	(Tries again to use the key. Fails again. Hands the toy to his father to wind up.)
FATHER:	(Takes the toy and winds it up.) Boy, that's a hard thing to do, isn't it? You tried real hard. That's great! But it didn't work. Here, let me do it for you. Dad can always help.

---

vantages and disadvantages of each, and (5) evaluating the merits of the selected solution after it has been implemented. It is rare for people, including adults, to be this deliberate in dealing with everyday problems. However, it is not difficult for clinicians, teachers, or parents to model this thought process for older children as they discuss everyday problems. In addition, clinicians and teachers can engage groups of children in these thought processes when genuine problems emerge or are contrived.

In working with cognitively impaired children, a learning trial need not involve the child's overt performance. Even with older children, the routine may look much like that presented in Table 22–4, in which the adult models most of the cognitive work. What is critical is that the child is engaged in the task and in solving the problem, thereby processing the adult's problem-solving activity and coming to appreciate the importance of problem-solving routines associated with any difficult task.

To be sure, a small number of these experiences cannot be expected to have a substantial impact on the development or redevelopment of the child's executive function. However, in rehabilitation, school, and home environments sensitive to the importance of executive functions, thousands of such learning trials are provided over the course of the developmental years. The cumulative effect of large numbers of learning trials in settings sensitive to the importance of executive system routines is what can be expected to have an impact, parallel to that of a positive parental interaction style on a young child's development of language and conversational skills.[75]

SELF-COACHING ROUTINES

The term *executive functions* is based on a metaphor: Thoughtful individuals can do for themselves what an executive does for a business organization. A more appropriate and equally accurate metaphor for adolescents with TBI is "self-coaching." Many adolescents know firsthand what a coach does for a team and can be encouraged to translate that knowledge into a meaningful executive function routine for themselves. In rehabilitation hospitals and schools, professionals can encourage adolescents to consider themselves both player and coach. As coach, they set goals for themselves, identify obstacles (weak areas of functioning), formulate game plans (e.g., what kind of activity or exercise might be useful to meet PT, speech, social, or academic goals), give themselves instructions, evaluate their own performance (analogous to a coach reviewing the game films), and make decisions about alternative strategies or types of practice. Therapists try to move into the background and play the role of consultant and cheerleader to the adolescent self-coach.

In contrast, when therapists hoard responsibilities like selecting goals for the individual, identifying strengths and weaknesses in relation to achieving the goals, planning how to achieve the goals, taking responsibility for initiating, monitoring, and evaluating performance, and solving problems when they arise, they are actively interfering with the individual's recovery and development of executive functions. Promoting self-coaching routines as part of therapy or academic tasks is a concrete and efficient way for therapists to avoid this destructive trap and to make executive function activities both concrete and attractive for adolescents with TBI.

A simpler executive function routine, appropriate for grade school children as well as adolescents, involves planning and producing customized "exercise videos" (analogous to commercial exercise videos featuring famous people like Jane Fonda). With whatever support is needed, children are videotaped giving themselves orientation to their therapy program, specific instructions, and a model of improved performance. With such a video, children can do required exercises, avoid nagging from adults, see themselves as leaders, and practice simple executive function routines at the same time. Furthermore, the process of developing the exercise video with a therapist can itself be a motivating executive system activity. This is one of the many ways in which members of the physical restoration team (e.g., physical and occupational therapists) can play a pivotal role in relation to cognitive and executive system goals.

ROUTINES FOR DEALING WITH CHANGES IN ROUTINE: COGNITIVE FLEXIBILITY

Frontal lobe injury, like early childhood, is associated with a relatively intense need for routine and with difficulty in accepting deviation from routine and failure to meet expectations. Attempts to train flexibility with decontextualized training tasks are often disappointing in their outcome. A more promising approach for people of any age with severe inflexibility is to establish acceptable "meta-routines" to deal with those times when routines must be broken or expectations cannot be met. Parents of young children understand this principle when they routinely prepare their children in advance for disappointments (e.g., losing the first Little League game) and promise them a positive alternative if they manage to maintain their composure in the face of disappointment.

Children with frontal lobe injury may need meta-routines that are more concrete and consistent than normal parent-child routines. For example, we have encouraged parents to create a choice board that lists desirable activities negotiated with the child. The meta-routine is then to take the child to the choice board so that the announcement of disappointing news or of a threatening change in routine is followed immediately by the child's choice of a desirable activity.[82] Implementation of this principle requires creativity in individual cases. However, for reasons presented earlier, this procedure is preferable to waiting for and then reacting to the child's response. As with other aspects of cognitive and behavioral development, the expectation is that this behavioral routine will gradually be internalized as covert self-regulatory activity that enables the child to negotiate unpredictable or disappointing events. However, even if the child is slow to internalize the self-regulatory routine, implementing the meta-routine script has the effect of reducing anxiety for the child, parents, and teachers.

TRANSITIONAL AND SELF-ADVOCACY VIDEOS

Table 22–5 presents a rationale and protocol for transitional and self-advocacy videos. The primary purpose of such videos is to provide children with a concrete and personally meaningful context in which to learn about their own strengths and needs and to take increasing responsibility for managing their own rehabilitation or special education. In summary, the children, with whatever help is necessary, make a statement about themselves, including strengths and interests, and also provide guidance for adults in how best to manage and teach them. This supported process of children teaching adults how to teach the child is unusual and reverses normal practices. However, there is great value in the message to the child—namely, that it is important to understand yourself and to take responsibility for helping others understand your needs. Collaborative and mutually respectful relationships with parents are also facilitated when the parents are involved in the development of the self-advocacy video. If the child is incapable of presenting himself or herself on video, a parent can make the presentation. It can be followed by short segments illustrating how best to teach, interact with, and manage the child.

Useful times for development of self-advocacy videos include transitions from rehabilitation to school and from one level of education to another. In our experience, institutionalizing this practice creates a culture in which professionals and other adults come to have appropriate sensitivity to the need for children's growth in the area of executive functions and ways to facilitate this growth. Furthermore, preparation of such a video helps professionals focus on *the child's* long-range goals and work through conflicts that may exist within the professional team. Ylvisaker and Feeney[81] illustrated the application of self-advocacy videos to adult brain injury rehabilitation.

EVERYDAY ORGANIZATIONAL ROUTINES

The section on executive function routines included the general outline of a goal-plan-do-review routine used to organize the day and any challenging activity over the course of the day. Organized people tend to implement such routines automatically (e.g., "What do I want to accomplish? How am I going to accomplish it? How did it turn out? What worked? What didn't work? What am I going to try next time?"). People with organizational impairment after TBI often need these organizational components of tasks made explicit as daily routines that are represented in a concrete way. In addition, the organization of specific tasks may need to be made explicit as part of a contextualized attempt to help children acquire or reacquire organizing schemes (knowledge structures) and, more important, to use these organizing schemes to guide their thinking, talking, and acting.

It is also critical for adults to help disorganized children by thematically integrating ac-

---

TABLE 22–5. Self-Advocacy Video: Transition/End-of-Year Routine

As part of an overall school focus on executive functions, it is recommended that children with disability, working collaboratively with staff and parents, create a videotape that has as its primary purpose to orient and train staff in how to teach, help, treat, and otherwise work with the student.

Goals

A. **Primary Goal: For Future Staff.** As part of their orientation to a new student, staff will have a video-tape that illustrates important aspects of the student's functioning in relation to teaching and class-room management (or anything else that would be useful to illustrate).

B. **For the Student.** The student will:
   1. Gain a sense of empowerment and control
   2. Gain progressively more insight into his or her strengths and needs
   3. Progressively become more strategic in relation to achieving success in his or her school career

C. **For the Parents.** Parents will:
   1. Gain a sense of empowerment
   2. Gain progressively more insight into their child's strengths and needs and also will share their insights with staff
   3. Gain an appreciation of the importance of executive functions and the student's participation in goal setting, planning, and strategic thinking

D. **For Current Staff.** Current staff will:
   1. Improve their collaborative relationships with other team members
   2. Gain greater appreciation for the perspective of students and parents

Procedures

A. At least 4–6 wk before the end of the school year (or other transitional time), staff, student, and parents begin to **plan the transitional video.** This could be done during a face-to-face meeting or through questionnaires. The purposes of this initial exploration are:
   1. To decide what **content** would be most important to demonstrate on video. It could include:
      a. **Physical** strengths, weaknesses, and management issues (e.g., seating, positioning, mobility, dressing, eating)
      b. **Cognitive** strengths, weaknesses, and management issues (e.g., What kind of advance organizers does the student need? What kind of environmental or materials modifications may be needed because of attentional, perceptual, or other processing problems? What kind of cues and prompts does the student need?)
      c. **Communication** strengths, weaknesses, and management issues (e.g., use of an augmentative communication system, demonstration of communication styles that facilitate comprehension)
      d. **Behavioral/social** strengths, weaknesses, and management issues (e.g., procedures for preventing behavior problems, ways to diffuse behavioral outbursts, ways to facilitate peer interaction)

It is critical that **strengths** be highlighted and that the **students' and parents' goals** be highlighted. This meeting could be part of an individualized education plan (IEP) meeting or standard parent conference. Alternatively, it could be a separate meeting.

   2. To decide what **format and scripts** would be most effective in demonstrating critical points:
      a. It is often effective to show the student (1) succeeding at a task that he or she is good at, (2) failing at an important but difficult task when appropriate procedures, modifications, or equipment are *not* in place, and then (3) succeeding when those procedures, modifications, or equipment are in place.
      b. It is often effective to communicate content by means of a **conversation** between student and staff or between staff and parents—as opposed to simply videotaping a "talking head."
      c. It is ideal to videotape the student's own orientation to and commentary about the video segments and then edit these into the tape as orientation for the viewer. This videotaping can be made after the student has watched the other segments.
   3. To decide **who should play what role** in the video. If possible, the student should play a leading role. This may require considerable support.
   4. To work out **logistics.**

The student and parents may be more or less involved in this planning, depending on many factors.

B. During the following month or so, the students can be engaged in planning this video project in many of their therapies and instructional sessions. For example, development of scripts can be part of language arts of speech-language therapy; development of presentation of strengths and needs can be part of counseling sessions; development of physical demonstrations can be part of PT, OT, ST, and other therapies; development of instructional demonstrations can be part of instructional sessions; summaries of performance data can be part of math class.
   1. Alternatively, if staff believe that these therapy and instructional times would not be wisely spent in these preparation activities, the video could be less carefully planned and still serve a useful purpose.

TABLE 22–5. *Continued*

C. The actual videotaping can be a simple matter of setting a camera up in a therapy or instructional session and proceeding with the demonstration. If other students are present, they must have signed releases. Ideally, the video will be edited (if staff have time and two VCRs). However, this is not necessary.

Advantages of this end-of-the-year or transitional routine

1. **Incidental learning: Student.** The student acquires important information about herself or himself and about her or his program by being engaged in a fun, product-oriented activity.
2. **Incidental learning: Staff.** Staff members acquire important information about the student, family, and their own program by being engaged in a fun, product-oriented activity.
3. **Incidental learning: Parents.** Parents acquire important information about the student and the program by being engaged in a fun, product-oriented activity.
4. **Efficient, nonthreatening, nonpunishing training and orientation:** Staff currently working with the child may learn important things without the stigma associated with being singled out for remedial instruction.
5. **Development of a shared conceptual framework:** The team refines its own shared conceptual framework by being engaged in a fun, product-oriented activity.
6. **Fun:** This can actually be fun.
7. **Permanent record:** If this practice becomes an annual routine, the student and family have an invaluable permanent record of the student's educational history.
8. **Student and parent satisfaction:** In general, student and parents are very pleased when staff accord them the respect that is implicit in this activity. Indeed, this can be a vehicle for overcoming an adversarial relationship if that exists.

Source: From Ylvisaker, M, Szekeres, S, and Feeney, T: Cognitive rehabilitation: Executive functions. In Ylvisaker, M (ed): Traumatic Brain Injury Rehabilitation: Children and Adolescents. Butterworth-Heinemann, Newton, Mass, 1998, with permission.

tivities over the course of the day and from day to day. Clearly, this thematic organization must make sense to the child so that he or she sees how events in life are connected. Thematic integration of activities is a staple of preschool and elementary education. Unfortunately, rehabilitation hospitals often fail to create obvious organization (from the child's perspective) from activity to activity and from day to day and thereby contribute to fragmentation and confusion rather than integration and orientation. This organizational mandate requires creativity and teamwork from the staff to ensure that what the child does in one therapy not only relates in obvious ways to what he or she did yesterday and will do tomorrow in tha therapy but also to what the child is doing at that time in other therapies and in the evening with family members. Clearly, there are limits to this organizational theme. However, staff should always ask themselves, "Do the activities in this child's life hang together in some meaningful way? If not, we need to make life more obviously and meaningfully organized." Furthermore, regular reviews of daily activities (supported with an efficient log or memory book system) help disorganized children maintain an anchor in the real world and understand connections among events in their lives. Ylvisaker et al.[67] developed these organizational themes in greater detail.

CONVERSATIONAL ROUTINES AND SOCIALLY COCONSTRUCTED NARRATIVES: COGNITIVE ORGANIZATION, LANGUAGE ORGANIZATION, AND AUTOBIOGRAPHICAL MEMORY

Recent research in developmental cognitive psychology has highlighted the usefulness of parent-child conversations about the past as the ideal context within which to promote the child's development of thought organization, language organization, and autobiographical memory.[70–74] Parents who take time to conversationally construct narratives about past experiences in a way that is both collaborative (e.g., "We will do this together; I am not making you perform for me; I enjoy chatting with you") and elaborative (e.g., "I will show you how to maintain topics and organize your thoughts in interesting ways") tend to have children who are effective at organizing their thoughts, organizing their expressive discourse, and remembering the past. Effective parents show their children how to think and talk and remember in an organized way, much as a master craftsperson shows an apprentice how to produce a beautiful piece of furniture. The product is an extended and organized narrative; the tools are the competencies associated with collaborative and elaborative style of conversational interaction. Ylvisaker et al.[87] described these conversational routines and listed the competencies associated with a collaborative and elaborative interactive style. The thesis that cognitive skills such as thought and language organization have their basis in interactive routines is analogous to the older and generally accepted hypothesis that conversational skills have their basis in prelinguistic interactive routines such as adult-child communication games,[69] with both the earlier and the later developmental phenomena supporting Yvgotsky's general hypothesis that cognitive skills are internalizations of social-interactive routines.

Unfortunately, many professionals adopt an unhelpful performance-oriented, directive, and nonelaborative style in interacting with children with cognitive disability. Similarly, parents, whose natural interactive style may be collaborative and elaborative, often move toward a less positive and less helpful style when their child has an acquired cognitive disability. Therefore, there is value in knowledgeable professionals helping parents and other everyday people acquire or reacquire the competencies associated with an elaborative and collaborative manner of conversing and encouraging them to engage the child as frequently as possible in such conversations. The goals of these positive conversational routines include the child's greater willingness to talk about and think about the past, acquisition or reacquisition of internal organizing schemes with which to organize thoughts, and growing use of those schemes in talking about events in an organized way. Ylvisaker et al.[67] presented a case that illustrated the effectiveness of this indirect, parent-focused approach to cognitive rehabilitation. In inpatient settings, nurses, child life staff, and others should possess the same interactive competencies and actively seek opportunities to socially coconstruct narratives with the child.

ORGANIZATIONAL ROUTINES AND EXTERNAL SUPPORT

Children with pronounced cognitive weakness profit from concrete external organizers that, in effect, give them a map for traveling through complex and potentially confusing conceptual territory. For example, the socially coconstructed narratives described in the previous section are facilitated by a sequence of photographs representing the events to be worked into the narrative. In addition, daily schedules should be represented as concretely as needed (e.g., a sequence of photographs for very concrete children); daily living tasks and household chores may need to be supported with easy to follow flow charts or photographs; expressive discourse tasks are easier to accomplish with a visual guide; reading comprehension may be facilitated with advance questions or other advance organizers. Ylvisaker et al.[67] described and illustrated a variety of advance organizers designed to meet this goal for children and adolescents with TBI. The general point is that many children with brain injury have organizational impairment and therefore require support that is much more concrete than might initially be suspected. In the absence of such support, the likely outcome is failure, followed by negative behavioral responses.[5]

EVERYDAY POSITIVE BEHAVIORAL ROUTINES

In a positive approach to behavior, the intervention targets are not negative behaviors targeted for extinction (e.g., hitting, yelling, refusing) but rather positive behaviors targeted for increases in frequency. Staff and family members work to increase the frequency of positive behavior and promote success as opposed to reacting to negative behavior. Training efforts focus primarily on teaching positive communication behaviors and preventing negative behavior. In addition, competence in crisis management is essential. However, managing crises and promoting positive behavior are considered entirely separate issues.[58,88–90]

The rationale for a positive, antecedent-focused approach to behavior management after TBI has pathophysiological, developmental, empirical, and general cultural components. First, from a pathophysiological perspective, the combination of orbital-prefrontal and ventromedial-prefrontal injury raises serious questions about the effectiveness of behavior management that focuses primarily on manipulation of consequences (i.e., rewards such as tokens for desirable behavior; punishment, time-out, or ignoring for undesirable behavior). Orbital prefrontal injury, if severe, can result in neurologically based disinhibition that makes it very difficult for the child to act on the basis of rules learned through consequences. In this respect, an individual with orbital prefrontal injury may be much like preschoolers, who know intellectually that it is important to share with peers but who cannot control the impulse to take more than their share in the real world of competing children.

Ventromedial prefrontal injury has only recently been explored in relation to behavioral self-regulation.[91,92] Studies of adults with selective lesions in this part of the brain suggest that they often fail to encode "somatic markers" along with the intellectual or dispositional representations that they store in memory as a result of their experiences. These somatic markers are believed to guide future behavior as a result of feedback from past experiences. For example, consistently losing at a game of chance leads most neurologically intact people to recognize that they cannot win and to therefore quit the game. In contrast, individuals with ventromedial prefrontal injury may understand with equal clarity that the game is unwinnable but continue to bet nonetheless, unable to explain why they are persisting; that is, the failure to add a somatic marker to the stored representation of the experience results in, at best, inefficient practical learning from feedback.

Combining these two loci of prefrontal damage (common in closed head injury) presents the clinical picture of an individual who can learn rules or remember them from before the injury, state the rules, and role play appropriate behavior in structured training contexts but who nevertheless behaves in ways that are unacceptable to others in real-world contexts—without intending to be oppositional. This status is consistent with the "riddle of the frontal lobes" described 30 years ago by Teuber—that is, "the curious dissociation between knowing and doing."[93] Behavior management focused primarily on manipulation of consequences is clearly ill advised for this group of people.

Second, placing the consequences of prefrontal injury in a developmental context yields great insight for behavior management. For example, although toddlers are clearly able to learn from experience, parents do not control their behavior primarily by manipulating consequences. To take an obvious example, parents do not eliminate priceless-crystal-vase-breaking behavior by praising the toddler who refrains from breaking the vase and, conversely, reprimanding the toddler who engages in vase-breaking behavior. Rather, understanding the child's impulsiveness and difficulty in following rules, parents simply remove the vase; that is, they eliminate the provocation for the unwanted behavior. In addition, they prepare the child for stressful activities. They try to make sure the child is in a good mood before presenting disappointing news or stressful tasks, they do not present the child with tasks that are too difficult, and they patiently coach the child to use words rather than obnoxious behavior to obtain what he or she wants. These common-sense, proactive, or antecedent-focused behavior management procedures are instinctively used by parents who understand the limited self-regulatory skill of very young children. Unfortunately, professionals working with older children with poorly regulated behavior

after TBI often neglect these simple but critically important procedures and opt instead for typically inefficient contingency management.

Third, experimental studies of individuals with developmental disabilities and behavioral disorders that do not have a neurological basis have established the effectiveness of giving choices,[94] ensuring positive setting events,[95] generating positive behavioral momentum,[96] providing alternative scripts,[97] and teaching communication alternatives to challenging behavior.[56,57] Feeney and Ylvisaker[5] provided experimental support for a combination of these antecedent-control procedures for adolescents with frontal lobe injury whose behavior had deteriorated badly over several years after their injuries.

Fourth, behavior management that emphasizes teaching positive behaviors and preventing negative behaviors contributes to a culture that is far more positive than one in which behavior programs emphasize procedures for reacting to challenging behavior. For example, when the goal is to reduce aggression (versus increase acceptable communication) and staff are authorized to use confrontational and provocative procedures with aggressive children, including physical restraints, the frequency of negative interaction between staff and child tends to escalate, and relationships with that child tend to deteriorate.[88,89]

POSITIVE BEHAVIORAL ROUTINES: ANTECEDENT APPROACHES TO BEHAVIOR MANAGEMENT

Positive Setting Events

Setting events are internal physiological and psychological states that influence an individual's response to stressful or difficult tasks, as well as the temporally distant events and environmental conditions that influence those internal states. Negative setting events in the case of a person with TBI often include (1) internal physiological states such as an overaroused limbic system, pain, and illness; (2) cognitive states such as confusion and disorientation; (3) emotional states such as anger, fear, depression, sense of loss, and frustration over lack of control; (4) perception or misperception of task difficulty; and (5) environmental stressors (e.g., presence or absence of certain people and ambient noise). In the presence of uniformly negative setting events, even mildly irritating or stressful stimuli can provoke seriously negative behavioral responses. In contrast, when setting events are uniformly positive (e.g., the individual is relaxed, comfortable, well oriented to surroundings and to the task at hand, confident of success, and feeling in control), the same level of demand is more likely to be met with positive and socially appropriate behavior.

The tradition in applied behavior analysis tended to avoid setting events on grounds that unobservable, internal states are not possible to measure or control. Increasingly, however, behavioral psychologists have recognized the importance of setting events[95,98,99] and have added attempts to control these events to the procedural armamentarium of behavior management.

Choice and Control

Life after brain injury is frequently dominated by externally imposed restrictions on physical and social activity, by overprotectiveness on the part of professionals and family members, and by a conviction that the individual is not capable of making responsible decisions. The need for control, particularly in the case of adolescents who were growing accustomed to increasing autonomy before their injury, commonly precipitates negative interaction between adults and individuals with TBI. When adults fail to create adequate opportunities for choice and control and, in contrast, engage in unnecessary battles over control, the child or adolescent is more likely to use challenging behavior as a means of acquiring some semblance of control over life. Unwary parents and professionals may then allow this conflict to escalate into the classic negative cycle of control, with ever-growing restrictions on behavior resulting in over-escalating negative behavior.[100]

Harchik et al.'s[94] review of more than 100 studies of the effects of choice making on behavior in individuals with developmental disabilities showed that, for that population, choice and control can (1) increase the individual's level of participation, (2) decrease the frequency of problem behaviors during participation, and (3) improve subjective ratings of the activity. Our experience suggests that these findings apply at least equally to children and adolescents with TBI.[5,101] Therefore, systems should be in place in rehabilitation hospitals, schools, and homes that create as many opportunities for choice and control as possible. Fortunately, this component of positive behavior management reinforces the everyday approach to executive function routines described earlier—that is, when everyday activities begin with a brief negotiation of a plan (i.e., an executive function routine) and that plan can easily contain some components of the child's choosing (i.e., a positive behavior management routine), both designed to promote the sense of control necessary for re-creation of a productive sense of self after brain injury.

Positive Behavioral Momentum

A recent history of positive and successful behavior increases the likelihood of subsequent positive and successful behavior, particularly if the backlog of successes is associated with tasks similar to the newly presented task. Conversely, a recent history of negative and unsuccessful behavior increases the likelihood of subsequent negative and resistive behavior.[96,102–104] This important behavioral principle captures the everyday observation that people who face a challenging task from the background of a rich history of success on similar tasks are likely to accept the challenge, work hard, and succeed. Because people with recent brain injury understandably carry with them a history of uninterrupted failure, *based on standards applicable to their preinjury profile of abilities,* the principle of positive behavioral momentum necessitates intensive and creative efforts from staff and family members. It is typically not enough to give the child extremely easy tasks or dramatically lower standards and then say, "Good job, have a sticker." Rather, adults should create systems of support so that the child can succeed at meaningful tasks, which increases the likelihood of engagement in future demanding tasks and decreases the likelihood of challenging behavior as a means of escape or expression of frustration.

Advance Organizers

In the section on organizational routines, we highlighted the importance of concrete advance organizers designed to help disorganized children successfully complete organizationally demanding tasks and to facilitate internalization of knowledge structures. It is also useful to think of advance organizers as antecedent-control behavioral procedures. If challenging behavior is a response to confusion, frustration, and ultimate failure, then appropriate help to succeed—and succeed independently—is a critical component of behavior management. For example, in the behavioral intervention described by Feeney and Ylvisaker,[5] adolescents with aggressive behavior after TBI were initially given concrete, photograph advance organizers because their organizational impairment was found to be a major contributor to their escalating behavior. This successful behavioral intervention serves as an excellent illustration of the need to integrate behavioral and cognitive rehabilitation after TBI.

Positive Behavioral Scripts

The life of a child with severe TBI is often dominated by activities that are chosen by others and that do not enable the child to excel or demonstrate special expertise. Under these circumstances, the implicit *role* choices are (1) to comply and try to succeed at (often difficult) tasks chosen by others or (2) to oppose and be defiant. Given these options, many young people with TBI, particularly adolescents who may have been somewhat oppositional before the injury, choose to be oppositional and defiant.

In an earlier section, we highlighted the importance of choice in preventing the negative control cycle. A second strategy for combating oppositional behavior is to give the child a desirable role that is associated with a script that is positive and incompatible with oppositional behavior. For example, in a rehabilitation hospital, children can be given simple but important jobs, like lunch assistant, group leader, and "buddy" for a newly admitted patient. Simple helper jobs in school include line leader, lunch counter, messenger, and scribe. It is particularly useful for these positive roles to include a helping dimension. Children with TBI are so consistently at the receiving end of help that it is easy for them to begin thinking of themselves as helpless or as victims and to retain a thoroughly egocentric perspective on life that often goes with being the constant recipient of others' help. To foster development of a more positive sense of self, children with adequate cognitive recovery can be engaged (with whatever support is necessary) in helping others.

When children return to school, this practice might continue by exploiting their expertise in brain injury, rehabilitation, and the like. For example, children with brain injury might assist the health teacher in teaching a curriculum on brains and injury prevention. Some children understandably react negatively to this ongoing focus on their injury and therefore resist such offers. The general point, however, is that staff and family should explore a variety of positive roles that the child might play, roles associated with scripts requiring positive behavior and roles that might be emotionally satisfying for children whose lives have been turned upside down by the injury.

Other Antecedent Approaches

People who remain extremely impulsive after frontal lobe injury may require ongoing "child-proofing" procedures—that is, elimination of predictable provocations for problem behavior. For example, adolescent boys who are both disinhibited and hypersexual may need to be educated in environments in which there are few young women and the women in the environment follow conservative rules about dress and physical proximity. For some students, system-

atic desensitization combined with relaxation exercises decreases the likelihood of challenging behavior. Self-instructing and self-monitoring can be taught to some children by means of frequently repeated scripts. Others may need ongoing orientation to the natural sequence of events associated with the current activity. In all of these approaches, the theme remains the same. What can be done before children act to ensure that they will behave positively versus how should we respond to the child's behavior, whether it is positive or negative?

POSITIVE COMMUNICATION
ROUTINES: COMMUNICATION
AND BEHAVIOR

Communication approaches to challenging behavior are based on the following premises:

1. All behaviors (including the apparent absence of behavior) communicate. Of course, not all behavior is deliberately or intentionally communicative. However, just as intentional communication in infants develops, in part, as a function of adults' responses to their preintentional communication, so also the use of negative behavior to communicate can evolve as a function of adults' responses to behavior that is initially reflexive, neurologically driven, or purely impulsive after brain injury.

2. There are very few truly maladaptive behaviors. When children persist in behaviors that others consider objectionable, it is reasonable to assume that the behavior is adaptive; that is, it is helping the child to achieve some goal.

3. If challenging behavior is used to communicate important messages, the primary focus of intervention is to teach communication alternatives to those challenging behaviors, not to simply extinguish the challenging behavior with no positive alternative.

4. The primary agents of intervention are everyday communication partners.

5. The primary goal is to modify communication routines, beginning with the behavior of communication partners, so that the child's most positive communication behaviors become routine.[57,101]

In its simplest form, the process of teaching communication alternatives has the following phases:

Phase 1: Collaboratively interpret challenging behavior.

Unwanted behavior is often used (consciously or subconsciously) to escape (e.g., a person, place, activity, or demand), to gain access (e.g., to a person, others' attention, a thing, a place, an activity), or to simply to express feelings (e.g., angry, frustrated, happy, excited, frightened). Substituting an acceptable communication alternative requires communication partners to know the meaning of the child's challenging behavior. Identifying this meaning may require collaborative hypothesis testing like that described earlier, sensitive to the fact that a specific behavior may have different meanings or intents on different occasions.

Phase 2: Collaboratively decide when escape and access are acceptable.

Assuming that the unwanted behavior is used (consciously or subconsciously) to communicate escape or access, staff and family members must collaboratively decide under what circumstances the child's communication alternatives are acceptable; that is, when is it acceptable for children to escape what they do not want and gain access to what they want. With the short-term goal of creating as many natural and significant teaching opportunities as possible, staff should agree to a wide domain of such circumstances early in training. Little progress will be made if the goal is to teach the child to say no or sign "stop" rather than hit as an escape signal and then therapists and others do not honor the refusal on grounds that their therapies are too important to disrupt.

At this phase of teaching, *battles must be chosen wisely.* For example, if a decision is made not to allow the child to escape physical therapy (however briefly), then staff must persevere in the face of possibly escalating behavior. The worst outcome is achieved if staff or family members allow themselves to be drawn into power struggles that they eventually lose. Such struggles are illustrated by the following exchange:

ADULT: Time for exercises.

CHILD: No (communicated in some way)

ADULT: Sorry, it's time for your exercises!

CHILD: No! No! No!

ADULT: We are going to do 10 exercises!

CHILD: Throws self on floor, hits, pulls hair, spits

ADULT: You are out of control now. You will need to spend some time in the time-out room to cool down. We will talk later about your exercises.

Communication routines of this sort teach a powerful lesson: Go directly to challenging behavior if you want to escape a demand! Clearly negative routines of this sort and the lessons that they teach must be avoided. The best way to avoid them is to train staff to engage in positive routines of the sort illustrated in Table 22–4.

Phase 3: Collaboratively ensure large numbers of positive communication routines daily.

Table 22–6 presents four illustrations of communication routines in which the child uses positive communication behaviors to communicate escape or access, either spontaneously or following a prompt. The goal of intervention at this phase is to ensure a large number of these positive routines in many communication contexts daily. A goal of 100 or more positive communication routines daily is desirable because children readily establish negative communication routines if the ratio of successful positive routines to successful negative routines is not high. Videotaping positive communication routines enables all everyday communication partners to see exactly what these routines look like. Using family members as the positive models in these training videos communicates respect and provides functional training for them at the same time.

Figure 22–2 illustrates a simple form that can be used to collect data about the communication and behavior program and also to provide general orientation to staff about the approach. We often photocopy illustrations of positive communication routines (Table 22–6) on the back side of the data collection form.

Phase 4: Gradually reintroduce normal demands.

The intensive teaching phase (phase 3) may last from a few days to many months for children with deeply habituated negative communication routines. Reintroducing normal demands—that is, decreasing the frequency with which requests for escape or access are honored—must occur in an environment in which the behavioral principles described earlier are implemented. If (1) the principles of positive setting events, choice, and positive behavioral momentum are not respected, (2) children are routinely expected to succeed at tasks beyond their level of ability, or (3) the positive communication alternative is inefficient or ineffective, then the child can be expected to return to challenging behavior as a means to escape undesirable situations or access desirable situations.

TABLE 22–6. Illustrations of Positive Communication Routines for Jon

Escape: Contrived communication situations

Context: Math instruction; assume that math is currently not a high priority and is not a desired activity.

ADULT: Here's your math book, Jon.
JON: (Looks unhappy, but hasn't yet acted.)
ADULT: It looks like you don't want to do this now. Here, show me "no" [or "break" or whatever].
JON: (Is prompted to use positive communication alternative.)
ADULT: OK! Thanks for telling me! Let's not do it now. We can come back to it later. It's great that you tell me that way that you don't want to do this. Let's do (*or* show me what you would like to do for a few minutes).

This teaching sequence could be repeated several times during a 20- or 30-min scheduled math period.

Escape: Natural communication situations

Context: Teacher wants Jon to carry his lunchbox as he walks down the hall.

ADULT: Here Jon, carry your lunch box.
JON: (Reacts negatively but does not yet fall to the floor or engage in any other negative communication.)
ADULT: I bet you don't want to carry the box, do you? Why don't you tell me no.
JON: (Is prompted to use positive communication alternative.)
ADULT: Oh! All right! I see you want me to carry it. Thanks for telling me so nicely. Of course I'll carry it when you ask like that.

Access: Contrived communication situation

Context: Jon is with other students and clearly wants to get a peer to interact with him. The peer has been alerted to respond when Jon uses the positive communication alternative.

ADULT: Jon, I bet you would like to talk with Tim. Why don't you tell him?
ADULT: (Prompts the positive communication alternative.)
JON: (Uses the positive communication alternative.)
PEER: (Responds to Jon's positive communication alternative.) Oh, hi, Jon. I didn't see you. Thanks for letting me know you want to talk.

Access: Natural communication situations

Context: Jon is at home, and it is time for him to do something he likes to do (e.g., watch TV).

ADULT: Jon, I wonder what you want to do. I bet you would like to watch TV. Can you let me know?"
ADULT: (Prompts the positive communication alternative.)
JON: (Uses the positive communication alternative.)
ADULT: (Responds to Jon's positive communication alternative.) OK, great, here's the remote. Thanks for telling me that you wanted to watch TV.

OBSTACLES TO SUCCESS

Success in teaching communication alternatives to challenging behavior often requires overcoming five natural obstacles to this approach:

1. Staff members' refusal to participate on grounds that their own goals for the child are too important to disrupt. Therapists and teachers often take their work seriously and therefore respond skeptically to the suggestion that they teach a child acceptable ways to escape their intervention. However, this obstacle can often be overcome by pointing out:

☐ That their current intervention may already be inefficient because of challenging behavior and may become much more efficient if the behavior is brought under control

☐ That honoring appropriate escape communication is compatible with returning to the activity after a short break

☐ That challenging behavior must be considered a priority because of its potentially devastating long-term effects on the developing life of the child

2. Staff or family members' fears that children will become thoroughly spoiled, escape what they want to escape, and acquire what they want to acquire. This natural objection is best met with the seemingly cavalier but accurate reply that the intervention, if appropriately implemented, will not have the effect of creating an "escape monster" or an "acquisition monster."[57] Routinely honoring escape and access communication is only the first phase of the teaching, and it is followed

Illustrations of Jon's Positive Communications:
ACCESS: reach, point, vocalize pleasantly, tap another's arm, point to picture/symbol, gesture/sign, _____,

_____, _____, _____

ESCAPE: shake head or hand "no", gesture "break" or "no", Say or sign "finished", _____, _____,

_____, _____

KEY:

A+S = access, positive communication, spontaneous	E+S = escape, positive communication, spontaneous
A+C = access, positive communication, cued/prompted	E+C = escape, positive communication, cued/prompted
A- = access, negative communication	E- = escape, negative communication

CHOICE: It is ACCEPTABLE for John to access or escape an activity, place, person, or demand.
NO CHOICE: It is NOT acceptable for John to access or escape an activity, place, person, or demand.

	CHOICE SITUATIONS					NO CHOICE SITUATIONS				
	A+S	A+C	A--	E+S	E+C	E--	Comply	Resist <1 min	Resist >1min	
Home AM										
Bus										
School #1										
School #2										
School #3										
School #4										
School #5										
School #6										
School #7										
School #8										
Home Pre Dinner										
Dinner										
HomePost Dinner										

FIGURE 22–2. Communication and behavior data collection form.

by a return to normal demands, ensuring appropriate sensitivity to the principles of positive setting events, positive behavioral momentum, and choice (described earlier) so that the child has little reason to resort to challenging behavior.

3. Staff or family members' response that there are times when escape or access is simply out of the question. For example, certain activities that the child would like to escape (e.g., taking medications) may be nonnego-

tiable. The appropriate script for these times includes preparing the child in advance (e.g., positive setting events, positive behavioral momentum), identifying the activity in question as a "no choice" activity, and proceeding through the activity as quickly and painlessly as possible while ignoring the child's challenging behavior.

4. Staff members' refusal to participate on grounds that behavior management is not their professional responsibility. Most professionals who work with children with brain injury understand that behavior management is everybody's responsibility. Behavior specialists must work patiently with staff and family members who do not understand so that they realize that challenging behavior will likely worsen unless all everyday communication partners work within the same general approach to communication and behavior.

5. Staff and family members' difficulty with timing, which thereby inadvertently reinforces unwanted behavior. A dangerous situation arises when staff and family members agree to honor appropriate escape and access communication but fail to respond before appropriate communication turns into challenging behavior, which is then unwisely rewarded with escape or access. Timing is critical. Training for staff and family members often includes clearly written scripts of positive communication routines (see Table 22–6), video illustrations of both positive models (to be imitated) and negative models (to be avoided) of interaction with the child, and, if necessary, situational coaching to improve timing.[105]

CRISIS MANAGEMENT

We have described a positive approach to behavior management designed to teach and promote positive behavior and to prevent negative behavior. Inevitably, times come in the lives of children with brain injury (and all other children) when positive behaviors are not yet well established and preventive efforts fail. The first line of reaction, particularly with children who are impulsive and possibly perseverative, is redirection. Simply ignoring behavior, when there is a threat of perseveration or escalation, is a mistake. Redirection (i.e., breaking the child's psychological set and reengaging him or her in ways that eliminate the behavioral provocation) can be effective in preventing escalation and avoiding crises. However, if redirection involves removing the child from a difficult or stressful activity (e.g., difficult physical therapy exercises) and engaging him in a desirable activity (e.g., eating chocolate ice cream), then it runs the risk of reinforcing and thereby increasing the likelihood of the original challenging behavior. Staff and family members must acquire the critical competency of redirecting the child *without reinforcing challenging behavior*.

When prevention and redirection both fail and problem behavior escalates into a crisis, the primary goal is to survive the crisis, keep everybody safe, and use a minimum of forceful restraint. Crisis management procedures and competencies are described in a variety of texts and manuals.[58] The important point here is simply that *crisis management is not behavior management, and times of crisis are not teaching times.* Staff and family members must avoid the temptation to "teach lessons," punish, or otherwise respond defensively during behavioral crises.

PREVENTION OF LONG-TERM BEHAVIOR PROBLEMS BY USING POSITIVE ANTECEDENT APPROACHES AND SUPPORTED COGNITION

Feeney and Ylvisaker[5] described a combined behavioral and cognitive intervention that successfully reversed a downward spiral of aggressive behavior in three adolescents whose behavior had deteriorated over several years after frontal lobe injury in early adolescence. All three students not only completed their educational programs but also, at follow-up, were employed and living independently. Although this intervention was successful, the main lesson to be derived is that the procedures used to intervene in severe and long-standing behavioral situations could have been used to prevent the challenging behavior from evolving in the first place. In addition to the antecedent behavior management procedures described in this section, prevention requires creative use of cognitive supports, including those described in the sections on executive system routines and organizational routines. Our current work with students with TBI and their staff members suggests that, in most cases, preventive efforts based on these principles have a positive outcome.

□ SENSORIMOTOR ASSESSMENT AND INTERVENTION

Critical Aspects of Pediatric Physical Rehabilitation

Elsewhere in this text, intervention for sensory and motor impairments following TBI in adults is discussed at length. Our primary goal in this section is to highlight dimensions of physical rehabilitation for children that necessitate special pediatric considerations. Virtually any combination of physical strengths and weaknesses is possible after TBI. Although cognitive and psychosocial problems tend to be more common than physical problems in this population, even an apparently minor physical disability can make a profound difference in the life of a child or adolescent because of the importance of physical appearance and prowess during these developmental years. This feature of childhood underscores the need for careful attention to mild deficits in coordination and speed[106] and for supportive counseling for those children and adolescents whose disability blocks return to activities that gave their lives meaning before the injury.

NEUROLOGICAL MATURATION AND PHYSICAL GROWTH

Children with TBI are injured during a time of neurological maturation and physical growth. From an assessment perspective, pediatric clinicians must have a clear understanding of age-related motor milestones against which to measure the effects of the child's injury. For example, reflexes that would indicate neurological dysfunction in older children and adults may be developmentally normal in infants. In addition, physical growth necessitates special planning for fitting a child for adaptive equipment and parceling out potentially limited funding over the developmental years. Equipment may need frequent adjustment and periodic replacement as the child grows and matures. Furthermore, long-term assessment and management must be sensitive to the possibility that mobility and orthopedic problems may worsen over time as the child grows, comes to have a higher center of gravity, and is required to exert greater force to remain upright against the increasing pull of gravity. Spasticity may also worsen as relatively larger muscles produce relatively greater resistance to passive stretch. Physical growth also increases the burden on caregivers, who may need increasing supports over the years after the injury. These developmental considerations are important not only for service providers but also for those responsible for managing resources for children injured during the developmental years.

GOALS OF PEDIATRIC PHYSICAL REHABILITATION

As with adults, central goals of physical rehabilitation for children include maximizing physical recovery and sensory and motor function in real-world activities and settings (possibly with compensatory equipment and procedures), while also reducing the burden on caregivers. For children, functional activities and real-world settings are different from those relevant to adults and may change over the course of development. For example, special attention must be paid to facilitating varied parent-child play activities for young children and to sports, social, educational, and vocational activities for older children. Therefore, pediatric rehabilitation pro-

grams should be designed to enable staff to assess and treat children in the context of activities and settings that are important for their specific age group. For example, a simulated classroom setting is useful for targeting functional mobility, fine motor function (e.g., handwriting), and communication (e.g., an augmentative communication device in the context of academic activities). Furthermore, it may be critical for therapists to have a flexible work schedule (e.g., begin and end their work day late one day every week) so that they can interact with parents who are available only in the evening and show them how to use developmentally appropriate activities to promote recovery of function and acquisition of new skills.

In contrast to adult rehabilitation, rehabilitation for children requires attention to achievement of new developmental milestones and acquisition of skills they did not possess before the injury. For example, treatment of infants and toddlers focuses on recovery of function, as well as acquisition of subsequent skills in normal developmental schedules (e.g., walking and talking in the case of children who did not do so before the injury). In this respect, goals of rehabilitation and habilitation merge.

In addition, the important goal of reducing caregiver burden is often more critical with severely injured children than with comparably injured adults. It is more common for family members to assume care of a child with very severe cognitive and motor impairment than is the case with adults with persistent severe impairment, who are often transferred from acute care to a long-term care facility.

Finally, facilitating an effective school reentry for children with physical disability requires specialized attention to the physical needs of children in school settings; to the types of intervention, equipment, and task and environment modifications needed for children to succeed in school; and to the training of school staff. In our era of managed care and dramatically shortened lengths of stay in rehabilitation hospitals, ensuring well-trained and well-supported family members and school staff is among the most important responsibilities of the acute rehabilitation team. For many clinicians, the changing professional climate requires a shift in professional role and self-image, from that of a person who primarily works directly with the patient to restore function to that of a person who is equally or even primarily a consultant to others (e.g., family members and school staff). The increased competence of those everyday people then puts them in the position to continue the child's rehabilitation indefinitely and in natural settings. This theme is developed by Ylvisaker and Feeney.[82]

ACTIVITIES USED IN PEDIATRIC REHABILITATION

In addition to preparing children to succeed in developmentally normal activities different from those of adults, clinicians also make use of different therapeutic activities. With young children, motivating play with toys should be a routine aspect of therapy sessions. In the case of older and fairly well-recovered children, it is wise to consider using natural, nonstigmatizing, and developmentally appropriate activities to achieve physical rehabilitation goals. For example, many physical restoration goals can be pursued in adaptive physical education class, therapeutic riding, art and dance classes, martial arts and swimming lessons, health club activities, coached vocational trials, and related activities, provided the staff in those settings are adequately oriented and trained. Similarly, choir, singing lessons, or a drama club may be a better choice than traditional speech therapy sessions as the context for ongoing voice and articulation therapy after acute rehabilitation. In addition to the increased motivation these activities afford, they may also yield natural occasions for social interaction and for ongoing assessment of the true functional limitations associated with the injury.

Assessment: Measurement of Outcome

To meet the need of payers, accreditors, and others for standardized, quantitative assessment of progress and outcome, adaptive behavior scales have been standardized for use with children, including the Wee Functional Independence Measure (Wee FIM)[107] and the Pediatric Evaluation of Disability Inventory (PEDI).[108] Functional measurement of progress and outcome should also include measures of performance and qualitative descriptions of activities that are particularly important to the child in question. For example, if specific chores on the family farm are central to the life of a child, functional rehabilitation should be oriented in part to successful performance of those chores, with measurement of that performance a critical indicator of success in rehabilitation. The functionality of rehabilitation tends to increase when the measurement of outcome includes function in tasks uniquely important to that child. Finally, because of the extreme importance of well-oriented and trained family members and school staff, an indicator of their level of preparedness to meet the child's ongoing needs after discharge should be included as a valid measure of the outcome of the rehabilitation program; that is, rehabilitation facilities should evaluate the success of their pediatric programs in part based on the competence of parents and school staff at the time of the child's discharge.

Assessment: Identifying Impairment and Planning Intervention

The key to assessment of children with brain injury for planning functional rehabilitation is to focus on the quality of movement and sensorimotor organization in relation to developmental expectations. Integration of sensory and motor systems, control over movement, the quality of those movements, and the way in which control is modified and augmented through therapeutic intervention form the foundation for the development of mature functional abilities. Developmental assessment identifies the components of movement that are prerequisites for acquiring functional, everyday skills. In the case of acquired brain injury, scattered sparing of functions may distinguish the assessment of these children from those with congenital neurological dysfunction. Parameters to be evaluated are:

- Range of motion
- Muscle tone
- Muscle length
- Reflexes
- Sensation (including visual, auditory, tactile, and vestibular sensation, proprioception, and kinesthesia)
- Posture
- Postural reflex mechanisms (righting, equilibrium, and protective reactions)
- Motor planning (praxis)

Assessment in each of these areas was discussed by Ylvisaker et al.[109] Consistent with a functional approach to treatment, assessment also includes observation and detailed description of motor functioning in the context of varied developmentally appropriate functional activities.

Intervention: Acute Care

As in the case of adults with TBI, physical rehabilitation of children begins during the acute phase of the injury at a time when medical stability and neurological condition are primary concerns. Responsible physicians and nurses must be consulted regarding necessary restrictions on the child's activity and stimulation, including the interventions of the physical restoration team, because of elevated intracranial pressure, fractures, or other injuries. These interventions are initially designed to prevent complications; to orient family members to appropriate stimulation activities from the perspective of physical, cognitive, and communication function; and to identify the possible need for services after discharge from acute care hospitalization. In general, early interventions provided to children are similar to those provided to adults. Positioning requirements may differ for young children, based on the relatively greater vulnerability of the occiput (versus sacrum in older children and adolescents) to pressure-related decubitus.

Intervention: Inpatient Rehabilitation

As with adults, the decision to transfer a child from acute care to inpatient rehabilitation is based in part on the child's medical condition, severity of the injury, and severity of physical and cognitive disability. However, because long-term beds for children are often unavailable, it is more common to refer children for active rehabilitation in the presence of severe cognitive and physical impairment and a guarded prognosis for functional improvement. The primary purpose of the admission may be to train family members and organize community supports so that the child can be cared for at home.

TEAM INTEGRATION: CONSIDERATION OF COGNITIVE AND PSYCHOSOCIAL FACTORS

Although team-based collaboration and integrated intervention are important for all age groups, they are particularly important for children. Children are less likely than adults to integrate their experiences and see the relation between one activity and another, which makes them vulnerable to confusion and the anxiety that confusion breeds. Furthermore, parents are often present during a child's therapies. A team-oriented approach also helps to reduce parents' confusion and thereby facilitate their acquisition of important competencies.

Following TBI, cognitive disability has a profound impact on physical functioning and physical intervention. Table 22–7 identifies cognitive deficits that are common after TBI and interventions that may be used by the physical rehabilitation team. Furthermore, members of the physical rehabilitation team may be in the best position to deliver the cognitive and behavioral interventions described earlier in this chapter. For example, because physical activities are concrete and important to children, the executive function routines described earlier may be most effectively employed during physical therapies. In addition, because physical rehabilitation activities are sometimes difficult, negative behaviors may emerge in these sessions, which are ideal occasions to use the positive, communication-based behavioral interventions described earlier. Table 22–8 illustrates a collaborative team approach to intervention, with joint physical therapy, occupational therapy, and speech therapy sessions as the focus of this collaboration.

SPECIFIC TYPES OF MOTOR DYSFUNCTION AND THEIR TREATMENT

Motor disorders, including rigidity, spasticity, flaccidity, ataxia, tremor, and apraxia, have similar presentations and treatment regimens in children and adults. Elsewhere in this text, a variety of specific interventions applicable to children and adults are described for each disorder.

Rigidity in all but the most severely injured children resolves over time, with attention to position and related primitive reflexes critical while rigidity is present.[110] Persisting spasticity is common after TBI in children. Interventions include passive range of motion, serial and inhibitory casts, functional activities designed to encourage normalization of tone and gains in strength and control, systemic medications, neurolytic blocks, and surgery (e.g., percutaneous tendo-Achilles lengthening). Because children in the early stages of cognitive recovery may become agitated with stretching, clever distraction may be necessary. Casting options for children (which may be accompanied by peripheral nerve blocks or motor point blocks) and medications to reduce spasticity are described by Russell et al.[111] Systemic medications, including dantrolene, diazepam, and baclofen, are used for children whose spasticity is sufficiently severe to interfere with positioning. Surgical intervention is generally not considered until at least 18 months postinjury.

Spasticity may create other problems for rehabilitative management, such as increased risk of malunion of long bone fractures. Comfort must be a critical consideration in prescribing external fixator devices (e.g., halo vest, Hoffman apparatus) for such injuries in young children. In addition, although heterotopic ossification occurs less frequently in children than in adults (especially if the child is under 10 years old), it is associated with severe spasticity in adolescents, particularly those in long-term coma. Deceptively elevated alkaline phosphatase levels occur in growing children and in patients who have sustained fractures. Treatment includes passive range of the affected joint to the point of

TABLE 22–7. Cognitive Interventions Commonly Used in Physical Rehabilitation

Area of Cognition	Possible Interfering Behavior	Possible Intervention
Attention/concentration	■ Becomes distracted; appears disinterested; interrupts frequently ■ Becomes agitated with excessive external stimulation ■ Is unable to complete tasks ■ Walks/looks away when talking	■ Provide high degree of structure; reduce environmental distractions ■ Treat in a quiet area; reduce length of sessions; redirect frequently ■ Give instructions in short, simple sentences; provide visual cues (e.g., photo routines) ■ Provide hand-over-hand guidance
Perception	■ Cannot identify common objects ■ Does not know what to do with common objects ■ Cannot locate objects within view ■ Does not understand verbal messages	■ Explore multimodality approach ■ Talk through the activity with the child ■ Have the child explore environment and objects with hands ■ Have the child visually scan the environment for cues; identify and use the child's optimum modality for processing information
Memory	■ Does not follow directions ■ Becomes disoriented ■ Forgets how and when to do daily tasks	■ Provide visual cues (e.g., photo cues or written cues) to guide the child through tasks ■ Use meaningful, familiar, functional objects, activities, and routines to achieve motor goals ■ Provide an easy-to-follow (e.g., photos) daily schedule; label areas (e.g., drawers) to facilitate independent activities of daily living; avoid nagging
Cognitive organization	■ Says ideas out of sequence ■ Fails to group items that go together; begins tasks without assembling needed materials ■ Is unable to identify main ideas or purposes of activities	■ Provide visual cues and talk through the organization of tasks with the child ■ Help the child to group necessary items before beginning an activity ■ Have the child identify the purpose of activities before beginning; have the child dictate a short summary of activities following completion
Judgment	■ Behaves in an unsafe manner; acts without recognizing possible consequences	■ Redirect the child before beginning an activity; with a safety net in place, allow the child to experience the effects of unsafe behavior; have the child view himself on videotape behaving in an unsafe manner

resistance. Disodium etidronate is used to treat only proven cases of heterotopic ossification in children because of a report of rachitic bone changes in a pediatric patient who had been treated with the drug.[112] Surgical excision of calcification may be considered approximately 2 years after the first appearance, as the calcifications are believed to be mature at that time.

Ataxia, with or without spasticity, is the most frequently observed motor dysfunction in children with TBI. It may become noticeable only as the child begins to move spontaneously or as spasticity resolves.[111] A reverse-style walker is often the most suitable for ataxic children. Pulling the walker behind the body encourages erect trunk posture and slows ambulation speed. Weights may be placed on the walker. Some children do relatively well with adapted tricycles. Those who walk independently but are vulnerable to falling may require a helmet for protection. Tremors, which may accompany ataxia, often subside spontaneously in children

---

TABLE 22–8. Illustration of Collaborative Team Intervention

Setting: Small gym area, which had diminished visual distractions.

Persons present: Patient's physical therapist, occupational therapist, and speech therapist. Parents, other family members, nursing staff, and school personnel occasionally observe and interact during therapy sessions, as part of a comprehensive effort to facilitate the development of their competence.

Patient and therapist positions: The patient was out of his wheelchair and seated on a mat, with the occupational therapist behind him for stabilization and facilitation. The physical therapist and speech therapist were in front of him. Only one person spoke to him at a time.

Goals for the session

1. Improve transfers
2. Improve trunk control, sitting balance, and head and neck control
3. Improve functional use of upper extremities
4. Improve functional eye-hand coordination
5. Improve breath control and support for speech
6. Investigate best immediate augmentative communication options (e.g., potential switch activation, use of spelling board)
7. Increased oral-motor control (e.g., lip closure, consistent control of saliva)
8. Improve orientation
9. Improve memory within a 30-min session

Activities of session

A. Therapists ask patient to identify them by eye gazing, pointing, or nodding his head.
B. Patient assists in transfer by:
    1. Helping to remove lap tray, splint, and Velcro attachments
    2. Holding arms up
    3. Preparing for transfer (e.g., leaning forward, scooting, lifting legs)
    4. Transferring (e.g., assisting in transition from sit to stand, pivoting, scooting back)
C. Patient readies himself physically for a sitting activity by:
    1. Positioning feet appropriately
    2. Aligning head and trunk
    3. Placing hands in weight-bearing position
    4. Swallowing saliva
D. Patient readies himself cognitively for the activity by:
    1. Acknowledging the purpose of the activity and his role in it
    2. Indicating his expectation regarding his level of success in the activity
    3. Indicating the materials that will be needed for the activity
E. Patient participates in sitting activities, including:
    1. Visually tracking a person moving throughout the room
    2. Pointing to a communication board in response to verbal questions and to indicate items needed for the activity
    3. Saying "yes" and "no" with maximum breath support and loudness
    4. Reaching for a pencil in a variety of planes, in order to complete a simple writing task
F. Patient assists in transfer back to wheelchair
G. Patient participates in a review of the session as a therapist records his words in his log book
    1. Identifies session goals and activities
    2. Identifies his accomplishments, comparing his prediction with his actual level of success
    3. Verifies log book note after it was written by a therapist

Source: From Russell, ML, et al: Intervention for motor disorders. In Ylvisaker, M (ed): Traumatic Brain Injury Rehabilitation: Children and Adolescents. Butterworth-Heinemann, Newton, Mass, 1998, with permission.

---

with TBI.[113] For residual tremor, propranolol (Inderol) has been successful in some cases.

Apraxia, including apraxia of speech, is common in children with TBI. Treatment, which is similar in children and adults, includes multiple repetition of tasks so that the movements become automatic (thereby avoiding the need for motor planning). Ensuring that the child has a concrete physical target for the movement (e.g., reaching for a ball versus simply reaching; directing the tongue to lick peanut butter versus simply directing the tongue) helps overcome the motor planning deficit during practice sessions.

AGE AND TASK-RELATED FUNCTIONAL INTERVENTION

Given that the goal of rehabilitation is ultimately to enable children to succeed in tasks that are developmentally appropriate and of their choosing, attention must be given to the importance of tasks and settings during rehabilitation. A goal of infant rehabilitation is to enable the infant to playfully explore objects and interact positively with caregivers. Interesting toys secured to a lap tray may enable the child to explore the world of objects without needing the constant presence of adults to retrieve the toys.

Preschoolers need to be able to play with a wider range of toys, master basic self-care, and interact effectively with peers. Electronically controlled toys (with appropriately adapted switches) may be a useful support for preschoolers with severe motor limitations. Adaptive devices and adaptations, such as special bath seats and Velcro fasteners, may enable preschoolers to be more independent in self-care. Because children as young as 3 have been taught to safely operate an electric wheelchair, such mobility options should be explored for preschoolers and older children with a guarded prognosis for functional motor recovery. Wheelchair training not only serves the obvious functional goal of improved mobility but also is an ideal context for facilitating improved safety judgment.

Success for schoolage children introduces academic settings and activities, such as handwriting (or alternatives), safe mobility in potentially busy corridors, and organized sports and other recreational activities. Providing inpatient rehabilitation in simulated school and recreational settings, with age-appropriate academic and recreational tasks, yields critical information needed to identify adaptations and equipment that will be useful as the child reenters school and social life. Teenagers begin to think about wider-ranging social activities, after-school jobs, career alternatives, and driving. During inpatient rehabilitation, safe community mobility should be explored, along with performance of household tasks (including safe operation of kitchen equipment). Referral to the Bureau of Vocational Services should be considered for all adolescents with residual disability after TBI. Ongoing physical intervention is more efficient and motivating if it is related to success in practical endeavors, such as a job.

Professionals accustomed to working with children with congenital cerebral palsy may be surprised by the strength of resistance to compensatory equipment observed in many children with TBI. Whereas a child who has never walked may greet an electric wheelchair with enthusiasm, a child who is accustomed to effortless walking and running may see the device as a lifelong sentence to inactivity. Similarly, whereas a child who has never spoken intelligibly may be pleased with an augmentative device that produces intelligible speech output at the rate of a few words per minute, a child who is accustomed to effortless speech at 150 words per minute may struggle emotionally with the device and ultimately reject it as too cumbersome, inefficient, and stigmatizing. These understandable reactions require the physical rehabilitation team to introduce compensatory equipment in a sensitive manner, possibly giving the child time to gain competence and comfort with the equipment before it is introduced into stressful social settings.

☐ REHABILITATIVE MEDICAL ASSESSMENT AND MANAGEMENT

The goal of rehabilitative medical management is to identify medical needs and provide medical services that promote recovery, ensure that the child benefits maximally from rehabilitation, and prevent complications that lead to further disability and disease. The importance of the medical component of rehabilitation is underscored by Kalisky et al.'s finding that 16 percent of the medical problems present in a series of 180 TBI admissions to rehabilitation (children and adults) were present but not identified in the acute care setting. An additional 18 percent of the medical difficulties occurred for the first time after admission to the rehabilitation center.

With dramatically decreased lengths of stay in children's hospitals and decreasing numbers of managed care providers willing to pay for prolonged inpatient rehabilitation except in cases of extreme need, the burden on pediatricians and other community physicians increases. In addition, school systems, which traditionally lack expertise in the medical and rehabilitative needs of children with TBI, have become a primary provider of these services. Therefore, rehabilitation physicians, as well as other rehabilitation professionals, have come to play an increasing role as consultants to school and community professionals who oversee the ongoing rehabilitation and medical management of the child.

Rehabilitation units that are an integral part of an acute care hospital can admit children who have not yet achieved medical stability and can therefore begin intensive rehabilitation while continuing treatment for serious medical conditions. Free-standing rehabilitation hospitals require a greater degree of medical stability. However, because children are being transferred to rehabilitation earlier in their recovery, tracheostomy, gastrostomy, and nasogastric tubes and orthopedic devices such as stabilizing halos and body jackets should not be an obstacle to admission.

The primary care physician in a pediatric rehabilitation facility must have special expertise in the pathological sequelae of brain injury, all aspects of child development, and the interaction of brain injury and development. Successful comprehensive management requires attention to interactions among preinjury status, genetic background, stage of development, severity and location of brain injury, associated multiple system injuries, and complications prior to admission.[111] Therefore, the initial rehabilitation medical evaluation includes a thorough history (sensitive to the fact that children with preexisting developmental conditions and environmental stressors are at increased risk for injury) and complete physical examination, focusing on the neurological and neuromuscular systems.[114] Findings are integrated with those of other rehabilitation team members, including nurse specialist, dietitian, physical therapist, occupational therapist, speech-language pathologist, child neuropsychologist, and social worker. Special medical consultations are obtained as needed throughout the admission. Repeated neurodiagnostic procedures are recommended only when indicated by neurological deterioration, changes in seizure patterns, or other alarming symptoms.[115] (See Chapter 21 for details of medical assessment and management.)

□ SUMMARY

Depending on varied preinjury, injury, and postinjury-related factors, virtually any combination of medical and rehabilitative needs is possible in children with severe TBI. This chapter reviewed issues that commonly require the attention of medical and rehabilitation professionals who serve these children. Our primary focus has been on cognitive, behavioral, and psychosocial themes because of their prominence in long-term outcome following TBI in children and adolescents. The approach to rehabilitation that we have described and illustrated features collaborative assessments and interventions, the creative use of natural activities and settings and the everyday people in those settings, an emphasis on executive or self-regulatory functions, and a proactive or antecedent-focused approach to challenging behavior. Consistent with the economic constraints that currently face rehabilitation, we have highlighted the increasingly important role of rehabilitation specialists in serving children indirectly through others, including family members and school and community professionals.

In many cases, assessment and intervention procedures appropriate for adults—and presented elsewhere in this book—are also useful for children. In addition, the habilitation and special education literatures are rich in assessment and intervention approaches that may, possibly with some modification, be appropriate for many children with TBI. Information about a population is important as a framework for approaching an individual who is a member of that population. However, when all is said and done, good clinical decision making is highly individualized and requires creative application and attentive monitoring of interventions with good potential for success.

REFERENCES

1. Lehr, E: Psychological Management of Traumatic Brain Injuries in Children and Adolescents. Aspen, Gaithersburg, Md, 1990.
2. Levin, HS, et al: The contribution of frontal lobe lesions to the neurobehavioral outcome of closed head injury. In Levin, HS, Eisenberg, HM, and Benton, AI (eds): Frontal Lobe Function and Dysfunction. Oxford University Press, New York, 1991, p 318.
3. Benton, A: Prefrontal injury and behavior in children. Developmental Neuropsychology 7:275, 1991.
4. Eslinger, PJ, et al: Developmental consequences of childhood frontal lobe damage. Arch Neurol 49:764, 1992.
5. Feeney, TJ, and Ylvisaker, M: Choice and routine: Antecedent behavioral interventions for adolescents with severe traumatic brain injury. J Head Trauma Rehabil 10:67, 1995.
6. Grattan, LM, and Eslinger, PJ: Frontal lobe damage in children and adults: A comparative review. Developmental Neuropsychology 7:283, 1991.
7. Grattan, LM, and Eslinger, PJ: Long-term psychological consequences of childhood frontal lobe lesion in patient DT. Brain Cogn 20:185, 1992.
8. Marlowe, WB: Consequences of frontal lobe injury in the developing child. J Clin Exp Neuropsychol 12:105, 1989.
9. Marlowe, WB: The impact of a right prefrontal lesion on the developing brain. Brain Cog 20:205, 1992.
10. Mateer, CA, and Williams, D: Effects of frontal lobe injury in childhood. Developmental Neuropsychology 7:359, 1991.
11. Thomsen, IV: Do young patients have worse outcomes after severe blunt head trauma? Brain Inj 3:157, 1989.
12. Ylvisaker, M: Communication outcome in children and adolescents with traumatic brain injury. Neuropsychological Rehabilitation 3:367, 1993.
13. Ylvisaker, M, and Feeney, T: Traumatic brain injury in adolescence: Assessment and reintegration. Seminars in Speech and Language 16:32, 1995.
14. Goldman, PS: Functional development of the prefrontal cortex in early life and the problem of neuronal plasticity. Exp Neurol 32:366, 1971.
15. Kolb, B: Brain Plasticity and Behavior. Erlbaum, Mahwah, NJ, 1995.
16. Asarnow, RF, et al: Behavior problems and adaptive functioning in children with mild and severe closed head injury. J Pediatr Psychol 16:534, 1991.
17. Brown, G, et al: A prospective study of children with head injuries. III. Psychiatric sequelae. Psychol Med 11:63, 1981.
18. Fletcher, JM, et al: Behavioral changes after closed head injury in children. J Consult Clin Psychol 58:93, 1990.
19. Greenspan, AI, and MacKenzie, EJ: Functional outcome after pediatric head injury. Pediatrics 94:425, 1994.
20. Williams, D, and Mateer, CA: Developmental impact of frontal lobe injury in middle childhood. Brain Cogn 20:196, 1992.

21. Ylvisaker, M, et al: School reentry following severe traumatic brain injury: Guidelines for educational planning. J Head Trauma Rehabil 10:25, 1995.

22. Ylvisaker, M, Feeney, T, and Mullins, K: School reentry following mild traumatic brain injury: A proposed hospital-to-school protocol. J Head Trauma Rehabil 10:42, 1995.

23. Bijou, SW, Peterson, RE, and Ault, MH: A method to integrate descriptive and experimental field studies at the level of data and empirical concepts. J Appl Behav Anal 1:175, 1968.

24. Dumas, JE: Let's not forget the context in behavioral assessment. Behavioral Assessment 11:231, 1986.

25. Iwata, BA, et al: Toward a functional analysis of self-injury. Analysis and Intervention in Developmental Disabilities 2:3, 1982.

26. Stokes, TF, and Baer, DM: An implicit technology of generalization. J Appl Behav Anal 10:349, 1977.

27. Singley, MK, and Anderson, JR: Transfer of Cognitive Skill. Harvard University Press, Cambridge, Mass, 1989.

28. Vygotsky, L: Mind. in Society: The Development of Higher Psychological Processes. Harvard University Press, Cambridge, Mass, 1978.

29. Bjorklund, DF: Children's Strategies: Contemporary Views of Cognitive Development. Erlbaum, Hillsdale, NJ, 1990.

30. Tranel, D, Anderson, SW, and Benton, AI: Development of the concept of executive functions and its relationship to the frontal lobes: In Boller, F, and Grafman, J (eds): Handbook of Neuropsychology. Elsevier, Amsterdam, 1995.

31. Welsh, MC, and Pennington, BF: Assessing frontal lobe functioning in children: Views from a developmental psychology. Developmental Neuropsychology 4:199, 1988.

32. Mann, L: On the Trail of Process: A Historical Perspective on Cognitive Processes and Their Training. Grune and Stratton, New York, 1979.

33. Hallowell, EM, and Ratey, JJ: Driven to Distraction. Pantheon, New York, 1994.

34. Kaplan, E: A process approach to neuropsychological assessment. In Boll, T, and Bryant, BK (eds): Clinical Neuropsychology and Brain Function: Research, Measurement, and Practice. American Psychological Association, Washington, DC, 1988, p 129.

35. Feuerstein, R: The Dynamic Assessment of Retarded Performers: The Learning Potential Assessment Device, Theory, Instruments, and Techniques. University Park Press, Baltimore, Md, 1979.

36. Bigler, ED: Frontal lobe damage and neuropsychological assessment. Archives of Clinical Neuropsychology 3:279, 1988.

37. Eslinger, PJ, and Damasio, AR: Severe disturbance of higher cognition following bilateral frontal lobe oblation: Patient EVR. Neurology 35:1731, 1985.

38. Stuss, DT, and Benson, DF: The Frontal Lobes: Raven, New York, 1986.

39. Dennis, M: Frontal lobe function in childhood and adolescence: A heuristic for assessing attention regulation, executive control, and the intentional states important for social discourse. Developmental Neuropsychology 7:327, 1991.

40. Welsh, MC, Pennington, BE, and Groisser, DB: A normative-developmental study of executive function: A window on prefrontal function in children. Developmental Neuropsychology 7:131, 1991.

41. Lezak, MD: The problem of assessing executive functions. International Journal of Psychology 17:281, 1982.

42. Denckla, MB: Research on executive function in a neurodevelopmental context: Application of clinical measures. Developmental Neuropsychology 12:5, 1996.

43. Dennis, M, et al: Appraising and managing knowledge: Metacognitive skills after childhood head injury. Developmental Neuropsychology 12:77, 1996.

44. Levin, HS, et al: Developmental changes in performance on tests of purported frontal lobe functioning. Developmental Neuropsychology 7:377, 1991.

45. Levin, HS, et al: Dimensions of cognition measures by the Tower of London and other cognitive tasks in head-injured children and adolescents. Developmental Neuropsychology 12:17, 1996.

46. Taylor, HG, et al: Executive dysfunction in children with early brain disease: Outcomes post *Haemophilus influenza* meningitis. Developmental Neuropsychology 12:35, 1996.

47. Delis, M, et al: California Verbal Learning Test. Psychological Corporation, New York, 1983.

48. Kern, L, et al: Using assessment based curricular intervention to improve the classroom behavior of a student with emotional and behavioral challenges. J Appl Behav Anal 27:7, 1994.

49. Wehman, P, et al: Critical factors associated with the successful employment of patients with severe traumatic brain injury. Brain Inj 7:31, 1993.

50. Ylvisaker, M, and Gioia, G: Cognitive assessment. In Ylvisaker, M (ed): Traumatic Brain Injury Rehabilitation: Children and Adolescents. Butterworth-Heinemann, Newton, Mass, 1998.

51. Roberts, RJ, and Pennington, BF: An interactive framework for examining prefrontal cognitive processes. Developmental Neuropsychology 12:105, 1996.

52. O'Neill, RE, et al: Functional Analysis of Problem Behavior. Sycamore, Sycamore, Ill, 1990.

53. Touchette, PE, MacDonald, RF, and Langer, SN: A scatterplot for identifying stimulus control of problem behavior. J Appl Behav Anal 18:343, 1985.

54. Treadwell, K, and Page, TJ: Functional analysis: Identification of environmental determinants of severe behavior disorders. J Head Trauma Rehabil 11:62, 1996.

55. Iwata, BA, Vollmer, TR, and Zarcone, JR: The experimental (functional) analysis of behavioral disorders: Methodology, applications, and limitations. In Repp, AC, and Singh, NN (eds): Perspectives on the Use of Nonaversive and Aversive Interventions for Persons with Developmental Disabilities. Sycamore, Sycamore, Ill, 1990, p 301.

56. Carr, EG, et al: Communication-based treatment of severe behavior problems. In VanHouten, R, and Axelrod, S (eds): Behavior Analysis and Treatment. Plenum, New York, 1993, p 231.

57. Carr, EG, et al: Communication-Based Interventions for Problem Behavior: A User's Guide for Producing Positive Change. Paul Brooks, Baltimore, Md, 1994.

58. Colvin, G, and Sugai, G: Managing Escalating Behavior. Behavior Associates, Eugene, Ore, 1989.

59. Dennis, M, and Barnes, M: Knowing the meaning, getting the point, bridging the gap and carrying the message: Aspects of discourse following closed head injury in childhood and adolescence. Brain Lang 39:428, 1990.

60. Prutting, CA, and Kirchner, DM: A clinical appraisal of the pragmatic aspects of language. Journal of Speech and Hearing Disorders 52:105, 1987.

61. German, DJ: Test of Word Finding. DLM Teaching Resources, Allen, Tex, 1989.

62. German, DJ: Test of Adolescent/Adult Word Finding. DLM Teaching Resources, Allen, Tex, 1990.

63. German, DJ: Test of Word Finding in Discourse. DLM Teaching Resources, Allen, Tex, 1991.

64. Gaddes, WH, and Crocket, DJ: The Spreen-Benton Aphasia Tests: Normative data as a measure of normal language development. Brain Lang 2:257, 1975.

65. Wiig, EH, and Secord, W: Test of Language Competence–Expanded Edition. Psychological Corporation, Antonio, Tex, 1988.

66. Ylvisaker, M, et al: Cognitive assessment. In Savage, R, and Wolcott, G (eds): Educational Dimensions of Acquired Brain Injury. Pro-Ed, Austin, Tex, 1994, p 69.

67. Ylvisaker, M, Szekeres, S, and Haarbauer-Krupa, J: Cognitive rehabilitation: Organization, memory, and language. In Ylvisaker, M (ed): Traumatic Brain Injury Re-

habilitation: Children and Adolescents. Butterworth-Heinemann, Newton, Mass, 1998.

68. Ylvisaker, M, Feeney, T, and Szekeres, S: Cognitive rehabilitation: Executive functions. In Ylvisaker, M (ed): Traumatic Brain Injury Rehabilitation: Children and Adolescents. Butterworth-Heinemann, Newton, Mass, 1998.

69. Ratner, N, and Bruner, J: Games, social exchange, and the acquisition of language. Journal of Child Language 5:391, 1978.

70. Fivush, R: The social construct of personal narratives. Merrill-Palmer Quarterly 37:59, 1991.

71. Fivush, R, and Reese, E: The social construction of autobiographical memory. In Conway, MA, et al (eds): Theoretical Perspectives on Autobiographical Memory. Kluwer, The Netherlands, 1992, p 115.

72. McCabe, A, and Peterson, C: Getting the story: A longitudinal study of parental styles in eliciting narratives and developing narrative skill. In McCabe, A, and Peterson, C (eds): Developing Narrative Structure. Erlbaum, Hillsdale, NJ, 1991, p 217.

73. Nelson, JA: Emergence of autobiographical memory at age 4. Human Development 35:172, 1992.

74. Reese, E, Haden, CA, and Fivush, R: Mother-child conversations about the past: Relationships of style and memory over time. Cognitive Development 8:403, 1993.

75. MacDonald, J: Becoming Partners with Children: From Play to Conversation. Riverside, Chicago, 1989.

76. Schneider, P, and Watkins, RV: Applying Vygotskyan developmental theory to language intervention. Language, Speech, and Hearing Services in the School 27:157, 1966.

77. Palinscar, AS, and Brown, AL: Classroom dialogues to promote self-regulated comprehension. In Brophy, J (ed): Teaching for Understanding and Self-Regulated Learning, vol 1. JIA Press, Greenwich, Conn, 1989.

78. Rogoff, B: Apprenticeship in Thinking: Cognitive Development in Social Context. Oxford University Press, New York, 1990.

79. Wood, D, Bruner, JS, and Ross, G: The role of tutoring in problem solving. J Child Psychol Psychiatry 17:89, 1976.

80. Meichenbaum, D: The "potential" contributions of cognitive behavior modification to the rehabilitation of individuals with traumatic brain injury. Seminars in Speech and Language 14:18, 1993.

81. Ylvisaker, M, and Feeney, T: Executive functions after traumatic brain injury: Supported cognition and self-advocacy. Seminars in Speech and Language 17:217, 1996.

82. Ylvisaker, M, and Feeney, T: Everyday people as supports: Developing competencies through collaboration. In Ylvisaker, M (ed): Traumatic Brain Injury Rehabilitation: Children and Adolescents. Butterworth-Heinemann, Newton, Mass, 1998.

83. Pressley, M, et al: Cognitive Strategy Instruction That Really Improves Children's Academic Performance. Brookline, Cambridge, Mass, 1990.

84. Hoffman, M, and Weikart, DP: Educating Young Children. High Scope Education Research Foundation, Ypsilanti, Mich, 1995.

85. Schweinhart, LF, and Weikart, DP: Success by empowerment: The High-Scope Perry Preschool study through age 27. Young Children 49:54, 1993.

86. Willatts, P: Development of problem-solving strategies in infancy. In Bjorklund, DF (ed): Children's Strategies: Contemporary Views of Cognitive Development. Erlbaum, Hillsdale, NJ, 1990, p 196.

87. Ylvisaker, M, Sellars, C, and Edelman, L: Rehabilitation following traumatic brain injury in preschoolers. In Ylvisaker, M (ed): Traumatic Brain Injury Rehabilitation: Children and Adolescents. Butterworth-Heinemann, Newton, Mass, 1998.

88. LaVigna, GW, and Donnellan, AM: Alternatives to Punishment: Solving Behavior Problems with Nonaversive Strategies. Irvington, New York, 1986.

89. Meyer, LH, and Evans, IA: Nonaversive Intervention Behavior Problems: A Manual for Home and Community. Paul Brookes, Baltimore, 1989.

90. Willis, TM, and LaVigna, GW: Emergency Management Guidelines. Institute for Applied Behavior Analysis, Los Angeles, 1989.

91. Damasio, AR: Descartes' Error. Avon, New York, 1994.

92. Damasio, AR, Tranel, D, and Damasio, H: Individuals with sociopathic behavior caused by frontal lobe damage fail to respond automatically to socially charged stimuli. Behav Brain Res 14:81, 1990.

93. Teuber, HL: The riddle of frontal lobe function in man. In Warren, JM, and Akert, K (eds): The Frontal Granular Cortex and Behavior. McGraw-Hill, New York, 1964.

94. Harchik, AE, et al: Choice and control: New opportunities for people with developmental disabilities. Ann Clin Psychiatry 5:151, 1993.

95. Fox, J, and Conroy, M: Setting events and behavioral disorders of children and youth: An interbehavioral field analysis for research and practice. Journal of Emotional and Behavioral Disorders 3:130, 1995.

96. Fowler, RC: Supporting students with challenging behaviors in general educational settings: A review of behavioral momentum techniques and guidelines for use. Oregon Conference Monograph 8:137, 1995.

97. Putnam, JW, et al: Collaborative skill instruction in promoting positive interactions between mentally handicapped and nonhandicapped children. Exceptional Children 55:550, 1989.

98. Kennedy, CH, and Itkonen, T: Setting events: Assessment and intervention to reduce the problem behavior of students with severe disabilities. J Appl Behav Anal 26:321, 1993.

99. Michael, J: Establishing operations. Behavior Analyst 16:191, 1993.

100. Feeney, TJ, and Ylvisaker, M: A positive, communication-based approach to challenging behavior after TBI. In Glang, A, and Singer, G (eds): Children with Acquired Brain Injury: The School's Response. Paul Brooks, Baltimore, Md, 1997.

101. Ylvisaker, M, and Feeney, T: Communication and behavior: Collaboration between speech-language pathologists and behavioral psychologists. Topics in Language Disorders 15:37, 1994.

102. Mace, FC, et al: The momentum of the human behavior in a natural setting. J Exp Anal Behav 54:163, 1990.

103. Mace, FC, et al: Behavioral momentum in the treatment of noncompliance. J Appl Behav Anal 21:123, 1988.

104. Nevin, JA: An integrated model for the study of behavioral momentum. J Exp Anal Behav 57:301, 1992.

105. Ylvisaker, M, Feeney, T, and Urbanczyk, B: Developing a positive communication culture for rehabilitation: Communication training for staff and family members. In Durgin, CJ, Schmidt, ND, and Fryer, LJ (eds): Staff Development and Clinical Intervention in Brain Injury Rehabilitation. Aspen, Gaithersburg, Md, 1993.

106. Chaplin, D, Deitz, J, and Jaffe, KM: Motor performance after traumatic brain injury. Arch Phys Med Rehabil 74:161, 1993.

107. Granger, CV, Hamilton, BB, and Kayton, R: Guide to the use of the Functional Independence Measure for Children (Wee-FIM) of the uniform data set for medical rehabilitation. Research Foundation, State University of New York, Buffalo, 1989.

108. Haley, SM, et al: Pediatric Evaluation of Disability Inventory, Examiner's Manual. Tufts University Department of Rehabilitation, Boston, 1989.

109. Ylvisaker, M, et al: Rehabilitative assessment following head injury in children. In Rosenthal, M, et al (eds): Rehabilitation of the Child and Adult with Traumatic Brain Injury. F A Davis, Philadelphia, 1990, p 558.

110. Molnar, GE, and Perrin, JCS: Head injury. In Molnar, GE (ed): Pediatric Rehabilitation. Williams & Wilkins, Baltimore, 1992, p 254.

ör

, et al: Intervention for motor disorders. In
1 (ed): Traumatic Brain Injury Rehabilitation:
nd Adolescents. Butterworth-Heinemann,
Mass, 1998.

n, SL, et al: Rachitic syndrome after disodium
te therapy in an adolescent. Arch Phys Med Re-
5:118, 1994.

on, SLJ, and Hall, DMB: Post traumatic tremor in
injured children. Arch Dis Child 67:227, 1992.

114. Chorazy, A, et al: Medical management. In Ylvisaker, M
(ed): Traumatic Brain Injury Rehabilitation: Children
and Adolescents. Butterworth-Heinemann, Newton,
Mass, 1998.
115. Jaffe, KM, and Hays, RM: Pediatric head injury: Rehabilitative medical management. J Head Trauma Rehabil
4:30, 1986.

CHAPTER 23

Managing Transitions for Education

ROBERTA DePOMPEI, PHD,
and JEAN L. BLOSSER, EDD

The job of children and adolescents is to play and to learn. After sustaining a traumatic brain injury (TBI), these youngsters are often faced with challenges that make playing and learning in home, school, and community much more difficult. Although all environments are important and contribute to development, growth, and adaptation, the school environment is usually the primary setting for long-term rehabilitation, education, and socialization of children and adolescents after brain injury.[1-6] As such, the focus in schools is to provide a dynamic, individualized, developmental, and age-appropriate approach to education that allows maximum growth and development.

This chapter is intended to assist service providers in understanding the unique challenges for children and adolescents and their families in planning appropriate transition, reintegration, and maintenance within a school program. It is based in our belief that proactive planning and treatment are central to successful involvement in school over the student's life cycle. A proactive stance enables planners in the school reintegration process to identify challenges that might affect success, formulate directions for change, establish priorities for education, define the roles of important individuals in the school environment, and develop strategies and plans for accomplishment of goals. It also allows equal partnerships with families in the planning and treatment process. To understand how to apply a proactive, quality-oriented approach to school transitioning, it is helpful to think in terms of planning a trip. To plan a trip, certain questions are asked, and the organization of the trip evolves from the answers. This chapter is based on 10 questions the planning team can ask as it develops an educational road map for the journey of the student with TBI.

◻ QUESTION 1: "WHAT BASIC INFORMATION DO WE NEED?"

To serve youngsters with TBI, knowledge about the laws, rules, and regulations that can affect service provision is essential.

Laws, Rules, and Regulations

Several initiatives through national and state legislation and international accreditation bodies have provided the impetus for developing procedures for treatment and community access for children and adolescents: the Americans with Disabilities Act (ADA),[7] Individuals with Disabilities Education Act (IDEA),[8] Section 504 of the Rehabilitation Act of 1973, Commission on Accreditation for Rehabilitation Facilities (CARF) new standards for TBI and children with medical conditions, and expanded definitions for mental retardation and developmental disabilities (MR/DD). The specifics of this section relate to legislation in the United States. Similar legislation in other countries can be obtained by contacting appropriate governmental agencies in the countries of interest.

AMERICANS WITH DISABILITIES ACT

The present ADA (1990)[7] provides individuals with disabilities with access and accommodation to employment, transportation, government activities, and communication. Children with TBI have access to all provisions of ADA. At the present time, ADA is under revision. Additional information about this law and forthcoming changes can be obtained from the U.S. Department of Justice, Civil Rights Division, P.O. Box 66118, Washington, D.C. 20035-6118.

INDIVIDUALS WITH DISABILITIES EDUCATION ACT

An amended and reauthorized IDEA (1990)[8] provided a special education category for youth with TBI. These children and adolescents, if qualified for special education, must be provided with appropriate education in the least restrictive environment, regardless of the severity of their injury. The law also provides for transitional planning to work, community, and independent living centers after graduation. There are two specific provisions for planning individual education programming: the individualized education program (IEP) and the individual transition plan (ITP).

Individualized Education Program

The IEP supports the entire educational program planning for students with special needs. It is the educational map that guides what is provided for the student and the contract between the family and school for the delivery of educational services to the child. After a student is assessed and educational modifications are made, a team consisting of the child, family, and representatives in education and health-related services is created. This team develops an integrated and coordinated action plan, which is updated as needed and designed to meet individual needs. Wolcott et al.,[9] Blosser and DePompei,[3] and Savage and Wolcott[4] have provided information about what should be covered in the IEP. DePompei and Blosser[10] have also provided specific information to prepare the family for their participation in the IEP process.

Individual Transition Plan

There is also provision for development of a transition plan to and from school for individuals with disabilities. This plan can be incorporated into the IEP or be written as a separate document. Information about how the school and other agencies will develop transition to community, vocation, or independent living should be included in the ITP. Wolcott and Pear-son[11] provided worksheets for planning transitions from hospital to school, grade to grade, and school level to level. These worksheets allow information to be transmitted to provide continuity of programming year after year.

Divisions of special education in state departments of education can be contacted for specific information about how they provide educational services to this population. However, the federal government is presently considering major revisions to IDEA that may affect youth with TBI.

SECTION 504 OF THE REHABILITATION ACT OF 1973

If a child is not eligible for special education services as provided under IDEA but does exhibit educational needs related to a physical or mental condition that substantially limits one or more life activities, appropriate services can be provided in accordance with Section 504.[12] Section 504 ensures that all students with disabilities have access to postsecondary education when appropriate and provides for schools to prepare these students for that opportunity.

COMMISSION FOR ACCREDITATION OF REHABILITATION FACILITIES STANDARDS

CARF has revised its requirements for individuals with TBI in organizations they accredit. The new standards, which became effective in July 1997, outline regulations for pediatric populations who have medical problems, including TBI. The issues related to education include:

1. Composition of staff requirements that specify inclusion of a developmental specialist and services of an education specialist.

2. Coordination of school reintegration services that require collaboration of hospital and school and knowledge of laws and regulations regarding special education services.

3. Inclusion of family in the school reentry process that designates them as planners and decision makers.

Specific regulations can be obtained from the Commission on Accreditation of Rehabilitation Facilities, 4891 E. Grant St., Tucson, AZ, 85712.

EXPANDED DEFINITIONS OF MENTAL RETARDATION AND DEVELOPMENTAL DISABILITIES

Several states have undertaken initiatives to develop new MR/DD definitions. These expanded definitions may provide opportunities for individuals injured prior to age 22. For example, in the state of Ohio, the qualifications for services now include a functional definition of developmental disabilities that states that people injured before age 22 may be eligible for services (such as therapy, case management, and group housing) under MR/DD boards if they have two or more handicapping conditions that interfere with normal life functioning. Although many children and adolescents with TBI would not qualify, service providers should be prepared to offer such alternative options to families.

☐ QUESTION 2: "WHAT SYSTEMS CAN HELP?"

Children and adolescents with TBI are continually confronted with transitions from situation to situation and from setting to setting. In school, these transitions occur whenever the youngster changes subjects, classrooms, buildings, teachers, or study groups. Students require a coordinated and integrated system of care that ensures the deliverance of comprehensive services in continuity from the emergency room through rehabilitation services, into the school, and into the community. To provide a system that is seamless[13] and appropriate to the individual needs and strengths of the child or adolescent and family, several factors regarding transition should be considered: developing a more coordinated networking process among agencies, ensuring policies and procedures suitable for aiding transitions, and planning for transitional programming over time.

The Networking Process

Traditionally, transitioning is thought of as the discharge from one facility, such as a hospital, and the new involvement of another, such as the school. In this traditional perspective, the referring facility often begins preparation for the next agency very close to the time of discharge. There may be little contact between agencies to determine the expectations and requirements of the receiving facility. DePompei and Blosser[14] found one of the major barriers to successful planning for school reentry to be networking among agencies that occurred too late in the transition process. One contributing factor to the poor timing of referrals to schools may be a systems misunderstanding. In contrast to hospitals, where evaluation and treatment usually occurs within 24 hours, special services in the schools can take up to 90 days for determination of eligibility for services. Contact with the school should be made as soon as the child's medical condition is stable. It is too late in the planning process to make contact when discharge from the hospital is imminent.

The child or adolescent and family members should be included in this networking process. Families are the constant in all transitions with their child over the life cycle of the family. Current literature[13,15] reinforces the concept that student choice, family choice, and self-determination are central to transition planning. With this viewpoint, the control for making decisions about goals and needs rests with the person with the disability and the family rather than with service providers. This perspective provides a family-centered approach to the process, which allows for input from service providers and choices by families.

Blosser and DePompei,[3] Savage and Wolcott,[1] and Ylvisaker et al.[16] provide useful suggestions for the transition process from hospital to school for children and adolescents with moderate and severe brain injury. Additionally, written policies and procedures are becoming more common for interaction among community agencies such as hospitals and schools.[17]

Planning Multiple Transitions for the Child or Adolescent

Transitioning and networking for the child or adolescent is necessary in multiple situations during the life of the individual. Although each situation is unique, certain procedures can remain the same. General guidelines for transitioning the child or adolescent into school, community, or vocational opportunities may include the following:

1. Include the child or adolescent and family as active participants in any transition. Prepare them for their role by providing them with needed information and skills.

2. Provide the child or adolescent with options and opportunities to participate in multiple community experiences.

3. After age 14, include vocational assessment in any evaluation process for developing an IEP or ITP.

4. State clearly the types of transitions the youngster is likely to encounter.

5. Develop a multiyear plan for transition that includes the child or adolescent's preferences, needs, strengths, interests, and potential in light of obstacles that may be encountered. Take steps to ensure that the child will gain the skills necessary for success and that the environment will be modified to accommodate for disability.

6. Specify (in writing) the individuals who will be responsible for the delivery of services to prepare the student for transition.

7. Establish interagency collaborative agreements to develop action plans to deliver transitional services. Persons from agencies that deal with vocational education, mental health, health and human services, adult education, and trade schools might be included.

8. Develop policies to ensure that treatment plans will be in place at the beginning of the transition. Clarify the roles and responsibilities of each person and agency, funding needed to make the transition succeed, and program evaluation issues.

9. Fully prepare staff to understand the unique needs of children or adolescents with TBI and the systematic transition planning that is needed.

10. Prepare the environment for the child or adolescent by removing obstacles to facilitate full inclusion and participation.

□ QUESTION 3: "WHERE IS THIS CHILD OR ADOLESCENT NOW?"

To understand the student's potential for performance in the classroom, it is necessary to know the impairment, strengths, and needs of the individual and how these behaviors may impact overall performance in the classroom. Team members may access this information by understanding the developmental issues of children, completing assessments of the youngster, and applying information about performance levels to classroom expectations.

Developmental Issues Affect Learning

In planning for community or school reintegration, developmental issues of children and adolescents distinguish them from adults. Children and adolescents are in periods of rapid change that affect physical and mental development.[6] They are undergoing the combined process of brain growth and development and experiential learning that shapes individual personality and the ability to deal with the environment. Alterations in the brain can affect a person's current and future ability to develop and learn. Service providers who do not have background from a developmental perspective should consult with developmental or educational specialists. Developmental factors that must be considered in the planning include:

1. The injury can affect the developing brain. Considerable neurophysiological change occurs in the normally developing brain of a young person. Each stage from infancy through adolescence provides specific expectations in terms of neurological development. For example, during elementary and middle school years, the child's brain is involved in rapid development for learning.[6] Interconnections between various portions of the brain are increased, and ease in learning academically related subjects such as reading and math is noted.[18] When a brain injury affects the developmental process, the ability of the brain to accommodate to the injury should be considered. In the case of preschool children, there is little previously learned information upon which they can rely in new learning situations. According to Savage,[19] preschoolers have some of the worst recovery records and great difficulty in adapting to brain injury because they have no base of experience from which to draw and because the brain itself is in such an early stage of development. Understanding brain injury in youth requires the appreciation of two simultaneously occurring processes: the recovery/improvement from injury superimposed on the overall process of the developing brain.[20]

2. Long-term effects may be cumulative. The injury can interfere with long-term capacity to develop, and there may be cumulative effects. For example, a 4-year-old may have developed an adequate vocabulary for his or her age. On vocabulary tests after the injury, the child may be able to rely on previously learned information and score within normal limits on the assessment. It could be assumed that the child's language capabilities are intact. However, as the child progresses into first or second grade, demands on vocabulary development and retention of new information may increase, and the child may begin to falter. It may take years to recognize the relationship of the brain injury and the decreased language-learning capacity.

3. There may be a delayed onset of disability. "Since an injury may affect parts of the brain that are in the process of developing or are not expected to be fully functioning for years to come, it is possible for the injury effects not to be apparent for many years after the time of injury (p. 302).[6] Various developmentalists such as Piaget[21] suggest that the child moves through a series of cognitive stages that influence those cognitive skills expected to be present at a particular age level. A child in elementary school may perform adequately during the first several years after an injury because she or he is in the same developmental stage as prior to the injury. When additional demands of deductive reasoning, organization, or interpretation of written materials are introduced in the upper grades, the adolescent begins to have difficulty. It is possible that the adolescent did not reach the next developmental plateau. Because so much time has passed between the injury and the onset of problems, parents and educators may not realize the connection between the earlier TBI and the lack of performance years later.

Assessment Provides Planning and Placement Information

Educational assessment is required to qualify students for special services in the schools. Standardized tests are often used to complete such evaluations. Telzrow[22] provided domain-specific tests that can be employed in such an assessment. Shurtleff et al.[23] suggested a screening method that can assist school reentry. Blosser and DePompei[3] outlined both formal and informal means of evaluating performances in cognitive-communicative areas, and Ylvisaker et al. discussed evaluation procedures in Chapter 22. Specific educational assessment for placement issues should be developed according to the needs of the individual and in conjunction with academic achievement and aptitude evaluation. Assessment should not be considered a one-time process but rather as ongoing for the duration of the education of the youngster. Reassessment may be necessary every few months during the first year or two after the injury.[2-4,20]

Applying Information about Performance Levels to Classroom Expectations

All the suggested evaluation procedures provide valuable information about the potential behavior of the youngster in the classroom. What sometimes is lacking in the report process is how these various needs and impairments look in the classroom and how the expectations of the classroom may not match the behaviors of the youngster. Terminology used to diagnose a child without relating a behavior to an educational need may not be appreciated as applicable to educational planning. For example, a report that states a child has slow processing time may not be as helpful as one that says the child may need extra time to complete homework assignments or to answer a question because of slowed information-processing abilities. Therefore, it becomes important to indicate how a relationship may exist between an impairment (such as poor attention) and the classroom behavior that may be anticipated as a result of the impairment (such as daydreaming) to facilitate the development of appropriate teaching techniques, strategies, and resources.[24] A chart such as Table 23-1 may assist team members to relate the impairment to the classroom behavior and then to suggest strategies that may be useful.

A further necessity is to learn from the teacher the performance expectations for that particular class. Some teachers work in small interactive groups; others teach in lecture style with expectations for questions to the large group to be answered. Some teachers give only verbal instructions and use few visual cues. Others use combinations of written, verbal, and homework sheets. Knowing the expectations for classroom performance and describing the strengths and needs of the student also aid the planning process.

Finally, the student should be asked to participate in the evaluation process. A questionnaire such as Table 23-2 is useful in gaining information from the student's perspective.[3]

TABLE 23–1. Relating Impairment to Classroom Behavior

Impairment	Classroom Behavior
Decreased judgment	Impulsive, easily persuaded by others; careless about safety
Poor attention	Distractible, daydreams; talks out
Less carryover for new learning	Information presented on day 1 not recalled or generalized on day 3; forgets to prepare for test or field trip
Decreased organization	Comes late to class; notebook disorganized; no text; can't read short story to find main idea
Poor memory	Requires large number of repetitions to learn classroom rules and routines
Poor self-initiation	Can't do homework; doesn't use class time to complete assignments; agrees to do more than is capable of completing

---

TABLE 23–2. Youngster's Opinion about Needed Changes

You are the best judge of how other people can cause problems for you or help you do better. Answer these 10 questions and let's work together to think of some helpful solutions.

1. What problems are you experiencing in class (at home, at work)? Briefly describe the problems you are having since you returned to school (your home, work, etc.).

2. How do you usually act when you are experiencing problems or frustrations in class (at home, at work)? List some of the ways you behave when you are having problems.

3. What classroom (home or work) situation causes you the most problems?
   □ Noise
   □ Temperature
   □ Pictures and wall decorations
   □ Other people in the room
   □ Other things

4. List several ways your teachers (family, classmates, coworkers) help you when you experience trouble in class (at home or work).

5. What do you think people should do to help you?

6. List several things your teachers (classmates, coworkers) do to frustrate you or cause you more problems.

7. What do you think people should *stop* doing when they are around you?

8. At what time of day do you do your best? Why do you feel this is your best time of day?
   □ Early morning
   □ Midmorning
   □ Around noon
   □ Midafternoon
   □ Early evening
   □ Late evening

9. If you could choose 3 skills to improve, what would they be?

10. Tell 5 things that are great about you that you wish other people would know.

Source: Reprinted with permission by Singular Publishing Group, Inc. From Blosser, JL, and DePompei, R: Pediatric Traumatic Brain Injury: Proactive Intervention. Singular Press: San Diego, 1994, p 133.

☐ QUESTION 4: "WHERE DO WE WANT THE YOUNGSTER TO GO?"

The long-term outcomes to be achieved should be discussed and agreed upon. The evaluation efforts must result in information about areas of critical concern, including academics, social acceptance and friendships, health and safety, self-concept and self-esteem, choice making, self-control and self-management, and inclusion in integrated activities.[25] Often, there is so much that needs to be accomplished. Planners are encouraged to focus the team's efforts on a few select priorities. For example, for children with cognitive-communicative impairments, treatment planners might ask if the services they are offering will help the student participate in social-interactive activities with family and friends, perform required classroom assignments, and prepare for work and adult responsibilities. Educational goals and activities should be designed to bring about the desired outcomes. All those who have a stake in the child's success need to participate equally in this discussion.

☐ QUESTION 5: "WHEN DO WE WANT THE CHILD TO GET THERE?"

An educational plan for children and adolescents with TBI is not just something that is developed and implemented and then is finished. Time lines should be established for implementing the program and achieving the desired outcomes. There must be continuing evaluation of the individual's performance, the strategies used, the people involved, and the desired outcomes. Because there are constant transitions, there is always a need to rethink and replan. Rather than view the child as "treated" and "cured," it is wiser to refocus efforts and strive for ongoing improvement in performance.

☐ QUESTION 6: "WHO DO WE WANT AND NEED TO HELP?"

Those individuals who hold the highest stake in the youngster's success should be involved in the program planning and implementation.

The people selected to participate should understand TBI, the child's strengths and needs, the policies that affect school placement and programming, the challenges the child is likely to face, and resources available for support. The team will need to function collaboratively. Multidisciplinary coordination is essential to ensure safe and successful classroom integration. Teachers, school administrators, family members, and rehabilitation and health care professionals can work as a team to plan effective educational programs for all students. Depending on the severity and diversity of the student's impairments, a wide variety of services may be necessary. For some youngsters, medical and emergency services will be a consideration. Team membership may change over time, depending on the needs of the student and the activities in which he or she will participate.[26]

☐ QUESTION 7: "HOW DO WE WANT TO PROCEED?"

The educational and interventive approaches used must be based on each youngster's characteristics and needs. After the planning team agrees upon the priority skill areas for focus, an analysis of where and how the student's needs can be met must be conducted. Discussion must include the most appropriate class placement and whether special education or related services are needed. Special modifications and instructional methods can then be selected and applied.

Sometimes special education services are needed for children with mild brain injury, but they may not be available because the disabilities are not considered "severe" enough to qualify for services. Ylvisaker et al.[27] outlined a protocol for school reentry following mild brain injury for children who appear to have no consequences immediately after an injury. They proposed a "safety net" that can provide for children who experience unexpected difficulty in school after initially appearing to have no problems. They suggested that a person such as the school nurse, psychologist, or special educator function as the TBI coordinator and provide necessary information to school personnel about consequences of TBI, short-term accommodations that may be needed, red flags indicating problems that might persist, and accommodations that may enable the education of the child with mild TBI if the problems appear to be more lasting in nature. By developing such a protocol, the team can work together to ensure these students do not slip through the cracks of the educational process.

Class Placement and Special Education Services

A variety of educational services, provisions, and modifications may be appropriate to the needs of students with TBI. All options should be considered, and families should be made aware of the choices that are possible. Recommendations should be a team effort, with family playing a pivotal role in the decision-making process.

The current trend in education is to fully serve the youngster in the general education setting and provide modifications and services to make the placement successful. Many educators believe the student should be removed from the general education classroom only when needs cannot be met. Some students can succeed in the general education or inclusive classroom setting; for others, homebound instruction, special education classes, or supplemental assistance outside the classroom is necessary. These services may include occupational therapy, physical therapy, speech-language therapy, audiological services, and mental health counseling. Infants and toddlers are eligible for early intervention services offered through their local school districts.[8]

A primary goal in education today is to educate students in the least restrictive environment (LRE). This policy keeps students with their age group so they can interact with their peers as much as possible. A word of caution: Placement selections should not be made at the expense of high-quality education and services. Placement decisions should be made by analyzing the education activities, determining skills required for success, and identifying performance demands and expectations in relation to the student's identified needs. Several authors have provided detailed explanations of procedures for exploring educational options and making educational decisions.[3–5,26,28,29]

Departments of education and local school districts have established protocols for making decisions about educational placement and modes of providing services. If a student has documented physical, cognitive-communication, or psychosocial needs that affect educational performance, the appropriate special services should be integrated into the student's daily school program to maximize the youngster's performance. Optimal classroom functioning with limited disruption should be achieved as the necessary services are provided. Schools have established procedures for qualifying students in differing ways and should be contacted for specific information. At a minimum, an educational assessment is required to qualify a youngster for services.

Special Modifications

Students with TBI may require special accommodations such as schedule adjustments or an abbreviated school day if they fatigue easily or if they require therapy services elsewhere in the community. When learning problems exist, students benefit from modifications in workload, performance requirements, evaluation criteria, or instructional materials. Those who demonstrate poor judgment and self-control need structure and supervision. All of these issues should be discussed during planning sessions. The planning team should clarify expectations for performance.

The learning environment can directly influence the performance of students with TBI. Educators need to consider the physical, social, and psychological environments and make modifications to maximize potential for learning. Blosser and DePompei[3] made the following suggestions: (1) identify aspects of the environment (physical, auditory, visual) that will restrict learning or pose barriers; (2) eliminate or modify barriers and decrease distractions; (3) convey a sense of order by structuring or manipulating the classroom environment to facilitate organization and identification of learning activities and materials; (4) consider the student's location in relation to the teacher's usual position; (5) permit ease of movement within the classroom; (6) make teaching resources, assistive devices, and materials accessible; (7) convey acceptance by treating the student fairly and consistently; and (8) promote group activities, peer interactions, and sharing to foster a positive social environment.

Instructional Methods

All instructional methods that can potentially bring about the desired functional outcomes should be explored. Thus, innovation, adaptation, and a continuing search for opportunities to improve programming are important planning concepts. A number of instructional strategies can be recommended to educators working with students with TBI. The strategies selected and role of the educator in implementing them should be discussed thoroughly and expressed in writing on the treatment and/or educational plan. Instructional strategies can be divided into four categories; teacher-to-student interactional instruction strategies, student-to-student interactional instruction strategies, classroom adaptation and modification techniques, and student learning techniques.[3] Many more could be added to each list. By suggesting examples such as these during planning meetings, others'

ideas will be generated. For each strategy, the question should be asked: "Will this tactic promote opportunities for better learning and understanding for this child?" Many of the strategies, especially the student learning techniques, can be made a part of home-based programming if family members are taught to implement them.[3]

TEACHER-STUDENT INSTRUCTIONAL STRATEGIES

Teachers are confronted daily by the challenges of the diversity of students in schools today. To meet these challenges, most teachers develop a number of teaching strategies for various situations they encounter. When a child with TBI is placed in the school situation, teachers should be helped to identify those instructional strategies that can be used to encourage the most positive learning response from the child. In addition, they must learn to identify exactly when to implement the strategy. Possible strategies include:

- Establish and clarify expectations for the student.

- Analyze the demands made upon the student by assigned tasks.

- Prioritize learning goals and tasks.

- Introduce information at a level that is commensurate with the youngster's developmental and mental capabilities.

- Individualize assignments and tests to accommodate special needs (reduce the number of questions, tape-record lectures, increase print size, modify the format or mode of response).

- Allow multiple opportunities for practice.

- Provide feedback and guidance to increase understanding of successful and unsuccessful attempts.

- Observe and measure performance frequently and systematically. Use information gleaned to modify teaching approaches.

- Provide incentives and consequences to stimulate motivation.

- Teach the student to recognize and measure personal success.

- Plan a specific time for rest and emotional release.

- Encourage the discussion and sharing of problems the child may be experiencing. Help the child understand the relationship between the TBI and problems.

- Discuss why some of the student's behaviors are inappropriate, and make suggestions for changing behavior.

- Be observant of stresses placed upon the child by others (teachers, peers, family, administrators). Reduce stresses as much as possible.

■ Implement holistic approaches to teaching content, involving the student actively in learning activities.

STUDENT-TO-STUDENT INTERACTIONAL INSTRUCTION ACTIVITIES

Peer tutoring and peer "buddy' systems have been successful strategies for improving the skills of children with disabilities. Preparing peers to play important roles in providing support and help to a classmate with TBI is paramount to successful reintegration. As a side benefit, these peer assistance interactions often lead to social friendships. Time should be taken to develop peers' sensitivity and awareness of their fellow student's problems and to establish student-to-student interactional instructional situations. Peer helpers need to learn how to provide assistance. English et al.[30] presented a valuable discussion of how to develop a buddy system for preschool children. Their suggestions have application for youngsters with TBI. Glang et al.[31] discussed developing social networks through peer supports at school.

CLASSROOM ADAPTATIONS AND MODIFICATIONS

The physical, social, and teaching climate can positively or negatively affect a child's success in the learning situation. Consequently, adaptations that make learning more efficient or effective should be identified and incorporated. Ideas include:

■ Encourage the use of assistive devices, including calculators, computers, tape recorders, and assistive listening devices.

■ Formulate a system to help the child maintain organization (schedule book, assignment notebook, "to do" lists).

■ Accompany textbooks and work pages with supportive materials (pictures, written or auditory cues, graphic illustrations).

STUDENT LEARNING TECHNIQUES

Youngsters with TBI often experience difficulty because they are unaware of their problems and lack the skills to implement the changes needed to improve their own performance. Asking children with learning difficulties to simply "try harder" or "do better" is generally ineffective. Unfortunately, there is not always a clear link between effort and success. Moreover, TBI often interferes with initiative and motivation. A more proactive approach is to provide youngsters with concrete strategies for improving their own performance. It provides students with the internal resources needed to make problem-solving efforts successful and permits some sense of control.

The ability to self-evaluate and self-monitor one's performance is essential if learning potential is to be achieved. Research with children with learning disabilities has shown that teaching self-regulation skills is particularly helpful for children who are described as inattentive, easily distracted, and off-task during classroom activities.[32,33] Teaching students to use problem-solving strategies for specific learning tasks such as writing has also proven to be a successful teaching approach for children with disabilities.[34]

Direct emphasis in treatment for TBI should include teaching students to initiate specific strategies to check and change their own performance of classroom work and when problematic social situations arise. It is not enough to simply teach strategies; they must learn to relate the successful outcome of their performance to the use of the strategy. For this procedure to be effective, there are several steps clinicians need to take. First, the learning strategies that will be most useful to the child must be identified. Second, the youngster should be taught to state what the strategy is and how it did (or can) lead to improved performance. This can be accomplished by modeling the strategy for the child through self-talk during teaching activities. (Clinicians or teachers talk about what they are doing as they are doing it during the completion of a task. This process may be presented to children as "thinking out loud about what to do.") Student learning can most reliably be used in association with work assignments from the classroom setting or job assignments. Examples of strategies that can be used to improve a student's schoolwork performance are provided by numerous authors.[2–4,9,29]

School to Work

Schools must provide specific transition plans for adolescents as they leave the school setting. The IEP should include a statement of transition services. Where appropriate, it should also identify interagency responsibilities or linkages that should occur before the student leaves the school setting. To that end, students should receive a wide variety of coordinated activities that lead to employment or further education. When developing plans for transition of the student from school to work, the team should base its recommendations on the student's needs, preferences, and interests.

The ITP that is developed for the student should be designed to help him or her focus on issues such as possible occupational interests and goals, independent living, interpersonal relations, social and recreational activities, and self-advocacy. Vocational testing and career exploration activities can provide excellent opportunities for determining students' options. Topics covered in the treatment plans or school curriculum for adolescents should include: managing finances, finding living quarters, making large purchases, completing job applications, interviewing, and participating in leisure activities. Transition planning at this point is strengthened if a person is designated to serve as the job coach or school-to-work liaison. Opportunities for students will be even greater if school personnel work collaboratively with vocational counselors from related community agencies to identify employment opportunities and promote successful participation in work-related activities. Examples of objectives that might be established for students include:

- To identify employment goals of at least one job that might be of interest (assistance provided by the school guidance counselor)
- To acknowledge employer's expectations for job performance and describe the job skills needed to succeed at the desired job (assistance provided by the school work-study coordinator)
- To demonstrate prerequisite job skills (skill acquisition monitored by teachers and work-study coordinator)
- To work or job shadow for 4 weeks (job training and monitoring provided by a job coach)

□ QUESTION 8: "HOW MUCH WILL THE TRIP COST?"

Adequate resources are necessary to meet the child or adolescent's needs. To appreciate the costs, the team should include finances as resource considerations. Laws of various countries determine the financial responsibility of the schools. Other considerations include:

- Personnel: There may be a need for related services such as physical therapy.
- Time: There may be a need to educate teachers about teaching methods that work with this population, planning team meetings, reassessment of goals, or modification of classroom expectations.
- Service options: There may be a need for services that require more collaboration and coordination of personnel.

Reasonable discussion about how the resources can be allocated is a means of furthering the services provided. Teaching family members to identify and access resources can strengthen their ability to advocate for programming needs.[35]

□ QUESTION 9: "HOW WILL WE KNOW WHEN THE GOAL HAS BEEN REACHED?"

It is helpful to establish benchmarks against which success can be measured. Helping the student achieve a better quality of life than would have been possible without the intervention is a good mark of success. The IEP should be reevaluated in an ongoing manner to determine its suitability for meeting the child's and family's needs. In the school setting, children with special needs must be reevaluated at least annually; students with TBI may experience frequent changes and transitions throughout their development and progress through school. At a minimum, the educational plan should be reevaluated at the following key points: movement to another grade, class, or school building; change in teachers; or significant change in performance or behavior. When planning for transitions such as these, the planning team should be reconstructed several months in advance of the transition to facilitate observations, data gathering, and dialogue between the sending and receiving teachers and other important service providers and family members. For example, for a student currently in sixth grade, the team might consist of the student, two classroom teachers, caretakers, the speech-language pathologist, and the physical therapist from the local rehabilitation center. Because students in seventh grade generally change classes for each subject, plans should be made for incorporating several of the student's seventh-grade teachers as well as an administrator from the middle school building. The new team can select subjects, formulate objectives, and develop a reasonable schedule. When school begins, the new seventh-grade team can feel free to consult with members of the sixth-grade team for advice and recommendations.

□ QUESTION 10: "HOW CAN FAMILIES HELP THEIR CHILD?"

Families are encouraged to accept equal responsibility in planning and implementing the educational program. With guidance, families of students who have sustained a TBI can experience meaningful involvement in the educational planning process. Families may help set the tone and climate for establishing a partnership with school personnel by informing educators of their desire to participate as equal team members. This should be done in the spirit of cooperation and collaboration rather than in an adversarial manner.

Families can expect educators to bring test results and recommendations for class placement, academic modifications, and ideas of appropriate instructional strategies to the planning meetings. Families should prepare for meetings in advance, just as the education team does. There are four key topics that families need to be prepared to discuss during planning meetings:

Topic 1: The nature of the child's TBI, the resulting impairments, and the effects the impairments may have on learning. The family can increase the education team's understanding of TBI and the youngster by discussing the following topics. This information can be solicited from written reports and discussion with health care, education, and rehabilitation professionals who have worked with the child:
□ The extent of the child's injury
□ The current medical, social, behavioral, and cognitive-communicative status of the child
□ Residual strengths and weaknesses
□ Functional skill areas that are impaired and how they will affect classroom performance

Topic 2: The family's expectations and goals for their child and their anxieties and concerns regarding school placement, the academic program, and special services. Planning teams need to understand the family's anxieties and concerns regarding the youngster's school placement, academic program, and therapy services. The following topics should be covered during planning sessions:
□ The family's expectations for the child
□ The degree of agreement among family members regarding expectations for the youngster and capabilities for success
□ Ideas for how personnel and educational programming appropriate for the child's needs might be selected
□ Descriptions of how the injury has affected the child, the family, and the future plans of all
□ The family's level of experience with the special education system
□ Contributions the family is capable of making toward implementing the education process
□ Other family problems and preexisting situations that may affect the school reintegration

□ Ideas regarding the type of special and support services needed and how much therapy (physical, occupational, and speech/language therapy) might be necessary within the school day

Some family members may have skills or talents that can contribute to their participation. Others may be limited in their ability to participate because of personal reasons or constraints. Family members who cannot take on responsibilities should voice their inability to do so to avoid misunderstandings with the education team members.

Topic 3: Resources and teaching strategies necessary for helping the child reach maximum potential. Family members should request clarification of strategies and resources known to benefit students with TBI. Sharing resources among family and education team members may be conducive to developing appropriate methodology for the child.

Topic 4: The structure of the local school district, the district's capabilities for providing needed services, and procedures for making inquiries, expressing needs, and accessing services. Families need to learn about how the educational system works, including special education requirements, placement options, and planning processes. This information can be obtained from administrators in local school districts or from specific state, province, or country divisions of education.

Families need to understand the pivotal role they can play in the educational process for their child. They should be made aware of their ability to present information about the child that will be beneficial for decision-making placements and for implementation of appropriate educational interventions. They should be made to feel like valued and welcome team members.

Case 1 ■ Angel, age 16, sustained a moderate brain injury in a car crash. Prior to her injury she was an A to B student and a cheerleader. She returned to school 3 months after her accident and was given no special accommodation in the classroom. She slept in most of her classes, produced failing work, was unable to retain what she heard or read in class, and eventually was withdrawn from school for poor attendance and attitude. Following several academic, neuropsychological, and cognitive-communicative evaluations, the educational team placed her back in school. By answering the 10 questions in this chapter, a roadmap (IEP/ITP) was developed. It focused on completing the credits necessary for graduation by use of modified reading assignments and verbal presentation of information learned, establishing computer skills, developing work skills by participating in a work-study program as a preschool aide, and creating study skills necessary for college participation. The individualized educational program is presented in the appendix at the end of this chapter.

◻ SUMMARY

Success is a journey, not a destination. This chapter was developed for individuals who desire to understand the special concerns associated with educational transitioning. It was designed to contribute to a better understanding of the educational process and the need for a collaborative effort to aid the child in continuing a journey of success within the educational system.

REFERENCES

1. Research and Training Center on Childhood Trauma: Children and adolescents with disability due to traumatic injury: A databook. Boston, Department of Rehabilitation Medicine, New England Medical Center, 1996.
2. Gerring, JP, and Carney, JM: Head Trauma: Strategies for Educational Reintegration, ed 2. Singular Press, San Diego, 1992.
3. Blosser, JL, and DePompei, R: Pediatric Traumatic Brain Injury: Proactive Intervention. Singular Press, San Diego, 1994.
4. Savage, R, and Wolcott, G: Educational Dimensions of Acquired Brain Injury. PRO-ED, Austin, Tex, 1994.
5. Urbanczyk, B, et al: Creating a workable education program. In Savage, R, and Wolcott, G (eds): An Educators' Manual. Brain Injury Association, Washington, DC, 1995, p 25.
6. Lehr, E, and Savage, R: Community and school integration from a developmental perspective. In Kreutzer, JS, and Wehman, P (eds): Community Integration following Traumatic Brain Injury. Paul H Brookes, Baltimore, 1990, p 301.
7. US Equal Employment Opportunity Commission: Americans with Disabilities Act. Government Printing Office, Washington, DC, 1991.
8. Individuals with Disabilities Education Act of 1990 (IDEA), PL 101-476. Title 20. USC 1400 et seq: US Statutes at Large, 104 (Part 2) October 30, 1990, p 1103.
9. Wolcott, G, et al: Signs and Strategies for Educating Students with Brain Injuries: A Practical Guide for Teachers and Schools. HDI Publishers, Houston, 1995.
10. DePompei, R, and Blosser, JL: Transition planning from hospital to special education placement in school. TBI Challenge, 3(2):9, 1995.
11. Wolcott, G, and Pearson, S: Transition planning worksheet. In Wolcott, G, et al (eds): Signs and Strategies for Educating Students with Brain Injuries: A Practical Guide for Teachers and Schools. HDI Publishers, Houston, 1995, p 73.
12. Federal Register: Rehabilitation Act of 1973, US Government Printing Office, Washington, DC, 1973.
13. Rosenkoetter, SE: Guidelines from recent legislation to structure transition planning. Infants and Young Children 5:21, 1992.
14. DePompei, R, and Blosser, JL: Professional training and development for pediatric rehabilitation. In Durgin, C, et al (eds): Staff Development and Clinical Intervention in Brain Injury Rehabilitation. Aspen, Gaithersberg, 1993, p 229.
15. Wehman, P: Life beyond the Classroom: Transition Strategies for Young People with Disabilities. Paul H Brookes, Baltimore, 1992.
16. Ylvisaker, M, et al: School reentry following severe traumatic brain injury: Guidelines for educational planning. J Head Trauma Rehabil 10(6):47, 1995.
17. Savage, R: Transitions for Children/Adolescents with TBI. Paper presented at Brain Injury Conference, San Diego, December 1995.
18. Hewitt, W: The development of the human corpus callosum. J Anat 96:355, 1962.
19. Savage, R: Shaken baby-sudden impact syndrome. Presentation to Pediatric Task Force of the Brain Injury Association. San Diego, December 1995.
20. Lehr, E: Community integration after traumatic brain injury: Infants and children. In Bachy-Rita, P (ed): Traumatic Brain Injury. Demos, New York, 1989, p 136.
21. Furth, H: Piaget for Teachers. Prentice-Hall, Englewood Cliffs, NJ, 1970.
22. Telzrow, C: The school psychologist's perspective on testing students with traumatic brain injury. J Head Trauma Rehabil 6(1):23, 1991.
23. Shurtleff, H, et al: Screening children and adolescents with mild or moderate traumatic brain injury to assist school reentry. J Head Trauma Rehabil 10(5):64, 1995.
24. Blosser, JL, and DePompei, R: The head injured student returns to school: Recognizing and treating deficits. Topics in Language Disorders 9:67, 1989.
25. Giangreco, M, et al: Perspectives of parents whose children have sensory impairments. Journal of the Association for Persons with Severe Handicaps 16:14, 1991.
26. Thousand, JS, and Villa, RA: Strategies for educating learners with severe disabilities within their local home schools and communities. Focus on Exceptional Children 23:1 (ERIC Document Reproduction Service No ED 361 977), 1990.
27. Ylvisaker, M, et al: School reentry following mild traumatic brain injury: A proposed hospital to school protocol. J Head Trauma Rehabil 10(6):64, 1995.
28. Williams, W, and Fox, TJ: Planning for inclusion: A practical process. Teaching Exceptional Children 28:6, 1996.
29. Blosser, JL, and Pearson, S: Transition in coordination for students with brain injury: A challenge schools can meet. J Head Trauma Rehabil 12(2):21, 1997.
30. English, K, et al: "Buddy skills" for preschoolers. Teaching Exceptional Children 28:62, 1996.
31. Glang, A, et al: Building social networks for children and adolescents with traumatic brain injury: A school-based intervention. J Head Trauma Rehabil 12(2):33, 1997.
32. Licht, B: Cognitive-motivational factors that contribute to the achievement of learning disabled children. Journal of Learn Disabilities 16:483, 1983.
33. Reid, R, and Harris, KR: Self-monitoring of attention versus self-monitoring of performance: Effects on attention and academic performance. Exceptional Children 26:34, 1993.
34. Stevens, DD, and Englert, CS: Making writing strategies work. Teaching Exceptional Children 26:34, 1993.
35. Williams, J: Supporting families after head injury: Implications for the speech-language pathologist. Seminars in Speech-Language 14:44, 1994

APPENDIX — Angel's Individualized Education Program

Present Levels of Development/ Functioning/Performance	Annual Goals	Objectives	Evaluation of Each Objective Procedure
[Refer to State of Ohio Model Policies and Procedures for the Education of Children with Disabilities or IEP Tourbook for specific information on procedures/process.] Step 1 Review the results of the evaluation team report or intervention-based multifactored evaluation or current IEP. In a narrative form, explain the child's/student's present levels of performance. Include progress, strengths, capabilities, interests, and needs displayed in school, at home, and in the community. Step 2 Determine the area(s) of the student's needs.	Step 3 Write goals and objectives in areas of need. (What will the student be able to do in 1 year?)	What are the intermediate/ sequential steps leading to the goal?	How?
Angel has normal range reading and writing skills, but she lacks computer skills.	Angel will understand basic computer skills.	Angel will be taught general word processing and general keyboarding skills.	Angel will utilize a computer at her work station in the Kearsley Building. She will use this technology for English, primarily; but it will generalize to other subjects as well.
Angel demonstrated delays in auditory memory on CELF-R3 testing.	Angel will recall verbal directions long enough to perform them or write them down.	Angel will rehearse verbal directions and remember them.	Angel will remember verbal instructions and do them in the tutoring session and in the work-study session with one or fewer prompts. She will write down in her daily planner instructions she received verbally from her tutors or work-study coordinator.
The Rainbow Babies and Children's Hospital Report and other behavior assessments noted delays in attention and stamina.	Angel will attend to seat work and assignments.	Angel's tutors and work-study coordinator will watch for signs of inattention and give her appropriate prompts. Angel will also have frequent breaks planned into her schedule.	Angel's tutors will use a range of appropriate prompts like verbal prompts, touching her shoulder, or making refocusing inquiries about her work. She may be given self-statements like "I am here now" to use when she notices herself drifting off task. Angel's tutors and work-study coordinator will provide periodic opportunities for Angel to get up, move around, get a drink, and interrupt her mood when attention and stamina begin to flag.

[This form can be used vertically or horizontally.]

Evaluation of Each Objective (Continued)				Services	Initiation/ Duration	LRE
Criteria	Schedule	Who	Review Progress			
What? How much?	When will we review?	Who is responsible?	Results?	Step 4 Determine special education, including related services, needed to implement each goal, as well as the amount of services. (*e.g., modifications, supplemental aids, assistive technology, providers*)		Step 5 Determine setting in which to deliver the service. (*Where will services be provided?*)
Angel will create, edit, save, and transfer text files within a hard disk, and to floppy disks for school assignments, business letters, and personal letters or files.	Her program will be reviewed biweekly.	Her work-study coordinator, and her tutors.		Angel will use a Macintosh computer using Microsoft Works 4.0.	03/11/96 through 08/30/96	Angel will work in her work station at the Kearsley Building.
Angel will begin working on oral instructions with one or fewer prompts 70% of the time.	This will be reviewed biweekly.	Her tutors and work-study coordinator.		Angel's tutors will use a standardized progress log to record this.	03/11/96 through 08/30/96	At her work station at the Kearsley Building.
Angel will accurately record all the essential items in oral instructions in her daily planner 70% of the time or more.	This will be reviewed biweekly.	Her tutors and work-study coordinator.		Angel will use a daily planner, and her tutors will use a standardized progress log.	03/11/96 through 08/30/96	At her work station at the Kearsley Building.
A baseline of attention and task endurance will be created and she will then be encouraged to stretch that endurance by a minute or two each week. If the baseline is 15 minutes, she should be encouraged to strive for 17 minutes, then 19. Ultimately, two 30- to 40-min stretches will be ideal.	This will be reviewed biweekly, but charted in her tutors' progress logs daily.	Her tutors and work-study coordinator.		Her tutors will note length of attention and number of breaks needed in their standardized progress logs.	03/11/96 through 08/30/96	At her Kearsley work station and on her work assignment.

Present Levels of Development/ Functioning/Performance	Annual Goals	Objectives	Evaluation of Each Objective
			Procedure
[Refer to State of Ohio Model Policies and Procedures for the Education of Children with Disabilities or IEP Tourbook for specific information on procedures/process.] Step 1 Review the results of the evaluation team report or intervention-based multifactored evaluation or current IEP. In a narrative form, explain the child's/student's present levels of performance. Include progress, strengths, capabilities, interests, and needs displayed in school, at home, and in the community. Step 2 Determine the area(s) of the student's needs.	Step 3 Write goals and objectives in areas of need. (What will the student be able to do in 1 year?)	What are the intermediate/sequential steps leading to the goal?	How?
The Rainbow Babies and Children's Hospital Report, past tutors, and Angel's mother have reported some difficulty with social judgment.	Angel will demonstrate age-appropriate social judgment.	Angel will rehearse appropriate social rules in various common settings.	As part of Angel's Social Studies coursework, and her work-study experience, she will be talked through various commonly occurring social/ethical dilemmas and will talk about the appropriate actions required in that setting.
On the Rainbow Babies and Children's Hospital Report, as well as the accounting of nearly everyone who has worked with Angel, she has been found to have anxieties about school generally and tends to doubt her abilities to do the work. She has a hard time getting started on tasks.	Her tutors, work-study coordinator, and her family will help her structure her work day so that she develops momentum and a routine.	Tutors will follow a routine in reviewing past work and introducing new work.	Tutors will follow a script for each tutoring session that will help Angel relax initially, rehearse past progress that she may not remember, review what will be done during the current tutoring session, do it, log what was done, and rehearse progress of the current session. The home support system will also provide prompts that include rehearsing progress, and assure her that the homework is well within her abilities. She will probably need to be guided through the "getting started" part of homework throughout the tutoring.
Angel expresses an interest in going to college for additional training after she graduates. She is not fully confident of the various steps involved in this process.	Angel will understand the process for going to college.	Angel will demonstrate how to get forms, catalogs, and admission books and use them.	Angel will write letters requesting the items needed for applying to a college and will transfer her records to college admission offices.

[This form can be used vertically or horizontally.]

Evaluation of Each Objective (Continued)				Services	Initiation/ Duration	LRE
Criteria	Schedule	Who	Review Progress			
What? How much?	When will we review?	Who is responsible?	Results?	Step 4 Determine special education, including related services, needed to implement each goal, as well as the amount of services. (*e.g., modifications, supplemental aids, assistive technology, providers*)		Step 5 Determine setting in which to deliver the service. (*Where will services be provided?*)
With respect to typical social/ethical situations, Angel will articulate a strategy for handling the situation and will discuss the implications for those actions with accuracy. That is, the implications that she articulates would be commonly agreed upon by most reasonable people of her age.	This will be reviewed biweekly.	Her tutors and her work-study coordinator.		Anecdotal progress notes will be kept in the tutors' standardized progress logs.	03/11/96 through 05/30/96	At her Kearsley work station, and on her work assignment.
The tutors will use the standardized protocol on the cover of their progress logs every session. The home may wish to utilize something very similar. It would be very helpful to have Angel verbalize her progress at the end of each session to ensure that she rehearses it and, perhaps, that it will impress itself on her.	This will be reviewed biweekly.	Her tutors and work-study coordinator. Her family support.		The standardized progress logs.	03/11/96 through 08/30/96	At Kearsley and at home.
Letters will be written to colleges of Angel's choosing.	Biweekly	Work-study coordinator.		Done at the study center of Kearsley.	03/11/96 through 05/31/96	

Special Topics

ERNEST R. GRIFFITH, MD,
and JEFFREY S. KREUTZER, PHD

CHAPTER 24

Ethical Dimensions of Severe Traumatic Brain Injury

JOHN D. BANJA, PHD

Ethical issues associated with severe traumatic brain injury (TBI) provoke an observation that would probably be uncontroversial among rehabilitation providers: More than any other disability group, people with severe TBI present an enormous array of ethical conundrums associated with their rehabilitation and their political status as rights holders. The problem that this observation presents in developing this chapter is that one can choose either to survey as many of these ethical situations as possible or to focus on a few rather fundamental ones that underlie many of the others and that have proven particularly difficult over the years.

The latter approach has been chosen in the hope that a more elaborate account of certain basic ethical problems in TBI not only gives these issues the space they deserve but also, because they are fundamental, sheds light on or suggests the diversity of other ethical problems that readers may have encountered and pondered. (Although *ethical* and *moral* have technically different meanings, in bioethical discussions they are frequently used interchangeably, which is the practice in this chapter.)

The first section of this chapter examines how severe TBI disrupts the core of an individual's "moral agency." Holding people morally accountable at least requires that they are able to exercise understanding, reasoning, and insight—the very cognitive abilities that are frequently compromised by severe TBI. On a deeper level, the "self" of the individual with TBI may have been profoundly disrupted by injury, which, in turn, creates wrenching existential issues about an individual's ability to develop, maintain, and enjoy a "meaningful" life. This section therefore treats the moral self not only as someone who makes calculations about right or wrong, but also as a self who struggles to realize his or her values in personal relationships, experiences, and attempts to live a good life.

◻ ETHICAL IMPLICATIONS OF THE DISRUPTED SELF

In the nineteenth and early twentieth centuries, philosophers began to explore certain ethical dimensions of human choice and how those choices affect the person who makes them. Existential thinkers like Nietzsche, Kierkegaard, and Sartre observed that morally adequate choices issue from an "authentic" self—that is, a self that is self-transparent, mature, insightful, and courageous enough to fashion a life based on the values he or she cherishes.[1] Pragmatist philosophers like John Dewey and William James were interested in how choices reflect back on and "constitute" the self.[2] They were intrigued by the ways human beings shape and are shaped by their choices. Indeed, philosophers at least since the time of Aristotle noted the important association of habituated behavior and the development of moral character.[3]

The great German phenomenologist Edmund Husserl took these speculations a step further to an "egological" level and asked about the "ultimate" or "primordial self," who performs cognitive acts and who is shaped by them.

Husserl's writings are extremely complex, but what they say about this ultimate self—which he called the *transcendental ego*—provides an excellent prototype for appreciating the intersections between severe brain injury and moral agency.

Philosophizing about an intact, reasonably functioning ego, Husserl observed that one of its most essential and critical aspects is its self-continuity of self-sameness over time.[4] He spoke about the ego as a primordial "ray" that connects its present life (i.e., its conscious acts) with its past and future moments. The transcendental ego provides the contents of my mind with a synthetic center (functioning like "psychical glue"), whereby the contents of my conscious life cohere in a familiar, accessible, ready-to-use way[5]: I am the unique person I am because of the way the transcendental ego organizes my experiences as my conscious life. Husserl would say that the transcendental ego accounts for my uniqueness because it (1) builds and has itself been built up by my experiences and (2) accounts for the unique, personal way that my conscious acts enable me to engage and give meaning to my experiences.

Brain Injury and the Disrupted Self

Although today's philosophers discuss transcendental egos only as historical artifacts, Husserl's egology provides a useful set of metaphors to understand the "rupture to the self" that is so typical of severe traumatic brain injury. The memory loss that invariably accompanies serious brain injury disconnects my past from my present. Confusion and confabulation disenable me from productively managing the world I encounter. Extremely important from an ethical perspective is the way profound TBI might compromise my ability to know and contemplate my moral beliefs and values. Indeed, a brain injury might not so much cause me to lose my premorbid set of values (my likes, interests, and notions of worth) as cause me to lose my ability to realize or integrate those values in action.

For example, many people with severe brain injury, especially those with the rather common impairments of the frontal lobes, may find themselves unable to execute actions that embody their intentions. They exhibit those "errors of action" deficits because of a variety of impairments (context dependency, inability to generate structure, attentional deficits, perseveration, confusion) associated with action sequencing or planning errors prevent them from operationalizing their values or from being "valuing selves."[6] Consider that the frontal lobes:

provide continuity and coherence to behavior across time . . . [and help] to integrate behaviors across much longer spans of time, allowing for such complex functions as "planning" and giving the coherency and predictability to behavior that we think of as part of the "personality." . . . Clients with significant frontal injury may appear unable to visualize themselves in the future, to grasp the relationship between long-term plans and the steps required to meet them, or to decide which actions fit most appropriately with a given goal. . . . The failure to appreciate one's performance in order to detect and correct errors, implement and fine tune novel ideas, and maintain an overall picture of oneself in one's social milieu leads to the classic descriptions of frontally injured clients as rigid, uninsightful, and unable to benefit from experience. (pp. 2–3)[7]

Notice that virtually every human choice looks to a backdrop of values that define appropriateness, goodness, desirability, attractiveness, satisfaction, adequacy, and so forth. Notice also that virtually all practically moral decision making ultimately requires analyzing, selecting, and applying values to real-world situations. If a person with severe brain injury is unable to initiate plans that realize his or her values in action or is unable to understand factual situations so that values can be applied in managing or resolving them, that person is severed from his or her sense of power or "self-actualization." I cannot be "my self" (i.e., a self that I can intend and control) because I cannot coherently realize my intentions in the world. If severe brain injury deprives me of my ability "to decide what is worth attending to and what is worth doing . . . [as well as my ability to assign] priorities or values to both stimuli and responses" (p. 2).[7] I am without a compass with which I could meaningfully shape my actions and vice versa. Tragically but not surprisingly, as I find myself deprived of the ability to value in a consistent and coherent way and unable to relate to the world or other human beings in ways reflecting those values, I might find my membership in the human community becoming tenuous or marginalized.

Moral Accountability and the Disrupted Self

The first moral dimension of severe brain injury, then, is precisely the loss of integrity or "wholeness" of the valuing self that contemplates and realizes worth, significance, importance, rightness, or goodness in the course of any—not just moral—decision making and action. As many commentators on brain injury have noted, the choices, thoughts, beliefs, and feelings that motivate or explain the choices of people with severe TBI may be uninsightful, uninformed, impulsive, inconsistent, unproductive, inflexible, hesitant, disorganized, or fragmentary because the self from which they issue is disrupted and fragmented.[6,8]

The diminished ability of people with TBI to value coherently and in socially approved ways has immediate implications for the degree to which they can be held morally accountable for their actions. As the section on competency demonstrates, to be a fully responsible moral agent, one has to act not only voluntarily but also knowingly and insightfully. I must be able to calculate the impact and consequences of my actions and determine whether those consequences are truly beneficial to me or others in ways that reflect how I or those others understand "benefits" and intend for them to occur. The essence of utilitarian approaches to moral decision making, for example, is to maximize benefits or minimize harms (if only harm will result).[9] Frequently, however, these benefits-versus-burdens calculations are considerably complex for persons with intact cognition, let alone for someone with serious cognitive impairments.

Another moral issue involving (un)insightful behavior among people with severe brain injury is their inability to live within certain behavioral limits. Aristotle lauded the life of moderation, temperance, and contemplation, prominent character traits of the virtuous individual.[3] People with severe brain injury, however, may simply be unable to discern the limits within which society expects they will orchestrate their behavior. Although brain injury does not usually cause an individual to exhibit emotional and character traits that were never part of his or her psychic reality, many people with brain injury become behaviorally disinhibited or disruptive to the point where they cannot even be effectively engaged in rehabilitative therapy.[10]

The remainder of this chapter focuses on certain more discrete and specifiable issues regarding rights, duties, and responsibilities relevant to persons with severe TBI. It is nevertheless important to recognize at the outset how the onset of severe TBI might usurp an individual's moral agency by disrupting that core or center of consciousness from which values and meanings originate and evolve. As those values and meanings become disconnected, fragmentary, or elusive, they are unavailable for valuative contemplation precisely because such contemplation requires comparisons, analyses, weighings, imaginings, and descriptions of *relevant, related* valuative notions and ideas.

Worst of all, the self that cannot value consistently and effectively may come to believe it is a self without value. As such, the effort to care for and rehabilitate the emotional and cognitive deficits of persons with severe brain injury often goes beyond any specific problem. Ultimately, what is being rehabilitated may well be the center of that person's being and his or her will to live.[11]

◻ MORAL ASPECTS OF FAMILIES WITH SEVERELY BRAIN INJURED MEMBERS

The moral significance of families in TBI rehabilitation cannot be overestimated. Many people with severe TBI, especially early in their rehabilitation, cannot demonstrate competent decision making. Close family members therefore find themselves recruited as significant decision makers and inevitably inject their values into situations requiring their opinions, preferences, and beliefs.[12]

A second reason for examining familial values is that it has become increasingly clear that parental and familial values are extremely influential in the valuative formation *of the patient*—as values that the patient has explicitly either accepted or rejected.[13] If "values" are ultimately ascriptions and beliefs about what is important, worthwhile, or desirable, then one needs only to point out that a person's values did not arise in a vacuum. All of us were born into a world of values that were adopted and practiced by our families and, frequently, our communities. The patient, then, may have appropriated many of those values as his or her own or may have rebelled against them in evolving a valuative framework. Either way, familial and community values represent important points of reference in understanding the values of the patient and in considering and negotiating how particularly value-laden decisions should proceed.

At this point, we might discuss in greater detail an observation made in the preceding section: that the moral dimensions of health care decision making can often be understood as an intersection of values with factual situations. For example, "What is the projected outcome of this treatment plan?" asks for a factual answer. "Will that outcome be sufficiently beneficial or not?" looks to values for a response. "How much will that regimen of treatment cost?" is a factual question. "Ought I spend that amount of money on an outcome that is not guaranteed?" requires a valuative opinion. "What will the patient's functional level be at discharge?"

is a factual question. "Will the patient's disability impose an unreasonable degree of burden on the family caregivers?" requires knowing the family's value-laden attitudes about what is a "reasonable" versus "unreasonable" burden.

A serious point in examining this intersection of values with fact is that neither family decision makers nor patients may have adequate understanding of either the factual situation they face or what values they might apply to that situation (i.e., what they believe *ought* to be done).[13] As a patient nears discharge, for example, the extent of his or her functional impairments may be obvious to family members, but they might be in turmoil as to how those functional impairments will alter the routine comings and goings of their family life. Equally unclear might be whether they ought to care for their loved one at home or seek another care setting if the caregiver burden is likely to be oppressive. Indeed, the degree of moral responsibility a family should assume in caring for their loved one is, at least in the United States, a decidedly personal choice. It is, nevertheless, the kind of choice whose gravity causes many families considerable anxiety and discomfort.

Another important moral aspect of the familial presence is that as the family begins to gather factual information about their loved one's condition and acquires greater familiarity with the patient's treatments and the professional staff, conflicts and disagreements among numerous parties might arise.[14] Perhaps the reason is primarily psychological because, in the early stage of acute rehabilitation, family members might feel helpless and frustrated by their inability to understand and control what is going on around them. As time passes and their knowledge of their loved one's clinical situation increases, family members might very well begin exerting some ownership and control of the situation by taking exception to or gainsaying clinical decisions made by the treatment team.

Although this behavior might upset some health providers who fear it will obstruct the patient's best interests, families with judgmentally incapacitated loved ones are frequently able to exert a moral and legal right to substantive information and participative decision making in their loved one's care. This right is based on the doctrine of informed consent, which the next of kin is usually able to exert by law on the judgmentally incapacitated patient's behalf. It also exists because, in so many instances, the family assumes the rehabilitation effort after their loved one is formally discharged from rehabilitation.[15] Their right to know, therefore, is more than just a legal entitlement; it is a clinically significant element in the patient's recovery.

The Family's Right to Information

Arthur Caplan has pointed out that informed consent in rehabilitation is different from its occurrence in more acute, especially surgical, scenarios.[16] There, the emphasis of the informed consent construct focuses on the (usually one-time) clinical intervention that is recommended, along with whatever benefits and risks it poses for the patient. Although the phrase "informed consent" seems to anticipate consent, the fundamental and somewhat paradoxical reason the right exists is to give the patient an opportunity to refuse the intervention; that is, armed with a knowledge of treatment benefits and its risks, the patient can then exercise his or her values in reasoning about whether the treatment's benefits outweigh the associated risks and whether the projected benefits justify proceeding with treatment.[17]

The delivery of rehabilitation services presents a markedly different decisional situation because rehabilitative care is processual and rarely poses the degree of risk that surgical interventions do.[18] Furthermore, successful rehabilitation absolutely requires the active engagement and motivation of its consumers, in contrast with the more passive, biologically based healing paradigm typical of a surgical intervention and its associated recovery course. Consequently, Caplan suggests that an educational model may be the most appropriate for rehabilitation. Some salient components of this model and the types of information that might be imparted to patients and their families include:

- The projected plan of rehabilitation treatments and fact that treatment will probably be delivered by a team of professionals for an extended period of time
- The responsibilities of the various treating professionals and who is responsible for the overall management of the team
- The patient's or family's right to request reasonable changes in the team composition or to refuse—as is legally allowable—certain therapies
- The probable need for significant familial interaction and familiarity with the rehabilitation process, given the likelihood of the patient's care needs continuing after formal rehabilitation discharge
- The fact that confidentiality in rehabilitation will be reasonably protected but that (1) a multiplicity of health professionals will need to access clinical information and (2) that family members might need to know otherwise confidential information, especially if they are to assume the patient's care after discharge

■ How discharge will be determined and what the patient's probable postdischarge needs will be[16]

Given the current era of cost constraints, other commentators have emphasized the importance of maintaining constant dialogue with patients and families on their health benefits coverage, the impact of the projected plan of care on that coverage, and the potential need for the patient or family to tap their personal financial resources to reimburse all the care that is needed.[19] Information with distinct economic implications that should be communicated to patients and families includes:

■ The overall rehabilitation benefits package the patient's insurer provides

■ Medical or rehabilitative treatments the patient might need that are not covered in the plan

■ Conflicts of interest (such as a rehabilitation or other health provider who has an ownership interest in some type of treatment or diagnostic service to which he or she would like to refer the patient)

■ How other services and referrals are economically structured by the patient's health care plan (e.g., the payer has an exclusive contract with a certain provider group to which the patient must go for services that the insurance plan will reimburse)

■ How denials of care might be appealed

If patients' and families' rights of informed consent are to be respected, it seems incumbent on health providers to impart this information. If, however, we are also to respect patient and familial values and the way those values are frequently interjected into interpreting the meaning and implications of the information they receive, then rehabilitation providers will also wish to discern what those values might be.

Ethnographic Considerations

Arthur Kleinman, a pioneering figure in medical anthropology, has suggested that health providers perform an "ethnographic assessment" of patient and familial values in view of how those values penetrate health care decisions.[20] Although Kleinman developed these thoughts from his work with culturally diverse groups of health consumers, the contemporary emphasis on acknowledging patient and familial values encourages the utilization of Kleinman's ethnographic questions in virtually any clinical encounter, especially if the provision of care is likely to be long-term. Included in Kleinman's suggestions are that health providers

learn their clients' and families' views on issues such as:

■ How they understand the illness or disability (e.g., do they think it analogous to a flu or virus from which they will entirely recover?)

■ What caused it (e.g., their irresponsibility, God's wrath)

■ What kinds of treatment should the patient receive (e.g., spiritual help, plenty of medicine, bed rest, chiropractic interventions)

■ What the patient or family fears most

■ How family members should respond to the patient's disability

■ What duties or obligations family members should assume in light of the patient's disabilities[20]

Kleinman makes the striking point that health providers experience disease but patients experience illness. He means that the health professional discerns the manifestations of sickness in terms of underlying pathophysiological processes, but patients experience the misery, functional disability, and a tremendous array of painful and sometimes self-destructive emotions deriving from their impairments. Professionals might do well to consider that conflicts or disagreements between them and families are frequently of psychogenic origin and may not revolve primarily about substantive moral points. Sometimes, families are angry or contentious only because they find the oppressiveness of their situations intolerable and project their rage on the nearest health professional. The health professional who is tuned into the family's psychic reality will not interpret these outbursts as inherently conflictual but rather as an expression of the family's trying to deal with their situation as best their coping mechanisms allow.[21,22]

Conflicts Involving Familial Values

Certain conflicts between professionals and families may indeed revolve about substantive valuative or moral points. Perhaps the most common—and frequently the most trying—is the family who refuses to comply with professional recommendations.

Family members or guardians do not have the right to make decisions that will predictably or foreseeably place the patient in harm's way,[23] but the moral problem occurs in defining *harm*. Not only do people differ in their definition of harmful situations or practices (e.g., is abortion or physician-assisted suicide "harmful"?) but also people routinely and voluntarily risk harming themselves by ignoring seat belts or motorcycle helmets, exceeding speed limits, eating a poor diet, smoking, and consuming alcohol.[24]

Nevertheless, certain instances of familial harm are unproblematic, such as the family who refuses to assume responsibility for their loved one's wound care at home. Assuming such neglect would place the individual in serious danger, the health provider in charge has a moral and legal responsibility to ensure that this patient receives appropriate care such as by a visiting home nurse or therapist. The provider who fails to do this is understood in law to have malpracticed by abandoning the patient if the patient experiences significant harm as a result.[25] For example, a pediatrician in the United States was recently ordered to pay $200,000 to the estate of a murdered girl and her half-brother. The jury said the doctor was guilty of malpractice when she failed to pursue her suspicions that her 16-month-old patient was being abused. The physician had seen this patient on multiple occasions, suspected her bruises were the result of abuse, and inquired about them from the girl's mother, who denied they were the results of abuse. Three months later, however, the girl was pronounced dead of massive head injuries. The mother's boyfriend was convicted of murder and sentenced to life in prison.[26]

Case 1 ■ All of this assumes that the health professional *knows* or *should know* about the potential for patient abuse but does not take reasonable measures to protect the patient.[25] Some cases, however, are not as straightforward. Suppose a young man with brain injury has a moderate swallowing problem and is receiving outpatient rehabilitation. The family has been informed of the patient's need for a soft or pureed diet, but they report that the patient refuses those foods at home and that they cannot control what he eats. The patient's noncompliance with the recommended diet places him at significant, possibly lethal risk of aspiration. What is the moral responsibility of the rehabilitation provider in this case?

If the family does not accommodate their loved one's need for a soft-textured diet after repeated instruction, the professional has to consider whether (1) they are cognitively unable to understand the situation and its risks, (2) they do understand but refuse to take even modest, reasonable measures to ensure the safety of their family member, or (3) the family is making a good-faith effort to carry through the professional's suggestions but find that the situation is beyond their control. (Of course, all of this assumes that the patient himself is unable to understand his need for a modified-consistency diet. As the next section illustrates, if the patient did

understand the risk and consequences of aspiration but refused to comply with the diet, then the ultimate responsibility for any adverse consequences resulting from his risky behavior would be his.)

Setting up a consultation with a speech-language therapist skilled in dysphagia management who might structure a home program is an obvious strategy, along with securing advice and recommendations from a counselor or psychologist on maintaining compliance. If these interventions fail and the patient continues to be at serious risk without the hope of regaining adequate swallowing ability, the family should be reminded that, as they are closest to the situation—temporally, geographically, and by the protective bonds of kinship—they might very well be held liable if serious harm befalls this patient and the health provider can demonstrate that he or she did everything reasonable to prevent that harm from occurring.[27] Making the family aware of their responsibility—and the possibility of prosecution by the state for abuse and neglect—might encourage them to try harder to enforce their son's diet. (And merely because the family is telling the health professional that they are making an honest effort does not mean they actually are.) Some rehabilitation providers might go so far as to contact their local adult or children's protective services to pressure the family, but this strategy should probably be a last resort. Although it might categorically relieve the provider from liability for any harm that befalls this individual, such a contact would almost certainly antagonize and probably alienate the patient's family.

Consequently, should this case proceed to a point of imminent danger, the rehabilitationist could face a difficult judgment call in weighing the dangers of the patient's risk of harm from aspiration against whatever psychological or emotional turbulence might occur to the family—which includes the patient—from a county or state agency investigation. The latter situation would be especially wrenching if the family was trying hard to have the patient comply with the diet but simply could not carry it through. In the event harm would transpire, one would want to know if the family did all they might reasonably have done to prevent the adverse event. If so—and especially if it could be demonstrated that it would have been beyond reason to anticipate the family could monitor the patient's eating habits 24 hours a day—it would seem inappropriate to hold the family morally or legally liable for any untoward events that might materialize from this situation. Indeed, if all parties took reasonable measures to prevent harm but harm transpired anyway, it would have to be attributed to tragedy, not irresponsibility.

The emphasis on reasonable actions is entirely congruent both with our society's legal expectations of health providers (i.e., that they act as "reasonable and prudent" health providers would) and with those liberal values common to most industrially advanced countries that refrain from insisting that persons perform unreasonably burdensome or "supererogatory" acts.[28] Our moral common sense tells us that it is simply wrong to hold someone to a standard of responsibility to which an average or reasonable individual could not adhere. Importantly, the reasonable standard in the case study would dictate that the health provider seek to protect both the patient's and the family's welfare (although the patient's welfare has primacy). And it should also suggest moral guidelines and limits for what we *ordinarily* ought to expect from people (whether they are families or professionals) who are responsible for their charges. If articulating a vision of "reasonability" proves difficult for some professionals, they might turn to organizational structures such as an ethics committee for help. If certain situations are commonly acknowledged to raise difficult problems about the nature or scope of a professional's moral obligations, they should be the focus of research and comment in the TBI literature and at national conferences.

Caring for a person with severe traumatic brain injury is enormously complicated by the unpredictability of the patient's needs, the adequacy of resources that families and their providers bring to the rehabilitation effort, and lingering uncertainties about the quality of the patient's outcome. What can be confidently asserted, however, is that the greater the congruence among patients, families, and providers regarding their understanding of what is happening, why it is happening, and what ought to be done as rehabilitation proceeds, the less one might expect moral argument or consternation.[20] Because family members are frequently unfamiliar with the nature of brain injury rehabilitation and may require as much or more help than the patient, the rehabilitationist must serve as a facilitator of knowledge, a skillful communicator who speaks to family members in a language they can understand, and a values negotiator who maintains a deep respect for the family's need to have their values recognized and respected.

☐ DECISION-MAKING ABILITY AND COMPETENCE

Whereas an earlier section of this chapter dealt with how brain injury might interfere with an individual's attempts to create and sustain meaning and value in life, this section discusses more task-specific impairments that people with moderately severe brain injury might experience. Also, whereas the immediately preceding section discussed the family's responsibility for the patient, this section discusses the extent of patients' responsibility for themselves. Because cognitive impairments involve important abilities of everyday life such that the person with the injury may be disposed to either self-harm or harming others, significant ethical and legal issues arise about the extent of curbing those potentially dangerous behaviors. Health providers are accustomed to recognizing these issues under the heading of "competency," although we sometimes speak about "decision-making capacity" or "judgmental ability."[29,30]

As has been frequently noted, *competency* is a legal construct meaning that decisions pertinent to the "incompetent" or questionably competent person come under the purview of the legal system. Commentators often point out that only a court can adjudicate someone as "incompetent."[31] This point hardly means, however, that health providers have no responsibility toward individuals who are obviously incompetent but have never been adjudicated so, like a delirious person admitted to an emergency room following an automobile accident, or a person with serious cognitive impairments just admitted to a brain injury facility. The health provider who complies with such an individual's refusal of care because a judge could not be located to adjudicate the patient incompetent will most certainly be liable for malpractice if the patient suffers harm as a direct result of not receiving treatment.[32,33] For that reason, many states have enacted statutes regarding who might provide consent to medical treatment if the patient is incompetent so that the health professional does not have to resort to the courts initially. (To the extent, however, that an adult will probably remain incompetent, a proxy decision maker or guardian should ultimately be appointed by the court.[34])

Much of the inspiration for our contemporary understanding of competency originated from two sources: (1) the state's concern about protecting individuals who could not care for themselves and (2) the state's desire to deal justly with those who broke the law.[35] Historical articulations prefiguring the contemporary notion of competency are found in eighteenth-century English legal commentaries arguing that "madmen" ought not be executed for their crimes and that the trial of insane defendants must be postponed until the defendants are able to appreciate the significance of their legal predicament and work with their lawyers in fashioning their defense.[35] In what has been called the "first of the historically significant" insanity defense trials, Judge Tracy in 1724 charged the jury with deciding whether the defendant:

> hath the use of his reason and sense? If he . . . could not distinguish between good and evil, and did not know what he did . . . he could not be guilty of any offence against any law whatsoever. . . . On the other side . . . it is not every kind of frantic humour or something unaccountable in a man's actions, that point him out to be such a madman as is to be exempted from punishment: *it must be a man that is totally deprived of his understanding and memory, and doth not know what he is doing, no more than an infant, than a brute, or a wild beast, such a one is never the object of punishment.* (p. 287)[36]

As society began to admit the moral impropriety of prosecuting those not responsible for their crimes or capable of defending themselves, so the state also came to believe it would violate its citizens' welfare by failing to protect citizens who could not care for themselves. Calling upon its *parens patriae* power—originating from the king's right to protect his subjects from danger—the modern liberal state customarily chooses to protect an incapacitated individual's best interest by appointing a guardian or having the individual institutionalized.[37]

The Competency Construct

The competency construct originated from society's need to remediate welfare problems associated with serious intellectual or judgmental impairments affecting some of its citizens. Indeed, the early connotations of competency were invariably linked to profoundly disabling mental dysfunction, such as madness, insanity, imbecility, or retardation.[34] Because of the global nature of cognitive or mental impairments that gave rise to the first guardianship and civil commitment statutes, guardians were usually appointed with "plenary" powers over their wards that extended to authority over decisions pertaining to both the ward and the ward's property. Today, however, incompetency is primarily understood not as global mental impairment but rather as dysfunction that is skill specific. As Buchanan and Brock note:

> Competence is always competence for some task—competence to do something. The concern here is with competence to perform the task of making a decision. Hence competence is to be understood as decision-making capacity. But the notion of decision-making capacity is itself incomplete until the nature

of the choice as well as the conditions under which it is to be made are specified. Thus competence is decision-relative, not global. A person may be competent to make a particular decision at a particular time, under certain circumstances, but incompetent to make another decision, or even the same decision, under different conditions. A competence determination, then, is a determination of a particular person's capacity to perform a particular decision-making task at a particular time and under specified conditions. (p. 18)[30]

Obviously, the individual with profound retardation, dementia, or catatonia is globally incompetent. However, the decisional specificity that Buchanan and Brock acknowledge is exceptionally apparent in lawsuits involving people with cognitive impairments, wherein courts have evaluated such individuals' competence to execute a will, sign tax returns, sign voter registration cards, sign checks, approve bills for payment, testify as a witness on their behalf, release a defendant from a lawsuit, and qualify for jury duty. Among states that have revised their guardianship laws and competency evaluations according to a "domain-specific" or functional capacity approach, the appointed guardians are empowered to make decisions in only those functional areas over which the ward is truly incapacitated. Quoting from the 1989 District of Columbia statute, Hommel et al.[34] write that courts shall "encourage the development of maximum self-reliance and independence of the incapacitated individual and make appointive and other orders only to the extent necessitated by the individual's mental and adaptive limitations or other conditions warranting the procedure" (DC Code 21-2044). The practical issue for health providers who perform competency evaluations is to respect the state's intention to maximally protect individuals whose competence might be suspect by ensuring that the individual does not lose decision-making authority over those areas *in which adequate capacity exists.* But in many instances, making these determinations is not straightforward. What does it mean to have "adequate" decision-making capacity? When do my actions "unduly" infringe upon the rights of others or pose an "unreasonable" danger or degree of risk to others? At what point ought the state decide that my actions pose a "significant" risk of harm to myself or others to the extent of justifying its interference? Because judicial intervention in such cases has enormous ramifications for individual freedom—Hommel et al.[34] point out that convicted felons have more rights than the individual for whom a plenary guardian is appointed—it has obvious moral import.

The Reliability of Competency Evaluations

Although a moral issue of first-order importance is for competency evaluators to exercise great care and scrutiny in conducting competency evaluations, some research has cast doubt on the reliability of such evaluations. In criminal law, defense lawyers, in a desperate eleventh-hour bid, sometimes secure psychiatric testimony that the death row prisoner is incompetent (i.e., so mentally compromised that he does not understand that he is going to be executed or the meaning of the execution) and therefore unavailable for execution.[38] The state then counters with its own psychiatric expert's findings that the prisoner exhibits some cognitive or psychological impairments but that enough understanding exists so that the execution can proceed. In the early 1980s, however, Kaufmann et al.[39] at Western Psychiatric Institute in Pitts-burgh published research showing a significant disparity among psychiatrists and lawyers on rating the competence of psychiatric patients to consent to or refuse electroconvulsive therapy. They found that lawyers were consistently more inclined than psychiatrists to rate patients competent. A more recent study on competency to consent to medical treatment found a statistically significant disparity between an expert panel of competency raters versus the competency ratings of rehabilitation therapists who treated those patients on a daily basis.[40]

This latter study raises important questions about certain professional and moral considerations in conducting competency assessments. A 14-member "expert" panel of physiatrists, psychiatrists, psychologists, and lawyers did not differ in a statistically significant way in rating 21 videotaped interviews of patients whose competency to consent to medical treatment was to be determined.[40] (The interview is reproduced in Table 24-1.) But their ratings—

TABLE 24–1. Competency Assessment

Preliminary content

- Discuss patient's premorbid functioning and relevant history (social, educational, and vocational information; preexisting physical or psychological problems; psychiatric diagnosis; learning disabilities; legal problems; general social history)
- Discuss patient's present medical condition (computerized tomographic or magnetic resonance imaging findings and severity indices); chronicity and medical course; current medical treatment, including rehabilitation therapies and goals; rehabilitation progress; length of stay determination; prognosis, including likely postdischarge disposition
- Mini–mental status examination

Structured interview

Personal information
    What happened to you? Why are you here? What do you do here? What are you working on? What are your deficits? What do you expect from treatment/recovery?
Treatment information
    Who is working with you? What are you working on in therapy? What do you wish to gain from therapy? What are your treatment goals? Are you making progress? Who makes decisions about what treatments you will have? What do you think would happen if you refused a certain treatment? Are there any risks associated with your treatment? Are there any benefits associated with your treatment? Are there any alternative treatments to the ones you are now getting? Do you have any problems here that aren't being taken care of? Are you taking any medications? What kind(s)? How much? Do you want to be here?
Emotional adjustment
    How are your spirits/mood? How does that affect you and your progress? How do you feel about therapy? How is your family coping? Do members of your family agree with your treatment plan? How does your disability affect you? How does your disability affect your family? What is the plan after discharge? What do you expect to be doing 5 years from now? Are there any questions you have? What would you do with $10,000?
Hypothetical scenario
    Present (hypothetical) problem. Describe treatment procedure.
    Explanation of risks, benefits (including probabilities), and treatment alternatives. Patient is asked what he/she would do in that situation, why, and to review the expected risks, benefits, and alternatives.

Source: Reprinted from NeuroRehabilitation, 6. Auerbach, VS, and Banja, JD, Assessing client competence to participate in rehabilitation decisionmaking, p 126, copyright 1996, with permission from Elsevier Science.

which tended toward finding patients competent—differed dramatically from the ratings of the patients' treatment team members, who very much inclined toward deeming the patients incompetent. For example, in one of the 21 interviews, all but 1 of the expert panel members determined the patient competent, whereas 8 of the 9 treating professionals believed the patient to be incompetent. Did the treating professionals not know what to look for, or were they, in fact, in a better position to rate the patient's competence, which they were observing every day during treatment? Can a competency assessment be accomplished by way of a brief, one-time interview (as exemplified in the videotape and, in fact, as it usually occurs in hospitals), or does it require a more elaborate examination of the patient's thinking and behavior, especially as they occur in ecologically relevant surroundings rather than in the sterile environment of a psychologist's testing room? Then again, did the treating team members incline toward rating patients incompetent because that rating accommodates the professional's narcissistically grounded need to feel wanted and valuable? The possibility that health care providers see what they want to see (as a projection of their psychic needs) can hardly be dismissed because a number of studies have corroborated the finding that rehabilitationists may differ dramatically in assessing the severity of a patient's impairments.[40,41]

What moral factors, then, ought to guide the assessment of competency? First, competency assessments must not be used to threaten noncompliant patients. Adults are presumed to be competent unless proven otherwise; indeed, "an individual's legal competency is not altered automatically by commitment to a mental facility" (p. 13).[42] If a patient's noncompliance or "orneriness" authentically derives from values that he or she knowingly and insightfully chooses, the patient's noncompliance should be honored. Health providers who disagree with a patient's values and choices have no right to override those choices unless they believe the patient lacks an adequate cognitive grasp of the choice situation and that serious harm may develop for the patient or others as a result of an ineptly made decision.[43] Consequently, the moral principle that should trigger a competency evaluation is the individual's *compromised autonomy*, meaning that the individual cannot meet a *de minimus* standard of understanding, reasoning, and insight into his or her decisions and might thereby be placing self or others at peril. The competency assessment, therefore, must be geared toward the following:

1. What is the competency domain under examination? Is it the individual's ability to make medical decisions, business decisions, care for his or her family, drive a car, stand trial, execute a will, live independently, or what?

2. Once the competency domain is identified, ask what relevant skills are required for adequate functioning in that domain. A person with brain injury might be able to execute a will but not manage a business or live independently but not drive.

3. Once the relevant skills are identified, determine the minimally adequate level of performance an individual needs to function "reasonably enough" in that domain and then assess the individual's skill according to that functional yardstick.

The testing instrument itself must be "ecologically valid"; that is, it must demonstrate valid and reliable measures of the skill being assessed. Certain individuals with brain injury, for example, might do well on paper-and-pencil tests but be unable to make a cup of coffee. Is what the instrument assesses, therefore, relevant to the skills under consideration?[31,44]

In the ideal testing situation, then, the conditions reasonably duplicate the skill domain under scrutiny, and professionally validated measures reliably distinguish "competent" from "incompetent" performance. This point is crucial as well as ironic because many commentators point out that no professional consensus exists on what such measures should be.[43,45] For example, although tests of competency to participate in medical decisions rely on assessing the patient's degree of ability to communicate, understand, reason, and exercise insight, no agreement exists on *how much* reasoning and insight the competent individual possesses. The absence of such a standard is particularly acute in organically based mental dysfunction as opposed to psychotic behavior because deficits of the latter sort frequently exhibit a more consistent texture or uniformity than the spotty, patchy, or inconsistent demonstrations of deficits common to persons with severe brain injuries. For example, people with TBI may be able to remember certain things like number of children but not their names, list all their physical impairments but believe they will be cured in a week, exhibit language problems (like anomia) along with thinking problems that might confound the evaluator's assessment of the quality of the reasoning and insight, and manifest considerable insight into certain decisional domains (like making medical decisions) but abysmal insight into others (like whether to drive).

Competence and the Ability to Manage Risk

What is of enormous valuative import in conducting competency evaluations is how great a level of risk the competency evaluator is willing to allow the patient to assume. Such an allowance seems to be wholly subjective—much akin to parental decisions about when a teenaged son or daughter is ready to drive an automobile unsupervised. Some competency assessors are liberal in allowing patients to assume risk and justify their stance by noting that cognitively unimpaired, judgmentally intact persons often make remarkably foolish and un insightful decisions and choices, which they nevertheless have an uncontroversial right to make. Other evaluators, perhaps most, assume a much more conservative stance and attribute risk-taking dispositions or inclinations toward unacceptably poor reasoning or insight. Their criterion of "competence" may be based on a reasonable person standard such that a reasonable person would not choose those behaviors.[40]

But because adopting a reasonable person standard often produces an unsubtle injection of values from the individual defining "reasonableness" (e.g., reasonable people do not race cars, eat or drink immoderately, or gamble), contemporary commentators on competence generally urge an *instrumental* approach to evaluating competency.[13] That is, the content of a person's decision or *what* he or she decides has little significance in the assessment process; rather, the evaluator should focus only on the *process* by which the decision occurs. Although my choice might be distasteful to many, as long as I make that choice by way of a cognitive process that does not appear excessively impaired, then I am responsible for that choice and its consequences.

Table 24–1 outlines a competency interview that developed from the aforementioned research study. This interview format (1) compares somewhat favorably with at least one other format for determining competency to consent to medical treatment,[29] (2) was developed specifically from a neurologically impaired (mostly TBI) patient population, and (3) was found to elicit competency assessments from the videotape raters that in the aggregate—over the course of the 21 subjects interviewed—did not ultimately differ in a statistically significant way.[40]

As research in competency assessment continues to evolve and instruments to test competency become more sophisticated, their superiority will depend on the degree that instruments and procedures (1) draw a bright line between acceptable and unacceptable cognitive functioning (i.e., "how much" memory, understanding, and insight a person should demonstrate to function competently), (2) validly test the competency domain under consideration, (3) eradicate as much as possible a rater's bias or prejudice that derives from irrelevant variables (such as the questionably competent individual's physical appearance, religious affiliation, or financial resources), and (4) embody a politically and socially thoughtful notion of allowable risk. Competency evaluations inevitably look to social decisions about the nature of human welfare and the extent to which a society might allow or sanction behaviors that threaten social welfare. Consequently, the theoretical underpinnings and ethical components of competency evaluations should be more than a professionally credible examination of a person's psychological functioning. They must also look to a community whose moral notions of harms, burdens, and risks define the meaning of personal and professional relationships and how "competence" is understood within those contexts.

□ PROFOUNDLY DIMINISHED CONSCIOUSNESS AND THE WITHHOLDING OR DISCONTINUATION OF LIFE-PROLONGING TREATMENT

In the 15 years between the onset of Karen Quinlan's vegetative state in 1975 and the U.S. Supreme Court decision in Cruzan in 1990, virtually every significant court case involving a person with permanent unconsciousness or terminal illness and a life-prolonging treatment had a common element: Patients or their families pleaded with health providers to withhold or discontinue life-prolonging treatment (WDLPT)—usually artificial ventilation or artificial nutrition or hydration—but the health professionals demurred.[46–51] A court was then asked to rule on the legal propriety of the patient's or family's request.

The appellate and occasionally state supreme courts rulings were extraordinarily uniform in at least one respect. If the patient or family could demonstrate to the court's satisfaction that the request for WDLPT was an authentic expression of the patient's wishes and there was no reasonable hope for the patient's recovery, the court granted the request, generally by finding that either (1) the patient had a constitutionally protected liberty interest under the due process clause of the Fourteenth Amendment that included the right to be free from unwanted medical treatment or (2) the common law right of informed consent included the right to refuse unwanted treatment.[46,51] In the historical course of these rulings, however, courts had to address numerous issues. Would, for example, WDLPT constitute homicide? In many cases, WDLPT would directly culminate in the death of the patient. What is the moral difference, then, between performing WDLPT and injecting the patient with a lethal dose of morphine?[52] And if ethics and law ultimately conclude that WDLPT is allowable under certain conditions, then what are the conditions enabling certain patients to be candidates but not others? Suppose an unconscious patient who is receiving aggressive measures has a reasonable chance for survival with a decent quality of life, but family members demand WDLPT. What criteria ought the health professional use to differentiate legitimate from perverse requests for WDLPT? If the patient manifests a condition whereby he or she might be a candidate for WDLPT, under what conditions might WDLPT be authorized if the patient has never executed a living will or durable power of attorney?

Most of these cases involved patients who could not make decisions for themselves. But when courts were confronted with requests for WDLPT from *competent* persons with serious physical disability, such as Elizabeth Bouvia or Larry McAfee, they uniformly ruled in favor of the requestor.[53,54] Although neither Bouvia nor McAfee carried through their lethal intentions, the general principle with which the court nevertheless accorded them the right to do so was that individuals who possess adequate insight and understanding into their medical conditions and quality of life are best positioned to determine if their lives should be medically prolonged. If they decide that the burdens of continued life outweigh the benefits, they have the authority to have life-prolonging treatment terminated. The courts also noted that a state's interest in preserving life wanes in proportion to the degree that the quality and vitality of a person's life diminishes. Last, the courts ruled that WDLPT in such cases would not unduly compromise the integrity of the medical profession.[53,54]

Nevertheless, apart from what a patient would or would not want a health professional to do, why is the health provider who performs WDLPT not guilty of murder or assisting a suicide? For a decisionally competent individual with high spinal cord injury who requests discontinuation from an artificial ventilator or for a survivor of TBI who has lived in a permanently unconscious state for a number of years and whose family secures a court's authoriza-tion to have gastric feeding discontinued, death as a result of WDLPT is assured in either instance. Is the health provider, therefore, an accomplice in that individual's death, and what criteria do we use to assess the moral and legal nature of that complicity?

The Ethical Propriety of Withholding or Discontinuing Life-Prolonging Treatment

The primary reason that health providers are allowed to perform WDLPT is that individuals are acknowledged to have the right—under the ethical principle of autonomy—not only to refuse unwanted medical treatment but also to die from their disease or disability as a result of that refusal. If a health provider, for instance, delivered a lethal dose of morphine to a person in the vegetative state, the courts rule that action a homicide because the provider's intention was to cause death and the patient died from causes unrelated to his or her neuropathology. When gastric feeding is discontinued, however, patients die from their neurologically based inability to ingest sufficient nutrition. The provider, moreover, did not intend the person to die but rather acted according to the duty to terminate a treatment the patient does not want. Likewise, individuals with high spinal cord injury who request disconnection from their ventilators and die as a result have their deaths attributed to respiratory insufficiency deriving from an inability to breathe on their own. Because death in these instances (1) would occur for pathophysiological reasons associated with the patient's underlying disease or disability and (2) the patient has a self-determinative right to refuse life-saving or life-prolonging medical treatment that (3) trumps whatever duty or power the health provider might otherwise have to preserve the patient's life, the general disposition of ethics and law interprets WDLPT in these instances as morally and legally allowable.[56,57]

Cases involving WDLPT become morally troublesome when patients become incompetent without having left written or oral instructions about the aggressiveness of their care, should they become catastrophically disabled. In these cases, legal and moral attention inevitably turns to questions about the individual's quality of life and best interests. Unfortunately but not surprisingly, without the patient's own testimony, arguments flare over what a "reasonable" person might want by way of life-prolonging measures, as well as what a just society ought to provide. Indeed, as the following shows, controversy now swirls around the value of the life of people with profoundly diminished consciousness who are minimally responsive. Are their lives valuable at all? If their families or guardians do not believe so, who is to protect—indeed, who is to determine—their "best interests"?

If a person has left no advance directives and becomes incompetent to make medical decisions, it is common practice to look to next of kin or others authorized to speak for the person to order WDLPT when the individual is terminally ill, in irreversible coma, or in a persistent vegetative state.[57] The moral notion driving this practice is that a "reasonable" person might very well not want to have aggressive measures continued under these circumstances and therefore familial requests to that effect are at least worthy of consideration. Not wanting to authorize permission for WDLPT solely for the sake of familial or caretaker convenience but acknowledging that people with profoundly diminished consciousness have an extremely low quality of life, the courts show a preference to leave these decisions in the hands of families and professional caretakers.[58] In these cases, a largely unspoken but compelling moral intuition seems to encourage shifting the gravity of moral considerations from those persons with catastrophic disability to whoever has responsibility for them, which is usually some next of kin. In effect, the intuition seems to say that if people with a catastrophic neurological impairment no longer have a life for themselves, our moral respect should favor the considerations of their loved ones, who, by virtue of their blood or legal ties, appear to have the strongest claim to make significant moral decisions about the person's future. Although we still try to make these decisions in the individual's "best interest," the best interest of the family inevitably seems to carry great weight.

Ethically Challenging Aspects of Withholding or Discontinuing Life-Prolonging Treatment

Figure 24–1 presents an algorithm that depicts ethical and legal stopping points in structuring WDLPT decisions. Despite the conceptual neatness of such a schema, the pathways it suggests are commonly but by no means universally accepted. For example, a strong, albeit minority, point of view is making itself felt—primarily through the medium of the Americans with Disabilities Act (ADA)—that interprets WDLPT in cases of people who never made their wishes known as an invidious capitulation to the convenience of the health provider or the eventual caretaker(s).

With the ADA as a backdrop, this viewpoint holds that "quality of life" criteria have no relevance whatsoever in WDLPT, only whether the individual was receiving services *equal* to what a person without disabilities would receive.[59] If health providers must not discriminate on the basis of a disability, then withholding, deescalating, or discontinuing life-prolonging treatment *because* a person was permanently unconscious or catastrophically disabled would seem to be a direct violation of the act's protections. Consequently, this argument could be extended to prohibit any request for WDLPT unless the individual has made advance directives. This view holds that the family who cannot show "clear and convincing" evidence to the court that their loved one would desire WDLPT should not expect the court to authorize a withholding or discontinuation request because such authorization would violate the act.[60]

Thus far, this argument has not by itself convinced the courts to gainsay a family's contention that their loved one would not want to continue to live in his or her compromised condition. At least one court, however, approvingly noted this argument in a case in which health providers deemed that life-prolonging artificial ventilation was futile but the patient's mother insisted that it be provided.

This 1994 case involved an infant with anencephaly. The child, known as Baby K, periodically required artificial ventilation, which a hospital opposed giving on the grounds that the infant's prognosis was terminal regardless of what treatment could be provided.[61] Although the hospital agreed to provide nutrition, hydration, and palliative care, it regarded the provision of artificial ventilation as a classic example of medical futility. Because Baby K's mother demanded that everything be done for her baby, the hospital went to court for authorization to withhold artificial ventilation from Baby K.

The court that originally heard this case declared that anencephaly is, indeed, a disability under the ADA and that the hospital's request to deny treatment to Baby K on the basis of her anencephaly was categorically prohibited: "denial of medical services to anencephalic babies as a class of disabled individuals . . . is exactly what the Americans with Disabilities Act was enacted to prohibit."[62]

This case has considerable implications for health providers who treat individuals with catastrophic TBI or other extremely serious neurological insults, whose death appears imminent. In the first place, many individuals with catastrophic TBI have not executed advance directives, and decisions about the aggressiveness of their care measures will probably turn to the person's next of kin or appointed guardian. If a fam-

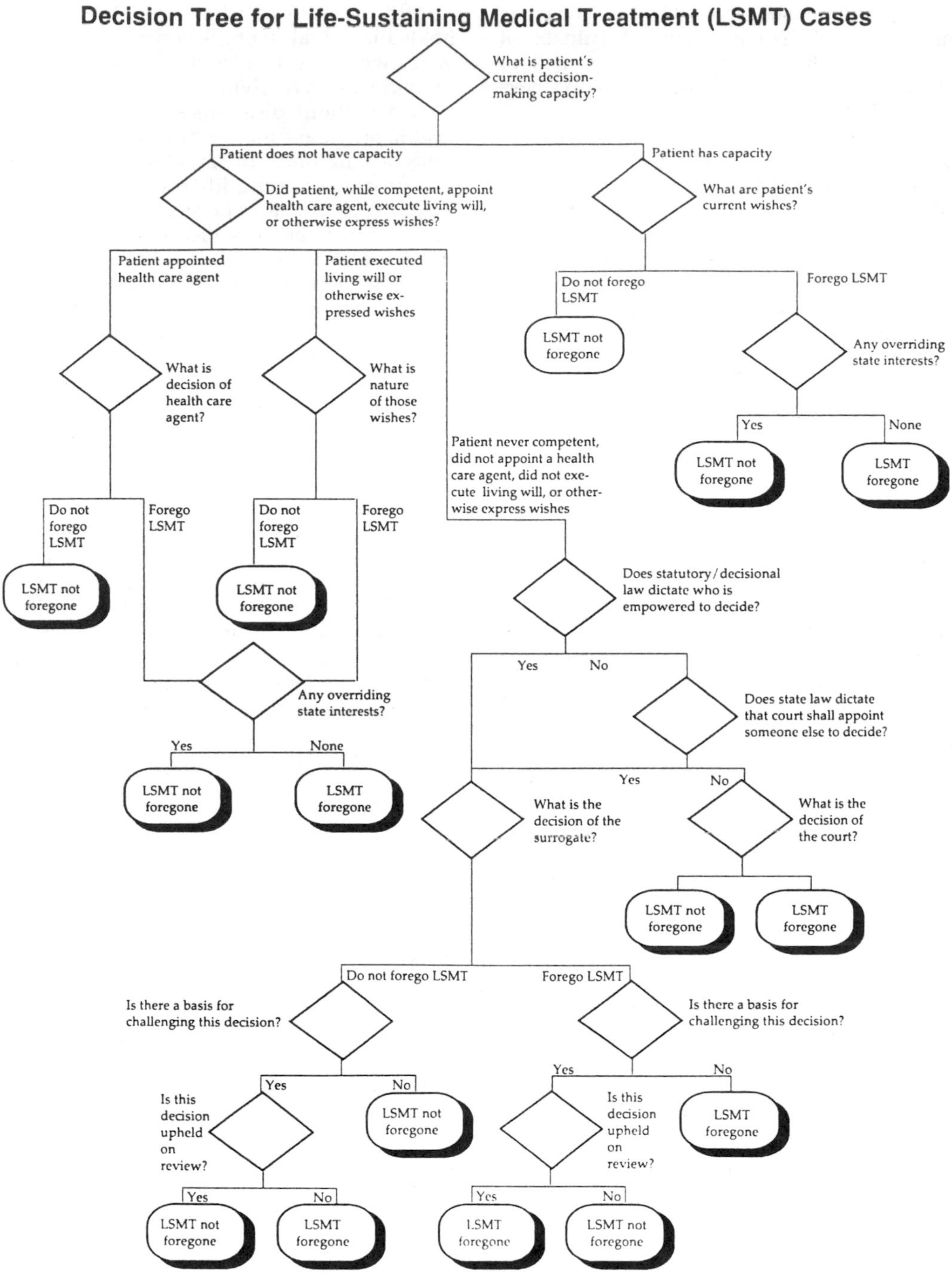

Decision Tree for Life-Sustaining Medical Treatment (LSMT) Cases

FIGURE 24–1. Decision tree for life-sustaining medical treatment (LSMT) cases. (From Coordinating Council on Life-Sustaining Medical Treatment Decision Making by the Courts. Williamsburg, Va, with permission.)

ily member insists that the patient receive life-prolonging care regardless of the perceived futility of the treatment, then because that patient certainly qualifies as disabled, he or she would be protected by the ADA, and the provider would have no recourse but to give it. In sum, an application of the ADA as cited in the Baby K case would appear to strip the provider of any authority to terminate a treatment deemed useless.[64]

The Tragedy of Michael Martin

Questions about "useless" treatment, however, intuitively look to the quality of life that such treatment may or may not preserve. Although some ideological groups believe that all human life, no matter how poor its quality, is worth preserving, they seem to be in a distinct minority. Much more troubling are those patients who appear to have an *arguably* poor quality of life. For example, what ought our moral sensibilities be toward Michael Martin, who sustained a catastrophic brain injury in 1987 that left him in a state of total physical dependency, although he can nod, smile, and grip with his right hand? In a nationally syndicated story in February 1996, his wife, Mary, was quoted as saying that "before the accident, Mike used to make me promise I would never keep him alive on machines."[64] By the time her husband's case became national news, it had been through a probate court,[65] the Michigan Court of Appeals,[66] and the Supreme Court of Michigan.[67] During February 1996, the U.S. Supreme Court declined to review the decision of the Supreme Court of Michigan, thus upholding that court's decision.[68]

Mrs. Martin's intention was to have her husband's gastric feeding discontinued, which she claimed would be his wish. In opposition was Mr. Martin's mother and sister, as well as certain advocacy groups, whose lawyer, Calvin Luker, claimed, "I've visited Mike and asked him what he wants, and he's indicated in a consistent way that he wants to live."[64] The case illustrates all the themes discussed up to now: the occasional obscurity connected with determining what a catastrophically impaired person "really wants"; the court's interest in balancing a respect for life with a respect for individual autonomy; ensuring that those who speak for the incompetent patient are truly representing the patient's interests and not mainly furthering their own; and concerns of disability groups about a judicial ruling setting what they believe might be a dangerous precedent by which family members are allowed to end the lives of those who are profoundly disabled. Perhaps more than anything else, however, this case illustrates the difficulty that legal stratagems have in providing directions in the midst of the remarkable idiosyncrasies that real-life tragedies present.

Michael Martin is not unconscious but is catastrophically cognitively and physically impaired. How explicit should someone like him be in directing next of kin about what conditions should dictate whether he should be a candidate for WDLPT? Mr. Martin did not leave a living will or durable power of attorney for health care, but Mrs. Martin brought forth considerable evidence that convinced both the probate and appeals courts that her husband would not want to have his gastric feeding continued and that he would want to die. Yet, when the Supreme Court of Michigan reviewed whether the evidence Mary Martin brought forward was "clear and convincing," they were unpersuaded. After ruling that individuals did have the right to decline life-sustaining treatment and that such individuals did not have to stipulate their wishes in writing, the court nevertheless remarked that "the amount of weight accorded prior oral statements depends on the remoteness (in time and place), consistency, specificity, and solemnity of the prior statement" (p. 411).[67] In effect, the court's definition of "clear and convincing" evidence was that the patient's declarations about WDLPT should have been made fairly recently rather than in the distant past, that those declarations should embody a consistent and unwavering desire or preference, that they should speak specifically to the physical or cognitive situation the patient now is in, and that these declarations should not have been made flippantly or cavalierly. Using these criteria to hand down its ruling, the court decided that:

> In the present case, appellants (i.e., Mary Martin) claim that Mr. Martin expressed a preaccident statement that he did not want to live like a vegetable. However, our review of the record reveals that virtually all the witnesses agreed that Mr. Martin is not in a vegetative state and is not suffering from the type of incapacitation referenced in his expression of a desire not to continue life-sustaining medical treatment. . . . Accordingly, we reverse the Court of Appeals determination because petitioner's testimony and affidavit do not constitute clear and convincing evidence of Mr. Martin's preinjury decision to decline life-sustaining medical treatment in the form of a gastrostomy tube that provides hydration and nutritive support. (pp. 411–413)[67]

In a stinging dissent, however, Justice Levin of the Michigan Supreme Court said that:

> As one physician testified, when laypersons express a desire not to be a "vegetable," they usually are not referring strictly to a persistent vegetative state. Rather, the popular understanding involves a "spectrum of things, but the commonality of that is, independence of life . . . things in terms of basic needs of human body,—bathing, eating and able to void. . . . As the Court of Appeals stated: "Prevalent throughout Michael's statements is the preference not to be maintained in a

condition where he was incapable of performing basic functions such as walking, talking, dressing, bathing, or eating, and, instead, was dependent upon others or machines for his basic needs. This is exactly the condition in which Michael now finds himself. (p. 415)[67]

What irked Justice Levin was that the majority's interpretation of clear and convincing evidence called for such specificity that the average (Michigan-residing) citizen—who could not be expected to appreciate the neurological nuances between the vegetative state, the minimally responsive state, and the commonly used simile "living like a vegetable"—simply cannot meet the court's evidentiary burden. Even though such persons might not desire to live in a minimally responsive state—as Justice Levin and the probate and appeals court were convinced about Michael Martin—they will not have their wishes honored in the absence of evidence envisaging *precisely the circumstances* in which they now find themselves. Consequently, by imposing such a high threshold of evidence in these cases, the Michigan Supreme Court might make it virtually impossible for (or easy to refute) a Michigan family's bringing forth evidence that their loved one had foreseen *precisely such an instance of disability* and clearly expressed to them his or her wishes for WDLPT. The court was not unaware of this possibility but said, "If we are to err, we must err in preserving life" (p. 409).[67] Justice Levin ended his dissent by lamenting that the majority decision "has sentenced Michael Martin to life in a helpless, degraded condition against his prior wishes. To quote the majority's own opinion, 'to condemn persons to lives from which they cry out for release is nothing short of barbaric' " (pp. 419–420).[67]

As these cases unfold, the phenomenon of WDLPT among people in the minimally responsive state may constitute the "new wave" of treatment discontinuation cases so that debates about WDLPT will probably intensify at the judicial level for an ever widening population of human beings with serious disease or disability. As they occur, we hope that the policy and regulation handed down will at least steer clear from imposing either a duty to live or a duty to die.

◻ WHO SHOULD PAY FOR CARE?

Health insurance reform was an item of national interest in the first 2 years of the Clinton administration and, despite the failure of that effort, will doubtlessly continue to have a place on the national agenda. Although the Clinton effort to nationalize health care delivery did not succeed, the landscape of health care nevertheless underwent unprecedented change in the early 1990s and is expected to continue to do so at least through the year 2000. The change is primarily in the form of "managed care," and this section examines some of the moral implications of this phenomenon.

First of all, it is morally important to note that an individual with traumatic brain injury might have care paid for by any number of sources, depending on the idiosyncrasies of the injury occurrence and other factors. For example, if an individual was elderly and injured at home, the payer source would most likely be Medicare. The individual who sustained a TBI from a work-related activity would probably be covered by workers' compensation insurance. Someone who was negligently struck by a vehicle that was owned and operated by a business would be able to sue the company in civil court. If the person was in an automobile accident that involved only that person, the health insurance would most likely derive from the group policy provided by his or her employer (assuming the employer offered such). And an individual who was indigent at the time of injury would ultimately be insured by Medicaid.

Of considerable moral significance is the fact that the generosity of these payer sources might vary dramatically. The lack of uniformity in the United States exhibited by third-party payers' willingness to pay for care—and the consequent heterogeneity of services and duration of treatment that patients receive on the basis of their insurance benefits—underlines perhaps the most discussed moral issue in health care today—namely, that health care in the United States is not allocated and reimbursed according to a notion of human entitlements that derives from a moral vision about what kind of life persons with disease or disability are owed or "should" enjoy. The fact that, in the United States, an insurance plan might or might not pay for more than 30 inpatient days in a rehabilitation hospital, a motorized wheelchair, various cognitive or behavioral therapies, psychological services, outpatient services, attendant care, or home health services means that neither one's potential for functional recovery nor the ways that these services might favorably affect a person's (or his or her family's) overall quality of life is dispositive in determining whether the patient receives them. What is dispositive are the particulars—in other words, the benefits and exclusions—of the individual's insurance plan. In moral terms, health insurers construe their responsibility to insureds as based in the contractual language of the insured's health policy. To the extent that attendant care or a motorized wheelchair is not allowed under the coverage, insurers disavow a moral responsibility to provide them because the insured is not contractually entitled to them.

The American health care system, unlike socialized health care systems in Europe, only partially and sometimes not at all authorizes treatment according to what an individual might *need;* rather, a primary determinant of allocation is what the plan will *reimburse.* Moral questions, then, about what the goal of rehabilitation should be in reference to what kind of life an individual deserves after catastrophic disability from TBI are at loggerheads with this kind of reimbursement paradigm. Treatments, therapies, durable medical equipment, and the like become ends in themselves because their allocation will derive from the plan's coverage.

Marketplace Economics and Allocation of Care

Americans have not settled on a collective vision or moral consensus on health care entitlements—just as previous sections of this chapter noted a similar absence of consensus on what qualifies as a "reasonable" caregiving burden that families should accept, who qualifies as a "reasonable" person for purposes of determining competency, and what the value of "sheer" biological survival is for purposes of determining WDLPT in cases of people who are permanently unconscious and have left no advance directives. The American insistence on individual freedoms—in which each person is granted as much latitude as possible to determine what shall count for him or her as benefits or burdens—opposes those more communitarian approaches that look to human nature, the nature of the "good" society, or some other generic or collective social construct to determine how much health care a person is owed.

The American spirit of individualism has largely accounted for a health care reimbursement system based on free market principles of private enterprise. Most Americans who are not covered by public insurance receive their health insurance through their employers, most of whom are self-insured.[69,70] This fact alone has enormous moral ramifications because employers are not primarily in business to provide health insurance to their employees but to succeed in the marketplace. Inevitably, employers regard their health care costs just as they regard any other cost of doing business. It seems obvious that employers do not ordinarily think of health care as a social good—as something on a par with education, national defense, police protection, or the economy—but rather as an *expense.*[71] It is hardly surprising, then, that as businesses seek to limit operating costs, they naturally seek to curb their health care costs.

Managed care has developed precisely as a response to the insurer's interest in reducing the rate of growth in health care expenditures. When employers, especially after World War II, increasingly offered to subsidize their employees' health care costs, those workers unwittingly ceded enormous authority to management to determine the nature and scope of health care benefits. The impact of that decision has become apparent only recently, as fee-for-service or indemnity reimbursement has given way to the "managed care" approach, and employers find themselves able to wield enormous power in directing insureds to provider groups, who contract with insurers for special rates. The essence of the managed care arrangement is that insureds are offered considerable incentives or simply required to use provider groups that either discount their fees or function as the exclusive provider group for the plan enrollees at a greatly reduced rate.[72,73]

Determining When Rehabilitation Is "Successful"

Rehabilitation professionals have become familiar with various managed care arrangements, especially those that impose limits on the reimbursement allowed or limit the number of hospital days or treatment sessions the patient might have.[74–76] Such a "capitated" approach has important moral ramifications in TBI rehabilitation, which can best be appreciated through a comparison with a surgical intervention. A person with appendicitis presents with a straightforward medical condition whose remediative measures are uncontroversial. Moreover, a "reasonable" outcome by which to judge the success of an appendectomy is likewise unproblematic. Much more complicated and obscure is what a "successful" rehabilitation would be for a person with serious brain injury. When generous financial resources existed and this individual could anticipate a lengthy rehabilitation, success was predicated on the person's reaching "maximal" functional recovery, which could only be known by determining that the patient had "plateaued." With reimbursements nowhere near that level now, the rehabilitationist works within the confines of the economic largesse or parsimony afforded by the patient's insurance plan. An extension of services beyond the reimbursement limit obviously contravenes the financial interests of the facility, whose fiscal administrators interpret such behavior as economically ruinous (and who are obviously correct, if such behavior becomes the norm at that facility). The rehabilitationist, however, might be chagrined at having to discharge a patient whose insurance ran out but who was making and would continue to make good progress.

Contrasting the goals of rehabilitation services with acute care services provides an important moral lesson. Where cure can reasonably be anticipated, people expect their insurers to pay for curative treatments or expect their health professional to provide them, even if they are not reimbursed. It would be ludicrous to expect a surgeon to "half-operate" on a fully curable malady and so allow it to continue to compromise or threaten the patient's life. With a disability whose handicapping effects can only be diminished, however, a rehabilitation effort analogous to a "half-cure" is not nearly so improbable. Despite being able to do far more for the patient, the rehabilitationist can easily be co-opted by the patient's insurance coverage because providing less than the degree of rehabilitation required for the patient to achieve his or her *maximal* level of recovery does not pose anywhere near the likelihood of disastrous consequences (or a malpractice suit) as a shoddy piece of surgery motivated by meager insurance dollars. If a patient's progress in rehabilitation is dependent on length or intensity of involvement in some therapeutic program, then rehabilitation consumers might see the quality of their treatment outcomes vary more with how much they can pay than would patients appearing for invasive surgeries from which cure can reasonably be expected.

Is, then, the deployment of rehabilitation services according to an insurance paradigm morally wrong? The question points toward the need to settle more fundamental ethical issues. First of all, rehabilitation commentators have frequently noted that many dimensions of rehabilitation, especially as they occur in TBI, are still without a reliable knowledge base that would encourage or discourage certain treatment interventions.[77,78] Until outcome studies have been produced with enough regularity, validity, and reliability to provide the rehabilitation community and its payer sources with an adequate notion of the quality and degree of functional recovery that might be expected from treatment, many payer sources might not be inclined toward generosity. Recall how the rehabilitation community was shocked some years ago by allegations of fraud and abuse directed at provider groups for maintaining patients' treatments or length of stay until their insurance was exhausted, irrespective of whether the patient continued or ceased to exhibit functional improvements.[79,80]

What about less problematic instances, in which it is clear to everyone that a patient can continue to improve but that care must be terminated because the insurance has been exhausted? On the one hand, like every other service that delivers a social good (e.g., education, defense, or police protection), the extent of that service delivery system is bounded by its economy. One cannot allocate what one does not have or cannot financially support. Consequently, allocating rehabilitation in each and every case on the basis of what a person with TBI "needs," regardless of what that person could pay for, would be a ruinous policy because the gravity of need would doubtlessly outstrip the financial capability of accommodating it.

Determining a "Decent Minimum" of Rehabilitation

Suppose, on the other hand, that the outcomes studies discussed earlier did exist, and a rehabilitationist would know the kind of outcome to expect from a patient engaged in a course of therapy. Here, our sense of moral fairness might say that everyone who sustains a serious disability should receive at least a *decent minimum* of services that would enable the person to live some kind of life with quality. The sentiment disposing toward a decent minimum is extremely common in discussions about universalized health insurance and access in which the necessity of imposing some kind of reasonable limits on allocation is admitted at the outset.[81]

Still, a moral inclination toward a decent minimum would be difficult to operationalize in rehabilitation because assessing the quality of a disabled person's life in terms of its functional potential—and, hence, the extent and nature of rehabilitation services needed to accommodate that functional potential—might be extremely subjective, depending on the unique ways that individual would wish to engage the world. For some persons, a "decent minimum" of rehabilitation might mean being able to return to work or care for their children; to others, it might mean being able to carry on meaningful conversations with friends and family; to others, it might mean their ability to live independently at home. Would a decent minimum mean to rehabilitate a gait impairment to the point that the individual could ambulate independently but not gracefully; or to speak intelligibly but not with particularly good pronunciation, intonation or inflection, or to be returned to gainful but menial employment rather than to better-paying and more interesting work? Somehow, these instances of a basic, decent minimum of rehabilitation seem morally dubious because they ignore the relationship between individual dignity and human function. As a number of commentators have pointed out,[21,22] the onset of a serious disability is a narcissistic injury of catastrophic proportions. To rehabilitate patients to a lesser functional level than they might be capable of maintaining seems demeaning to both patients and providers. Yet payers of rehabilitation services seem reluctant or unable to incorporate an ideology that envisions human dignity as meriting a serious place in the insurance plan's coverage.

Perhaps the marketplace ideology of profit and loss has not considered the intersection of functional recovery with quality of life as something all that valuable. Then again, certain insurers may remain unconvinced that rehabilitation therapies are sufficiently responsible for the functional gains that rehabilitation consumers frequently make and so remain reluctant to pay for them.

If so, then a number of items should occupy serious places on rehabilitation professionals' agenda. One is to continue to aggressively conduct outcome studies by which rehabilitation therapies can be deployed more efficiently with superior therapeutic results. Another is to maintain a national conversation with insurers, policy makers, nonrehabilitative health professionals, and the public at large about the nature of disability and the therapeutic and life-enhancing opportunities that are afforded by rehabilitation. A third is to educate health care consumers, the insureds of this nation, about the tenuousness and vulnerability of their health care benefits. Americans, especially in this age of managed care, need to appreciate how the scope and content of their health benefits are not designed according to a paradigm of need but rather according to what a third-party payer is willing to subsidize. And further, for most Americans, the loss of health benefits is as close at hand as loss of their jobs.

Last, Americans should be impressed with how nearby lurks the specter of disability itself—if not through a traumatic injury, then through some disease process like heart disease or cancer or just through the process of aging. Some form of disability awaits virtually all of us—and, if not us, then someone we love. Because of its extraordinary gravity and penchant for befalling the youth of our society, the onset of severe brain injury is a unique horror—so horrible, perhaps, that our society's insurers and policy makers are revolted by its ugliness and so retreat to a position of indifference about its remediation. To cause a favorable turn in attitude will require a continued commitment from the research, clinical, and advocacy echelons of the rehabilitation community. With enough prodding and advocacy—especially on legislative and public policy levels—along with empirically based reasons to support the value of rehabilitation, payers of health care will be better positioned to understand that life is nearly always stronger than disability and that a rehabilitation effort that has a reasonable chance to secure a life worth living is certainly worth paying for.

❑ CONCLUSION

Although this chapter has examined certain prominent issues in severe traumatic brain injury, the specter of TBI invites dozens more moral problems. For example, the ways the incidence of head injury might be reduced—such as a state's mandate of motorcycle helmet and seat belt usage—require actions that many political groups interpret as infringements on their personal liberty.[82] There are issues about the use of therapies and treatments whose efficacy has not been substantiated. Indeed, even if such efficacy was known with statistically sophisticated measures, we would still be left with the moral question of whether that level of success—in terms of its nature and its frequency—should merit the deployment of treatment and its reimbursement.[83,84] Other issues focus on the person with TBI who is engaging in dangerous or risk-taking behaviors. Should guardians be appointed if individuals with brain injury are obviously hurting themselves through noncompliance with therapy but seem to understand the risk they are taking and refuse further help?[85] A plethora of social issues encourage health professionals to recognize the powerful role that culture plays in the incidence of TBI, especially its association with people of lower academic and socioeconomic achievement, not to mention those involved in criminal activity. Ought health professionals, then, move beyond the purely clinical dimensions of their jobs and advocate for the eradication of these culturally driven causal factors of TBI?[86]

A contemporary movement in philosophy encourages conceptualizing the notion of thinking from something that represents reality (i.e., whether my beliefs correspond to what is "out there") to something that enables me to adapt to my environment (i.e., whether my beliefs enable me to survive and live an acceptable life).[87] Although TBI clearly affects "representational" thinking, its devastating effects involve adaptive thinking and emphasize the point so fre-

---

TABLE 24–2. Considerations in Resolving Ethical Dilemmas

1. What is the ethical dilemma at issue? Can it be explained in terms of clashes or conflicts among values or rights? Here are some general parameters:

   □ *Autonomy:* Is the client's right to be heard respected? Are the client's civil rights imperiled by the way the decision-making process is being managed? Does the client have decisional capacity? Might the fact that the client has a brain injury be used against him or her to justify overriding what would otherwise be an acceptable decision or preference?

   □ *Nonmaleficence:* Is any outright or immediate harm threatened by the situation at hand or by the outcomes of the modes of action being contemplated? If harm is an inevitable outcome of any available strategy, will the ultimate decision pose the least amount of harm?

   □ *Beneficence:* How does one define goodness in the particular case at hand? How can one accomplish the most good? What reasons are there to think that the client's version of goodness is unacceptable?

   □ *Justice:* Is the locus of decision-making power fair and just? Whose version of goodness ought to prevail? Why? Might decisions be made in a prejudicial or biased manner? Is the right of all relevant parties to engage in the ethical decision-making process acknowledged, and is the input of all relevant parties evaluated fairly and objectively?

2. Has objective information been obtained? How much is known with certainty? How much is reasonable to believe? How much is sheer guesswork or speculation? How much speculation over the consequences ensuing from the various resolutional strategies is reasonable?

3. Do all parties understand the ethical language being used and agree on the ethical principles at stake? Might concrete examples or references to actual cases be used to clarify points at issue?

4. Will the decision makers be willing to have the decisional process and outcome serve as a precedent? If faced with a future dilemma similar to the one they now face, will they be willing to decide it in the same way?

5. Is the reasoning of the decision makers logical, objective, fair to facts, and consistent, or is it partisan, subjective, and ideologically biased to the point where it risks corrupting the interests of fairness and justice?

6. Are there professional standards or norms that might be useful to consider in resolving the dilemma? Would the decision makers be willing to exhibit the major elements of their decisional approach as emblematic of such standards?

Source: From Banja, J: Ethical issues in staff development. In Durgin, CJ, Schmidt, ND, and Fryer, LJ: Staff Development and Clinical Intervention in Brain Injury Rehabilitation. Aspen, Gaithersburgh, Md, 1993, with permission.

---

quently made that serious cognitive deficits are much more disabling than only physical ones.

Table 24–2 provides a series of questions to which individuals confronted with ethical dilemmas might refer in resolving these challenges. But if we return to certain opening thoughts of this chapter, the task in TBI seems to be to mend two fissures in our mechanisms of adaptation: one affecting the interface of mind and body, the other affecting the person with TBI and his or her physical and social environment. As such, advocacy efforts must at least be two-pronged. One set must continue to improve clinical modalities that return persons to themselves—that enable them to have sovereignty over their bodies and minds so that they can harness their will, interests, and skills in a coherent way to live the kinds of lives they desire. The other set must remove those socioeconomic and attitudinal obstacles that can compromise a productive rehabilitation. A society that is poorly disposed, fiscally and ideologically, to assist the lives of persons with disability negatively affects us all. We must appreciate the fact that what we do for persons with disability, we ultimately do for ourselves. As political columnist George Will pointed out, "All of us are, potentially, in the antechamber of the disability community."[88] Because our country does not impose a constitutional obligation on its citizens to do good to and for one another, we might find in Will's observation a national rallying point for diminishing the handicapping effects of disability. To the extent that the body politic becomes impressed with the ubiquity of disability, we have reason to be optimistic about the future of rehabilitation, its ability to provide benefits to its consumers, and the quality of life that may accrue to persons with TBI and other serious disabilities.

REFERENCES

1. Barrett, W: Irrational Man. A Study in Existential Philosophy. Doubleday, New York, 1962, pp 149–263.
2. Thayer, HS: Meaning and Action: A Critical History of Pragmatism. Bobbs-Merrill, Indianapolis, 1968, pp 133–204.

3. MacIntyre, A: After Virtue. University of Notre Dame Press, Notre Dame, Ind, 1981, pp 123–153.
4. Husserl, E: Cartesian Meditations: An Introduction to Phenomenology, trans. Dorion Cairnes. Martinus Nijhoff, The Hague, 1970, pp 65–88.
5. Husserl, E: The Crisis of European Sciences and Transcendental Phenomenology, trans. David Carr. Northwestern University Press, Evanston, Ill, 1970, pp 170–172.
6. Schwartz, MF, et al: Cognitive theory and the study of everyday action disorders after brain damage. J Head Trauma Rehabil 8:59, 1993.
7. Hart, T, and Jacobs, HE: Rehabilitation and management of behavioral disturbances following frontal lobe injury. J Head Trauma Rehabil 8:1, 1993.
8. Prigatano, GP: Anosognosia, delusions, and altered self-awareness after brain injury: A historical perspective. BNI Quarterly 4:40, 1988.
9. Beauchamp, TL, and Childress, JF: Principles of Biomedical Ethics, ed 3. Oxford University Press, New York, 1989, pp 26–36.
10. Treadwell, K, and Page, TJ: Functional analysis: Identifying the environmental determinants of severe behavior disorders. J Head Trauma Rehabil 11:62–74, 1996.
11. Prigatano, GP: Disordered mind, wounded soul: The emerging role of psychotherapy in rehabilitation after brain injury. J Head Trauma Rehabil 6:1, 1991.
12. Nelson, JL: Taking families seriously. Hastings Cent Rep 22:6–12, 1992.
13. Kuczewski, MG: Reconceiving the family: The process of consent in medical decisionmaking. Hastings Cent Rep 26:30–37, 1996.
14. Maitz, EA, and Sachs, PR: Treating families of individuals with traumatic brain injury from a family system perspective. J Head Trauma Rehabil 10:1–11, 1995.
15. Hosack, KR, and Rocchio, CA: Serving families of persons with severe brain injury in an era of managed care. J Head Trauma Rehabil 10:57–65, 1995.
16. Caplan, AL: Informed consent and provider patient relationships in rehabilitation medicine. Arch Phys Med Rehabil 69:312–317, 1988.
17. Meisel, A, Roth, LH, and Lidz, CW: Toward a model of the legal doctrine of informed consent. Am J Psychiatry 134:285–289, 1977.
18. Banja, J, and Wolf, S: Malpractice litigation for uninformed consent: Implications for physical therapists. Phys Ther 67:1226–1229, 1987.
19. Council on Ethical and Judicial Affairs, American Medical Association: Ethical issues in managed care. JAMA 273:330–335, 1995.
20. Kleinman, A, Eisenberg, L, and Good, B: Culture, illness and care: Clinical lessons from anthropologic and cross-cultural research. Ann Intern Med 88:251–258, 1978.
21. Gunther, M: Countertransference issues in staff caregivers who work to rehabilitate catastrophic-injury survivors. Am J Psychother 48:208–220, 1994.
22. Gans, J: Facilitating staff/patient interaction in rehabilitation. In Caplan, B (ed): Rehabilitation Psychology Desk Reference. Aspen, Rockville, Md, 1987, pp 185–217.
23. Superintendent of Belchertown School v Saikewicz, 370 NE2d 417 (Mass 1977).
24. Banja, J: When we have to pay for someone else's risk taking. Case Manager 7:32–34, 1996.
25. King, JH: The Law of Medical Malpractice in a Nutshell. West, St Paul, 1986, pp 23–28.
26. Jury Says Malpractice after Doctor Ignored Abuse of Child. Georgia Healthcare News 4(1):19, 1997.
27. Banja, J, Ashley, CJ, and Taylor, JS: The case manager's duty to act in problematic situations. Case Manager 3:28–30, 1992.
28. Beauchamp, TL, and Childress, JF: Principles of Biomedical Ethics, ed 3, supra note 9, pp 366–374.
29. Janofsky, JS, McCarthy, RJ, and Folstein, MF: The Hopkins Competency Assessment Test: A brief method for evaluating patients' capacity to give informed consent. Hosp Community Psychiatry 43:132, 1992.
30. Buchanan, AE, and Brock, DW: Deciding for Others: The Ethics of Surrogate Decision Making. Cambridge University Press, Cambridge, 1989, pp 17–86.
31. Searight, HR: Assessing patient competence for medical decisionmaking. Am Fam Physician 45:751, 1992.
32. John F Kennedy Memorial Hosp v Heston, 58 NJ 576, 279 A2d 670 (1971).
33. Steele v Woods, 327 SW2d 187, 198 (Mo 1959).
34. Hommel, PA, Wang, L, and Bergman, JA: Trends in guardianship reform: Implications for the medical and legal professions. Law Med Health Care 18:213, 1990.
35. Robitscher, J: The Powers of Psychiatry. Houghton Mifflin, Boston, 1980, p 25.
36. Perlin, ML: Mental Disability Law: Civil and Criminal, vol 3. Michie, Charlottesville, Va, 1989, p 287.
37. Perlin, ML: Mental Disability Law: Civil and Criminal, vol. 1. Michie, Charlottesville, Va, 1989, pp 139–158.
38. Sargent, DA: Treating the condemned to death. Hastings Cent Rep 16:5, 1986.
39. Kaufmann, C, et al: Informed consent and patient decisionmaking. Int J Law Psychiatry 4:345, 1981.
40. Auerbach, VS, and Banja, JD: Assessing client competence to participate in rehabilitation decision making. NeuroRehabilitation 6:123, 1996.
41. Wanlass, RL, Reutter, SL, and Kline, AE: Communication among rehabilitation staff: "mild," "moderate," or "severe" deficits. Arch Phys Med Rehabil 73:477, 1992.
42. Rozovsky, F: Consent to Treatment: A Practical Guide. Little, Brown, Boston, 1984, p 13.
43. Rosenthal, M, and Lourie, I: Ethical issues in the evaluation of competence in persons with acquired brain injuries. NeuroRehabilitation 6:113, 1996.
44. Auerbach, VA, and Banja, JD: Competency determinations. In Stoudemire, A, and Fogel, BS (eds): Medical Psychiatric Practice, vol 2. American Psychiatric Press, Washington, DC, 1993, pp 515–535.
45. Stanley, B, Sieber, J, and Melton, G: Empirical studies of ethical issues in research. Am Psychol 42:735, 1987.
46. In re Quinlan, 355 A2d 647, cert denied, 429 US 922 (1976).
47. Application of Eichner, 423 NYS2d 580 (1979).
48. In the Matter of Claire C Conroy, 486 A2d 1209 (NJ 1985).
49. Corbett v D'Alessandro, 487 So2d 368 (Fla App 2Dist 1986).
50. Brophy v New England Sinai Hosp, 497 NE2d 626 (Mass 1986).
51. Cruzan v Director, Missouri Dept of Health, 110 SCt 2841 (1990).
52. Rachels, J: Active and passive euthanasia. N Engl J Med 292:78, 1975.
53. Bouvia v Superior Court of State of California, 195 Cal Rptr 484 (Cal App 2Dist, 1983).
54. State v McAfee, 385 SE2d 651 (Ga 1989).
55. Stradley, B: Elizabeth Bouvia v Riverside Hospital: Suicide, euthanasia, murder: The line blurs. Golden Gate University Law Review 15:407, 1985.
56. Meisel, A: Legal myths about terminating life support. Arch Intern Med 151:1497, 1991.
57. Areen, J: The legal status of consent obtained from families of adult patients to withhold or withdraw treatment. JAMA 258:229, 1987.
58. Council on Ethical and Judicial Affairs, American Medical Association: Decisions near the end of life. JAMA 267:222, 1992.
59. Avila, D: The Americans with Disabilities Act and unconsciousness: A rejoinder. J Head Trauma Rehabil 9:103, 1994.
60. Reply brief of Appellant Daniel Avila, temporary limited guardian for Sue Ann Lawrence. In the Matter of Sue Ann Lawrence. In the Supreme Court of Indiana. No. 29SO4-9106-CV-00460.
61. In re Baby K, 16 F3d 590 (4th Cir), cert denied, 115 SCt 91 (1994).
62. In re Baby K, 832 FSupp 1022 at 1029.
63. Darr, JF: Medical futility and implications for physician autonomy. Am J Law Med 21:221, 1995.

64. Lewin, T: Bitter fight to Supreme Court over the life of a man who can only smile. New York Times, Feb 19, 1996.

65. Broder, AJ, and Cranford, RE: "Mary, Mary, quite contrary, how was I to know?" Michael Martin, absolute prescience, and the right to die in Michigan. University of Detroit Mercy Law Review 72:787–832, 1996.

66. In re Martin, 517 NW2d 749 (Mich App 1994).

67. In re Martin, 538 NW2d 399 (Mich 1995).

68. Dresser, R: Still troubled: In re Martin. Hastings Cent Rep 26:21–22, 1996.

69. Cmiel, AJ: Who is the self-insurance market? Case Manager 3:30, 1992.

70. Kass, NE: Insurance for the insurers: The use of genetic tests. Hastings Cent Rep 22:6, 1992.

71. Klerman, JA, and Goldman, DP: Job loss due to health insurance mandates. JAMA 272:552, 1994.

72. Iglehart, J: Health policy report: The American health care system: Managed care. N Engl J Med 327:742, 1992.

73. Iglehart, J: Health policy report: Physicians and the growth of managed care. N Engl J Med 331:1167, 1994.

74. Eazell, DE: Managed care and rehabilitation in the 90s. REHAB Management February–March, 1992, p 79.

75. Thomas, MB (ed): Rehabilitation consortium finds profits in capitated contracts. Hospital Rehab 4:129, 1995.

76. DeJong, G, Wheatley, B, and Sutton, J: Perspective and analysis. BNA's Managed Care Reporter 2:138, 1996.

77. Banja, J, and Johnston, MV: Outcomes evaluation in traumatic brain injury. Part III: Ethical perspectives and social policy. Arch Phys Med Rehabil 75:SC19, 1994.

78. Keith, RA: The comprehensive treatment team in rehabilitation. Arch Phys Med Rehabil 72:269, 1991.

79. Zimmerman, D: Brain injury rehabs under fire. Probe 1:1, 1991.

80. Centers for head injury accused of neglect. New York Times, March 16, 1992, A1.

81. Daniels, N: Just Health Care. Cambridge University, Cambridge, 1985, pp 74–85.

82. People v Kohrig, 498 NE2d 1158 (Ill 1986).

83. Banja, J: Outcomes and value. J Head Trauma Rehabil 9:111, 1994.

84. Banja, J: Values, function and managed care: An ethical analysis. J Head Trauma Rehabil 12:60–70, 1997.

85. Banja, J, Adler, RK, and Stringer, AY: Ethical dimensions of caring for defiant patients: A case study. J Head Trauma Rehabil 11:103–107, 1996.

86. Banja, J: Ethics, values and world culture: Their impact on rehabilitation. Disabil Rehabil 18:279–284, 1996.

87. Rorty, R: Introduction: Antirepresentationalism, ethnocentrism, and liberalism. In Rorty, R: Objectivity, Relativism and Truth: Philosophical Papers, vol 1. Cambridge University Press, Cambridge, 1991, pp 1–17.

88. Will, GF: For the handicapped, rights but no welcome. Hastings Cent Rep 16:5, 1986.

CHAPTER 25

Assessment and Treatment of the Vegetative and Minimally Conscious Patient

JOHN WHYTE, MD, PHD,

ANDREA LABORDE, MD,

and MADELINE C. DIPASQUALE, PHD

Coma is the starting point for all patients with severe traumatic brain injury (TBI). Some of these patients begin to regain consciousness within a few days or weeks. Those survivors whose unconsciousness persists beyond 2 to 4 weeks evolve into the vegetative state,* in which spontaneous control of bodily ("vegetative") functions, such as respiration, cardiovascular function, and sleep-wake cycles return, under the control of recovering brain stem mechanisms. Both coma and the vegetative state are characterized by "absence of function in the cerebral cortex, as judged behaviorally,"[1] and consciousness can reemerge from either state, or the vegetative state may be permanent. Unlike depictions in the popular media, evolution from unconsciousness to consciousness is not sudden. Rather, conscious behavior emerges gradually, with the pace of reemergence related to the severity of the injury and the duration of unconsciousness.

Some patients spend considerable time with very restricted behavioral repertoires that suggest some limited conscious processing. Until recently, there was no specific term for this clinical subgroup, who are clearly no longer comatose or vegetative and yet have very limited cognitive abilities. To merely classify them as severely disabled by the Glasgow Outcome Scale (GOS) would fail to distinguish them from the many patients who are "conscious but disabled" in terms of their ability to live independently.[1] In 1995, members of the Brain Injury Interdisciplinary Special Interest Group of the American Congress of Rehabilitation Medicine recommended a set of terms for describing patients with "severe alterations of consciousness" and introduced, for the first time, an official term for this group: the min-

We would like to thank Monica J. Vaccaro, MS, for supplying data on some of the cases, Etienne Phipps, PhD, for consultation on ethical issues, and our other clinical collaborators who have worked with us in caring for minimally conscious patients. Many thanks to Joseph T. Giacino, PhD, James P. Kelly, MD, and Christopher M. Filley, MD, for their leadership at the Aspen Neurobehavioral Conference. We also extend our thanks to our patients and their families, from whom we continue to learn.

*The term *vegetative state* is objectionable to many families of brain injury survivors because of its association with "vegetable." Other terms such as "wakeful unconsciousness" have been suggested as less pejorative alternatives but have yet to make their way into the mainstream medical literature.

imally responsive state.[2] Subsequently, participants at the 1996 Aspen Neurobehavioral Conference, a consensus conference of invited experts from a variety of disciplines that dealt with the issue of management guidelines for this state, recommended that it be renamed the "minimally conscious state."[3]

The minimally conscious state is distinguished from both coma and the vegetative state by one or more of the following: visual fixation and/or tracking; the emergence of out-of-pattern, nonstereotypical movements, which may occur in response to stimulation or spontaneously; or stereotypical movements (such as blinking and affective behaviors) *if* they occur in a meaningful relationship to the eliciting stimulation and are not attributable to reflex activity. It is distinguished from patients with higher function (albeit still severely disabled by GOS criteria) by the ability to follow complex commands, the ability to communicate intelligibly, and/or the appropriate use of objects.[3] The minimally conscious state must also be distinguished from the locked-in syndrome. In the latter, the neuropathology is generally focal in the pons and vascular in nature. Furthermore, careful examination with eye movements as signals will reveal that the patient's consciousness is largely preserved.[2]

TBI typically produces a combination of diffuse axonal injury (DAI) and focal cortical contusions.[4] DAI is believed to initiate coma through disruption of the arousal functions of the midbrain ascending reticular activating system.[4] It is now generally believed that the transition from coma to the vegetative state signals return of brain stem arousal mechanisms[5] and that persistent unconsciousness reflects damage to the thalamus and/or global cortical and subcortical damage.[6,7]

The functional prognosis after TBI is related to the duration of unconsciousness. Adult patients who remain vegetative at 1 month after TBI have approximately a 52 percent probability of regaining some degree of consciousness by 1 year.[7] The comparable figure for children is 62 percent. When the mechanism of injury is nontraumatic, the probability of recovery of consciousness is considerably less, and the functional plateau occurs earlier. As the duration of unconsciousness lengthens, the probability of ever regaining consciousness diminishes, and the ultimate functional plateau that might be reached is diminished. Although evoked potential testing has been used to predict prognosis acutely, little attention has been given to the predictive value of such assessment done later (e.g., 1 month postinjury), to know whether it may add to behaviorally based prognostic predictions.

The minimally conscious state can be either a transitional state on the way to higher levels of function or a functional plateau in its own right. As expected, the longer postinjury that a patient remains in the minimally conscious state, the less likelihood there is of major functional changes, but specific functional improvements may still occur. Because this patient subgroup has only recently been operationally defined, no good outcome statistics yet exist.

The treatment priorities differ for patients in the vegetative and minimally conscious states and evolve over time for both groups. For patients who are in the vegetative state (VS), the initial priority is to maintain or attain physical health so that there is a useful body for the brain to control if recovery ensues. Patients who fail to evolve out of the VS by 12 months (in trauma) or 3 months (in anoxia) are extremely unlikely ever to do so. It has been suggested that the conditions be referred to as "permanent" after these time points, even though the probability of some limited functional recovery is not absolutely zero (similarly, it has been recommended that the designation "persistent" vegetative state be abandoned). Once the VS is judged to be permanent, it is appropriate to consider withdrawal of active treatments and (in discussion with caregivers) life-sustaining treatments, such as fluids, nutrition, and resuscitation. For patients in the minimally conscious state soon after injury, aggressive rehabilitation efforts should be applied across multiple goal areas. As time passes, those patients who remain minimally conscious should have their treatment focused toward specific functional areas where there appears to be potential for improvement or where no previous treatment has been attempted.

Clear-cut evidence of consciousness is easy to recognize: Patients interact meaningfully with their examiner and the rest of their environment and produce behaviors that are far too complex to have occurred by chance. However, it is sometimes difficult to distinguish minimally conscious patients from those who are truly vegetative. Reports from experienced centers document high rates of misdiagnosing minimally conscious patients as vegetative.[8] Both groups have periods of eye opening and spontaneous movement of the limbs and eyes, and neither performs any complex behaviors that can be easily recognized. Thus, establishing that a patient has some degree of conscious processing rests on establishing a *contingent relationship* between very rudimentary behaviors and conditions in the environment. For example, simple eye blinking clearly does not indicate consciousness, but if it can be shown that the rate of eye blinking is lower after the command "Keep your eyes open" than in its absence, this behavior does suggest conscious processing of the command.

Several standard instruments have been developed to track the subtle changes that signal emergence from coma or the vegetative state and that signal increasingly reliable and complex behavior as improvement occurs within the minimally conscious state. The strengths and weaknesses of the Coma Near Coma Scale, Coma Recovery Scale, Sensory Stimulation Assessment Measure, and Western Neuro Sensory Stimulation Profile have recently been discussed.[9] In addition, we have applied the methods of single-subject experimental design to the evaluation of vegetative and minimally conscious patients.[10,11] This latter method lacks the benefits of standardization but has the advantage that it can be tailored to answer individualized diagnostic (e.g., does the patient have a hemianopsia?) or treatment (e.g., does that patient communicate more reliably on a particular drug than without it?) questions.

☐ MEDICAL ASSESSMENT

Rationale

Many complications in minimally conscious brain injured patients also occur in those with less severe injury. Medical stabilization is important for every patient, and medical instability may slow or prevent emergence from unconsciousness or interfere with valid assessment of consciousness. In the minimally conscious patient, medical evaluation is challenging because of the patient's inability to participate in the examination or report symptoms.

Tachycardia

Careful review of vital signs is important on first presentation. Tachycardia may be caused by hypovolemia, anemia, cardiac abnormalities (premorbid or secondary to cardiac trauma in the injury), or pain. Assessment of blood pressure for orthostasis, laboratory studies (such as complete blood cell count and electrolytes), and electrocardiography may be beneficial on admission. The patient should be examined carefully to rule out causes of pain such as pressure sores, abdominal abnormalities, and sores caused by lip biting. Only when all other etiologies have been ruled out should beta-blockers be entertained for symptomatic treatment. If used, a beta-blocker with low lipophilic properties should be chosen to minimize crossing of the blood-brain barrier.[12]

Fever

Fever can be caused by infections, medications, atelectasis, aspiration without pneumonia, pancreatitis, and thrombophlebitis. Information from acute care charts regarding previous evaluations is often incomplete. Central fever is most common in minimally conscious patients with increased temperatures and normal white blood cell counts. However, a fever workup and an infectious disease consult may be needed before declaring a central cause. Patients diagnosed with central fever can be treated symptomatically with cooling blankets, bromocriptine,[13] or indomethacin.[14]

Hypertension

Hypertension is particularly common in vegetative and minimally conscious patients because of the location and severity of their brain damage (see Chapter 4 for further discussion of hypertension) and often resolves with sufficient recovery. Occult causes should be sought. Because of the associated tachycardia, hypertonia, and sweating, treatment with a beta-blocker with both β-1 and β-2 properties may be preferred. Propranolol has been proposed in the past,[15,16] but nadolol, which has reduced lipophilic properties, may minimize cognitive side effects.

Medications

Medication side effects may be particularly problematic in minimally conscious patients for several reasons. First, such patients are not able to report subjective sedation. Second, a side effect that may be relatively minor in a higher-level patient can have significant effects on cognition in a low-level patient.

It is now generally accepted that seizure prophylaxis is not indicated in most cases of TBI after the first week of injury.[17,18] Therefore, fewer patients are transferred to a rehabilitation setting on anticonvulsants. If a review of records does not reveal an active seizure disorder, weaning of the anticonvulsant should be discussed with the family. If weaning is not possible, either because of a clear seizure disorder or because of a family member's reluctance, the least sedating medication should be chosen (generally carbamazepine or a valproate).[19] As for all patients on anticonvulsants, careful monitoring of therapeutic levels should be maintained, utilizing the minimally effective dose.

Many patients are placed on H_2 blockers, as well as metoclopramide, during their acute management. Once they are discharged from intensive care, these medications may no longer be indicated but are often continued. If there is a clear indication for such drugs (e.g., documented peptic ulcer disease, reflux esophagitis, or aspiration caused by reflux), efforts should be made to use those that are less sedating, such as sucralfate and cisapride.[20]

Post-Traumatic Epilepsy

Minimally conscious patients are at high risk for development of post-traumatic epilepsy (PTE) because of the severity of injury and prolonged periods of unconsciousness.[21] Although prophylaxis is not advocated, treatment of PTE is. The difficulty lies in detection. Eye deviations during seizures may be confused with random eye movements; motor manifestations of simple or complex partial seizures may be difficult to distinguish from hypertonia or movement disorders, and seizure-induced depression of consciousness may be difficult to recognize in a patient whose consciousness is already marginal.

Routine electroencephlograms (EEGs) may or may not be of benefit. Twenty-four-hour EEGs may be more helpful but still may not be diagnostic unless a seizure is captured by the recording. Alerting staff and family to signs of seizures may increase detection. Unless seizures are generalized seizures, it may take several episodes before a clear pattern is determined (e.g., eye fluttering as a manifestation of seizures).

Once PTE is clearly diagnosed, treatment with an anticonvulsant should be initiated. As previously discussed, carbamazepine is currently the medication of choice. Prior to initiation, appropriate baseline studies should be obtained. Laboratory monitoring of drug levels can be minimized through use of a rational algorithm.[22] Clinical determination of an appropriate level may be more difficult because side effects are not reported, but if the lowest levels are maintained with adequate control, side effects should be minimized.[23]

Post-Traumatic Hydrocephalus

Post-traumatic hydrocephalus (PTH) may be responsible for maintaining a low level of responding in a minimally conscious patient but is very difficult to diagnose, as discussed in Chapter 4. A diagnostic lumbar puncture (LP; "tap test") with withdrawal of cerebral spinal fluid (CSF) may be helpful to differentiate communicating hydrocephalus from hydrocephalus ex vacuo. In the minimally conscious patient, it is recommended that staff determine behavioral indices to be monitored during sev-

eral days of baseline data collection prior to the LP and in the few hours immediately after. A clear indication of improvement should be seen.[24]

Case 1 ■ RL is a 28-year-old woman with TBI sustained in an assault. She had severe spastic quadriparesis, dysphagia, dysarthria, and significant cognitive impairments. Repeat computed tomography (CT) scans several months postinjury revealed large ventricles, but it was difficult to determine if this was caused by communicating hydrocephalus or by hydrocephalus ex vacuo. Data were collected regarding various aspects of grooming (toothbrushing, hairbrushing, and application of Chapstick). Time to initiate and persistence in these tasks were monitored. If the patient did not initiate the task after 3 minutes of cuing, the therapist initiated the activity for the patient. A tap test was performed and data were collected within several hours of the lumbar puncture. As illustrated in Figure 25–1, application of Chapstick, which had always required the therapist's assistance after 3 minutes of cuing, occurred spontaneously after the tap test. This aided in the decision to place a lumboperitoneal shunt. Postoperatively, the patient had increased verbal communication, allowing her to express her needs and interact with her family.

Even after diagnosis and shunting, the recovery course may be complicated by clinical decline in as many as 40 percent of cases.[25] Complications include shunt malfunction, seizures, infection, undershunting, overshunting, and subdural collections.[26] In the minimally conscious patient, complications may be particularly difficult to recognize because cognitive decline is likely to be subtle. Again, careful documentation of predetermined behavioral indices may be beneficial. If the patient has no improvement or declines postoperatively, a follow-up CT scan can be obtained.

Though diagnosis and treatment of PTH remain controversial, diagnostic studies and surgical intervention should be considered in minimally conscious patients, particularly those with early onset and clear findings on CT scan. Gross outcome may remain the same (i.e., maximal care), but quality of life may be improved by greater alertness and more reliable responding. Complications, however, should be anticipated, particularly in the older population.

Case 2 ■ HT is a 63-year-old man who sustained diffuse axonal injury and multiple contusions as a result of a bicycle accident. On admission to our service, he was able to follow some instructions and had limited ability to communicate through writing. CT scan revealed findings consistent with post-traumatic hydrocephalus. A

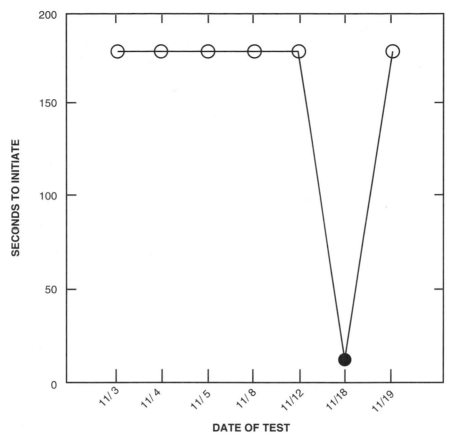

FIGURE 25–1. Behavioral assessment of response to the "tap test." The time to initiate a grooming task is shown on the *y* axis for several assessment days (180 sec was the cutoff if no initiation occurred). The filled circle represents the trial conducted within a few hours of the tap test.

low-pressure shunt was placed with improvement in functional status when coupled with dopaminergic agents. However, later the patient began to show evidence of clinical decline despite an increase in medication dose. A follow-up CT scan revealed a subdural hematoma.

The patient underwent closure of the shunt and drainage of the hematoma. As would be expected, he had enlargement of his ventricles and further decline in clinical function. Once adequate scarring of the area of the hematoma was felt to be achieved, a high-pressure shunt replaced his prior valve. Immediately following the procedure, there was dramatic improvement in the patient's performance. However, the improvement was not maintained. The clinical team hypothesized that the high-pressure shunt still allowed excessive fluid accumulation. Despite presentation of the behavioral data, the neurosurgeon was reluctant to revise the shunt because of previous failure.

Several months after discharge, the patient developed pneumonia and complications of ventri-

culitis. Because of infection, the shunt was again revised, with a low-pressure valve resulting in improved function. The patient developed seizures requiring carbamazepine and refractory hiccups requiring treatment with baclofen. Subsequent CT scans showed slitlike ventricles, which predispose to major increases in intracranial pressure with minor clinical illnesses (such as infection with fever).[26] The patient continues to have functional fluctuations, with days when he can move all extremities and speak, contrasted with days of limited communication and need for maximal assistance. Though it is clear that PTH is a major factor in his clinical status, further shunt revision is not feasible at this time.

Heterotopic Ossification

Vegetative and minimally conscious patients are at high risk for development of heterotopic ossification (HO) because of prolonged unconsciousness and frequently associated spastic quadriparesis and are at high risk for recurrence after resection.[27] Diagnosis and treatment of this condition are discussed in detail in Chapter 4. If, despite treatment, rigid deformity develops, surgery can be considered, but very clear goals must be established because of the high rate of recurrence in this population. In the minimally conscious patient, passive treatment goals may include improving seating position in the wheelchair, decreasing risk or improving healing of pressure sores, increasing ease of transfers, improving access for hygiene, and increasing joint mobility.

When addressing improved mobility about a joint, one has to carefully review the functional goal. Improvement of motion for motion's sake may not be worth the risks of surgery or recurrence, but when HO appears to limit the patient's active motion, treatment may be indicated. For example, increased active elbow motion may enhance the use of an augmentive communication device. Even when a goal is clear, one should proceed cautiously with surgery and discuss potential complications with family members.

Case 3 ■ ER is a 23-year-old woman who was minimally conscious because of injuries sustained in a motor vehicle accident. She had complications of heterotopic ossification at the posterior right elbow, which impaired flexion. Despite this contracture, it was her most functional limb and was the best mechanism for communication through a yes-no communication board. Because she was 16 months postinjury and radiological studies showed maturity of bone, staff felt that surgical resection might enhance further communication and encourage other functions, such as self-feeding, for which she showed promise.

Postoperatively, the patient had difficulties with pain, despite the liberal use of pain medications, and constantly moved her elbow. This led to development of a seroma and then to severe skin breakdown requiring surgical treatment with a pedicle graft. During this 10-week period, the patient was unable to participate in her usual therapy program. She did ultimately have increased range of motion at the elbow, but whether this will lead to furthering of function remains to be determined.

Hypertonia and Motor Control

Hypertonia, both focal and diffuse, is commonly seen in minimally conscious patients and may follow no particular pattern. In addition to limb involvement, truncal tone may also be present. Hypertonic posturing may lead to contracture, difficulties in positioning, poor hygiene management, and masking of underlying motor function.

Oral medications may be used to address global hypertonia but, because of sedative side effects, may impair cognitive function while inadequately controlling tone.[28] Also, systemic treatment may improve global tone without targetting specific motor goals. Focal management with phenol nerve or motor point blocks, botulinum toxin injection, or surgical tendon lengthening or release may be more effective in the minimally conscious population.[29–31] As with other functional management, goals need to be clearly defined. For example, reduction of finger flexor tone may improve hygiene in a macerated palm or use of a manual communication device. Surgery may be helpful to reduce ankle deformities to maintain skin integrity or allow for stand-pivot transfers.

Clarification of these goals may be obtained through dynamic electromyography as discussed in more detail in Chapter 29. Proper placement of electrodes may help to differentiate spasticity from contracture and reveal which muscles are the chief offenders. It may also demonstrate the presence of some volitional activity. The pattern of electromyographic (EMG) activity can suggest further appropriate therapeutic interventions. The presence of some volitional control may lead the surgeon to choose tendon lengthening versus release.

Timing of these interventions is not clearly defined. There is a reluctance to perform surgery in the early stages because of its permanence. Phenol or botulinum toxin blocks are more temporary but may not adequately address the issue, particularly when multiple muscle groups are involved or contractures are present that fail to respond to conservative stretching.

Case 4 ■ KT is a 50-year-old man who had significant extensor tone in the lower extremities because of a TBI sustained in an assault. Three months postinjury, he developed a pressure sore at the base of his fifth toe, which was not responsive to local care. EMG testing of his calf musculature revealed inappropriate activation of his tibialis anterior on the left and tibialis posterior on the right, despite the fact that his ankle deformities appeared symmetrical. Phenol motor point blocks were performed to the left tibialis anterior and right tibialis posterior, which helped reduce his tone, but tone reappeared 4 weeks later. The patient underwent split anterior tibialis tendon lengthening and transfer (SPLATT) and lengthening of the right posterior tibialis muscle with resultant improvement in wound healing postoperatively.

Decannulation

Most minimally conscious patients have a tracheostomy tube in place at rehabilitation admission unless they are being evaluated several years postinjury. Maintenance of tracheostomy tubes is controversial. Minimally conscious patients may be at risk for respiratory complications with decannulation because of suppressed ability to clear secretions with coughing.[32] Then again, these patients are exposed to complications of prolonged tracheostomies such as fistulas, dysphagia, stenosis, and introduction of organisms into the lungs.[33]

> **Case 5** ■ KS was a 44-year-old woman who was minimally conscious because of injuries sustained in a motor vehicle accident. She developed tracheal stenosis very quickly from endotracheal intubation. A custom tracheostomy tube was placed beyond the site of stenosis. She developed stenosis at the new site, requiring an even longer tracheostomy tube. This series of events continued until the length of the tube made pulmonary toilet exceedingly difficult. The patient ultimately died of airway obstruction.

Tracheal tubes may also be a source of irritation that leads to increased respiratory secretions. This irritation, coupled with the fact that most tubes are colonized, makes it difficult to differentiate benign secretions from infection. Although cultures taken through the tracheostomy tube may assist in antibiotic selection, the decision to treat should be based on chest x-ray and/or white blood cell results.

Once the decision is made to decannulate, various methods are available, as discussed in Chapter 4 and elsewhere.[34,35] We have found it helpful to combine nebulizer treatments, expectorants, increased fluids, and chest percussion to aid in mobilization of secretions to expedite the process. One may or may not wish to continue any or all of these interventions postdecannulation, depending on clinical indications (thick secretions, rhonchi on auscultation).

Feeding

Most minimally conscious patients are admitted with an enteral feeding tube (either gastrostomy or jejunostomy). Although meeting nutritional needs orally may not be an early goal (as team members may be more involved in assessment of arousal or communication), oral intake of some form may be expressed as a goal by family members or indicated by the patient when more aroused. Assessment of ability to swallow safely should proceed as with other brain injured patients. Assessment of oral motor and sensory function and gag and cough reflexes can be performed at bedside.[36] Often, minimally conscious patients are mute, so laryngeal evaluation may not be possible. If the tracheostomy tube is still present, a modified blue dye study can be performed first with saliva and then with purees (keeping in mind that a single negative dye study does not rule out aspiration). If aspiration of the dye occurs, further oral feeding should be postponed, and reassessment performed periodically. If further clarification regarding the mechanism of aspiration is needed or the patient does not have a tracheostomy tube (as might be the case in a patient being evaluated several years postinjury), a videofluoroscopy can be performed. Positioning these patients for evaluation and feeding can be difficult because of hypertonic posturing and poor head control, making it difficult for one clinician to position, give feeding cues, and assess oral motor function. We have found that cotreating with speech and physical or occupational therapists is helpful.

Gastroesophageal reflux may be a contributing factor to aspiration and an obstacle to advancement of feeding.[37] Treatment in the past consisted of metoclopramide in addition to acid suppressants, but it has the potential for cognitive and motor side effects.[38] A newer medication, cisapride, increases gastrointestinal sphincter tone without such side effects.

If good oral function is present and there is no evidence of aspiration, recreational feeding may be considered until functional improvement allows more intensive work on feeding as a route to nutrition. Favorite foods with appropriate consistencies are introduced in small quantities. Often, recreational feeding is found to be beneficial for family members, as it provides a way for them to interact with the patient or have the patient participate in a social or holiday function. The family should be instructed in appropriate feeding techniques, as in other TBI cases.[39]

During feeding assessment, enteral feedings should be maintained. It is unlikely that a patient who remains minimally conscious will be discharged without tube feedings as the major source of nutrition. Bolus feedings or continuous feedings can be chosen, depending on the patient's need for mobility, risk for aspiration, response of the gastrointestinal tract (such as ileus or diarrhea), and family resources and sophistication.[40]

Bruxism

Bruxism is a severe grinding of teeth found in both normal and brain injured individuals. Because it is thought to improve with recovery of consciousness, treatment in early stages may not be worth the expense, risks, and side effects.[41] However, in the minimally conscious patient, treatment may be beneficial to reduce loosening of teeth and destruction of dental surfaces. The challenge is finding an effective treatment. Traditional mouth guards may be destroyed by the strong patient bite. This repetitive biting may also cause damage to mucosal tissue, gums, jaw, and lips. Effective medications, such as phenothiazines, may cause further sedation.

We have found a lip "bumper" to be helpful when serious destruction of the lips accompanies bruxism. The bumper is placed via braces on the incisors. A soft wire arced in a convex position is attached to the braces, which causes a jutting of the lip outward, beyond the teeth, thereby reducing damage. Occasionally, motor point blocks to the masseter muscles may be helpful when severe tooth loosening or destruction continues. If bruxism persists, a thorough oral exam and a dental medicine consult, if necessary, are in order to rule out noxious inciting stimuli (such as cavities and abscesses).

> **Case 6** ■ TG is a 20-year-old man who sustained both anoxia and TBI when he fell after overdosing on drugs and alcohol. On admission, he was noted to have persistent bruxism. Dental evaluation revealed oral abscesses secondary to loosened teeth, combined with poor hygiene. His teeth were extracted, and he was treated with intravenous antibiotics. His bruxism persisted. He was treated with masseter motor point blocks, with some improvement. Dental x-rays to evaluate the status of remaining teeth revealed osteomyelitis and jaw fracture. The fracture was reduced and the osteomyelitis was treated with further antibiotics, with a significant reduction in bruxism.

Sensory and Cognitive Issues

As mentioned previously, the ultimate priority for vegetative and minimally conscious patients is cognitive improvement; physical health in the absence of consciousness is of little value, whereas a severely limited body can be helped to function adaptively in service of a good mind. To maximize the chances of cognitive recovery, arousal must be maximized, which means giving attention to the withdrawal of sedating (e.g., narcotics and benzodiazepines) and potentially sedating (e.g., certain antihistamines and antihypertensives) medications and consideration of stimulant, dopaminergic, and noradrenergic drugs that may increase alertness and cognitive function.

The sensory capacities of a patient are equally important to know because failure to follow verbal commands means something quite different in a deaf patient than in one who hears. Our initial evaluation of a patient includes careful review of the mechanism of injury, serial neuroimaging studies, associated injuries, and evoked potential testing, if conducted. Knowing that a patient had an anoxic episode, for example, raises the likelihood of cortical blindness and reduces the likelihood that hearing has been impaired by trauma to the eighth nerve. Finding a large focal lesion in the left hemisphere would induce us to consider aphasia as a possible reason for a patient's failure to follow verbal commands rather than global deficits in consciousness. Knowing that a patient had an orbital fracture raises the question of whether vision may have been impaired focally. Finding that auditory and visual pathways are grossly intact from an electrophysiological perspective gives us greater confidence that responses (or lack thereof) to auditory or visual stimuli can be interpreted unambiguously. Assessment of these sensory functions is discussed later.

Once we have established that a degree of visual or auditory processing is possible, the next priority is generally to assess cognitive function via one or more sensory pathways. The initial issue is whether the patient can comprehend verbal commands. If there is concern about a hearing deficit, commands can be given in writing or by gesture; if there is a concern about aphasia, gesture is most appropriate. If there is evidence that the patient can follow commands, one can proceed to determine whether the patient can follow the specific command to use a yes-no signal, whether by looking at yes-no signs, pointing to yes-no cards, or nodding yes-no. If this attempt is successful, one can then assess use of yes-no signals to respond to meaningful factual questions, the answers to which are known by caregivers (e.g., "Do you like lasagna?). Once a functional yes-no system is available, it can be used as a window to explore cognitive function more generally because, in principle, any neuropsychological examination can be transformed into a series of yes-no questions. Thus, the types of assessment issues a minimally conscious patient presents generally unfold in a logical, chronological sequence.

Methods of Assessment and Evaluation

There are several problems unique to the evaluation of minimally conscious patients. Traditional clinical methods, such as a mental status evaluation, interviews, and brief neuropsychological screens, fail to elicit meaningful information because they assume a consistency of performance; that is, a patient who is able to exhibit a particular behavior or response once is assumed to have the ability to consistently demonstrate that behavior on demand. Additionally, examiners often rely on the complexity of patients' responses to evaluate cognitive status; if patients can perform "serial 7s," an examiner may conclude that they are able to hear and understand the command, hold information in working memory, perform mental manipulations with speed and accuracy, and attend and concentrate. Minimally conscious patients, however, lack these complex behaviors. In addition, the examiner may attribute meaning to a spontaneous or reflexive movement, or the reverse may be true, in that an examiner who is unable to identify any consistent response over the course of a brief evaluation may conclude that the patient is vegetative. Consequently, minimally conscious patients should be evaluated *over time* to determine level of arousal, consistency of response, and temporal change.

Several behavioral observation and classification systems are currently available to assess coma, the vegetative state, and emergence from them. However, scales commonly used to categorize persons with traumatic brain injury generally, such as the Disability Rating Scale,[42] Glasgow Outcome Scale,[1] and the Rancho Los Amigos Levels of Cognitive Functioning Scale,[43] are less appropriate for minimally conscious patients because these scales are unable to identify the initial subtle changes that such patients are likely to make. Scales developed specifically for this population include the Coma Recovery Scale,[44] the Western Neuro Sensory Stimulation Profile,[45] and the Coma/Near Coma Scale.[46]

These standardized scales can evaluate a range of behaviors in a patient who may or may not be vegetative at the time the assessment begins, and they provide scores that can be examined programwide and used for prediction of prognosis and program evaluation. Administration time for the standardized scales varies from about 15 to 50 minutes.[9] Thus, in most programs, it is possible to administer these scales only once or twice per week. However, because of their standardized nature, they lack the flexibility to focus on specific questions that may be raised in the course of caring for a minimally conscious patient. For example, if it becomes clear that patients are following verbal commands on some occasions, clinicians may wish to assess which motor behavior provides the highest response rate, whether they can make a movement once versus twice on command, and whether they can learn to use one

movement to signal yes and two movements to signal no. Using such a system, are they able to accurately answer personal biographical questions?

In addition, the directions for administering the standardized scales often lack clear operationalized methods for administering the stimuli and defining the responses. For example, if the command is to demonstrate a "thumbs up," how many times should the command be given, how long should the observer wait, and how much movement constitutes a valid response? Our experience suggests that, unless these factors are specified, clinicians will disagree about their observations.

In our experience, the broad overview provided by standardized scales should be supplemented with individually tailored quantitative assessments that can be administered several times a day and that focus on particular questions of clinical interest. Single-subject methodology—the systematic collection and analysis of quantitative information to answer a question about the individual—lends itself to such evaluation. The treatment team can design individualized protocols, based on initial observations and interactions, with clear operational definitions of stimuli and responses, and assess interrater reliability to assure consistency in the data.

Visual Function

Visual function is difficult to assess in minimally conscious patients but highly important in view of the fact that many conclusions about general responding are based on response to visual inputs. Some clarification of visual function can be obtained through visual evoked potentials (VEPs), which are the recordings of the cortical electrical response to a visual stimulus (usually a patterned stimulus or luminance change).[47] In the patterned stimulus method (usually reversal of a checkerboard pattern), a positive deflection occurs, and its amplitude and latency are measured. Pattern stimuli are most useful in assessing optic nerve integrity but are rarely feasible in the minimally conscious patient because they require patient cooperation and good visual acuity to focus.[48]

Luminance VEPs are primarily used for assessment of cortical function. They are obtained with a photic flash or pulse. The primary response probably represents the striate visual cortex, with the secondary response representing association areas.[49] Luminance VEPs require little patient cooperation but have limited ability to evaluate visual acuity or visual attention. Despite these limitations. VEPs may be beneficial as an adjunct to clinical exam, particularly when abnormal extraocular movements preclude the use of visual orienting as a marker of vision. However, we have evaluated patients with absent VEPs in whom we could demonstrate some visual function behaviorally and vice versa.

We have developed a behavioral assessment of vision and visual attention suitable for administration to vegetative and minimally conscious patients, which has been described in detail elsewhere.[10] The protocol makes use of colorful photographs and a blank white card, which are raised abruptly into one or both visual fields. The first horizontal eye movement within a 5-second interval is taken as a potential indication of visual orienting to the stimulus. Patients with dysconjugate gaze are assessed with one eye patched. Typically seven trials, representing seven different conditions, are run in each administration (Table 25–1), and the total number of trials needed to develop a definitive conclusion is related to both the frequency of orienting to stimuli (as opposed to response failures) and the frequency of spontaneous eye movements in the no-stimulus control condition. Complete absence of visual orienting could mean either blindness or the vegetative state, whereas some degree of visual discrimination is evidence for the minimally conscious state.

In Table 25–1, the results of one such assessment are shown. In condition 7, it can be seen that the patient has eye movements on every trial, although no specific visual stimulation is provided and there is a highly significant gaze preference to the right. When a unilateral photo or card is displayed on the right side (conditions 2 and 4), the proportion of right-sided eye movements is nearly identical to the control condition (percentages are most easily interpreted because the number of trials is not the same for each condition). In contrast, when the photo or card is displayed on the left, the number of left-sided movements is significantly greater than in the control condition, providing clear evidence of vision in the left hemifield

and a tendency to orient to the left, which only partially counteracts the baseline gaze preference. The fact that the patient orients to the left more consistently to a photo than to a blank card is also evidence of some degree of cortical visual discrimination. Whether the patient is blind in the right hemifield or simply has such a strong right gaze preference that no increase in right-sided movements can be documented is unclear. However, the fact that the patient shows increased left-sided orienting in condition 6 is evidence for a right hemianopsia because, if he could see the right-sided photo, his gaze should preferentially orient to it rather than the card, which it does not.

Auditory Function

Intact auditory processing is necessary to interpret responses to auditory commands. Because even vegetative patients can generate a brain stem startle reflex to loud noise, however, it is difficult to evaluate higher-level auditory processing before the patient can respond in more meaningful ways. If startle responses are absent or equivocal, brain stem auditory evoked responses (BAERs) can be obtained.

BAERs are a series of positive and negative wave forms in response to a repeated auditory stimulus (usually a calibrated click that can be varied in intensity). The sources of these wave forms are believed to represent function at the eighth nerve and brain stem. These wave forms are unaffected by level of consciousness or medications[50] and thus are helpful in the minimally responsive patient. They can assist therapists in determining whether auditory stimulation is an appropriate assessment modality or whether there is a hearing asymmetry. Abnormal BAERs should be approached with caution, as hearing impairments may be of mixed origin. Also, injury to the peripheral auditory system (including tympanic membrane, ossicles, and eighth nerve) can be misinterpreted as evi-

Stimulus Condition	Responses		
Left / Right	Left-sided Orienting	Right-sided Orienting	Failures to Respond
1. Photo / —	21 (49%)	22 (51%)	0 (0%)
2. — / Photo	2 (5%)	42 (95%)	0 (0%)
3. Card / —	8 (20%)	33 (80%)	0 (0%)
4. — / Card	2 (5%)	40 (95%)	0 (0%)
5. Photo / Card	13 (30%)	30 (70%)	0 (0%)
6. Card / Photo	7 (16%)	35 (84%)	0 (0%)
7. — / —	6 (7%)	77 (93%)	0 (0%)

TABLE 25–1. Results of Visual Assessment in an Individual Patient

dence of central auditory pathology. Impedance audiometry and pure tone audiometry should accompany "abnormal" BAERs.[51]

Following Commands

Following commands is a key element in assessment of consciousness because it provides evidence that the commands are perceived and that the patient has control over their execution. Indeed, command following appears on virtually every assessment scale for severe brain injury. However, not all scales provide clear guidance on how an examiner is to determine whether a behavior that occurs in proximity to a command is to be judged as evidence for command following rather than as coincidence.

Evaluation of command following can be assessed differently, depending on whether the patient has only one possible behavior available on a voluntary basis or whether two or more such behaviors are under consideration. Our study of a single behavior such as hand squeezing typically includes three conditions: "squeeze my hand" (the target command); "relax your hand" or "hold still" (the incompatible command); and simple observation. Each command condition is administered an equal number of times, and the patient is allowed a set time to respond. If the patient is able to follow the command, the frequency of squeezes should be higher in the target command condition than in either of the others. A comparison of the incompatible command and the simple observation condition helps control for the nonspecific effects of noise on random movement. An example of such a protocol is shown in Table 25–2. Although the patient responds only inconsistently to the command, it is clear that the rate of responding is significantly higher to the command than in either of the other conditions.

Evaluation of response to two different commands often centers around yes and no signals,

which, if demonstrated, have great functional utility. Signals chosen might be eye movements to yes-no cards, yes-no head nods, or specific finger, hand, or foot signals that may be able to indicate yes and no. Here, an equal number of "show me yes" and "show me no" conditions are run in random order, and a differential frequency of responses to the two categories serves as evidence for command following. An example of such a protocol is shown in Table 25–3, in which a minimally conscious patient was asked to hit one of two buzzers that were labeled with the large printed words "Yes" and "No." It can be seen that responding is not entirely reliable (14% response failures) or accurate (69% accuracy when considering only responses) but significantly greater than chance, indicating that the patient differentially processed the commands.

Assessment results may indicate the presence of some conscious processing but may not provide evidence of functionally useful behavior. For example, we have evaluated a number of patients whose rates of yes and no signals were different in response to yes and no commands, which provided unequivocal evidence that they, at some level, distinguished between the two commands. However, some of these patients might respond to a yes command with 90 percent yes signals and 10 percent no signals and respond to a no command with 75 percent yes signals and 25 percent no signals. Although the patient has a different pattern of results for the two commands, attempts to use such a system functionally will be thwarted by the fact that the patient usually responds yes, no matter which command is given.

Establishing a Communication System

One of the highest functional priorities in minimally conscious patients is the development of some type of communication system. If successful, the patient can indicate care needs, engage in limited social interaction with caregivers, and provide further information about his or her cognitive function by answering other assessment questions. A simple yes-no communication system is almost always the initial step in augmentative communication because it requires only two simple motor responses. Although scanning systems also require only one or two motor responses to halt the system at the appropriate target letter or symbol, we rarely find patients at this level who can master scanning systems and anticipate the target arrival so that they can stop the system before the target is passed. However, al-

---

TABLE 25–2. Evaluation of a Patient's Ability to Hit a Buzzer on Command		
	Patient Responses	
Stimulus Condition	Buzzer Hits	Nonresponses
"Hit the buzzer"	40 (50%)	41 (50%)
"Hold still"	11 (14%)	70 (86%)
Observation	8 (10%)	73 (90%)

TABLE 25–3. Evaluation of a Patient's Ability to Hit a "Yes" or "No" Buzzer on Command

Stimulus Condition	Responses		
	Hit Yes Buzzer	Hit No Buzzer	Nonresponses
"Hit the Yes"	43 (72%)	9 (15%)	8 (13%)
"Hit the No"	11 (19%)	39 (66%)	9 (15%)

---

though yes-no systems are both simple and useful, they may pose particular problems for some patients with aphasia who have specific confusion between yes and no, despite better preservation of other language concepts. Thus, failure on a yes-no system should not necessarily be taken to mean complete absence of language function.

Once a patient can be shown to follow commands to indicate a yes-no response, it is appropriate to begin to incorporate this skill into a communication assessment. Our approach has typically been to gather a series of factual questions and their correct answers from family members. We try to avoid questions that relate to recent history because retrograde amnesia may confound the assessment. Ideally, we collect a sample of approximately equal numbers of yes and no questions, without telling team members what the correct answers are. This practice avoids bias in interpreting ambiguous eye or finger movements. The questions are administered in random order, and the patient's response is recorded. We then calculate the frequency of responding (patients often simply fail to respond to some questions) and the percentage of correct responses out of those trials on which a response occurred. An accuracy rate that is significantly greater than 50 percent provides evidence that the patient is successful at using such a system for communication. Accuracy rates close to 100 percent clearly support a viable system. Intermediate accuracy rates provide evidence of conscious processing but may not be functionally useful. However, in some such cases, we have been successful in using paired questions (e.g., "Are you a man?" and

"Are you a woman?") and counting the response as correct only if it switches when the question is transformed.

We evaluated a patient who demonstrated the ability to signal yes and no on command by using two different movements of his thumb. During this initial evaluation, his response rate was 83 percent, and his accuracy was also 83 percent. We went on to apply this thumb-signaling system to answering biographical questions, as shown in Table 25–4. As can be seen, although his response rate was even higher than in the prior protocol (94%), his accuracy dropped to 71 percent, presumably because of the increased cognitive demands of the question content. Also, note that he showed a preference for yes responses, which interfered with his accuracy. Although he was significantly more accurate than chance, the team compensated for this relatively poor accuracy by asking each question twice, once in the affirmative and once in the negative, as discussed previously.

To use such a system functionally, one must know its limits. If the communication system was assessed by using short declarative factual questions, it cannot necessarily be assumed that the patient can also answer longer or more complex questions. Thus, whenever complexity is to be increased, some reassessment is in order. In addition, some patients who are initially assessed with, for example, an eye movement system are later noted to begin to spontaneously nod yes and no, to point, or to mouth words. As the patient gives indications of increasing ability, new and more functional alternatives should be evaluated.

TABLE 25–4. Evaluation of a Patient's Ability to Answer Biographical Questions

Type of Question	Patient's Response		
	"Yes" Movement	"No" Movement	Nonresponses
"Yes"	38 (79%)	7 (15%)	3 (6%)
"No"	18 (43%)	22 (52%)	2 (5%)

Psychopharmacology

As mentioned previously, every effort should be made to wean vegetative and minimally conscious patients from sedating or potentially sedating drugs or to substitute less sedating alternatives. However, if patients fail to improve in their level of consciousness in a reasonable period, it may be appropriate to consider a trial of a stimulant or cognition-enhancing medication. Although no drugs are formally indicated for this purpose, there are many that may be beneficial on the basis of theoretical arguments and several that have been shown in case reports and single-subject evaluations to be beneficial to at least some patients.[52,53] In our experience, it is rare to find a vegetative patient who becomes minimally conscious in response to drug administration, but it is more common for minimally conscious patients to become more reliable with drug treatment.

The two neurotransmitter systems that have been most studied and advocated for improving function and recovery are norepinephrine and dopamine. The former is believed to be particularly useful for selecting environmental stimuli to attend to; the latter appears more involved in initiation of responding.[54] Psychostimulants such as methylphenidate and dextroamphetamine, which affect both neurotransmitter systems, may increase eye opening and alertness and, in some cases, may improve the accuracy of responding. Dextroamphetamine, specifically, has been reported to enhance neurological recovery.[55] Drugs with noradrenergic activity, such as desipramine (a relatively pure noradrenergic drug) or amitriptyline (a drug with mixed actions), are also believed to enhance neurological recovery and have shown some utility in minimally conscious patients. Several drugs with dopamine agonist activity have also been advocated. Those that function as dopamine precursors (e.g., L-dopa) may actually increase both dopamine and norepinephrine levels; direct agonists such as bromocriptine and pergolide have more specific dopaminergic activity.[55]

Because of the relative dearth of research on the efficacy of these drugs in TBI, one is left to choose a drug partly based on side effect profile (e.g., seizure risk is increased with tricyclics but not with methylphenidate)[56,57] and partly based on practicality (e.g., bromocriptine must be increased and tapered slowly, so its evaluation is quite time-consuming). Whatever drug is chosen, it is critical that some form of objective evaluation of its effects be undertaken. Otherwise, the random variation in behavior that is so typical of minimally conscious patients will leave team members confused about whether the drug had any useful effects.

Our approach to drug evaluation nearly always involves gathering baseline data on patient function prior to any drug changes to allow the target behaviors to be clearly understood and to enable the team to estimate how much data will be required after the drug change to provide a clear assessment. In our experience, medications are most often used in minimally conscious patients to increase alertness or to increase the reliability with which commands are followed or communication is engaged in. Thus, baseline data on eye opening (or other indices of alertness), command following, and yes-no accuracy are required. Review of baseline data allows the team to assess the day-to-day variability and to determine whether there is any spontaneous change over time in the absence of drug intervention. Greater variability indicates the need for more data both before and after drug intervention to get a clear answer. Spontaneous improvement may lead the team to postpone drug intervention. If drug interventions are planned despite an upward trend in the baseline data, then a more dramatic upward trend will be required to support the effectiveness of the intervention.

Short-acting drugs such as methylphenidate and dextroamphetamine are ideal for this type of assessment because they can be introduced and withdrawn every day or two, allowing a single-subject placebo-controlled trial. Even if there is some underlying recovery taking place, it will be distributed equally across drugs. Longer-acting drugs, such as bromocriptine or tricyclic antidepressants, generally cannot be studied in this way. However, if the team develops a clear pattern of baseline data, it is generally possible to detect a change in that pattern as the drug in introduced. Lingering uncertainty about the drug's effects can be answered by withdrawing the drug later to see if regression occurs.

Drug-induced increases in alertness may not always translate into improvements in meaningful function. We have repeatedly seen patients in the vegetative state increase their eye opening on medication while remaining at chance in terms of following commands. Minimally conscious patients often increase the proportion of responses that they produce in response to commands or questions during drug treatment, but the drug's effects on accuracy are more variable. Thus, it is generally important to evaluate not only alertness and ability to respond but also accuracy or quality of response.

Case 7 ■ We performed a baseline evaluation on a patient who was several years post-TBI and who appeared to be in the vegetative state, with intermittent eye opening and no clear evidence that finger movements could be used to answer biographical questions, despite his family's belief that this was occurring. In view of his frequent eye closure, we hypothesized that he might be underaroused and might benefit from a dopaminergic drug both to increase alertness and to improve command following. Five degrees of eye opening were drawn and circulated to staff, who were asked to rate his eye position at the beginning of each treatment session. We also performed a protocol similar to the one discussed previously in which yes and no finger movements were assessed in response to biographical questions. As shown in Table 25–5, the patient showed a clear increase in eye opening, compared to placebo, on amantadine, as well as an increased rate of finger movements. His accuracy, however, remained at chance, suggesting that arousal was not at the root of his vegetative state.

Assessing Change

Few vegetative patients are seen in acute rehabilitation programs, and those who are generally receive brief treatment courses unless they begin to develop more active treatment goals. Similarly, minimally conscious patients do not benefit from ongoing active rehabilitation unless their clinical status evolves and new behavioral capacities emerge. Thus, for both patient groups an essential question is whether their behavioral repertoires are changing over time. In addition to the practical importance of this question, detection of behavioral change has been suggested as one of the most important indices of a positive prognosis for further clinical improvement.[44]

Behavioral change can be assessed in much the same way that the effects of a drug might be evaluated. A standardized assessment tool is particularly useful for vegetative patients because there are not yet any specific behaviors of interest to follow. Scores are collected 1 to 3 times a week and plotted against time. After a number of such scores are collected, whether there is merely random variation from day to day or whether a temporal recovery trend is present should be evident. In some cases, such evaluation shows behavioral regression, which can signal the need to look for adverse medical events such as hydrocephalus or metabolic abnormalities.

In some minimally conscious patients, it may be more useful to track specific behaviors of importance, such as command following or communication, to see if they are showing any improvement. By plotting both response rate and accuracy over time, a clear interpretation of clinical change is possible. Figure 25–2 presents a patient who showed the ability to nod yes and no in response to commands or questions but did so very inconsistently. We developed an assessment to determine whether her ability to communicate in this way was improving over time. As can be seen, accuracy when she did respond was high from the beginning and showed little further change. Her consistency of responding, however, showed steady improvement. It should be kept in mind that some new behavior, not currently being assessed, could emerge and reveal positive change, so the team must be prepared to incorporate newly emerging behaviors into the assessment as needed.

An assessment of a vegetative patient soon after injury that reveals no recovery over time does not mean that such recovery will never occur. Because some recovery is possible at least until 1 year after injury, however, it is generally not feasible to continue intensive rehabilitation and assessment for that length of time. Our approach has been to train caregivers in the assessment that we are using so that, should additional recovery become evident in the future, a reevaluation can be triggered. Lack of documented change in a vegetative patient nearing the 1-year anniversary of injury can be taken to indicate a very low probability that meaningful recovery will ever occur.

In minimally conscious patients, the interpretation of temporal trend is more complex and more flexible. Lack of spontaneous change in a specific behavior does not necessarily mean that such a change cannot be induced by a treatment intervention (drug or device). If spontaneous change is not seen across a range of tar-

TABLE 25–5. Drug Effects on Eye Opening and Answering Questions

	Measure of Drug Response		
Drug Condition	Eye Opening Rating (1–5) (Median, range)	Finger Movement Response Rate	Finger Movement Accuracy
Baseline	1 (1–3)	18%	52%
Amantadine	2 (1–3)	37%	45%

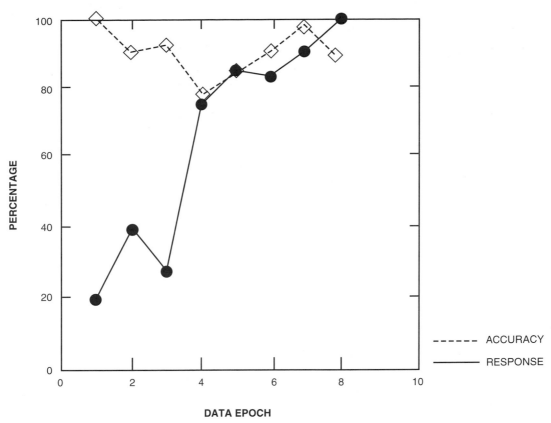

FIGURE 25–2. Changes in response rate and accuracy over time. A patient's percentage of responses and percentage accuracy are shown on the y axis, in a protocol involving nodding yes or no on command. The x axis represents different data-gathering epochs of several days each.

get behaviors, however, then one must begin to conclude that a behavioral plateau is arriving and that only very specific treatment-related gains are likely in the future.

Psychosocial and Ethical Issues

The response of a family to a severe traumatic brain injury changes over time. It is important for clinicians to think about how a family constructs beliefs about severe traumatic brain injury. Their experience with it is probably limited, and they are thrust into a crisis without having any knowledge base. In the emergency room and initial days following the injury, the issues of concern are literally life and death. If the patient survives, the family feels some sense of relief that their loved one "beat the odds" and, having beat them once, can do it again. Although knowing what information is shared between the medical staff and the family during the initial emergency stages is impossible, it is probably most important to understand the family's perception of what they have been told. During family sessions, we have heard remarks such as "Don't worry, they told me the lobotomies were minor" and "The neurologist told us our mom would come back 90 percent, 40 percent the first year and 50 percent the second year."

Many have the idea, supported by the popular media, that people with severe TBI "wake up" from their comas ready to resume life as they knew it. Of course, some do resume a meaningful activity pattern, which can include gainful employment, school, volunteer and leisure interests, and successful social and personal relationships. For the patient who remains minimally conscious for a significant period, however, the prognosis is limited. Clearly, families are confronted with information that challenges their beliefs about recovery and the cognitive status of their family member. In our work with minimally conscious patients, we are often asked whether the patient's lack of responsiveness is caused by depression or boredom. In effect, the family projects a variety of complex feelings and thoughts onto the patient, in the absence of observable behavior, whereas it is unlikely such patients have the cognitive ability to understand, introspect, and grieve over their present circumstances.

Although family education is difficult, time-consuming, and costly work, it is time well spent because long-term treatment and care options need to be solidified. The information gained from quantitative assessment can provide some content for family meetings. During the initial sessions, the focus should be on providing some basic brain injury education, including some of the consequences of the pathology. Families typically have many questions. Although the "harder facts" may not be discussed in extensive detail, the message of a severe injury should be communicated. As the team's relationship with the family continues to evolve and as more information about the patient is gathered, extrapolations about the functional implications of the brain injury can be made. The focus moves from a more generalized model about brain injury to the more specific ramifications of the patient's pathology and disability. Although strong attempts are made to do this in a supportive manner, families are likely to be angry and defensive on hearing this information. The role of the clinicians is to provide some foundation of information for the family, to be used at the time when the family is more emotionally ready, rather than force the family to adjust. Honesty is a critical factor because decisions need to be made, based specifically on the quantitative assessment and the medical status, regarding treatment direction and destination planning.

A quantitative evaluation of responses to stimulation over time can help to remove some of the ambiguity of the diagnosis. One possible outcome of the evaluation is that the patient shows no evidence of consciousness. This, paired with information about the etiology of the injury, length of time since injury, age of the patient, and knowledge of the patient's wishes, can be used to guide decisions about the direction of future treatment and care. Recent cases, like that of Nancy Cruzan,[58] have brought the ethical dilemmas faced by families, medical staff, and the legal system into the public arena. When the vegetative state is considered irreversible, the question may arise as to whether to continue medical treatment of the patient, including do not resuscitate (DNR) status, administering medication to treat conditions like infection, and artificial hydration and nutrition. Highly publicized cases, like that of Karen Ann Quinlan and Cruzan, evoke public and personal debate over treatment of patients in the vegetative state. Clinicians may feel uncomfortable about discussing these issues with families, and there is always some uncertainty about the label of "permanent" because of a few highly publicized cases about people who emerged after the diagnosis of a permanent vegetative state had been made. We suggest an initial time-limited assessment, followed by a tracking system that would allow for detection of change following discharge from the acute rehabilitation setting. Considering recent data on outcome of the vegetative state,[7] people who sustained their injury secondary to trauma have a longer window for recovery than those with an anoxic event. Such an assessment and tracking system can facilitate discharge of those patients who fail to show early progress, while minimizing the chance that later improvements will be overlooked.

For those diagnosed as minimally conscious rather than vegetative, it is likely that they will remain dependent on others for a variety of needs, including 24-hour supervision, even if some improvement occurs. Although some issues, like decisions about DNR status and aggressive medical treatment, are similar to those for people diagnosed as vegetative, families of minimally conscious patients may be more likely to pursue aggressive treatment or, even if they wish not to, may have more difficulty with decisions to withdraw treatment from a family member who is able to engage in some limited interaction. Additionally, without a living will or advance directives, the rehabilitation team may have difficulty assessing what the patient's desires might have been and what the family's motivations for treatment withdrawal are. Thus, a physician who fears a legal challenge may be reluctant to participate in withdrawal of treatment.

This multifaceted issue, involving medical, ethical, legal, and often religious opinions, has typically been argued by those wanting to discontinue life support measures for their family member in a vegetative state. A suggestion has been made to shift the burden of that decision from those who want to discontinue treatment to those who want it to continue.[59] This argument supports the establishment of a standard of care that would include stopping treatment after a specified time, considering the results of clinical evaluations, for those diagnosed in a permanent vegetative state.[59] This standard of care should include a more concrete method of evaluation for these patients that would eliminate, in part, the ambiguity for clinicians and families alike.

□ SUMMARY

Vegetative and minimally conscious patients present clinical and emotional challenges to those who care for them. Yet, particularly for those with traumatic brain injuries, there is potential for substantial functional progress. Clinicians who commit themselves to aggressive and sensitive care of these patients and their families will be gratified by their ability to substantially reduce complications and to achieve meaningful function for a considerable number of those they treat.

REFERENCES

1. Jennett, B, and Bond, M: Assessment of outcome after severe brain damage: A practical scale. Lancet 1:480–484, 1975.
2. Giacino, J, et al: Recommendations for use of uniform nomenclature pertinent to patients with severe alterations in consciousness. Arch Phys Med Rehabil 76:205–209, 1995.
3. Aspen Neurobehavioral Conference: Draft consensus statement. 1996.
4. Auerbach, SH: The pathophysiology of traumatic brain injury. Physical Medicine and Rehabilitation: State of the Art Reviews 3:1–11, 1989.
5. The Multi-Society Task Force on PVS: Medical aspects of the persistent vegetative state (part 1). N Engl J Med 330:1499–1508, 1994.
6. Kinney, HC, et al: Neuropathological findings in the brain of Karen Ann Quinlan: The role of the thalamus in the persistent vegetative state. N Engl J Med 330:1469–1475, 1994.
7. The Multi-Society Task Force on PVS: Medical aspects of the persistent vegetative state (part 2). N Engl J Med 330:1572–1579, 1994.
8. Childs, NL, Mercer, WN, and Childs, HW: Accuracy of diagnosis of the persistent vegetative state. Neurology 43:1457–1458, 1993.
9. O'Dell, MW, et al: Standardized assessment instruments for minimally-responsive, brain-injured patients. NeuroRehabilitation 6:45–55, 1996.
10. Whyte, J, and DiPasquale, MC: Assessment of vision and visual attention in minimally responsive brain injured patients. Arch Phys Med Rehabil 76:804–810, 1995.
11. Whyte, J: Toward rational psychopharmacological treatment: Integrating research and clinical practice. J Head Trauma Rehabil 9:91–103, 1994.
12. Cruikshank, JM, and Neil-Dwyer, G: Beta blocker brain concentrations in man. Eur J Clin Pharmacol (suppl)28:21–23, 1985.
13. Horn, LJ, and Glenn, MB: Update on pharmacology: Pharmacological interventions in neuroendocrine disorders following traumatic brain injury, part I. J Head Trauma Rehabil 3(2):87–90, 1988.
14. Benedek, G, et al: Indomethacin is effective against neurogenic hyperthermia following cranial trauma or brain surgery. Can J Neurol Sci 14:145–148, 1987.
15. Sandel, ME, Abrams, P, and Horn, LJ: Hypertension after brain injury: A case report. Arch Phys Med Rehabil 67:469–472, 1986.
16. Feibel, JH, Balwin, CA, and Joynt, RJ: Catecholamine-associated refractory hypertension following acute intracerebral haemorrhage: Control with propranolol. Ann Neurol 9:340–343, 1981.
17. Hauser, WA: Prevention of post-traumatic epilepsy. N Engl J Med 323:340–341, 1990.
18. Yablon, SA: Postraumatic seizures. Arch Phys Med Rehabil 74:983–1001, 1993.
19. Meador, KJ, et al: Comparative cognitive effects of anticonvulsants. Neurology 40:391–394, 1990.
20. Cisapride for nocturnal heartburn. Med Lett Drugs Ther 36:11–13, 1994.
21. Jennett, B, and Teasdale, G: Management of Head Injuries. FA Davis, Philadelphia, 1981.
22. Pellock, JM, and Willmore, IJ: A rationale guide to routine blood monitoring in patients receiving antiepileptic drugs. Neurology 41:961–964, 1991.
23. Commission on Antiepileptic Drugs, International League against Epilepsy: Guideline for therapeutic monitoring of antiepileptic drugs. Epilepsia 34:585–587, 1993.
24. Wikkelso, C, et al: Normal-pressure hydrocephalus: Predictive value of the cerebral spinal fluid tap test. Acta Neurol Scand 73:566, 1986.
25. Drake, JM: The Shunt Book. Cambridge, Mass, Blackwell Science, 1995.
26. Black, P: Idiopathic normal-pressure hydrocephalus: Results of shunting 62 patients. J Neurosurg 52:371–377, 1980.
27. Garland, DE, et al: Resection of heterotopic ossification in the adult with head trauma. J Bone Joint Surg 67:1261–1269, 1985.
28. Young, RR, and Delwaide, PJ: Drug therapy, spasticity (2 parts). N Engl J Med 304:28–33, 96–99, 1981.
29. Glenn, MB: Nerve blocks. In Glenn, MB, and Whyte, J (eds): The Practical Management of Spasticity. Lea & Febiger, Philadelphia, 1990, pp 227–258.
30. Keenan, MA: Orthopedic management of spasticity. J Head Trauma Rehabil 2(2):62–71, 1987.
31. Jankovic, J, and Brin, MF: Therapeutic uses of botulinum toxin. N Engl J Med 324:1186–1194, 1991.
32. Nowak, P, Cohn, AM, and Guidice, MA: Airway complications in patients with closed-head injuries. Am J Otolaryngol 8:91–96, 1987.
33. Akers, SM, Bartter, TC, and Pratter, MR: Respiratory care. Physical Medicine and Rehabilitation: State of the Art Reviews 4:527–542, 1990.
34. Heffner, JE, and Sahn, SA: The technique of weaning from tracheostomy. Chest 96:186–189, 1989.
35. Klingbeil, GEG: Airway problems in patients with traumatic brain injury. Arch Phys Med Rehabil 68:79–84, 1987.
36. Logemann, JA: Evaluation and treatment planning for the head-injured patient with oral intake disorders. J Head Trauma Rehabil 4(4):24–33, 1989.
37. Vane, DW, et al: Reduced lower esophageal sphincter (LES) pressure after acute and chronic brain injury. J Pediatr Surg 17:960–964, 1982.
38. Metoclopramide (Reglan) for gastroesophageal reflux. Med Lett Drugs Ther 27:21–22, 1985.
39. Hutchins, BE: Establishing a dysphagia family intervention program for head-injured patients. J Head Trauma Rehabil 4(4):64–72, 1989.
40. Parathyras, AJ, and Kassak, LA: Tolerance, nutritional adequacy, and cost-effectiveness of continuing drip vs. bolus and/or intermittent feeding techniques. Nutritional Support Services 4:576–577, 1983.
41. Andrews, K: Medical management. Physical Medicine and Rehabilitation: State of the Art Reviews 4:495–508, 1990.
42. Rappaport, M, et al: Disability rating scale for severe head trauma: Coma to community. Arch Phys Med Rehabil 63:118–123, 1982.
43. Hagen, C, Malkmus, D, and Durham P: Levels of Cognitive Functioning. Rancho Los Amigos Hospital, Downey, Calif, 1972.
44. Giacino, J, et al: Monitoring rate of recovery to predict outcome in minimally responsive patients. Arch Phys Med Rehabil 72:897–901, 1991.
45. Ansell, BJ, and Keenan, JW: The Western Neuro Sensory Stimulation Profile: A tool for assessing slow to recover head injured patients. Arch Phys Med Rehabil 70:104–108, 1989.

46. Rappaport, M, Dougherty, A, and Kelting, D: Evaluation of coma and the vegetative states. Arch Phys Med Rehabil 73:628–634, 1992.

47. American Electroencephalographic Society: Guideline for clinical evoked potential studies. J Clin Neurophysiol 11:48–59, 1994.

48. Celsia, G: Anatomy and physiology of visual evoked potentials and electroretinograms. Neurol Clin 6:657–679, 1988.

49. Weinstein, G, Odom JV, and Cavender, S: Visually evoked potentials and electroretinography in neurologic evaluation. Neurol Clin 9:225–242, 1991.

50. Epstein, C: The use of brain stem auditory evoked potentials in the evaluation of the central nervous system. Neurol Clin 6:771–790, 1988.

51. Davis, H, and Owens, J: Auditory evoked potentials. In Owen, J, and Hallowel, D (eds): Evoked Potential Testing. Grune and Stratton, Orlando, Fla, 1985.

52. Wroblewski, BA, and Glenn, MB: Pharmacological treatment of arousal and cognitive deficits. J Head Trauma Rehabil 9(3):19–42, 1994.

53. Reinhard, DL, Whyte, J, and Sandel, ME: Improved arousal and initiation following tricyclic antidepressant use in severe brain injury. Arch Phys Med Rehabil 77:80–83, 1996.

54. Whyte, J: Attention and arousal: Basic science aspects. Arch Phys Med Rehabil 73:940–949, 1992.

55. Boyeson, MG, and Harmon, RL: Acute and postacute drug-induced effects on rate of behavioral recovery after brain injury. J Head Trauma Rehabil 9(3):78–90, 1994.

56. Wroblewski, BA, et al: Incidence of seizures with tricyclic antidepressant treatment in a brain-injured population. J Clin Psychopharm 10:124–128, 1990.

57. Wroblewski, BA, et al: Methylphenidate and seizure frequency in brain injured patients with seizure disorders. J Clin Psychiatry 53:86–89, 1992.

58. Weir, R, and Gostin, L: Decisions to abate life-sustaining treatment for non-autonomous patients. JAMA 264:1846–1853, 1990.

59. Angell, M: After Quinlan: The dilemma of the persistent vegetative state. N Engl J Med 330:1524–1525, 1994

The Older Adult with Traumatic Brain Injury

JEFFREY ENGLANDER, MD,
and DAVID X. CIFU, MD

☐ DEMOGRAPHICS OF AGING

The older adult or geriatric population includes all individuals aged 65 years and older. This chronological cutoff is arbitrary and more related to federal statues (Medicare eligibility) than scientific standards. Currently, 12 percent (25 million people) of the U.S. population are aged 65 or older. This percentage of older adults is projected to rise to 21 percent (64 million people) of the population by the year 2050. In addition, those 85 and older will increase from 1 percent (2 million) to nearly 5 percent (15 million) in that same time frame.[1-3] In the brain injury literature, the term *older adults* often refers to individuals as young as 50 or 55. In fact, differences in demographics and outcome have been noted between individuals who are 55 and older and those younger than 50; therefore, this demarcation may be more functional. However, for this text, older adults are those aged 65 or older, unless otherwise noted.

☐ DISABILITY IN THE OLDER ADULT

More than three quarters of older adults living in the community have no deficits in everyday functional abilities. The functional limitations reported by the 23 percent with deficits are walking (19%), bathing (10%), getting outside (10%), getting in and out of bed (8%), dressing (6%), toileting (4%), and eating (2%). Of note, only 10 percent of these individuals actually receive assistance with functional activities.[4] The need for assistance increases with increasing age, and nearly 40 percent of individuals 80 years and older require help.[5] The brain injury literature indicates that, after hospitalization for traumatic brain injury (TBI), 95 percent of older adults require assistance.[6]

☐ GERIATRIC REHABILITATION

Maximizing function of the older adult following brain injury involves an understanding of the specialized principles of geriatric medicine, in addition to an appreciation of brain injury rehabilitation. Factors that must be taken into consideration include concomitant conditions (arthritis, cardiovascular disease, pulmonary disease, diabetes mellitus), decreased functional reserves, and age-related cognitive and sensory impairments.[7] The central nervous system of the healthy older adult is highly sensitive to anything that affects its homeostasis,

This work was supported by the U.S. Department of Education, National Institute on Disability and Rehabilitation Research Grants No. H1331-2002 (Santa Clara Valley Medical Center) and H133A-20012 (Medical College of Virginia). Thanks to Maureen Cervelli and Pamela Slaughter for assistance in manuscript preparation.

whether altered flow of blood or cerebral spinal fluid, decreased oxygenation, central-acting medications, or excessive environmental stimuli. This sensitivity is compounded in the face of acute brain injury. Available information indicates that structured, interdisciplinary rehabilitation for the older adult with disabilities can be well tolerated and effective.[1]

◻ INJURY PREVENTION

Unlike younger age groups, the elderly sustain a majority of TBIs in domestic falls.[8–11] Tinetti and Speechley[12] have stratified fall risk factors to the following groups: (1) chronic, such as neurological disease, sensory impairment, or musculoskeletal disease, especially in the lower extremities; (2) short-term, such as episodic postural hypotension, acute illness, alcohol use, or medication effects; (3) activity-related, such as tripping while walking, climbing ladders, or descending stairs; and (4) environmental, such as throw rugs, poor lighting, or ill-fitting shoes or trousers. The risk factors for falls also predispose the elderly to motor vehicle, pedestrian, and recreational accidents, all of which may result in TBI.[11,13,14] Geriatric rehabilitation programs can address these risk factors and provide appropriate interventions.

◻ EPIDEMIOLOGY

The incidence of TBI in the geriatric population is not clearly defined; however, it is estimated at approximately half the rate of the 16 to 34 age group, or approximately 200 per 100,000.[8,15] Thus, there are an estimated 50,000 TBIs per year in the older adult population in the United States. The overall gender distribution of TBI in the elderly is 1.4 to 2 men for each woman, al-

---

TABLE 26–1. Mechanism of Injury and Pathology

	TCDB (n = 19)	Haifa (n = 263)	Braintree (n = 46)	NDB (n = 37)
Age (yr)	55+	65+	60+	65+
Glasgow Coma Scores	3–8	3–15	3–15	3–15
Sex (% male/female)	60/40	67/33	52/48	62/38
Mechanism				
Fall	45%	72%	55%	35%
Pedestrian accident	20%	19%	see below[f]	16%
Vehicle crash	17%	5%	41%[f]	27%
Assault	8%	2%	2%	11%
Bike or motorcycle	3%	1%		5%
Other	7%	1%	1%	5%
Pathology				
Contusions		28%	34%	
Intraparenchymal hemorrhage	68%[d]			19%
Acute SDH	72%[e]	21%	36%[c]	49%[c]
Chronic SDH		29%		
Acute EDH		3%	0%	8%
Concussion		13%		8%
Diffuse axonal injury[a]		7%[a]	51%[b]	
Hypoxic/ischemic injury			12%	
Subarachnoid hemorrhage	61%			49%

TCDB = Traumatic Coma Data Bank, all closed head injury, prospective data collection[23]; Haifa = Rambam (Maimonides) Medical Center, Neurosurgical Referral Center, prospective and retrospective data collection[21]; Braintree = Braintree Hospital, private rehabilitation center, consecutive admissions[22]; NDB = National Data Base consecutive admissions of patients receiving acute care and rehabilitation within NIDRR TBI Model Systems[28]; SDH = subdural hematoma; EDH = epidural hematoma.
[a]Defined by Levy as one or more small, nonexpansive, hemorrhagic lesions at corticomedullary or nuclear-medullary junction, corpus callosum, or cerebellum.[22]
[b]Defined by deceleration injury, coma without lucid interval; radiological findings: petechial hemorrhages, isolated subarachnoid or intraventricular hemorrhage, diffuse swelling or no pathology.[22]
[c]Any SDH, acute or chronic.[22,28]
[d]Includes contusions and hemorrhages 42% <5 cc, 26% >15 cc.
[e]Includes any extra-axial lesion (SDH acute or chronic, EDH): 26% <15 cc, 46% >15 cc.
[f]Includes pedestrian and motor vehicle driver and passenger injuries.

though in the subset over age 80, women predominate 3:2[9,16–18] (Table 26–1). Data on racial distribution of TBI in the older adult population are not available.

❏ MECHANISM AND PATHOLOGY OF INJURY

Severe trauma in individuals over 70 is 6 times more likely to cause intracerebral lesions than severe chest, abdominal, or pelvic injury. This finding is the extreme end of the trend that starts at age 40.[19] All studies confirm that older individuals are most commonly injured as a result of falls, both on level surfaces (78%) and stairs (22%).[20] Falls tend to result in focal brain injuries, most commonly frontal and temporal lobe contusions and/or subdural hematomas (SDH). Contusions tend to occur in multiple foci and often appear radiologically several days after injury.[21] Immediate loss of consciousness implies some degree of diffuse axonal injury (DAI), which can also occur with falls, and, when combined with focal injury, portends a worse prognosis.

Motor vehicle crashes that injure the elderly are not typically high-speed encounters, like younger individuals, but nevertheless can result in DAI.[22] Focal contusions and SDH are also common with this mechanism of injury.

Pedestrian injuries in the elderly can result in DAI, focal contusions, and/or extra-axial lesions, most commonly SDH. Individuals with these injuries are the most likely to have other skeletal trauma, especially visceral injuries and pelvic and lower extremity fractures.

Although assaults are the most frequent cause of injury in the middle-aged group, at least in North American urban areas, they are a less common cause of injury in the elderly. These injuries invariably result in focal contusions, SDH, and/or skull fractures, with bone or bullet fragments.

The demography of the patient population served by a given practitioner, medical center, or rehabilitation center plays a large role in determining the causes and pathological findings that may be seen in association with TBI (see Table 26–1). Urban areas see more injuries from violence and to pedestrians. Suburban and rural areas see more injuries from motor vehicle crashes. Falls are the most common in the older adult, regardless of demography.

❏ MORTALITY

The largest reported group of older individuals with TBI is from Rambam Medical Center in Haifa, Israel, and consisted of 263 individuals. The mortality rate was 18 percent; however, many patients were transferred to that facility from other centers and had thus survived their initial injuries. The highest mortality group were those with SDH (33%), most of whom suffered multiple brain lacerations. Those with contusions had a 27 percent mortality rate; DAI, 11 percent; and chronic SDH, 3 percent.[21]

The Traumatic Coma Data Bank (TCDB) reported mortality in 80 percent of individuals over age 55 who presented with severe closed head injury, defined as Glasgow Coma Score (GCS) of 3 to 8. More than 80 percent of the deaths were primarily attributable to the head trauma itself, usually because of cerebral mass lesions that required evacuation. These deaths tended to occur in the first 10 days postinjury. Only 17 percent of those over 55 had severe cardiac complications.[23] Further analysis from the TCDB emphasized the critical role of hypotension (60%), hypoxia (33%), or both (75%) for predicting mortality, regardless of age. The older group (>40 years) was not more sensitive to the secondary effects of hypotension, hypoxia, or both.[24] However, given the same kind of injury, the older individual is at more risk for hypotension or hypoxia because of limited cardiopulmonary reserve.

In another study, older (>60 years) individuals with severe TBI (admission GCS 3–5) had 79 percent mortality compared with 36 percent of a younger group, when reviewed retrospectively. Whereas all deaths in the younger group were attributed to the brain injury itself and occurred within the first 5 days of hospitalization, 67 percent in the elderly group died primarily of brain injuries. The remaining deaths were attributed to pulmonary, cardiac, and multisystem failure. Ninety percent of the deaths in the elderly occurred in the first 2 weeks postinjury.[25]

Cagetti et al.[26] reported a series of 28 individuals over age 80, all of whom required surgical evacuation of a subdural (n = 26) or epidural (n = 2) hematoma. Mortality was 88 percent and 100 percent, respectively, with a median survival of 6 days from injury. All 19 individuals with GCS less than 10 died; four of five with GCS 10 to 12 died; two of four with GCS 13 to 15 died. The authors noted multiple system failure in those who died. They postulated that individuals older than 80 should be treated aggressively if their GCS is 10 or greater, but that those with lower levels of awareness should perhaps be spared such interventions.

None of these reports mentions suicide in analyzing etiology of injury. The U.S. Centers for Disease Control and Prevention (CDC) reported that suicide ranks third as a cause for injury-related mortality, after unintentional falls and motor vehicle crashes, in individuals over age 65. Seventy-four percent of men and 31 percent of women used firearms as the means of suicide, so that most of these would have suffered TBI. Divorced or widowed men are in the highest risk group.[27] Such desperate acts must be considered in investigating precipitating causes for TBI in this population.

The low likelihood of surviving with a good outcome evokes ethical considerations when individuals do not recover over a reasonable period of time.

Case 1 ■ GS was a 75-year-old retired machinist with non-insulin-dependent diabetes mellitus who lived with his wife in a retirement home. As a pedestrian, he collided with a car going 25 mph, was thrown onto the hood, and struck the windshield. He briefly lost consciousness but had recovered to a GCS of 12 (eyes 4, verbal 3, motor 5) in the emergency department. Head computed tomography (CT) scan revealed subarachnoid hemorrhage and right temporal and parietal lobe contusions, with no midline shift or midbrain swelling. No other fractures or injuries were present. Three days later, he exhibited left hemibody seizures that were treated with intravenous phenytoin. A repeat CT scan showed the interval development of bifrontal contusions and a small, right SDH. Phenobarbital was added for breakthrough seizures. Rehabilitation services started on the fifth hospital day in the intensive care unit. He acquired a staphylococcal urinary tract infection and bacteremia, requiring intravenous antibiotics. As the phenobarbital was successfully weaned and infection resolved, he became more alert, was able to speak in short sentences, and began to participate in self-care.

He entered the rehabilitation unit 3 weeks postinjury oriented to person, month, year, his family members, and address but was still in post-traumatic amnesia (PTA) and incontinent. Despite aggressive medication and rehabilitation management, he made little progress. Six weeks postinjury, he had recurrent seizures, requiring transfer to the intensive care unit (ICU) for intubation and monitoring. He had acquired an aspiration pneumonia but was able to come off the ventilator within 1 week. Stating that he had never wanted to be on life support if there was little chance for recovery, his wife requested no reintubation at this point. He continued to require maximum assistance for self-care and mobility and gradually became less responsive, dying in his sleep 10 weeks postinjury.

The initial prognosis for this man was fair, given his previous level of activity, family support, initial GCS of 12, and lack of associated injuries and complications. Recurrent seizures, a

late SDH, infections, and lack of progress became apparent within the first 3 to 4 weeks postinjury. Fortunately, he and his wife had previously discussed possible health care scenarios, and, when she realized that his future looked dim, she was able to honor his wishes of no long-term life support.

◻ MORBIDITY

Multiple Trauma and Hypotension

Severe multiple trauma as measured by the Abbreviated Injury Severity (AIS) score is less common in older (>40 years) than in younger (<40 years) age groups. Hypotension and multiple trauma are closely associated. Severe multiple trauma without hypotension or hypoxia has not been associated with worse outcome as measured by the Glasgow Outcome Scale (GOS).[24] Cerebrovascular events can occur as a result of hypotension in the peritraumatic period; strokes caused by thromboembolism, thrombosis, or ischemia from massive swelling are uncommon causes of peritraumatic stroke in older individuals.

Fractures

Skull fractures occurred in 22 percent of individuals over 65 in the National Institute on Disability and Rehabilitation Research (NIDRR) TBI Model Systems Data Set. In descending order, the next most common fracture sites were ribs (22%), upper extremity (11%), pelvis (5%), femur (5%), and spinal column (5%). Only 8 percent required open reduction and internal fixation. Combinations of TBI and spinal cord injury (SCI) are more common among younger individuals. Surviving with this combination of injuries is unusual in the elderly; only one such individual over 65 years is represented in the TBI national data base.[28]

Medical Complications

Respiratory failure requiring mechanical ventilation for more than 7 days and/or pneumonia has been reported in 39 percent of all individuals with TBI who go to acute rehabilitation.[29] In the elderly population, respiratory failure occurs in 22 percent and pneumonia in 30 percent.[28] Gastrostomies or jejunostomies are placed in more than 40 percent of individuals with TBI who go into acute rehabilitation. Twenty-seven percent of elderly patients have gastrostomies or je-junostomies placed.

Acute anemia occurs in nearly all individuals who incur trauma. Older individuals' tolerance for blood loss is less than younger individuals'. Anemia may affect energy level, tolerance for activity, appearance, and overall sense of well-being. It may not be apparent until after rehydration occurs following discharge from the intensive care unit, where therapeutic dehydration and diuresis may be implemented to decrease brain swelling. Coagulopathy requiring transfusion of platelets or fresh frozen plasma occurred in 5 percent.[28]

Post-traumatic seizures (PTS) occurred in 19 percent of elderly individuals, a slightly higher percentage than the 17 percent reported for the entire population aged at least 15.[29] Of those elderly individuals who had seizures, 43 percent occurred in the first 24 hours and 57 percent in the first 7 days.[28]

Documented acute alcohol intoxication is present in approximately 10 percent of individuals over 65 admitted with TBI, as compared with 39 percent of individuals aged 18 to 64; however, the TBI national data base indicated that less than half of older individuals are even tested for substance use.[28] Intoxicated individuals are more likely to require intubation, intracranial pressure monitoring, ventilatory assistance, and treatment for pneumonia, even though their length of stay is not longer.[30]

Those who are able to survive the sequelae of trauma are therefore a select group.

Case 2 ■ RP is a 70-year-old married rancher who fell off his horse while riding at high speed. He had had at least one previous concussion and broken ribs from similar falls. He was initially unconscious. His GCS at the scene was 10 (verbal 3, eyes 3, motor 4) with blood pressure (BP) 74/50. His GCS improved to 12 (verbal 4, eyes 3, motor 5), and his BP fluctuated from 83 to 166/39 to 93 en route. He could not move his left arm or leg to command. In the emergency department, his GCS was 12 with systolic BP of 70 mm Hg; he remained hypotensive and required emergent splenectomy and left nephrectomy. Initial head CT scan showed cerebrospinal fluid (CSF) adjacent to the clivus. During the next week, CT scans showed bifrontal subdural hygromas, left parietal lobe contusion, and 1 right parietal lobe infarction in a watershed distribution. He also fractured his left scapula and fourth through sixth ribs. Postoperative complications included bacteremia, a wound abscess, nephrostomy tube placement, urinary sepsis, and hypercalcemia. He required a tracheostomy and mechanical ventilation for 5 weeks.

Two months postinjury, he transferred to acute rehabilitation. Within the first 24 hours, he exhibited a brief focal seizure. The following day, he developed recurrent focal seizures that required intravenous diazepam and phenytoin to stop. He was reintubated through his healing tracheostomy site and weaned off the ventilator in 2 weeks.

He returned to acute rehabilitation 11 weeks postinjury. His hypercalcemia resolved with mobilization and a change of diet from enteral tube feedings to regular food. He had developed exposure band keratopathy on one eye, which was treated with eye patching and antibiotic ointment. PTA resolved 15 weeks postinjury. His tracheostomy and bladder catheter were discontinued, and he was discharged continent, ambulating with a cane, and performing self-care with standby assistance. Nine months postinjury, he had passed the state driving exams, independently made travel arrangements for a hunting trip with his friends, and successfully shot a large deer. Sixteen months postinjury, he had two mild car accidents on the ranch, prompting referral for further driving evaluation and training.

This individual had multiple poor prognostic signs, including previous TBI, hypotension resulting in an ischemic infarct, severe abdominal trauma, sepsis, recurrent PTS, metabolic problems, and prolonged PTA. No one would have predicted such a successful outcome, except his wife, who was confident he would recover and return to his independent lifestyle. He illustrates the benefits of a coordinated system of care for individuals with TBI and associated injuries and the tenacity that can sometimes lead to successful outcomes, defying the great majority of reports in the literature.

❑ FACTORS AFFECTING OUTCOME

Age

Most of our knowledge about outcome in older adult brain injury patients comes from studies involving all age groups. These investigations report the positive association between increasing age and mortality.[6,17,18,25,31–33] Several studies have examined the functional outcome of older adults who survive a traumatic brain injury.[6,20,22,34–36] The majority show poorer prognosis for the older than the younger adult, with a correlation noted as young as 40 years. In one study, fewer than 5 percent of older adults with TBI made a "good" recovery.[6] This study is supported by recent analyses of the NIDRR TBI

Model Systems Data Set, which revealed that individuals aged 55 and older had significantly longer, more costly stays on rehabilitation units, recovered approximately half as quickly, and had greater cognitive impairment at discharge than a group of individuals aged 50 and younger who were matched for similar injury severity.[37] The association between increased age and outcome is complex and appears closely related to duration of coma, duration of PTA, alcohol intake, postinjury behavior (e.g., presence of depression or agitation), and social support factors.[11,22,25,32,38] In contrast, some studies have demonstrated that good outcomes are achievable in the older adult with similar costs.[39–41] In the NIDRR Model Systems sample, return to the community rates (>90%) and physical function were comparable for the older and younger groups.

Injury Severity

The impact of injury severity on functional outcome in the older adult with TBI has not been well studied. It appears that the relationship between outcome and injury severity, as measured by duration of coma or PTA, which exists in younger adults after TBI, also exists in the older adult subgroup.[11,22,25,32,38,42,43] No investigations have examined the impact of mechanism of injury, neuropathology, and associated injuries.

□ REHABILITATION

Assessment

Some areas of rehabilitation assessment are unique to the geriatric TBI patient. Clearly, an understanding of preinjury activity levels and major acute and chronic medical issues is vital. It assists in determining the degree of physiological reserve, which then allows a more specific structuring of the rehabilitation program. Direct communication with the individual's primary care physician (PCP) can help integrate her or his management recommendations directly into the rehabilitation treatment program. This step is crucial for patients in managed care networks, in which the PCP is often a gatekeeper for current and future medical resource management.

Of equal importance is a comprehensive review of the social network, which involves an understanding of the formal and informal support systems available.[40] Formal support systems include federal (Medicare, Social Security), state (Medicaid, disability, welfare), and local (adult day health programs, transporta-

tion, Meals on Wheels) resources. Informal support systems include family and friends. Older adults tend to have greater involvement of extended families in their systems of support. Daughters and female caregivers in general are more likely to play a major support role than sons.[44] Early involvement of family and friends in planning and implementing the rehabilitation program is vital.

Other social factors to consider are the older adult's role in the family unit, the role of organized religion in the individual's life, the patient and caregiver's goal for rehabilitation, and any applicable advance directives. Although an understanding of these components of a person's life is important at any age, they become increasingly relevant for the older adult (see previous case studies).

Knowledge of the most common funding mechanisms available for post-TBI care of the older adult is vital. For example, 98 percent of the older adults in the United States are primarily funded by a single source, Medicare. Secondary or copayment insurance ("medigap") varies greatly in coverage but typically does not pay for extensive rehabilitation services. Similarly, in Canada, Australia, and most European countries, the government funds the overwhelming majority of medical care for the elderly. Straight Medicare is a federally sponsored program, so its coverages are uniform throughout the United States. With the recent inclusion of managed care in Medicare, benefits may vary. Any individual who has paid into the federal tax system for 40 quarters and meets any of the following three criteria is covered free by Medicare part A: (1) age 65 or older, (2) disabled for longer than 2 years, or (3) end-stage renal disease. Medicare part A reimburses for durable medical equipment and inpatient, nursing home, and home health services. Medicare part B, which is available for a monthly fee (currently $32), reimburses for outpatient and physician services. Medicaid (e.g., Medi-Cal in California) is a state-sponsored and, therefore, state-specific program to provide health insurance to the medically indigent. Medicaid inpatient and outpatient rehabilitation benefits thus vary from state to state. Medicaid pays for more than 85 percent of all nursing home care in the United States. Older adults who continue to work or who have been federal employees typically have private or managed care insurance as their primary funding source.[45–47]

Settings

Older adults with acute physical impairments caused by TBI should receive rehabilitation services in the least restrictive environment. Al-

TABLE 26–2. Levels of Care and Types of Service Options for the Older Adult with Traumatic Brain Injury

Level of Care	Intensity/Frequency	Therapy Services	Reimbursement	Type of Setting	Duration of Program	Comments
Acute care services	5–6 days/wk; 0.5–2 hr/day	Multidisciplinary (MD, N, PT, OT, SLP, SW)	Medicare*, Medicaid	Acute care hospital	3–21 days	Acutely after injury to prevent complications, allow comprehensive rehabilitation assessment
Home health services	3 days/wk; 0.5–2 hr/day	Oligodisciplinary (N, PT, OT, SLP, HHA)	Medicare*, Medicaid (sometimes)	After acute care hospital, subacute or inpatient rehab services	6–12 wk	Homebound for physical or cognitive reasons
Outpatient services	2–3 days/wk; 0.5–3 hr/day	Multidisciplinary (PT, OT, SLP)	Medicare*, Medicaid	After acute care hospital, inpatient rehabilitation or home health	2–4 wk	High-functioning individuals who have very focused needs (e.g., cognitive, balance deficits)
Day rehabilitation services	3–5 days/wk; 3–5 hr/day	Interdisciplinary (PT, OT, SLP, SW, PSY, TR)	Medicare*, Medicaid	After acute care hospital, inpatient rehab or day rehabilitation	4–6 wk	Sufficient endurance to travel and good informal support systems; may allow shorter acute hospital or inpatient rehab length of stay

TABLE 26–2. *Continued*

Level of Care	Intensity/Frequency	Therapy Services	Reimbursement	Type of Setting	Duration of Program	Comments
Day care services	5 days/wk; 4–10 hr/day	Multidisciplinary (N, PT, OT, SLP, SW, TR)	Medicaid (partial)	Custodial care of community-dwelling older adults	Indefinite	High-functioning individuals who are independent or supervised for self-care (e.g., feeding, toileting)
Subacute rehabilitation services	5–7 days/wk; 1–2.5 hr/day	Multidisciplinary (MD, N, PT, OT, SLP, SW)	Medicare*, Medicaid in some states	Located in acute care hospitals or freestanding skilled nursing facilities; may progress to level of inpatient rehabilitation	3–10 wk	Severely impaired individuals who are expected to make slow gradual recovery, significant medical issues, limited informal support systems; before or after inpatient rehab
Geriatric evaluation and management	5–7 days/wk; 3–5 hr/day; 24-hr nursing care	Interdisciplinary (MD, N, PT, OT, SLP, SW, TR, PSY)	US Veterans Administration	Geriatric nursing unit; utilized primarily in Europe; model adopted by US Veterans Admin Medical System	4–8 wk	Outcomes shown to be superior to nongeriatric settings[49]; moderate to severely impaired individuals with acute medical needs[50–52]
Inpatient rehabilitation services	6–7 days/wk; 3–5 hr/day; 24-hr nursing care	Interdisciplinary (MD, N, PT, OT, SLP, SW, TR, PSY)	Medicare*, Medicaid (most states)	Hospital-based	2–4 wk	Moderate to severely impaired individuals requiring 2 therapies, nursing

MD = Physician; PT = physical therapist; OT = occupational therapist; SLP = speech-language pathologist; SW = social worker; PSY = psychologist; N = nursing; HHA = home health aide; TR = therapeutic recreation specialist.
*Medicare generally pays 80% allowable charges up to deductible; many individuals carry supplemental benefits.

though all patients may benefit from some type and intensity of therapy services, patients who are appropriate for intensive inpatient or day rehabilitation must demonstrate the following characteristics: (1) acute or new disability (i.e., significantly worse than baseline), (2) supportive family who can assist with return to home, (3) ability to participate and improve in acute care therapies, and (4) appropriate funding source. A return to a noninstitutional living environment as soon as feasible is usually the goal. Common rehabilitation options are outlined in Table 26–2.[7,48,50–52] The chosen rehabilitation pathway(s) will depend on medical and nursing acuity needs, endurance for therapeutic activities, formal and informal support systems, and funding options.

◻ MANAGEMENT OF THE OLDER INDIVIDUAL WITH TRAUMATIC BRAIN INJURY

Medical Issues

A number of rehabilitation modifications can facilitate recovery. These alterations help to maximize participation by gradually increasing tolerance to activity and encouraging full individual and family involvement.

Early assessment of rehabilitation issues should be initiated in the intensive care unit. Early, controlled mobilization out of bed minimizes the effects of immobilization, including muscle weakness, cardiac deconditioning, venous thrombosis, constipation, and confusion. Scheduled rest periods and up-down schedules may be required to gradually increase tolerance to activity. Improved participation and motivation can be facilitated by involving the individual with TBI and family in goal setting and focusing on functional tasks that are similar to his or her home routines.[16]

Day-to-day medical management of the elderly individual recovering from acute trauma must be diligent and thorough. When a team of rehabilitation professionals is working with an individual, changes in medical status and performance are often discovered earlier than they would be noticed by a smaller team of a physician, nurse, and family member. Newly identified problems must be evaluated efficiently and appropriate treatment instituted so that these problems interfere minimally with progress toward rehabilitation goals. If the identified problem is unlikely to resolve quickly, the entire team must be informed so that goals can be reformulated[16] or the patient transferred to different level of care.

◻ MEDICATION MANAGEMENT

More than 90 percent of the entire population over age 65 takes at least one prescription medication daily; most take two or more.[53] During the acute traumatic period, previously prescribed medications may be inappropriate, not feasible to administer, or unknown to the acute management team. Invariably, medications are added to treat or prevent conditions associated with acute trauma. Common medications include histamine-2 (H_2) blocking agents to prevent stress ulceration, anticonvulsants to prevent seizures, sedatives and/or hypnotics for agitation, antiarrhythmics for transient cardiac conduction events, narcotics and/or analgesics for pain control, aerosolized inhalers for respiratory problems, and antibiotics for diagnosed or presumed infection.

Medication review with the acute treatment team is crucial as the individual is transitioned from emergent and acute care to rehabilitation. Ideally, this process begins during the rehabilitation medicine evaluation in the acute setting. Nonessential medications should be tapered or discontinued as soon as feasible. Medications that must be continued should be prescribed in the simplest form—that is, the lowest frequency with fewest pills, during normal waking hours so as not to disturb sleep-wake cycle. Principles of drug absorption, distribution, metabolism, excretion, interaction, and compliance should guide the physician's choice of medications for any given condition.[54]

◻ PAIN

Narcotic analgesics have very limited indications as the individual begins to be mobilized for rehabilitation; they invariably cause constipation and lethargy in older people with TBI. Physical activity and modalities such as positioning, heat, ice, ultrasound, and massage are the preferred interventions. If pain is occurring at predictable times of the day or with predictable activities, then analgesic medication can be used in conjunction with them on a regular, not as-needed basis. Scheduled dosing of acetaminophen is preferable to as-needed narcotics or nonsteroidal anti-inflammatory drugs (NSAIDs) as a therapeutic blood level may be established. In cognitively impaired older adults, as-needed pain medications are often ineffective or not requested, and scheduled-dose acetaminophen has been demonstrated to be safer and as effective as NSAIDs.[55] Musculoskeletal pain that disturbs sleep may be addressed with bed positioning and nonnarcotic analgesia at bedtime.

□ SEIZURE RISK

Although seizures occur in about one fifth of older persons with TBI, more than half of these occur during the first week postinjury. Most PTS are focal and self-limiting in nature. Therefore, anticonvulsant medication can be stopped abruptly (phenytoin, carbamazepine) or weaned (barbiturates, benzodiazepines) in the great majority of persons after the first week postinjury.[56] For those with higher risk (i.e., penetrating injuries, large SDH, or intraparenchymal hemorrhages requiring surgical removal, earlier seizures), the use of padded side rails or enclosure beds can protect the person from further injury, should seizures occur. The continued usage of anticonvulsant medication for persons in the higher-risk groups is controversial[57]; practice parameters issued by the American Academy of Neurological Surgeons and the American Board of Physical Medicine and Rehabilitation support withdrawal of prophylactic anticonvulsants in penetrating and nonpenetrating TBI after the first week.[58–60] We and others are currently investigating this issue.

□ DEEP VENOUS THROMBOSIS AND PULMONARY EMBOLISM RISK

Despite some agreement regarding the acute management of deep venous thromboses (DVTs), there is no consensus in the use of DVT prophylaxis after TBI, although this population is at moderate to high risk for DVT occurrence. Sequential compression devices (SCDs) and thigh-length antiembolism stockings are considered safe if they are initially applied within the first 2 to 3 days postinjury. Data support their use for DVT and pulmonary embolism (PE) prevention if they can be applied 23 hours per day.[61] This amount of SCD use is feasible only in the ICU setting; as soon as patients are mobilized out of bed for more than an hour a day, consistent usage is not feasible. Practitioners continue to prescribe them, however, because there is often no safe alternative. Low-dose (10,000–15,000 units/day in divided doses) unfractionated subcutaneous heparin use is contraindicated with recent intracranial surgery or SDH. No consensus exists as to the time that postinjury prophylaxis is relatively less risky than intracranial rehemorrhage. Insufficient data exist with regard to safety of subcutaneous heparin with intracerebral contusions. It is probably safe for those individuals with DAI.[62–64] Low-molecular-weight heparin, which reportedly has fewer bleeding complications than unfractionated heparin, has not been studied sufficiently in individuals with intracerebral hemorrhage to recommend routine usage.

□ NUTRITION AND SWALLOWING

Older individuals with TBI are just as likely as younger individuals to have neurogenic dysphagia and more likely to have some preexisting gastrointestinal motility problem that affects effective feeding. They are more likely to have premorbid problems with dentition than the younger population; dentures may no longer fit after being removed for even several days during acute care.

Establishing adequate nutrition is an important step in facilitating health and optimal recovery. Determining an elderly individual's ideal body weight from their preinjury weight and eating habits is a start, although many older people have a tendency to have inadequate baseline intake. Serum albumin less than 3 g/dl or cholesterol less than 160 mg/dl are laboratory indicators of inadequate nutrition. Low serum ferritin or iron levels are also common posttrauma because blood loss is common and many enteral and parenteral formulas do not contain supplemental iron. If accurate weights are difficult to obtain, serial midarm circumference measurements are more accurate than monitoring skin fold thickness in older individuals.[65] Other medications frequently used in this population can decrease appetite (digoxin, L-dopa, selective serotonin reuptake inhibitors (SSRIs), NSAIDs, thyroxine, alcohol, furosemide) or decrease psychomotor skills for self-feeding (antipsychotics, sedatives, and the injury itself).

Evaluation of swallowing capabilities should start as soon as an individual is sufficiently alert to tolerate a bedside swallowing examination, so that aspiration pneumonia can be avoided. Further evaluation with videofluoroscopic studies of swallowing is best a joint clinical decision between the swallowing evaluator, physician, and those helping with feeding. Frequent monitoring for aspiration by lung auscultation, listening for laryngeal wetness in speech and breathing patterns, and using blue dye in food and liquids that can be suctioned from tracheostomies are effective bedside monitoring techniques.

Until oral feeding can occur, appropriate enteral formulas are necessary. The smallest-gauge feeding tube should be used for optimal patient comfort. A gastrostomy may be preferable if prolonged enteral feeding is projected. Using formulas with fiber and starting with half-strength dilutions are less likely to cause diarrhea. Bolus feeding with or without gastric motility agents that corresponds with future mealtimes makes transition to an eating routine easier and facilitates gastrocolic reflexes that aid in regular elimination. Iron supplements may be necessary as long as the primary nutrition is provided by formula, until iron deficiency anemia resolves and iron stores are repleted, which usually takes 6 months.[66] Supplemental enteral feeding has been associated with decreased mortality and better rehabilitation outcome after hip fractures.[65]

☐ SUBSTANCE ABUSE

After dementia and anxiety disorders, alcoholism is the third most common mental disorder among elderly men in the United States.[67] Chemical abuse ties with depression as the most common mental health problem for individuals in their 60s.[68] Alcoholism in the elderly is closely associated with tobacco abuse, other drug dependence, organic mental disorders (including dementia, delirium, amnestic disorders, and head trauma), hypertension, and liver disease; in younger age groups, high alcohol tolerance, antisocial behavior, and job-related problems are the common associations.[69] Ascertaining the history of alcoholism and other substance abuse in TBI is a challenge in and of itself. The CAGE questionnaire is perhaps the easiest and quickest screening tool.[70]

Treatment of substance abuse in the older individual is also a unique challenge. Most programs are designed for younger people, and therefore the group experience may be less attractive. Living alone postinjury is less likely than preinjury, so caretakers or living partners must be clear on the consequences of ongoing substance use, such as increased risk of recurrent injury and lowered alcohol tolerance and seizure threshold, and the advisability of a substance-free environment. Their codependence in the process must be addressed and confronted directly. Hurt et al.[71] recommend equally intense treatment of the older individual with alcoholism as the younger one. Follow-up of their cohort from 2 to 11 years postinpatient treatment showed that 25 percent were able to remain sober, 41 percent had returned to alcohol use, and 32 percent were dead, nearly half from alcohol-related illnesses.

☐ CONTINENCE

Bladder

Effects of normal aging on bladder function include (1) prostatic hypertrophy in men causing relative outlet obstruction and diminished bladder capacity with symptoms of increased frequency, hesitancy, and/or diminished stream; (2) pelvic relaxation in women with uterine prolapse or cystocele, causing stress incontinence of small volumes of urine when intra-abdominal pressure exceeds the internal and external sphincter pressures; (3) increased urinary frequency from a diminished bladder size and capacity; and (4) increased urgency from delayed or decreased ability to suppress detrusor contraction at low bladder volumes.[72]

Individuals with TBI may have increased frequency because of difficulty with inhibiting the parasympathetic nervous system from firing once the bladder fills to a minimal volume. Increased frequency can also be caused by urinary tract infection. Medications that affect bladder emptying include anticholinergics, calcium channel blockers, and narcotics. Bowel impaction or prostatic hypertrophy may also cause a relative obstruction. Functional incontinence can occur if the individual has insufficient mobility or self-care skills to reach the toilet in a timely manner. Preinjury voiding patterns and physical examination are helpful in discerning any underlying pathology, independent of the effects of TBI.

The first step in achieving continence is removal of the indwelling bladder catheter or diaper that invariably accompanies the individual with TBI from the acute care or skilled nursing settings. Many practitioners prescribe a single intravenous or intramuscular dose of an aminoglycoside (1.3–1.7 mg/kg of gentamicin or tobramycin) just before catheter removal; others note that antibiotic prophylaxis is unnecessary with catheter change.[73] Elimination of medications that may affect bladder emptying is helpful. Encouraging the individual to void on a toilet or commode or standing and then measuring postvoid residual (PVR) by portable ultrasound or with a one-time catheterization can provide a quantitative measurement of bladder emptying. If the PVR is less than 50 cc, then the measurement need not be repeated unless the individual becomes symptomatic. If it is 50 to 100 cc, it is advisable to repeat the measurement to make sure that residual volumes are not sufficient to result in infection. Consistent PVRs greater than 50 percent of total voiding bladder volumes (spontaneous void plus PVR) indicate poor detrusor contraction or outlet obstruction and should be managed with intermittent catheterization once or twice daily until PVR is consistently less than 50 percent of bladder volume.

A timed voiding schedule may be necessary to help individuals achieve urinary continence. This schedule may be necessary as long as mobility is impaired or the individual can reliably call for help with sufficient lead time to avoid functional incontinence.[16] Using these techniques can often eliminate the need for indwelling catheters, diapers, or condom catheters, none of which is well tolerated in older individuals.

Bowel

A patient's bowel routine is invariably disrupted during hospitalization for trauma and is often a low priority in acute care settings. In older individuals, this disruption often becomes a preoccupation, unless it is promptly addressed. Ascertaining a person's preinjury habits is helpful in reestablishing routines, but following them may be unrealistic until safe swallowing, mobility, and gastrointestinal motility are restored.

Fecal impaction often occurs from bed rest and anticholinergic or narcotic medications. With impaction, a one-time laxative or suppository dose often relieves the problem. Stool softeners may be needed for some time because of other constipating medications or dietary supplements, especially iron replacement.

Diarrhea or loose stool is common with antibiotic usage or certain enteral feedings given by feeding tubes. Infectious causes of diarrhea, especially infection with *Clostridium difficile*, should be eliminated; fiber-containing enteral formulas or dilution with water can improve stool consistency. Bolus feedings can encourage a normal gastrocolic reflex and more regular bowel evacuation. Once an acceptable pattern is reestablished, interventions should be weaned one at a time to determine if each is still necessary.[16]

☐ SENSORY HEALTH

Vision

It is a rare person over 65 who does not use glasses at least for reading. Cataracts, glaucoma, and dry eyes are very common. Glasses or contact lenses may be lost or broken during the acute traumatic event and probably are not used in ICU settings. Easily correctable visual problems, such as resumption of glaucoma medication, natural tears, or a useful pair of glasses can aid the rehabilitation process greatly.

Hearing

High-frequency hearing loss occurs as a consequence of aging. Hearing can be altered with injury to the middle ear or cranial nerve VIII

from basilar skull fractures. Use of preinjury hearing aids is sometimes difficult because the injured individual is often the only one who is familiar with their adjustment. Yet accurate communication is crucial to progress through the acute confusional state and to communication with caretakers in rehabilitation settings. Until hearing aid use can be reestablished, written communication, direct eye contact to facilitate lip reading, and an environment without extraneous noise are helpful alternatives.

Smell

Anosmia is probably the most frequent sensory loss associated with TBI. Diminished olfactory acuity also occurs in older individuals without TBI. It may result in decreased appetite for a hospitalized person. More important for safety in the home environment, it may impair the individual's ability to detect smoke when something is burning on the stove or elsewhere. Presence of smoke detectors in the discharge environment is therefore part of the safety check that should accompany home visits or review of the home situation with eventual living mates.

Taste

Diminished sense of taste is related to sense of smell. It is easy to test the basic elements of salty, sweet, sour, and bitter tastes. However, it is often necessary for friends or family members to bring in the individual's favorite foods when it is safe for swallowing to ascertain whether appetite is actually going to be affected.

Touch, Vibration, and Joint Position Sense

Vibratory sense diminishes with age. Conditions that cause an underlying peripheral neuropathy are more frequent in the elderly population, although acute peripheral nerve, brachial, or lumbosacral plexopathies are less frequent. Correctable causes of peripheral neuropathy, such as folic acid, vitamin B_{12}, thyroid deficiencies, or neurotoxic medications, should be identified and treated. Less reversible causes such as diabetes mellitus, alcoholism, uremia, and syphilis are still worth identifying so that their progression can be altered by better glucose control, alcohol abstinence, or definitive treatment of the underlying condition. Compensation techniques, good lighting in dark places, and assistive devices for mobility and self-care may help the individual adapt to these deficits.

❑ GENERAL MEDICAL HEALTH

Space does not permit discussion of the common medical problems of the elderly. If the injured individual has a primary care physician, comanagement of medical problems is advisable. Many individuals who suffer trauma have neglected routine medical care, particularly treatment of asymptomatic hypertension, osteoporosis, hyperglycemia, mammograms and pap smears, rectal examinations for detection of masses or occult blood, screening for glaucoma, tuberculosis, and other common treatable problems. If these problems cannot be diagnosed or cared for efficiently during acute or rehabilitation stays, referral to a primary care practitioner on discharge is even more urgent. Older individuals are more likely to have insurance (e.g., Medicare part B coverage for outpatient care) than younger individuals.

Behavior and Cognition

As a result of physiological and pathological changes that accompany aging, one would anticipate age-specific differences in the incidence and appropriate management of most common cognitive and behavioral issues seen after TBI.[16,40,74] The level of arousal in the older adult with a brain injury may vary greatly, depending on the degree and type of injury, concomitant illness, pharmacological agents, alcohol intoxication and withdrawal, secondary insults to the recovering brain, psychological factors, premorbid factors, and environmental stimulation. The typical pattern of recovery includes initial diminished level of arousal, followed by some degree of hyperarousal, and culminating in a return to a premorbid level of arousal. The treatment team can influence the safe and successful progression through these levels of arousal by limiting secondary insult, addressing concomitant illness, appropriately managing pharmacological interventions, and regulating environmental stimulation.

❑ ATTENTION

Hypoarousal and hypoattention are common after DAI, hypoxic ischemic injury (HII), and frontal lobe focal cortical contusion (FCC) injuries. Hypoarousal is characterized by the inability to remain awake and alert, despite adequate sleep and appropriate stimulation. Hypoattention is characterized by appropriate or increased alertness, but an inability to focus or attend to conversation or self-care tasks. Varying degrees of hypoarousal and hypoattention are especially common after brain injury in older adults. Both deficits limit the ability of individuals to progress in rehabilitation programs. Management is similar to that of the younger patient and includes limiting environmental distractions, normalizing sleep/wake patterns, scheduling rest periods, establishing a reasonable up-down schedule, eliminating centrally acting medications, and treating concomitant medical illness. When medications are needed, methylphenidate is an excellent first-line agent.[75] Amantadine, selective serotonin reuptake inhibitors (fluoxetine, sertraline, paroxetine, fluvoxamine), levodopa-carbidopa, and bromocriptine are also used.[76]

❑ AGITATION

Some degree of agitation has been documented in one third to one half of individuals with TBI, and it often interferes with their participation in rehabilitation efforts.[77–80] The Agitated Behavior Scale (ABS) is the most useful tool to define and monitor agitation in the older adult.[81] Agitated people with TBI are more likely to require supervision after discharge, to require alternative institutional care, and to have psychological adjustment difficulties.[80] There are no studies that specifically define the incidence or outcome of agitation in the older adult with TBI. Management is similar to that of the younger population and includes behavioral strategies, environmental modifications like cubicle or enclosure beds, structured therapy sessions, appropriate medical management, and neuropharmacological interventions. Commonly used medications include amantadine, carbamazepine, and propranolol.[82]

❑ ALTERATION IN MOOD

Depression may occur in more than 25 percent of individuals with TBI in the first 12 months after injury. Major depression is less frequent than in younger people, but depressive symptoms are more common.[83–85] There is typically no correlation of depression with degree of impairment or disability.[86] Normalizing sleep-wake cycles is vital. Psychological counseling is appropriate initially for the majority of individuals. For those who are refractory to nonpharmacological techniques, methylphenidate is an excellent short-term activating agent that improves arousal and attention and may assist with depression. Insomnia may be a side effect if methylphenidate is given near bedtime.[75] SSRIs are common first-line antidepressant medications in the older adult.[76] Insomnia and anorexia may be side effects of these medications. Psychiatric monitoring is recommended for anyone on these medications; however, because of the complexity of medical, functional, and behavioral issues involved, physiatrists often manage these conditions.

□ SLEEP-WAKE DISTURBANCE

Insomnia often occurs acutely after brain injury and may persist long-term, resulting in decreased daytime arousal, diminished cognitive skills, and impaired performance. Contributing factors include alterations in neurotransmitter levels, disturbed sleep-wake cycles from acute hospitalization, sleep interruption by hospital personnel, anxiety, and lingering effects from sedating or stimulating medications taken at other times. It is important to adjust the individual's day-night schedule (lights off at night, medications scheduled to maintain daytime awakening, up-down schedule, minimizing daytime naps).[82] Low doses of trazodone or zolpidem are first-line medications when behavioral and environmental interventions are ineffective. Dosing is usually 1 hour before desired sleep time and is limited to 1 to 2 weeks duration for zolpidem. Therefore, if longer usage is anticipated, trazodone is a better choice. Diphenhydramine and hydroxyzine are often used as second-line agents. Benzodiazepines and tricyclic antidepressants with marked anticholinergic activity should be avoided in the elderly because they may cause persistent sedation, hypotension, and other undesirable side effects.

□ MOTIVATION

Motivation is a multifactorial issue that is especially difficult in the brain injured older adult with significant cognitive and physical limitations that preclude full participation in therapy programs. Although lowered expectations may lead rehabilitation team members to accept a decreased performance level in the elderly,[87] a more therapeutic solution is to anticipate initial difficulty with full participation and modify the treatment program. Scheduled rest periods and up-down schedules, improved sleep-wake cycles, optimized medical management, judicious use of neurostimulants, realistic patient-oriented goals, task-specific ("functional") therapy, and early therapeutic outings to assess function in the home are appropriate interventions.

□ MEMORY

Significant premorbid memory deficits are present in nearly 10 percent of community-dwelling older adults. The prevalence in the oldest old is greater than 20 percent.[88,89] Additionally, prolonged post-traumatic amnesia is more common in older adults after TBI.[11,42,90] These two factors, in combination with the increased sensitivity of the aged brain to alterations in homeostasis and medications, result in significant cognitive deficits. Family members and consistent staff members are essential components of the treatment team. Additionally, rapid return to a more familiar environment (i.e., home) is very important. For these reasons, home-based rehabilitation services for the individual with severe memory problems may be preferable if the medical and social situations permit.

□ SAFETY JUDGMENT

Premorbid or newly acquired limitations in cognition, sensation, strength, and balance often challenge individuals' safety. Many elders have a difficult time adjusting to these limitations and therefore pose a significant risk in safety judgment. Falls are common in the hospitalized and nonhospitalized elderly population, and this risk increases with an acute TBI.[11,91]

□ COMPETENCE AND CAPACITY

The acute cognitive, behavioral, and communication deficits commonly following TBI, in combination with the mild cognitive slowing inherent to aging, make issues of self-determination difficult. *Competence* is a legal term focusing on the right of self-determination; *capacity* is a medical term focusing on cognitive and physical abilities to convey and carry out one's wishes. An interdisciplinary evaluation by an appropriate physician, psychologist, occupational therapist, and/or speech-language pathologist is recommended to provide a comprehensive assessment that includes topographical and verbal orientation and money management, as well as attention, memory, language, reasoning, and affective components.[92]

◻ LANGUAGE

Limitations of hearing and seeing complicate language and communication deficits secondary to the brain injury. Additionally, dentures (often loose-fitting) and the inability to clear oral secretions often complicate dysarthrias in the older adult. Aphasia with combinations of dysnomia, auditory comprehension deficits, dysgraphia, and dyslexia also affect communication abilities. Compensation for these deficits is crucial for a person to be safe in the home environment. Interventions should be practical and simple—for example, a simple "pocket talker," instead of a new hearing aid, and working with caretakers on functional communication techniques.

◻ SEXUALITY

Sexuality encompasses a sense of self, interaction with others, and many levels of expression and affection, in addition to sexual relations. Physiological and pathological alterations that are seen with aging often limit the ability and enjoyment of sexual function in the older adult but affect sexuality less so. The cognitive and physical sequelae of TBI further impair sexual function and also may impair other aspects of sexuality. Open discussion of these issues should be initiated in the acute rehabilitation setting and then monitored over time. Counseling is appropriate for individuals with sexual dysfunction of any age.[93]

◻ SELF-CARE

Standard rehabilitation principles to recover self-care abilities are often effective in the older adult with TBI. Older adults may have difficulty with attempts to utilize the concept of transfer of training skills (i.e., breaking down functional tasks into smaller components); therefore, very functional therapy is recommended. Automatic or overlearned activities often return rapidly, but new learning or significant adaptations may be more slowly integrated than in younger adults. A firm understanding of the individual's preinjury characteristics and habits is vital. Adaptive equipment may be useful; however, acceptance of and ability to effectively utilize it will also be more difficult. Typical equipment recommendations include built-up utensils and devices to accommodate hand weakness, decreased dexterity, and joint limitations; long-handled devices and reachers to accommodate decreases in flexibility and poor truncal balance; bathroom safety aids (grab bars, tub benches, hand-held showers, raised commode chairs) to accommodate balance deficits and decreased strength. Home management skills must often be modified. Particular emphasis must be placed on the limited physical and cognitive endurance of the older adult.

◻ MOBILITY

Special considerations necessary to address mobility in the older adult with TBI include alterations in vision, decreased peripheral sensation, imbalance, decreased strength, and limited physical endurance. Motor and balance functions tend to recover more slowly in the older adult because of premorbid limitations, decreased tolerance for intensive therapy sessions, and joint and musculoskeletal pain. Household-level mobility may be facilitated with a home evaluation by members of the rehabilitation team to assess architectural barriers (doorways, stairs), spacing of furniture, appropriateness of floor coverings, appropriateness of natural and artificial lighting, and available modifications. Community mobility goals must include the ability to get to different areas in the community (transportation and route finding) and to get around safely in different settings (e.g., malls, restaurants, golf courses, homes). Public transportation for individuals with disabilities is becoming increasingly available throughout the world, and so physical limitations are becoming less important as barriers to community mobility. Deficits in higher-level cognitive skills remain as barriers to successful use of public transportation systems, which are often complex to negotiate. Funding for adapted transportation systems is usually provided by federal and local resources and is therefore at risk for reallocation at any time.

Driving

Driving after TBI must take into account the older adult's preinjury abilities and new limitations. Some jurisdictions require physicians and other health care practitioners to report to public health authorities or the department of motor vehicles (DMV) physical and cognitive conditions that may affect an individual's ability to drive.[94] The DMV's response also varies by location. California revokes licenses from individuals with moderate or severe cognitive deficits reported by a physician or other health care practitioner. Interviews and more rigorous testing procedures are given to those with mild cognitive deficits, with a schedule for reexamination if the applicant is considered at risk for further cognitive decline.[94] Comprehensive driving evaluations may be helpful, although third-party funding for these programs is rarely available. Testing of range of motion, muscle strength, proprioception, light touch, pathological reflexes, vision, sitting balance, transfer skills, attention, judgment, perception, memory, information processing, and psychomotor speed is important but cannot replace the on-the-road evaluation.[95,96]

☐ RECREATION AND VOCATION

A clear understanding of an older adult's preinjury recreational level is necessary to recommend options after TBI. Often, the elderly have had sedentary activities that can easily be resumed with minor modifications. Socialization may have been the primary leisure activity prior to TBI and is often the most appropriate leisure skill after injury. Thus, involvement in group experiences in both the rehabilitative setting and in more informal community settings is appropriate. Return to work rates are poor for older adults after TBI. Realistic goals need to be established and, if appropriate, referral to supported employment programs made. In general, early retirement or part-time or volunteer work is recommended for older adults who are unable to return to premorbid function.[6,97,98]

☐ CONCLUSION

Traumatic brain injury in the older adult occurs primarily as the result of falls, pedestrian accidents, and low- to moderate-speed motor vehicle crashes. The aging of the entire population in industrialized countries points to increasing incidence and prevalence of TBI in the elderly. Most injuries result in subdural hematomas and intracerebral contusions, although some may produce DAI. Severe injuries are rarely survivable, but individuals who do survive can have favorable functional outcomes.

Caring for the older individual with TBI requires implementation of principles of geriatric medicine and brain injury rehabilitation, with particular attention to the timing, setting, and intensity of therapeutic interventions. Therefore, models for care of TBI in younger individuals or care of disabling conditions like stroke or dementia in older individuals must be adjusted to the unique needs of this population.

Older people with TBI require more time to recover cognitively and physically than younger individuals with TBI and older individuals with common disabling conditions like stroke. Removal or simplification of medications is more helpful than adding new ones. Therapeutic interventions should be tailored to the individual and family's needs in their postdischarge environment, with early training of caretakers and environmental modifications for safety. This chapter provides a framework for continuing development of that model as more experience and research accumulate with the care of the older individual with TBI.

REFERENCES

1. Cifu, DX, and Lorish, TR: Stroke rehabilitation: Stroke outcome. Arch Phys Med Rehabil 75:S56, 1994.
2. American Medical Association: White paper on elderly health. Arch Intern Med 150:2459, 1990.
3. US Senate Special Committee on Aging: Developments in Aging. US Government Printing Office, Washington, DC, 1988, p 1:2.
4. National Center for Health Statistics: NCHS advance data (No 133). Department of Health and Human Services, Washington, DC, 1987.
5. Williams, TF: The aging process: Biological and psychosocial considerations. In Brody, SJ, and Ruff, GE (eds): Aging and Rehabilitation: Advances in the State of the Art. Springer, New York, 1986, p 13.
6. Heiskanen, H, and Sipponen, P: Prognosis of severe brain injury. Acta Neurol Scand 46:343, 1970.
7. Weber, DC, Fleming, KC, and Evans, JM: Rehabilitation of geriatric patients. Mayo Clin Proc 70:1198, 1995.
8. Kraus, JF, et al: The incidence of acute brain injury and serious impairment in a defined population. Am J Epidemiol 119:186, 1983.
9. Wilson, JA: The functional effects of head injury in the elderly. Brain Inj 1:183, 1987.
10. Horn, LJ, and Cope, DN: Demographics. In Horn, LJ, and Cope, ND (eds): Traumatic Brain Injury. Hanley and Belfus, Philadelphia, 1989.
11. Katz, DI, Kehs, GJ, and Alexander, MD: Prognosis and recovery from TBI: The influence of advancing age. Neurology 40:276, 1990.
12. Tinetti, MD, and Speechley, M: Prevention of falls in the elderly. N Engl J Med 320:1055, 1989.
13. Kraus, JF: Injury to the head and spinal cord. J Neurosurg 53:S3, 1980.
14. Lehman, LB: Head trauma in the elderly. Postgraduate Geriatrics 83:140, 1988.
15. Frankowski, RF: Descriptive epidemiologic studies of head injury in the United States: 1974–1984. Adv Psychosom Med 16:153, 1986.
16. Goodman, H, and Englander, J: Traumatic brain injury in elderly individuals. Physical Medicine and Rehabilitation Clinics of North America 3:441, 1992.
17. Amacher, AL, and Bybee, DE: Toleration of head injury by the elderly. Neurosurgery 20:954, 1979.
18. Sosin, DN, Sacks, JJ, and Smith, SM: Head injury-associated deaths in the U.S. from 1979–1986. JAMA 282:2251, 1989.
19. Gutman, MB, et al: Relative incidence of intracranial mass lesions and severe torso injury after accidental injury: Implications for triage and management. J Trauma 31:974, 1991.
20. Braakman, R, et al: Systematic selection of prognostic features in patients with severe head injury. Neurosurgery 6:362, 1980.
21. Rakier, A, et al: Head injuries in the elderly. Brain Inj 9:187, 1995.
22. Katz, DI, and Alexander, MP: Traumatic brain injury: Predicting course of recovery and outcome for patients admitted to rehabilitation. Arch Neurol 51:661, 1994.
23. Vollmer, DG, et al: Age and outcome following traumatic coma: Why do older patients fare worse. J Neurosurg 75:S37, 1991.
24. Chesnut, RM, et al: The role of secondary brain injury in determining outcome from severe head injury. J Trauma 34:216, 1993.

25. Pennings, JL, et al: Survival after severe brain injury in the aged. Arch Surg 128:787, 1993.
26. Cagetti, B, et al: The outcome from acute subdural and epidural intracranial hematomas in very elderly patients. Br J Neurosurg 6:227, 1992.
27. CDC: Suicide among older persons: United States, 1980–1992, Morb Mortal Wkly Rep 46:1, 1996.
28. Traumatic Brain Injury Model Systems National Data Base Syllabus. Traumatic Brain Injury Model Systems National Data Center. Rehabilitation Institute of Michigan, Detroit.
29. Bontke, C, et al: Medical complications and associated injuries of persons treated in the Traumatic Brain Injury Model Systems programs. J Head Trauma Rehabil 8(2): 34, 1993.
30. Gurney, JG, et al: The effects of alcohol intoxication on the initial treatment and hospital course of patients with acute brain injury. J Trauma 33:709, 1992.
31. Morrison, RG: Medical and public health aspects of boxing. JAMA 255:2475, 1986.
32. Herneasniemi, J: Outcome following head injuries in the aged. Acta Neurochir (Wien) 49:67, 1979.
33. Jennett, B, et al: Predicting outcome in individual patients after severe head injury. Lancet 1:1031, 1976.
34. Born, JD, et al: Relative prognostic value of best motor response and brainstem reflexes in patients with severe head injury. Neurosurgery 16:595, 1985.
35. Choi, S, et al: Temporal profile of outcome in severe head injury. J Neurosurg 81:169, 1994.
36. Luerssen, T, Klauber, M, and Marshall, L: Outcome from head injury related to patient's age. J Neurosurg 68:409, 1988.
37. Cifu, DX, et al: Functional outcomes of older adults with TBI: A prospective, multicenter analysis. Arch Phys Med Rehabil 77:S888, 1996.
38. Galbraith, S: Head injuries in the elderly. BMJ 294:325, 1987.
39. Reeder, K, et al: Impact of age on functional outcome following traumatic brain injury. J Head Trauma Rehabil 11:22, 1996.
40. Gershkoff, AM, Cifu, DX, and Means, KM: Geriatric rehabilitation: Social, attitudinal and economic factors. Arch Phys Med Rehabil 74:S402, 1993.
41. Saywell, RM, et al: The value of age and severity as predictors of costs in geriatric head injury trauma patients. J Am Geriatr Soc 37:625, 1989.
42. Carlsson, CA, von Essen, C, and Losgren, J: Clinical factors in severe head injuries. J Neurosurg 29:242, 1968.
43. Galbraith, S, et al: The relationship between alcohol and head injury and its effects on the conscious level. Br J Surg 63:128, 1976.
44. Brody, SJ, and Paulson, LG (eds): Aging and Rehabilitation II: The State of the Practice. Springer, New York, 1990, p 139.
45. France, AC, Schultz, AK, and Nanney, MT: Medicare, geriatrics and the family physician. Am Fam Physician 44:754, 1991.
46. Maloney, FP, and Means, KM (eds): Rehabilitation and the Aging Population. Hanley and Belfus, Philadelphia, 1990, p 143.
47. Sherman, FT: Physician reimbursement for the care of the elderly: Concerns of a practicing geriatrician. Bull N Y Acad Med 63:732, 1988.
48. Walker, WC, Kreutzer, JS, and Witol, AD: Level of care options for the low-functioning brain injury survivor. Brain Inj 10:65, 1996.
49. Applegate, WB, Miller, ST, and Graney, MJ: A randomized, controlled trial of a geriatric assessment unit in a community rehabilitation hospital. N Engl J Med 322: 1572, 1990.
50. Applegate, WB, et al: Geriatric evaluation and management: Current status and future research directions. J Am Geriatr Soc (suppl)39:25, 1991.
51. Rubenstein, LZ, et al: Impacts of geriatric evaluation and management programs on defined outcomes: Overview of the evidence. J Am Geriatr Soc (suppl)39:85, 1991.
52. Stewart, DG, and Cifu, DX: Rehabilitation of the old, old stroke patient. Journal of Back and Musculoskeletal Rehabilitation 4:135, 1994.
53. Chutka, DS, et al: Drug prescribing for elderly patients. Mayo Clin Proc 70:685, 1995.
54. Montamat, SC, Cusack, BJ, and Vestal, RE: Management of drug therapy in the elderly. N Engl J Med 321:303, 1989.
55. Bradely, J, et al: Comparison of an antiinflammatory dose of ibuprofen, an analgesic dose of ibuprofen, and acetaminophen in the treatment of patients with osteoarthritis of the knee. N Engl J Med 325:87, 1991.
56. Temkin, N, et al: A randomized, double-blinded study of phenytoin for the prevention of post-traumatic seizures. N Engl J Med 323:497, 1990.
57. Jennet, B: Post traumatic epilepsy. In Rosenthal, M, et al: Rehabilitation of the Adult and Child with Traumatic Brain Injury, ed 2. FA Davis, Philadelphia, 1990, p 89.
58. Yablon, SA: Posttraumatic seizures. Arch Phys Med Rehabil 74:983, 1993.
59. Bullock, R, et al: Guidelines for the Management of Severe Head Injury. Brain Trauma Foundation, San Francisco, 1995.
60. Brain Injury Special Interest Group of the American Academy of Physical Medicine and Rehabilitation: Practice parameter: Antiepileptic drug treatment of posttraumatic seizures. Arch Phys Med Rehabil 79:594, 1998.
61. Weinmann, EE, and Salzman, EW: Deep-venous thrombosis. N Engl J Med 331:1630, 1994.
62. Hamilton, MG, Hull, RD, and Pineo, GF: Venous thromboembolism in neurosurgery and neurology patients: A review. Neurosurgery 34:280, 1994.
63. Kaufman, HH, et al: Deep venous thrombosis and pulmonary embolism in head injured patients. Angiology 34:627, 1983.
64. Office of Medical Applications of Research, NIH: Consensus conference: Prevention of venous thrombosis and pulmonary embolism. JAMA 256:744, 1986.
65. Morley, JE, and Miller, DK: Malnutrition in the elderly. Hosp Pract (Off Ed) 7:95, 1992.
66. Schafer, AI, and Bunn, HF: Anemias of iron deficiency and iron overload. In Braunwald, E, et al: Harrison's Principles of Internal Medicines, ed 11. 1987, p 1497.
67. Myers, JK, et al: Six-month prevalence of psychiatric disorders in three communities: 1980–1982. Arch Gen Psychiatry 41:959, 1984.
68. American Psychiatric Association: Diagnostic and Statistical Manual of Mental Disorders, ed 3, revised. American Psychiatric Association, Washington, DC, 1987.
69. Finlayson, RE, et al: Alcoholism in elderly persons: A study of the psychiatric and psychosocial features of 216 inpatients. Mayo Clin Proc 63:761, 1988.
70. Ewing, JA: Detecting alcoholism: The CAGE questionnaire. JAMA 252:1905, 1984.
71. Hurt, RD, et al: Alcoholism in elderly persons: Medical aspects and prognosis of 216 inpatients. Mayo Clin Proc 63:750, 1988.
72. Chutka, DS, et al: Urinary incontinence in the elderly population. Mayo Clin Proc 71:93, 1996.
73. Polaski, F, et al: Absence of significant bacteremia during urinary catheter manipulation in patients with chronic indwelling catheters. J Am Geriatr Soc 38:1203, 1990.
74. Cifu, DX, et al: Geriatric rehabilitation: Diagnosis and management of acquired disabling disorders. Arch Phys Med Rehabil 74:S406, 1993.
75. Kaelin, D, Cifu, DX, and Matthies, B: Methylphenidate effect on attention deficit in the acutely brain-injured adult. Arch Phys Med Rehabil 77:6, 1996.
76. Cardenas, D, and McLean, A: Psychopharmacologic management of traumatic brain injury. In Berrol, S (ed): Physical Medicine and Rehabilitation Clinics of North America. Saunders, Philadelphia, 1992.
77. Sandel, ME, and Mysiw, WJ: The agitated brain injured patient. Part I: Definitions, differential diagnosis, and assessment. Arch Phys Med Rehabil 77:617, 1996.

78. Brooke, MM, et al: Agitation and restlessness after closed head injury: A prospective study of 100 consecutive admissions. Arch Phys Med Rehabil 73:320, 1992.

79. Levin, HS, and Grossman, RG: Behavioral sequelae of closed head injury: Quantitative study. Arch Neurol 35:720, 1978.

80. Reyes, RL, Bhattacharyya, AK, and Heler, D: Traumatic head injury: Restlessness and agitation as prognosticators of physical and psychological improvements in patients. Arch Phys Med Rehabil 62:20, 1981.

81. Corrigan, JD: Development of a scale for assessment of agitation following traumatic brain injury. J Clin Exp Neuropsychol 11:261, 1989.

82. Cifu DX, Anderson, JC, and Lopez, E: Agitation in the older adult with traumatic brain injury. Neurorehabilitation 5:245, 1995.

83. Martin, LM, Fleming, KC, and Evans, JM: Recognition and management of anxiety and depression in elderly patients. Mayo Clin Proc 70:999, 1995.

84. Koenig, HG, and Blazer, DG: Mood disorders and suicide. In Birren, JE, Sloane, RB, and Cohen, GD (eds): Handbook of Mental Health and Aging, ed 2. Academic Press, San Diego, 1992, p 383.

85. Blazer, DG: Affective disorders in late life. In Busse, EW, and Blazer, DG (eds): Geriatric Psychiatry. American Psychiatric Press, Washington, DC, 1989, pp 370–373.

86. Whyte, J, and Rosenthal, M: Rehabilitation of the patient with traumatic brain injury. In DeLisa, J (ed): Rehabilitation Medicine Principles and Practice, ed 2. JB Lippincott, Philadelphia, 1993.

87. Hesse, KA, and Champion, EW: Motivating the geriatric patient for rehabilitation. J Am Geriatr Soc 31:586, 1983.

88. Beard, CM, et al: The prevalence of dementia is changing over time in Rochester, Minnesota. Neurology 45:75, 1995.

89. Skoog, I, et al: A population-based study of dementia in 85-year-olds. N Engl J Med 328:153, 1993.

90. Levati, A, et al: Prognosis of severe brain injuries. J Neurosurg 57:779, 1982.

91. Rubenstein, LZ, et al: Falls and instability in the elderly. J Am Geriatr Soc 36:266, 1988.

92. Callahan, CD, and Hagglund, KJ: Comparing neuropsychological and psychiatric evaluation of competency in rehabilitation: A case example. Arch Phys Med Rehabil 76:909, 1995.

93. Roughan, PA, Kaiser, FE, and Morley, JE: Sexuality and the older woman. Clin Geriatr Med 9:87, 1993.

94. Reuben, DB, and St George, P: Driving and dementia: California's approach to a medical and policy dilemma. West J Med 164:111, 1996.

95. Hunt, LA: Evaluation and retraining programs for older drivers. Clin Geriatr Med 9:439, 1993.

96. Galski, T, Bruno, RL, and Ehle, HT: Prediction of behind-the-wheel driving performance in patients with cerebral brain damage: A discriminant function analysis. Am J Occup Ther 47:391, 1993.

97. McMordie, WR, Barker, SL, and Paolo, TM: Return to work after head injury. Brain Inj 4:57, 1990.

98. Wehman, PH, et al: Return to work for persons with TBI: A supported employment approach. Arch Phys Med Rehabil 71:1047, 1990.

CHAPTER 27

Mild Head Injury: Current Research and Clinical Issues

JEFFREY T. BARTH, PHD,
STEPHEN N. MACCIOCCHI, PHD,
and PAUL T. DIAMOND, MD

As Karl Menninger once suggested, "The teacher is faced with the eternal dilemma, whether to present the clear, simple but inaccurate fact, or the complex, confusing, presumptive truth." A similar dilemma becomes apparent when considering the neurobehavioral issues associated with mild head injury. Nonetheless, in our discussion of mild injury we attempt to avoid simplicity without lapsing into confusing complexity. Our discussion initially focuses on a brief review of the history of mild head injury. Subsequently, we summarize relevant empirical findings and clinical problems, including a pragmatic approach to treatment.

At the present time, the scientific and clinical communities have no genuine consensus regarding the etiology of symptom presentation and duration following mild head injury. In fact, controversy has been endemic to mild head injury for more than 30 years. In the early 1960s, Miller[1,2] suggested that most patients with mild head injuries who reported persistent postconcussion symptoms were actually suffering from "accident" or "compensation neurosis," characterized by unsubstantiated complaints or exaggeration of symptoms that were unrelated to genuine neurologic injury. Miller concluded that mild head injury did not result in permanent "organic" damage yet could produce "functional," psychiatric conditions or symptoms consistent with factitious disorder or malingering. In con-

trast, Oppenheimer[3] documented postmortem microscopic lesions in patients who had suffered a significant concussion but evidenced no overt postconcussive symptomatology. Moreover, as early as 1943, Holbourn[4] thought that damage to axons caused by "shear-strain" injury occurred in mild forms of concussion. Somewhat later, Symonds[5] concurred with Holbourn's findings and stated that it was "questionable whether the effects of concussion, however slight, are ever completely reversible" (p. 5).

□ DEFINITION

The term *minor head injury* became popular in the early 1980s in association with popular press exposés on "the silent epidemic." To avoid minimization and create a greater appreciation for the potential problems associated with this pathology, *mild head injury* emerged as the central terminology. Today, consensus is lacking on a single definition of *mild head injury,* and other terms such as *mild concussion* are often viewed as synonymous. Gennarelli[6] has defined *classical cerebral concussion* as "temporary, reversible neurological deficiency caused by trauma that results in temporary *loss of consciousness* for less than six hours" (p. 108). Gennarelli adds that some forms of mild concussion may occur with a mere *alteration* rather than complete loss of *consciousness*. As is apparent, Gennarelli's definition is quite broad, and, in fact, most clinicians and investigators have relied on vague clinical criteria to define *mild concussion* and *mild head injury*. For example, head trauma without prolonged unconsciousness followed by a typical constellation of postconcussive symptoms and normal radiological studies is frequently classified as mild. The typical research definition of *mild head injury* or *trauma* considers duration of unconsciousness (<20 min), Glasgow Coma Scale (GCS) score (>12), length of hospitalization (<48 hr), and negative radiological findings. This definition does not necessarily imply physiological alteration in brain function; underlying histological damage; permanent alteration in brain structure, physiology, or function; or permanent disability. In other words, mild head injury does not necessarily imply *any brain* injury.

Recently, the American Congress of Rehabilitation Medicine, Head Injury Special Interest Group on Mild Traumatic Brain Injury[7] defined *mild traumatic brain injury* as an injury to the head or mechanical forces applied to the head involving loss of consciousness for less than 30 minutes (possibly no loss of consciousness) with posttraumatic amnesia for less than 24 hours. The definition does imply physiological impairment and possible histological damage, at least at the time of injury. Temporary or permanent altered mental or neurological state is required. Symptoms (including physical, cognitive, behavioral, emotional, and psychosocial deficits) of brain injury may or may not persist, and symptoms can result in temporary or permanent disability, which implies that mild head injury can cause a persistent postconcussion syndrome (headache, dizziness, vomiting, depression, sleep disturbance, memory impairment, irritability, personality change, decreased speed of mental processing, impaired new problem solving, and inattention).

The American Congress of Rehabilitation Medicine's definition is similar to the concept of "complicated mild head injury." *Complicated mild head injury* was a term originally used to denote a mild injury by GCS criteria, associated with a documented lesion, skull fracture, or other factor that complicated recovery. Both definitions suggest flexibility regarding the presence and permanence of underlying histological damage and subsequent disability. Use of the term *brain injury*, however, does *imply* permanence and potential disability related to identifiable neurological impairment. Although we could argue that the term *mild traumatic brain injury* brings medical recognition and flexible interpretation to this disorder, use of the term *brain injury* remains controversial.

Kibby and Long[8] suggest that there is significant confusion over the lower limits of mild head injury. As noted previously, it is possible to be diagnosed with a "mild traumatic brain injury despite minimal or no neurological damage being present" (p. 159). The authors suggest that there are degrees of mild head injury that have yet to be defined. Increased precision in defining mild head injury has solved some problems associated with documenting the nature of the injury, but unfortunately clinicians still face considerable uncertainty, particularly at the mildest end of the spectrum, where very brief or nonexistent periods of interrupted consciousness are apparent.

Given the vague and at best variable definition of the terms *minor head injury, mild head injury, mild concussion,* and *mild traumatic brain injury*, we propose that the terms *mild head injury* or *mild head trauma* continue to be utilized as generic terms for mild trauma to the head with no specific implication for brain injury. In this way, identifiable brain injury and cognitive-behavioral sequelae would be described separately from the level of impact to the head. Until more sophisticated classification methods and alternative functional radiological techniques are available, clinicians must document all parameters of mild head injuries as accurately as possible. At a minimum, clinicians should document duration of unconsciousness (if any), duration of posttraumatic amnesia, and symptom type and duration of an injury, which may facilitate neurobehavioral indexing of injury severity. Injury severity is also viewed as being dependent on symptom etiology. The following section discusses the psychogenic-physiogenic issue and presents some guidelines for clinicians.

☐ PHYSIOGENIC VERSUS PSYCHOGENIC

To examine whether mild head trauma causes identifiable central nervous system (CNS) damage, Ommaya and Gennarelli et al.[9,10] tested Holbourn's shear-strain model with primates. In these studies, the investigators used an acceleration-deceleration model rather than the traditional animal impact injury design (weighted object striking the head from a calculated distance at a determined velocity) because most mild head injuries in humans are caused by motor vehicle accidents that involve deceleration and rotational forces. These mild injuries in humans are often the result of the shaking and abrupt movement of the head and brain, particularly when the victim is restrained by a cross-chest and lap seat belt. Direct impact to the head resulting in mild head injury is less common in clinical populations (yet more common in moderate and severe brain trauma). In the primate studies, an apparatus caused the monkey's head to move rapidly forward in a linear plane from a stationary, upright position and come to a complete stop less than 1 second later (acceleration-deceleration forces). At autopsy, Gennarelli et al. discovered stretched and broken axons (shear-strain) in the brain stems of monkeys who had suffered less than 2 minutes of unconsciousness and had returned to normal cage activities within 30 minutes. These findings documented axon damage following mild acceleration-deceleration injuries and argued for a possible neurological basis for symptoms experienced by patients with mild head injury. Povlishock et al.[11] and Dixon et al.[12] have also described axonal changes, release of excessive neurotransmitters, and diffuse deafferentation as additional underlying pathophysiology associated with mild closed head injury.

Recent human studies addressing symptom presentation following mild head injury, such as the investigations of Gronwall, Wrightson, and Sampson[13-16] found significant neuropsychological deficits (particularly in speed of mental processing) in approximately 20 percent of their population with mild head injuries. Similar findings were documented by investigators at the University of Virginia[17,18] in a study of such patients as part of a larger research project on the full spectrum of closed head injury. Using inclusion criteria of documented emergency department visits, GCS above 12, loss of consciousness less than 20 minutes, and less than 48 hours of hospitalization, the authors found that 34 percent of patients with mild head injuries had not returned to their previous employment at 3 months postinjury and that 24 percent of this population demonstrated significant neuropsychological deficits at that time.[18]

Despite animal studies and correlational findings in human subjects, most of the early human research did not control for such factors as previous head injury, substance abuse, or involvement in litigation.[19] Control groups were also absent in most of these studies, thus limiting interpretation of the contribution of organic versus functional (psychosocial) factors in symptom presentation and duration following mild head injury. Subsequent attempts to address these research deficiencies led to more controlled neuropsychological studies of mild head injury. Several studies excluded persons with previous head injury, psychiatric disorder, or substance abuse histories or pending litigation. These investigations by Dikman, Levin, McLean, et al.[20-22] involved neu-

rocognitive testing at 1 and 3 months after mild head injury. The results revealed neuropsychological deficits at 1 month posttrauma in many patients, as compared with matched controls. At 3 months, the vast majority of these patients evidenced normal neuropsychological functioning on the tests administered.

Although these data indicate that selected patients evidence good recovery within 3 months after mild head injury, there was no control for practice effects; in at least one study, a different control group was used for each assessment. Although patients with mild head injuries generally returned to the baseline level of the control group after 3 months, the control group may also have shown improved performance if tested a second time.[23] In addition, a small number of patients in each study did not return to control group baseline levels of neuropsychological functioning, indicating a few poor outcomes. More important, subsequent analysis of a subset of data from one of these studies noted memory impairment in a portion of this population at 3 months postinjury.[24]

Following these clinical investigations, a large study of college football players ($n = 2350$) addressed symptom presentation and duration in very mild acceleration-deceleration head injury.[25,26] In a prospective, repeated measures design, players presumably experiencing a mild head injury characterized by momentary confusion or altered consciousness were tested at 24 hours, 5 days, and 10 days postinjury, along with matched control subjects. When compared with controls, these athletes with mild head injuries demonstrated neuropsychological deficits (attention, concentration, and speed of mental processing) at 24 hours and 5 days postinjury. By 10 days postinjury, head injured athletes evidenced neuropsychological skills comparable to controls.

In another study of a selected sample of mild head injury patients, Leininger et al.[27] assessed neuropsychological functioning in patients who complained of postconcussion symptoms 6 to 8 months postinjury. When compared with controls, most of these patients exhibited neuropsychological deficits. Because of potential selection bias and other factors, these results must be placed in the context of later research. Symptoms of postconcussion syndrome (headache, dizziness, memory impairment, depression, sleep disturbances, slowed mental processing, decreased tolerance, and apathy) can (and often do) occur in the absence of identifiable brain injury.[28,29] In addition, Alves, et al.[30] documented the incidence of postconcussion symptoms in a large, nonselected sample of mild head injury patients. The authors found that one to two symptoms were common 3 months postinjury but that more than two complaints were uncommon and that the overwhelming majority of patients were asymptomatic at 1 year. Again, "a small percentage of patients experienced extended post concussive symptoms" (p 55).

Although most of the studies reviewed principally focused on neurobehavioral functioning following mild head injury, Levin, Ruff, and Varney et al.[31–33] correlated neuroradiological findings with neurobehavioral test scores in patients with mild head injuries. Levin et al.[31] studied mild and moderate head injuries and found that lesions observed on magnetic resonance scans correlated with neuropsychological deficits. Unfortunately, in this investigation, these authors did not distinguish between mild and moderate injuries in their analyses but rather combined data across injury severity. Subsequently, Ruff, et al.[32] published a study focusing on neuropsychological functioning and positron emission tomography (PET) results in patients with symptomatic mild head injuries and controls. The investigators found correlations between neuropsychological deficits and abnormalities in glucose metabolism (mainly focused in anteriotemporofrontal areas) at 1 to 49 months postinjury in all nine patients with mild head injuries. These findings were in sharp contrast to the normal presentation observed in the controls.

More recently, Varney et al.[33] obtained results similar to Ruff et al.[32] in 14 symptomatic mild head injury patients (and 5 control subjects) studied with single-photon emission computed tomography (neuroSPECT) imaging. Results showed significant anterior mesial temporal hypoperfusion and less striking dominant (left) orbitofrontal abnormalities. The authors conclude that "mild head injuries with unusually catastrophic psychosocial consequences can produce regional abnormalities in cerebral perfusion that are apparent with neuroSPECT, even in the absence of abnormalities seen on CT or MRI" (p. 18).

The conclusions suggested by the research reviewed may appear contradictory, but these contradictions are caused, in large part, by varying methodological approaches and the limitations inherent in any correlational study. In all the studies mentioned, there was variability in subject inclusion criteria (injury severity and description), subject characteristics, assessment procedures, outcome measures, time since injury, control groups, time of testing, statistical analyses, and treatment history. Despite problems, these studies do suggest several tentative conclusions. First, mild head and/or brain injury can cause neuropsychological symptoms. Second, although the presence, pattern, and duration of symptoms are generally consistent across patients, variability in clinical presentation is apparent. Although most mild head injury patients make an apparently complete recovery within days or weeks of trauma and never require medical or neuropsychological intervention, a small subset of these patients experience neurocognitive deficits that can last weeks, months, or, in some cases, years. Finally, the pattern and duration of extended post-traumatic symptoms are most likely related to variability in injury dynamics, CNS integrity, and psychological factors yet to be clearly elucidated.

In terms of clinical application, clinicians should be aware that, in most cases, people who present for assessment and intervention experience symptoms of extended duration. In such cases, it is tempting to generalize from these patients to all those who sustain mild head injury, but to do so invites problems. Also,

---

TABLE 27–1. Clinicians' Checklist

Age
Education
Occupation

History

Medical
  Systemic diseases
  Chronic diseases
  Traumatic illnesses
Medications
  Past
  Present
Psychiatric
  Diagnosed
  Undiagnosed
  Substance abuse
Medications
  Past
  Present
Neurological
Educational
Occupational

Injury

Glasgow Coma Scale
Post-traumatic amnesia
  Duration
Retrograde amnesia
  Degree
Symptoms
Computed tomography/magnetic resonance
  imaging
Neuroexam
Symptom onset
Symptom duration
Symptom intensity
Legal history
Test results
Treatment history

assuming that all people who present with extended postconcussion symptoms have a psychogenic disorder is a clinical strategy fraught with difficulty. When faced with uncertainty regarding the etiology of postconcussive symptoms, clinicians would be wise to remain neutral and note all factors—patient age, education, history (medical-psychiatric-neurological, educational, occupational), injury dynamics (physical forces), symptom presentation, duration, evolution-resolution, existence of comorbid disorders (see Table 27–1)—potentially contributing to the symptom presentation. In all cases, a balanced, thoughtful, and methodical approach to diagnosis and treatment yields more accurate test findings and treatment results than a frantic search for confirmation of a psychogenic or physiogenic hypothesis. The neuropsychological literature is replete with examples of clinicians on a psychogenic or physiogenic witch hunt, often motivated by forensic bias. In cases like mild head injury, where science is often equivocal, hard-line approaches do not appear prudent. In any case, because variability in outcome following mild head injury is apparent, a brief discussion of the basis for variable outcomes is in order.

□ VARIABILITY IN OUTCOME

One of the most critical variables for outcome after mild head injury is individual vulnerability to trauma.[34,35] Although the severity of head injury or actual brain trauma is of great importance, additional factors such as head, neck, and back pain; age; general health; premorbid intellectual abilities; previous neurological, psychiatric, and substance abuse history; the availability of family, psychosocial, economic, and vocational support systems; treatment; and pending litigation are all critically important to individual vulnerability and outcome after mild head injury.[34–38]

An example of variability in outcome is provided by Ruff et al.[39] In a study using standardized behavioral criteria for diagnosis, longitudinal assessment of memory revealed three recovery curves. One recovery curve was flat over time (no change); another showed improved memory at 6 months but a decline at 12 months. A final pattern demonstrated decline at 6 months with improvement at 12 months. The variability in memory functioning over time is likely caused by a number of factors yet to be determined, but mild head injury seems to produce variable outcomes like more severe injury. In other words, the same injury produces different outcomes, and different injuries may produce the same outcome. These findings underscore the need for caution in approaching assessment and treatment problems following mild head injury. In many cases, prolonged symptoms may be physiogenically based or have a significant psychogenic component. Accordingly, we discuss the most prominent presumed basis for psychogenic symptoms, malingering.

□ MALINGERING

There is considerable debate in the scientific literature regarding the etiology, symptoms, and assessment of malingering in the mild head injury population. The *Diagnostic and Statistical Manual of Mental Disorders,* fourth edition,[40] defines malingering as follows:

The intentional production of false or grossly exaggerated physical or psychological symptoms, motivated by external incentives such as avoiding military duty, avoiding work, obtaining financial compensation, evading criminal prosecution, or obtaining drugs. . . . Malingering should be strongly suspected . . . [in the] medicolegal context . . . [when] marked discrepancy between the person's claimed stress or disability and the objective findings [are observed]. . . . [There is] lack of cooperation during the diagnostic evaluation and in complying with the prescribed treatment regimen . . . [or there is] the presence of Antisocial Personality Disorder. (p. 683)

Portions of this definition may apply to a small percentage of patients with mild head injuries, some of whom are involved in litigation with implications for secondary gain, but only a very limited segment of the population with mild head injuries actually seeks or requires medical or neuropsychological intervention, and the vast majority of them make rapid recoveries and have good outcomes that do not require forensic solutions.

In some cases requiring medicolegal solutions, malingering could account for the clinical presentation, yet at present there are no credible scientific data to support or refute such contentions. Several studies have shown the potential for "motivational" problems in some with mild head injuries.[41,42] These "motivational" problems, often documented via symptom validity testing, are presumed to reflect malingering, although other explanations (malingering-like disorders) are possible.[43] For example, people with mild head injuries may have psychiatric disorders such as general symptom exaggeration (hypochondriasis), factitious disorders, Ganser syndrome, Munchausen syndrome, conversion and somatoform disorders, and post-traumatic stress disorder (PTSD). Even though some of these disorders, like PTSD, are thought by some to be clinically distinct from postconcussive syndrome,[44] finding "motivational problems" on symptom validity testing is not a litmus test for malingering.

Although tests have been developed to evaluate motivation and test consistency,[44,46] determining whether an individual is malingering is extremely difficult without direct covert observation of the behavior the patient claims to be unable to perform. Although such observations may someday provide us with sufficient data to correlate with neurological, neuropsychological, and psychosocial findings, the solution for measurement problems is thorough and comprehensive evaluation of all relevant factors within each individual case.[47] Accordingly, clinicians should accept patients' statements of their deficits, encourage them to provide their best performances during the examination, and explain the clinician's obligation to report their level of motivation, which can be extrapolated from their test performance. Such statements usually promote compliance and honesty.

Clinicians should be attentive to symptom clusters or deviations in test performance that are statistically rare and atypical for persons with mild injury. The key here is substantive knowledge of clinical and research findings in mild head injury. As previously recommended, clinicians should remain neutral in their approach to assessment and treatment. Unfortunately, in most cases, the perceived etiology of symptoms may be determined by clinicians' individual practices and philosophical orientations to the problem. Personal experience suggests that, for example, clinicians who examine patients for plaintiffs tend to view malingering as rare; clinicians who are experts for the defendants typically view malingering as more common. The demands of the forensic arena have made us more sensitive to this issue, although it is not clear how accurate neurologically trained clinicians (neuropsychologists, neurologists, psychiatrists) are at identifying this disorder or assessing its impact on outcome. In any case, further refinement in assessing motivation, factitious disorders, and malingering is needed.

□ TREATMENT

In addition to definitional and diagnostic issues, treatment of people with mild head injury is frequently indicated. Accordingly, treatment of mild head injury must consider physical, neurological, psychological, objective cognitive, subjective cognitive, and psychosocial-environmental factors.[48] Kay[48] has developed a treatment model based on experience with hundreds of patients with mild head injuries. This model includes the following clinical guidelines for early intervention and prevention of post concussion syndrome (PCS) and interventions initiated at a later date: Early in the recovery process, interventions should be designed to prevent development of dysfunctional adjustment. The intervention may include an educational component focused on symptoms and their resolution. Clinicians can provide cognitive therapies as needed. Clinicians should also actively manage a gradual process of return to functioning and, when possible, a return to work. In addition, the patient's family or significant other(s) can be involved in treatment planning and referral to extended treatment (e.g., cognitive therapy) for specific symptoms that do not improve spontaneously.

When symptoms have been present for some time, clinicians should validate the experience of the person and not prematurely confront emotional factors as having etiological significance. Attempts to reestablish self-efficacy via psychotherapy are recommended and may include the patient's family. Clinicians should treat emotional problems along with cognitive problems and eventually begin the process of sorting out primary from secondary deficits.

Assessment and treatment of all factors associated with individual vulnerability are crucial to effective intervention in mild head injury. Factors that contribute to individual vulnerability to mild head injury are severity of injury, pain, age, education, premorbid intellectual ability, general physical health, employment security, psychosocial support systems, information provided immediately following the injury, and premorbid psychiatric, neurological, or substance abuse problems. Whenever possible, prevention of the development or entrenchment of PCS symptoms is highly desirable.[49] Prevention is best accomplished by rapid recognition of potential problems, followed by immediate educational intervention focused on symptom development and resolution.

Encouragement and positive expectations for a speedy recovery, via weekly emotional and medical support until the patient is symptom-free, may be very effective.[48,49] At the same time, clinicians should seek to reduce stress (and vocational or educational load) and obtain appropriate treatment for noncognitive symptoms (pain) to decrease the risk of poor outcome. Factors that preclude an immediate return to work or school should be fully evaluated, and specialists in vocational and educational counseling should be consulted to determine need for specific remediation, consideration of alternative careers, or placement in special education. Neuropsychologists and rehabilitation specialists are trained in determining the need for compensation strategies and in cognitive retraining.

Postinjury emotional changes often include depression, anxiety, irritability, low frustration tolerance, and lack of motivation and initiative. These symptoms typically resolve as part of the natural recovery process over a few days or weeks, but persistent emotional sequelae can be treated by traditional psychotherapeutic techniques, especially if the clinicians are aware of the potential etiology and offer education, support, and cognitive-behavioral therapy to the patient and family who must live with these problems during recovery.

Use of alcohol at the time of injury may be a negative prognostic sign because it can prolong medical complications and recovery in some head injuries.[50] More important, those who suffered an injury secondary to alcohol abuse are likely to continue abusing alcohol postinjury. Preinjury and postinjury substance abuse is also common in the mild head injury population, and it must be diagnosed and then treated. The Brain Injury Association (formerly the National Head Injury Foundation) in its white paper on the dual problems of substance abuse and head injury[51] suggests a comprehensive evaluation of the extent of substance use and abuse. It recommends education, alternative socialization models, and a modified Alcoholics Anonymous 12-step approach whenever necessary

In the preceding discussion, we have attempted to present current research and clinical issues in mild head injury. As is apparent, much is yet to be learned about traumatic head injury, particularly the outcomes of those who experience significant and extended postconcussive symptoms. Until we can adequately link injury parameters to neurological dysfunction and associated clinical syndromes, clinicians must be comfortable with some uncertainty in the diagnostic and treatment process.

REFERENCES

1. Miller, H: Accident neurosis. BMJ 1:919, 1961.
2. Miller, H: Mental sequelae of head injury. Proceedings of the Royal Society of Medicine 59:257, 1966.
3. Oppenheimer, RD: Microscopic lesions in the brain following head injury. J Neurol Neurosurg Psychiatry 31:299, 1968.
4. Holbourn, AHS: Mechanics of head injury. Lancet 2:438, 1943.
5. Symonds, C: Concussion and its sequelae. Lancet 1:1, 1962.
6. Gennarelli, TA: Cerebral concussion and diffuse brain injury. In Cooper, PR (ed): Head Injury, ed 2. Williams & Wilkins, Baltimore, 1987, p 108.
7. Kay, T, et al: Definition of mild traumatic brain injury. J Head Trauma Rehabil 8(3):86, 1993.
8. Kibby, MY, and Long, CJ: Minor head injury: Attempts at clarifying the confusion. Brain Inj 10:159, 1996.
9. Gennarelli, TA, Adams, GH, and Graham, DI: Acceleration induced head injury in the monkey: The model, its mechanism and physiological correlate. Acta Neuropathol (Berl) (supp)7:23, 1981.
10. Ommaya, AK, and Gennarelli, TA: Cerebral concussion and traumatic unconsciousness: Correlation of experimental and clinical observations on blunt head injuries. Brain 97:633, 1974.
11. Povlishock, JT, et al: Axonal change in minor head injury. J Neuropathol Exp Neurol 42:225, 1983.
12. Dixon, EC, Taft, WC, and Hayes, RL: Mechanisms of mild traumatic brain injury. J Head Trauma Rehabil 8(3):1, 1993.
13. Gronwall, D, and Sampson, H: The Psychological Effects of Concussion. Auckland University Press, Auckland, 1980.
14. Gronwall, D, and Wrightson, P: Delayed recovery of intellectual function after minor head injury. Lancet 2:604, 1974.
15. Gronwall, D, and Wrightson, P: Duration of post-traumatic amnesia after mild head injury. Journal of Clinical Neuropsychology 1:51, 1980.
16. Wrightson, P, and Gronwall, D: Time off work and symptoms after mild head injury. Inquiry 12:445, 1980.
17. Rimel, RW, et al: Disability caused by minor head injury. Neurosurgery 9:221, 1981.
18. Barth, JT, et al: Neuropsychological sequelae of minor head injury. Neurosurgery 13:529, 1983.
19. Dikmen, SS, and Levin, HS: Methodological issues in the study of mild head injury. J Head Trauma Rehabil 8(3):30, 1993.
20. Dikmen, S, McLean, A, and Temkin, N: Neuropsychological and psychological consequences of minor head injury. J Neurol Neurosurg Psychiatry 48:1227, 1986.
21. Levin, HS, et al: Neurobehavioral outcome following minor head injury: A three center study. J Neurosurg 66:234, 1987.
22. McLean, A Jr, et al: The behavioral sequelae of head injury. Journal of Clinical Neuropsychology 5:361, 1983.
23. Macciocchi, SN: Practice makes perfect: Retest effects in college athletes. J Clin Psychol 5:628, 1990.
24. Ruff, RM, et al: Recovery of memory after mild head injury: A three center study. In Levin, HS, Eisenberg, HM, and Benton, AL (eds): Mild Head Injury, Oxford University Press, New York, 1989, p 476.
25. Barth, JT, et al: Mild head injury in sports: Neuropsychological sequelae and recovery of function. In Levin, HS, Eisenberg, HM, and Benton, AL (eds): Mild Head Injury, Oxford University Press, New York, 1989, p 257.
26. Macciocchi, SN, Barth, JT, Alves, W, Rimel, RW, and Jane, JA: Neuropsychological functioning and recovery following mild head injury in collegiate athletes. Neurosurgery 39(3):510, 1996.
27. Leininger, BE, et al: Neuropsychological deficits in symptomatic minor head injury patients after concussion and mild concussion. J Neurol Neurosurg Psychiatry 53:293, 1990.
28. Fox, DD, et al: Base rates of postconcussive symptoms in health maintenance organization patients and controls. Neuropsychology 9:606, 1995.
29. Lees-Haley, PR, and Brown, RS: Neuropsychological complaint base rates of 170 personal injury claimants. Archives of Clinical Neuropsychology 8:203, 1993.
30. Alves, WA, Macciocchi, SN, and Barth, JT: Post concussion symptoms after uncomplicated mild head injury. J Head Trauma Rehabil 8(3):48, 1993.
31. Levin, HS, et al: Magnetic resonance imaging and computerized tomography in relation to the neurobehavioral sequelae of mild and moderate head injuries. J Neurosurg 66:706, 1987.
32. Ruff, RM, et al: Selected cases of poor outcome following a minor brain trauma: Comparing neuropsychological and positron emission tomography assessment. Brain Inj 8:297, 1994.
33. Varney, NR, et al: NeuroSPECT correlates of disabling mild head injury: Preliminary findings. J Head Trauma Rehabil 10(3):18, 1995.
34. Kay, T: Neuropsychological diagnosis: Disentangling the multiple determinants of functional disability after mild

traumatic brain injury. In Horn, LJ, and Zalser, ND (eds): Rehabilitation of Post-Concussive Disorders. Hanley & Belfus, Philadelphia, 1992, p 109.

35. Kay, T, et al: Toward a neuropsychological model of functional disability after mild traumatic brain injury. Neuropsychology 6:371, 1992.

36. Barth, JT, Diamond, R, and Errico, A: Mild head injury and post concussion syndrome: Does anyone really suffer? Clin Electroencephalogr 27:183, 1996.

37. Smith, R, Barth, JT, and Diamond, R, and Giuliano, AJ: Evaluation of head trauma. In Goldstein, G, Nussbaum, PD, and Beers, SR (eds): Neuropsychology. Plenum, New York, 1998, pp 135–170.

38. Gregsby, J, and Rosenberg, NL: Chronic pain is associated with deficits in information processing. Percept Mot Skills 81:403, 1995.

39. Ruff, RM, et al: Verbal learning deficits following severe head injury: What recovery occurs after one year? J Neurosurg 75:50, 1991.

40. Diagnostic and Statistical Manual of Mental Disorders, ed 4. American Psychiatric Association, Washington, DC, 1994, p 683.

41. Binder, LM, and Willis, SC: Assessment of motivation after financially compensable minor head trauma. J Consul Clin Psychol 3:175, 1991.

42. Youngjohn, JR, Burrows, L, and Erdal, K: Brain damage or compensation neurosis? The controversial post-concussion syndrome. Clinical Neuropsychologist 9:112, 1995.

43. Ruff, RM, Wylie, T, and Tennant, W: Malingering and malingering-like aspects of mild closed head injury. J Head Trauma Rehabil 8(3):60, 1993.

44. Rattok, J, and Boake, C: Do patients with mild brain injuries have posttraumatic stress disorder too? J Head Trauma Rehabil 11(1):95, 1996.

45. Binder, LM: Assessment of malingering after mild head trauma with the Portland Digit Recognition Test. J Clin Exp Neuropsychol 15:170, 1993.

46. Hiscock, M, and Hiscock, CK: Refining the forced-choice method for the detection of malingering. J Clin Exp Neuropsychol 11:967, 1989.

47. Millis, SR, and Putnam, SH: Evaluation of malingering in the neuropsychological examination of mild head injury. NeuroRehabilitation 7:55, 1996.

48. Kay, T: Neuropsychological treatment of mild traumatic brain injury. J Head Trauma Rehab 8(3):74, 1993.

49. Mittenberg, W, et al: Cognitive-behavioral prevention of post concussive syndrome. Archives of Clinical Neuropsychology 11:139, 1996.

50. Sparadeo, FR, Strauss, D, and Barth, JT: The incidence, impact, and treatment of substance abuse in head trauma rehabilitation. J Head Trauma Rehabil 5(3):1, 1990.

51. National Head Injury Foundation: Substance Abuse Task Force White Paper. NHIF, Southborough, Mass, 1988, p 1.

Sexuality and Sexual Dysfunction

AMY HERSTEIN GERVASIO, PHD,
and ERNEST R. GRIFFITH, MD

In the Western world, sexual mores have changed more rapidly in the last century than at any other time in history.[1] The effects of this change on society at large are debated in academic fields, in legislative bodies, and in the media. The field of scientific sex research has also grown. Yet, the empirical literature on sexual health after catastrophic injury such as brain injury is rather sparse.

Current scholarship emphasizes the interplay of biological, psychological, and social factors in sexual health and sexual dysfunction.[2] Only recently has research addressed the sexual problems of chronically ill people. In the case of the person with traumatic brain injury (TBI), physical disability coupled with cognitive losses may contribute to a multitude of difficulties in sexuality and intimacy after injury.

This chapter is divided into four major parts. We first present an overview of the scope of research on sexuality after TBI, including the prevalence and types of sexual problems, with particular reference to brain and behavior relationships. A section on functional issues and the psychological responses of the person and partner follows. The third section describes assessment and treatment methods. Fourth, we integrate sexual concerns with a developmental model of sexuality across the lifespan, paying special attention to problems arising in people with brain injury and institutionalized populations.

□ PREVALENCE AND TYPES OF SEXUAL DYSFUNCTION AFTER TRAUMATIC BRAIN INJURY

Definitions

Sexuality encompasses more than the ability to perform sexual acts. It includes a person's capacity to love and maintain relationships, attitudes and beliefs about sex and reproduction, and implicit knowledge of the social context of sexual behavior and gender roles. Forms of sexual expression may vary with the age and cultural background of the individual.[3] For our purposes, the term *sexual behavior* includes verbal, visual, and tactile communication as well as auditory, gustatory, and olfactory experiences that express love and intimacy between two people,[4] or solitary behavior such as masturbation. *Gender identity* refers to a person's subjectively experienced sense of self as male or female. This subjective sense may develop from participation in the social roles and habits commonly ascribed to men and women in a given culture, including emphasis on certain physical features, dress, mannerisms, interpersonal dynamics, nurturing roles, and occupations. In a circular fashion, gender identity may be predicated upon engaging in specific kinds of sexual behavior. For example, men traditionally initiate sexual relationships, and vaginal sexual intercourse is viewed as the basic goal of sexual

Thanks go to Adrienne Witol, Psy D, for her editorial comments and suggestions for case material.

behavior. A man who cannot participate in these events may view himself as unmanly and question his gender identity.

Most authors in the area of sexual dysfunction identify four broad classes of difficulty: desire, arousal, orgasm, and pain. Infertility may also be classified as a type of "sexual problem." The actual diagnostic categories of sexual dysfunction are shaped by our society's definitions of functional sex: problems with erection in men, vaginal lubrication and painful intercourse in women, and difficulties achieving orgasm through sexual intercourse.[1] The *Diagnostic and Statistical Manual of Mental Disorders* (DSM-IV) lists nine kinds of dysfunction, corresponding to the four major categories.[5] Complaints about the level of sexual satisfaction are not part of this diagnostic schema. However, an individual's subjective reports of the overall level of sexual satisfaction may not correlate well with the presence of a diagnosed "sexual dysfunction."[6] Similarly, the presence of a particular kind of dysfunction does not necessarily correlate with a particular etiology. Thus, several multiaxial systems of classification have been developed. For example, LoPiccolo's[7] system specifies information such as whether a person can achieve orgasm through masturbation, whether the problem has been lifelong, and whether it is situational.

Prevalence of Sexual Dysfunction

The prevalence and incidence of sexual dysfunction in the general population are hard to estimate because research relies heavily on self-report data. One study estimated that the lifetime incidence of sexual dysfunction is 24 percent.[8] The hallmark of sexual dysfunctions associated with brain injury is their diversity. Preexisting dysfunctions can persist or be aggravated by the injury, associated injuries, medical complications, and subsequent physical or psychosocial events. Dysfunctions may appear *de novo* at various times after the injury. Although many sex researchers prefer to think in terms of biopsychosexual health rather than focus on physiological dysfunction, the neurological literature has tended to discuss the latter. Case studies of exotic problems such as Klüver-Bucy syndrome abound in the literature, emphasizing symptoms that do not seem to apply to the majority of people with TBI.

It is hard to estimate the true prevalence of sexual dysfunction after TBI. In a population of more then 700 veterans with TBI, Walker and Jablon[9] estimated that 8.1 percent experienced decreased potency. Yet Meyer[10] reported that 81 subjects in a sample of 100 men with a variety of neurological problems had experienced erectile dysfunction after illness. A study of men with postconcussive head injuries reported that 58 percent of subjects experienced reduced sexual drive.[11] Few empirical data exist on the sexual dysfunction of women with TBI or on the sexual dysfunction of the partners of people with TBI. Family studies focusing on the interpersonal relationships of spouses suggest that the sexual relationship is altered in the majority of cases.[12–15] Using a very detailed questionnaire comparing sexual behavior before and after injury, Garden et al.[16] found that 47 percent of the 15 couples in the sample were dissatisfied with the frequency of intercourse and overall marital sexual adjustment. In a slightly different vein, the staff sample polled in Davis and Schneider[17] reported that "less access to intimacy" was a major barrier to sexuality in a rehabilitation setting.

Zasler's[18] review of 13 studies of sexual functioning following TBI concludes that most of the studies report declines in frequency of intercourse, "altered libido," and other unspecified negative changes. A number of studies report increases in erectile dysfunction. Fewer studies considered changes in expression of affection or subjective feelings of reduced sex appeal. Because nearly all of these studies follow patients for a very limited time, they do not reflect the ultimate course of sexual difficulties over a lifetime after a traumatic brain injury.

Primary Sexual Dysfunction

Sexual disorders after brain injury can be categorized as organic or functional.[19] Organic disorders are those caused by physical or medical conditions; functional disorders are those in which psychosocial impairments are the basis of disability. As in other areas of TBI, attempting to designate sexual disorders as organic versus functional presents the problem of differentiating psychological deficits directly related to organic brain injury from those related to secondary psychological reactions to organic deficits or to the responses of others. For example, depression may be directly related to brain injury (organic) or arise secondary to negative consequences of recovery from injury (functional). In practice, it is often difficult to clearly distinguish between organic and functional disorders. Frequently, the survivor's dysfunctions are multiple, and many are of mixed etiology.

There are five major etiologic categories of organic sexual dysfunctions after TBI: neurological, endocrinological, musculoskeletal, craniofacial, and medical complications. Neurological factors involve the brain itself, concomitant spinal cord injury, and conditions affecting the peripheral nervous system. Endocrine disorders usually involve the hypothalamic-pituitary–end organ axis. Preexisting medical conditions or sequelae of postinjury medical complications and conditions are also factors in dysfunction. Finally, the side effects of a host of medications taken by the person with brain injury can cause sexual dysfunctions.[19–21] Functional etiologic factors include behavioral and emotional reactions to the injury and its consequences, psychosocial sequelae of cognitive-perceptual-executive deficits, post-traumatic stress disorders, and psychological responses to postinjury stresses. Table 28–1 relates types of sexual dysfunction to sites of brain injury.[19]

The most universally reported sexual problems are decreased libido, decreased frequency of sexual activity, erectile dysfunction (impotence), and inappropriate behaviors. Erectile dysfunction is probably more often identified as a problem for survivors of mild brain injury. There is insufficient research on the relative frequency of organic versus functional etiology in erectile dysfunction. Similarly, we have inadequate data concerning the integrity of the stages of sexual response after injury. Clinically, it appears that the sexual responses of excitement, vaginal lubrication, ejaculation, and orgasm are generally intact unless there are problems such as medication side effects, endocrine disorders, or spinal cord and peripheral nerve or nerve root injuries.

NEUROLOGICAL AND ENDOCRINOLOGICAL FACTORS

Neurological and endocrinological factors have been recently described by several researchers.[19,22] Hypothalamic or pituitary injury can affect sexual functions by inducing hypofunction of ovaries, testes, thyroid, or adrenal glands.[19] Occasional reports of precocious puberty appear in the literature.[23] Temporolimbic epilepsy (TLE) is associated with endocrine disorders.[24] In women, polycystic ovarian syndrome is associated with predominantly left-sided interictal epileptic discharge and hypogonadism with right-sided discharges. About half of the males with temporolimbic epilepsy are impotent or hyposexual. Bilateral anteromedial temporal lobe injuries can result in the Klüver-

TABLE 28–1. Relations Between Nature and Sites of Injury and Types of Sexual Problems

Function	Impairment	Effect on Sexuality
	Prefrontal	
Emotion/behavior	Dorsolateral lesions: abulia	Inability to fantasize Lack of initiation, indifference but sex responses intact
	Orbital-inferior lesions: disinhibition, discontrol, and rage-violence	Impulsive, inappropriate, disrupted sexual responses
	Combined lesions: diminished executive skills, diminished attention	Selfish, childish, vulnerable to seduction, pregnancy
	Temporal lobe and limbic	
Sensation	Taste, smell, hearing	Loss of components of arousal
Language	Aphasia, apraxia, poverty of thought	Inability to express affection Diminished social skill
	Problems in receptive speech	Inability to follow instruction re contraception
Perceptual	Decreased musical awareness	Decreased expression, fantasy arousal
	Limbic seizures with endocrine disorder	
Emotion/behavior		Interictal: bizarre behaviors
	Cerebellar injuries	
Motor	Dyscoordination, balance	Clumsiness, poor positioning
	Dysarthria, nystagmus	Communication problems, oral control, cosmesis
	Other brain stem injuries	
Motor	Cranial nerve deficits: diplopia, facial paresis, vocal paresis	Cosmesis, oral control, communication deficits
Sensory	Cranial nerve deficits: vision, taste, hearing, smell loss, vertigo	Loss of arousing stimuli, nausea with head movements
Behavior	Locked-in syndrome	Helplessness, vulnerable to abuse
	RAS damage	Lethargy; disturbed sleep-wake cycle

Bucy syndrome, which is characterized by sexual and oral activity with inappropriate objects.[25]

Seizures can be related to sexual function in other respects. Hyperventilation during sexual excitement is a potential inducer of seizures. Elevations of estrogen blood levels in pregnancy and during the menstrual cycle lower seizure threshold. Seizures during sexual activity are disruptive, frightening to an unsuspecting partner, and embarrassing to the person who experiences them. On rare occasions, temporolimbic seizures are accompanied by sensations of genital arousal and autonomic changes associated with arousal. TLE events may not have sexual manifestations, but in the postictal period sexual arousal can be heightened. More often the postictal state is marked by decreased sexuality and bizarre practices such as fetishism, transvestism, exhibitionism, and occasionally change in gender preference.[26]

Frontal lobe injuries produce syndromes that can greatly influence sexual functions. Dorsolateral injuries induce varying degrees of sexual indifference, along with reduced sexual initiation. In extreme cases, the patient may show near-total inertia, but physical sexual responses usually are intact and coitus is possible. Orbital injuries can result in impulsive, disinhibited behavior leading to coprolalia, sexual propositioning, and other inappropriate acts. However, with rare exceptions, people with orbital injuries are "all talk." Their sexual activity may be compromised by erectile dysfunction and ejaculatory difficulties. The extreme of hypersexual arousal has been described as "sexual rage." Although uncommon, it has been associated with orbital injuries.

Frontal lobe injuries also affect executive functioning, attention and concentration, imagination and fantasizing, and abstract thinking. These problems, coupled with childish, dependent, selfish, and silly behaviors, disrupt capacity for intimacy and fragment interpersonal relationships.[27] Such injuries may lead to the "secondary" or functional sexual dysfunctions of partners. Finally, frontal injuries, particularly those involving the left hemisphere, have been implicated in organic depression. In turn, depression—regardless of its source—is a major cause of reduced libido and erectile dysfunction.

Sensory deficits can involve primary and secondary sexual organs, the hands, face, and other erogenous or explorative sites. The sensory organs of smell, touch, taste, vision, and hearing potentially contribute to enhancement of sexual pleasure. When they are damaged, changes in degree of sexual arousal or intensity may occur. Perceptual deficits may affect any modality of sensation. Visual-perceptual losses can produce hemineglect and misidentifications of distance, speed of movement, and shapes and sizes of ob-

jects. Thus, the person with brain injury may not be able to coordinate parts of the body during sex or properly apply contraceptive devices. Tactile disturbances may include hemineglect and bizarre or unpleasant sensations during sex. Lack of time sense and spatial distortions may have implications for courting and dating activities.

PERIPHERAL AND OTHER INJURIES

Spinal cord injury (SCI) coexists with traumatic brain injury in about 3.2 percent of head injury cases.[28] In addition, some researchers have suggested that 30 to 40 percent of SCI patients also experience concussion.[29] Upper and lower motor neuron lesions lead to various neurogenic sexual disorders, accompanied by neurogenic bowel and bladder dysfunction. Bowel and bladder problems may lead to urgency or incontinence during sex acts, poor personal hygiene, poor self-image, and embarrassment. Catheters and drainage bags can be formidable obstacles to intimacy.

Peripheral nervous system injuries such as lumbosacral plexus lesions may also produce bladder, bowel, and sexual dysfunctions. Genital sensation and sexual responses can be involved. Although rare in brain injury, vascular injuries such as aortic rupture or pelvic arterial damage can result in genital vascular compromise, another cause of erectile insufficiency.

MUSCULOSKELETAL AND CRANIOFACIAL FACTORS

Motor problems can directly affect sexual activity and indirectly affect "cosmesis," sexual attractiveness, and self-image. Increased spasticity may disrupt sexual acts. Hemiparesis, ataxia, apraxias, and involuntary movement disorders such as chorea, athetosis, tremors, dystonias, and myotonia may affect mobility and positioning. The poor oral-labial function associated with many of these disorders leads to drooling and difficulties with kissing, oral sexual stimulation, and speech, not to mention problems in dining. Musculoskeletal sequelae such as contractures and bony deformities (e.g., hip contractures) may preclude comfortable positioning, make intromission difficult, and cause distracting pain.

The residua of craniomaxillofacial injuries are mainly cosmetic problems. Facial nerve injuries, squints, depressions of the skull, laceration scars, and dental defects are among the deformities that are so damaging to self-image and self-esteem.

PHARMACOLOGICAL FACTORS

Medication is probably one of the most implicated yet overlooked factors in sexual dysfunction after brain injury. The list of potential offenders is impressively long, as Table 28–2 suggests. Chief among them are anticonvulsants, antipsychotics, antidepressants, and serotoninergics—all of which are commonly prescribed for people with TBI.

Secondary Sexual Dysfunctions after TBI

People with TBI sustain a host of functional or "secondary" sexual dysfunctions stemming from cognitive and behavioral difficulties. Despite a lack of systematic research on the relationship between cognitive deficits and the maintenance of sexual and interpersonal relationships, clinical experience suggests that these deficits may pose

more problems for people with TBI than actual physical disabilities. Because these difficulties are not usually thought of as "sexual," both the practitioner, the individual, and the partner may misattribute problems to primary neurological disorders. Chief among these difficulties are deficiencies in self-care, executive functioning, emotional regulation, and behavior.[21]

DISORDERS IN SELF-CARE

Maintenance of sexual attractiveness requires activities of daily living (ADL) skills, including good hygiene and grooming. Dressing and undressing are an important part of foreplay in our society. Use of contraceptive devices requires memory, planning, and often physical

---

TABLE 28–2. Drugs That May Cause Sexual Dysfunctions

Drug Class	Clinical Effect
Anorexics Amphetamines	Decreased libido, impotence, ejaculatory dysfunction, anorgasmia
Anticholinergics Oxybutynin Scopolamine	Inhibited erection and ejaculation, decreased libido
Anticonvulsants Carbamazepine Phenytoin	Impotence and decreased libido, secondary hypogonadism (phenytoin)
Antidepressants Nortriptyline Doxepin	Decreased libido, delayed female orgasm, ejaculatory and erectile dysfunction
Antihypertensives Beta-blockers Methyldopa Clonidine	Impotence, decreased libido, and ejaculatory dysfunction
Nonsteroidal anti-inflammatory drugs Naproxen	Erectile problems, anejaculation
Noradrenergic agonists Yohimbine Activating TCSs	Increased libido in both sexes
Phenoxybenzamine	Ejaculatory dysfunction
Progestins Medroxyprogesterone Cyproterone	Decreased libido, impotence
Serotoninergic agonists Trazadone Sertraline Paroxetine	Decreased libido, reports of increased libido in females

Source: Adapted from Zasler, N: Traumatic brain injury and sexuality. In Monga, T (ed): Sexuality and Disability. Hanley & Belfus, Philadelphia, 1995, p 371, with permission.

coordination. Deficiencies in any of these skills can jeopardize a new relationship.

EXECUTIVE FUNCTIONING AND SEXUALITY

Sexual problems related to frontal lobe syndromes can be particularly dramatic. People with executive functioning problems may have difficulty in orchestrating the complex planning involved in dating and social skills. Impulsivity and poor judgment are not conducive to sustaining relationships or to providing a good sexual experience for one's partner. Conversely, the person with TBI who is lethargic and uninterested is also unrewarding as a partner.

Many people with brain injury seem to lose their imaginative capacities, including the capacity to fantasize. Because fantasy seems to be a crucial component of romantic and sexual experience, brain injured people may find romantic and sexual relationships less satisfying without knowing why. Partners may complain of "lack of spontaneity" after an injury. The person with brain injury may be capable of sexual behavior only after a certain routine has been satisfied (e.g., only at night or only in a particular room). People who have deficits in executive functioning are also at risk for sexual exploitation; they may quickly agree to sex with strangers but lack the skills to disentangle themselves from abusive situations.

Memory deficiencies also have consequences for sexual relationships. The person with TBI may forget how often sex has occurred or may perseverate in making sexual requests or comments, which can prove embarrassing for relatives, as well as for the patient.

COMMUNICATION

Communication to a partner of sexual wants and comfort level is presumed to be essential in sex therapy.[1] However, the person with TBI may be impaired by aphasia, dysarthria, or other communication disorders. Reduced ability to abstract and decreased ideation may also inhibit communication. Inability to generalize may make it more difficult for a person to perform newly learned but appropriate verbal behavior in different settings or with different people. Nonverbal communication is also crucial in sexual relationships. Because of physical or perceptual difficulties, the person may not be able to use touch, gestures, or facial cues in the same manner as before injury, or the person may misjudge the nonverbal behavior of others, assuming that it is sexual in tone when it is not. Failure to express desires, to utter a compli-

mentary phrase, or to refuse certain sexual advances may lead to frustration for both partners.[21]

EMOTIONAL REGULATION AND BEHAVIORAL DISORDERS

In brain injury, emotional disorders are often related to behavioral problems. The person who is easily frustrated or prone to the "catastrophic reaction" may throw things or verbally berate others. Disorders of the limbic system can also have a "secondary" impact on sexual expression. People with emotional lability may cry during heightened periods of emotional expression such as sex. Vituperative outbursts may follow a slight rebuff during lovemaking, which may halt the act altogether. More often, the frequent temper tantrums that the person with brain injury directs toward the spouse diminish the partner's desire to engage in sexual behavior in the first place.

PSYCHOLOGICAL RESPONSES OF THE BRAIN INJURED PERSON AND THE FAMILY

Other psychological reactions to TBI may increase sexual dysfunction. People with brain injury may suffer a loss of self-esteem. They may be able to recognize, but not articulate, changes in reasoning abilities, memory, and functional capacities. They may be aware of changes in their appearance and in their sexual attractiveness. They may not feel in control of their sexual organs or desires. A man may be embarrassed by spontaneous erections. Especially in the early stages of recovery, the caregiver's provision of intimate personal genital care or bowel and bladder care may make the person feel infantilized.[21] Similarly, the partner of a person with brain injury may have to delegate bowel and bladder care to others to emotionally "decouple" it from sexual behavior.

The survivor who went through a phase of agitation that included exhibiting sexual behavior may be newly embarrassed when reminded of "how crazy you acted" by family. Discriminating between previous unsuitable behavior and currently acceptable discussion of sexual feelings may be difficult.

The family members of the person with brain injury may be equally troubled and embarrassed by the person's sexual behavior. Many family members assume that the swearing, public masturbation, and obscene gestures found in the early phases of recovery are a result of "bad upbringing and parenting." Their own embarrassment further distances them from the relative with brain injury.

Responses of the Partner

The person with brain injury and the spouse experience role changes almost immediately. Even in the hospital setting, partners often become caregivers. This role demands more parental than spousal behavior. It places the injured patient in the role of the child; the spouse may feel as though the relationship is nonreciprocal and inequitable. The tired, overburdened spouse may find the injured person sexually unattractive, perhaps even repulsive. Even after months in the hospital, neither the injured person nor the spouse may feel the need for sex. Even if they do feel sexual desire, they may not express it for fear that engaging in sex would physically harm the patient in some way.[27] Thus, it may come as a surprise to the partner when the patient makes a first tentative but appropriate sexual overture.

On occasion, the spouse may use the brain injury as an excuse to curtail an already unhappy sexual relationship. Other spouses find that the very real headaches of the person with brain injury preclude comfortable sex. When the healthy spouse directs anger at the patient for "causing" the accident, decreased sexual feelings may ensue.

The injured person and the partner may also have to overcome religious or cultural taboos to resume their sex life. Use of contraception may pose religious problems for Catholics. Oral sex, mutual masturbation, or use of sexual aids may violate religious tenets as well as strongly held personal beliefs. The diminution in the capacity for fantasy, coupled with societal taboos, may also make partners feel awkward when engaging in new kinds of sexual behavior.

Responses of Parents

Parents of the injured person may also have negative responses to the adult child's sexual behavior. Many parents deny that their single children have sexual partners. If the parents exercised the "not in my house" option prior to injury, they will be less likely to feel comfortable condoning sexual behavior after injury. Even when the injured person is married, the parents may be involved in caretaking. Asking parents to handle their adult child's genitals may be understandably difficult for both parent and child.

RESPONSES OF THE PROFESSIONAL STAFF

Hospital staff may have difficulty conceiving of the person with brain injury as a potentially competent adult. "Patients" are often viewed as asexual.[30] Thus, the brain injured person's unsuitable sexual behavior can create great tension among staff and between the person and staff. Even experienced staff find it difficult to respond consistently to the brain injured person's inappropriate sexual behavior, without embarrassment. The problem is compounded when staff can not agree on the acceptability of specific public or private behaviors or on what constitutes appropriate touch or verbal affection. In fact, the behaviors that are inappropriate may change during the course of the rehab stay. For example, how should a nurse who enters a single room without knocking respond when she finds a patient masturbating? The environmental context would seem to be an important determinant.

RESPONSES OF THE COMMUNITY

Community reentry is difficult for the person with brain injury. A double, even paradoxical, standard exists in America regarding sexual display in public. Sexual exhibitionism and sexually charged language are not tolerated in legally sanctioned public settings such as malls, theaters, and parks. On the one hand, bars and restaurant chains flaunt the sexual attractiveness of their employees; on the other, overt sexual display on the part of the customers is discouraged. Underground sexual communities have always existed, as in the case of gay bath houses; these, too, have their own "rules."

The emotional aftermaths of sexual abuse and sexual harassment have been well publicized. What is considered verbally appropriate has changed in recent years, as well. Women who might previously have tolerated unwelcome sexual behavior from men are now quite properly encouraged to speak up. Research shows that men and women consistently differ in their perceptions of what constitutes verbal sexual harassment.[31] For the person with brain injury, however, disentangling the paradoxical messages becomes even harder. Training in social skills and the generalization of these skills to a variety of community settings become very important.

□ ASSESSMENT OF SEXUAL DYSFUNCTION

The clinician who attempts to gain information about sexual functioning from cognitively intact clients can often assume the following: The client will be embarrassed, may not understand medically correct terms, and may be misinformed about sexual functioning.[3] Clinicians working with people with TBI may find it doubly difficult to elicit accurate information from people with memory losses, distractibility, reduction in executive functioning, and impulsivity. For these reasons, it is often crucial to involve a spouse or partner in the assessment process, with the recognition that the partner may also unwittingly provide erroneous or otherwise biased information. On occasion, a parent or close friend may be able to corroborate information about the sexual experiences of the patient.

The essentials of the assessment have been well described in several rehabilitation publications.[19–21] The three components are the sexual history interview, the physical examination, and selected laboratory studies as indicated by conclusions reached from history and examination. The interview is a critical method of assessment for understanding sexual dysfunction. The clinician may propose separate interviews with both partners as well as a conjoint interview. We have found that a coassessment method of separate interviews by a physiatrist and another professional—usually a psychologist or social worker—is effective.

Because one member of the couple may provide information that he or she does not wish to disclose to the partner, issues of confidentiality must be resolved before beginning the assessment and therapeutic relationship. In our experience, complete information about sexual history is not usually obtained in one or even several interviews. It is more likely furnished over time as rapport between patient or partner and interviewer(s) grows.

The Interview and Sexual History

Topics to be covered in the interview should first include the patient's own presentation of the problem. A detailed psychosexual and medical history is also indicated. The sexual history should include sections covering childhood, adolescence, and adulthood. Information about messages concerning sex, religion and guilt, sexual abuse or neglect, body image, and relationships with peers can be as useful as information about menarche, menopause, or the memory of one's first sexual experience. Dating practices are also important. The clinician should ask about frequency and intensity of specific sexual acts, foreplay, masturbation, and both heterosexual and homosexual experiences. The role of alcohol or drugs in sexual arousal should also be explored. When dealing with married adults, knowledge of extramarital affairs may prove important for understanding current sexual and relationship issues. Finally,

the sexual history should include a thorough discussion of current medications the person with TBI is taking because many commonly used medications may affect sexual arousal and performance.

Clinicians may be almost as uncomfortable asking sexual questions as the patient is in answering them. By isolating sexual questions from questions about relationships, professionals may inadvertently reinforce a medical model of sexual functioning. Therefore, we first embed discussions about sex in questions about relationships[1,2] and then ask very direct questions about genital function, such as the occurrence of diurnal and nocturnal erections and ejaculation in men or vaginal lubrication and arousal for women.[19] It is also informative to ask questions about interpersonal behavior other than sexual intercourse. Besides assessing sexual history, the interview can also be used to assess the person's sexual knowledge of reproductive cycles, fertility, contraception, or the risks for sexually transmitted diseases.

Regardless of the context of questioning, it is imperative to use correct sexual terminology and to ensure that the patient understands the terminology. By using noneuphemistic language, the clinician models a more precise way to communicate about sex for the client and partner. Later, as the clinician gets to know the client, he or she may judiciously use slang or euphemistic language to develop rapport. Different professionals working with the same client should clarify their use of terms. For instance, psychologists and psychiatrists follow the DSM-IV[5] in using the term *erectile dysfunction,* while the more familiar but deconnotative term *impotence* is often used by urologists.

Self-Report Inventories

In addition to the interview, self-report questionnaires for the client and partner may be useful. The partner or significant other may have to complete the surveys alone if the patient has cognitive difficulties. If the clinician must read the inventories to the client, the validity of the information will depend in part on the rapport between clinician and client.

Two representative inventories used in the field of sexual dysfunction are the Sexual Interaction Inventory (SII) and the Derogatis Sexual Functioning Index (DSFI). The SII[7] asks respondents to indicate how pleasant they find 17 sexual behaviors as well as their beliefs about the partner's view of the experience. The DSFI[32] contains 245 items scored as contributing to 10 domains: information, experience, drive, attitudes, psychological symptoms, affect, gender-role definition, fantasy, body image, and sexual satisfaction. The Sexual Opinion Survey (SOS)[33] assesses the respondent's positive and negative affective and evaluative responses to a range of sexual stimuli, including descriptions of fantasy and visual stimuli. The SOS takes about 10 minutes to complete.

To our knowledge, only one research report on sexuality after TBI used an instrument previously validated on the general population.[34] Only Kreutzer and Zasler[35] specifically devised a sexual functioning inventory for a TBI population. They incorporated a variety of items from standard interviews used in brain injury and other sex inventories. Additional frequently used inventories may focus on the marital relationship in general rather than on sexual behaviors per se. For example, some sex therapists use the Dyadic Adjustment Scale,[36] in which sex is only one of many areas of agreement and conflict assessed.

The advantage of using standardized inventories originally designed for the general population is that their reliability has been fairly well established, and scores can be compared to non-TBI groups. People often find it easier to answer printed questions than to talk face to face. Inventories can be useful to provide guidance for therapy, but they should not be used alone to "diagnose" sexual dysfunction. During a feedback session focusing on the results of the assessment, discussion with the client and partner should emphasize the importance of their participation in an intimate or sexual relationship that is satisfactory to them rather than comparing themselves to a mythical "average."

Medical Examination and Diagnostic Studies

The physical examination is directed to the neurological, endocrine, genitourinary, gynecologic, and musculoskeletal systems and any other systems as indicated by the history. Consultations with other specialists such as a gynecologist or endocrinologist may be indicated. The neurological evaluation should include testing for intactness of sacral reflexes and genital sensation. Mobility, communication, and self-care skills pertinent to preparations for and engagement in sexual activities can be evaluated by therapists or the physiatrist. Hygienic and cosmetic aspects should be noted. Elements of the medical evaluation are listed in Table 28–3.

Based on the conclusions derived from history and physical examination, appropriate diagnostic studies can be pursued. Penile erectile insufficiency can be further assessed by noctur-

---

TABLE 28–3. Elements of the Medical Examination

Intactness of sacral reflexes
Intactness of genital sensation
Penile tumescence testing
Penile dorsal nerve somatosensory evoked potentials
Endocrine study of serum hormones
Cytological study of vaginal secretions
Radiographic studies of inhibiting contractures
Urodynamic studies

---

nal penile tumescence testing. Endocrine studies may include measurement of serum hormones secreted by the hypothalamus, the pituitary gland, and its end organs. Cytological study of vaginal secretions can be informative. Contractures and musculoskeletal deformities may require up-to-date radiographic studies. Electromyography and nerve conduction studies such as penile dorsal nerve somatosensory evoked potentials are an extension of the neurological examination. Urodynamic studies may add further information concerning genital innervation.

Information gleaned from the interview, inventories, medical exam, and behavioral assessment may reveal that the sexual problem is directly related to the brain injury or, conversely, that its onset predated the injury and is part of larger relationship or social skills issues. Findings from all assessment sources should be shared with the TBI survivor, partner, and, when indicated, family and caregivers. Illustrations, handouts, and other informational aids will clarify the discussion and provide ongoing resources to the partners. Recommendations for remediation should be offered, and the partners should be afforded ample opportunity for asking questions and participating in further planning.

☐ MANAGEMENT AND TREATMENT OF SEXUAL PROBLEMS

Comprehensive treatment of the many diverse forms of sexual dysfunction and facilitation of intimacy require an extended continuum of care and a professional team approach during the lifetime of the survivor. Physical-medical treatment must be blended with educational training and counseling expertise. Education of professional staff can be integrated into the total rehabilitation program, but practically speaking, only a few professional specialties routinely focus on the sexual concerns of the patient. At the outpatient level, the person with TBI and the partner are more likely to express their concerns to physicians, nurses, psychologists, and social workers, who historically are known to "be interested in sex." Nevertheless, all rehabilitation disciplines have roles to play in the management and treatment of sexual dysfunction. But before they can do so effectively, the professionals' sensitivity to and expertise in dealing with sexual dysfunction must be assessed. Consideration of the training of professional staff should precede attempts to institute sex therapy for patients.

Research on Sexuality Education and Disability

Research suggests that few professionals in occupational and physical therapy have extensive training in how to provide sex education.[38] Clinical experience suggests that one cannot take for granted the comfort level of staff from any discipline, including nursing, when discussing sexual concerns of patients.

Recent research in disability and sexuality has found that, compared with studies in the early 1980s, staff have more liberal, if vague, attitudes about the importance of sexuality and sex education with disabled populations such as the mentally regarded.[37] Gill[38] found that rehabilitation professionals agreed that sexual adjustment was important but only 9 percent of the staff indicated that they felt comfortable discussing sexual issues with patients. Rarely did staff initiate discussion of sexual issues; most waited for patients to ask questions. Staff feel that lack of pertinent training precludes their ability to bring up sexual issues comfortably.[39,40]

Davis and Schneider[17] found that staff attitudes, discomfort, and biases were a barrier to successful discussion of sexual issues with patients. Ducharme and Gill[38] speculate about the reasons why staff avoid discussions about sexuality: general anxiety about sexual issues, myths that sex education may increase the patient's sexual inappropriateness, myths that people with TBI are either hypersexual or asexual, overprotection of the patient, lack of inclusion of patients in setting rehabilitation goals, and a tendency to moralize. In addition, they perceptively note that anger at the patient's generally inappropriate behavior may lead to overly restrictive limit setting on sexual behavior.

Boundaries between professionals and patients are sorely taxed when dealing with problems of a sexual nature. Some professionals may overidentify with patients. Others may rightly demonstrate self-awareness of boundaries and limitations when they choose *not* to discuss sexual issues with patients (e.g., when a staff member strongly disapproves of premarital sex).[41]

Finally, several authors note that in the majority of TBI rehabilitation settings, young female staff work with young male patients.[38,41] This "imbalance" puts female staff at risk for being perceived as sexual objects by patients who are chronological peers. Inexperienced female staff are liable to ignore unsuitable sexual behavior or half-flirtatiously respond to it. Conversely, staff are wary of sexual advances made by patients and may be concerned that broaching a sexual issue with a patient will be misperceived as a sexual overture.

Educating the Rehabilitation Professional about Sexual Issues

Several models from the sex education and sex therapy literature, as well as from the work on sexuality after disability, can be applied to education of professionals who work with a TBI population. The PLISSIT model is a widely cited guideline that identifies four levels of staff involvement in sexual concerns.[42] In the first level, "permission giving," staff convey to patients that their concerns are normal and encourage open discussion. They may direct patients to others who can better help them find remedies for their concerns. At the second level, "limited information," staff may give information by using diagrams and charts. The third level, called "specific suggestions," may involve suggesting specific sexual exercises, viewing more explicit training videos, referring to support groups, or communication training. The last level, called "intensive therapy," involves referral to experts in sexual counseling or in medicosurgical aspects of sexual dysfunction. The PLISSIT model also applies to the actual process of counseling the patient. For example, early in rehabilitation, persons with TBI or relatives may desire only a brief discussion of sexuality; several months into outpatient treatment, they may request specific suggestions or intensive therapy.

Training procedures for professionals are varied. They range from 1-day workshops to multiweek courses.[1] Intensive workshops often involve both didactic presentation and experiential exercises in which participants present a guided fantasy concerning the impact of chronic illness on their sexual life. Later in the workshops, they are also asked to write down and discuss their biases and judgments regarding sexual fantasies or experiences. In specialty courses, the topics range from strategies to deal with prevalent sexual dysfunction, such as premature ejaculation or anorgasmia, to the impact of sexuality after cancer, renal disease, and chronic pain. Other programs include presentations by disabled people. Smith,[43] a disabled nurse, describes a "sociosexual" discussion of misconceptions about sexuality after disability that includes his own experiences as a patient.

Regardless of the methods of training, educators from all disciplines agree that awareness of one's own sexual values and biases is crucial to becoming an effective educator on sexual matters.[44,45] Formal sexual attitude reassessment (SAR) workshops,[46] which may include role-playing exercises, are encouraged, but personal reflection concerning one's own sexual milestones and attitudes is a must.[41]

Treatment Roles of Staff

Each professional on the rehabilitation team has a role to play in functional retraining of sexual behavior. Nurses can be involved in teaching people to use contraception and prostheses as well as helping increase hygienic skills such as skin care, oral hygiene, and bowel and bladder preparation. Physical therapy can extend instruction in bed transfers and balance to include helping people identify the proper support they will need for sexual positioning. The mobility needed for sexual activity may be enhanced by attention to such details as pelvic thrust capabilities and more flexible use of arms and legs in sexual positions. Occupational therapy may provide adaptive equipment to help in dressing and undressing or provide assistance in modifying bathrooms and bedrooms. A variety of therapists can involve themselves in pain management or relaxation training.

Cognitive and social skills retraining can also be directed toward providing appropriate sexual information. For instance, genitalia should be included in body orientation training. Later, sensory and perceptual retraining may help the person identify intact areas of tactile or erotic stimulation. The speech pathologist may help with mouth, tongue, and lip control essential for controlling drooling and engaging in kissing or orogenital activity.

The psychologist, speech-language pathologist, therapeutic recreation specialist, and even a pastoral counselor may be involved with social skills training. Communication training may include focusing on appropriate expressions of love and sexual desire, with attention to both verbal and nonverbal communication. Commu-

nity reintegration can include developing leisure activities as part of dating and relationship enhancement skills. Regardless of discipline, all staff can be involved in helping the person with brain injury to regain self-esteem and self-efficacy by providing a warm atmosphere, reinforcing the concept of progress, and emphasizing the relationship between one's actions and outcomes.

Varieties of Treatment

Treatment for sexual dysfunction after brain injury can be as narrowly focused as hormone replacement therapy or as broad as social skills training. Rarely does one component remediate the problem. Most sex therapists advocate a program that includes education, behavioral therapy and social skills training, elements of family therapy, and participation in community activities. Medication, pain management, mobility, and sensory retraining may be included, depending upon the problem. A unique form of communications training, called Symbolic Sexual Vocabulary,[47] may require the expertise of speech-language pathologists.

EDUCATION AS A FIRST STEP

Education about sexuality and reproduction is the first phase of treatment. Among the earliest interventions of rehabilitation professionals is the provision of information concerning the interpretation of sexual responses of the patient aroused from coma. Many patients "discover" their genitalia on arousal from coma, much to the consternation of family and staff. Staff should provide information to family about the usefulness of self-stimulation during the acute stages of recovery.[38] Early vocalizations may consist of coprolalic utterances. The patient's confused, disoriented gropings of staff and visitors may involve any part of the body. Indiscriminate solicitations of sexual favors can be directed at anyone of either sex. Staff and visitors can be coordinated to apply consistent behavioral approaches to deal with such responses. Family can be reassured that these activities are often a part of the transitional process of early recovery and are not indicative of perversion, "bad character," poor parenting, or ill omens of past or future sexual deviations.[21]

As the patient's recovery proceeds, more formal education, either inpatient or outpatient, can be directed at the survivor. Education in a small group setting helps people realize that others also have difficulties. Sometimes same-sex groups are more cohesive than mixed-sex groups. However, to ensure that people feel comfortable discussing sexual issues, individual sessions may be more appropriate. Although a person with TBI probably will not retain detailed physiological information, basic concepts can be presented with models, diagrams, and films. Information must be presented at a slower pace with a brain injured population, and therapists may have to pay more attention to turn-taking issues, client distractibility, and memory loss. Simple written materials or written homework assignments are helpful for those people with memory deficits. The therapist should verify comprehension by periodically asking the client to paraphrase information.[41]

In the education phase, it is important to convey the idea that sexuality encompasses more than sexual intercourse. Sex education should also encompass information about sexually transmitted diseases and high-risk sexual behaviors. The relationship of drugs and alcohol to sexual assault and unwanted pregnancy can also be discussed here. Finally, basic information about sexual aids or medications to increase libido can be presented.

MEDICAL-SURGICAL APPROACHES

Earlier we noted that sexual dysfunction after TBI could be associated with neurological, endocrinological, and musculoskeletal problems, among others. Medical-surgical treatment logically follows from these difficulties. Remediation of sexual dysfunction after TBI often requires the expertise of a specialist who is willing to collaborate with the physiatrist.

Endocrine Disorders

The need for physician cooperation is especially salient when dealing with endocrinological problems. For instance, replacement hormonal therapy must be combined with supportive counseling and education for optimal results.[20] Polycystic ovary syndrome (PCO) includes symptoms of oligorrhea or amenorrhea, galactorrhea, hirsutism, acne, reduced libido, obesity, repeated spontaneous abortions, and infertility. Most women with PCO respond to androgen-blocking agents.[19,20] Clomiphene or pulsatile gonadotropin release hormone is used to induce ovulation in PCO and in hypothalamic injury causing infertility, provided the pituitary gland is responsive. With severe pituitary damage, gonadotropin analogue therapy is indicated; however, severe pituitary damage is less common in TBI than hypothalamic injury.

Children with endocrine problems can be treated in a number of ways. Boys with delayed puberty require human chorionic gonadotropin for 1 to 2 years, followed by testosterone maintenance therapy. Girls with this disorder respond to cyclic estrogen-progesterone. Precocious puberty is effectively treated with long-acting luteinizing hormone–releasing hormone-agonist analogues.[23] Postpubertal hypogonadism should respond to the appropriate replacement hormone: intramuscular testosterone for males and cyclic estrogen-progesterone for females.[19] Bromocriptine can be used with hyperprolactinemia, which is another variant of hypothalamic-pituitary axis dysfunction characterized by male gynecomastia, galactorrhea, impotence, amenorrhea, infertility, and osteoporosis.

Anticonvulsants

Temporolimbic seizures and their associated sexual disorders respond to antiseizure therapy, particularly carbamazepine or valproic acid.[18,20] Klüver-Bucy symptomatology also responds well to these drugs. Efforts to control seizures with anticonvulsants must take into account the fact that the potential side effects of some of these drugs produce sexual problems.

Erectile Dysfunction

Erectile insufficiency has multiple organic and functional causes.[48] Endocrine disorders, medication, and drug effects and their treatment have already been discussed earlier. Vascular causes resulting from associated trauma are rare but require surgical management.[18,19] Neurogenic causes must be sorted out to differentiate central from peripheral neurological disorders. Treatment considerations include noradrenergic agonists (e.g., yohimbine) and dopamine agonists.[18] Intracavernosal injections of papaverine, phentolamine, prostaglandin-E, in either mono-doses or mixed doses, have been used in brain injured males. Medication can also be used for functional causes in erectile insufficiency. Anxiety and depression are the most prevalent psychological causes and should respond to specific treatment combinations, such as anxiolytics, antidepressants, and counseling.

Medications that are highly suspect as causes of sexual dysfunctions should be reduced, withdrawn, or replaced. Alcohol and drug abusers with TBI should be strongly encouraged to participate fully in substance abuse treatment, including detoxification.

Prosthetics

Penile prostheses of several designs are available. Implantable devices should be reserved for men who have had medical and psychological screening, with partners included in the latter. With proper training and precautions, entrapment of blood within the penis can be done by tourniquet. Vacuum devices for enhancing erection have gained currency by virtue of their convenience, reversibility, noninvasiveness, and relative inexpense. Along with prostheses, a person should be encouraged to experiment with various means of stimulation, including visual provocative stimuli; mental imagery; tactile, taste, olfactory, oral, and auditory stimulation; and prolonged foreplay. The partner can also be taught the technique of stuffing a semierect penis into the vagina. Any of these methods are best integrated with counseling and behavioral approaches.

Ejaculatory Remediation

Premature ejaculation should be treated by behavioral methods, which can be efficacious as the primary form of treatment in functionally based cases and can be of supportive help in organic disorders.[2] The squeeze technique is a useful and efficacious method that requires application of pressure just proximal to the glans at the moment of imminent ejaculation. Topical anesthetics can be applied to the penile shaft to retard sensation leading to ejaculation. Imipramine and phenoxybenzamine are oral agents reported to be beneficial in some cases. In contrast, hypersexuality may require suppression with medroxyprogesterone or cyproterone.[19,20] Finally, neurogenic ejaculatory failure occurring with spinal cord injury is treated by electroejaculation for purposes of insemination.[19]

Treatment for Women

Women with inadequate vaginal lubrication, whether organic or functional, should use a water-soluble lubricant. Topical or systemic estrogen is helpful when this hormone is deficient. Arousal and orgasmic difficulties of both sexes may improve with imagery and body exploration or "sensate focus" training, as discussed later. Vaginismus and dyspareunia are commonly treated using a combination of masturbation, relaxation exercises, and a series of graduated dildos.

Musculoskeletal Remediation

Motor problems can be approached in a number of ways. Antispasticity drugs, phenol neurolysis, botulinum toxin injections, and physical therapy modalities, including casting, are nonsurgical options for managing spasticity.[18,20] Positional variations may reduce tone and provide for increased use of nonspastic limbs during sex. Orthopedic or neurosurgical proce-

dures may be indicated in severely resistant cases. Movement disorders may respond to certain medications or, in extreme cases, to neurosurgical procedures. In addition, physical therapy techniques and adaptive devices may be useful.

Contractures resistant to physical modalities such as progressive casting may require surgical correction. Heterotopic ossification may be curtailed early in its formation by diphosphonates or nonsteroidal anti-inflammatory drugs; if mature, it can be surgically excised.

Sensory problems call for identification of alternate sites of intact sensation as foci of erotic stimulation. The clinician may suggest stimulation enhancement by means of electrical vibrators, dildos, French ticklers, or other devices.

Cases of nongenital pain or discomfort during sex may call for broad pain management techniques such as topical or systemic analgesics, antidepressants, antiseizure agents, or imagery and relaxation training.

If bowel and bladder problems occur during sex, a review of a comprehensive program to ensure consistency and predictability of these functions is in order. Remedies include stool softeners, hydration, dietary measures, timed suppository stimulation, and timed voiding. The person with TBI may need reminders to ensure that bowel and bladder are empty prior to sexual activity, as well as training in scrupulous hygiene. Ensuring the proper care and unobtrusiveness of urinary and bowel collecting devices also adds to a more conducive atmosphere for sex.

Craniofacial Remedies

Craniomaxillofacial defects may require secondary surgical repair. These defects may become more accentuated with time because of soft tissue contractures and atrophy. Upon returning to community life, the injured person may encounter less tolerant responses to his or her appearance than those experienced in the hospital and rehabilitation milieus. Thus, with heightened sensitivity to cosmesis, there may be an increased desire for plastic surgery.

PSYCHOTHERAPY
AND BEHAVIOR THERAPY

Maintaining effective use of medical and surgical treatment often involves counseling and behavioral treatment, but psychotherapy alone is useful. Sometimes specific sexual and interpersonal skills need to be taught in individual psychotherapy sessions. Usually sexual retraining includes a discussion of attitudes toward particular sexual acts. In such cases the clinician faces an ethical dilemma about suggesting that the client reassess attitudes toward sex. For instance, prior to injury, clients may have had religious scruples concerning masturbation or oral sex. The clinician should acknowledge potential clashes in values rather than pretend that sexual activity is value-neutral.[41]

COUNSELING AND SPECIFIC TRAINING

The aims of sex therapy may not necessarily be to achieve satisfying sexual intercourse. Most counseling focuses on helping people achieve alternative forms of physical and psychological intimacy, including masturbation and oral-genital sex. Blackerby[49] contends that clients often have misinformation about the ills of masturbation. People who were brain injured in childhood and who suffer from physical deficits may have to be taught to masturbate. Posting a list in the client's bedroom of "OK and not OK" behavioral guidelines for masturbation can be a component of treatment.[41] Masturbation training is also commonly used in sex therapy as a technique to enhance orgasm in nonorgasmic women.[2]

"Sensate focus" is a commonly used technique that deemphasizes the insistence that orgasm through sexual intercourse is the ultimate goal of sexual behavior.[2,50] This technique shapes sexual behavior through a series of carefully constructed steps. For example, a couple may be instructed to go out to dinner and express positive statements about their love for each other. The next step may involve spending a few evenings caressing each other, without attempting to have intercourse. A third step may include mutual masturbation. Performance anxiety lessens as communication, sensuality, and intimacy are enhanced. People with healthy sexual lives seem to participate spontaneously in sensate focus. Couples who regularly reached noncoital orgasm before chronic illness were more likely to resume sexual activity after illness than those whose repertoire included intercourse exclusively.[51]

Learning to communicate about sexual desire and feelings of love is an important part of sexual retraining and rebuilding intimacy. "Symbolic sexual vocabulary" is a unique approach for helping clients with severe speech impairment.[47] Special symbols and gestures relating to sexual desires and levels of comfort can be taught to the patient or placed on a communication board.

Massage classes have been advocated as a method to enhance physical intimacy.[49] Trained physical therapists can teach both patients and family members massage techniques. Not only do the classes provide an atmosphere of relaxation but also they afford people experience in giving and receiving nonsexual touch and pleasure.

COUPLES COUNSELING

Ideally, sexual counseling for people with TBI involves marital or couples counseling. Empirical research documents the number of role changes experienced by people with brain injury.[52] Couples may need to reassess their role expectations as marital and sexual partners. Decreased sexual contact may be related to unexpressed anger, resentment, fatigue, or depression on the part of the spouse or injured person. However, some of the traditional confronting techniques used in marital therapy are not suitable for people with brain injury. One of the authors (AHG) had several experiences where marital counselors unfamiliar with the behavioral manifestations of TBI referred clients with "tremendous unresolved anger surrounding sexual issues." Usually these clients exhibited the impulsivity and quick temper associated with brain injury, regardless of whether sexual issues were involved. Anger management and empathy training, rather than "anger expression," was more appropriate for these clients.

Although the cognitive losses of many brain injured people preclude their ability to theorize about the meaning of relationships, they can still itemize concrete behaviors and experiences that constitute "a happy marriage." Even listing two or three items to change helps the couple reassess their assumptions about marriage.

BUILDING INTIMACY

Most people with TBI do not have difficulties in the physical performance of sex. Rather, they have difficulty initiating and maintaining healthy relationships and achieving intimacy. Intimacy requires love and respect for the self and for others. People with brain injury cannot easily assess their own attributes, deficits, and strengths. Out of their confusion and despair, they may even demean themselves. At an existential level, we teach people to respect the self by first providing respect and unconditional positive regard toward them. On a behavioral level, clients can be taught very specific social skills focusing on building intimacy, including role plays to teach appropriate eye contact, voice tone, and friendly body language. Practice in "making social conversation" is useful. Nonverbal cues to decrease social intrusiveness can also be taught to the client and relatives.[41] Clients can learn to remind themselves how to act in social situations by using "self-talk" statements such as "compliment, don't criticize." These instructions can also be written down and posted around the house. Teaching the partner to provide genuine, positive feedback when small changes occur is also crucial. Theoretically, respect for the self will increase as (1) the client recognizes his or her capacity to change and to learn concrete skills and (2) as these skills in turn trigger positive, more intimate responses from others.

Assertiveness training is an important component in both rebuilding intimacy and sexual counseling because it helps a person identify and communicate about desired and unwanted behaviors. In assertiveness training, all interpersonal communication, whether verbal or nonverbal, is categorized as passive, aggressive, or assertive.[53] Most importantly for the person with TBI, assertiveness is distinguished from both aggressive, impulsive behavior and from mere acquiescence. A variety of role playing and rehearsal techniques can be used to teach a person to use more assertive, yet polite communication. When a person with TBI finds it difficult to refuse to engage in risk-taking behavior, assertiveness training can be used to help the person say no. Consider the following case.

Case 1 ■ AB was a 24-year-old woman who had suffered a brain injury in a motor vehicle accident when she was 16. She had been sexually active prior to the injury. After rehabilitation, AB began work in a sheltered workshop. As one of the few women in the work program, she found herself being approached for sexual favors by men in the workshop and on the bus to work. Assertiveness training was one component of psychotherapy. First, the therapist presented the concept of "assertive rights," including the "right to her own body." The therapist and client identified firm but polite "refusal phrases" such as "Please don't touch me that way; it's not polite" and "I don't feel ready to have sex yet." AB practiced saying the phrases in several therapy sessions and at home. During the course of therapy, she successfully rebuffed the verbal sexual comments of a coworker and attempts at fondling. Neither perpetrator bothered her again.

Sexual Surrogates

Many people with TBI lack sexual partners and therefore cannot benefit from some aspects of the educational and therapeutic programs described here. In the 1970s, a small but significant and controversial portion of the sex therapy literature focused on the use of sexual surrogates. Yet, 20 years later, there is no index listing for surrogacy in a book devoted entirely to the topic of sex after disability.[3] The ethical and legal issues involved, as well as a more conservative moral climate, have perhaps diminished interest in sexual surrogacy. No literature specifically addresses the efficacy or ethicality of sexual surrogates for people with TBI. To advocate sexual surrogacy in inpatient settings would contradict the caveats about staff and patient boundaries presented in this chapter. Nevertheless, people in outpatient psychotherapy sometimes request referrals to sex therapists. The decision to refer to a sexual surrogate must be explored with the family and injured person on a case-by-case basis.

Even when an actual sexual surrogate is not an option, the concept of "surrogate" may prove useful. In a sense, any caregiver who teaches social skills or community integration is a kind of surrogate friend or, at the very least, a coach.[21] Day programs, de facto, provide social settings in which people can learn to care for each other. Initially, the intimacy needed for deep friendship may only indirectly relate to sexuality but may nevertheless prove important for sustaining sexual relationships in the long run.

Appropriateness of the Setting

As noted earlier, both patients and staff agree that lack of access to privacy and opportunity for intimacy during acute rehabilitation is a major sexual concern. The design of most hospital rooms, even "single" ones, discourages sexual behavior. Nevertheless, we all know patients who have been found in sexual embraces by shocked staff members. It is crucial for all rehabilitation settings to have easily stated, official policies regarding sexual behavior of patients on the unit. Some hospitals have "closed-door policies" by which a patient may request conjugal visits. Experience suggests that these official channels are hardly ever discussed with either staff or patients. Even when patients are aware of the possibility for closed-door privacy, they may feel embarrassed to request it: "everyone will know what we're doing." Methods of using a private hospital room to enhance sexual intimacy are discussed in the section of sex in institutional settings.

The recent emergence of transitional living programs suggests a sanctioned and more comfortable alternative to "pulling the drapes closed" when sexual contact is desired. Patients may spend a weekend with family practicing many kinds of household skills in special transitional rooms with acute rehabilitation facilities; programs need to have rules governing closed-door privacy in these apartments. Similarly, full-fledged transitional or apartment living programs can provide more "ecologically valid" settings for sexual intimacy. There is usually less supervision and a more pleasant atmosphere. In fact, preparing the apartment for having a date or spouse over for a meal may be a helpful part of the patient's rehabilitation. However, the person and families attending these programs must be informed about the "sexual policy," including rules governing sexual behavior with other patients.

Home settings may also be changed to make them conducive for sexual behavior. Rearranging the home is sometimes harder when the person with TBI is a single adult and living with his or her parents. The physically disabled person may be confined to the first floor or take up a room that used to be the living room, with her or his living space divided by a screen. A sexual partner may have to walk past a parent's bedroom, thus advertising his or her presence. (The parent's own sexual partner may also feel uncomfortable.) Sexual behavior can be heard through thin walls. There may not be enough bathroom space. Younger children may live in the house as well. Obviously, open communication about general day-to-day arrangements, as well as about sex, becomes even more essential when the patient returns home to parents.

In summary, there are a variety of efficacious treatments for the multitude of sexual difficulties that people with TBI encounter. Survivors and their partners should be encouraged to discuss sexual issues as a normal part of rehabilitation and be provided with appropriate kinds of help at each stage of recovery.

☐ SEXUALITY ACROSS THE LIFESPAN

Sexuality and its expression change throughout the lifespan. Sex education and the techniques for the remediation of sexual dysfunction must be adapted to the age and stage of life of the person with TBI.

Childhood Sexuality

Some theorists argue that the framework for all future relationships, including sexual relationships, is formulated in the first 6 months of life.[54] Babies learn to use all the senses to bond with their caregivers. By the time children are 2 years old, they have some conception of gender identity, although it may be separate from sexual identity. For example, children identify hairstyle or clothes as determining factors in deciding whether someone is a boy or girl. Preschoolers often explore their genitals and are taught words for the penis and vagina. By the time children enter school, they begin to recognize that descriptions of genitalia and sex are "different" and taboo topics, even though they may share their limited and often incorrect information.

A discussion of sexual development and TBI must be extrapolated from the sparse research on development and disability.[55] Neurological damage frequently results in a regression to previous levels of development. Presumably, TBI in children can disrupt psychosexual development in a number of ways. Cognitive deficits may preclude the ability of children to be socialized at the same pace as their peers. The development of gender-based behavior as well as sexual knowledge may be slowed. Impulsive children with TBI may require extensive supervision from adults. Interaction with peers may be diminished not only because of increased parental involvement but also because the child with TBI may lack age-appropriate social skills.

In addition, frequent painful examinations or physical therapy can teach the child that touch is unpleasant and that the body as a whole is an agent of pain rather than pleasure.[56] Physical disability may hinder the child from exploring his or her genitalia in a healthy, typical fashion. However, after TBI, inappropriate masturbation may pose problems.

Early sex education becomes important for the child with TBI. Information should be paced at the child's cognitive level, but it is essential that the child learn the correct words for genitalia. Although children may appear uninterested or even disgusted about sex, sex education should continue throughout the elementary years. Brief, spontaneous discussion may be more helpful than formal education.[56] Self-esteem issues should be embedded in these discussions. The elementary school child with TBI should also be involved in activities that build self-esteem, including sports, social activities, and social skills training.

Puberty and Adolescence

Adolescent children are expected to begin separating themselves from the family. Part of this separation includes emotional attachments to members of the opposite sex. Children begin to show interest in sex around the time of puberty. Teenagers may be uncomfortable with the changes in their bodies; cultural standards for attractiveness loom very large. Often teenagers experiment with masturbation and both heterosexual and homosexual genital stimulation. For many teens, sexual behavior "proves" that they are physically attractive. Engaging in sex confers an adult identity on teenagers that they otherwise may not have. However, many young teenagers appear outwardly sophisticated about sexual matters, even though they may not have sexual experience.

Teenagers with physical disabilities may feel especially unattractive because our culture places extreme emphasis on the perfect face and body.[55] Disabled teenagers often wonder if their bodies will function sexually, yet they almost never speak with doctors or other adults about these concerns.[56] Even parents who encourage impressive educational goals for their disabled children do not expect them to be socially active. Disabled teenagers date less than their compatriots. Few teenagers know disabled adults who can serve as role models for healthy interpersonal relationships.

Teenagers with brain injury probably have the same social difficulties as their physically disabled peers. Parents of brain injured children with behavioral and cognitive deficits may struggle with allowing their children social independence, especially in light of the teenager's vulnerability to abuse by others. On occasion, the child with brain injury who reaches puberty may exhibit sexual acting out, including sexual behavior toward the parent or other siblings. We recommend that siblings be taught to discourage sexual play with the TBI child because it is more difficult for the injured child to discriminate between inappropriate and appropriate sexual partners than for other children.

Many teenagers have had sexual relationships by the time they become brain injured. Clinical experience suggests that a fair number of car accidents occur while the teenager was on a date or out with a group of mixed-sex peers. Given that a large number of these teenagers engage in high-risk behavior, it would not be surprising to discover that, as a group, teenagers who incur TBI are proportionately more sexually active than their same-age counterparts. A previously sexually active teenager with TBI may find it more difficult to control sexual desires than the teenager who was not previously sexually active. Parents may find it difficult to supervise or forbid the teenager's behavior, as well. To the teenager with TBI, not being allowed to date or to have sex appears to be another infantilizing result of the brain injury. Cognitive deficits and lack of self-awareness may make feelings of rejection more acute; the teenager may fail to understand why the boyfriend or girlfriend no longer is interested. Teenagers may also fail to use contraception.

Sometimes the teenage sexual partner feels guilty and continues the relationship with the injured person longer than she or he might have otherwise. We have known several cases in which the driver who sustained the motor vehicle accident married the teenage passenger with TBI out of a sense of responsibility. As might be predicted, the marriages were not happy in the long run.

Young Adulthood

In young adulthood, sex life can be affected by the task of establishing a family and building a career. Work, household tasks, and parenting leave little leisure time for adults to spend together. Physically healthy couples who complain of sexual dysfunction often report a lack of "adult time." Adult time also decreases dramatically when one partner becomes chronically ill because of the number of role changes incurred by the healthy spouse.[1] In a vicious circle, the spouse of the person with TBI may then use increased chores to avoid sexual encounters. We have already alluded to the research findings that spouses of people with TBI feel overwhelmed and burdened with the care of the ill relative.[13] Inequitable relationships make many spouses feel as though they are married to children; one does not wish for sexual relations with a child. Paradoxically, the brain injured man's poor, childlike social skills may decrease his ability for romance but not his desire for sex. Because women, more than men, rely on romance and fantasy to foment sexual desire, the female spouse's sexual interest may become further diminished.

As discussed earlier, the single person with TBI is at a distinct disadvantage in sexual relationships. Odd and eccentric behavior make him or her unattractive to peers. Lack of employment, so common after TBI, not only adds to unsuitability as a mate but also hinders meeting appropriate people. For the person who suffers a TBI as a child, achieving mature adult sexuality poses even more problems. The person may lack social skills and sexual experience or appear immature and generally "ineligible" as a mate. Thus, counseling that focuses on relationship building and intimacy is particularly important for the younger adult.

Under most circumstances, deciding to have children is a developmental task of young adulthood. People with brain injury need to consider whether it is feasible for them to become parents. If not, then reinforcing the consistent use of contraception becomes a crucial component of sexual counseling and education. For those people who cannot or choose not to have children, counseling must also focus on the survivor's and partner's sense of loss or grief concerning the decision.

CONTRACEPTION

Methods of contraception are an integral topic for any sexuality education and training program for survivors, partners, families, and staff. Education about contraception may begin in adolescence and continue in young adulthood. Methods of contraception fall into two categories: reversible and irreversible.[21,57] Within the first category, choices include condoms for either sex, diaphragms, spermicides, intrauterine devices, cervical caps, oral cyclic female hormones, and long-term injectable or implantable female hormones. The latter two provide contraceptive protection for 3 months and 5 years, respectively.

Because some contraceptives have side effects, the advantages, disadvantages, relative effectiveness, side effects, and contraindications for each of these methods must be weighed and discussed with survivor, partner, and family before asking them to reach a decision. Female hormones are contraindicated in women with breast cancer, liver disorders, cerebrovascular disease, or a history of thromboembolic disease. The latter two diseases occasionally may be induced by these hormones. They can create side effects such as headache, irregular or unpredictable uterine bleeding, and weight gain. Intrauterine devices may produce infection or perforate the uterus. Compromised patient compliance because of cognitive or behavioral problems may require that the partner either supervise or perform condom or diaphragm application or administer oral contraceptives.

Permanent, usually irreversible contraceptive measures are surgical procedures: tubal ligation and vasectomy. In cases of severe mental deficits, legal guardianship and psychiatric or psychological consultation may be necessary before surgery.[58] The rhythm method may be the choice of some couples, even though it is much less effective than any of the other methods and requires careful counting and memory skills. Nevertheless, it should be mentioned in the education curriculum as an option. Abstinence from sexual intercourse is a legitimate alternative to contraceptive methods and should be included in discussions.

PREGNANCY AND CHILDBIRTH

At the time of their brain injury, women of childbearing age routinely should be tested for pregnancy.[58] Fetal death can result not only from maternal death but also from maternal abdominal-pelvic injuries involving the uterus. Knowledge of pregnancy necessitates certain precautionary measures during the emergency care of the woman. The uterus must be shielded from x-radiation. The supine position is avoided in women at or beyond 20 weeks of gestation. The left lateral position is an alternative position that does not cause uterine compression of the large abdominal blood vessels. Drugs and anesthetics known to cause birth defects or severe side effects to the fetus are avoided if possible. Pregnancy warrants cautious use of hyperventilation as treatment for elevated intracranial pressure to avoid maternal alkalosis and consequent fetal hypoxia.

Patel and Bontke[58] have provided a detailed review of medications frequently used in brain injured patients. They emphasize that the teratogenic potential of many drugs is not established; therefore, drugs should be used only when definite indications for their use exist. For the use of anticonvulsants during pregnancy, they recommend single-drug therapy whenever possible, frequent monitoring of blood levels, maintenance of drug levels in the low therapeutic range, and prophylactic use of folic acid with phenytoin, primidone, or barbiturates. Interpretation of laboratory values in managing fluid-electrolyte balance involves appreciation of physiological alterations in the pregnant woman.

Depression is of concern in the event of miscarriage, especially in the cognitively aware woman. Postpartum depression is another potentially distressing complication that requires vigorous intervention.

The woman who becomes pregnant after brain injury should not normally encounter undue medical complications. Anticonvulsants should continue to be monitored. Newborns whose mothers are taking antiepileptic drugs, particularly barbiturates, should receive vitamin K.

The social and legal issues regarding abortion during the acute phases of recovery, as well as parenting after brain injury, are beyond the scope of this chapter. Mothers (and fathers) with mild, moderate, or even severe brain injury may continue to care for their children, with training, help of the family, and community resources. Parents with severe cognitive residua require assistance in child care. If family and community support services are not adequate, temporary or permanent placement of the child may be necessary. Legal counsel and guardianship should be obtained before this decision is made.

Middle Age

Researchers note that under ordinary circumstances middle age can bring a renewal of interest in sex.[1] With children out of the house, couples increase their amount of leisure time. Menopause often brings women a sense of freedom from worries about pregnancy. However, middle age sparks the beginning of chronic illness for many people. Any illness, including TBI, can hamper a newly renewed sex life. Illness tends to impair men's sexual functioning more than women's. Although chronically ill men often stop initiating sex, their partners may still expect them to take the initiator role. People who sustained brain injury in middle age are probably less likely to be risk takers or to have multiple sexual partners and are more likely to have developed intimacy skills. When brain injury occurs at age 45, as opposed to age 25, stable couples may be better able to cope with disruption to their sexual lives, although their occupational and financial difficulties may increase. Although dealing with a childlike spouse can be just as devastating to the middle-aged adult as to the younger adult, the middle-aged spouse, especially the wife, is more likely to remain with the injured person. Divorce of a chronically ill spouse is probably more common in younger people. However, living arrangements sometimes have to change. For example, one man with brain injury moved to a supervised adult home because his difficult and unsafe behavior made it impossible for him to stay home alone, and his wife had to work. The couple remained married and visited each other several times a week at her apartment.

Thorough medical management of sexual dysfunction is particularly important for the middle-aged adult because there may be undiscovered endocrinological causes for changes in sex drive. In addition, sexual retraining and attitude reassessment can help the couple change long-standing patterns of sexual behavior.

Old Age

It is now a cliché to reiterate that sexuality does not end with old age. However, health care providers, the younger population, and even the elderly themselves seem to have negative attitudes toward sex among the aged.[59] Although many older adults report sexual dysfunction, few seek services from sexual dysfunction clinics.[1] Older people may not mention problems unless specifically asked about sex by their physicians.

Both men and women experience change in the sexual response cycle with age.[60,61] Briefly, women experience increased vaginal irritation and decreased lubrication and pelvic contractions during sex. Menopause has been associated with both lowered and increased sexual activity. Men experience slower erection time and take longer to climax. Ejaculatory volume may be decreased, and the refractory period may last for several days. After the sixth decade, there is an accelerated decline in the

production of testosterone.[59] Diminished sex drive may also be related to alterations in sensation, hearing, vision, and smell.

In the healthy individual, declining sexual activity appears to be more related to psychological and cultural factors than to physiological factors.[60] In fact, chronic illness accounts for much of the decline of sexual activity in the elderly, with genitourinary and endocrine disorders having the foremost negative impact, followed by cardiovascular and respiratory disorders.[60]

Cross-sectional studies show that sexual activity and interest decline somewhat with age, with about 70 to 80 percent of older people still reporting sexual interest.[61] These patterns seem to be the same for heterosexuals and homosexuals. In general, more older men than women report sexual interest, and single older women report the least sexual activity. Longitudinal studies of sexual activity find that the aging individual's level of interest and participation in sexual activity are highly correlated to his or her activity and interest in previous years. Among long-married couples, sexual interest is stable across age, but the choice to engage in sex usually rests with the male partner.[61]

Declining sexual activity in older women may have a number of social causes. Because elderly husbands are usually several years older than their wives, they are more likely to be ill or suffer sexual dysfunction. Consequently, wives may appear to show a decrease in sexual activity at earlier ages than their husbands. Also, more older women are single, and fewer partners are available. Older women may feel unattractive and less desirable, so they pursue sexual relationships less often. The double standard castigates older women for engaging in sex outside marriage even more than it does younger women. Finally, there are no social institutions, whether legally sanctioned or otherwise, that allow older women to meet much younger men; older women do not typically buy the services of male prostitutes.

IMPACT OF AGING ON SEXUALITY AFTER TRAUMATIC BRAIN INJURY

Although younger males are more likely to suffer a TBI than females, elderly women with TBI outnumber elderly men.[62] The elderly are rarely asked about their sexual concerns after TBI, especially if they are unmarried or widowed. Elderly people with TBI who make sexual remarks or use foul language during the early phases of recovery may be tolerated less by staff and family than younger people. Rather than viewing such behavior as typical of brain injury, the elderly person may be labeled as "a dirty old man" who "shouldn't be interested in that kind of thing." At later stages of recovery, the legitimate sexual concerns of the older person may be ignored or even attributed to dementia. Interestingly, there is no research evidence of an increase of sexual acting out in older, institutionalized, demented people. Rather, the lack of privacy and general affection (including nonsexual touch) in nursing homes may encourage residents to express angry and frustrated feelings, which are then labeled as verbal symptoms of "dementia."[1]

It is important for the clinician to ask an elderly person and the significant other if they have any sexual concerns. One way of doing this is to place the question in the context of other questions: "We've talked about many effects of brain injury. One question some people have is about sex. Do you have any concerns relating to sex?" Although a decrease in sexual desire is more likely after illness, occasionally after TBI the older person may show an increased desire, which comes as a surprise to the elderly spouse. The clinician or counselor may need to explore with the couple their attitudes about sex in old age, as well as the level of tenderness involved in the sexual advances. As with sexual desire at any age, the spouse may be less troubled by sexual desire itself than by the impulsive, egocentric quality and the insensitivity of the "demands" of the person with TBI. Thus, techniques to enhance relationships are as crucial for the elderly as they are at any other stage of life.

☐ SPECIAL TOPICS IN SEXUALITY

Homosexuality

Approximately 10 percent of the population are predominantly homosexual.[63,64] There appear to be more male homosexuals than female, and homosexual lifestyles vary greatly.[65,66] Thus we should surmise that a similar percentage of brain injured survivors are homosexuals. Homosexuality per se is not classified as a mental disorder.[5] Homosexual *behavior* is not always equated with homosexuality as a sexual identity. As a phase of normal sexual development, homosexual experimentation is very common, and the sexual assessment for people with TBI must differentiate such experimental encounters from homosexuality.[19] For example, early recovery may include periods of confusion concerning sexual identity or indiscriminate overtures to persons of the same gender. Teenage TBI survivors who have homosexual experiences may not have developed a definitive choice of gender preference or expression of that choice. Some heterosexuals may turn to homosexual activities when there are no opportunities for heterosexual intimacy. None of these situations should be confused with a lifelong homosexual orientation. In any event, the sexual assessment must be inclusive of potential or actual gay or lesbian lifestyle and practices.

As professionals, we are obligated to treat this delicate subject in a tolerant, nonjudgmental manner or to ensure that other professionals who are free of prejudice and discomfort serve in our stead. Homophobia is a major factor in the continuing discrimination against homosexuals, often leading to their loss of self-esteem, distrust of health care professionals, anxiety, depression, guilt, and internalized homophobia.[67] *Internalized homophobia* is a term used to describe the self-directed fear and hatred of being homosexual. Its consequences may include reckless sexual behavior, avoidance of intimacy, and drug abuse—behaviors already prevalent in a large proportion of the heterosexual TBI population.

The treatment team should be knowledgeable of the lifestyles of gay and lesbian survivors. We should be sensitive to the barriers imposed by a homophobic society, including the attitudes of the family, which may vary from acceptance to rejection of the survivor's sexual preference and lifestyle. We should be aware that relationships, particularly of gay males, are often serial or multiple. If we advise monogamy, whether for heterosexuals or homosexuals, we should acknowledge the implicit values presented in our therapy.

The sexual dysfunctions of gay and lesbian individuals are very much the same as those of heterosexuals. Problems of sexual partner incompatibilities, decreased libido, and erectile dysfunction are among the most frequent dysfunctions of male homosexual couples.[67]

Families may insist on "protecting" their relative from a homosexual partner.[68] They may assume custody of the survivor against the will of the partner, leading to legal and ethical controversies. Although many professionals agree that the homosexual partner of a recovering person with brain injury should be afforded the same consideration and central role as a heterosexual partner, only one state recognizes homosexual marriage. The reality of the situation is that the partner may have no legal standing if there are next of kin. Obviously, the homosexual partner may have the same variety of responses as a heterosexual companion to the condition of the injured person: continuing devotion, a wait-and-see attitude, or frank rejection and abandonment. The partner is entitled to the same nonjudgmental treatment as the survivor and should be fully involved in an education-training program that addresses the particular issues and concerns of the homosexual couple. Community and other gay-oriented resources can be made available to the team, survivor, and partner. Among these resources, gay and lesbian professionals and peers are especially valuable extensions of the rehabilitation team. SAR programs are particularly useful in helping the team incorporate openly gay professionals.[46]

Another ominous shadow for homosexuals is the epidemic of AIDS. A gay man in this thirties may have lost a staggering number of friends to AIDS. For men particularly, the fear and oppression of this disease may be overwhelming, resulting at times in an irrational fear of imminent death.[67] Homosexuality is a major risk factor in the transmission of other sexually transmitted diseases as well.[69]

Sexually Transmitted Diseases

The incidence of sexually transmitted diseases (STDs) in the United States has been increasing in recent years.[69] There is no published information concerning the incidence and prevalence of STD among survivors of brain injury. People initially at risk for STDs in the general population include the poor, minorities, urban dwellers, prostitutes, male homosexuals, people engaging in sex with multiple or casual partners, those having careless or indifferent health care practices, and substance abusers.[70] Sadly, a large proportion of the brain injury population includes people who fall into one or more of these groups. The cognitive and consequent psychosocial difficulties of these survivors create additional risks for STDs, although there may be countervailing factors such as loss of mobility, lack of opportunity for sexual contact, or lack of interest.

The deadliest of the diseases is AIDS, still an incurable and almost invariably fatal affliction. Besides AIDS, there are epidemic increases of venereal warts, genital herpes, and chlamydial infections. Resistant gonococcal strains have created difficulty in treating gonorrhea. Those infected with one STD may have others. The clear implications for brain injury survivors, their families, and their treatment teams are that education and training must be directed toward prevention and early detection of STDs.[21] In the face of the survivor's uninhibited behaviors, poor judgment, poor safety awareness, impulsivity, and forgetfulness, the focus of education and training may fall largely upon family, partner(s), or caretakers. Training sessions, at the minimum, should stress the proper use of condoms, avoidance of blood and blood products, the dangers of vaginal secretions and semen, and use of sterile products for IV drug users.[70] Discussion should include avoidance of other high-risk sexual behavior such as soul kissing, anal intercourse, and multiple sex partners. Finally, teaching about the warning signs of STDs is imperative because patients are likely to procrastinate about consulting a physician.

Sexual Abuse

People with traumatic brain injury may become either perpetrators or victims of sexual abuse. This aspect of sexual dysfunction has not been discussed to any extent in rehabilitation publications.[18] Among the general population, sexual abuse is inadequately and belatedly reported. Young children, more often girls, are most vulnerable to abuse.[71] Sexual aggression may take various forms: verbal threats and abuse, stalking, grabbing, fondling, exhibitionism, and voyeurism. In rarer cases, sadism, sodomy, rape, and gang rape may occur. A relative may commit incest, but strangers and friends may also be perpetrators.

People with TBI may be targeted as victims for several reasons. First, those with cognitive deficits may be passive, indecisive, and gullible. Brain injured survivors may be lonely, eager for attention, and lacking in self-esteem, thus increasing their susceptibility to abusers. Second, people with physical impairments are less able to fend off aggressors and may provoke overtures from persons who find such individuals sexually enticing.

Brain injured persons may be the aggressors. As noted earlier, they frequently direct sexual overtures indiscriminately to any available person in the early period of recovery, most often in the form of sexual solicitations and demands without physical abuse.[19] However, grasping and fondling of buttocks and genital areas by the person with brain injury is a common problem in the hospital. Staff must remove the person's hand and firmly state, "No, that's not appropriate."

A small proportion of brain injured people may suffer from syndromes that increase the chance that they will be perpetrators of sexual abuse. The sexual rage of orbitofrontal injuries is a rare form of hypersexuality that can lead to physical violence. Hypersexual behavior with limbic and temporal lobe injuries is seldom physically abusive. In the case of Klüver Bucy syndrome, excessive masturbation and indiscriminate oral stimulation are the usual manifestations, rather than sexual behavior directed at others. For the brain injured abuser, the treatment modalities of choice are medroxyprogesterone, antiseizure and antiagitation drugs, and counseling.[20]

The consequences of sexual abuse may appear soon after the abuse, whether it occurs as a solitary episode or as repeated insults. Physical signs of injury are often present in the facial area.[72] Victims can become further alienated, angry, anxious, fearful, depressed, and lacking in self-esteem. Children may resort to precocious, overt sexual activities. Sexually transmitted diseases and pregnancy may also result from abusive encounters.

Long-term consequences of abuse may appear in adult life in the form of sexual dysfunctions such as decreased libido, rejection of foreplay or any other form of physical intimacy, and propensity toward participation in recurrent abusive relationships—as either abuser or victim. Personality "styles" such as alienation from others and hostility, as well as multiple personality disorder, are thought to be linked to extreme sexual abuse.[73,74]

Management and treatment of the person with TBI who is sexually abused must focus on the medical, legal, and psychological ramifications of the abuse. Early recognition of the abuse and prosecution and/or treatment of abusers are encouraged. The victim should be screened for STDs and pregnancy. Appropriate prophylaxis should be offered, with consideration of abortion in the event of pregnancy.

With guidance from legal sources, alteration of the environment, such as removal of the abused person from the setting, or supervised visits may be proposed. The victim can be protected through restraining orders. Victims and their families or caretakers should receive counseling and education.

Sexuality in Institutions: A Dilemma

Consider the many institutions where people with TBI may encounter sexual behavior: hospitals, transitional living centers, group homes, skilled nursing facilities, long-term care centers, behavioral training centers, special educational programs, mainstream educational institutions, and vocational training centers. Sexual dysfunctions of all varieties may continue, appear, or reappear in any of these institutional settings. Sexual abuse is a daunting concern of institutional life, threatening those in hospitals, education and training centers, and long-term care facilities. Fellow patients, clients, and staff may be victims or aggressors, regardless of sexual orientation. Yet not all sexual behavior occurring in institutions is abusive. Health care professionals must walk a fine line when determining when noncoercive sexual expression in an institution is acceptable and when it is exploitive or, if not exploitive, illegal. Even the terminology used to discuss sex in institutions bespeaks our discomfort with it: Is sexual behavior a "problem" or a "dysfunction"?

Although personnel in some institutional settings, such as acute rehabilitation facilities, are well educated and trained to recognize and deal with these dilemmas, in other settings such preparation is nonexistent. The resulting crises may mean expulsion of the "offending" individuals from the institution. Therefore, it is incumbent on institutions that serve people with brain injury to adequately prepare their staff and to adopt philosophies, missions, goals and objectives, policies, and procedures relating to issues of sexuality and sexual dysfunction.[75] Institutions must be concerned about the legal ramifications of their stance regarding sexuality and should have germane policies and practices reviewed by legal counsel.

At the core of institutional attitudes regarding sexuality is the acknowledgment that people with brain injury are sexual beings who have the right to seek ways to express their sexuality, provided that their expressions do no harm to others. Too often, prevailing attitudes either deny or ignore the sexuality of the survivors. Infantilization is one way of supporting such attitudes. Creating an environment where intimacy of any sort is impossible is another.

Despite physical and attitudinal barriers, coercive sex may yet "rear its ugly head." But "nonassaultive" liaisons between clients and staff occur, even in the face of dire consequences, such as expulsion or firing. From a moral standpoint, it is arguable that a person who lives in an institution never "freely" enters into a relationship with a staff member, by virtue of the power that the staff member holds, even if the relationship is not technically physically abusive.

Client-client relationships, consenting or otherwise, also occur in institutions. The unavailability of heterosexual partners may result in homosexual overtures among brain injured people not previously homosexual. Mobile clients, such as those who leave adult homes daily to work, seek opportunities for interpersonal relationships outside the institution. These often naive and innocent contacts with others may be misconstrued as sexual liaisons by caregivers. At the other extreme, staff may badger clients into participating in social activities and dating or courting others, under the guise of "mental health" or treatment.

When an institution has policies regarding the sexual behavior of its clients and staff, sexual needs and dysfunctions can be identified as part of the admissions plan for each person. If abuse occurs, family and guardians know to whom to report. Institutions may recognize the sexuality of their clients in a variety of ways. The concept of the private room can be extended beyond the hospital setting as a means of permitting various expressions of intimacy, including sexual activity, within the institution.[76] The room can be reserved, its door locked, and its privacy assured by staff. The room can be used as a treatment site for sexual dysfunctions, a place to practice techniques alone, with a partner, or with trained staff. It can serve simply as a place for quiet, confidential conversation. Instead of reserving a private room, institutions can provide connubial visiting privileges or reserve nearby apartments or motels. As always, it is essential for institutions to provide opportunity for social surrogates, peer groups, and community outings because the opportunity for pursuing interpersonal relationships, apart from sexual behavior, remains crucial for the TBI survivor's emotional well-being.

◻ SUMMARY AND CONCLUSIONS

Research on the implementation and success of sexuality training with TBI is scant. Clinical experience suggests that most sexual disabilities stem from the "secondary" sequelae of brain injury: personality, emotional, cognitive, and behavioral deficits. However, many primary sexual dysfunctions, especially those related to endocrinopathies, probably go undiagnosed. Questions for future research include the relative incidence of primary versus secondary dysfunctions and the efficacy of adapting different treatment modalities with a brain injured population.

The interdisciplinary rehabilitation team is uniquely qualified to provide sexual training to TBI survivors at all levels of recovery. Where sexual behavior is concerned, ascertaining the needs, feelings, and attitudes of the person with TBI and the partner become even more important. Recognizing that the expression of sexuality differs across the lifespan and among people of different backgrounds is crucial for the ethical and compassionate delivery of treatment in this most intimate area of our lives.

REFERENCES

1. Schover, LR, and Jensen, SB: Sexuality and Chronic Illness: A Comprehensive Approach. Guilford, New York, 1988.
2. Wincze, JP, and Carey, MP: Sexual Dysfunction: A Guide for Assessment and Treatment. Guilford, New York, 1991.
3. Monga, TN, and Lefebvre, KA: Sexuality. An overview. In Monga, TN (ed): Sexuality and Disability. Hanley & Belfus, Philadelphia, 1995, p 299.
4. Thorn-Gray, B, and Kern, L: Sexual dysfunction associated with physical disability: A treatment guide for the rehabilitation practitioner. Rehabilitation Literature 44:138–144, 1983.
5. American Psychiatric Association: Diagnostic and Statistical Manual of Mental Disorders, ed 4. American Psychiatric Association, Washington, DC, 1994.
6. Bansal, S, et al: Sex-steroid levels in chronic alcoholic males: Relationship to sex and liver functions. Unpublished manuscript. Brown University, 1990.
7. LoPiccolo, J, and Heiman, JR: Sexual assessment and history interview. In LoPiccolo, J, and LoPiccolo, L (eds): Handbook of Sex Therapy. Plenum, New York, 1978, p 103.
8. Robins, LN, et al: Lifetime prevalence of specific psychiatric disorders in three sites. Arch Gen Psychiatry 41:949, 1984.
9. Walker, AE, and Jablon, S: A followup of head injured men of World War II. J Neurosurg 16:600, 1959.
10. Meyer, J: Sexual disturbances after cerebral injuries. Journal of Neuro-visceral Relations (suppl 10):519, 1971.
11. Kosteljanetz, M, et al: Sexual and hypothalamic dysfunction in post-concussional syndrome. Acta Neurol Scand 63:169, 1981.
12. Lezak, M: Living with the characterologically altered brain injured patient. J Clin Psychiatry 39:592, 1978.
13. Romano, M: Family response to traumatic head injury. Scand J Rehabil Med 6:1, 1974.
14. Thomsen, IV: The patient with severe head injury and his family. Scand J Rehabil Med 6:180, 1974.
15. Thomsen, IV: Late outcome of severe blunt head trauma. A 10–15 year follow-up. J Neurol Neurosurg Psychiatry 47:260, 1984.
16. Garden, FH, Bontke, CF, and Hoffman, M: Sexual functioning and marital adjustment after traumatic brain injury. J Head Trauma Rehabil 5(2):52, 1990.
17. Davis, DL, and Schneider, LK: Ramifications of traumatic brain injury for sexuality. J Head Trauma Rehabil 5(2):31, 1990.
18. Zasler, ND: Traumatic brain injury and sexuality. In Monga, TN (ed): Sexuality and Disability. Hanley & Belfus, Philadelphia, 1995, p 361.
19. Griffith, ER, Cole, S, and Cole, T: Sexuality and sexual dysfunction. In Rosenthal, MJ, et al (eds): Rehabilitation of the Adult and Child with Traumatic Brain Injury, ed 2. FA Davis, Philadelphia, 1990, p 206.
20. Zasler, ND, and Horn, LJ: Rehabilitative management of sexual dysfunction. J Head Trauma Rehabil 5(2):14, 1990.
21. Griffith, ER, and Lemberg, S: Sexuality and the person with traumatic brain injury. FA Davis, Philadelphia, 1993.
22. Sandel, ME: Sexuality and reproduction after traumatic brain injury. In Horn, L, and Zasler, N (eds): Medical Rehabilitation of Traumatic Brain Injury. Hanley & Belfus, Philadelphia, 1996, p 557.
23. Blendonohy, P, and Puliyodil, AP. Precocious puberty in children after traumatic brain injury. Brain Inj 5(1):63, 1991.
24. Terzian, H, and Ore, G: Syndrome of Kluver and Bucy. Neurology 5:373, 1962.
25. Herzog, A, et al: Reproductive endocrine disorders in women with partial seizures of temporal lobe origin. Arch Neurol 43:341, 1986.
26. Miller, BL, et al: Hypersexuality or altered sexual preference following brain injury. J Neurol Neurosurg Psychiatry 9:867, 1986.
27. Blackerby, WA, and Porter, S: Psychosocial aspects of sexual dysfunction in head injury. In Horn, LJ, and Cope, DN (eds): Traumatic Brain Injury. Hanley & Belfus, Philadelphia, 1989, p 143.
28. O'Malley, KF, and Ross, SE: The incidence of injury to the cervical spine in patients with craniocerebral injury. J Trauma 28:476, 1988.
29. Stutts, M, et al: Cognitive impairment in persons with recent spinal cord injury: Findings and implications for clinical practice. NeuroRehabilitation 1:79, 1991.
30. Comfort, A (ed): Sexual Consequences of Disability. George F. Stickly, Philadelphia, 1978.
31. Gervasio, AH, and Ruckdeschel, K: College students' judgments of verbal sexual harassment. Journal of Applied Social Psychology 22:190, 1992.

32. Derogatis, LR, and Melisaratos, N: The DSFI: A multidimensional measure of sexual functioning. J Sex Marital Ther 5:244, 1979.

33. Fisher, WA: The sexual opinion survey. In Davis, CM, Yarber, WL, and Davis, SL (eds): Sexuality-related Measures: A Compendium. Graphic, Lake Mills, Iowa, 1988, p 34.

34. O'Carroll, RE, Woodrow, J, and Maroun, F: Psychosexual and psychosocial sequelae of closed head injury. Brain Inj 5:303, 1991.

35. Kruetzer, J, and Zasler, N: Psychosexual consequences of traumatic brain injury: methodology and preliminary findings. Brain Inj 3:177, 1989.

36. Spanier, G: Measuring dyadic adjustment: New scales for assessing the quality of marriage and similar dyads. Journal of Marriage and the Family. 38:15, 1976.

37. Murray, JL: Staff attitudes towards the sexuality of persons with intellectual disability. Australia and New Zealand Journal of Developmental Disabilities 19:45, 1994.

38. Ducharme, S, and Gill, KM: Sexual values, training and professional roles. Head Trauma Rehabil 5:38, 1990.

39. Hough, S: Sexuality within the head-injury rehabilitation setting: A staff's perspective. Psychol Rep 65:745, 1989.

40. Ducharme, S: Providing sexuality services in head injury rehabilitation centers: Issues in staff training. International Journal of Adolescent Medicine and Health 7:179, 1994.

41. Medlar, TM: Sexual counseling and traumatic brain injury. Sexuality and Disability 11:57, 1993.

42. Annon, JS: The PLISSIT model: A proposed conceptual scheme for behavioral treatment of sexual problems. Journal of Sex Education and Therapy 2:1, 1976.

43. Smith, D: Sex and disability: Sociosexual education presentation format. In Tallmer, M, et al (eds): Sexuality and Life-Threatening Illness. Charles C Thomas, Springfield, Ill, 1984, p 160.

44. Cole, TM: Gathering a sex history from a physically disabled adult. Sexuality and Disability 9:29, 1991.

45. Boyle, PS: Training in sexuality and disability: Preparing social workers to provide services to individuals with disabilities. Journal of Social Work and Human Sexuality 8:45, 1993.

46. Halstead, L, and Halstead, K: Disability SARs and the small group experience: A conceptual framework. Sexuality and Disability 6:183, 1983.

47. Ziff, SF: Symbolic sexual vocabulary for the severely speech impaired. Journal of Sexuality and Disability 7:3, 1984–1986.

48. Droller, M (conference chair): Impotence. NIH Consensus Statement 10:1, 1992.

49. Blackerby, WF: A treatment model for sexuality disturbance following brain injury. J Head Trauma Rehabil 5(2):73, 1990.

50. Kaplan, HS: The New Sex Therapy. Brunner/Mazel, New York, 1974.

51. Schover, LR, Evans, RB, and von Eschenbach, AC: Sexual rehabilitation in a cancer center: Diagnosis and outcome in 384 cases. Arch Sex Behav 16:445, 1987.

52. Hallett, JD, et al: Role changes after traumatic brain injury in adults. Am J Occup Ther 48:241, 1984.

53. Gervasio, AH: Assertiveness techniques as speech acts. Clinical Psychology Review 7:105, 1987.

54. Wolman, BB, and Money, J (eds): Handbook of Human Sexuality. Jason Aronson, London, 1993.

55. Nelson, MR: Sexuality in childhood disability. In Monga, TN (ed): Sexuality and Disability. Hanley & Belfus, Philadelphia, 1996, p 451.

56. Cromer, BA, et al: Knowledge, attitude and behavior related to sexuality in adolescents with chronic disability. Dev Med Child Neurol 32:602, 1990.

57. Shane, J: Evaluation and treatment of infertility. Clinical Symp 45:2, 1993.

58. Patel, M, and Bontke C: Impact of traumatic brain injury on pregnancy. J Head Trauma Rehabil 5(2):60, 1990.

59. Garden, FH, and Schramm, DM: The effects of aging and chronic illness on sexual function in older adults. In Monga, TN (ed): Sexuality and Disability. Hanley & Belfus, Philadelphia, 1995, p 463.

60. Silny, AJ: Sexuality and aging. In Wolman, BB, and Money, J (eds): Handbook of Human Sexuality. Jason Aronson, London, 1993, p 123.

61. George, LK, and Weiler, SJ: Sexuality in middle and late life: The effects of age, cohort, and gender. Arch Gen Psychiatry 38:919, 1981.

62. Goodman, H, and Englander, J: Traumatic brain injury in elderly individuals. Physical Medicine and Rehabilitation Clinics of North America 3:441, 1992.

63. Kinsey, AC, et al: Sexual Behavior in the Human Female. WB Saunders, Philadelphia, 1953.

64. Kinsey, AC, Pomeroy, WB, and Martin, CE: Sexual Behavior in the Human Male. WB Saunders, Philadelphia, 1948.

65. Fay, RE, et al: Prevalence and patterns of same gender sexual contact among men. Science 1243:338, 1989.

66. Rogers, SM, and Turner, CF: Male-male sexual contact in the USA: Findings from five sample surveys, 1970–1990. Journal of Sex Research 28:491, 1991.

67. Coleman, E, Rosser, B, and Strapko, N: Sexual and intimacy dysfunction among homosexual men and women. Psychiatric Medicine 10:257, 1992.

68. Mapou, RL: Traumatic brain injury rehabilitation with gay and lesbian individuals. J Head Trauma Rehabil 5(2):67, 1990.

69. Holmes, K, et al (eds): Sexually Transmitted Diseases. McGraw-Hill, New York, 1990.

70. American Medical Association: Information on AIDS for the Practicing Physician, vol 3: Recommendations to Family, Friends and Household Contacts, and Guidelines for the General Public. American Medical Association, Chicago, 1987.

71. Slusser, M: Manifestations of sexual abuse in preschool aged children. Issues in Mental Health Nursing 16:481, 1995.

72. Jessee, S: Orofacial manifestations of child abuse and neglect. Am Fam Physician 52:1829, 1989.

73. Ross, CA: Multiple Personality Disorder: Diagnosis, Clinical Features and Treatment. Wiley, New York, 1989.

74. Meyer, RG, and Osborne, YH: Case Studies in Abnormal Behavior, ed 2. Allyn & Bacon, Boston, 1987.

75. Ghusn, H: Sexuality in institutionalized patients. In Monga, TN (ed): Sexuality and Disability. Hanley & Belfus, Philadelphia, 1995, p 475.

76. Griffith, E, and Trieschmann, R: Use of a private hospital room in restoring sexual function to the physically disabled. Sexuality and Disability 13:179, 1978.

CHAPTER 29

Limbs with Restricted or Excessive Motion after Traumatic Brain Injury

NATHANIEL H. MAYER, MD,

MARY ANN E. KEENAN, MD,

and ALBERTO ESQUENAZI, MD

Diffuse axonal injury, multifocal vascular pathology, and diffuse hypoxic encephalopathy lead to a large variety of post-traumatic motor phenomena with many functional consequences. In this chapter, we present a way of organizing the somewhat bewildering array of motor phenomena that are seen after brain injury. Lesions of the central nervous system, the peripheral nervous system, and the musculoskeletal system and lesions causing pain may lead directly or indirectly to two types of motion syndromes: restricted motion or excessive motion.

Restricted limb motion is manifested by limbs with impaired access to environmental targets during voluntary movement production. Restricted limbs are limited in their ability to move toward objects or places because motion across joints is restricted by central or peripheral factors. For example, spastic elbow flexors restrain reaching; spastic finger flexors impair access to the hand for washing; heterotopic bone at the hip restricts step and stride length during gait. Limbs with restricted motion lose their operating range. The general treatment strategy for limbs with restricted motion is to reduce sources of limb restriction by means of medications, surgery, mobilization strategies, and orthotic and assistive devices.

In contrast, syndromes of excessive limb motion are characterized by poor control in the production of voluntary movement parameters such as movement amplitude, accuracy, timing, and force. Limbs with excessive motion are limited in their ability to maintain parameters of voluntary movement and posture within a general operating range (tolerance) of performance. Consider, for example, a patient with cerebellar dysfunction who misses an elevator button when he or she tries to reach out and press it. Button-pressing accuracy is impaired because the patient's dysmetria causes the finger to fall outside the tolerance of the elevator button as a target of specific diameter. Syndromes of excessive motion lead to unreliable and unpredictable performance, postural instability, spatial errors, timing errors, and misapplication of forces. Syndromes of excessive motion generally reflect pathologies affecting control systems or actuator systems. Rehabilitation strategies for limbs with excessive motion have favored environmental modification and orthotic and assistive devices to augment stability. Clinical conditions and phenomena that are associated with restricted or excessive motion after traumatic brain injury (TBI) are presented in Table 29–1.

TABLE 29–1. Clinical Conditions and Phenomena Associated
with Restricted or Excessive Motion after Traumatic Brain Injury

Limbs with Restricted Motion	Limbs with Excessive Motion
1. Spasticity, stiffness, and contracture	1. Cerebellar ataxia
2. Upper motor neuron patterns of dysfunction	2. Brain stem syndrome
3. Heterotopic ossification	3. Clonus
4. Bony malalignment/fracture malunion	4. Ballismus
5. Pain syndromes	5. Chorea
6. Pseudobulbar athetoid syndrome	6. Tremors
7. Brain stem syndrome	7. Myoclonus
8. Rigidity and bradykinesia	8. Tics
9. Dystonia, torticollis, bruxism, locked jaws	9. Ligament and capsular laxities, fractures
10. Decerebrate and decorticate posturing	10. Sensory disturbance

□ PRINCIPLES AND CONSIDERATIONS REGARDING RECOVERY FROM BRAIN INJURY

From the perspective of movement recovery, rehabilitation approaches differ according to the characteristics of each of three distinct time periods: acute injury, motor recovery, and functional adaptation to residual motor deficits. The period of acute injury is characterized by a volatile physiology requiring rehabilitation strategies that are preventive, diagnostic, and supportive. The next period of motor recovery is characterized by changing levels of sensorimotor performance as the patient recovers use of musculoskeletal actuators. In the period of motor recovery, we recommend conservative strategies that temporize rather than surgical ones that produce irreversible changes because the final level of recovery has not yet materialized. The third time period is characterized by a loss of functionality based on permanent motor deficits that may, however, be remediable through rehabilitation strategies influencing the adaptive aspects of movement systems rather than their "normal" physiological functioning.

The Period of Acute Injury

The initial phase of rehabilitation occurs in the acute care hospital immediately after injury. Head trauma is frequently the result of a high-velocity accident. Multiple injuries are common. Diagnosis is difficult. Life-saving resuscitation efforts often detract from complete examination. Patients who are disoriented or who are in coma are unable to assist in the history or physical examination.

A number of principles may be described. The first requirement, with respect to movement problems, is to make the diagnosis. Eleven percent of patients have missed fractures or dislocations[1]; 34% of patients have missed peripheral nerve injuries.[2] A second principle is to assume that the patient will make a good neurological recovery.[3] Basic treatment principles are often waived on the erroneous assumption that the patient will not survive. For example, a patient whose fractures are left untreated on this assumption poses a much greater treatment problem in later periods of recovery. A third consideration is to anticipate uncontrolled limb motion and lack of patient cooperation for reasons of impaired behavior, attention, or cognition.[4] The patient often goes through a period of restlessness and agitation as neurological recovery progresses. During the acute care period, traction and external fixators are best avoided for extremity injuries. Open reduction and internal fixation of fractures and dislocations diminish complications, require less nursing care, allow for early mobilization, and result in fewer residual deformities.[5]

A fourth principle is prevention and containment of deformity.[6] Severe problems with hypertonia are typical in the acute care phase. Range of motion exercises are indicated but often difficult to accomplish when tone is severe. Triggerable reflex phenomena such as the asymmetric tonic neck reflex for the upper limbs and the pinch-induced triple flexion reflex in the lower limbs may be helpful in accomplishing range of motion exercises.[7] These "tricks of the trade" may enable ranging of a limb that otherwise has so much tone that it is virtually impossible to range directly. Temporary nerve blocks, performed bedside, are a consideration when excessive tone restricts motion and the potential for contracture is high.[8] Pulmonary, bowel, bladder, and skin care go a long way toward reducing afferent triggers of hypertonia.

The Period of Motor Recovery

Recovery in the nervous system occurs over a time period ranging from months to years for many different types of functions. In addition, the skeletal system, particularly fractures and related soft tissue injuries, will show recovery from injuries over a somewhat narrower but variable time course. In contrast, heterotopic ossification—abnormal bone forming near proximal joints—may take years to mature, and clinical experience requires that surgical removal be delayed until maturity has been reached.[9] The period of motor recovery may extend to 12 months or more.

During motor recovery, deformities caused by unbalanced muscle forces may reverse themselves as recovery proceeds. Surgery done to rebalance these forces when recovery is still occurring may later result in a renewed imbalance of muscle forces and opposite deformity as the situation changes. During motor recovery, a key principle of managing limbs restricted by excessive tone and resistant to aggressive range of motion therapy is the use of temporizing measures, such as nerve and motor point blocks with serial casting.[10] The effect of blocks with neurolytic or chemodenervating agents will wear off months later, at which time motor issues may have changed and new treatment plans can be formulated. Systemic medications, inherently reversible, sometimes help, but patients with TBI are vulnerable to central side effects that compromise their budding functionality during the period of motor recovery. The newer technique of intrathecal instillation of baclofen, using a programmable drug pump, may be a better technique for reducing central side effects because of the reduced drug concentrations that the technique allows.[11] Definitive surgical procedures such as muscle transfers, lengthenings, or releases are not recommended during motor recovery, although early surgical intervention is sometimes considered if contractures are severe and unyielding to conservative treatments and the patient's functional progress is seriously impeded.

The Period of Functional Adaptation to Residual Motor Deficits

After motor recovery has ended, residual deficits often remain. The ability of an individual to function in the real world does not necessarily correlate with the degree of residual clinical deficits. A patient's function may be improved even if neurological and musculoskeletal deficits are permanent because conservative and surgical interventions may be used to remediate motor problems for adaptive purposes by manipulating musculoskeletal actuators. An adaptive functional result may be produced, even though the period of spontaneous motor recovery has long since ended.[12] For example, a patient who has severe equinovarus deformity in the lower extremity will have a poor base of support that significantly impedes walking. This deformed and nonfunctional base of support can be corrected surgically by suitable muscle transfers, lengthenings, and releases. This type of intervention can be performed any time after physiological recovery has ended, and it is not unusual for such an intervention to be successful a decade after the original brain insult. For equinovarus, the key to functionality is providing a plantigrade base of support that allows stability in the stance phase of gait. In general, strategies that enhance adaptation of movement systems by remediating restricted or excessive motion may be useful in improving functionality, even though neurological deficits from brain injury remain.

☐ PRINCIPLES OF EVALUATION

Patients with restricted motion often give a functional history that describes difficulty acquiring target objects or locations in space. They describe effortful movement as they try to overcome restraining forces such as spasticity, stiffness, and contracture. They complain of impaired access to the axilla, hand, and perineum because of restricted joint motion. Patients with excessive motion typically give a history of spillage including its cosmetic consequences, instability, self-injury, breakage, and other errors when performing daily tasks. The functional history aims at defining the practical circumstances in which patients with restricted or excessive motion need help.

A history and direct observations of the functional usage, reports by family, other collateral sources, and staff may be organized under the categories of passive function and active function.[13] Issues of passive function refer to functional needs that depend on passive manipulation of limbs to achieve functional ends, typically by caregivers, though patients may also manipulate their limbs passively during functional effort. Problems of passive function typically relate to activities in which a limb is passively manipulated for purposes such as washing, dressing, bathing, sitting, and transfers. Issues of active function, by contrast, refer to a patient's direct use of a limb to carry out a functional activity. Categorizing problems of function as being either passive or active, in nature, is a useful construct for treatment goals. For example, when a patient has had no voluntary recovery in a spastic muscle that is causing deformity, surgical release of that muscle is considered. However, if the muscle had recovered some degree of volitional control, surgical lengthening would be considered rather than release. A lengthening procedure preserves continuity of the muscle tendon system and allows for voluntary movement even as it reduces spastic reactivity.

Sensory Evaluation

An important principle of evaluation is testing sensory function. Limb weight-bearing awareness is critical for lower extremity functioning. Retained sensation is essential to functional usage of the hand. Basic modalities such as pain, light touch, and temperature must be present at least to a moderate degree. Two-point discrimination is a valuable predictive test.[14] A patient rarely uses the hand for functional activities if the discrimination between two points is greater than 10 millimeters. Proprioception and kinesthetic awareness of the limb in space are important. Kinesthetic awareness may be tested in an individual by passively moving joints of the involved part and asking the patient, with eyes closed, to duplicate these positional movements with the contralateral limb. We have not found stereognosis to be a practical test in patients who lack the fine motor control necessary to manipulate an object.

Kinesiological Considerations Underlying Functional Examination

Motion at the shoulder and hip have many degrees of freedom; as a consequence, these are the only joints that can place the hand and foot in a large volume of spatial locations. Pathologies that restrict shoulder motion characteristically lead to inadequate placement of the hand in space. In the lower extremity, restricted motion at the hip impairs step length, stride length, and base width. When disorders of excessive motion occur at the shoulder or the hip, the length of the limb (from hip to foot or shoulder to hand) magnifies the absolute error of shoulder and hip at the hand and foot. For example, a 5-degree error at the shoulder translates into an error of several centimeters for the outstretched arm when measured at the fingers. A 5-degree

error at the finger metacarpophalangeal joint results only in a few millimeters of linear error on an absolute basis. The more proximal the joint, the greater the absolute linear error one finds distally. As a consequence, dysmetria at the shoulder produces significant error at the hand, even if there is no dysmetria at the elbow, wrist, or finger joints. Ataxia at the hip joint results in great variability in the width of the base of support, as well as in step and stride length. Hemiballismus produces great bodily perturbation, primarily because it originates proximally at the shoulder. Flinging shoulder movements catapult the arm and shake the body as well.

Kinesiologically, the elbow and knee are length change elements. Flexion and extension of the elbow result in shortening or lengthening of the moment arm of the upper extremity about the shoulder. Lengthening the upper extremity serves functional purposes for reaching, acquiring targets away from the body, or pushing targets away. Flexion at the elbow enables bringing objects or the hand to the body. Flexion and extension of the knee change the moment arm of the lower extremity in a similar manner. Flexion of the knee is critical to clearance of the lower extremity because it effectively shortens the limb, enabling the swinging limb to clear the floor at the level of the foot. Lengthening the lower extremity by extending the knee contributes to step and stride length. In patients with "stiff knee" gait, the relatively longer lower extremity has difficulty clearing the floor during swing phase. Similarly, restricted motion at the elbow, seen in cases of heterotopic ossification, results in a limb that is unable to shorten or lengthen. The patient is unable to bring hand to mouth or to reach out. Excessive motion at the elbow or knee leads to instability. For example, ligamentous and soft tissue laxity behind the knee may lead to hyperextension thrust during stance phase, which may produce pain and instability of the body as it advances over the stance phase limb. Severe elbow clonus may lead to inaccurate reaching in the upper extremity. Elbow tremor has an effect on object transport and usage.

In the upper extremity, the forearm orients the hand toward the body by means of supination or away from the body toward the environment by means of pronation. The foot articulates with uneven surfaces by means of inversion and eversion. Pathologies that restrict forearm motion result in restricted hand orientation to or from the body. For example, pronation deformity impairs supination of the hand as it proceeds toward the mouth during self-feeding. In the lower extremity, a foot deformed in supination causes painful weight bearing during stance phase. Excessive motion of a forearm or a foot, seen in tremor, clonus, or choreiform movements, often produces spillage, inaccurate target acquisition, or articulatory instability.

The wrist allows for local adjustment of the hand during target acquisition. Small amplitude adjustments are made by the wrist as the trajectory of reaching for an object is finalized. A similar function is attributed to the ankle, which allows for articulation with the ground, particularly on inclines but also when the tibia translates forward or backward during standing. When the body's center of gravity moves short distances, ankle motion is usually sufficient to compensate for anteroposterior shifts in superincumbent body weight. Larger excursions of the center of gravity typically elicit compensatory flexion or extension of the hip or taking a step forward to prevent falling. When ankle motion is restricted by severe equinus, the tibia cannot advance forward during stance phase. As a result, the contralateral step length shortens because the body is unable to advance forward over the stance phase limb. Restricted motion at the wrist, secondary to flexor spasticity results in weakened grasp and impaired finger manipulation. Excessive motion at the wrist secondary to clonus, chorea, or tremor leads to unstable use of objects, particularly those needing precision grip.

The hand functions to grasp, release, and manipulate objects. Restricted motions of fingers and thumb have obviously deleterious effects on upper limb usage as a whole. For example, spastic finger flexors that result in a clenched fist deformity restrict the hand's ability to open prior to grasping an object; once the object is grasped, there is an impairment in the ability to release the grasped object. Excessive motions affecting thumb and fingers may be seen with choreiform movements, tremor, or clonus. Such movements impair object usage, object stabilization, accuracy of manipulation, and precision of use. The major function of the foot is to articulate with the ground and with shoe wear. Restricted motion impairs ground reaction forces that are transmitted through the foot. For example, spastic toe flexors contribute to an impairment of rollover during terminal stance. Hitchhiker's great toe (resulting from a spastic extensor hallucis longus) can result in a painful toe dorsum that abrades against the anterior toe box of the shoe. Excessive motion at the foot also interferes with the stability of the foot and hence compromises stability of superincumbent body mass.

Laboratory Studies

For patients with head injury who may be noncompliant, radiographic examination is especially useful in the diagnosis of structural problems. Occult fractures, malunion, and heterotopic ossification are important diagnostic entities that are found frequently as causes of restricted motion after brain injury. Radiographic appearance is singularly important in determining the maturity of heterotopic ossification prior to its surgical removal, along with a normal alkaline phosphatase. Because peripheral nerve injuries are common, electrodiagnostic testing is a useful laboratory modality. In upper motor neuron syndromes, multichannel dynamic electromyography (EMG) studies, kinesiologic in nature, allow the examiner to evaluate relationships between agonist and antagonist muscles across individual joints and limb segments. Voluntary capacity and spastic reactivity are examined and interpreted in light of clinical and functional complaints. The laboratory examination supplements clinical examination because the latter alone may not identify all offending muscles. Dynamic EMG examination often provides details of analysis that give direction and confidence for therapeutic interventions. In addition to dynamic EMG studies, gait laboratories may examine ground reaction forces, joint motion, and foot pressures to further enhance movement analysis.[15]

Treatment Considerations

Five treatment considerations are useful in dealing with movement related to TBI:

1. Treatment varies as a function of the period of recovery.

2. Treatment differs for focal versus diffuse problems.

3. Many pharmacological agents that are useful in treating movement disorders also produce side effects that are dysfunctional. A balance needs to be struck between benefits and side effects, and a useful method is to target specific results that the drug agent is expected to produce.

4. The ability to comply with treatment is an important consideration in selecting treatment for persons with TBI.

5. In an era of managed care, resource considerations may play a specific role in therapeutic selection.

In the period of motor recovery, temporizing interventions are used because permanent changes may result in chronic imbalance of forces across joints. Thus, neurolytic agents such as phenol and chemodenervation agents such as botulinum toxin A are used because they "wear off" in approximately 3 to 5 months.[16–19] These agents are used when restricted motion is a result of focal spasticity. When these agents wear off, reevaluation determines whether additional recovery has taken place and whether there is further indication for reblocking. Oral antispastic agents may be helpful in this period, but surgical corrections are generally not performed. For patients with pathologies causing excessive motion, environmental modification and, in some cases, weights, bracing, or oral medications may be considered during the period of physiological recovery.

During the period of residual deficits and functional adaptation, definitive orthopedic interventions may be indicated in patients with restricted motion. Passive and active function are targeted as goals of surgical intervention. Neurolytic and chemodenervation blocks may be performed, but we note that repeated blocks may be less effective for botulinum toxin because of the possibility of antibody formation and for phenol blocks because of the possibility of fibrosis after many previous injections. Oral antispastic agents may be used when spasticity is diffuse.[20] In patients with excessive motion, environmental modification, orthotics, and weights may be considered. Neurosurgical interventions such as stereotactic thalamotomy are sometimes used for specific conditions.[21]

Treatment approaches vary, depending on whether spastic or dystonic restrictions in motion are related to many muscles diffusely or localized to only a few. In general, when restricted motion can be attributed to small numbers of muscles, localized muscle blocks become feasible. If widespread muscles are involved, however, oral or intrathecal antispastic agents may be considered. Patients with attentional deficits or memory disorders may be further compromised by antispastic agents such as baclofen, diazepam, and clonidine that have sedating properties. Even drugs such as dantrolene sodium, with a peripheral mechanism of action, may also cause drowsiness. Though also sedating, the drug tizanidine, newly available in the United States, has been reported to be tolerable and useful in cases where exacerbation of weakness was a concern.[22–24] The recent arrival of baclofen pump technology, allowing small intrathecal concentrations that minimize central side effects and provide continuous delivery, may play a larger role in the future. Our preference for patients with TBI is to use focal injections of neurolytic or chemodenervating agents to treat problems of restricted motion secondary to spasticity (if the functional problems of the patient can truly be linked to specific muscles). Even if many muscles in a limb are involved, a number of focal injections may ameliorate function without central side effects. For patients

with focal excessive motion, compensatory use of other limbs is one strategy that is often adopted. In addition, bracing may be used in situations of ligamentous or capsular laxity. When the problem of excessive motion involves many joints diffusely, environmental modifications, adaptive strategies, and customized solutions based on specific goals, knowledge of family resources, and living arrangements are often helpful.

The patient's cognitive and behavioral ability to comply with treatment plays a key role in many of the decisions regarding treatment of movement-related disturbances. A number of concepts apply:

1. Patients with TBI often forget to take pills because they have difficulty organizing themselves to do tasks that unfold over time, among which is the medication schedule.

2. Surgical interventions require postoperative mobilization, and, for best results, patients must be able to participate in the therapy program from cognitive, behavioral, and motivational perspectives.

3. Patients need some modicum of pain tolerance, and they have to work hard to make and consolidate gains after surgery. For example, those who undergo excision of heterotopic ossification must endure physical and occupational therapy to mobilize joints that have been severely restricted by the pathological process. Patients with poor compliance preoperatively do not do well in the postoperative therapy phase because they are not compliant with the rigor of the therapy regimens.

4. Procedural techniques play a role in decision making for patients with TBI. For example, the technique of botulinum toxin injection overall appears to be quicker and easier than phenolization techniques for patients with TBI. Both techniques may be more practical to rely on for some patients than a daily oral medication regimen.

5. The cost of treatment needs to be factored in because there are choices. For example, the cost of phenol is negligible, and botulinum toxin is expensive (though the cost for 3 months of some oral agents may be similar). When a patient is hospitalized and the hospital is reimbursed on a per diem basis, the cost of botulinum toxin is a significant percentage of the overall per diem that the hospital may be reimbursed under certain insurance plans. This fact is often a disincentive for using this medication in hospitalized patients. It is often easier to obtain coverage and use botulinum toxin on an outpatient basis. Many patients with movement-related problems and consequences have skin problems and may require specialized and expensive beds. Again, the availability of funding through insurance or family sources varies in such cases. Orthotic solutions to limb positioning are frequently used as a clinical strategy. The type of orthosis that is used, however, is also a resource consideration. "High tech" solutions such as molded orthoses are usually the most expensive; "off the shelf" orthoses are less expensive and hence might be generally more available. When there are virtually no resources, sometimes ad hoc solutions such as hightop sneakers may be a "low tech" solution. In all situations in which resources are a concern, clinical judgment is needed to determine whether a less expensive treatment will suffice and, therefore, may be prescribed in good conscience. Health care providers have an ethical obligation to provide the care needed by their patients. Once they undertake the care of a specific patient with specific circumstances, care appropriate to the specific needs of that patient must be given.

◻ LIMBS WITH EXCESSIVE MOTION: SPECIFIC CLINICAL CONDITIONS AND APPROACHES

Cerebellar Pathway Ataxia

Although many different clinical terms have been coined to capture observable features of cerebellar pathway ataxia, excessive variability in movement parameters such as accuracy, force, rhythm, and timing lies at the essence of the problem.[25] Terms such as *dysmetria, past pointing,* and *dysdiadochokinesia* exemplify movements whose amplitude varies in excess of what is normally expected. When reaching for a target, an ataxic limb may undershoot the target on one trial and overshoot the target on another. The development of force is similarly plagued by underdevelopment or overdevelopment of force, ultimately resulting in inappropriate application of force. It is not unusual for a patient with cerebellar ataxia to crush a styrofoam cup by exerting too much force during gripping. From a functional perspective, patients with cerebellar ataxia spill liquids, break objects, mishandle actions that require precision, and generally do poorly with actions that require target accuracy. For the lower extremities, ataxic motions produce variability in step length and base width. It is often difficult for patients with lower limb ataxia to maintain their center of gravity within their base of support, and they easily lose balance as their center of gravity moves outside of the support base. When the trunk but not the legs are ataxic, the patient tends to compensate for an ataxic center of mass by abducting the lower extremities to widen the base of support. Patients with a wide-based gait are actually compensating for an ataxic trunk. If the lower extremities were also ataxic, they would not be able to regulate the base width to keep it wide but rather would suffer from variability in base width as well as step and stride lengths. In addition to variability in amplitude and force generation, ataxic limbs lose rhythmicity when performing repetitive movements. The common test of finger tapping reveals variability in rhythm as well as amplitude when the patient is requested to maintain rhythmic, repetitive action. Functional tasks that require rhythmicity, such as brushing and wiping, are typically impaired in the ataxic patient.

Controlling the length of a limb is important to treatment strategy for the patient with cerebellar ataxia. As previously noted, proximal joint ataxia magnifies the absolute arc of error at the end of a limb. Consequently, an ataxic shoulder causes significant dysmetria at the hand. When the arm is fully extended, accuracy is most impaired. A similar observation can be made for the lower extremity: Ataxia at the hip is magnified in terms of absolute arc of foot movement. Clinical strategies that emphasize shortening of the limbs, such as holding objects close to the body, are functionally more adaptive for the patient with limb ataxia. It is not uncommon to observe a patient with upper limb ataxia attempt to stabilize a bent elbow on a table throughout a feeding cycle, scooping food from a plate and bringing the mouth to the utensil to avoid lifting the elbow off the table (Fig. 29–1). In such an adaptive strategy, the patient attempts to reduce the degrees of freedom by minimizing movement of the ataxic limb; at the same time, the length of the upper limb is "cut down" by flexion at the elbow. Aids such as weighted jackets, wrist cuffs, and shoes have been recommended to improve accuracy, but in our experience weighting is inconsistently helpful. For some patients, the benefit of a weighted cuff may result more from their avoidance of full elbow extension because of the weight's heaviness than for any other reason. The use of isoniazid and beta-adrenergic blockers has been reported for intention tremor in patients with multiple sclerosis, but there is little experience with this medication in patients with brain injury.[26,27] In the lower extremity, wide-based walkers help stability. We prefer a two-wheeled walker that rolls on the ground at all times. Otherwise, a patient who must lift the walker may lose balance when the walker is in the air. Bilateral platform walkers may give added stability, when needed.

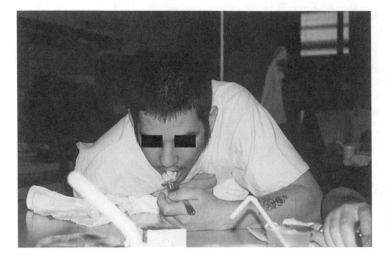

FIGURE 29–1. This 19-year-old patient with TBI minimizes ataxic errors by stabilizing his upper limb on the table, scooping eggs from his plate with small movements, and bringing his mouth to the fork rather than the fork to his mouth.

Brain Stem Syndrome

Twenty percent of patients in Roberts's[28,29] series demonstrated combined hemiataxia with contralateral spastic hemiparesis. The usual cause was uncal herniation that compressed the brain stem, causing damage to ipsilateral cerebellar pathways and the contralateral corticospinal tract. Concerning the upper extremity, a decision usually has to be made with regard to which upper limb should be selected for dominance retraining. When the hemiparetic limb has greater control over accuracy (even if movement is restricted), it may be more suitable than the ataxic limb to perform everyday skills. For instance, if the upper motor neuron limb can produce a movement pattern that can bring a spoon to the mouth, feeding training should probably be focused on using this limb instead of the ataxic one. In some situations, however, it may be desirable to have the hemiparetic limb "guide" the ataxic limb by grasping it and moving with it, which may have the effect of damping oscillatory ataxic movements and improving accuracy. For example, the accuracy of transporting food to mouth with a spoon may be improved if the hemiparetic hand grasps the ataxic limb at the wrist and helps guide the hand-held spoon toward the mouth. Transfers, ambulation, and sitting balance pose unique problems for patients with a brain stem syndrome because restrictive movement on the hemiparetic side is commingled with excessive and highly variable movement production on the ataxic side. Patients who ambulate typically do so with the aid of a walker. A platform is usually necessary on the hemiparetic side. Sometimes weights placed around the ankle help to provide some additional stability during gait. The use of locked ankle-foot orthoses to reduce the degrees of freedom may also be considered. When using a wheelchair, the patient typically wheels it with the ataxic limb. Inaccuracy is observed when the patient attempts to grasp the rim of the wheel, but once it is grasped, the patient has much less difficulty pushing the wheel forward. Dysmetria is usually not sufficient to perturb the heavy wheelchair system.

Clonus

Clonus, an oscillatory phenomenon usually at a frequency of 5 to 7 Hz, reflects stretch reactivity in the upper motor neuron syndrome.[30,31] Muscle clonus may be induced by the examiner with rapid stretch, and clonus may be sustained or unsustained. Clonus may be induced by the patient as well. For example, calf muscle clonus may be induced at initial contact with the ground or later in stance phase or when the tibia attempts to roll forward. Clonus may also be induced by afferent stimuli that cause reflexive movement in a limb. The resulting stretch generated by afferent-induced movement leads to a clonic episode. Eletromyographically, clonus is manifested by bursts of EMG activity at the frequency rate of the clinically observed clonus. Alternating activity between agonists and antagonists may be seen in many patients, and under these circumstances clonus is often sustained.

Clonus induced by an examiner in a single muscle or muscle group is inconsequential to function; however, when patients develop sustained clonus during functional activities, major functional interference may result. Some patients report that they have been literally knocked off their feet by violent clonus, often induced by episodic afferent input such as a cold blowing wind. A history of frequently occurring disabling episodes is a good indication for treatment. Clonus may be aborted by placing clonic muscles on slack. Patients may be taught how to diminish their own clonus with this technique. If a small number of muscles can be identified as a major source of clonic activity, focal injections with neurolytic or chemodenervating agents may be utilized. However, when clonus involves many muscles diffusely, especially if two or more limbs are clonic, a systemic agent is useful. We prefer dantrolene sodium is such cases because this agent is particularly useful in weakening the force developed by low-frequency, nontetanic stimulation of muscle.[32] Smooth contraction of muscle requires tetanic neural input to muscle, usually in excess of 20 Hz. Dantrolene inhibits release of calcium within the sarcoplasmic reticulum, and this inhibition is maximized at low frequencies of stimulation. At tetanic frequencies, calcium literally floods the sarcoplasmic reticulum, rendering dantrolene inhibition much less effective. Because dantrolene's physiological effect is peripheral, it has a favorable profile with respect to central side effects, although central side effects can occur.[33] It is a reasonable choice for mild to moderate spasticity, especially for patients with clonus. Clonus often remits at a dose level of 50 mg 4 times a day. The maximum recommended dose is 600 mg a day in divided doses. Patients with preexisting liver disease need to be scrutinized more closely because this medication may cause toxic liver cell reactions.

Hemiballismus

Ballismus is descriptively defined as involuntary limb movements that are flinging or ballistic in nature.[34] Typical movements begin suddenly, often without warning, and they originate proximally within the limb. They are most extreme in shoulder and hip girdle musculature. Movements usually have a rotatory component that is more evident in the arms than in the legs. The arm is usually affected first, and most often both arm and leg contribute to rapid, flinging movements that occur at irregular intervals. Many patients have abnormal facial movements, and a small percentage exhibit glossal and palatal movements. Generalized arousal increases the frequency and the amplitude of movements, and those movements are strikingly reduced when the patient is relaxed. Movements are not present when the patient is asleep. Functionally, ballismic movements may be violent enough to cause lacerations and bruises on the limb that bangs against objects. The limb is not functionally useful during a ballismic episode. Hemiballismus, involving extremities on one side of the body, is the most common form.

Hemiballismus is most commonly seen after injury to the contralateral subthalamic nucleus of Luys, but it has also been noted with lesions in the striatum, the thalamus, and even the cerebellum.[35] Animal studies have generated ballismic movements with lesions in the subthalamic area, but no ballismic movements were noted with lesions in the globus pallidus alone, which suggests that the subthalamic nucleus has an inhibitory influence on the globus pallidus. Consequently, it has been thought that decreased inhibitory outflow to the globus pallidus from the subthalamic nucleus may lead to dopamine overactivity in the striatum, resulting in ballismic movements. Clinicians have tried to alleviate this excess dopamine activity with neuroleptics such as haloperidol and other drugs such as reserpine and tetrabenazine.[36,37] In addition, γ-aminobutyric acid (GABA) is thought to mediate outflow from the subthalamic nucleus to the striatum; therefore, GABAnergic agents have been used to treat hemiballismus. Kant and Zeiler reported a post-traumatic case of hemiballismus that was successfully treated with a combination of haloperidol (a dopamine antagonist) and clonazepam (a GABAnergic agent).[34] The incidence of hemiballismus after TBI is very small, and only a handful of case reports are present in the literature. Valproic acid, a drug that is believed to enhance GABA transmission, may also be useful in treating hemiballismus.[38]

Chorea

Chorea reflects involuntary, dancelike movements characterized by rapid jerks without a specific rhythmic or regular pattern. Movements can involve arms, legs, face, neck, and trunk, but, in contrast to patients with ballismus, whose movement patterns are more often determined by proximal muscle involvement, patients with chorea show distal muscle involvement.[39] Some have described chorea as "semipurposeful."

Because choreiform movements are usually situated more distally and are generally small in amplitude, they pose their greatest functional interference in tasks that require fine accuracy and precision. Only a small number of cases have been reported after TBI, typically associated with athetosis.[40] (The latter is characterized by involuntary slow, sinuous movements of any muscle group, including the tongue and face, often presenting prominently in the hand and foot.) Chorea has been attributed to lesions in the contralateral subthalamic nucleus, striatum, and thalamic nuclei. The disorder may respond to valproic acid and phenobarbital.[41,42] Stereotactic destruction of part of the dentate nucleus has been reported as a neurosurgical intervention for this condition.[43]

Tremor

Tremor is an involuntary movement characterized by rhythmic oscillations, usually produced by alternating activity of agonist and antagonist muscle groups. Tremor may occur at rest; during the initiation, course, or end of a movement; during the maintenance of a limb posture; during position-specific or task-specific circumstances; or during the course of voluntary isometric contraction. The functional consequences of tremor relate to its excessive motion in circumstances that impair accuracy and precision. Resting tremors, most commonly of the pill-rolling finger movement variety seen in parkinsonian syndromes, do not really pose a functional problem, except for its cosmetic appearance. Postural tremor is typically induced by having the patient extend an upper limb and hold it in that sustained posture. It becomes functionally problematic when a task requires a postural hold. For example, pouring liquids requires just such a postural set and thus is problematic for patients with postural tremor. The most functionally disabling type is kinetic tremor, in which oscillations are induced and may get progressively worse as the limb moves through a trajectory. Especially problematic are movements to specific targets requiring end-point accuracy that elicit a specific type of tremor known as *intention tremor.* Clinicians typically attempt to elicit such tremor by asking the patient to do finger-to-nose testing. It is not advisable to ask a patient who truly has an intention tremor to touch her or his nose because the excessive oscillations induced by this maneuver are likely to result in facial or ocular injury. Patients with intention tremor have significant difficulty using the upper extremities for activities of daily living.

The literature on tremor after traumatic brain injury is relatively small.[44] Treatment has generally been difficult. Medications that have been tried in the management of tremor include propranolol, valproic acid, and clonazepam.[45–47] Drugs such as valproic acid and clonazepam, which have influence in GABAnergic transmission pathways, have been used empirically to treat tremor. Cerebellar pathway damage is probably implicated in many types of tremor after TBI, and medications affecting cerebellar pathway lesions have been particularly unrewarding thus far. A peripheral approach may be taken to try to control tremor because muscle contraction is the ultimate expression of central lesions causing tremor. If a relatively small number of muscles can be identified as tremorous or as causing the major part of a dysfunction, chemodenervation agents such as botulinum toxin or phenol blocks may be considered.[48] Weighting of a limb sometimes reduces the magnitude of a tremor, though muscle fatigue may ultimately result. Neurosurgical interventions that have been tried include thalamic stimulation and stereotactic thalamotomy, especially for tremors of cerebellar origin.[21] Medical-surgical treatments of tremor are still problematic. Strategies that urge compensatory behaviors and avoidance of tasks that are vulnerable to tremor are probably of greatest benefit.

Myoclonus

Myoclonus is an abrupt, shocklike, fine or gross involuntary movement that may be irregular or rhythmic in its timing.[49] When it is secondary to muscle contraction, the term *positive myoclonus* may be applied. When actively contracting muscles sustaining a limb posture suddenly have their contraction briefly interrupted, the limb may drop briefly to produce the phenomenon of negative myoclonus. Asterixis, most often seen with liver failure, is an example of this type of jerklike relaxation phenomenon. Myoclonus activated by voluntary (rapid, fine) movement is termed *action myoclonus.* The causes and sites of pathological lesions associated with myoclonus are diverse.[50] Action myoclonus can be functionally disabling because the excessive movements that are produced generate inaccuracies during target acquisition. Palatal myoclonus, not infrequently seen after head injury, may affect vocal quality; however, many of these patients are anarthric or severely dysarthric. The cholinergic system may be relevant to palatal myoclonus, and occasional improvements may be seen with anticholinergic medications.[51] Action myoclonus, by contrast, may be sensitive to drugs such as clonazepam. Medications such as valproic acid that increase the level of GABA at nerve terminals may also be empirically useful in these conditions. Some types of myoclonus, particularly after hypoxic damage to the brain, may be responsive to serotonin precursors such as 5-hydroxytryptophan. All such medications have central sedating properties and must be used with caution in patients with TBI.

Tics

Tics are sudden, intermittent, habitual, usually complex sequences of coordinated automatic movements. Vocal tics such as coprolalia and echolalia are extremely common following brain injury. Examples of motor tics include head and bodily shakes, grimacing, and shoulder shrugs. Sniffing and snorting behaviors are seen. Tics may be interposed between normal behaviors, and they disappear during sleep. Stress may make them worse.

Medications such as clonazepam (a GABA agonist) and clonidine (a noradrenergic agonist) have been suggested for their management. Tics are often perceived as peculiar behaviors and thus bring the patient to the attention of others. Bodily tics may cause problems during activities of daily living. A small number of post-traumatic tics have been described in the literature. It is of note that methylphenidate (or amphetamine), frequently used in patients with TBI to improve attention and arousal, may exacerbate tics.[52]

Capsular and Ligamentous Laxity

Inferior subluxation of the shoulder, fairly common in patients with stroke, is not seen as often in patients with TBI, perhaps because patients with TBI do not typically go through a hypotonic stage as often as patients with stroke do. However, brachial plexopathy with flaccid paralysis of the shoulder does occur as part of brain injury with multiple trauma, and inferior subluxation of the shoulder is a common occurrence in such patients.[53] Subluxation is usually self-limiting, but, occasionally, the shoulder becomes chronically subluxed and painful. Patients typically have little or no use of the involved extremity. Because the sensory deficit does not match the motor deficit, patients complain of greater pain when seated or standing. The pain may be caused by chronic stretch of the shoulder capsule or from traction on the brachial plexus. Physical examination shows a positive sulcus sign with little to no active motion of the involved shoulder. There is a prominence of the acromion and atrophy of the deltoid. There may be contracture of the shoulder in adduction and internal rotation. The symptoms are not relieved by either subacromial or intra-articular injections of anesthetics. Radiographs show inferior subluxation of the humerus on the glenoid. Brachial plexopathy must be ruled out by electromyography. Conservative treatment may include electrical stimulation to the deltoid and supraspinatus muscles, but commonly and pragmatically the arm is placed in a sling. This relieves symptoms by reducing stretch on neurovascular and joint structures. Although usually successful in the short run, it is frequently unacceptable to the patient as a permanent solution. Dynamic shoulder orthoses are also available but tend to be cumbersome and rejected by patients. A surgical solution for the problem of excessive laxity is the biceps suspension procedure. A drill hole is made in the humerus, posterior and parallel to the biceps groove. The detached tendon of the long head of the biceps is then passed through this channel, pulled back, and sutured to itself to provide a loop to hold the humeral head in reduced position. It is helpful to suture the biceps tendon to the bicipital groove. The repair is protected in a sling for 3 months to allow healing of bone to tendon. This technique theoretically keeps the glenohumeral joint reduced while allowing motion.

Excessive motion at the shoulder is also associated with various types of clavicular fracture with acromioclavicular ligamentous disruption. Although clavicular fracture might otherwise be treated with closed methods, this procedure may be difficult to manage if spasticity or paralytic muscle imbalance is also present and, in particular, if severe deformity is produced by muscle imbalance. Open reduction and internal fixation in such situations should be considered. The most common injuries in the upper extremity are fractures about the clavicle and scapula and also separation of the acromioclavicular joint. A high index of suspicion is needed to recognize peripheral nerve injuries in this setting. It is not unusual for brachial plexus injury to be present, especially when the upper extremity appears to be flail while other extremities are spastic.

In the lower extremity, joint and ligamentous disruption can occur anywhere because of multiple trauma, but the knee, in particular, is usually vulnerable. Cruciate and collateral ligament strains and disruptions may produce excessive joint motion. Patients with brain injury may not provide discernible symptoms or behavioral compliance with examination. Superimposed spasticity of muscles may also complicate the picture. Mobilizing a patient with a damaged knee may be aggravated by a spastic equinus at the ankle, which results in hyperextension thrust at the knee. Pressure on the posterior capsule of the knee as well as on impaired ligamentous and meniscal structures exacerbates the situation. The use of knee, ankle, and/or foot orthoses to control excessive motion may be indicated. Operative intervention is usually necessary, but the timing of such intervention is artful because behavioral compliance with postoperative rehabilitation is especially important.

Fractures, of course, intrinsically create excessive limb motion. Five general principles in the acute management of fractures in patients with TBI are usefully kept in mind:

1. Anticipate the presence of musculoskeletal injuries in high- and low-velocity injuries. Initial radiographs should include anteroposterior (AP) and lateral views of the cervical spine and AP views of the pelvis, hips, and knees.

2. Treat all fractures based on the view that the patient will recover neurologically.

3. Anticipate uncontrolled limb motion in the patient with a severe injury. Stable internal fixation of fractures is usually justified.

4. Avoid casting joints in the flexed position or in equinus because spasticity may result in contractures. Open reduction, internal fixation of a fracture should be seriously entertained if muscle spasticity is present.

5. Avoid skeletal or skin traction in the confused and agitated patient,[54] which adds difficulty to nursing care and may result in patient self-injury.

Sensory Disturbance

Though peripheral nerve injury is common after TBI, profound sensory loss of an entire limb is usually not seen (except in massive root avulsions). However, occasionally an insensate limb may be secondary to a severe parietal lobe lesion. Lesions of the parietal lobe affect the patient's kinesthesis on the contralateral side of the body. Such patients lose passive and active position sense, and, if blindfolded, their limb movement toward a target is severely disturbed. These patients lose their spatial frame of reference, and, without visual guidance, they operate "blindly." They may quickly adapt to lack of kinesthetic awareness by using visual compensation strategies, but they get into trouble when vision is occluded in the course of performing ordinary particular tasks. Most often these patients prefer to use the uninvolved limb.

◻ LIMBS WITH RESTRICTIVE MOTION: SPECIFIC CLINICAL CONDITIONS AND APPROACHES

Spasticity, Stiffness, and Contracture

In a literal sense, *spasticity* connotes the increasing resistance felt by an examiner stretching a muscle group across a joint at increasing velocities of stretch.[55] (In contrast, *rigidity* shows little or no velocity sensitivity, meaning that the examiner experiences just about the same resistance to stretch, irrespective of whether a muscle group is stretched at slow, medium, or rapid rates.) Spasticity is a component of the upper motor neuron syndrome (UMN), whose larger context is more important to our understanding of movement problems in this syndrome. According to Lance, the distinguishing features of UMN syndrome include enhanced phasic (ten-

don jerk) and tonic (spastic) stretch reflexes, released flexor reflexes in the lower extremities, weakness, and loss of movement dexterity.[56] The UMN syndrome is commonly associated with increased stiffness and contracture of spastic muscle. Herman has shown that the rheologic (viscoelastic and plastic) properties of muscle change in the direction of increased stiffness when spasticity is severe, especially if contracture has already begun to develop.[57] Changes in the rheologic properties of muscle and soft tissues restrain motion. In persons with spasticity, the development of force and control over force, amplitude, and timing of movement is reduced not only by paresis of agonist muscles and spastic reactivity of antagonist muscles but also by changes in the rheologic properties of spastic antagonists.

"Muscle tone" is not a simple construct. It depends upon complex mechanisms, of which hyperexcitable reflexes are just one part. The biomechanics of joint motion, the active contractile and passive rheologic properties of muscle, tendon, skin, subcutaneous connective tissue, blood vessels, and nerves, all contribute to the resistance the examiner appreciates as "muscle tone," and they also contribute to the resistance that the patient with UMN works against when trying to generate a voluntary movement. For rehabilitation clinicians, manifestations of spasticity, muscle stiffness, and contracture become intertwined with the issue of how much motor control has been spared and how much will recover. These factors are important determinants of how the patient will function with the involved limbs. They are also pertinent to the clinical goals—namely, whether the clinician is trying to improve passive function or active function.

Functional problems linked to the consequences of an upper motor neuron lesion take on a context that is broader than the circumscribed phenomenon of spasticity. For example, many complications can occur in the presence of spasticity. Restrictive contractures are common. Limited positioning and myotatic contracture, combined with a patient's diminished nutritional status, can result in pressure sores or hygiene problems. When fractures are present, malunions can occur in the face of uncontrolled muscle tone and accelerated fracture healing. Joint subluxation can also occur from prolonged spasticity or the attempts to range a joint in the face of severe spasticity. If a ligament injury occurred, frank dislocation of a joint can be caused by hypertonicity. Spasticity also appears to be one of several etiologic factors in the formation of heterotopic ossification in periarticular locations.[58] Another common complication of spasticity is acquired peripheral neuropathy. The most common peripheral neuropathies acquired with severe spasticity and contracture are ulnar neuropathy at the elbow from severe flexion and continuous pressure on the ulnar nerve and carpal tunnel syndrome secondary to severe wrist flexion and pressure on the median nerve by the edge of the transverse carpal ligament.[59]

DIFFUSE SPASTICITY AND SYSTEMIC ANTISPASTIC DRUGS

When problems of passive or active function are rooted in spasticity spread across many muscle groups, systemic drugs are often considered. Two oral agents, baclofen and dantrolene sodium (discussed earlier), are more commonly used than diazepam and some recent mention has been made of clonidine and tizanidine.[60] Baclofen, a GABA analogue, supports presynaptic inhibition in the spinal cord and suppresses release of excitatory neurotransmitters.[20] Baclofen ultimately appears to have an inhibitory effect on alpha motor neuron activity that leads to a reduction in skeletal muscle spasticity. Clinically, it has well-documented effects in patients with spinal cord injury and multiple sclerosis. Experience in patients with TBI is not wide, and central side effects have been a concern. Oral baclofen may be initiated at 15 mg/day in divided doses and increased to 80 mg/day as needed. It may have a distinct role in patients who are permanently vegetative; whose spasticity is a hindrance to caregivers performing passive functions such as bathing, dressing, toileting, and skin care; and who can tolerate high doses of the drug without penalty of central side effects such as drowsiness, confusion, and hallucinations. Withdrawal symptoms may appear if the drug is not tapered when discontinued.

Diazepam, a centrally acting and highly sedating drug of the benzodiazepine class, increases the inhibitory effects of GABA.[61] Ultimately, inhibition of alpha motor neuron excitability results in diazepam's antispasticity effect, but some of its muscle-relaxant properties may be caused by its generalized sedating properties. Diazepam is not used much in people with TBI because of sedation and memory impairment. However, patients who have persistent flexor spasms that disturb sleep and activities of daily living may benefit from small doses appropriately timed to reduce the frequency and intensity of such spasms. The drug is available in 2, 5, and 10 mg and generally is titrated upward slowly in 2- or 2.5-mg steps, beginning at an initial dose of 4 mg/day.

Clonidine is thought to act centrally as an α_2-noradrenergic receptor *agonist.* Its mechanism of action in spasticity may be related to suppression of polysynaptic reflexes in the spinal cord. Clonidine has been reported as useful in treating supraspinal "brain stem" spasticity, although its effectiveness has largely been studied in patients with spinal cord injury.[62] In patients with stroke, tizanidine, an imidazoline derivative similar to clonidine but without the same cardiovascular effects, is reported to be as effective as diazepam but with fewer central side effects.[60] The role of these α_2-agonist drugs in spasticity associated with TBI is still uncertain. Of related interest are reports that α-adrenergic *blocking* agents, such as chlorpromazine, may reduce spasticity.[63] Chlorpromazine reduces decerebrate rigidity in cats, probably by means of α-adrenergic blockade. Our observation of people receiving this drug is that they become very sedated, and we therefore think that chlorpromazine should be considered only for an extremely spastic patient who is permanently vegetative and unresponsive to other systemic agents.

FOCAL SPASTICITY AND LOCALIZED INTERVENTIONS

Treatment of focal problems lends itself well to interventions that can target small numbers of muscle groups. Injection of specific nerves or muscles with neurolytic or chemodenervating agents or surgical lengthening, transfer, or release of targeted muscles can provide very effective solutions to focal problems of function.[13] We commonly use three techniques: neurolytic blocks with phenol, chemodenervation with botulinum toxin A, and orthopedic surgical interventions. Because the first two are temporizing agents and their effects cease after a period of months, injections of phenol and botulinum toxin have their greatest usefulness during the period of motor recovery. Orthopedic surgical interventions have their greatest usefulness in the period of functional adaptation after significant spontaneous motor recovery is no longer expected. A newer technique, intrathecal baclofen, provides regional control of spasticity.

Phenol

Phenol, a derivative of benzene known to our grandparents as carbolic acid, denatures the protein membrane of peripheral nerves in aqueous concentrations of 5 percent or more.[63] Phenol's neurolytic action on the myelin sheath of the axon reduces neural traffic along the nerve, and hence it is useful in treating spasticity. The onset of the destructive process occurs several days after injection, but phenol also has a local anesthetic feature that allows a clinician and the patient to see "results" shortly after a block is performed. In our experience, the effect of a phenol block typically lasts 3 to 5 months. The time course of recovery is probably related to the duration of Wallerian degeneration and the rate of regeneration. For example, a nerve injected 3 inches from its neuromuscular junction may regenerate in approximately 4 months: 1 month for Wallerian degeneration, 3 months for regeneration. Histologically, phenol destroys axons of all sizes, probably in a patchy distribution but more so on the outer aspect of the nerve. Interior axons within the nerve bundle are theoretically spared more than their sibling axons located on the outer aspect of the nerve, where phenol has more access to denature them. Thus, a phenol block is likely to be incomplete, a finding especially useful when it is desired to preserve voluntary control but still reduce spasticity. Technical aspects of injection are reviewed by Glenn.[8]

There has been concern that phenol applied to sensory or mixed nerves may yield troublesome dysesthesias. We do not recommend injecting mixed peripheral nerves except perhaps in vegetative patients who are indifferent to sensory consequences. Most often, we inject motor "points," which are distal *motor* branches entering a muscle. Because a certain amount of needling is required to find the best place for injecting the motor nerve, we prefer not to use phenol in patients who are anticoagulated with coumadin. The technique for botulinum toxin injection may be preferable in this circumstance. If a phenol block seems ineffective after several weeks, it may be repeated (in contrast to botulinum toxin, for which a 12-week interval is used before reinjection. With repeated phenol injections, an increase in fibrous tissue at the site of injection may occur, making repeat injections more difficult. This is not problematic when phenol is used during the period of motor recovery because it is unlikely that more than two or three phenol blocks will be required in this period. In summary, phenol injected into motor nerves and motor points is a good temporizing agent during motor recovery. It facilitates serial casting and range of motion exercises, improves passive function, and may improve active function. Phenol is inexpensive and may be reinjected as soon as it becomes clear that the desired effect has not been obtained. In this sense, it is a titratable drug.

Botulinum Toxin

Ordinarily, an action potential propagating down a motor nerve to the neuromuscular junction triggers the release of acetylcholine (ACh) into the synaptic space from presynaptic storage sites in the nerve terminal. The released quanta of ACh, after traversing the synapse and attaching onto receptors located on the postsynaptic muscle membrane, cause depolarization of muscle membrane and activate a biochemical sequence that ultimately leads to muscle contraction and the development of force. Botulinum toxin type A is a protein produced by *Clostridium botulinum* that inhibits this calcium-mediated release of ACh at the neuromuscular junction.[64] The toxin attaches onto the presynaptic nerve terminal and divides into light and heavy components. The light component interferes with "fusion proteins" affiliated with vesicles of ACh, thereby preventing the release of ACh from their storage vesicles.

Botulinum toxin injection has been used to treat a variety of dystonias and is currently approved by the U.S. Food and Drug Administration for the treatment of blepharospasm, facial spasm, and strabismus.[65] Studies have reported its use in treating spasticity in individuals with cerebral palsy, stroke, acquired brain injury, and multiple sclerosis.[66–68] Clinical benefit lasts 3 to 5 months but may be more variable. Botulinum toxin is injected directly into an offending muscle, and, depending on the size of the muscle being injected, dosing has ranged between 10 and 200 units (U) (Fig. 29–2). Greene and Fahn[69] found that patients with torticollis who became resistant to the effects of the toxin after repeated injections were likely to have received more than 250 U in a single treatment session or to have been injected at intervals of less than 12 weeks. Current practice is to wait at least 12 weeks before reinjection and not to administer a total of more than 400 U in a single treatment session. When proximal and distal muscles require injection, an upper limit of 400 U may be reached rather quickly. In this circumstance, a strategy of phenol for the larger proximal muscles combined with botulinum toxin A for the smaller distal muscles may be considered.

A 3- to 7-day delay between injection and the onset of clinical effect is typical, and a follow-up visit is usually arranged to check the result. The ability to "titrate" the dose is not available to the physician until the 12-week mark. Neurological recovery and variability in the site of muscle reinjection are factors in titration. O'Brien[70] has indicated that the "dose chosen must be sufficient to produce the desired amount of weakness without excessive weakness in the injected or nearby muscles." Because botulinum toxin is the most potent biological toxin known and the cost is relatively high, it is desirable to use the smallest possible dose to achieve a desired result. Thus far, the cost of this agent has not been covered easily by insurance companies, who often require that physicians justify its use in advance with time-consuming documentation. Nevertheless, the undoubted biological effect of the drug and the ease and speed of the injection technique are fa-

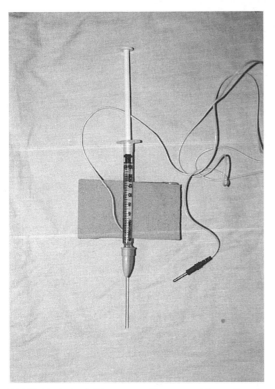

FIGURE 29–2. A 25-gauge teflon-coated hypodermic needle used for injecting botulinum toxin. The pin jack of the wired needle may be connected to an EMG machine or to an electrical stimulator to verify location of needle tip in the target muscle. Reconstituted toxin is drawn in a 1cc syringe with unit markings of 0.1cc equivalent to 10 U of toxin.

vorable factors that recommend its use to busy clinicians.

Orthopedic Interventions

The origin of limb deformity in patients with UMN syndrome is based on the idea that findings such as paresis, spasticity, stiffness, contracture, and impaired motor control generate a net imbalance of muscular forces affecting joint position statically and joint movement dynamically.[13] Orthopedic interventions have responded to this conceptual model with the idea of surgically rebalancing static and dynamic forces across joints to achieve a more functional alignment of forces. Surgical options for rebalancing forces across joints include tendon lengthening, muscle release, tendon transfer, neurectomy, release of joint contracture, and joint fusion. The concept of surgical rebalancing of muscle and other soft tissue restrictive forces is particularly germane *after* motor recovery has ended. Procedures performed too early may lead later to new imbalances as added motor recovery occurs.

As part of the focal strategy for treating spasticity, we believe that surgical interventions should be based on explicit functional goals. Functional goals may be classified as passive or active. *Passive function* refers to passive manipulation of limbs to achieve functional ends, typically by caregivers, though patients may do likewise. Passive functions may include activities such as dressing, bathing, and grooming that are affected by conditions restricting passive motion and positioning. *Active function,* by contrast, refers to a patient's direct use of a limb or body segment in performing functional activities. Orthopedic approaches differ markedly when clinical goals are aimed at improving active rather than passive functions (Table 29–2).

Intrathecal Baclofen

In recent years, an intrathecal delivery system[71] has successfully been used to treat spasticity of spinal cord origin, and currently multicenter trials for management of spastic hypertonia in cerebral disorders are under way as well. The delivery system consists of a programmable pump that is placed subcutaneously with a reservoir that is refilled periodically. The system concentrates baclofen in the lower area of the spinal cord at a much higher concentration than is attainable by the oral route. The pump's drug delivery rate to the intrathecal space is controlled by the clinician. When medication is concentrated intrathecally, cognitive side effects are greatly contained. In addition, intrathecal delivery by means of a programmable pump allows titration of dosage so that predictable changes in spasticity over the course of the day may be addressed more effectively.

From the perspective of focal treatment strategy, the baclofen pump potentially might find its greatest use in patients with diffuse regional spasticity in the lower extremities. Prior to making a decision to implant the pump, bolus assessment of the effect of intrathecal baclofen is performed through a temporarily inserted catheter. This serves as a diagnostic trial to gauge potential longer-term effects of this medication on the clinical problem at hand. Recent studies have begun to look at the effect of intrathecal baclofen on the upper extremities as well by threading the delivery catheter more cephalad than the T10 level. Of interest is that baclofen pump technology has been applied fairly late after spinal cord injury. Meythaler[72] has recommended that most patients should probably not be evaluated for placement of a pump for at least 1 year after injury because "spastic hypertonia may be variable during this

TABLE 29–2.

Clinical and Laboratory Findings for Muscle X			Period of Functional Adaptation
As a movement Agonist	As a movement Antagonist		
VOLUNTARY CONTROL	SPASTICITY	CONTRACTURE	LOCALIZED TREATMENT OPTIONS
			General surgical strategy: to improve passive function
Poor	Yes	No	Surgical release
Poor	Yes	Yes	Surgical release with 50% correction of contractured tissues, followed postop by serial casting, aggressive range of motion therapy
			General surgical strategy: to improve active function
Fair to good	Yes	No	Surgical lengthening
Fair to good	Yes	Yes	Surgical lengthening with 50% correction of contractured tissues, followed postop by serial casting, aggressive range of motion therapy
Fair to good	No	Yes	Surgical lengthening with 50% correction of contractured tissues, followed postop by serial casting, aggressive range of motion therapy

period." From the perspective of active function, doses of intrathecal baclofen do seem to significantly decrease motor strength in patients with spinal cord injury who have retained some residual active function in their muscles below the level of the lesion. However, Meythaler specifically reports that he has seen no reduction of voluntary motor function in patients with brain injury treated with continuously delivered intrathecal baclofen. The ease of titration with programmable technology might be relevant to the issue of weakness because the clinician should be able to titrate medication delivery according to clinical findings. Complications related to the procedure include headaches, temporary atelectasis, orthostatic hypotension, and postsurgical pseudomeningocoeles. Longer-term complications may relate to miscalculated dosing and the possibility of pump malfunction, catheter disruptions, and exhausted pump reservoirs.

Patterns of Upper Motor Neuron Dysfunction

Common patterns of upper and lower extremity motor dysfunction are seen in patients with TBI who have a UMN syndrome (Table 29–3). These patterns of dysfunction are amenable to strategies of focal evaluation and localized treatment[10] (Table 29–4). Clinically relevant questions regarding a given muscle, targeted for localized intervention, include the following: Does the patient have selective voluntary control over the given muscle? Is the muscle activated dyssynergically (i.e., in antagonism to movement) when the patient attempts to move the relevant joint? Is the muscle resistive to passive stretch? Does the given muscle have fixed shortening (i.e., contracture: limited range of motion that is attributed, in large measure, to fixed shortening of the given muscle crossing

TABLE 29–3. Common Patterns of Upper Motor Neuron Dysfunction

1.	Adducted internally rotated shoulder	7.	Intrinsic plus hand
2.	Flexed elbow	8.	Flexed hip
3.	Pronated forearm	9.	Adducted thigh
4.	Flexed wrist	10.	Stiff knee
5.	Clenched fist	11.	Flexed knee
6.	Thumb-in-palm deformity	12.	Equinovarus foot with curl toes or claw toes
		13.	Hitchhiker's great toe

TABLE 29–4. Deformities, Commonly Spastic Muscles, and Authors' Guidelines for Dosing

COMMON DEFORMITIES	MUSCLES/NERVES FOR POTENTIAL INJECTION	Botulinum Toxin A*†		Aqueous Phenol 5–7%	
		TOTAL UNITS PER MUSCLE (U)	# INJECTION SITES	# MOTOR "POINTS"‡	VOLUME PER POINT or nerve (cc)
Adducted/ internally rotated shoulder	Pectoralis major	50–100	3	2	3–5
	Latissimus dorsi	80—160	4	1	
	Teres major	25–50	1	1	4–5
	Subscapularis	25–50	1		
	Thoracodorsal nerve				4–6
Flexed elbow	Biceps	50–100	4	1	4–6
	Brachioradialis	25–75	2	1	4–6
	Musculocutaneous n.				4–6
Pronated forearm	Pronator teres	25–50	1	1	4–6
	Pronator quadratus	20–50	1	1	3–5
Flexed wrist and clenched fist	Flexor carpi radialis	25–75	2	1	4–6
	Flexor carpi ulnaris	20–50	1	1	3–4
	Flexor dig sublimis	80–160	4	4	2–3
	Flexor dig profundus	80–160	4	4	2–3
Thumb-in-palm	Flexor pollicis longus	10–25	1	1	3–4
	Adductor pollicis	10–25	1	1	2–3
	Flexor pollicis brevis	10–20	1		
	Ulnar motor branch (palm)				2–3
	Recurrent median n. (palm)				2–3
Intrinsic plus hand	Dorsal interossei	40–60	4	4	2–3
	Ulnar motor branch (palm)				2–3
Flexed hip	Iliacus	50–150	1	3–6	
	Rectus femoris	75–200	2	1	5–7
	L2,L3 motor n. to psoas				2–4cc/root
Adducted thighs	Adductor longus	100–150	2	1	
	Adductor magnus	75–150	2	1	
	Obturator nerve				4–6
Flexed knee	Medial hamstrings	50–150	2	2	4–6
	Lateral hamstrings	50–150	2	1	4–6
	Motor branches to hams				4–6
Stiff (extended) knee	Rectus femoris	75–200	2	1	5–7
	Vastus lateralis	25–50	2	1	3–5
	Vastus medialis	25–50	2	1	3–5
	Vastus intermedius	25–50	1		3–5
	Medial gastrocnemius	50–100	2	1	3–5
	Lateral gastrocnemius	50–100	2	1	3–5
	Soleus	50–100	2	2	4–6
Equinovarus	Tibialis posterior	25–100	1	1	3–5
	Tibialis anterior	25–100	2	1	2–4
	Flexor digitorum longus	25–100	2	1	2–4
	Flexor hallucis longus	25–100	1	1	2–4
Hitchhiker's great toe	Extensor hallucis longus	25–100	1	1	2–4

Source: From Warfel, JH: The Extremities: Muscles and Motor Points, ed 5, Lea & Febiger, Philadelphia, 1985, with permission.
*Botox A (Allergan).
†Use larger doses for passive dysfunction.
‡Motor "point" = distal branch of motor nerve.

its joint)? Given the degree of clinical effort, patient morbidity, and procedural costs involved in treating complicated movement dysfunction in patients with TBI, clinical examination alone may not suffice to answer these questions with a high degree of confidence. Laboratory assessments that may be helpful include formal gait and motion analysis, dynamic EMG studies, and nerve blocks. Dynamic multichannel EMG is acquired with simultaneous measurements of joint motion (kinematics) in the upper and lower extremities. For the lower extremities, kinetic information regarding ground reaction forces are obtained from force plate sensors. Kinetic, kinematic, and dynamic EMG data assist the clinician in interpreting whether voluntary function (effort-related initiation, modulation, and termination of activity) is present in a given muscle and whether that muscle's behavior is also dyssynergic ("out of phase" and/or "spastic"). In addition, responses to different rates of passive stretch of muscle before and after local anesthetic nerve block can help the clinician distinguish between the dynamic, velocity-sensitive reflex resistance of spasticity versus passive muscle tissue stiffness and contracture. Combined with clinical information, laboratory measurements of muscle function often provide the degree of detail and confidence necessary for making conservative and surgical treatment decisions. How to apply strategies of focal evaluation and localized treatment is illustrated in the next section with a joint-by-joint approach in spastic patients with familiar patterns of UMN dysfunction.

THE ADDUCTED AND INTERNALLY ROTATED SHOULDER

The arm is adducted tightly against the lateral chest wall, and shoulder internal rotation causes the forearm to lie against the middle of the chest anteriorly. The tendon of pectoralis major is prominent when the examiner abducts and externally rotates the shoulder, but other muscles may contribute to resistance. When patients attempt to reach forward, spastic adductors and internal rotators may severely restrict acquisition of targets in the environment and on the body. From the perspective of passive function goals, restricted motion may impair dressing, washing, and bathing and promote skin irritation and maceration. Passive manipulation of the shoulder during personal care may cause pain when skin contact and joint motion trigger spastic resistance in reactive muscles (Fig. 29–3).

Muscles that may contribute to spastic adduction and internal rotation dysfunction of the shoulder include latissimus dorsi, teres major, pectoralis major, and subscapularis. Antagonistic activity in latissimus dorsi and/or teres major may be masking a patient's potential for active flexion. Diagnostic lidocaine block to the thoracodorsal nerve and/or lower subscapular nerve may unmask that voluntary potential. Subscapularis may also be a source of spastic internal rotation.

During the period of motor recovery, large spastic shoulder muscles are amenable to phenol neurolysis or botulinum chemodenervation. We prefer to use phenol for large proximal muscles because the doses of botulinum toxin required for injecting a number of these spastic muscles quickly approaches the current maximum dose of 400 U, and little is left over for distal muscles that are inevitably spastic as well. The motor points of pectoralis major and teres major and the thoracodorsal nerve innervating latissimus dorsi are convenient for blocking. Upper and lower subscapular nerve blocks have been reported as a treatment for

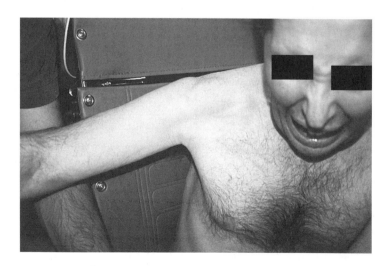

FIGURE 29–3. This patient has prominent adductor spasticity of the shoulder. Pectoralis major and latissimus dorsi are visibly taut. Passive motion to gain access to the axilla is limited and painful. The patient's cooperation in washing and dressing the arm and shoulder regions is not easily gained.

subscapularis-driven spastic internal rotation of the shoulder.

During the period of functional adaptation, surgical approaches are considered, especially for young people with brain injury who have many years to live and benefit from permanently improved functionality. When the goal is to improve passive functions that aid caregiving, release of pectoralis major, subscapularis, latissimus dorsi, and teres major is usually necessary. Release of the subscapularis muscle is performed without violating the joint capsule to prevent instability or intra-articular adhesions. If adhesive capsulitis is present, the joint can be passively manipulated. An aggressive mobilization program is instituted following wound healing to correct remaining contracture. Careful positioning of the limb in abduction and external rotation is necessary for several months to prevent recurrence.

Overactivity of the supraspinatus muscle can cause spastic abduction posturing, which is especially troublesome during walking. Patients complain their balance is off and that they bump into furniture, doorways, and people in crowds. Dynamic EMG raises suspicion regarding excessive activation of the supraspinatus, and relief of the abducted posture with a diagnostic motor point block of the supraspinatus helps to confirm the diagnosis. Surgically, a

slide procedure is used, and the patient is allowed full, unrestricted postoperative motion.

THE FLEXED ELBOW

Upright posture favors hypertonia in the "antigravity" elbow flexors. Severe flexion posturing can lead to skin maceration in the antecubital fossa, malodor, and breakdown. Many patients complain that their elbows "ride up" when they stand up and walk. They also complain that a flexed elbow hooks door frames and people and that putting on a shirt or jacket is a struggle. Active dysfunction is characterized by impaired reaching for objects in the environment and inability to bring those objects to the body or elsewhere. Muscles that potentially contribute to elbow deformity include biceps, brachialis, and brachioradialis (Fig. 29–4). Dynamic EMG studies have indicated that brachioradialis is often more spastic than biceps and brachialis. During motor recovery, therapeutic blocks with phenol or botulinum toxin are used. If the patient has moderate or severe contracture, these blocks may be combined with serial casting.

In the period of functional adaptation, dynamic EMG and diagnostic blocks help determine voluntary capacity, spastic reactivity, and the presence of contracture. When patients have little ability to activate muscles voluntarily, sur-

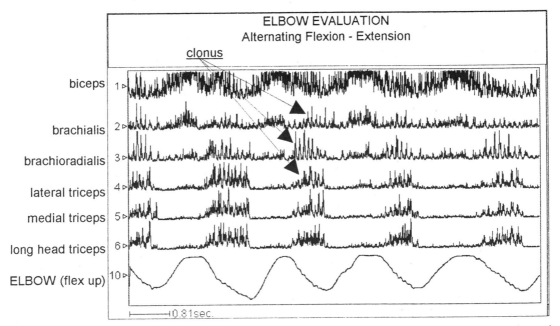

FIGURE 29–4. In this patient with an upper motoneuron syndrome, the elbow flexors demonstrate volitional activation during flexion phase. However, they are also active dyssynergically ("out of phase") during extension. In particular, clonus during extension phase is seen in brachioradialis and brachialis, alternating with clonic activity in all three heads of the triceps. Elbow motion is correspondingly ratchety and prolonged.

gery aims at improving passive function related to antecubital skin care, malodor, dressing, ulnar nerve compression, and standing and walking balance. Compression neuropathy of the ulnar nerve frequently occurs because the flexed elbow stretches this nerve, which is also vulnerable to external compression by lap boards and bed rails. Surgical release of contractured muscles and gradual reextension of the elbow corrects the preoperative deformity. Brachioradialis and biceps tendon are transected outright. The brachialis is fractionally lengthened at its myotendinous junction to keep dead space in the wound small, lessening the incidence of wound hematoma and infection. Brachialis continuity also helps prevent extension contracture by an otherwise unopposed triceps. Anterior transposition of the ulnar nerve may be necessary. Anterior capsulotomy is avoided because of increased stiffness and intra-articular adhesions postoperatively. Approximately 50 percent correction of the deformity can be expected at surgery without causing excessive tension on the contracted neurovascular structures. Serial casting or drop out casts can be used to obtain further correction of contracture over the ensuing weeks.

PRONATED FOREARM

Pronation deformity of the forearm in UMN appears to be more common than supination deformity. Pronation bias makes it difficult for a person to reach for a target underhand, whereas supination deformity impairs reaching for targets that require overhand reach. Using feeding and grooming utensils and clothes fasteners becomes problematic when supination is restricted by spastic or contractured pronators.

Physical examination reveals a fully pronated "resting position" of the forearm. When passive supination range of motion exceeds active supination range, muscle dyssynergy during active supination should be suspected. Muscles that may contribute include pronator teres and pronator quadratus. Dynamic EMG studies of pronator teres, pronator quadratus, and biceps greatly augment clinical examination. Clinical examination does not easily predict which pronators retain volitional capacity and which may be spastic.

During motor recovery, phenol or botulinum toxin may be injected into either or both pronators. In the period of functional adaptation, surgical lengthening of pronator teres and pronator quadratus may be performed when the clinical goal is to improve active supinatory function by reducing pronator dyssynergy. The possibility of lengthening pronator teres has long been recognized, but fractional lengthening of pronator quadratus is of recent vintage.

THE FLEXED WRIST

A flexed wrist is most common after TBI, but hyperextension deformity is also seen. Patients complain of difficulty inserting their hand into shirts, jackets, and other narrow openings, and they frequently have pain on passive motion. Patients may have symptoms of carpal tunnel syndrome secondary to compression of the median nerve against the transverse carpal ligament by taut flexor tendons. In severe cases, wrist subluxation may be present. Radial or ulnar deviation and a clenched fist are often present as well.

Muscles that potentially contribute to wrist flexion include flexor carpi radialis (FCR), flexor carpi ulnaris (FCU), flexor digitorum sublimis (FDS), and flexor digitorum profundus (FDP). FCR, FCU, or both may bowstring across the wrist, and radial or ulnar deviation suggests their respective involvement. A clenched fist points to extrinsic finger flexors as playing a role. If fingernails dig into the palm, FDP is likely to be involved. If the proximal interphalangeal (PIP) but not the distal interphalangeal (DIP) joint is markedly flexed, involvement of FDS is likely. Distinguishing between limitations attributable to wrist versus finger flexors is one aim of passive range of motion testing (Fig. 29–5). By allowing the fingers to remain flexed in the palm, passive extension of the wrist provides preferential information about wrist flexors. When finger flexors are tight, simultaneous passive stretch of the wrist and finger flexors restricts wrist motion more markedly.

Observing even a small degree of active wrist extension may be important because surgical interventions that alleviate muscle contracture and spasticity on the flexor side may unmask more voluntary extension on the extensor side. When a patient has more overt extension it may be useful to observe the patient's effort in performing repetitive flexion/extension movements of the wrist. Smoothness of motion, speed, effort, and decrement in movement amplitude over time and fatigue may be observed (Fig. 29–6).

Singly or in combination, the wrist and finger flexors may have variable findings of spasticity, contracture, and voluntary control. Despite a net balance of forces favoring flexion, the extent to which a patient may have voluntary control over wrist extensors should be investigated. Dynamic EMG studies and temporary diagnostic motor point blocks are helpful in this regard. Temporary chemical "weakening" of a dyssynergic wrist flexor may unmask strength in the wrist extensors sufficient to improve active wrist movement. A similar hypothesis can be formulated for the extrinsic finger flexors after dynamic EMG reveals whether FDS, FDP, or

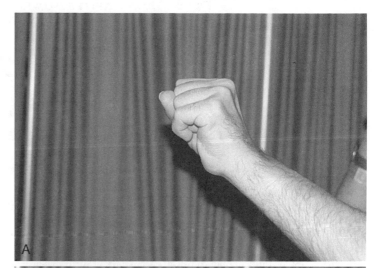

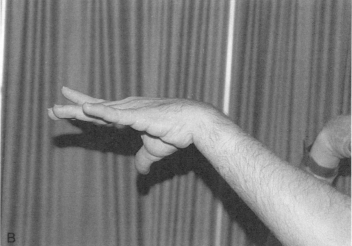

FIGURE 29–5. This patient is able to extend his wrist when his fingers are flexed into the palm (*A*); this suggests that the wrist flexors are not restricting extension of the wrist. When attempting to extend his wrist *and* fingers maximally (*B*), the flexed wrist posture suggests that the extrinsic finger flexors are tight enough to restrict wrist extension. In the period of functional adaptation, lengthening finger flexors would be indicated.

both are generating activity in antagonism to wrist extension. Motor point block of the target muscle group or median and/or ulnar nerve blocks at the elbow may be performed to examine for active wrist extension during reach. When wrist hyperextension deformity is present, wrist extensors are typically volitional and spastic, wrist flexors are often poorly volitional and mildly spastic, and the fingers are tightly clenched into the palm.

During the period of motor recovery, phenol or botulinum toxin may be injected into wrist flexors and/or the various muscle slips of FDS and FDP, depending on clinical and laboratory identification of the offending muscles. In the period of functional adaptation, surgical options include muscle lengthenings and releases. When a patient has underlying voluntary control, surgical options for bent and hyperextended wrists may include myotendinous frac-

tional lengthenings. Selective muscle releases, wrist fusion, proximal row carpectomy, and superficialis to profundus tendon transfer (discussed later) may be considered when the goal is to improve passive function only.

THE CLENCHED FIST

The fingers are flexed into the palm. Fingernails may dig into palmar skin, and access to the palm for washing is typically compromised. When access is chronically restricted, skin maceration, breakdown, and malodor develop (Fig. 29–7). Patients complain of pain when they or their caregivers attempt to pry fingers open to gain palmar access. Some relaxation of finger tightness may occur if the wrist is positioned by the examiner in extreme flexion. Muscles that contribute to the clenched fist deformity include FDS and FDP. The intrinsics may also be

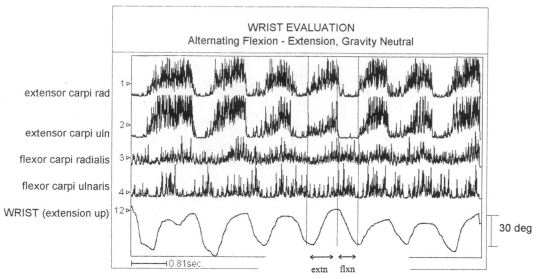

FIGURE 29–6. A multichannel dynamic EMG study of wrist extensors and flexors in a patient with an upper motoneuron syndrome who is actively moving his wrist in a gravity neutral position. Note the distinct activity of wrist extensors during extension (*extn*) phase with relative silence during flexion (*flxn*) phase. In contrast, the wrist flexors are active during both phases, suggesting that they have volitional *and* spastic characteristics.

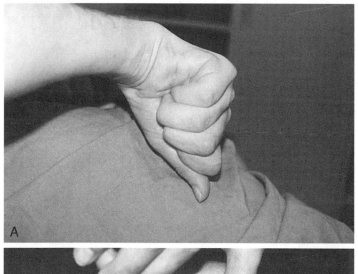

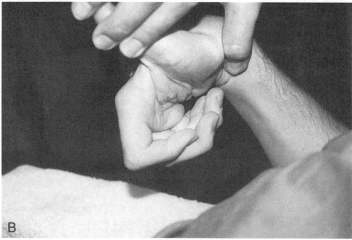

FIGURE 29–7. (*A*) Five months after head injury, this patient has a spastic clenched fist deformity with finger nails digging into the palm. Both the superficial and the deep finger flexors are involved. (*B*) Following 7% phenol motor point blocks to the deep and superficial finger flexors, the palm opened up sufficiently to reveal malodorous, excoriated, and callused skin. Ten months after the injury, the patient regained fair control over the finger flexors. Neurolytic and chemodenervating agents are best used as temporizing measures during the period of motor recovery.

spastic, but an intrinsic plus posture (i.e., combined metacarpophalangeal flexion and PIP extension) is not seen because spastic extrinsic flexors dominate by flexing all joints. Some degree of contracture of the extrinsics is typical of patients with a chronically clenched fist.

Some degree of volitional control may be present in either or both sets of extrinsic finger flexors. Spastic finger flexors may override and mask the patient's potential to extend the fingers. Dynamic EMG and differential lidocaine blocks may help. Sometimes a patient presents with spasticity in just one or two muscle slips of either FDP or FDS. For example, isolated index finger flexion is not uncommonly seen secondary to spastic FDP and/or FDS muscle slips to that finger alone. These patients complain that their flexed index finger gets in the way of picking up objects with the radial side of the hand (Fig. 29–8).

During the period of motor recovery, focal neurolysis or chemodenervation is a useful intervention. Treatment of spasticity in the extrinsics may unmask spasticity in the intrinsics, potentially converting an extrinsic deformity into an intrinsic plus deformity. Chemodenervation with botulinum toxin is an excellent remedy for treating spasticity of the intrinsics because these small muscles of the hand are readily accessible for injection and require only small amounts of toxin to be effective.

During the period of functional adaptation, a variety of surgical options are available. When volitional control is present in the extrinsic flexors and extensors, fractional lengthening is indicated. Lengthening of the FDS, FDP, and flexor pollicis longus tendons is performed by transecting the flexor tendon as it overlies the muscle belly at the musculotendinous junction. The hand is not immobilized postoperatively. The patient is allowed to actively flex and extend the fingers on the first postoperative day to allow each muscle tendon unit to lengthen as much as needed.

When a patient has a malodorous, macerated fist, devoid of useful voluntary movement, more significant lengthening of the flexor tendons is required to improve passive function. In this situation, a superficialis to profundus (STP) tendon transfer is performed. The flexor superficialis tendons are cut distally while the flexor profundus tendons are transected proximally. The distal ends of the superficial flexors are then sewn to the proximal ends of the deep flexors. This procedure allows for extensive lengthening in a severely spastic, contractured hand. A wrist arthrodesis is usually done to stabilize the wrist and eliminate the need for an orthosis. The median nerve is decompressed in the carpal canal, and a neurectomy of the motor branches of the ulnar nerve is performed to prevent an intrinsic plus deformity from developing.

When spastic intrinsics dominate hand posture, metacarpophalangeal (MCP) joints are typically flexed 90 degrees, and PIP joints are fully extended. Hyperextension of the PIP joints combined with DIP joint flexion produces a swan neck deformity representing intrinsic

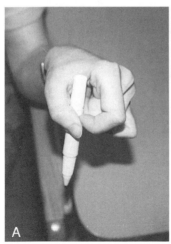 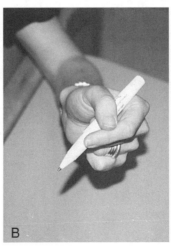 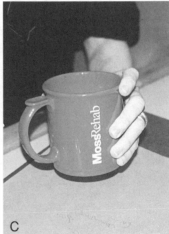

FIGURE 29–8. (*A*) This patient has spastic *index* finger flexors. She grips small objects poorly because the index finger flexes past the best contact point for gripping. The flexed index finger also cannot surround a cup sufficiently to allow her to hold it to her lips and drink, so she uses a straw to drink. (*B*) At 14 days after injection of FDS and FDP of the *index* finger with 25 U of Botox A in each, the index finger no longer flexes past good contact points for gripping. The patient was now able to write. (*C*) At 14 days after injection of the index finger flexors with Botox A, the patient discovered she was now able to drink directly from a cup, and she no longer had to use a straw.

and extrinsic overactivity. For spastic, noncontracted intrinsics with poor volition, neurectomy of the palmar motor branch of the ulnar nerve may be considered. If contracture is present, intrinsic releases may be performed. However, when spasticity coexists with voluntary function, intrinsic lengthening is performed by stripping them off their metacarpal origins and allowing them to slide distally (Fig. 29–9).

THE THUMB-IN-PALM DEFORMITY

The thumb is held within the palm, the DIP joint of the thumb is commonly flexed along with MCP flexion, and the thumb is unable to function during key grasp or three-jaw chuck pattern. Some patients may be able to extend the thumb if the wrist is flexed, suggesting that a spastic flexor pollicis longus (FPL) may be impeding active thumb extension when the wrist is more extended and FPL is stretched. The thumb-in-palm deformity may result from spastic activity in FPL, adductor pollicis (AP), and/or the thenar muscles (particularly flexor pollicis brevis (Fig. 29–10). Contracture of the skin of the web space and interphalangeal joint contracture of the thumb may also develop in time. If some volitional potential in thumb extensors or thumb

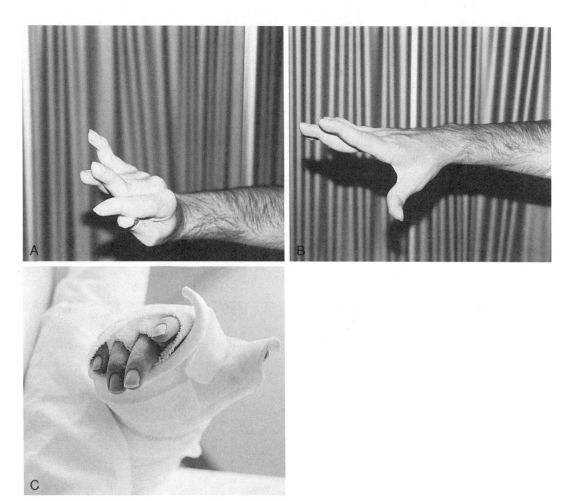

FIGURE 29–9. This 27-year-old man, two years after TBI, has a spastic intrinsic plus deformity. (*A*) The MCP joints remain flexed at 90 degrees; hyperextension is present at the PIPs of digits 3,4,5; swan-neck deformities generated by combined tightness of intrinsics and extrinsics are visible. Note narrowed web space and contact between thumb pad and index finger. (*B*) The effect of a diagnostic ulnar nerve block at the wrist (2% lidocaine, 4cc). Note that the web space is now actively opened and the fingers extend fully at the MCP joints. Dynamic EMG revealed that this patient had good underlying control of the hand extrinsics and intrinsics, although they were also spastic. He was judged to be a good candidate for lengthening procedures of offending muscles. (*C*) The positioning of the hand in a soft splint, one day after having lengthening of the interossei, flexor digitorum profundus, and a thenar slide that lengthens the thumb intrinsics. The patient starts active motion exercises almost immediately. Lengthening procedures preserve anatomical continuity and are done to improve active movement.

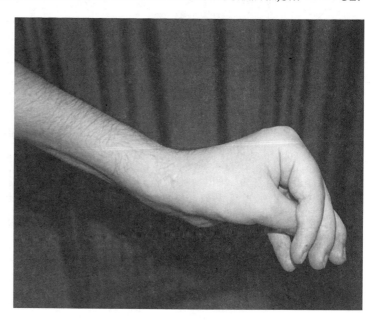

FIGURE 29–10. This patient has a thumb-in-palm deformity. Dynamic EMG helps identify contributions of adductor pollicis, thenar intrinsics, and flexor pollicis longus to this deformity.

abductors is present, treatment of spastic FPL and AP may facilitate active grasp, usually in the form of a modified type of key grasp. Dynamic EMG and lidocaine blocks may be helpful in this regard. During the period of motor recovery, treatment of spastic muscles by chemodenervation may allow application of hand orthoses for passive or active purposes.

In the period of functional adaptation, orthopedic treatment consists of fractional lengthening of the FPL at the myotendinous junction combined with a thenar muscle slide in which the origins of the thenar muscles are detached from the transverse palmar ligament while preserving the neurovascular pedicle. This allows the thenar muscles to be repositioned with the thumb in a more abducted and functional position. The origin of the AP muscle is detached from the shaft of the third metacarpal to allow it to slide radially. Occasionally a Z-plasty of the thumb web space may be required if shortening of the skin has occurred.

EQUINOVARUS

Equinovarus is the most common posture seen in the lower extremity. The foot and ankle are turned down and in. Toe curling or toe clawing may coexist. The lateral border of the foot is often compressed against mattress, bed rail, floor, or foot rest. Skin breakdown over the fifth metatarsal head may develop from such unrelieved pressure. During stance phase of gait, contact with the ground occurs first at the forefoot, weight is borne primarily on the lateral border, and toe flexion is typically present. The patient often complains of pain over the lateral

border of the foot in the region of the fifth metatarsal head during weight bearing, and skin breakdown can be seen. Equinovarus limits dorsiflexion motion during early and midstance and prevents forward progression of the tibia over the stationary foot, resulting in hyperextension thrust of the knee and dysrhythmic and restrained forward translation of body mass. During early swing phase, foot drag associated with equinovarus may make limb advancement and floor clearance difficult.

Muscles that can potentially contribute to equinovarus deformity include tibialis anterior, tibialis posterior, the long toe flexors, medial and lateral gastrocnemius, soleus, and flexor and extensor hallucis longus. Clinical examination, diagnostic lidocaine blocks, and dynamic EMG may all be helpful in teasing apart the role of the various muscles. For example, when it is difficult to differentiate between the varus contributions of tibialis anterior and tibialis posterior, a diagnostic tibial nerve block that narcotizes tibialis posterior but not anterior allows the clinician to assess the role of tibialis anterior in producing varus deformity. (If the block is complete, it also reveals whether equinus contracture—fixed shortening of posterior compartment muscles—is present.) Equinovarus produces an inadequate base of support with instability of the whole body and is, therefore, a key deformity that makes or breaks even limited functional ambulation.

During motor recovery, the use of neurolytic and chemodenervation agents in targeted muscles helps control this deformity and makes bracing, serial casting, manual stretching, and therapeutic exercise easier to apply. In the period of functional adaptation, equinovarus is corrected surgically to provide a stable base of support for transfers and ambulation (Fig. 29–11). Lengthening the Achilles tendon is performed first to correct equinus. Long and short toe flexor tendons are then divided at the base of each toe to correct toe curling. Foot repositioning in plantigrade position accentuates toe flexion if this is not done. Forefoot varus is corrected by a split anterior tibial (AT) tendon transfer (SPLATT), in which half of the AT tendon is transferred to the lateral side of the foot, thereby equalizing the pull of this muscle. If dynamic EMG demonstrates that tibialis posterior contributes to the varus deformity, it is lengthened at its myotendinous junction. Spastic leg muscles are usually weak, and lengthening of the Achilles tendon further weakens the pull of gastrocnemius and soleus muscles. To supplement the power of the weakened gastrocnemius and soleus muscles, the flexor hallucis longus and flexor digitorum longus mus-

cles can be transferred to the os calcis, thereby converting them to calf muscles. This additional transfer has resulted in 70 percent of patients being able to walk brace-free after surgery.

HITCHHIKER'S GREAT TOE

Persistent Babinski-like extension of the great toe is not uncommon, and the patient may complain of being unable to wear a shoe (Fig. 29–12). Sometimes the patient presents with the toe box of the shoe cut out. When wearing shoes, the patient complains of pain at the tip of the shoe and under the first metatarsal head during stance phase of gait. The main offender appears to be a hyperactive extensor hallucis longus (EHL) but cocontraction of flexor hallucis longus (FHL) may be present and masked. During motor recovery, chemodenervation or neurolytic agents applied to EHL relieve the problem. However, cocontraction in FHL may reverse the deformity, requiring additional intervention for that muscle. Diagnostic blocks of EHL, FHL, or both may be helpful in this regard.

During functional adaptation, orthopedic intervention is useful for permanent correction of the deformity. EHL is lengthened at the myotendinous junction. If this is the only foot deformity being treated, no immobilization is needed after surgery. Commonly, hitchhiker's toe is seen in combination with an equinovarus foot. In this case, EHL is lengthened in conjunction with the SPLATT procedure.

STIFF KNEE

In stiff knee, the knee usually remains extended throughout the gait cycle. It is a particular problem during swing phase of gait. Toe drag in early swing may cause tripping and falling. The limb appears to be functionally longer because it remains extended throughout swing phase. The patient attempts to compensate for this relative length by ipsilateral circumduction or hiking of the pelvis and/or contralateral vaulting to clear the floor. The result is an increase in energy consumption. Muscles that potentially contribute include iliopsoas, gluteus maximus, rectus femoris, vastus intermedius, vastus medialis and lateralis, and the hamstrings. Dynamic EMG studies help identify overactive muscles. If the quadriceps group is overactive during swing, the knee remains extended. If the hamstrings are overactive, the patient may be guarding against the possibility of knee flexion collapse. Weak iliopsoas may decrease inertial momentum for knee flexion. Dynamic EMG may demonstrate activity in one or more heads of the quadriceps or in the

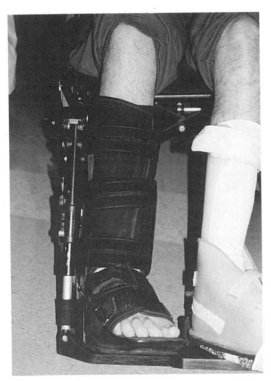

FIGURE 29–11. This patient had right and left foot surgeries for equinovarus deformities. After surgery, he is placed in a CAM boot for 6 weeks, then a rigid MAFO for 3 months. A clinical decision is then made to let him walk brace free or to use a flexible orthosis. The CAM boot (seen on the right foot) has front-closing Velcro that allows wounds to be inspected. Patients walk on it a day after surgery. The left foot is in the rigid MAFO stage.

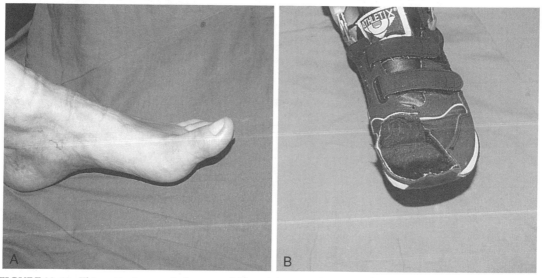

FIGURE 29–12. This patient presented to one of the authors complaining of great toe pain. (*A*) An extended, inflamed hitchhiker's great toe is evident. Motor point block with 4cc of 7% aqueous phenol to EHL relieved the problem. (*B*) He had a positive Esquenazi sign: The removal of the toe box performed by the patient before seeing the physiatrist, to relieve painful shearing of the extended toe against the undersurface of the shoe's toe box.

various hamstrings. Lidocaine motor point blocks to identified muscles may reveal whether "weakening" strategies will be helpful in reducing stiff knee gait. During motor recovery, chemodenervation or neurolytic agents may be used when diagnostic blocks are successful.

In the period of functional adaptation, orthopedic intervention is employed for permanent correction of the gait deformity. Previously, standard treatment was selective release of rectus femoris or rectus and vastus intermedius muscles when they were determined by dynamic EMG to be acting dyssynergically. This required that the vastus medialis and vastus lateralis muscles be appropriately activated during gait. Only 25 percent of patients with a stiff knee gait deformity met these criteria. Selective release of the rectus femoris tendon from the patella eliminated it as a deforming force and resulted in a mean gain of 15 degrees of knee flexion during swing phase.[73] An improved treatment has been the transfer of the rectus femoris to the gracilis tendon on the posteromedial aspect of the knee. This tendon transfer relies on rectus femoris activity in early swing to flex the knee.

FLEXED KNEE

The knee remains flexed throughout swing and stance. A flexed knee during stance phase elicits compensatory ipsilateral hip flexion and con-

tralateral hip and knee flexion (crouch gait pattern). A lack of full knee extension in terminal swing severely limits limb advancement, resulting in a short step length. Muscles that potentially contribute to this deformity include medial and lateral hamstrings and the quadriceps. Dynamic EMG studies may demonstrate prolonged activation of hamstrings, medial more often than lateral. The quadriceps group may be overactive to compensate for deforming flexor forces, or they may have decreased activity, requiring upper extremity stabilization with an assistive device to guard against knee collapse. Hamstrings contracture is likely when the deformity has been present chronically. Chemodenervation of targeted hamstrings during the period of motor recovery may allow stretching, serial casting, and other modalities aimed at reversing static deformity while the block is active.

During functional adaptation, orthopedic treatment is aimed at permanent correction of the flexed knee. It is critical to evaluate the hip for a concomitant flexion contracture. When both deformities are present, which is generally the case, they should be corrected simultaneously. The flexed knee deformity is surgically treated by lengthening or release of the hamstring muscles at the knee. If the knee flexion deformity is less than 50 degrees and the patient exhibits volitional hamstring activity, lengthenings are done. The biceps femoris, gracilis, and semimembranosus muscles are fractionally lengthened at the myotendinous junction. The semitendinosus can be released or Z-lengthened. When more severe knee flexion contractures are present, the hamstring tendons are transected distally. Release of the posterior knee joint capsule should be reserved for rigid, recurrent flexion contractures. Significant flexion contractures cannot be fully corrected at the time of the initial surgical release because of shortening of the joint capsule as well as the neurovascular structures. Serial casting is done to correct the residual deformity.

ADDUCTED THIGHS

The patient with adductor spasticity sits with scissoring thighs or walks with a scissoring pattern characterized by medial thigh contact throughout the gait cycle. Scissoring thighs may interfere with hygiene, dressing, sexual intimacy, sitting, transfers, standing, and walking. During swing phase, severe hip adduction interferes with limb advancement. The base of support is narrow during stance, potentially impairing balance. When adductor spasticity is also complicated by hip flexor spasticity, toileting functions and perineal access are markedly impeded, and positioning in a chair is problematic. Muscles that potentially contribute include adductor longus and brevis, adductor magnus, gracilis, iliopsoas, and pectineus. Diagnostic obturator nerve block helps to establish whether contracture is present. Unmasking of voluntary hip abduction may also be revealed. The patient's base of support may widen and advancement of the swing limb may improve following obturator block, suggesting that the spastic deformity is dynamic. The use of chemodenervation or neurolytic agents may be helpful in providing passive access for perineal care. Active function during gait may also improve. Chemodenervation of the spastic iliacus is feasible during motor recovery. Translumbar instillation of neurolytic agents to block a spastic psoas major muscle is also reported.

In the period of functional adaptation, limb scissoring is corrected surgically. If there is a dynamic hip adduction deformity with little or no contracture, denervation of the hip adductor muscles is done by transecting the anterior branches of the obturator nerve. When contracture has occurred, hip adductors are released near their proximal origin. Severe adduction contractures require release of the adductor longus, adductor brevis, and gracilis muscles. Moderate degrees of contracture can be treated with release of the adductor longus and gracilis muscles, combined with obturator neurectomy. The minimal amount of release needed to achieve 30 degrees of passive abduction under anesthesia is done to minimize the amount of "dead space" in the wound, which predisposes to hematoma formation and potential postoperative infection in the groin.

EXCESSIVE HIP FLEXION

Persistent hip flexion may interfere with positioning, perineal care, sexual intimacy, and gait. Severe hip flexion deformity may contribute to knee flexion deformity. During stance, excessive hip flexion interferes with advancement of the body over the stance phase limb, resulting in a shortened contralateral step. Muscles that potentially contribute to an excessively flexed hip include iliopsoas, rectus femoris (also a knee extensor), and pectineus (also a thigh adductor). The adductor longus and brevis may also contribute to hip flexion. Adductor and hip flexor spasticity often coexist and consequently pelvic obliquity may occur. Clinical examination, dynamic EMG studies, and diagnostic nerve and motor point blocks may be helpful in sorting out various muscle contributions. During motor recovery, a combination of neurolytic and chemodenervation agents is often helpful in dealing with discrete muscle groups that cause complex hip and knee deformities. When clinical judgment indicates that localized treatment is not feasible, intrathecal techniques and systemic oral medications are considered.

In the period of functional adaptation, orthopedic treatment consists of releasing or lengthening hip flexors. Care is taken to preserve as much hip flexor function as possible for limb advancement during walking and for stair climbing. For flexion deformities of 30 to 45 degrees, the iliopsoas tendon is released from its insertion at the lesser trochanter and allowed to slide proximally. Because the iliopsoas has multiple insertions on the anterior hip joint capsule, it does not retract very far and then reattaches. Release of the tendon from the lesser trochanter weakens but does not totally eliminate its action as a hip flexor. In a patient with a hip flexion deformity greater than 45 degrees, it is advisable to release the pectineus by transecting it through its muscle belly, along with release of iliopsoas. Though the pectineus is transected, hip flexion is still served by rectus femoris, sartorius, and a weakened iliopsoas.

In nonambulatory patients with severe hip flexion contractures, surgical release is indicated to improve passive positioning of the patient, prevent decubitus ulcers, and facilitate perineal care. In this situation, it is necessary to transect the iliopsoas through its muscle belly at the rim of the pelvis to completely eliminate its activity as a hip flexor. The pectineus, rectus femoris, and sartorius muscles are also released. Generally, it is also necessary to release the hip adductor muscles and to perform concomitant distal hamstring releases.

Heterotopic Ossification

Heterotopic ossification (HO) causes restriction of proximal joint motion in persons with severe TBI, particularly when there have been skeletal fractures. Although HO is seen in spastic patients with paresis, surprisingly, good underlying motor control may often be present but cannot be expressed because of the severe restriction of motion imposed by the HO. Thorough clinical examination, sometimes aided by dynamic EMG that evaluates control of the isometric contraction, distinguishes restricted motion on a structural basis (HO) from neurologically restricted motion.

The early treatment of HO consists of drug therapy using diphosphonates (etidronate sodium 20 mg/kg/day) to inhibit calcium crystal deposition in the underlying collagen matrix. Anti-inflammatory agents (indomethacin 75 mg daily) are used to control the intense inflammatory process that occurs secondary to the formation of HO. Spasticity is aggressively treated with phenol nerve blocks or botulinum toxin. Physical therapy with gentle range of motion exercises is used to maintain joint motion, though the battle is often uphill.

Surgical excision is the definitive treatment of heterotopic bone.[74] Surgical excision should be delayed until the heterotopic bone is fully mature to prevent recurrence. A true bone cortex with mature trabeculae should be visible radiographically, and serum alkaline phosphatase should be normal. We do not rely on triple-phase bone scan findings to determine full maturity. If the patient has voluntary motion about the joint, the surgical excision predictably results in an increased range of motion. Patients should have sufficient cognitive recovery and behavioral compliance to cooperate with an arduous physical therapy program after surgery.

Bony Malalignment or Fracture Malunion

Because the majority of TBI cases are associated with high-velocity motor vehicle accidents, multiple trauma is common, and fractures may be inadequately treated or even remain undiagnosed. Secondary discovery of undiagnosed fractures is not uncommon in an acute rehabilitation setting. Initial musculoskeletal injuries should be treated aggressively with operative stabilization on the assumption that eventual neurological recovery will occur. Otherwise, secondary consequences such as body angular deformities, malunited fractures, severe leg length discrepancies, and soft tissue contractures will require additional reconstructive surgery. Unfortunately, fracture malunions continue to be prevalent in the TBI patient and contribute to significant loss of function. Moore[75] recently reviewed cases of five male patients with TBI who had malunited tibial fractures that required reconstructive surgery. Four patients required correction of bony angularities, and one patient needed extensive soft tissue releases. One patient had residual shortening of 6 cm and required bone-lengthening procedures. The brain injured individual is less able to accommodate residual limb deformities such as leg length discrepancy than a neurologically intact person.

Pain Syndromes

The paretic shoulder deserves special attention as a common source of pain. Different factors contribute to the painful, immobile shoulder: reflex sympathetic dystrophy, brachial plexitis, inferior subluxation, spasticity with adduction, internal rotation contracture, adhesive capsulitis, spastic abduction, heterotopic ossification, and traumatic lesions such as rotator cuff tears or fractures and dislocations.[76]

Diagnosis can be difficult in the patient with pain from reflex sympathetic dystrophy (RSD). The classic clinical signs of RSD may not be apparent. If the arm is painful and no etiology is apparent, a technetium bone scan will assist in establishing the diagnosis. Treatment should be instituted immediately. Treatment options include medications such as amitriptyline (Elavil), physical therapy, and nerve blocks (stellate ganglion blocks, brachial plexus blocks, or Bier IV regional blocks). Each of these techniques is successful with some patients; however, none is reliable for all patients.

Adhesive capsulitis or "frozen shoulder" may be seen after TBI but is more often seen in patients following stroke or in those with RSD. The shoulder is characteristically painful, and glenohumeral motion is limited. Three clinical and four arthroscopic stages have been identified. Treatment in this group of patients is similar to that for the general population: nonsteroidal anti-inflammatory drugs, physical therapy, and intra-articular injections of steroids with a local anesthetic. Selected cases may benefit from manipulation under anesthesia. The role of arthroscopy in the treatment of this disorder has not been established.

Pseudobulbar Athetoid Syndrome

Roberts[28] attached the term *pseudobulbar athetoid syndrome* to patients who had evidence of severe bilateral pyramidal damage with postural dystonia and fragmentary athetosis. The athetoid pseudobulbar pattern was seen in approximately 5 percent of patients in his follow-up series. In some patients, there was a remarkable discrepancy between the severity of physical disability and preservation of intellect and personality traits that Roberts thought might have been the result of secondary infarction rather than primary diffuse axonal injury. He commented on the similarities between these patients and many cases of congenital diplegia. We have seen only an occasional patient fitting Roberts's original description of the athetoid pseudobulbar syndrome, but those patients did have striking preservation of intellect and personality in the face of severe bradykinesia and athetoid movements. They moved slothlike and much too slowly to be functional without assistance. These patients were unresponsive to dopaminergic agents. Adaptive devices were helpful for communicating; they predominantly used yes-no scanning systems, smiles, and head nods. These individuals read books and magazines with the aid of page turners and personal attendants. They could walk but only with assistance to prevent loss of balance. Although they displayed athetoid movements, athetosis as a consequence of TBI is unusual.

Brain Stem Syndrome

Brain stem syndrome, resulting from brain stem compression, is characterized by ipsilateral ataxia and contralateral spastic hemiparesis. It was discussed in association with ataxia in the section on excessive motion. In addition to ataxia, this syndrome also produces spastic limbs, whose management is similar to that discussed previously on patterns of dysfunction after UMN lesions. However, solutions to the combination of ataxia and spasticity—mixing problems of excessive motion and restricted motion—must be thoughtfully individualized, especially because the severity of each set of findings can vary significantly within the same patient.

Rigidity and Bradykinesia

The resistance of rigidity experienced by an examiner moving a joint passively persists throughout the entire range, and, within certain limits, the resistance feels the same, regardless of range or velocity of movement. Classically, this type of resistance has been likened to bending a piece of solder or a lead pipe. Lead pipe rigidity usually indicates a lesion of extrapyramidal pathways and is one of the cardinal features of Parkinson's disease, which also includes bradykinesia, tremor at rest, and a loss of postural reflexes. Post-traumatic parkinsonism, however, is an unusual complication of TBI.[45] In this regard, one syndrome with Parkinson-like features results from cumulative head blows in boxers. Years after their boxing careers have ended, boxers develop symptoms of progressive neurological injury associated with dementia. Histologically, degeneration of substantia nigra and medial temporal cortex is found. Beta-amyloid plaques are also found, resembling findings in Alzheimer's disease. Lewy bodies, found in the substantia nigra in classic parkinsonism, are not found in the syndrome of "pugilistic" parkinsonism.

In our experience, the production of slowed movement in patients with TBI is usually a function of the UMN syndrome rather than a true extrapyramidal bradykinesia.[77] Severe spasticity may communicate a "rigid feel" to the examining clinician, but closer attention often reveals a clasp-knife response, typical of spasticity. In this regard, a patient who presents with decerebrate "rigidity," a postural syndrome associated with rostral brain stem lesions (as may be seen after transtentorial herniation), typically reveals extended and internally rotated arms with flexed wrists and fingers, extended and internally rotated legs, and equinovarus feet. During muscle tone testing in such an individual, the extremities are usually seen as rigidly extended, but a limb segment that is bent yields like a clasp knife and hence the disturbance in tone is spastic, with the term *rigidity* used as a colloquial descriptor of the posture. Thus, decerebrate "rigidity" is very unlike extrapyramidal lead pipe rigidity. (Historically, Sherrington applied the term *rigidity* to limb posturing of cats who underwent rostral brain stem transections. Their limbs had a rigid feel but yielded to pressure in a sudden, clasp-knife manner, very unlike a lead pipe.) Finally, patients with dystonia, a very slow, alternating contraction-relaxation of agonist and antagonists, also present to the examiner as having "a rigid feel." In this situation, the constant writhing movements of these individuals literally strengthens the involved muscles and disables the examiner's efforts at passive motion when the dystonia actively occurs during examination. Spastic and lead pipe rigid muscles are quiet at rest. Patients with dystonia or decerebrate rigidity actually do not afford the examiner a starting point of "rest." They are actively in contraction before the examiner begins testing.

Treatment of true post-traumtic parkinsonism, like idiopathic parkinsonism, relies on dopamine precursors and anticholinergic medications. Details of management are extensive and beyond the scope of this chapter, except that anticholinergic medications, often useful in treating rest tremor, may produce undesirable sedation in patients with TBI. Interestingly, dopaminergic agents such as L-dopa, carbidopa, and amantadine have been used effectively to improve arousal and attention in patients with TBI. These medications do not particularly improve "slow movement," which suggests that slow movement seen in TBI is probably not of extrapyramidal origin. Decerebrate rigidity is commonly seen in the intensive care unit shortly after acute injury and is difficult to control. Barbiturate coma, when used as a neurosurgical treatment for acute brain injury, may influence severe tone of decerebrate rigidity. In the future, programmable pumps may be used with such medications as baclofen. Decorticate rigidity may indicate a lesion of cortical white matter, internal capsule, cerebral peduncle, basal ganglia, or thalamus. Clinically, the lower extremities are extended in both rigidities, but the upper extremities are flexed at the elbow in decorticate rigidity in contrast to the elbow extension of decerebrate rigidity. The significance of either posture lies in the potential for developing contracture. Sometimes a patient has had neurological recovery, but the limb remains in decerebrate or decorticate "posture" because of residual contractures. Clinicians should not assume that continuing problems with dynamic tone are actually causing these fixed postures.

Dystonia, Torticollis, Bruxism, and Locked Jaws

We have already described the slow alternations of contraction and relaxation of agonists and antagonists that lead to contorsional movements described as dystonia. Some clinicians seem to use the term more broadly to describe fixed abnormal postures, such as "dystonic hemiplegia," but spastic muscles of hemiplegia are quiet at rest and end postures are static, not dynamic. We prefer to limit the term *dystonia* to dynamic cocontraction of agonists and antagonists that varies in time to produce slow, writhing or repetitive twisting types of movements or actively sustained, contorted postures. Post-traumatic dystonia is not uncommon and is more often focal and distal than proximal or diffuse in one or more limbs. Treatment of dystonia re-

quires identification of the muscles that are involved in generating dystonic postures and movement. Because many muscles appear to be involved, treatment focally aimed at only one muscle group will almost surely result in a new deformity dominated by actively dystonic muscles that were not included in the treatment. Dynamic EMG may be helpful in this regard. Diagnostic motor point blocks with lidocaine to suspected muscle groups may in fact simulate what a longer-term intervention might accomplish. Botulinum toxin A is currently the drug of choice for focal dystonias.[65] Theoretically, phenol motor point or nerve blocks may be useful, but, practically speaking, it is difficult to perform a phenol block in a muscle that is contracting because the phenol technique involves electrical stimulation to localize the nerve or motor point. Twitch contractions induced by electrical stimulation are typically masked by the constant contraction of dystonic muscle. Botulinum toxin injection technique utilizing clinical or EMG verification of needle electrode placement obviates this problem.

Torticollis as a manifestation of dystonia may also be treated with botulinum toxin. Because botulinum toxin wears off, repeated injections are necessary. The possibility of immunological resistance is of some concern. The problem of persistent torticollis, unrelieved, may be so disabling that surgical neurectomy, if feasible, may have to be considered. More typically, torticollis occurs because of a combination of spasticity and contracture in the sternocleidomastoid muscles. These muscles may be studied with dynamic EMG, as may the upper trapezii, which are sometimes involved in torticollis. The sternocleidomastoid muscles are powerful neck flexors, and they develop contracture easily. Treatment is aimed at reducing the spastic component by focally injecting this muscle with botulinum toxin or by phenolizing their motor points. Stretching exercises are very important in reducing stiffness and contracture of this powerful muscle group. Occasionally some of the splenius muscles may also be involved in spastic torticollis, and blocks are potentially useful for these muscles as well.

The functional problems attributed to bruxism (persistent jaw grinding) and to "locked jaws" (jaws kept closed by spasticity and contracture) are not uncommon. Muscles that potentially contribute include the masseters, the temporalis muscles, and the medial and lateral pterygoids. The last group is difficult to access intraorally for dynamic EMG studies or for blocks, but the masseters and the temporalis muscles are readily available for study. EMG activity may be seen in both masseters and/or both temporalis muscles. Asymmetrical findings are possible. Findings help the clinician decide which muscle groups need to be injected. Phenol blocks to the masseteric nerves are difficult to perform, but application of botulinum toxin is satisfactory. Phenol blocks to the motor point of the temporalis muscle is often effective in relieving a locked jaw. The condition can be quite disabling because the separation between the front teeth can be as narrow as several millimeters and the time course of prying open the jaw can be prolonged (weeks to months), even if spastic temporalis and masseter muscles are blocked chemically. Radiographs of the temporomandibular joints should be undertaken prior to neuromotor interventions to rule out subluxation or dislocation or even occult fractures.

□ SUMMATION

TBI leads to motor phenomena that functionally may produce restricted or excessive motion. Restricted motion has two types of consequences: limitations of access to body parts for personal care and activities of daily living and limitations on performing active movements for a variety of functional purposes. The consequences of excessive motion are the instability, spatial and temporal errors, and misapplication of forces when the patient attempts to perform tasks in real life. The functional classification of restricted versus excessive motion may be useful for categorizing and managing the great variety of motor phenomena that emerge from a damaged nervous system after TBI. At present, there are more medical and surgical treatment options available for the consequences of restricted motion than for excessive motion.

REFERENCES

1. Garland, DE, and Bailey, S: Undetected injuries in head-injured adults. Clin Orthop 155:162, 1981.
2. Stone, L, and Keenan, MAE: Peripheral nerve injuries in head-injured adults. Clin Orthop 233:136, 1988.
3. Botte, MJ, and Moore, TJ: The orthopaedic management of extremity injuries in head trauma. J Head Trauma Rehabil 2:13, 1987.
4. Keenan, MAE, and Botte, MJ: Traumatic brain injury. In Nickel, VL, and Botte, MJ (eds): Orthopaedic Rehabilitation. Churchill Livingstone, New York, 1992.
5. Garland, DE, and Waters, RL: Extremity fractures in head injured adults. In Meyer, MH (ed): The Multiply Injured Patient with Complex Fractures. Lea & Febiger, Philadelphia, 1984.
6. Guanche, C, and Keenan, MAE: Principles of orthopaedic rehabilitation. Physical Medicine and Rehabilitation Clinics of North America 3:417, 1992.
7. Gans, BM: Rehabilitation of the pediatric patient. In De Lisa, et al (eds): Rehabilitation Medicine: Principles and Practice. J B Lippincott, Philadelphia, 1988.
8. Glenn, M: Nerve blocks. In Glenn, M, and Whyte, J (eds): The Practical Management of Spasticity in Children and Adults. Lea & Febiger, Philadelphia, 1990.
9. Garland, DE, et al: Resection of heterotopic ossification in the adult with head trauma. J Bone Joint Surg Am 67: 1261, 1985.
10. Mayer, NH, Esquenazi, A, and Keenan, MAE: Evaluation and management of spasticity, contracture and impaired motor control. In Zasler, N, and Horn, L (eds): Medical Rehabilitation of Traumatic Brain Injury. Hanley & Belfus, Philadelphia, 1996.
11. Penn, RD: Intrathecal baclofen for severe spasticity. Ann N Y Acad Sci 531:157, 1988.
12. Keenan, MAE: The orthopaedic management of spasticity. J Head Trauma Rehabil 2(2):62, 1987.
13. Mayer, NH, Esquenazi, A, and Wannstedt, G: Surgical planning for upper motoneuron dysfunction: The role of motor control evaluation. J Head Trauma Rehabil 11(4): 37, 1996.
14. Keenan, MAE: Management of the spastic upper extremity in the neurologically impaired adult. Clin Orthop 233: 116, 1988.
15. Sutherland, DH, and Kaufman, KR: Motion analysis: Lower extremity. In Nickel, VL, and Botte, MJ (eds): Orthopaedic Rehabilitation. Churchill Livingstone, New York, 1992.
16. DeLateur, BJ: A new technique of intramuscular phenol neurolysis. Arch Phys Med Rehabil 53:179, 1972.
17. Garland, DE, Lucie, RS, and Walters, RL: Current uses of open phenol nerve block for adult acquired spasticity. Clin Orthop 165:217, 1982.
18. Keenan, MAE, et al: Percutaneous phenol block of the musculocutaneous nerve to control elbow flexor spasticity. J Hand Surg [Am] 15:340, 1990.
19. Borg-Stein, J, and Stein, J: Pharmacology of botulinum toxin and implications for use in disorders of muscle tone. J Head Trauma Rehabil 8(3):103, 1993.
20. Whyte, J, and Robinson, K: Pharmacologic management. In Glenn, M, and Whyte, J (eds): The Practical Management of Spasticity in Children and Adults. Lea & Febiger, Philadelphia, 1990.
21. Andrew, J, Fowler, CJ, and Harison, MJ: Tremor after head injury and its treatment by stereotaxic surgery. J Neurol Neurosurg Psychiatry 45:815, 1982.
22. Bass, B, et al: Tizanidine versus baclofen in the treatment of spasticity in patients with multiple sclerosis. Can J Neurol Sci 15:15, 1988.
23. Bes, A, et al: A multi-centre, double-blind trial of tizanidine, a new antispastic agent, in spasticity associated with hemiplegia. Curr Med Res Opin 10:709, 1988.
24. Kaplan, MS: Tizanidine: Another tool in the management of spasticity. J Head Trauma Rehabil 12(5).
25. Holmes, G: The cerebellum of man. Brain 62:21, 1939.
26. Koller, KC: Pharmacological trials in the treatment of cerebellar tremor. Arch Neurol 41:280, 1984.
27. Edwards, RV: Nadolol use for cerebellar tremor. Am J Psychiatry 139:1522, 1982.
28. Roberts, AH: Severe Accidental Head Injury: An Assessment of Long-Term Prognosis. Macmillan, London, 1979.
29. Tomlinson, BE: Brain stem lesions after head injury. J Clin Pathol (supp 4)23:154, 1970.
30. Dimitrijevic, MR, Nathan, PW, and Sherwood, AM: Clonus: The role of central mechanisms. J Neurol Neurosurg Psychiatry 43:329, 1980.
31. Rack, PMH, Ross, HF, and Thilman, AF: The ankle stretch reflexes in normal and spastic subjects. Brain 107:637, 1984.
32. Herman, R, Mayer, N, and Mecomber, SA: The pharmacophysiology of dantrolene sodium. Am J Phys Med 51:296, 1972.
33. Mayer, N, Mecomber, SA, and Herman, R: Treatment of spasticity with dantrolene sodium. Am J Phys Med 52:18, 1973.
34. Kant, R, and Zeiler, D: Hemiballismus following closed head injury. Brain Inj 10:155, 1996.
35. Whittier, JR, and Mettler, FA: Studies on the subthalamus of the rhesus monkey: Hyperkinesia and other physiological effects of subthalamic lesions, with special reference to the subthalamic nucleus of Luys. J Comp Neurol 90:319, 1949.

36. Gilbert, GJ: Response of hemiballismus to haloperidol. JAMA 233:535, 1975.
37. Jankovic, J, and Orman, J: Tetrabenazine therapy of dystonia, chorea, tics and other dyskinesias. Neurology 38:391, 1988.
38. Chandra, V, Wharton, S, and Spunt, AL: Amelioration of hemiballismus with sodium valproate. Ann Neurol 12:407, 1982.
39. Dewey, RB, and Jankovic, J: Hemiballismus, hemichorea: Clinical and pharmacological findings in 21 patients. Arch Neurol 46:862, 1989.
40. Robin, JJ: Paroxysmal choreoathetosis following head injury. Ann Neurol 2:447, 1977.
41. Chandra, V, Spunt, AL, and Rusinowitz, MS: Treatment of post-traumatic choreoathetosis with sodium valproate (letter). J Neurol Neurosurg Psychiatry 46:963, 1983.
42. Katz, DI: Movement disorders following traumatic head injury. J Head Trauma Rehabil 5:86, 1990.
43. Jankovic, J, and Tolosa, E (eds): Parkinson's Disease and Movement Disorders, ed 2. Wiliams & Wilkins, Baltimore, 1993.
44. Koller, WC, Wong, GF, and Lang, A: Post-traumatic movement disorders: A review. Mov Disord 4:20, 1989.
45. Ivanhoe, CB, and Bontke, CF: Movement disorders after traumatic brain injury. In Zasler, N, and Horn, L (eds): Medical Rehabilitation of Traumatic Brain Injury. Hanley & Belfus, Philadelphia, 1996.
46. Ellison, PH: Propranolol for severe post-head injury action tremor. Neurology 28:197, 1978.
47. Biary, N, et al: Post-traumatic tremor. Neurology 39:103, 1989.
48. Jankovic, J, and Schwartz, K: Botulinum toxin treatment of tremors. Neurology 41:1185, 1991.
49. Adams, RD, and Victor, M: Abnormalities of movement and posture. In Adams, RD, and Victor, M (eds): Principles of Neurology, ed 4. McGraw-Hill, New York, 1989.
50. Fahn, S, Marsden, CD, and Van Woert, M: Definition and classification of myoclonus. In Fahn, S, Marsden, CD, and Van Woert, M (eds): Advances in Neurology, vol 43, Myoclonus. Raven Press, New York, 1986, p 265.
51. Lapresle, J: Palatal myoclonus. In Fahn, S, Marsden, CD, and Van Woert, M (eds): Advances in Neurology, vol 43, Myoclonus. Raven Press, New York, 1986, p 265.
52. Appel, SA (ed): Movement disorders. Neurol Clin 3, 1981.
53. Stone, L, and Keenan, MAE: Peripheral nerve injuries in the adult with traumatic brain injury. Clin Orthop 233:136, 1988.
54. Young, S, and Keenan, MAE: Extremity fractures in the brain-injured patient. In Nickel, VL, and Botte, MJ (eds): Orthopaedic Rehabilitation, ed 2. Churchill Livingstone, New York, 1992.
55. Nathan, P: Some comments on spasticity and rigidity. In Desmedt, JE (ed): New Developments in Electromyography and Clinical Neurophysiology. Karger, Basel, 1973, p 13.
56. Lance, JW: Pyramidal and extrapyramidal disorders. In Shahani, BT (ed): Electromyography in CNS Disorders: Central EMG. Butterworth, Boston, 1984.
57. Herman, R: The myotatic reflex. Brain 93:273, 1970.
58. Garland, DE, Razza, BE, and Waters, RL: Forceful joint manipulation in head-injured adults with heterotopic ossification. Clin Orthop 169:133, 1982.
59. Keenan, MAE, et al: Late ulnar neuropathy in the brain-injured adult. J Hand Surg [Am] 13:120, 1988.
60. Medici, et al: A double-blind, long-term study of tizanidine in spasticity due to cerebrovascular lesions. Curr Med Res Opin 11:398, 1989.
61. Yourn, RR, and Delwaide, PJ: Spasticity. N Engl J Med 304:28, 1981.
62. Yablon, SA, and Sipski, ML: Effect of transdermal clonidine on spinal spasticity: A case series. Am J Phys Med Rehabil 72:154, 1993.
63. Mai, J: Depression of spasticity by alpha-adrenergic blockade. Acta Neurol Scand 57:65, 1978.
64. Black, JD, and Dolly, JO: Interaction of I-labelled botulinum neurotoxins with nerve terminals. II, Autoradiographic evidence for its uptake into motor nerves by acceptor-mediated endocytosis. J Cell Biol 103:535, 1986.
65. Brin, MF, et al: Disorders of excessive muscle contractions: Candidates for treatment with intramuscular botulinum. In Das Gupta, BR (ed): Botulinum and Tetanus Neurotoxins: Neurotransmission and Biomedical Aspects. Plenum, New York, 1993.
66. Cosgrove, AP, and Graham, HK: Botulinum toxin A in the management of children with cerebral palsy. J Bone Joint Surg BR (supp 2)74:135, 1992.
67. Snow, BJ, et al: Treatment of spasticity with botulinum toxin: A double-blind study. Ann Neurol 28:512: 1990.
68. Konstanzer, A, et al: Botulinum toxin A treatment in spasticity of arm and leg. Mov Disord (supp 1)7:137, 1992.
69. Greene, P, and Fahn, S: Development of antibodies to botulinum toxin type A in torticollis patients treated with botulinum toxin injections. Mov Disord (supp 1)7:134, 1992.
70. O'Brien, C: Clinical pharmacology of botulinum toxin. In O'Brien, C, and Yablon, S (eds): Management of Spasticity with Botulinum Toxin. Postgraduate Institute for Medicine, Littleton, Colo, 1995.
71. Penn, RD: Intrathecal baclofen for severe spasticity. Ann N Y Acad Sci 531:157, 1988.
72. Meythaler, JM: Intrathecal baclofen for spastic hypertonia in brain injury. J Head Trauma Rehabil 12(1):87, 1997.
73. Waters, RL, et al: Stiff-legged gait in hemiplegia surgical correction. J Bone Joint Surg Am 61:927, 1979.
74. Kolessar, DJ, Katz, SD, and Keenan, MAE: Functional outcome following surgical resection of heterotopic ossification in patients with brain injury. J Head Trauma Rehabil 11(4):78, 1996.
75. Moore, TJ: The treatment of malunion of tibial fractures in patients with traumatic brain injury. J Head Trauma Rehabil 11(4):31, 1996.
76. Gellman, H, Keenan, MAE, and Botte, MJ: Recognition and management of upper extremity pain syndromes in the patient with brain injury. J Head Trauma Rehabil 11(4):23, 1996.
77. Freund, JH: The pathophysiology of central paresis. In Stuppler, A, and Seindl, A (eds): Electromyography and Evoked Potentials. Springer-Verlag, New York, 1985.

Pharmacology in Traumatic Brain Injury: Fundamentals and Treatment Strategies

ROSS D. ZAFONTE, DO,
ELIE ELOVIC, MD,
W. JERRY MYSIW, MD,
MICHAEL O'DELL, MD,
and THOMAS WATANABE, MD

Over the past several decades, there has been a tremendous improvement in the fundamental understanding of the acute mechanisms of traumatic brain injury. Additional knowledge has been gained about recovery of the traumatic brain injury (TBI) survivor. Recently, interest has grown in the potential positive and negative roles pharmaceuticals can play in the recovery process. Although this chapter aims to present state-of-the-art practice, our overall understanding of this topic is in its infancy. Clinicians are often forced to turn to a sparse literature and limited clinical experience to assist the patient with TBI. To best present this topic, we have chosen to first review the fundamental neurochemical issues that are germane to the clinical care of the patient with TBI, next discuss those medications that may have a negative impact on recovery, and concentrate on pharmacotherapy for sleep disturbance, behavioral and mood dysfunction, and cognitive enhancement.

◻ NEUROTRANSMITTERS

Medications are used to treat TBI to either facilitate or inhibit specific neurotransmitter activity. Table 30–1 summarizes the significant neurotransmitter pathways.

Acetylcholine

Acetylcholine (ACh) is the neurotransmitter most keenly involved with memory. There are two groups of central nervous system (CNS) acetylcholine pathways (Fig. 30–1). The forebrain pathways originate from cell bodies in the nucleus basalis of Meynert and the basal forebrain and the striatum; those innervating the brain stem and diencephalon originate in the laterodorsal and pedunculopontine tegmental nuclei.[1] ACh is synthesized within cholinergic neurons from the precursor choline.[2] Acetyl

TABLE 30–1. Neurotransmitters		
NEUROTRANSMITTER	NUCLEUS OR SITE OF ORIGIN	PRIMARY FUNCTION
Serotonin	Raphe nuclei	Sleep, mood, behavior
Acetylcholine	Nucleus basalis of Meynert	Memory
Norepinephrine	Locus caeruleus	Sleep, arousal, attention, processing
Dopamine	Substantia nigra, ventral tegmentum	Motor control, arousal, mentation
GABA	Diffuse pathways	General inhibition

coenzyme A is also required for the synthesis of ACh from choline. The enzyme choline acetyltransferase facilitates the formation of acetylcholine.[3] Although most neurotransmitters are inactivated by reuptake of the neurotransmitter, ACh inactivation occurs predominantly by enzymatic degradation.[4] The enzyme that degrades acetylcholine is acetylcholinesterase. This is the site of action of most drugs used to increase ACh activity following TBI.

Norepinephrine

Epinephrine, dopamine, and norepinephrine are referred to as *catecholamines*. Norepineph-

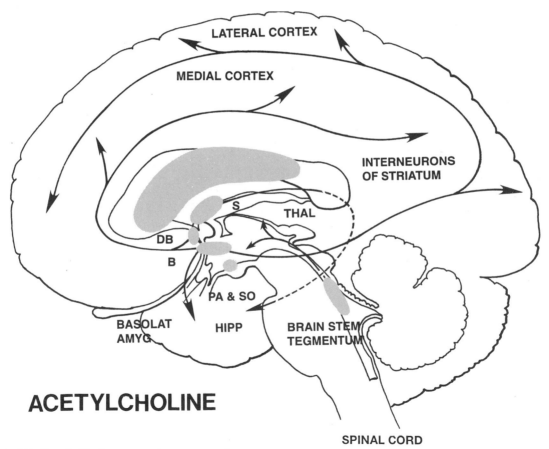

FIGURE 30–1. The location and projections of acetylcholine neurons are illustrated. Areas containing cell bodies are shaded. HYPO = hypothalamus; IPN = interpeduncular nucleus; THAL = thalamus. (From Gilman, S, and Newman, SW: Manter and Gatz's Essentials of Clinical Neuroanatomy and Neurophysiology, ed 9. FA Davis, Philadelphia, 1996, with permission.)

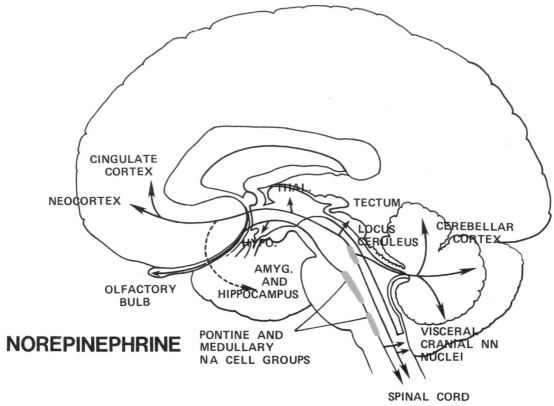

FIGURE 30–2. The locations and projections of noradrenergic neurons are illustrated. Cell groups are shaded. AMYG = amygdala; HYPO = hypothalamus; NA = norepinephrine; THAL = thalamus. (From Gilman, S, and Newman, SW: Manter and Gatz's Essentials of Clinical Neuroanatomy and Neurophysiology, ed 9. FA Davis, Philadelphia, 1996, with permission.)

rine (NE) is associated with noradrenergic neurons in the brain. These noradrenergic neurons are located primarily in the locus caeruleus and the lateral tegmental system (Fig. 30–2).[5] These neurons have a diffuse set of projections that extend toward the forebrain. Tyrosine is converted to dopamine via a hydroxylation reaction.[6] Dopamine is then transformed to norepinephrine via dopamine β-hydroxylase. NE in the central nervous system has been found to be involved in sleep regulation, arousal, mood, aggression, and perception of sensation.[7] Medications employed in the treatment of TBI that treat TBI increase NE release, block NE reuptake, or both.

Dopamine

Dopamine (DA) is a catecholamine with rather diffuse effects on the cardiovascular, renal, and central nervous systems. Most dopaminergic neurons have their cell bodies in the substantia nigra or the hypothalamus (Fig. 30–3). The major dopaminergic pathways are the nigrostriatal, tuberoinfundibular, mesocortical, and mesolimbic systems. DA is derived from the hydroxylation of tyrosine and is also an intermediate compound in norepinephrine synthesis.[8] Five types of DA receptors (D-1, D-2, D-3, D-4, D-5) have been described and provide for the specificity of action of various medications for TBI.[9] D-1 appears to act via activation of adenyl cyclase and the increase of cyclic adenosine monophosphate, whereas D-2 receptors are effective via the inhibition of adenyl cyclase. The D-4 receptor is largely found in the limbic system and has been implicated in the etiology of schizophrenia.[10] The D-3 receptor is somewhat less well understood and is also found in the limbic areas of the brain.[11] Traditional antipsychotic agents work by blocking the D-2 receptor; however, the newer atypical antipsychotics such as clozapine employ part of their action at the D-4 receptor. Dopamine activity can be increased pharmacologically by increasing synthesis and release, decreasing reuptake, and/or postsynaptic stimulation.

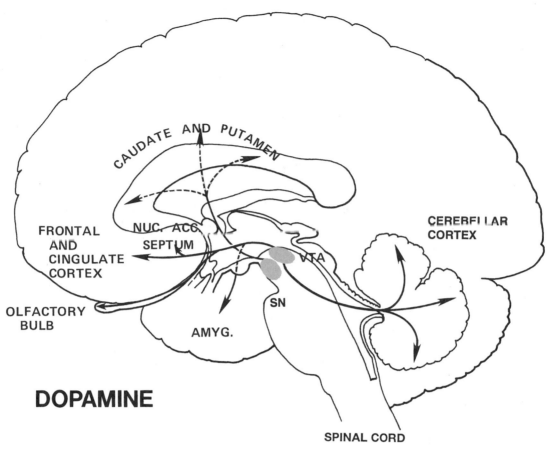

DOPAMINE

FIGURE 30–3. The locations and projections of dopaminergic systems are illustrated. Cell groups are shaded. AMYG = amygdala; NUC ACC = nucleus accumbens; VTA = ventral tegmental area. (From Gilman, S, and Newman, SW: Manter and Gatz's Essentials of Clinical Neuroanatomy and Neurophysiology, ed 9. FA Davis, Philadelphia, 1996, with permission.)

Serotonin

Serotonin (5HT or 5-hydroxytryptamine) is classified as an indolamine. The cell bodies that produce serotonin are located in the raphe nuclei of the brain stem (Fig. 30–4). These neurons have a rather diffuse distribution and project forward to innervate the forebrain. 5HT is derived from the amino acid precursor tryptophan.[12] Tryptophan is converted to 5HT via tryptophan hydroxylase. Typically, serotonin is inactivated by reuptake from the neuron and by degradation via the enzyme monoamine oxidase. Serotonin receptors have been a focus of much interest and research. There are four well-known families of 5HT: 5HT-1 through 5HT-4. Recently, three new classes of receptors have been identified: 5HT-5 through 5HT-7; however their physiological activity has not been fully identified. The subtypes 5HT-1 through 5HT-4 differ in their method of action, function, agonist, and antagonist properties.[13] The 5HT-1 family (5HT1a, 5HT1b, 5HT1c, 5HT1d, 5HT1e) is negatively coupled to adenyl cyclase. Agents that selectively stimulate these receptors have alleviated aggression in animals.[14] Medications with a high affinity for 5HT1a, 5HT1b, and 5HT1c receptors appear to have antiaggressive properties in humans. Serotonin activity is most commonly enhanced by inhibiting reuptake or interfering with degradation.

☐ AMINO ACIDS

Certain amino acids have been shown to be active neurotransmitters—some inhibitory and some excitatory. γ-aminobutyric acid (GABA) and glycine are two of the most common inhibitory neurotransmitters in the brain. GABA is widely distributed throughout the mammalian central nervous system, with almost none located

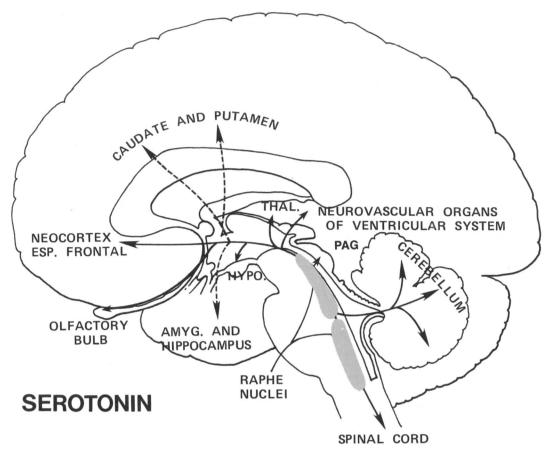

SEROTONIN

FIGURE 30–4. The locations and projections of serotoninergic neurons are illustrated. Cell groups are shaded. AMYG = amygdala; HYPO = hypothalamus; SUB NIGRA = substantia nigra; THAL = thalamus. (From Gilman, S, and Newman, SW: Manter and Gatz's Essentials of Clinical Neuroanatomy and Neurophysiology, ed 9. FA Davis, Philadelphia, 1996, with permission.)

in the peripheral nervous system. Areas of function include inhibition between cerebellar neurons and Deiters' nucleus, interneurons, and the output of the cerebellar cortex, olfactory bulb, cuneate nucleus, and hippocampus. GABA is also the mediator of inhibition in the cerebral cortex and the basal ganglia. There are two separate GABA receptors, GABA a and GABA b, in addition to a GABA transporter. GABA a receptors are more prevalent and act by opening chloride channels, making depolarization more difficult.[15] This action results in membrane hyperpolarization and thus inhibition, with benzodiazepine the prototypical agents. GABA b is less ubiquitous than GABA a and does not have an effect on chloride channels but rather acts by increasing potassium or decreasing calcium conductance, dampening excitability. GABA b is the receptor where baclofen has its major effect. GABA b receptors have been identified in the hippocampus and the spinal cord.[16–18]

Glycine, the simplest amino acid, has been shown to be active in the spinal cord and brain stem. It is an inhibitory neurotransmitter that is found only in vertebrates. Our knowledge of its mode of action is limited, but it appears similar to the GABA a receptors.

Glutamate and aspartate are found throughout the central nervous system; glutamate and also possibly aspartate are believed to function as classic fast excitatory neurotransmitters. Originally, excitatory receptors were divided into N-methyl-D-aspartate (NMDA) and non-NMDA; however, more recent work has identified four separate receptor types: NMDA, AMPA, kaniate, and ACPD (metabotropic receptors). NMDA receptors are found throughout the CNS, with increased concentrations within the hippocampus and the cerebral cortex.

AMPA distribution within the central nervous system parallels that of the NMDA, with their principal function long-term potentiation in various excitatory pathways. The kaniate receptors are concentrated in the hippocampus. The ACPD receptors, in contrast to the other pathways, manifest their function via guanosine triphosphate (GTP) mediated intermediates, whereas the other pathways work through ion channels and have been implicated in brain plasticity. Excitatory amino acids (EAA) have been linked to numerous activities, including long-term memory potentiation, brain plasticity, and cell death. An enormous amount of study is still needed to fully understand their importance in the mammalian brain.

□ NEUROTRANSMITTERS AND BRAIN TRAUMA

A comprehensive description of the neurophysiological dysfunction that occurs after TBI is beyond the scope of this chapter. Observations have, however, led to the belief that monoamine metabolites are decreased after TBI. Having diffuse projections, neurons containing these neurotransmitters are vulnerable to post-traumatic dysfunction. Feeney et al.[19] have demonstrated that brain lesioned rats that receive amphetamine (a monoamine agonist) show an enhanced recovery. Monoamine infusions have been demonstrated to promote plasticity in brain lesioned kittens.[20] In addition, those agents that decrease monoamines have been associated with slower progress. The role of ACh in both the acute and postacute phases of TBI has not yet been completely clarified.[21]

□ MEDICATIONS THAT CAN IMPAIR RECOVERY

Pharmacological management of the brain injury survivor requires an assessment of medications that may impede recovery. Many medications may induce sedation or memory dysfunction or decrease overall arousal. Table 30–2 is a partial list of potentially cognitively inhibitory medications. Those medication classes of particular relevance are discussed in greater detail.

Anticonvulsants

Recent recommendations have advocated that anticonvulsant prophylaxis may be warranted for only the first week after injury.[22,23] Although anticonvulsant prophylaxis remains a point of discussion, no clear evidence supports long-term prophylaxis.[24] Practice guidelines from several societies have advocated against prolonged anticonvulsant prophylaxis in an as-

---

> **TABLE 30–2. Medications That Can Impair Cognition**
>
> Aminophylline
> Anticholinergic agents
> Anticonvulsants
> Antiemetics
> Antipsychotics
> Beta-blockers
> Benzodiazepines
> Barbiturates
> Cardiac glycosides
> Centrally acting antihypertensive agents
> Chloral hydrate
> Gastric motility agents (metoclopramide)
> H_2 Blockers
> Hypnotics
> Opiates
> Propofol

---

symptomatic population. The role of anticonvulsant prophylaxis in those patients with penetrating head trauma remains controversial. Long-term use of phenytoin has been reported to have adverse cognitive effects.[25] The deleterious impact of phenobarbital on cognition is well documented, and this medication should not be a first choice as anticonvulsant therapy in the TBI survivor. Glenn and Wrobleski[26] have advocated carbamazepine or valproic acid to treat post-traumatic seizures because of the suggestion of lower cognitive side effects. However, controversy remains as to the relative cognitive disturbance each one of these agents may cause.[27]

Second-generation anticonvulsants such as gabapentin and lamotrigene are now available and are thus far approved only as adjuvant agents, not monotherapy.[28] Recent reports have discussed the potential role of these medications in behavioral regulation and pain syndromes. Vigabatrin carries unique NMDA antagonist qualities but is not yet available in the United States. The effects of these agents on cognition in brain injury are not well described.[29]

Antihypertensive Agents

Central antihypertensives such as methyldopa may have a significant sedating effect. Clonidine is an α_2-agonist with central activity that may produce impaired cognition.[30] Clonidine has been advocated for treatment of spasticity and agitation. Lipophilic beta-blockers that cross the blood-brain barrier have been useful in the treatment of agitation; however, they may also produce significant sedation.[31] A decrease in dopaminergic neurotransmission has been implicated with calcium channel antagonists.[32] No direct effect of calcium channel antagonists on motor or cognitive recovery has been established.[33]

Benzodiazepines

Benzodiazepines work via action at the GABA a receptor. These agents bind to the GABA a site and increase the rate of chloride channel opening.[34] Benzodiazepines readily cross the blood-brain barrier and produce antegrade amnesia and anxiolysis. These agents are employed to produce sedation but also decrease new learning and memory and have been reported to produce increased confusion and agitation.[35] Therefore, their routine use in the TBI survivor is generally not recommended.

Gastrointestinal Agents

Histamine-2 blockers (cimetidine, ranitidine, famotidine, and nizatidine) have been implicated as having sedating potential in the patient with central neurological injury and in the elderly.[36] Metoclopramide is commonly employed to enhance gastrointestinal motility. This agent enhances gastric contraction, raises esophageal pressure, and promotes relaxation of the pylorus. Metoclopramide has significant DA (D-2) antagonist effects and can produce impaired cognitive responses.[37] It has also been associated with extrapyramidal side effects. Agents such as cisapride and erythromycin can be used in place of metoclopramide to facilitate gastrointestinal motility.

Neuroleptics

Neuroleptics block DA in addition to serving as cholinergic and adrenergic antagonists. Because monoamines such as DA appear to be decreased after brain injury, use of agents that also decrease monoamine activity is somewhat concerning. As previously discussed, Feeney et al.[19] first raised concerns that neuroleptics may impair recovery after brain injury. Potential neuroleptic side effects include extrapyramidal symptoms, the neuroleptic malignant syndrome, anticholinergic side effects, a lowered seizure threshold, and detrimental effects on new learning and memory. The majority of neuroleptic agents act at the D-2 receptor, which may in part explain some of their side effect profile.[38] In a small study, Rao et al.[39] noted little impact on recovery by the neuroleptic haloperidol. Yet many experimental clinicians remain concerned with

the potential side effect profile of haloperidol. A reasonable recommendation is that neuroleptic medications not be considered agents of first choice in the treatment of TBI patients with behavioral disturbance.

Atypical antipsychotics (risperidone and clozapine) are newer agents with both dopaminergic and serotoninergic blocking properties.[40] Clozapine has unique action at the D-4 and D-1 receptors, as well as action at the 5HT-1 site.[41] Risperidone has action at the D-2 receptor as well as the 5HT-2 receptor. Olanzapine is another atypical antipsychotic that is a member of the thienobenzocliazepine class. Atypical antipsychotics appear to have a lower potential for extrapyramidal side effects, yet their effect on cognitive outcome in the brain injury survivor is not well described.[42]

◻ PHARMACOTHERAPY OF SLEEP DISTURBANCE

Prigatano et al.[43] have shown that sleep disturbance is relatively common in the TBI population. Accurate clinical evaluation of this problem is often necessary and requisite when considering pharmacological intervention. A significant amount of sleep pathology can be accounted for by neurophysiological and environmental alterations that occur after TBI.

Basic Concepts in Sleep

Sleep-wake cycles have been studied extensively over the past 75 years. Elegant work by Aserinsky and Kleitman[44] has helped us establish the conceptual issues of alternating sleep cycles and REM (rapid eye movement) and non-REM sleep. Quite simply, REM sleep is the active brain in the paralyzed body, and non-REM sleep is the inactive brain in the active body. Individuals go though so-called slow wave sleep (stages 1–4) prior to entering REM sleep. Humans alternate between REM and non-REM sleep in cycles throughout the night. Studies appear to indicate that in humans the sleep-generating centers are located in the lower brain stem.[45] Medullary and pontine lesions have been associated with states of chronic wakefulness on electroencephalography, and lesions of the midbrain have been associated with arousal deficits. Clearly, caudal solitary tract nucleus stimulation appears to induce sleep. A sleep inhibitory center is located in the posterior hypothalamus, and a sleep facilitory center has been demonstrated in the anterior hypothalamus.[46] These regions have neocortical projections. Previous studies of diencephalic cats have shown that those animals without neocortex did not sleep normally. Bilateral frontal lesions in animals have been demonstrated to result in permanent sleep dysfunction.[47] Forebrain and brain stem interconnections thus act to form a rather complex network that participates in sleep generation. Sleep modulation occurs over a diffuse area; thus it is understandable why those who have sustained a TBI are likely to experience sleep disturbances.

Neurochemistry of Sleep

Serotonin has been implicated as a primary agent in sleep induction. A lesion in the region of the raphe nucleus has been noted to cause chronic insomnia in humans. However, whereas serotoninergic neurons are active in onset of slow wave (non-REM) sleep, their activity is almost absent during REM sleep.[48] Thus the major role of serotonin may be in sleep initiation. Less clear is the neurochemistry of REM sleep. It has been observed that ACh concentration is increased during REM sleep in the cat. Critical doses of physostigmine, a cholinergic agonist, facilitate REM sleep in the rat.[49] NE in small doses also tends to increase REM sleep. There exists a fine balance in the neurochemistry of sleep initiation and sleep regulation that can easily be perturbed by neurological lesions and external influences.[50]

Medications to Enhance Sleep

A key component prior to any pharmacological intervention is the evaluation for any potential neuromedical cause of sleep disturbance. In addition, a measurement tool to evaluate for disorders of sleep maintenance or initiation is warranted. Scales such as the Pittsburgh Sleep Quality Index questionnaire or simple nursing observation can be extremely helpful.[51,52] Traditionally, sleep disturbance has been treated with benzodiazepines or hypnotic agents. Although useful in the general population, these agents may have distinct limitations for a population in which sedation needs to be avoided and new learning and memory concerns are paramount.

As noted, benzodiazepines work via modulation of GABA neurotransmission. This benzodiazepine receptor GABA–chloride channel complex is effective in inhibiting neuronal cell discharge.[34] These agents classically reduce phasic interruptions of sleep.[53] Total sleep time is increased. However, the latency to REM sleep may be increased, and REM sleep appears to decrease in the first third of the night.

Hypnotic benzodiazepines are rather widely available and are generally employed to shorten sleep onset or decrease the number of wakeful episodes throughout the night. There has been a move toward agents that are ultrarapidly eliminated. Care must be taken to avoid adverse effects that may play a significant role in the TBI population: sedation, anterograde amnesia, and impaired performance on motor tasks.[35] A concern in the TBI survivor is the fact that rapidly discontinuing these medications may result in rebound insomnia.

Partial benzodiazepine agonist medications such as clonazepam appear to have similar effects on sleep. Clonazepam can decrease number of wakeful episodes yet does have some inhibitory effect on REM sleep.[54] Later stages of slow wave sleep (stage 4) increase with the administration of clonazepam. A newer agent, zolpidem, is a partial benzodiazepine-like agent that also appears to increase stage 4 sleep.[55] The overall cognitive effects of this agent are not yet clear; however, anecdotal reports in the TBI population seem to indicate a more favorable profile than the more traditional sleep-enhancing agents.

ANTIDEPRESSANTS

Antidepressants have been used not only to relieve depression but also to improve sleep. Typical antidepressants present along a spectrum of sedating activity and noradrenergic activity. The tricyclic antidepressants (TCA) are typically divided into the tertiary and secondary amines. Those medications with increased anticholinergic activity have an increased tendency to produce sedation. In the small nighttime doses necessary to produce sleep, excess sedation is not an overwhelming problem. Because these agents may have a proadrenergic action, they may be most useful when sleep regulation or cycling is found clinically to be the most pronounced concern.[56] Antidepressants decrease REM sleep. However, REM duration may be increased in the depressed patient.[50] When sedation is sought, amitriptyline is preferred and, in contradistinction, desipramine is the medication most likely to avoid sedating potential. These agents also can lower the seizure threshold.

SEROTONINERGIC AGENTS

As discussed earlier, serotoninergic neurons play a primary role in the early stages of sleep initiation. Thus, agents that increase serotonin may be a principal therapy for sleep initiation deficits. Trazodone is a competitive reuptake inhibitor of serotonin whose effect is particularly good in those depressed patients with chronic insomnia.[57] Trazodone has a relative dearth of cardiovascular and anticholinergic side effects. Priapism is a concern, but it is relatively rare (1 in 7000) and has been associated with other medications. Boyeson and Harmon have raised concerns regarding the potential effects of trazodone on recovery in the rodent model.[58] These potential effects may be lessened by utilizing this medication in low doses at night. Nefazodone is a sedating serotoninergic medication that also appears to enhance sleep initiation. Mirtazapine is a new antidepressant with 5HT1a activity that may also be useful in the treatment of sleep disturbance.

☐ POST-TRAUMATIC AGITATION

Post-traumatic agitation is the neurobehavioral consequence of severe TBI that receives the greatest attention in the medical rehabilitation literature. This attention is likely secondary to both the high incidence of post-traumatic agitation and its implications for the safety of patients and staff, which, in turn, necessitate an intensive commitment of resources for appropriate and prompt management.

The incidence estimates of post-traumatic agitation range widely from 11 percent to 50 percent, largely because of the lack of a consistent definition of the term.[59–61] The absence of a consistent definition has, in turn, hindered development of effective treatment strategies. A definition for *post-traumatic agitation* was, therefore, recently proposed that encompasses the components of aggression, restlessness, emotional discontrol, and cognitive changes described in many of the earlier definitions. This definition suggests that post-traumatic agitation is (1) a subtype of delirium unique to survivors of TBI in which (2) the survivor is in the state of post-traumatic amnesia and (3) there are excesses of behavior that include some combination of aggression, akathisia, disinhibition, and/or emotional lability.[62] The subsequent discussion of pharmacological intervention for post-traumatic agitation is largely predicated on this definition. In 1990, the Omnibus Budget Reconciliation Act (OBRA) by the Health Care Financing Administration published guidelines for neuroleptic use in long-term care facilities.[63] Briefly stated, the guidelines suggest that dementia and delirium are among the appropriate indications for neuroleptics if there are concomitant psychotic or agitated behaviors. Specifically, these OBRA guidelines state that neuroleptics are warranted in the management of dementia and delirium with associated psychotic and/or agitated behaviors that are (1) quantitatively and objectively documented, (2) where preventable etiologies are excluded, and (3) when

there is evidence of danger to the patient or others caused by the behaviors.[63] These guidelines do not directly apply to all pharmacological decisions concerning the management of post-traumatic agitation because the neuroleptics represent only one of several pharmacological intervention options. In the past, the management of agitated severe TBI survivors was primarily provided during acute care and subsequent acute rehabilitation hospitalizations; an ever larger amount of TBI rehabilitation is now provided in skilled nursing facilities, which fall under OBRA jurisdiction.

Familiarity with the OBRA guidelines is, however, salient to this discussion in that they provide a useful conceptual framework for considering pharmacological intervention for post-traumatic agitation; that is, the OBRA guidelines suggest that the extent and severity of target behaviors should be objectively quantified. The obvious implication of this guideline is that the outcome of the intervention is likely to be enhanced if there is an objective measure of the target behaviors. Toward that goal, the Agitated Behavior Scale remains the only instrument that is both reliable and validated as a measure of post-traumatic agitation in severe TBI survivors.[64] This instrument is easy to administer, and its subscales remain consistent with the previously described definition for post-traumatic agitation. The second OBRA recommendation suggests that reversible etiologies for the target behaviors should be considered before pharmacological intervention is initiated. Corrigan et al.[65] documented that cognition improved before post traumatic agitation decreased, providing support for the clinical observation that medical complications and pharmacological interventions that impair cognition are likely to exacerbate post-traumatic agitation. Hence, patients with persistent post-traumatic agitation deserve an evaluation to exclude all sources of pain and reversible causes of impaired cognition if the differential diagnosis is essentially the same as one would consider with most delirium evaluations.[66]

The third OBRA guideline, suggesting that the severity of target behaviors should warrant the use of pharmacological intervention, is relevant to this discussion in that there are no studies documenting the impact of the pharmacological intervention on long-term outcome. Animal studies have, for example, suggested that catecholamine, serotonin, and cholinergic manipulation does affect the quality of outcome after CNS injury, but corroborating human studies are still needed.[67] Until these issues are better understood, the use of neuropharmacological strategies as an adjunct in the management of TBI survivors deserves caution.

There are virtually no prospective evaluations of pharmacological interventions for the management of post-traumatic agitation. Despite this serious limitation in the TBI literature, a recent survey of rehabilitation professionals suggests a clear pattern of practice preferences[68] (Table 30–3).

Specifically, the pharmacological agents used by these rehabilitation professionals in the management of post-traumatic agitation were described in decreasing order as carbamazepine, tricyclic antidepressants, beta-blockers, haloperidol, benzodiazepines, methylphenidate, buspirone, trazodone, and amantadine.[68] The medical rehabilitation literature is reviewed in the subsequent section concerning the relative merits of these pharmacological strategies. Where no substantial rehabilitation literature exists, other prospective studies describing the efficacy of that agent in the management of behavioral disturbances are described.

Carbamazepine

Carbamazepine is described as the most commonly used pharmacological agent in the management of post-traumatic agitation, but there is comparatively little published evidence to support its efficacy in ameliorating the target behaviors of post-traumatic agitation. Several case studies have described the efficacy of carbamazepine in the management of agitation and aggression after acute brain injury.[69] Carbamazepine has also been described as effective in the management of manic-depressive illness precipitated by TBI.[70]

The adverse effects of carbamazepine that are unique to traumatic brain injured survivors are relatively minor. Carbamazepine has been suspected of having adverse cognitive consequences for TBI survivors. It has, in fact, been shown to adversely affect motor and speeded performance tasks; these effects are reversible after cessation of the drug.[71] One series involving TBI patients in a rehabilitation setting described the replacement of phenytoin, phenobarbital, and primidone with carbamazepine with little consequence or a slight improvement in seizure control in 20 of 21 patients.[72] The pharmacokinetics of carbamazepine in TBI survivors are atypical in that months following observed evidence of autoinduction, an increase in the dose-to-serum concentration was observed, warranting closer drug monitoring.[73] However, carbamazepine used solely for neurobehavioral purposes should be titrated on the basis of clinical response rather than rigidly adhering to "therapeutic" drug levels.

Valproic Acid

Recent work has begun to demonstrate the efficacy of valproic acid in the treatment of behavioral disturbance. The mechanism of action of valproic acid is not yet clear. Theories focus on GABA-ergic activity and "antikindling activity." Valproic acid has been advocated for disorders such as mania, bipolar disorder, and schizoaffective behaviors.[74] Geracotti[75] reported a case in which valproic acid was an instrumental therapy for post-traumatic episodic explosive disorder. Wrobleski et al.[76] have reported a case series of post-traumatic patients with destructive and aggressive behaviors treated with valproic acid, which was effective when other

TABLE 30–3. Pharmacological Agents to Treat Post-traumatic Agitation: Summary of the Literature

Drug	Studies	Design	Response Rate	Dose (maximum)
Carbamazepine	1[66]	Case report	100%	800 mg
Amitriptyline	2[77,78]	Case report Retrospective	65%	75 mg
Propranolol	1[87]	Double-blind, placebo-controlled	Uncertain	420 mg
Haloperidol	1[39]	Retrospective	Uncertain	2–15 mg
Benzodiazepines	None			
Methylphenidate	None			
Amantadine	2[100,101]	Case reports	80%	400 mg
Valproic acid	2[75,76]	Case reports	100%	2250 mg
Buspirone	2[102,103]	Case report Retrospective	90%	40 mg
Trazodone	1[104]	Case report	83%	400 mg
Lithium	1[105]	Case report	70%	1200 mg

agents appeared to fail. Potential side effects of valproic acid include tremor, dizziness, pancreatitis, and elevated levels of ammonia.

Tricyclic Antidepressants

Tricyclic antidepressants (TCAs) were first suggested as effective interventions for post-traumatic agitation in a 1985 case report of a patient functioning at Rancho level IV.[77] A subsequent larger series supported this observation in that 13 of 20 patients with agitation responded favorably within 1 week of initiating amitriptyline.[78] Target behaviors of patients functioning at Rancho level IV were more likely to respond to amitriptyline than patients functioning at Rancho level V or VI; still, 60 percent of patients at Rancho level V or VI responded to amitriptyline therapy at an average daily dose of 75 mg. Several potential adverse effects of TCAs for TBI survivors warrant consideration. The negative impact of the anticholinergic properties of TCAs on cognitive recovery during post-traumatic amnesia has been at least partially addressed with amitriptyline. The previously described series of 20 patients receiving amitriptyline for agitation were compared with 38 TBI survivors who were similar in demographics and coma duration but who were not sufficiently agitated to warrant pharmacological intervention.[78] Both patient populations demonstrated similar rates of cognitive improvement based on gains in their weekly aggregate Orientation Group Monitoring System score, but the amitriptyline-treated group had more patients who never cleared post-traumatic amnesia. This observation has not been corroborated, but these data may reflect the possibility that severe agitation is a predictor of poorer cognitive recovery, that these TCAs have an adverse effect on cognitive recovery, or that the retrospective design could not control for inherent bias. Cases describing improvement in arousal and initiation in severe TBI survivors after initiating amitriptyline, protriptyline, and desipramine would argue against adverse effects on cognitive recovery after severe TBI.[79,80] The impact of TCAs on motor recovery is less certain because no human studies involving TBI survivors are available. Animal studies suggest that desipramine, with epinephrine reuptake inhibition and anticholinergic properties, may enhance motor recovery. Amitriptyline, with its prominent noradrenergic, serotoninergic, and anticholinergic properties, does not appear to affect motor recovery acutely but may transiently reinstate motor deficits in a stable CNS injury.[81,82]

Beta-Blockers

Beta-blockers have been used effectively to manage behavioral disturbances in patients with diagnoses that include mental retardation, autism, dementia, and organic brain syndrome.[83–86] Only one study has examined the effects of a beta-blocker, propranolol, for the treatment of agitation after severe TBI.[87] That study included 21 survivors of severe TBI in a double-blind, placebo-controlled trial in which the treatment group received a maximum dose of 420 mg of the long-acting variant of propranolol. That study documented that the number of episodes of agitation was unchanged by the use of propranolol, but the intensity of agitation significantly decreased in the propranolol-treated group. However, the instrument utilized was not validated as a measure of agitation in TBI survivors.

The previously described prospective study involving propranolol indicated that no adverse effects occurred that necessitated subjects to withdraw from the study.[87] Animal studies suggest that early intervention with propranolol has no impact on motor recovery if it is administered acutely or after recovery has stabilized.[88] However, animal studies do suggest that propranolol may adversely affect the recovery of learning after CNS injury.

Haloperidol

Post-traumatic agitation that is severe in intensity would fall within the OBRA guidelines of appropriate indications for neuroleptics. Only one study has described the efficacy of this intervention for the management of post-traumatic agitation.[39] That retrospective study of 26 consecutive patients admitted to acute rehabilitation compared the use of haloperidol in 11 severely agitated survivors versus 15 less severely agitated patients. Both groups were similar in demographics and length of coma. Treatment consisted of haloperidol doses that ranged between 2 and 15 mg per day, for a period of 14 to 61 days. No significant differences in outcome were found between the two populations, based on the Patient Evaluation Conference System (PECS), except the duration of post-traumatic amnesia was longer in the haloperidol-treated group. The only adverse affect to haloperidol described in this study was an episode of oculogyric crisis. However, animal and human studies raise serious concerns about the negative impact of dopamine antagonists on motor recovery. A recent study of stroke survivors supported the clinical relevance of previous animal studies by demonstrating that pharmacologic agents such as dopamine receptor blockers impaired the recovery of both motor function and functional independence.[89]

Benzodiazepine

The benzodiazepines represent the fifth most common category of agents utilized in the management of post-traumatic agitation. However, there are no published studies or cases supporting their efficacy in this population. These agents have been effectively utilized for the management of acute and chronic agitation secondary to dementia.[90,91] Most studies use lorazepam for acute agitation. In chronic agitation with dementia, the efficacy of benzodiazepines compares favorably with the neuroleptics.[92] The adverse effect of benzodiazepines, of particular concern to the TBI survivor, is the fact that they are amnestic. Animal studies have suggested persistent sensory asymmetry in animals allowed to recover for several weeks after CNS injury before their exposure to diazepam.[93] The previously mentioned human study exploring the impact of various drugs on recovery after stroke suggested that benzodiazepines contributed to the observed impaired recovery of motor and functional skills.[89]

Methylphenidate

Methylphenidate for the management of post-traumatic agitation is perhaps initially counterintuitive in that a stimulant is utilized to diminish behaviors that include restlessness and aggression. However, its use is consistent with the conceptual framework of the post-traumatic agitation definition described earlier in which post-traumatic amnesia and cognitive deficits were an important component of that definition.[62] Studies that suggest that aggressive behaviors are predicted by the extent of disorientation and that cognition improves before agitation diminishes would support the utilization of agents that improve cognitive performance for the management of post-traumatic agitation.[65,94] Methylphenidate has been shown to improve cognitive performance—specifically, attention—in acute TBI survivors.[95,96]

There are no published studies to support the use of methylphenidate in the management of post-traumatic agitation. One intriguing randomized, pretest–post-test, placebo-controlled group in a single-blind-designed study of severe TBI survivors demonstrated that methylphenidate significantly diminished anger.[97] However, the study population was an average of 2 years postinjury, and all had cleared post-traumatic amnesia; therefore, the anger described in this study may have limited relevance to the target behaviors of post-traumatic agitation as defined in this chapter. Animal studies involving methylphenidate in the management of TBI are also lacking, whereas a number of animal studies utilizing amphetamines suggest that these agents enhance recovery; the extent to which this positive outcome is ascribable to methylphenidate is uncertain.[19,98]

The dose of methylphenidate described in the previously mentioned prospective studies peaked at 15 to 30 mg per day.[96,97] The adverse effects, secondary to methylphenidate in TBI survivors, appear relatively minor. One of the studies described a patient with paroxysmal tachycardia, whereas a second study demonstrated no difference in adverse effects compared with the control group. The issue of methylphenidate's adverse effect on seizure control does not appear to be of significant concern because one study documented a trend toward a lower seizure incidence in TBI patients with active seizure disorders while on methylphenidate.[99]

Amantadine

Amantadine is similar to methylphenidate in that it has been advocated as an effective pharmacological regimen in the treatment of both cognitive and neurobehavioral disorders after TBI. Cognitive benefits attributed to amantadine primarily include various aspects of attention, such as improving arousal.[100] A number of case reports describe amantadine as effective in doses of up to 400 mg per day in decreasing target behaviors consistent with post-traumatic agitation, even when other pharmacological interventions have failed.[100,101] It is believed that the beneficial effects of amantadine on cognition and behavior are mediated through its dopamine-enhancing properties.[100] This agent may also have NMDA receptor antagonist activity. The adverse effects of amantadine described in TBI survivors include seizures, irritability, anxiety, hypomania, hallucination, and livedo reticularis.

Alternative Agents

Buspirone and trazodone are among the previously described list of pharmacological agents frequently utilized in the management of post-traumatic agitation, but there is very little literature to support their efficacy. Buspirone has been described as effective in the management of post-traumatic agitation in several case studies.[102,103] These case studies describe doses of up to 20 mg twice a day with positive responses observed within days. These findings imply that the therapeutic effects of buspirone are different from its anxiolytic properties, which are typically observed several weeks after the initiation of the drug.[102] No significant adverse effects have been attributed to buspirone utilized to manage post-traumatic agitation.

Trazodone efficacy in the management of post-traumatic agitation is described in only one abstract, which describes trazodone as effective in decreasing agitation in a group of brain injury survivors who failed to respond to amitriptyline.[104] Significant improvement in agitated behavior scores were noted within 7 days at doses of trazodone that approached 400 mg per day. As previously stated, animal studies of trazodone have raised concerns about transient impairments in motor skills.

Lithium represents a potentially important intervention for post-traumatic agitation. One particular series described 10 patients given lithium for agitated behavior; 7 patients responded favorably at doses as high as 1200 mg per day, whereas 3 patients developed neurotoxic effects.[105] An intriguing aspect of these cases is the fact that a number of patients were several years postinjury, with a range of 1 to 66 months. Lithium has also effectively treated episodes of mania precipitated by brain injury.[106]

The pathogenesis and prognostic significance of post-traumatic agitation remain poorly understood. Until recently, there was no attempt to establish a consistent definition. Similarly, the literature describing appropriate pharmacotherapy is sparse and lacking in prospective blinded studies (Table 30–3).

◻ MEDICATIONS TO ENHANCE AROUSAL AND MEMORY

The use of neuropharmacological agents to remediate specific cognitive impairments represents one of the most exciting therapeutic modalities in the rehabilitation of people with TBI.[107–109] Despite the dearth and limitations of TBI-specific empirical research,[110] clinicians can make logical, if strictly unproven, drug choices based on theoretical rationale and literature in related, nontraumatic brain disorders.[108,109] This discussion overviews pharmacological treatment of deficits in arousal, attention, initiation, and memory following TBI.

Before drug therapy is initiated, several considerations are warranted. Not all cognitive

deficits after TBI are caused by organic brain damage. As stated earlier in the chapter, CNS side effects from other medications are among the most common remediable, secondary etiologies for cognitive deficits in TBI.[108,111] Three principles should guide medication management. *Minimalization* requires stopping all unneeded, potentially detrimental drugs,[111] such as discontinuing histamine-2 blockers when stress ulcer prophylaxis is no longer needed and phenytoin when seizure prophylaxis is no longer appropriate. Assuming that certain medical conditions do require treatment, *substitution* stresses changing potentially detrimental medications to equally effective drugs with fewer, or no, cognitive side effects, for example, substituting cisapride for metoclopramide to treat gastroparesis[112] and substituting centrally acting antihypertensive medications with angiotensin converting enzyme inhibitors or atenolol.[113] Only after minimalization and substitution is *functional augmentation*—the addition of cognitively enhancing medications—applied.

Maximizing medical stability and treating neurological complications should precede any consideration for drug intervention.[111] Cognitive dysfunction can occur secondary to mood disorders, depression, and/or anxiety. Neuropsychology input can be valuable both in estimating the relative contribution of mood disorders to cognitive dysfunction and in assessing response to treatment. The lesser degree of sedation associated with buspirone treatment of anxiety and serotonin-specific reuptake inhibitors (SSRI) treatment of depression make these agents particularly suited to people with TBI.[108] At times, cognitive dysfunction is secondary to other cognitive deficits, for example, memory dysfunction caused by poor attention.[114] In these cases, the primary cognitive deficit should be treated first. Finally, many people with TBI have premorbid histories of attention deficit disorder, learning disabilities, drug and alcohol abuse, and previous brain injuries, and expectations for drug response might be more modest.[115,116]

Treatment of Hypoarousal

Arousal is the most basic cognitive function on which other higher-level neurobehavioral functions are predicated.[108] Despite the separate discussions here, arousal, attention, and initiation can be considered constructs along the same continuum. Whyte[117] has defined *arousal* as the "general state of readiness of an individual to process sensory information and/or organize a response." Although the neurochemical substrates of arousal are many, dopamine may be more involved in response preparation, whereas noradrenergic and acetylcholine influence perceptual processing.[117] Anatomically, the reticular activating and limbic systems are implicated in "general" and "goal-directed" arousal, respectively.[108]

The data on drug treatment of hypoarousal are limited by lack of controlled studies, standardized outcome measures, and detailed dosing regimens and the small sample sizes.[109,111] Given Whyte's observations, the dopaminergic agents such as levodopa/carbidopa, bromocriptine, pergolide, amantadine, and selegiline might best be applied with minimally conscious patients in need of "response preparation."[108,118] Others have suggested that drugs enhancing norepinephrine, serotonin, and acetylcholine might be beneficial.[79,109,110,119] The use of serial standardized or idiographic assessments may be helpful to document clinical response.[110,111] Even with the favorable side effect profiles of these drugs, efficacy in treating hypoarousal remains unclear. Clinicians should carefully establish clinical end points and document discussions of potential benefits and risks with patients and families before treatment.

Treatment of Attention Deficits

The medical literature is somewhat more encouraging with regard to psychostimulant treatment of attention deficits after TBI.[108,109] First popularized by Evans et al.,[120] treatment with various agents, especially methylphenidate, has gained widespread acceptance. Recent suggestions that methylphenidate also affects the speed and ultimate degree of functional recovery provide additional incentive for its use.[98,121]

Evidence for the efficacy of psychostimulants in those with brain injuries includes case reports,[120,122] case series,[123] and a few small prospective group studies.[96,97,121] In addition to the case reports and series, two recent studies are worth expanded consideration here. Kaelin et al.[96] reported data using a single case (multiple baseline) methodology comparing methylphenidate (maximum dose of 30 mg/day) and placebo in 11 patients with severe brain injuries (3 nontraumatic) in an inpatient rehabilitation setting (mean time from injury = 19.8 days). One patient who developed paroxysmal tachycardia was discontinued. Statistically significant treatment effects were noted in simple neuropsychological tests of attention with trends toward improvement in overall functional status according to the Disability Rating Scale (DRS). Drug effects were noted to extend beyond the treatment period. Relative weakness of the study include mixed etiologies for injuries,

small sample size, nonfunctional measures of attention, and lack of follow-up beyond inpatient rehabilitation. Plenger et al.[121] reported a double-blind, placebo-controlled, two-group trial of methylphenidate (maximum dose of 0.3 mg/kg per day) in 23 persons with TBI. Significant differences were found between the active and placebo groups on DRS and measures of attention, concentration, vigilance, and motor memory at 30 days but not 90 days. The authors concluded that methylphenidate may affect the rate of recovery from TBI but not the final degree. However, only 9 of 23 patients completed the study at 90 days, which introduces the potential for substantial bias. Few side effects were noted in either study. Refuting these data are cross-over design studies by Speech et al.,[124] which found no significant differences in standardized tests of cognition between methylphenidate and placebo in 12 TBI patients. It should be noted that most patients and family members did note a subjective improvement, and mean time from injury was just over 4 years. Similar results were noted by Gualtieri et al.,[125] whereas Mooney and Haas[97] noted improvement in anger control but not in cognitive testing in comparisons of placebo and methylphenidate. These studies, once again, noted few side effects.

Agents other than methylphenidate described as beneficial in treating attention deficits following TBI include protriptyline amantadine and bromocriptine, dextroamphetamine, and dexedrine.[109,122,123,126]

In general, these studies suggest a modest treatment effect and, with other data, are remarkable for the relative lack of significant side effects.[127] Taken as a whole, there appears to be an acceptable risk-benefit ratio to warrant expanded research and clinical use.

Treatment of Initiation Deficits

A number of CNS lesions can produce the clinical picture of "apathy" or "lack of motivation" occasionally seen after TBI. Frontal lobe injury, especially of the dorsolateral region, and lesions of the limbic and hippocampal systems can be manifested as a lack of initiation.[128,129] This alteration of personality is also seen with subcortical pathology, including lesions of the midbrain reticular activating system, substantia nigra, and locus caeruleus.[130] Given the number of structures and associated neurotransmitters involved in this neurological deficit, it is not surprising that a wide variety of "rational" attempts at pharmacological intervention have been implemented. They have primarily focused on modulating the previously described dopaminergic and noradrenergic pathways.

Stimulants have been used to treat deficits in initiation, as well as the related problem of inattention, in patients with TBI. Amphetamine and methylphenidate are catecholamine agonists that primarily increase DA activity. Among other actions, DA modulates mesolimbic tone.[131] Stern,[132] who treated with dextroamphetamine 11 patients with frontal lobe lesions and decreased initiation, reported subjective improvement in 8 of the 11, without side effects. Weinstein and Wells[133] reported good results in a patient treated with methylphenidate 5 years after TBI. Finally, the possible effect of stimulants in improving overall functional recovery from brain injury in animals and humans deserves mention.[39,96,122]

Although stimulants are thought to exert their action through dopaminergic pathways, other dopaminergic agents have also been employed to improve initiation in patients with TBI. Bromocriptine was reported to decrease apathy in a patient with bilateral thalamic infarcts and other types of brain injury.[134,135] Amantadine has also been reported to improve initiation, possibly through multiple, incompletely defined, primarily dopaminergic actions. Nickels et al.[100] reported subjective improvement in arousal and initiation in a retrospective study of 12 patients with TBI treated with amantadine. Van Reekum et al.,[136] using a randomized, double-blind, placebo-controlled, single-case methodology, reported improvement with amantadine in a patient with TBI. Gualtieri et al.[125] described one case of abulia that responded to amantadine among 30 patients with TBI treated with this agent for a variety of clinical indications.

The TCAs exert their CNS effects primarily through noradrenergic pathways, although they also affect serotonin, acetylcholine, and dopamine levels.[137,138] In addition to modulating function of the locus caeruleus, noradrenergic systems have been implicated in neurological recovery.[139,140] Wrobleski et al. presented eight cases in which protriptyline use was associated with subjective improvement in initiation.[126] Reinhard et al.[79] reported improved arousal and initiation after TCA therapy in three patients who had suffered brain injuries. Two of these patients worsened when the medications were discontinued or tapered and then improved again after they were resumed.

Overall, studies regarding improvement of initiation have been handicapped by small subject numbers, subjective outcome measures, and inadequate controls and the lack of blinding, not unlike pharmacological research aimed at treating other cognitive sequelae of TBI. In addition, lack of precise neuroanatomic localization of the injury will hinder efforts aimed at implementing rational pharmacological therapy based on neurophysiology. More studies are needed to clarify the efficacy and physiological action of these agents.

Treatment of Memory Deficits

Because memory deficits are so common, much effort has been put forth, utilizing a diverse set of neuroactive medications, to enhance recovery of memory after brain injuries. This diversity should not be surprising because memory encompasses and is dependent on a variety of mental tasks, from the basic states of arousal and initiation to the higher-level processes of acquisition, storage, and recall. The scope of activities involved implicates multiple areas of the nervous system (frontal and temporal lobes, thalamus) and therefore many biochemical modulators.[141] This discussion is not a comprehensive review of pharmacological enhancement of memory; rather, it is a broad survey of the various exogenous and endogenous substances hypothesized to affect memory. This survey includes animal and human models and both normal and diseased states.

The cholinergic system is one of the best-known and most thoroughly studied components in memory.[142,143] Evidence for the role of ACh in memory enhancement has come from studies in Alzheimer's patients and primates as well as in memory-impaired TBI patients.[144–148] There is evidence that ACh precursors and cholinergic agonists such as physostigmine can improve memory.[147,149] For example, in Cardenas's study,[147] 36 men with TBI were enrolled to compare physostigmine (2–4 mg/day) with placebo and scopolamine (a cholinergic antagonist) in a double-blind clinical trial. Forty-four percent of the subjects demonstrated improved memory as demonstrated by a more than 50 percent increase of the Long-Term Storage or Sum Consistent Long-Term Retrieval of the Selective Reminding Test. Tacrine, a centrally acting anticholinesterase inhibitor, has been implicated in memory improvement for people with Alzheimer's disease.[150] Tacrine may be useful in TBI patients who have lost some presynaptic neurons by maximizing the function of the neurons that remain. Donepezil is a new acetylcholinesterase inhibitor that has been shown to have a positive impact on the function of Alzheimer's disease patients. Donepezil's minimal side effect profile make it an option for further study in the TBI population.

A number of neuropeptides, especially ACTH and vasopressin, have also been implicated in memory. Regarding vasopressin, possible modes of action include increased excitation of limbic neurons and enhancement of neuronal response to the excitatory neurotransmitter glutamate.[151,152] Using a rat model, Rigter et al.[152] demonstrated reversal of retrograde amnesia with vasopressin and ACTH. Kovacs and DeWied[151] provided a comprehensive review of the effects of many of the neuropeptides in memory processes.

Catecholamine agonists have been utilized to improve memory. They are thought to work primarily by improving attention and initiation to facilitate encoding and retention. DA and NE are the main endogenous catecholaminergic neurotransmitters. Methylphenidate increases release of catecholamine, whereas the TCAs primarily decrease reuptake. Bromocriptine acts as an agonist, and amantadine is thought to work both presynaptically and postsynaptically.[125] All of these drugs have, to a varying degree, been clinically implicated in improving memory in people with TBI.[97,120] Evans et al., in a controlled, double-blind case study, demonstrated a dose-dependent improvement in memory (using the Selective Reminding Test) in a patient who suffered a severe TBI. He improved with both methylphenidate and, to a greater degree, dextroamphetamine.[120]

Nootropes are another class of pharmacologically active compounds that have been shown to have some cognition-enhancing properties. Their mechanisms of action are not well understood, but they may also affect cholinergic or excitatory amino acid pathways.[153] In any event, there are data suggesting that these chemicals do enhance memory.[154] McLean et al.[155] conducted a double-blind, placebo-controlled trial of pramiracetam in four brain injured patients and described improvement in memory (Wechsler Memory Scale and Selective Reminding Test) over several months, even up to 1 month after the drug was discontinued. This study was hampered by a small number of subjects with varied diagnoses and times from injury. It is also unclear whether the improvements in memory were statistically significant. This class of drugs has been studied to a greater extent in senile organic brain syndrome with mixed results.[156]

Central and peripheral opioid peptides have also been implicated in memory, primarily in patients with dementia. This concept has been supported by studies that have demonstrated improvement in memory in patients treated with naloxone, an opioid antagonist,[157] although similar studies have not yielded consistent results.[158] Substance P, a compound found both in the brain (striatonigral pathways, hypothalamus, septum, nucleus basalis magnocellularis) and the spinal cord, has been identified as having a role in memory. Enkephalins, found

peripherally, also have effects on memory, perhaps by modulating incoming information.[159]

Treatment of Mood and Affective Disorders

Problematic mood and affective disorders are prominent after TBI. In fact, TBI is considered a risk factor for subsequent psychiatric symptomology.[160] The presence of these sequelae is significant in that they contribute to suboptimal outcomes. For example, presence of major depression at 1 year postinjury adversely affects social outcomes; when the major depression has persisted for more than 6 months, function in activities of daily living is additionally adversely affected.[161,162]

The longitudinal study by Jorge et al.[163] appears to provide the most reliable incidence estimates of depression after TBI. These investigators performed structured psychiatric examinations on a group of 66 consecutive survivors at 0, 3, 6, and 12 months postinjury. The incidence of major depression at each of these time points ranges between 19 percent and 26 percent; the incidence of minor depression ranges between 3 percent and 7 percent.[164]

Despite the importance of pharmacological intervention in the treatment of major depression and the anxiety disorders, there has been little work directed at developing treatment strategies for these disorders after TBI. To date, there are no controlled studies exploring the efficacy of pharmacological interventions in the treatment of depression or the anxiety disorders after TBI.

Experience seems to indicate that SSRI agents are useful in treating depression and emotional lability after TBI. Additional agents that the authors have found helpful in the treatment of post-traumatic depression include protriptyline, desipramine, nortriptyline, venlafaxine, and bupropion. All these agents have been noted to lower the seizure threshold.

◻ SUMMARY

In summary, many different areas of the brain are involved in behavior and memory formation, production, and retrieval. Therefore, it is perhaps not surprising that various compounds have been suggested to enhance performance following brain injury. Nor is it surprising that there have been inconsistencies in studies examining the effectiveness of these compounds. We have sought to discuss the rationales, side effect profiles, limited scientific evidence, and potential indications for pharmacological intervention after traumatic brain injury in an attempt to provide some guidelines for their use.

The medical literature concerning pharmacological treatment of cognitive deficits following TBI is less than ideal, at best. There are substantial overlaps in clinical syndromes and treatment regimens and, where any exists, conflicting data regarding efficacy. Yet, the influence of cognitive and behavioral deficits on quality of life, community integration, and return to work following TBI, in addition to the risk-benefit ratio of the medications discussed, would weigh in favor of their continued, intelligent clinical and research use. Open and honest communication is suggested with patients and family members regarding evidence for efficacy, or lack thereof, and potential benefits and risks. Consistent implementation of validated objective measures of the effectiveness of these agents is also essential if we are to progress beyond the anecdotal stage of research.

REFERENCES

1. Cooper, J, Bloom, F, and Roth, R: The Biochemical Basis of Neuropharmacology, ed 6. Oxford University Press, New York, 1991.
2. Wurtaman, R: Choline metabolism as a basis for the selective vulnerability of cholinergic neurons. Trends Neurosci 15:72–84, 1992.
3. Richard, J, Araujo, D, and Quirion, R: Modulation of cortical acetylcholine release by cholinergic agents in an in vivo dialysis study. Society of Neuroscience Abstracts 15:1197–1204, 1989.
4. Marshall, I, and Parsons, S: The vesicular acetylcholine transport system. Trends Neurosci 4:174–182, 1987.
5. Moore, R, and Bloom, F: Central catecholamine neuron systems: Anatomy and physiology of the norepinephrine and epinephrine systems. Annu Rev Neurosci 2:113, 1979.
6. Weiner, N, and Molinkoff, P: Catecholamines. In Agranoff, B, Albers, R, and Molinkoff, P (eds): Basic Neurochemistry, ed 4. Raven, New York, 1989.
7. Graham, D, and Langer, S: Advances in sodium-ion coupled biogenic amine transporters. Life Sci 51:631–635, 1992.
8. Seeman, P, and Van Tol, H: Dopamine receptor pharmacology. Trends Pharmacol Sci 15:264–270, 1994.
9. O'Dowd, B: Structures of dopamine receptors. J Neurochem 60:804–817, 1993.
10. Van Tol, H, et al: Cloning of the gene for a human dopamine D4 receptor with high affinity for the antipsychotic clozapine. Nature 350:610–623, 1991.
11. Sokoloff, P, et al: Molecular cloning and characterization of a novel dopamine receptor D3 as a target for neuroleptics. Nature 347:146, 1990.
12. Molliver, M: Serotonergic neuronal systems: What their anatomic organization tells us about function. J Clin Psychopharmacol 7:35–41, 1987.
13. Schmidt, A, and Pertouka, J: 5-Hydroxytryptamine receptor families. FASEB J 3:2242–2249, 1989.
14. Sijbesma, H, Schipper, J, and de Kloet, E: Postsynaptic 5-HT1 receptors and offensive aggression in rats: A combined behavioral and autoradiographic study with clozapine. Pharmacol Biochem Behav 38:447–458, 1991.
15. Barnard, E, Darlison, M, and Seeburg, P: Molecular biology of the Gaba a receptor: The receptor/channel superfamily. Trends Neurosci 10:502–515, 1987.
16. Olsen, R, and Tobin, A: Molecular biology of the Gaba a receptor. FASEB J 4:1469–1478, 1990.
17. Sieghart, W: Gaba a receptor ligan gated Cl-ion channels. Trends Pharmacol Sci 13:446–453, 1992.
18. Bowery, N: Gaba b receptors and their significance in mammalian pharmacology. Trends Pharmacol Sci 10:401–409, 1989.
19. Feeney, D, Gonzalez, A, and Law, W: Amphetamine, haloperidol, and experience interact to affect rate of recovery after motor cortex injury. Science 217:855–857, 1982.
20. Kasumatsu, T, and Pettigrew, J: Preservation of binocularity after monocular deprivation in the striata cortex of kittens treated with 6-hydroxydopamine. J Comp Neurol 185:139–162, 1979.
21. Hayes, R, Jenkins, L, and Lyeth, B: Neurotransmitter-mediated mechanism of traumatic brain injury: Acetylcholine. J Neurotrauma 9:S73–S87, 1993.
22. Yablon, S: Postraumatic seizures. Arch Phys Med Rehabil 74:983–1001, 1993.
23. Temkin, N: A randomized double blind trial following severe head injury: Implications for clinical trials and prophylaxis. N Engl J Med 323:497–502, 1990.
24. Guidelines for the Management of Severe Head Injury. Brain Trauma Foundation Guidelines, New York, 1995.
25. Dimken, S, Temkin, N, and Miller, B: Neurobehavioral effects of phenytoin prophylaxis for postraumatic seizures. JAMA 265:1271–1277, 1991.
26. Glenn, M, and Wrobleski, B: Anticonvulsants for prophylaxis of postraumatic seizures. J Head Trauma Rehabil 1:73–74, 1986.
27. Masagli, T: Neurobehavioral effects of phenytoin, carbamazepine, and valproic acid: Implications for use in traumatic brain injury. Arch Phys Med Rehabil 71:219–226, 1991.
28. Britton, J, and So, E: Selection of antiepileptic drugs: A practical approach. Mayo Clin Proc 71:778–786, 1996.
29. Rogawski, M, and Porter, R: Antiepileptic drugs: Pharmacologic mechanisms and clinical efficacy with consideration of promising developmental compounds. Pharmacol Rev 42:223–227, 1990.
30. Donovan, W, et al: Clonidine effect on spasticity, A clinical trial. Arch Phys Med Rehabil 69:193–194, 1988.
31. Yudofsky, S, and Silver, J: Propranolol in the treatment of rage and violent behavior in patients with chronic brain syndromes. Am J Psychiatry 138:218–220, 1981.
32. Horn, L: "Atypical" medications for the treatment of disruptive aggressive behavior in the brain injured patient. J Head Trauma Rehabil 2(4):18–28, 1987.
33. Mena, M, Garcia de Yebenes, M, and Tabernero, C: Effects of calcium antagonists on the dopamine system. Clin Neuropharmacol 18:410–426, 1995.
34. Masumoto, R: Gaba receptor: Are cellular differences reflected in function? Brain Res Rev 14:203–209, 1989.
35. Block, R, and Berchou, R: Alprazolam and lorazepam effects on memory acquisition and retrieval processes. Biology, Biochemistry and Behavior 20:233–241, 1984.
36. Sedman, A: Cimetidine: Drug interactions. Am J Med 76:109–112, 1984.
37. Meyers, MA: Gastrointestinal complications of traumatic brain injury. In Horn, L, and Zasler, N (eds): Medical Rehabilitation of Traumatic Brain Injury. Hanley and Belfus, Philadelphia, 1996.
38. Killian, G, Holzman, P, and Davis, J: Effects of psychotropic medication on selected cognitive and perceptual measures. J Abnorm Psychol 93:58–70, 1984.
39. Rao N, Jellinick, M, and Woolstion, D: Agitation in closed head injury: Haloperidol effects on rehabilitation outcome. Arch Phys Med Rehabil 66:30–34, 1985.
40. Elovic, E: Atypical antipsychotics: Risperidone and clozapine. J Head Trauma Rehabil 11:89–92, 1996.
41. Criswell, H, Mueller, R, and Breese, G: Clozapine antagonism of D1 and D2 dopamine receptor-mediated behaviors. Eur J Pharmacol 159:141–147, 1988.
42. Kane, J: Newer antipsychotics drugs: A review of their pharmacology and therapeutic potential. Drugs 46:585–593, 1993.

43. Prigatano, G, et al: Sleep and dreaming disturbances in closed head injury patients. J Neurol Neurosurg Psychiatry 45:78–80, 1982.
44. Aserinsky, E, and Kleitman, N: Regularly occurring periods of eye motility, and concomitant phenomena during sleep. Science 273:274, 1953.
45. Freemaon, F, Salinas-Garcia, R, and Ward, J: Sleep patterns in a pattern with a brain stem infarction involving the raphe nucleus. J Clin Neurophysiol 36:657–663, 1974.
46. Nauta, W: Hypothalamic regulation of sleep in rats: An experimental study. J Neurophysiol 9:246–249, 1946.
47. Villablanca, J, Marcus, R, and Omstead, C: Effects of frontal cortex ablation in cats: Sleep wakefulness, EEG, and motor activity, Exp Neurol 53:31–39, 1976.
48. Markland, O, and Dyken, M: Sleep abnormalities in patients with brain stem lesions. Neurology 26:769–775, 1976.
49. Donio, E, Yamamoto, K, and Dren, A: Role of cholinergic mechanisms in states of wakefulness and sleep. Prog Brain Res 28:113–133, 1968.
50. Galliard, J, Kafi, S, and Justafre, J: On the role of brain alpha adrenergic systems in the production of paradoxical sleep. Encephale 8:413–434, 1982.
51. Edwards, G, and Shuring, L: Pilot study: Validating staff nurses observations of sleep and wake states among critically ill patients using polysomonography. Am J Crit Care 2:125–131, 1993.
52. Bussye, D, et al: The Pittsburgh Sleep Quality Index: A new instrument of psychiatric practice and research. Psychiatry Res 28:193–213, 1989.
53. Belyvan, A, and Nicholson, A: Rapid eye movements in man: Modulations by benzodiazepines. Neuropharmacology 26:485–491, 1987.
54. Zafonte, R, Mann, N, and Fichtenberg, N: Sleep disturbance in traumatic brain injury: Pharmacologic options. NeuroRehabilitation 7:189–195, 1996.
55. Merlotti, L: Clinical effects of zolpidem. J Clin Psychopharmacol 9:9–14, 1989.
56. Kupfer, D, Spiker, D, and Coble, P: Sleep and treatment of endogenous depression. Am J Psychiatry 138:429–434, 1981.
57. Nirenberg, A, et al: Trazodone for antidepressant associated insomnia. Am J Psychiatry 151–160, 1991.
58. Boyeson, M, and Harmon, R: Effects of trazodone and desipramine on motor recovery in brain injured rats. Am J Phys Med Rehabil 72:286–293, 1996.
59. Levin, H, and Grossman, R: Behavioral sequelae of closed head injury: A quantitative study. Arch Neurol 35:720–727, 1978.
60. Reyes, R, Bhattacharyya, A, and Heller, D: Traumatic head injury: Restlessness and agitation as prognosticators of physical and psychological improvement in patients. Arch Phys Med Rehabil 62:20–23, 1981.
61. Brooke, M, et al: Agitation and restlessness after closed head injury: A prospective study of 100 consecutive admissions. Arch Phys Med Rehabil 73:320–323, 1992.
62. Sandel, M, and Mysiw, W: The agitated brain injury patient. Part 1: Definitions, differential diagnosis and assessment. Arch Phys Med Rehabil 77:617–623, 1996.
63. Druckembrod, R, Rosen, J, and Cluxton, R: As-needed dosing of antipsychotic drugs: Limitations and guidelines for use in the elderly agitated patient. Ann Pharmacother 27:645–648, 1993.
64. Corrigan, J, and Bogner, J: Factor structure of the agitated behavior scale. J Clin Exp Neuropsychol (in press).
65. Corrigan, J, et al: Agitation, cognition and attention during postraumatic amnesia. Brain Inj 6:155–160, 1992.
66. Mysiw, W, and Jackson, R: Differential diagnosis of agitation following brain injury. NeuroRehabilitation 5: 197–204, 1995.
67. Mysiw, W, and Sandel, M: The agitated brain injury patient. Part 2: Pathophysiology and treatment. Arch Phys Med Rehabil 78:213–219, 1997.
68. Gvoic-Fugate, L, et al: Definitions and pharmacological intervention for agitation following traumatic brain injury (abstract). Arch Phys Med Rehabil 75:1036, 1994.
69. Porcher, E, et al: Efficacy of the combination of buspirone and carbamazepine in early postraumatic delirium. Am J Psychiatry 151:150–151, 1994.
70. Stewart, J, and Hemsath, R: Bipolar illness following traumatic brain injury: Treatment with lithium and carbamazepine. J Clin Psychiatry 49:74–75, 1988.
71. Smith, K, et al: Neurobehavioral effects of phenytoin and carbamazepine in patients recovering from brain trauma: A comparative study. Arch Neurol 51:653–660, 1994.
72. Wroblewski, B, et al: Carbamazepine replacement of phenytoin, phenobarbital and primidone in a rehabilitation setting: Effects on seizure control. Brain Inj 3:149–156, 1989.
73. Rivery, M, et al: Alteration of carbamazepine pharmacokinetics in patients with traumatic brain injury. Brain Inj 9:41–47, 1995.
74. McElroy, S, Keck, P, and Pope, H: Sodium valproate: Its use in primary psychiatric disorders. J Clin Psychopharmacol 7:16–24, 1987.
75. Geracotti, T: Valproic acid treatment of episodic explosiveness related to brain injury. J Clin Psychiatry 150: 916–921, 1993.
76. Wrobleski, B, et al: Effectiveness of valproic acid on destructive and aggressive behaviours in patients with acquired brain injury. Brain Inj 11:37–47, 1997.
77. Jackson, R, Corrigan, J, and Arnett, J: Amitriptyline for agitation in head injury. Arch Phys Med Rehabil 66:180–181, 1985.
78. Mysiw, W, Jackson, R, and Corrigan, J: Amitriptyline for posttraumatic agitation. Am J Phys Med Rehabil 67(1): 29–33, 1988.
79. Reinhard, D, Whyte, J, and Sandel, M: Improved arousal and initiation following tricyclic antidepressant use in traumatic brain injury. Arch Phys Med Rehabil 77:80–83, 1996.
80. Wroblewski, B, et al: Protriptyline as an alternative stimulant medication in patients with brain injury: A series of case reports. Brain Inj 7:353–362, 1993.
81. Boyeson, M, Harmon, R, and Jones, J: Comparative effects of fluoxetine, amitriptyline and serotonin on functional motor recovery after sensorimotor cortex injury. Am J Phys Med Rehabil 73:76–83, 1994.
82. Boyeson, M, and Harmon, R: Effects of trazodone and desipramine on motor recovery in brain-injured rats. Am J Phys Med Rehabil 72:286–293, 1993.
83. Greendyke, R, et al: Propranolol treatment of assaultive with organic brain disease. J Nerv Ment Dis 174:290–294, 1986.
84. Greendyke, R, Schuster, D, and Wooton, J: Propranolol in the treatment of assaultive patients with organic brain disease. J Clin Psychopharmacol 4:282–285, 1984.
85. Ratey, J, et al: Beta blockers in the severely and profoundly mentally retarded. J Clin Psychopharmacol 6:703–707, 1986.
86. Ratey, J, et al: Brief report: On trial effects of beta-blockers on speech and social behaviors in 8 autistic adults. J Autism Dev Disord 7:439–446, 1987.
87. Brooke, M, et al: The treatment of agitation during initial hospitalization after traumatic brain injury. Arch Phys Med Rehabil 73:917–921, 1992.
88. Feeney, D, and Westerberg, V: Norepinephrine and brain damage: Alpha noradrenergic pharmacology alters functional recovery after cortical trauma. Canadian Journal of Psychology 44:233–252, 1990.
89. Goldstein, L: Sygen in acute stroke study: Common drugs may influence motor recovery after stroke. Neurology 45:865–871, 1995.
90. Yudofsky, S, Silver, J, and Hales, R: Pharmacologic management of aggression in the elderly. J Clin Psychiatry 51:22–28, 1990.
91. Beber, C: Management of behavior in the institutionalized aged. Diseases of the Nervous System 26:591–595, 1965.
92. Kirven, I, and Montero, E: Comparison of thioridazine and diazepam in the control of nonpsychotic symptoms

associated with senility: Double-blind study. J Am Geriatr Soc 21:546–551, 1973.

93. Schallert, T, Hernandez, T, and Barth, T: Recovery of function after brain damage: Severe and chronic disruption by diazepam. Brain Res 379:104–111, 1986.

94. Galski, T, et al: Predicting physical and verbal aggression on a brain trauma unit. Arch Phys Med Rehabil 75:380–383, 1994.

95. Weinberg, R, Auerbach, S, and Moore, S: Pharmacologic treatment of cognitive deficits: A case study. Brain Inj 1:57–59, 1987.

96. Kaelin, D, Cifu, D, and Maitthes, B: Methylphenidate effect on attention deficit in the acutely brain-injured adult study. Arch Phys Med Rehabil 77:6–9, 1996.

97. Mooney, G, and Haas, L: Effect of methylphenidate on brain injured-related anger. Arch Phys Med Rehabil 74:153–160, 1993.

98. Feeney, D, and Sutton, R: Pharmacotherapy for the recovery of function after brain injury. Crit Rev Neurobiol 13:135–197, 1987.

99. Wroblewski, B, et al: Methylphenidate and seizure frequency in brain injured patients with seizure disorders. J Clin Psychiatry 53:86–89, 1992.

100. Nickels, J, et al: Clinical use of amantadine in brain injury rehabilitation. Brain Inj 8:809–818, 1994.

101. Chandler, M, Barnhill, J, and Gualtieri, C: Amantadine for the agitated head-injury patient. Brain Inj 2:309–311, 1988.

102. Levine, A: Buspirone and agitation in head injury. Brain Inj 2:165–167, 1988.

103. Stanislav, S, et al: Buspirone's efficacy in organic-induced aggression. J Clin Psychopharmacol 14:126–130, 1994.

104. Rowland, T, Mysiw, W, and Bogner, J: Trazodone for post-traumatic agitation (abstract). Arch Phys Med Rehabil 73:963, 1992.

105. Glenn, M, et al: Lithium carbonate for aggressive behavior or affective instability in 10 brain-injured patients. Am J Phys Med Rehabil 68:221–226, 1989.

106. Joshi, P, Capozzoli, J, and Coyle, J: Effective management with lithium of a persistent, postraumatic hypomania in a 10-year-old child. J Dev Behav Pediatr 6:352–354, 1986.

107. Cope, DN: An integration of psychopharmacological and rehabilitation approaches to traumatic brain injury rehabilitation. J Head Trauma Rehabil 9:1–18, 1994.

108. Cope, DN: Psychopharmacologic aspects of traumatic brain injury. In Horn, L, and Zasler, N (eds): Medical Rehabilitation of Traumatic Brain Injury. Hanley and Belfus, Philadelphia, 1996, pp 573–611.

109. Wroblewski, BA, and Glenn, MB: Pharmacological treatment of arousal and cognitive deficits. J Head Trauma Rehabil 9:19–42, 1994.

110. Whyte, J: Integration of research and clinical practice for drug use. J Head Trauma Rehabil 9:101–123, 1994.

111. O'Dell, MW, and Riggs, RV: Management of the minimally-responsive patient. In Horn, L, and Zasler, N (eds): Medical Rehabilitation of Traumatic Brain Injury. Hanley and Belfus, Philadelphia, 1996, pp 103–131.

112. Altmeyer, TA, O'Dell, MW, and Jones, M: Cisapride to treat gastroparesis following traumatic brain injury. Arch Phys Med Rehabil 77:1093–1094, 1996.

113. Glenn, M: Update on pharmacology: Chronic hypertension after traumatic brain injury: Pharmacologic options. J Head Trauma Rehabil 2:87–89, 1987.

114. Mateer, KA, and Mapou, RL: Understanding, evaluating, and managing attention disorders following traumatic brain injury. J Head Trauma Rehabil 11:1–16, 1996.

115. Kruetzer, JS, et al: Alcohol use among persons with traumatic brain injury. J Head Trauma Rehabil 5:9–13, 1990.

116. Salcido, R, et al: Recurrent severe traumatic brain injury: Series of six cases. Am J Phys Med Rehabil 70:215–219, 1991.

117. Whyte, J: Attention and arousal: Basic science aspects. Arch Phys Med Rehabil 73:940–949, 1992.

118. Haig, AJ, and Ruess, JM: Recovery from vegetative state of six months' duration associated with sinemet (levodopa/carbidopa). Arch Phys Med Rehabil 71:1081–1083, 1990.

119. Zasler, N: Advances in neuropharmacologic rehabilitation for brain dysfunction. Brain Inj 6:1–14, 1991.

120. Evans, R, Gualtieri, T, and Patterson, D: Treatment of chronic closed head injury with psychostimulant drugs: A controlled case study and appropriate evaluation procedure. J Nerv Ment Dis 175:106–110, 1987.

121. Plenger, PM, et al: Subacute methylphenidate treatment for moderate to moderately severe traumatic brain injury: A preliminary double-blind placebo-controlled study. Arch Phys Med Rehabil 77:536–540, 1996.

122. Bleiberg, J, et al: Effects of dexedrine on performance consistency following brain injury. Neuropsychiatry Neuropsychol Behavior Neurol 6:245–248, 1993.

123. Hornstein, A, et al: Amphetamine in recovery from brain injury. Brain Inj 10:145–148, 1996.

124. Speech, TJ, et al: A double-blind controlled study of methylphenidate treatment in closed head injury. Brain Inj 7:333–338, 1993.

125. Gualtieri, T, et al: Amantadine: A new clinical profile for traumatic brain injury. Clin Neuropharmacol 12:258–270, 1989.

126. Wroblewski, B, et al: Protriptyline as an alternative stimulant medication in patients with brain injury: A series of case reports. Brain Inj 7:353–362, 1993.

127. Barr, K, Goddard, M, and O'Dell, MW: Side-effects of methylphenidate in inpatient rehabilitation (abstract). Arch Phys Med Rehabil 76:1069, 1995.

128. Fuster, JM: The Prefrontal Cortex: Anatomy, Physiology, and Neuropsychology of the Frontal Lobe, ed 2. Raven, New York, 1989, pp 100–102.

129. Auerbach, SH: Neuroanatomical correlates of attention and memory disorders in traumatic brain injury: An application of neurobehavioral subtypes. J Head Trauma Rehabil 1:1–12, 1986.

130. Albert, M, Feldman, R, and Willis, A: The "subcortical dementia" of progressive supranuclear palsy. J Neuron Neurosurg Psychiatry 37:121–130, 1974.

131. Glenn, M: Update on pharmacology: CNS stimulants: Applications for traumatic brain injury. J Head Trauma Rehabil 1:74–76, 1986.

132. Stern, J: Craniocerebral injured patients: A psychiatric clinical description. Scand J Rehabil Med 10:7–10, 1978.

133. Weinstein, G, and Wells, C: Case studies in neuropsychiatry: Posttraumatic psychiatric dysfunction: Diagnosis and treatment. J Clin Psychiatry 42:120–122, 1981.

134. Catsman-Berrevoets, CE, and Harkskamp, F: Compulsive pre-sleep behavior and apathy due to bilateral thalamic stroke: Response to bromocriptine. Neurology 38:647–649, 1988.

135. Barrett, K: Treating organic abulia with bromocriptine and lisuride: 4 cases. J Neurol Neurosurg Psychiatry 54:718–721, 1991.

136. Van Reekum, R, et al: N of 1 study: Amantadine for the amotivational syndrome in a patient with traumatic brain injury. Brain Inj 9:49–53, 1995.

137. Richelson, E: The newer antidepressants: Structures, pharmacokinetics, and proposed mechanisms of action. Psychopharmacol Bull 20:213–223, 1984.

138. Hornstein, A, et al: Amphetamine in recovery from brain injury. Brain Inj 10:145–148, 1996.

139. Morrison, JH, Molliver, ME, and Grzanna, R: Noradrenergic innervation of cerebral cortex: Widespread effects of local cortical lesions. Science 205:313–316, 1979.

140. Boyeson, M, and Feeney, D: Intraventricular norepinephrine facilitates motor recovery following sensorimotor cortex injury. Pharmacol Biochem Behav 35:497–501, 1990.

141. McGuire, BE: Pharmacological treatment for memory impairment. Clin Rehabil 4:235–244, 1990.

142. Deutsch, J: The cholinergic synapse and the site of memory. Science 174:788–794, 1971.

143. Klopeman, M: The cholinergic neurotransmitter system in human memory and dementia. Q J Exp Pscyhol (A) 38: 535– 573, 1986.

144. Thal, J: Chronic oral physostigmine without lecithin improves memory in Alzheimer's disease. J Am Geriatr Soc 37:42–48, 1989.

145. Daives, P, and Maloney, A: Selective loss of central cholinergic neurons in Alzheimer's disease. Lancet 3:1403, 1976.

146. Bartus, T: Physostigmine and recent memory: Effects in young and aged nonhuman. Science 206:1087–1089, 1979.

147. Cardenas, D: Oral physostigmine and impaired memory in adults with brain injury. Brain Inj 8:579–587, 1994.

148. Goldberg, E, et al: Effects of cholinergic treatment on posttraumatic antegrade amnesia. Arch Neurol 39:581, 1982.

149. Little, A: A double blind placebo controlled trial of high dose lecithin in Alzheimer's disease. J Neurol Neurosurg Psychiatry 48:736–742, 1985.

150. Knapp, M: A 30 week controlled trial of high dose tacrine in patients with Alzheimer's disease. JAMA 271: 985–991, 1991.

151. Kovacs, G, and DeWied, D: Peptidergic modulation of learning and memory processes. Pharmacol Rev 46:269–291, 1994.

152. Rigter, H, van Riezen, H, and DeWied, D: The effects of ACTh and vasopressin analogues on Co1-induced retrograde amnesia in rats. Physiol Behav 13:381–388, 1974.

153. Pugsley, TA, et al: Some pharmacological and neurochemical properties of a new cognition activator agent, pramiracetam (CI-879). Psychopharmacol Bull 19:721–726, 1983.

154. Ito, I, et al: Allosteric potentiation of quisqualate receptors by a nootropic drug aniracetam. J Physiol (Lond) 424:533–543, 1990.

155. McLean, A, et al: Placebo-controlled study of pramiracetam in young males with memory and cognitive problems resulting from head injury and anoxia. Brain Inj 5:375–380, 1991.

156. Suletu, B, et al: Double-blind, placebo-controlled, clinical, psychometric and neurophysiological investigations with oxiracetam in the organic brain syndrome of later life. Neuropsychobiology 13:44–52, 1985.

157. Reisberg, B, et al: Effects of naloxone in senile dementia: A double-blind trial (letter to the editor). N Engl J Med 308:721–722, 1983.

158. Panella, JJ, and Blas, JP: Lack of clinical benefit from naloxone in a dementia day hospital. Ann Neurol 15: 308, 1984.

159. Schulteis, G, and Martinez, JL: Peripheral modulation of learning and memory: Enkephalins as a model system. Psychopharmacology (Berl) 109:347–364, 1992.

160. Van Reekum, R, et al: Psychiatric disorders after traumatic brain injury. Brain Inj 10:319 327, 1996.

161. Jorge, R, et al: Influence of major depression on 1-year outcome in patients with traumatic brain injury. J Neurosurg 81:726–733, 1994.

162. Mclean, A, Dimken, S, and Temkin, N: Psychological recovery after head injury. Arch Phys Med Rehabil 74: 1041–1046, 1993.

163. Jorge, R, et al: Depression following traumatic brain injury: A 1 year longitudinal study. J Affect Disord 27:233–243, 1993.

164. Robinson, R: Depression and antidepressants in patients with brain injury. Clin Neuropharmacol 15(S):638–639, 1992.

Substance Abuse and Brain Injury

JOHN D. CORRIGAN, PHD,
JENNIFER A. BOGNER, PHD,
and GARY L. LAMB-HART, MDIV

Substance abuse is more prevalent among persons with disabilities than in society in general,[1] yet research and treatment specific to this segment of the population have been minimal.[2] Among disability groups with unique issues of substance abuse are those individuals who have experienced traumatic brain injury (TBI). Prior to publication of the *White Paper* on substance abuse and brain injury by the Substance Abuse Task Force of the Brain Injury Association (formerly the National Head Injury Foundation),[3] there was acknowledgement of the relationship between intoxication and brain injury but little mention of substance abuse as a mediating factor in rehabilitation outcomes. Subsequent studies have sensitized the rehabilitation community to substance abuse in this population,[4–6] but significant gaps persist in our understanding of its incidence, impact, and treatment following brain injury. This chapter reviews the scope of the problem and describes approaches to intervention during rehabilitation.

◻ SCOPE OF THE PROBLEM

To fully understand how alcohol and other drug use affects rehabilitation requires consideration of at least three facets of the problem. Minimally, the frequency with which the use of substances causes injury or results in greater mortality or morbidity is one dimension. Second, alcohol and other drug use can affect recovery as a preexisting condition that changes the likelihood of attaining certain rehabilitation outcomes. A third dimension is the consequences of use following a brain injury and how such behavior interacts with outcomes that might be expected otherwise.

Incidence of Intoxication and Abuse

How many adolescents and adults hospitalized after TBI are intoxicated at the time of injury? Most studies have excluded children from any questions related to intoxication or history of abuse because of lack of available data. However, the age at which substances are being used has continued to decline in the United States, which may call into question the exclusion of preadolescent youth. Numerous studies[7–15] have examined the frequency of intoxication at time of injury in adolescents and adults. Using the presence of a blood alcohol concentration greater than 0.10 percent (the legal limit to operate a motor vehicle in most states) as the criterion for intoxication, studies[8–15] have found

Preparation of this manuscript was supported in part by Grant #H 235L20001 from the U.S. Department of Education, Rehabilitation Services Administration, to the Ohio Valley Center for Head Injury Prevention and Rehabilitation.

from one-third to one-half of persons injured were intoxicated. The TBI Model Systems project reported that 39 percent of their subjects were intoxicated at time of injury.[15] There has been little or no systematic study of intoxication caused by drugs other than alcohol; yet, there is growing concern that intoxication from marijuana and cocaine may be greater than expected causes of injury.[7] Better data regarding the presence of drugs other than alcohol could increase estimates of the incidence of intoxication at time of injury; however, the high frequency with which alcohol is used in conjunction with other drugs results in considerable overlap between intoxication caused by alcohol and that caused by other drugs.

How many adolescents and adults who experienced TBI have a preexisting history of substance abuse? This question has also been studied, though not as often as intoxication.[7,10–12,16–20] Two caveats are necessary prior to examining the available data. First, the methods used to determine a history of substance abuse are not as sound as those used to determine intoxication caused by alcohol. In most cases, researchers have either relied on subjective judgments by significant others as to whether a person's pattern of use was problematic or drawn inferences from standardized self-report measures of the amount consumed. Some research has used retrospective reviews of medical records for an indication of a history of abuse, usually without a contemporaneous means of inquiring about use. Thus, the methods for determining history of abuse are much more questionable and would in general appear to underestimate the frequency of this problem. A second caveat in understanding this question is to appreciate what substance abuse is. The American Psychiatric Association's *Diagnostic and Statistical Manual* (DSM-IV)[21] defines *substance abuse* as any of the following consequences of use recurring within a year: (1) failure to fulfill

major obligations at home, work, or school; (2) engaging in potentially hazardous behavior, including driving under the influence; (3) legal problems; or (4) social or interpersonal problems. A substance abuse problem can be present regardless of income, social class, familial support, vocational attainment, or physical appearance. Many rehabilitation professionals, like the general public, visualize an unkempt, social outcast with signs of withdrawal when they hear the term *substance abuse,* a stereotype more consistent with advanced stages of *substance dependence.*

These caveats in mind, studies have found a higher degree of variability in the incidence of a history of abuse, ranging from 16 percent to 66 percent for alcohol.[10–12,16–20] However, Corrigan[7] further investigated differences among studies and suggested that two factors may account for the wide range of findings. Table 31–1 shows the setting, method of detection, and rate of occurrence reported in several studies. Systematic differences appear to be present for samples drawn from admissions to trauma centers versus those composed of individuals involved in rehabilitation. In particular, the rehabilitation samples tended to consist of higher proportions of individuals with a history of alcohol abuse. At the same time, the method of detection appeared to influence results, with those studies that used prospective methods finding higher percentages of history of alcohol abuse then those studies that relied on retrospective medical record review. Thus, the studies of rehabilitation samples that used either relatives' reports or clinical interview found the highest percentages of people with a history of alcohol abuse.[16,18–20] The one study conducted in a rehabilitation setting that used medical record review found a significantly lower proportion.[17] Similarly, among trauma center admissions, the one study that used a prospective method[12] was significantly higher than the two

TABLE 31–1. Setting, Method of Detection, and Incidence of a History of Alcohol Abuse

Source	Authors	Method of Detection	Incidence
Trauma center admissions			
	Rimel et al.[11]	Not reported	16%
	Sparadeo & Gill[10]	Medical record review	25%
	Ruff et al.[12]	Relatives' reports of use	44%
Rehabilitation programs			
	Wong et al.[17]	Medical record review	37%
	Kreutzer ct al.[18]	Relatives' reports of use	66%
	Kreutzer et al.[19]	Relatives' reports of use	58%
	Drubach et al.[16]	Clinical interview	62%
	Corrigan et al.[20]	Clinical interview	64%

that either used retrospective methods[10] or did not report the method used.[11]

Again, only a small number of studies considered a history of other drug abuse.[12,16–20] Among these, a higher incidence rate in rehabilitation samples was again evident,[16–20] with the single study that did not use a prospective method finding the lowest incidence.[17] Although consistent screening for all forms of substance abuse might increase estimates of incidence, the impact would be moderated by the frequent occurrence of polysubstance abuse that includes alcohol. Based on findings from his review, Corrigan[7] concluded that nearly two-thirds of adolescents and adults admitted for rehabilitation following TBI have histories of alcohol and/or other drug abuse.

At Ohio State University, we have attempted to study these two questions as part of a prospective, longitudinal study of patients receiving acute, inpatient rehabilitation following acquired brain injury. Other findings have tended to support conclusions drawn from the earlier literature. Table 31–2 shows results for the first 100 patients treated on the traumatic brain injury unit and enrolled in our suboptimal outcomes study.[20] Consistent with previous studies, we found 43 percent of those tested had blood alcohol concentrations greater than 0.10 percent. Of those subjected to a screen for the presence of other drugs, 44 percent were positive. Overall, 53 percent of our sample had a blood alcohol concentration greater than 0.10 percent, a positive drug screen, or both. In terms of a history of abuse, 62 percent of our sample had a history of alcohol abuse and 34 percent had a history of other drug abuse. Most of those with a history of other drug abuse were positive for alcohol abuse; thus, the history of either was 64 percent. These histories were based on prospective interviews of both individual and family, when available, as well as a review of contemporaneous and historical medical records. The percentage found is consistent with the estimation that about two-thirds of the adolescents and adults we work with in brain injury rehabilitation have a history of alcohol or other drug abuse.

Morbidity and Mortality

Given that there appears to be a high incidence of both intoxication at time of injury and a history of substance abuse, the second dimension of the scope of the problem is the extent that these conditions affect the consequences of the injury itself—the mortality and morbidity. In studies that have identified an effect for intoxication, associations have been found with respiratory function,[8] overall severity of neurological impairment,[9,10] and agitation.[10] However, several studies have not found a relationship between intoxication and outcome.[9,12,14,22] In contrast, studies that examined the relationship between a prior history of substance abuse and mortality and morbidity have consistently identified associations, including likelihood of mass lesions[12] and poorer neurological outcome.[12,23,24] Indeed, in the only study that examined both history and intoxication to determine how each phenomenon contributed to the observed effects, Ruff et al.[12] concluded that history of abuse was far more related to the mortality and morbidity observed than intoxication at time of injury. The relationship between a history of abuse and morbidity and mortality may be caused by a subset of those abusing with the most severe histories.[11,23] Furthermore, because people with a history of abuse also tend to have multiple brain injuries,[16,17] the extent to which there is a direct effect of history or that the association results from consequences of previous injuries has not been determined.

In our longitudinal study at Ohio State University, we have examined the effects of both intoxication and history; however, our findings are not completely consistent with the previous literature. First, we found only few indices of morbidity with which either intoxication or history of abuse was associated. (Mortality cannot be studied effectively in a prospective sample from a rehabilitation setting because most deaths occur prior to that admission.) Indeed, among acute consequences, the only association we found was between intoxication and the presence of agitation. Sparadeo and Gill[10] had observed a relationship between intoxication and the duration of agitation, though not its presence. Our results seem to be consistent with those of Drubach et al.,[16] whose findings were also based on a prospective study of rehabilitation inpatients. At least one postulation might be

TABLE 31–2. Results from the Ohio State University Suboptimal Outcomes Study

Abuse Indicators	Percentage of Patients
Intoxication	
Blood alcohol	43%
Positive drug screen	44%
Either	53%
Prior history of abuse	
Alcohol abuse	62%
Other drug abuse	34%
Either	64%

that the effects of intoxication and/or history are masked in rehabilitation inpatients because of the more severe nature of their brain injuries.

Consequences of Use Following Brain Injury

A third dimension of the scope of the problem is the long-term consequences of use following the injury. There is probably the least amount of information available from the existing literature about this question, and as a result conclusions have to be tentative. Dunlop et al.[24] conducted an archival study from Social Security Disability files of people who had experienced TBI and shown deterioration in neurobehavioral functioning 6 months to 1 year following injury. From 193 files of persons with TBI, 34 such cases of deterioration were identified. These 34 were then matched with 34 cases of individuals with TBI who showed the same level of functioning at 6 months postinjury. Those who deteriorated were twice as likely to have a history of alcohol abuse; however, this study was not designed to identify causal factors.

Kreutzer et al.[18,19] at the Medical College of Virginia have looked at alcohol and other drug use among people with TBI whom they evaluated several years postinjury. Additionally, Kreutzer et al.[25] in the TBI Model Systems project have reported alcohol use among subjects in their data base. These studies have consistently found that preinjury moderate and heavy alcohol use is significantly more frequent among people who have incurred TBI than among peers matched for gender and age. Use declines postinjury to rates consistent with comparison groups. The proportion of individuals who abstain postinjury is higher than peers; however, recent studies have suggested that use increases with time postinjury.[25,26] For adolescents and young adults, consumption approaches preinjury levels by 2 years postinjury.[27] Males and those with higher preinjury use are at greater risk for postinjury moderate and heavy consumption.[18,19,26] Those with greater use also have a greater likelihood of having engaged in criminal activity.[28] In the Model Systems sample, those younger and with higher blood alcohol levels at admission consumed more, and those with greater disability tended to have lower levels of alcohol use.[25]

Our studies at Ohio State University have found that people with a history of alcohol or other drug abuse are less likely to be working or back in school 1 year following discharge from rehabilitation and are more likely to be socially isolated.[20] Causes of reduced productivity have not been determined, but the relationship may be multifaceted and include premorbid work history, greater neuropsychological impairment as a result of injury, or resumption of use. Causes of isolation may be multifaceted as well. An unexpected finding has been that people with an alcohol history are more likely to be living independently at 1 year follow-up. We have also found that among those we are not able to locate for follow-up at 1 year, those with a history of substance abuse are significantly more represented than those without a history. In our initial sample, 50 percent of those we were able to follow up at 1 year had a history of substance abuse, whereas 80 percent of those we were not able to find had a history. We have concluded that we must be tentative in any conclusions about either the long-term effects of a history of abuse or long-term outcomes from TBI because of the potential systematic bias introduced by this subset of the population that is lost to follow-up.

One additional source of information may indirectly shed light on the long-term consequences of alcohol and other drug use after brain injury. Corrigan, et al.[26] reported on characteristics of more than 200 individuals who had been referred to a specialized treatment program for people with substance abuse problems following brain injury, the "TBI Network." Approximately 50 percent of these referrals were in the acute phase of recovery from TBI, and the other half were longer postinjury and tended to be referrals from various community-based providers. Ninety percent of those referred had a diagnosis of either substance abuse or substance dependence. The drug of choice for 83 percent of this sample was alcohol, 72 percent of whom indicated that beer was their primary alcohol consumed. Thus, 61 percent of all those referred had beer as their drug of choice. For all subjects, alcohol was a primary, secondary, or tertiary drug of choice for 98 percent.

After alcohol, marijuana was the next most frequently abused substance, with little more than half reporting it as a primary, secondary, or tertiary drug of choice. The frequency of abuse of other substances dropped considerably after alcohol and marijuana, though cocaine, including crack, was abused by approximately one-quarter of those evaluated. Similar to findings reported by Kreutzer et al.,[18,19] this population drank considerably more alcohol prior to injury than same-aged peers. Afterward, consumption tended to match same-aged peers, who themselves consumed more alcohol than other adult age groups. Corrigan et al.[26] also reported that approximately 20 percent of those who abstained or were light drinkers preinjury became high-volume users afterward. Additionally, the volume of alcohol consumed increased dramatically as time postinjury increased, with 2 years postinjury appearing to be a point of significantly increased use. At least two additional studies have found an increase in use 2 to 3 years postinjury.[25,27]

Among costs to society observed in clients of the TBI Network, 69 percent were not working or in school at the time of their referral, even though more than half of those referred were several years postinjury. In this sample, 41 percent had their primary income through government supports; the next most frequent source of financial support was family. These individuals tended to have multiple injuries, with the medium- and high-volume alcohol users almost 3 times more likely to have use-related injuries. There also appeared to be both high medical utilization and a high number of arrests among individuals who were well past their acute injury. Those more than 12 months postinjury averaged one hospital admission every 2 years, and half of those more than 2 years postinjury had at least one arrest.

This section has attempted to look at the scope of the problem of alcohol and other drug use in brain injury rehabilitation. We have concluded that this behavior presents a significant challenge to rehabilitation, for multiple reasons. Both intoxication and a history of abuse are common in those we treat. Although the effects on morbidity and mortality in a rehabilitation population may not be as great because of the greater severity of injury, the likelihood that long-term outcomes from rehabilitation will be affected seems evident. We believe that resuming alcohol or other drug use presents a significant cost to a person's recovery. Clinically, we have found that the effects are insidious, and the impact of periodic use may not be readily apparent to individuals or others in their environment. However, once a person does abstain for a period of time, dramatic changes in personality and cognitive ability are observed. Although the cost to individuals and their recovery is reason enough to be concerned with alcohol and other drug abuse in this population, there are also significant costs to society. In the current climate of shrinking social programs, this cost is not insignificant. Finally, from a completely self-serving point of view as professionals, our ability to prove the effectiveness of rehabilitation is compromised if we ignore a person's alcohol and other drug use. Thus, from every perspective, it is important to take steps to minimize the impact of substance abuse on recovery. In the following sections, we describe systematic programming for secondary prevention of and intervention for substance abuse following brain injury.

□ SECONDARY PREVENTION IN REHABILITATION

Early rehabilitation has changed dramatically in the past 5 years. Lengths of stay are significantly shorter, and resources are more closely managed. Unfortunately, initiating new programming in this environment can be very difficult, especially given the need to surmount institutional barriers. Though the economics of rehabilitation have changed, the needs of the persons we care for have not. Further, the substance abuse risks of individuals who experience brain injuries have not diminished. In response to these needs, a model was developed at Ohio State University through the Ohio Valley Center for Brain Injury Prevention and Rehabilitation to facilitate the development of systematic prevention and intervention programs that meet both the current needs and the current resources of rehabilitation programs.[29] Three fundamental assumptions guided the development of this methodology: (1) Systematic programming is important, regardless of a person's readiness to change behavior; (2) any substance use following a brain injury is detrimental to optimum recovery; and (3) all rehabilitation centers should offer at least basic programming in prevention and intervention for substance use and can do so with minimal additional resources.

Early educational initiatives lay a groundwork for individuals to reconsider their use of alcohol and other drugs after brain injury. If the entire rehabilitation team presents a consistent attitude toward substance use after brain injury and information about it, then the process of change can start. Dissonance is created between the desire to use and the desire to achieve goals that cannot be reached while using. Later, cognitive-behavioral approaches can be effective in assisting individuals who are recognizing the negative consequences of substance abuse to readjust expectancies and improve coping, decision-making, and other requisite skills. Though not directly related to our first assumption that systematic programming is important regardless of readiness to change, educational and cognitive-behavioral approaches are far preferable to confrontation, which is ineffective for those persons with brain injury, who have an inability to self-reflect, experience poor control of emotions, or have difficulties with abstract thought.

Prochaska et al.'s[30] stages of change theory is particularly useful for working with individuals who have not recognized they have a problem or have not committed to changing their behavior. They describe five *stages* of change and numerous *processes* of change that are differentially effective, depending on the stage. Some individuals have no idea that there is a problem (pre-contemplative stage), whereas others may be aware of a problem but feel ambivalent about the need to change (contemplative stage). These individuals benefit from education and exploration of negative consequences of continued use, as well as potentially positive implications of behavior change. When people have recognized that there is a problem they want to change but have not set specific goals (preparation stage), then assistance and support in planning for change are appropriate. In the action stage, individuals may need encouragement to sustain the steps they have taken to attain a specific goal and incorporate changed behavior into their lifestyle. If successful change is attained for 6 months, people enter the maintenance stage, when the changed behavior has become a part of the regular routine, and the focus is on maintaining the new lifestyle rather than the change itself. Setbacks are common at every stage in the process of change, creating a pattern of recycling through previous stages until desired goals are reached.

Our second basic assumption is that any substance use following a brain injury is detrimental to optimum recovery. Although light or occasional alcohol use normally does not create a substance abuse problem, multiple factors necessitate different criteria for assessing any substance use after brain injury. There are at least eight risk factors unique to individuals with brain injury: (1) the young age of the population, (2) the frequency of a prior history, (3) unknowns regarding the healing processes of the brain, (4) the likelihood of decreased tolerance for any drugs, (5) the potential for interaction with prescribed medications, (6) the possibility of seizures, (7) the interaction between sequelae of brain injury and intoxicants, and (8) the stresses of prolonged recovery from serious brain injury. A "safe" amount to drink for the general population of healthy adults can be recommended, but the risk factors associated with brain injury make it difficult to identify a level of consumption, other than abstinence, that definitely would not be detrimental. Indeed, we believe that a palatable message for persons who have had brain injury is that no matter the extent of use before an injury, the occurrence of a brain injury dictates a reexamination of whether they put toxic substances like alcohol and illicit drugs in their bodies.

A final assumption is that all rehabilitation centers should offer at least basic programming in prevention and intervention for substance use, and can do so with minimal additional resources. The model described next proposes that all brain injury rehabilitation programs provide at least patient and family education,

screening, and referral to additional resources. In-service training for all rehabilitation staff should address the need for consistent messages about the problems of alcohol and other drug use after brain injury. Incorporating substance abuse prevention can be a relatively simple procedure, just as programs have added other issues based on the changing state of the art. Except for some initial staff training, a basic program of education, screening, and referral does not require additional resources. Figure 31–1 illustrates the components of basic programming (the "good" version) for the minimum level of service that should be available in specialized brain injury programs. After describing educational efforts, screening, and referral, enhancements to basic prevention programming (the "better" and "best" versions) are detailed.

Staff Education

Obstacles to the success of a substance abuse prevention program often revolve around staff acceptance. The institution itself must cooperate for programming to be developed and maintained and, more important, for a consistent message to be conveyed to individuals and their families. Staff members need to understand the importance of substance abuse programming and its place in rehabilitation. Sparadeo has advocated that ongoing education of all staff, including administrators, program directors, therapists, and ancillary staff, is necessary to ensure the most effective program.[31] Top-level management also often need to be convinced of the necessity of substance abuse programming, and some resistance to eduction efforts may be encountered because of lack of accurate knowledge of the seriousness of the problem. Administrators, like everyone else, may require information about the effects of substance use on the success of rehabilitation and may need to be encouraged to allocate resources for staff training and development.

Among direct service staff, program directors need information regarding treatment models and the necessary components of an effective program, including training of clinical and support staff. Clinical staff need to learn the skills necessary for each of the program elements. Equally important, they need to learn to work as a team in providing information, despite differences in attitudes and values regarding substance use. Support staff must receive training on how to recognize behavior changes associated with substance use, education regarding the importance of abstinence in this population, and assistance in improving their ability to communicate with both patients and therapists.

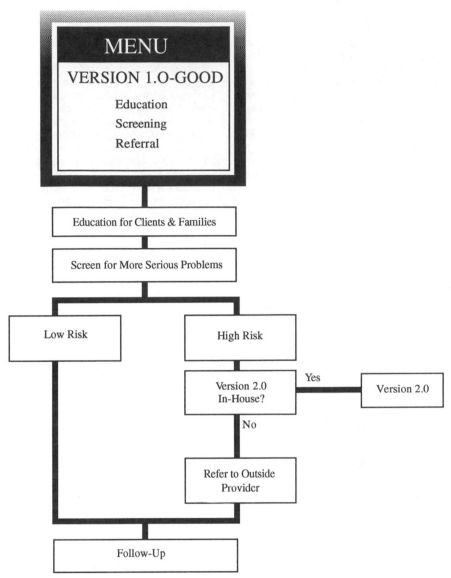

FIGURE 31–1. Basic elements for secondary prevention: "good" programming. (From the Ohio Valley Center for Brain Injury Prevention and Rehabilitation: Substance Use and Abuse after Brain Injury: A Programmer's Guide. Ohio Valley Center for Brain Injury Prevention and Rehabilitation, Columbus, Ohio, 1997, p 6, with permission.)

Staff members at all levels may be ambivalent toward systematic substance abuse programming because they do not understand the differences between use and abuse or recognize that the presence of a brain injury makes even modest use questionable. Some staff members may experience internal conflicts regarding their own or significant others' use of substances, which will be exacerbated by staff education and attempts to develop programming. These staff may require counseling to address their personal issues.

Client Education

All persons with brain injury, regardless of their prior history or potential risk, should receive education regarding the risks of substance use after brain injury. The information provided should include the effects of alcohol and other drugs on recovery, the detrimental impact on cognition and behavior, and health risks associated with substance use. Langley et al.[32] emphasized that educational efforts should be tailored to the individual's level of cognitive impairment and should include feedback that will help the individual learn through personal experience. Others have suggested that an educational component presented in a group format is effective, with various forms of media used to communicate the information.[33,34] In inpatient rehabilitation, the educational package must be compact to fit into short periods between the reacquisition of minimal cognitive abilities and hospital discharge.

For efficiency of staff time, we have recommended that the patient education program be presented in a group format, though with adaptations it can be conducted individually. Group members should be at a Rancho level V or higher and no problems with expressive or receptive aphasia that would make group participation frustrating. Although members who have not cleared post-traumatic amnesia may not remember the details of the material presented, in our experience they may retain a greater openness to reconsidering alcohol and other drug use. Some attention to awareness of deficits should be given prior to enrollment in the group, as individuals who have difficulty understanding that they have a brain injury and associated deficits have significant problems understanding why the consequences of alcohol or other drug use to recovery from brain injury applies to them. Awareness of deficits can, however, be at a very basic level—the individual may simply be acknowledging that something significant has happened.

Patient education groups should include a variety of presentations and discussions that can be of benefit to individuals with varying areas of cognitive deficit. Because many individuals will have difficulty remembering details of the discussion, each session should have a central idea expressed in a clear statement repeated several times during the discussion and again when summarizing at the end of a session. At each subsequent session, group members should be asked to repeat the statement given during the previous session. In addition, to aid in compensation for attention deficits, the material presented should vary in media format as well as content during each session. Finally, group members should be provided with various levels of cues to aid memory, attention, and problem solving and encouraged to keep a journal. To provide some basic information about potential negative consequences of substance use after brain injury, the Ohio Valley Center developed *A User's Manual for Faster, More Reliable Operation of a Brain after Injury."*[35] The pamphlet presents eight core messages, listed in Table 31–3, in written and pictorial form.

We have proposed a group patient education program organized into five 30- to 45-minute sessions.[29] Although additional sessions would be useful and encouraged, the basic goals can be accomplished in this time frame, which is adaptable to the shorter lengths of rehabilitation stay. During the first session, group members are exposed to the idea that the information to be presented in subsequent sessions is important for all people in the group, regardless of their history of alcohol or other drug abuse. The link between substance use and the occurrence of brain injury is also introduced. The second session focuses on the impact of substance use on brain functions and how this impact is similar to the impact of the brain injury itself. The third session introduces the *User's Manual* as a method for further illustrating the effects of substance use on brain injury

---

TABLE 31–3. Eight Messages about Consequences of Substance Use after Brain Injury

1. People who use alcohol or other drugs after they have had a brain injury don't recover as much.
2. Brain injuries cause problems in balance, walking, or talking that get worse when a person uses alcohol or other drugs.
3. People who have had a brain injury often say or do things without thinking first, a problem that is made worse by using alcohol and other drugs.
4. Brain injuries cause problems with thinking, like concentration or memory, and using alcohol or other drugs makes these problems worse.
5. After brain injury, alcohol and other drugs have a more powerful effect.
6. People who have had a brain injury are more likely to have times when they feel low or depressed, and drinking alcohol and getting high on other drugs makes this worse.
7. After brain injury, drinking alcohol or using other drugs can cause a seizure.
8. People who drink alcohol or use other drugs after a brain injury are more likely to have another brain injury.

Source: Adapted from the Ohio Valley Center for Brain Injury Prevention and Rehabilitation: A User's Manual for Faster, More Reliable Operation of a Brain after Injury. Ohio Valley Center for Brain Injury Prevention and Rehabilitation, Columbus, Ohio, 1994, with permission.

recovery. An active problem-solving and decision-making process is encouraged during the fourth session through a discussion of the pros and cons of substance use after brain injury. Through a discussion of why people use after an injury and how this decision results in negative consequences, members may reconsider their own use or be inoculated against future use. The final session extends this discussion to include potential obstacles to a person's ability to abstain from use and potential resources that can help overcome these obstacles. The information is presented in a nonjudgmental manner, with emphasis on the general applicability to all persons who have had a brain injury. Exploration of individuals' substance abuse problems should not be prohibited but is best deflected to individual sessions or groups designed to address abuse rather than use.

Family Education

All families also need basic education about the risks of substance use after brain injury and additional information about how to support prevention efforts. The family needs to know the general effects of alcohol and other drugs on brain functioning, as well as the effects of use on their particular family member.[36] Again, information should be presented in a nonjudgmental manner that encourages the family's participation and cooperation in the education efforts. The appropriate atmosphere is most easily accomplished in a group format, with discussions of the specific client and family substance use patterns conducted individually outside the group. Handouts similar to those used for client education, such as the *User's Manual*, can be referred to after family members return home.

When necessitated by their loved one's previous use, family members will also need help in determining their role in supporting behavior change. The social support network provided by family and friends should be carefully evaluated to determine how previous roles and behaviors may have supported substance use prior to the injury. The family can then be helped to identify potential barriers to sobriety and how to change their behavior to support a substance-free lifestyle. How active each person in the support network is in the intervention effort will depend not only on their desire to participate but also on the individual with a brain injury's reaction to that person's involvement. Despite best intentions, some family members may evoke oppositional behavior, which can undermine the intervention effort. Frequently, a family member's own use may prevent support of an environment that promotes abstinence. Furthermore, the patient's

awareness of deficits and stage of change will further determine the extent of structure and cueing that will be required from the family. For a more detailed discussion of family participation, Sparadeo has provided an excellent summary of family involvement in changing substance abuse behaviors after brain injury.[31]

Screening

Screening is conducted to determine the level of risk for substance abuse in the future so that additional interventions can be provided. It is a preliminary indicator of risk that can be administered by almost any professional. In contrast, assessment is a detailed process administered by a professional trained to identify substance abuse and dependency and formulate treatment plans. Because of the significant consequences of substance use after brain injury, all individuals receiving rehabilitation services should be screened for potential risk. We recommend screening early in the treatment process but after the person has cleared post-traumatic amnesia.

All methods of defining risk include consideration of characteristics of the person and the environment that may be barriers to abstinence. Is the individual currently using or making plans to use after discharge? Was the patient using immediately prior to hospitalization? Does the person live in an environment that encourages use? Even an individual without a previous history of abuse may be at risk after the injury. Though there are objective measures for detecting alcohol abuse and dependence (e.g., The Brief Michigan Alcohol Screening Test,[37] The Trauma Index,[38] or the CAGE[39]), we believe there is no substitute for a sensitively conducted, structured interview for gaining the information necessary to make a determination of risk. ABUSE, shown in Figure 31–2, is a screening tool developed at the Ohio Valley Center to guide the interview process. ABUSE outlines areas to be explored, not necessarily in the order listed, and preferably in a natural flow of conversation. A positive response in any of the areas indicates a risk of substance abuse.

Although the ABUSE screening tool can be used by any staff member who has a primary relationship with the person served, we recommend that a formal policy be developed and a single team member be given responsibility for this screening. In addition, other treatment professionals should be trained to support the screening process by reporting relevant information about the individual's use or abuse history. This information may come from statements made spontaneously, statements made by family members in the course of interactions, or from medical records. Ultimately, the problem of substance abuse affects all aspects of a person's recovery, and all staff members should be a part of the identification process.

Referral

Those patients and clients with risk for specific abuse after injury need additional attention. If specialized services are not available through the brain injury rehabilitation program, then a referral to community resources needs to be made. Referral is not just providing a name and phone number; it is an intervention process. Every brain injury program should have a method for making a referral in such a way that patients find the community resource accessible, acceptable, and useful. The program should develop a referral network of providers who, through experience and training, have some understanding of the unique issues of brain injury. Community providers can be most effective when they are adequately prepared for the client. The rehabilitation center should provide educational materials or in-service training regarding brain injury in general, as well as common characteristics of persons who may be re-

ABUSE Screening

A quick reference to identify the need for further screening and/or assessment for substance abuse problems or risk to develop substance abuse problems.

User note: This form is designed to provide non-substance abuse professionals with an awareness of issues that should become a natural part of your interactions with persons who have sustained a brain injury. Questions do not need to be asked directly or in this order and can be included in the regular course of conversation. Screening may also include information obtained outside the formal interview. **A positive response in any category indicates the need for a formal assessment**. For interpetation of positive responses, see ABUSE Interpetation on the following page.

*A*mount
Type, quantity and frequency of current (or most recent) use

*B*ackground (history of use)
Positive Blood Alcohol Level (BAL) or Blood Alcohol Content (BAC) at time of injury
Age at first use, first intoxication and abuse
Previous substance abuse treatment

*U*se related effects
Injury was use related
Use has resulted in consequences in important life areas such as:

Legal	Medical
Family/Social	Emotional
Job/School	Spiritual
Financial	

*S*ocial
Social engagements involving alcohol/other drugs
Friends' type, quantity and frequency of use
Recreational activities have alcohol/other drugs present
Alcohol/other drugs are used to relax, unwind or feel comfortable with others

*E*nvironment
Family history of substance abuse/dependence
Use is a regular part of family activities or get-togethers
Use is a regular part of job or job-related activities either during or after work

A

FIGURE 31–2. The ABUSE screening tool. (From the Ohio Valley Center for Brain Injury Prevention and Rehabilitation: Substance Use and Abuse after Brain Injury: A Programmer's Guide. Ohio Valley Center for Brain Injury Prevention and Rehabilitation, Columbus, Ohio, 1997, pp 30–31, with permission.)

ABUSE Interpretation

Reminder: A positive response in any category is indication of the need for a formal assessment

*A*mount:

- indication of polysubstance use (more than one chemical or substance used)
- intoxication or "getting high" as goal or result on a regular or consistent basis
- daily or binge type use
- increasing use or changing drug use to get the same effect (i.e. switching from beer or wine to hard liquor, mixing drugs, switching to crack or cocaine)

*B*ackground:

- BAL's above the legal limit for intoxication (.1 in most states) at the time of injury
- first use or intoxication prior to the age of 15
- reports of prior treatments for alcohol or other drug related problems

*U*se related effects:

- injury is use related
- arrests for DUI or OMVI, public intoxication, open container, disorderly conduct, possession/distribution of illegal substances, or other use related arrests
- giving up social activities, avoiding family gatherings, repeated arguments, fights, separation, divorce, and relationship problems as a result of use
- poor job or school performance, reprimands, attendance problems, terminations, demotions, suspensions or quitting/dropping out as a result of use
- financial problems due to poor decisions, gambling, fines, jail time, lost jobs, or poor credit as a result of use
- ulcers, high blood pressure, strokes, injuries, certain cancers, and cirrhosis as a result of use
- depression, paranoia, aggression, crying or anger outbursts when using
- sense of hopelessness or worthlessness, reducing usual spiritual practices or attacking religious practices of others when of using

*S*ocial:

- preference for or attendance only at social activities where alcohol and/or other drugs are present
- most friends are reported to use frequently or heavily
- recreational activities are planned around use
- reports of feeling unable to relax, unwind or be with others without using

*E*nvironment:

- one or more family members, substance dependent in the current generation or two preceding generations
- identification of using being a regular part of family get togethers and activities
- job-related using such as after-work get togethers, lunches, meetings, or customer relations

---

CAUTION:

Interpretation of questions is not meant to replace a comprehensive assessment by a qualified professional. It is an indicator of the need for such an assessment.

B

FIGURE 31–2. Continued

ferred. Cultural congruence should play a role in choosing an appropriate resource, whether Alcoholics Anonymous group, individual counselor, or culturally specific treatment programs (if available) in the home community. When

possible, staff should visit referral sources to gain a better appreciation of the culture of the program.

Equally important, patients must be prepared for the first meeting with a provider to increase the likelihood that they will accept the services offered. Through the educational efforts previously discussed, the individual may begin to appreciate why, as brain injury professionals, we believe that a change in substance use is needed. Reiterating risks associated with use after brain injury may help the individual who does not understand why a referral is being made. At the same time, pragmatic issues significantly influence whether a referral is successful. Deficits in planning and problem-solving skills create barriers to making an appointment, arranging transportation, or finding a facility. Assistance should be provided to accomplish these tasks. Funding issues should also be addressed. A rehabilitation program's responsibility for referral is not complete until at least an initial contact has occurred. Better yet, follow-up communication with either the person served or the provider should ascertain that premature termination did not result.

The family should also be provided with information about possible resources within the community that can help them avoid enabling behaviors and find support during difficult times. Not all resources are useful for all people, and families should be assisted in determining what assistance might be most effective for their situation. Again, knowledge of the substance abuse resources in the communities served by a rehabilitation program is necessary, and this knowledge must involve more than the address and phone number.

❑ APPROACHES TO INTERVENTION IN REHABILITATION

Given the impact of substance abuse on the effectiveness of rehabilitation and on long-term outcomes, it is imperative that the onset of resurgence of substance abuse following brain injury be addressed. Although there has been some improvement in awareness of substance abuse services in rehabilitation settings, a substantial percentage of facilities do not provide routine screenings of clients or engage in systematic education about the harmful effects of substance use.[40] In recent years, several models have been proposed for addressing substance abuse by persons with disabilities, three specifically for brain injury rehabilitation. Additionally, a program Krause[34] described for use in acute spinal cord injury rehabilitation contained important elements applicable across injury populations. Langley et al.[32,41] described a skills-based model for acute rehabilitation facilities. Sparadeo et al.[31,36] adapted this model by including methods for addressing substance abuse issues from the time of injury

through community reentry and incorporating the family into intervention strategies. Blackerby and Baumgarten[42] proposed a cognitive-behavioral model for treating persons with a dual diagnosis of brain injury and substance abuse, intended for the postacute phase of treatment; the other three programs were designed to be integrated into acute rehabilitation, with substance abuse intervention becoming one of the goals in the individual treatment plan. These programs were proposed prior to recent dramatic declines in the length of stay for acute rehabilitation, which have dictated more compact approaches to systematic intervention, at least during inpatient care. Still, a brief review may be useful to highlight both similarities and differences in targeted populations and underlying treatment philosophies.

Target Populations

Two of the three models for addressing substance abuse after brain injury described schemes for assessing risk of future abuse to determine which individuals should receive attention, as well as the type and intensity of intervention. The third, Blackerby and Baumgarten's[42] postacute model, also incorporated differential risk, but the method of determining it was not described. Langley et al.[32,41] suggested a three-tiered classification system: low risk, high risk, and chemically dependent. Those with high risk for future substance abuse had a history of such behavior in the past but were not currently dependent, whereas those at low risk had no such history. Those who were dependent could be expected to experience serious withdrawal symptoms and cravings, leading them to seek alcohol or other drugs after, if not during, acute rehabilitation.

Sparadeo et al.[31,36] distinguished individuals as low risk, high risk, or currently using. Those at low risk for future use were not currently using and did not have a substance abuse history. They did not crave alcohol or other drugs or associate certain situations or activities with substance use. These individuals received information regarding the consequences of substance abuse following brain injury but did not receive any other form of intervention. Those at high risk were not currently using but met at least one of the following criteria: experienced a significant number of triggering situations, had cravings for a substance, or had an ineffective support system, or a substance abuse history existed for the individual or a family member. For high-risk individuals, in addition to an educational program, substance abuse treatment was integrated into the overall rehabilitation program. Those who were currently using received the same program as those at high risk, with the possible addition of drug testing.

Treatment Philosophies

Generally, acute intervention programs have adopted the goal of increasing the occurrence of adaptive behaviors that are incompatible with substance abuse.[31,34,41] Langley et al.'s[32,41] skill-based model increased "effective coping behaviors"; Krause[34] described improving "health maintenance behaviors" to avoid medical complications. These approaches were consistent with behavior management research, which has demonstrated that the most effective method for promoting behavior change is reinforcement of appropriate behaviors rather than attention to and punishment of maladaptive behaviors.

To varying degrees, each intervention program emphasized that effectiveness was dependent upon the individual's readiness for change. On one end of the continuum, Blackerby and Baumgarten's[42] postacute program excluded individuals who did not demonstrate at least a minimal level of insight into the difficulties wrought by substance abuse, though participants without awareness were integrated into programming via progressive staging. Krause[34] proposed to improve readiness through individual and group counseling sessions, confrontations in team meetings, denying opportunities for achieving goals such as a driving evaluation, and threats of early discharge.

Krause's more confrontational approach was dramatically different from both Langley et al.[32,41] and Sparadeo et al.,[31,36] perhaps in part because of salient differences in cognitive and emotional functioning between persons with spinal cord injuries and those with brain injuries. Langley et al.[32,41] noted that traditional approaches for improving readiness, such as insight-oriented therapies and confrontation, are ineffective for people with brain injury who have cognitive and behavioral deficits, including an inability to self-reflect and difficulties with abstract thought. Instead, they proposed utilizing cognitive-behavioral approaches to assist the individual by experiencing dissonance between the desire to use and the desire to achieve goals that cannot be reached if using. For similar reasons, Sparadeo et al.[31,36] recommended educational approaches that facilitate movement through the stages of change proposed by Prochaska et al.[30]

Even when individuals with brain injury want to make a change in behavior, they have difficulty sustaining this intention, in part because of problems with impulse control.[32,41] Training in appropriate coping skills, as proposed by Langley et al.[32,41] and supported by Sparadeo et al.[31,36] was suggested for countering this difficulty. The client learned appropriate responses to high-risk situations and how to control impulsivity though verbal mediation techniques that encourage the individual to think before acting. Blackerby and Baumgarten[42] also recommended a cognitive-behavioral approach that encouraged identification of triggering stimuli, appropriate responses to peer pressure, and methods of restructuring one's lifestyle.

All programs emphasized the role of the family in sustaining sobriety after discharge. Sparadeo et al.[31,36] noted that the approach taken with the family should vary according to how the family functions. Issues unique to each family should be identified early to anticipate any special problems that may interfere with the family's ability and willingness to assist in the process. Treatment should include education of the family and, in some cases, family therapy. A case manager also may be critical to the process to assist the family and the client through rehabilitation and arrange for adequate support after discharge.[36]

All programs proposed that generalization could be facilitated through the use of community resources. In Blackerby and Baumgarten's[42] postacute program, the Alcoholics Anonymous and Narcotics Anonymous (AA/NA) philosophy provided a foundation for the program, thus preparing the individual to use these resources after discharge. Clients attended community-based meetings with staff members to assist in understanding new material, learning how to participate in the group, and integrating material into the rehabilitation program. Krause's[34] program also emphasized the AA/NA philosophy, but clients attended in-house meetings.

Although differences in approach among these four programs were apparent, the similarities were more striking. Traditional treatment approaches (i.e., AA/NA) were not eschewed; however, cognitive-behavioral approaches were emphasized. Most of the programs gave some attention to the individual's readiness to change, including the prospect of no readiness at all. Except for Krause's[34] program designed for person's with spinal cord injuries, confrontation was avoided; instead, dissonance was created via presentation of information and individual exploration of the consequences of use. Finally, all programs valued family involvement.

Enhancing Basic Programming

The secondary prevention program outlined earlier in this chapter involves only the most basic elements required to begin to address substance abuse issues during rehabilitation. As management and clinical staff begin to better recognize the impact of substance abuse on rehabilitation outcomes, resources to increase the comprehensiveness of programming can be sought. Elaboration of the "good" version of programming recommended by the Ohio Valley Center first involves an increase in time allotted to substance abuse intervention (the "better"

version) and then, to attain a truly comprehensive approach, the addition of a staff member who is a specialist in chemical dependency (the "best" version). Figure 31–3 illustrates the programming components that could be included with additional time and staff.

The better version of programming includes the education, screening, and referral elements of the good version and adds capability for indepth assessment and motivational interview-

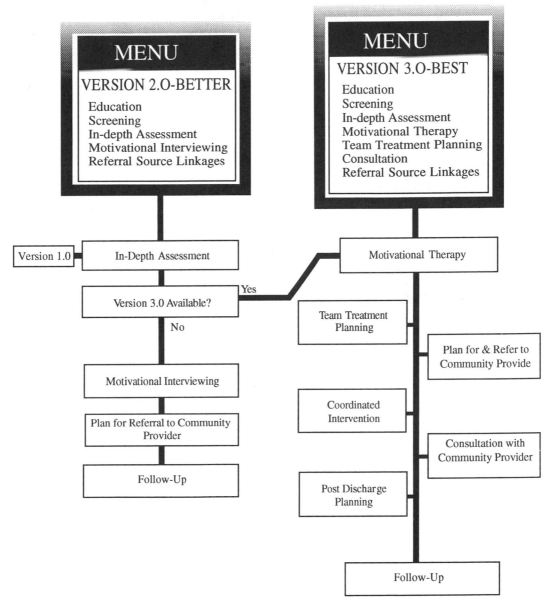

FIGURE 31–3. Enhancing substance abuse interventions: "better" and "best" programming. (From the Ohio Valley Center for Brain Injury Prevention and Rehabilitation: Substance Use and Abuse after Brain Injury: A Programmer's Guide. Ohio Valley Center for Brain Injury Prevention and Rehabilitation, Columbus, Ohio, 1997, p 7, with permission.)

ing,[43] techniques that require special training for some existing staff. In-depth assessment of substance abuse can help to tailor the program to the individual and contribute to more effective referrals for additional intervention in the community. Motivational interviewing is intended to increase the likelihood that people will follow through with community-based services. Motivational interviewing is based on the underlying principle from motivational psychology that people make the most effective and long-lasting changes when their motivation is internal rather than external. This technique fits nicely within the stages and processes of change described by Prochaska et al.[30] and is most useful with precontemplative and contemplative individuals.[43] Better programming also involves more aggressive identification and evaluation of community resources, as well as preparation of providers for referral. This bridging between the person served and the substance abuse treatment resources further facilitates successful referral, enhances continuity of services, and promotes successful intervention and generalization.

The best version of programming adds a staff member trained in chemical dependency treatment. Dedicating staff for this purpose significantly expands the capability of the program to provide a holistic approach to substance use issues. A dedicated staff member has responsibilities for all activities previously described in the good and better versions, as well as expanding motivational interviewing as indicated by the person's readiness to change. This staff member also facilitates a unified treatment plan, implemented by the entire team, based on issues identified in the assessment. Consultation with treatment team members allows adaptation of therapies to incorporate substance use issues (e.g., ways to reinforce messages from motivational interviewing or strengthen self-motivation statements). Perhaps it is idealistic to be proposing new staff when specialists are being pruned from the rehabilitation effort; however, based on the available information, a chemical dependency specialist may be an essential team member for enhancing long-term, if not short-term, outcomes. Furthermore, this expertise can sometimes be efficiently added to the rehabilitation team via collaborative relationships with substance abuse agencies.

❑ CONCLUSIONS

Substance abuse is a significant problem for persons with brain injury. Between one-third and one-half of adolescents and adults are intoxicated at time of injury. Almost two-thirds of adolescents and adults admitted for rehabilitation have histories of alcohol and/or other drug abuse. Males and younger people are more likely to have been moderate and high-volume consumers of alcohol before injury. Although alcohol consumption declines after injury, as time proceeds, so does the resumption of use; a critical point of departure from abstinence appears to be 2 years postinjury. As many as 20 percent of those who have substance abuse problems after injury had no prior history. Individuals who are more severely disabled may be less likely to resume use, perhaps because of their inability to carry out the behavior without assistance.

Alcohol and other drug use appears to affect recovery, both as a mediating factor in severity of neurological impairment and as a preexisting condition that changes the likelihood of attaining certain rehabilitation outcomes. The observed relationship with severity of neurological impairment may be complex and reflect a subset of individuals with preexisting neurological compromise caused by use, prior brain injury, and/or other sources, as well as a facilitative effect on initial brain damage and/or spontaneous healing. As a preexisting condition, a history of substance abuse may have affected familial, financial, or other personal resources that, in turn, diminish opportunities for recovery. Clinical experience also suggests that the resumption of alcohol or other drugs appears to have a deleterious effect on recovery, in all likelihood both spontaneous healing and learned behaviors.

It has been 10 years since the Substance Abuse Task Force *White Paper* from the National Head Injury Foundation called for inclusion of interventions for substance abuse in brain injury rehabilitation.[3] Although we may be more aware of the problem than we were 10 years ago, systematic programming for prevention and intervention is infrequent, at best. Every rehabilitation program serving people with brain injuries should provide patient and family education, conduct screening for risk of substance abuse, and have an effective method for making appropriate referrals. Beyond this minimum, the rehabilitation setting offers an important opportunity for intervention with substance abuse problems that can be capitalized upon without significant additional resources.

We have summarized recommendations for "good," "better," and "best" programming developed by the Ohio Valley Center for Brain Injury Prevention and Rehabilitation.[29] Three fundamental assumptions guided the development of these recommendations and merit reiteration: (1) Systematic programming is important, regardless of a person's readiness to change the behavior; (2) any substance use following brain injury is detrimental to optimum recovery; and (3) all rehabilitation programs should offer at least basic programming in prevention and intervention for substance use and can do so with minimal additional resources. Whether one agrees with our specific recommendations or not, incorporation of these assumptions into the methods of rehabilitation would be beneficial for people who have had brain injuries.

REFERENCES

1. Moore, D, and Polsgrove, L: Disabilities, developmental handicaps, and substance misuse: A review. Int J Addict 26:65, 1992.
2. Moore, D: Substance abuse assessment and diagnosis in medical rehabilitation. NeuroRehabilitation 2:7, 1992.
3. National Head Injury Foundation Substance Abuse Task Force: White Paper. National Head Injury Foundation, Southborough, Mass, 1988.
4. Sparadeo, FR, Strauss, D, and Barth, JT: The incidence, impact and treatment of substance abuse in head trauma rehabilitation. J Head Trauma Rehabil 5(3):1, 1990.
5. Kreutzer, JS, Marwitz, JH, and Wehman, PH: Substance abuse assessment and treatment in vocational rehabilitation for persons with brain injury. J Head Trauma Rehabil 6(3):12, 1991.
6. Langley, MJ: Preventing post-injury alcohol-related problems: A behavioral approach. In McMahon, BT, and Shaw, LR (eds): Work worth doing: Advances in brain injury rehabilitation. Paul M Deutsch, Orlando, Fla, 1991, p 251.
7. Corrigan, JD: Substance abuse as a mediating factor in outcome from traumatic brain injury. Arch Phys Med Rehabil 76:302, 1995.
8. Gurney, JG, et al: The effects of alcohol intoxication on the initial treatment and hospital course of patients with acute brain injury. J Trauma 33:709, 1992.
9. Kraus, JF, et al: Blood alcohol tests, prevalence of involvement and outcomes following brain injury. Am J Public Health 79:294, 1989.
10. Sparadeo, FR, and Gill, D: Effects of prior alcohol use on head injury recovery. J Head Trauma Rehabil 4(1):75, 1989.
11. Rimel, RW, et al: Moderate head injury: Completing the clinical spectrum of brain trauma. Neurosurgery 11:344, 1982.
12. Ruff, RM, et al: Alcohol abuse and neurological outcome of the severely head injured. J Head Trauma Rehabil 5(3):21, 1990.
13. Gordon, WA, Mann, N, and Willer, B: Demographic and social characteristics of the traumatic brain injury model system database. J Head Trauma Rehabil 8(2):26:1993.
14. Kaplan, CA, and Corrigan, JD: Effect of blood alcohol level on recovery from severe closed head injury. Brain Inj 6:337, 1992.
15. Harrison-Felix, C, et al: Descriptive findings from the Traumatic Brain Injury Model Systems National Data-Base. J Head Trauma Rehabil 11(5):1, 1996.
16. Drubach, DA, et al: Substance abuse as a factor in the causality, severity, and recurrence rate of traumatic brain injury. Md Med J 42:989, 1993.
17. Wong, PP, et al: Statistical profile of traumatic brain injury: A Canadian rehabilitation population. Brain Inj 7:283, 1993.
18. Kreutzer, JS, et al: Substance abuse and crime patterns among persons with traumatic brain injury referred for supported employment. Brain Inj 5:177, 1991.
19. Kreutzer, JS, et al: Alcohol use among persons with traumatic brain injury. J Head Trauma Rehabil 5(3):9–20, 1990.
20. Corrigan, JD, et al: Systematic bias in outcome studies of persons with traumatic brain injury. Arch Phys Med Rehabil, 1997.
21. American Psychiatric Association: Diagnostic and Statistical Manual of Mental Disorders, ed 4. American Psychiatric Association, Washington, DC, 1994.
22. Lehmkuhl, LD, et al: Factors that influence costs and length of stay of persons with traumatic brain injury in acute care and inpatient rehabilitation. J Head Trauma Rehabil 8(2):88, 1993.
23. Dikmen, SS, et al: Alcohol use and its effects on neuropsychological outcome in head injury. Neuropsychologia 7:296, 1993.
24. Dunlop, TW, et al: Comparison of patients with and without emotional/behavioral deterioration during the first year after traumatic brain injury. J Neuropsychiatry Clin Neurosci 3:150, 1991.
25. Kreutzer, JS, et al: A prospective longitudinal multicenter analysis of alcohol use patterns among persons with traumatic brain injury. J Head Trauma Rehabil 11(5):58, 1996.
26. Corrigan, JD, Rust, E, and Lamb-Hart, GL: The nature and extent of substance abuse problems among persons with traumatic brain injuries. J Head Trauma Rehabil 10(3):29, 1995.
27. Kreutzer, JS, Witol, AD, and Marwitz, JH: Alcohol and drug use among young persons with traumatic brain injury. Journal of Learning Disabilities 29:643, 1996.
28. Kreutzer, JS, Marwitz, JH, and Witol, AD: Interrelationships between crime, substance abuse, and aggressive behaviors among persons with traumatic brain injury. Brain Inj 9:757, 1995.
29. Ohio Valley Center for Brain Injury Prevention and Rehabilitation: Substance Use and Abuse after Brain Injury: A Programmer's Guide. Ohio Valley Center for Brain Injury Prevention and Rehabilitation. Columbus, Ohio, 1997.
30. Prochaska, JO, DiClemente, CC, and Norcross, JC: In search of how people change: Applications to addictive behaviors. Am Psychol 47:1102, 1992.
31. Sparadeo, FR: Substance use: A critical training issue for staff in brain injury rehabilitation. In Durgin, D, Schmidt, N, and Fryer, LJ (eds): Staff Development and Clinical Intervention in Brain Injury Rehabilitation. Aspen, Gaithersburg, Md, 1993, p 189.
32. Langley, WJ, et al: A comprehensive alcohol abuse treatment programme for persons with traumatic brain injury. Brain Inj 4:77, 1990.
33. Kreutzer, JS, and Harris, JA: Model systems of treatment for alcohol abuse following traumatic brain injury. Brain Inj 4:1, 1990.
34. Krause, JS: Delivery of substance abuse service during spinal cord injury rehabilitation. NeuroRehabilitation 2:45, 1992.
35. Ohio Valley Center for Brain Injury Prevention and Rehabilitation: A User's Manual for Faster, More Reliable Operation of a Brain after Injury. Ohio Valley Center for Brain Injury Prevention and Rehabilitation, Columbus, Ohio, 1994.
36. Sparadeo, FR, Strauss, D, and Kapsalis, KB: Substance abuse, brain injury, and family adjustment. NeuroRehabilitation 2:65, 1992.
37. Pokorney, AD, Miller, BA, and Kaplan, HB: The Brief MAST: A shortened version of the Michigan Alcoholism Screening Test. Am J Psychiatry 129:342, 1972.
38. Skinner, H, et al: Identification of alcohol abuse using laboratory tests and history of trauma. Ann Int Med 101:847, 1984.
39. Ewing, JA: Detecting alcoholism: The CAGE Questionnaire. JAMA 252:27, 1984.
40. Kiley, DJ, et al: Rehabilitation professionals' knowledge and attitudes about substance abuse issues. NeuroRehabilitation 2:35, 1992.
41. Langley, MJ, and Kiley, DJ: Prevention of substance abuse in persons with neurological disabilities. NeuroRehabilitation 2:52, 1992.
42. Blackerby, WF, and Baumgarten, A: A model treatment program for the head-injured substance abuser: Preliminary findings. J Head Trauma Rehabil 5(3):47, 1990.
43. Miller, WR, and Rollnick, S: Motivational Interviewing: Preparing People to Change Addictive Behavior. Guilford, New York, 1991.

Therapeutic Recreation

SUSAN POPEK-BOEVE, CTRS

Recreation activity involvement is most likely the last thing a patient or family member is concerned with immediately following a traumatic brain injury (TBI). Yet, as recovery begins, "leisure" and the myriad related issues (including the ability to plan, social skills, peer involvement, excess time, boredom, family impact, adaptive recreation, and community integration) begin to emerge and must be addressed as an integral part of the rehabilitation process. Deficits resulting from TBI that directly affect leisure have been reported. In outcome studies assessing individuals who had survived a TBI (from 2 to 8 years postinjury), difficulties with interpersonal relationships, pursuit of meaningful recreation, and problems with excess time caused by return-to-work issues are consistently reported.[1-5] These studies support the view that recreation and leisure must be addressed if rehabilitation is to be truly comprehensive.[6] The pursuit of meaningful involvement in a recreation activity often keeps a person motivated toward the overall goal of restoring an optimal level of function. Pursuit of and involvement in recreation activity may give an individual a sense of control and empowerment. Patients often benefit from assistance with modifying and adapting activity, as well as an opportunity for growth. "Recreational therapy interventions result in significant health outcomes in the process of treatment and rehabilitation, making them crucial services with a truly comprehensive continuum of health care."[7]

□ THERAPEUTIC RECREATION

Therapeutic recreation service is described as a "process which utilizes recreation services for

purposive intervention in some physical, emotional and/or social behavior to bring about a desired change in that behavior and to promote the growth and development of the individual" (p. 11).[8] In a joint statement released by the American Therapeutic Recreation Association (ATRA) and the National Therapeutic Recreation Society (NTRS), it was noted that:

> The most effective rehabilitation services that exist today are individualized and include therapies that address psychosocial needs as well as physical functioning . . . recreation therapy utilizes various interventions to treat physical, social, cognitive and emotional conditions associated with . . . injury. Recreational therapy includes an educational component which helps people become more informed and active partners in their health care by using activity to cope with the stress of illness and disability, and to acquire knowledge, skills, and abilities to manage their disability so they may achieve and maintain optimal levels of independence, productivity and well being.[9]

These definitions and descriptions of therapeutic recreation illustrate the similarity between the overall purpose of rehabilitation and this discipline.

Therapeutic recreation services should be provided by professionals with training and education in therapeutic recreation who are certified by the National Council for Therapeutic Recreation Certification (NCTRC). The professional certification designation is CTRS (certified therapeutic recreation specialist).

The therapeutic recreation specialist works to address the individual needs of the patient, which, in turn, determine the specific program goals, activities, and implementation. For the individual with TBI, physical, cognitive, and behavioral deficits may affect recreation participation, family and peer relationships, and overall feelings of satisfaction. During the rehabilitation process, the therapeutic recreation specialist works to structure, control, direct, and prescribe recreation activities.[8] Emphasis is on improving capability relating to patient goals. Recreational therapy addresses general rehabilitation goals (e.g., improved ambulation and communication) and goals specifically designed to address improved leisure functioning, including ability to plan, community integration skills, social skills, resource awareness, adapted skills, and leisure education.

□ THE TREATMENT TEAM

The therapeutic recreation specialist works as an integral member of the rehabilitation team. Insurance case managers and adjusters may also be involved in team decisions. Crucial to the rehabilitation team are the family members. Although they are not *treating* the patient, they provide invaluable information and will most likely be the primary caregivers following discharge from the rehabilitation program.

The therapeutic recreation specialist assesses the patient with TBI and, after designing a program incorporating patient goals, rehabilitation focus, and input from family members, provides feedback and recommendations to the team members. Communication among team members is vital to facilitate a smoother rehabilitation process and avoid unnecessary distress for the patient and family.

The therapeutic recreation specialist incorporates the treatment focuses of other disciplines in the sessions, both in-house and during community outings.[10] For example, during a community outing trip to a bowling alley, the therapeutic recreation specialist encourages the patient to self-propel his or her wheelchair (physical therapy focus), recall the planned activity and record the bowling score in a journal (speech therapy focus), and learn how to use a bowling ramp (leisure education focus). The therapeutic recreation specialist follows up by providing team members with information on the patient's ability to incorporate and carry over strategies to a "real-life" situation or activity. Through this valuable feedback, the treatment team is able to evaluate the effectiveness of the program and modify goals or focus areas accordingly. Therapeutic recreation specialists may also work with members of other disciplines to cofacilitate therapy groups. Examples include therapeutic recreation with physical therapy facilitating a fitness group (hospital or community based), with occupational therapy facilitating a basic or advanced community skills group, and speech-language pathology facilitating a social skills group.

□ FAMILY INVOLVEMENT

Burton and Volpe state that "the impact of head injury reverberates throughout the entire family system."[11] The literature continues to report that the caregivers experience psychological distress because of a high level of subjective burden.[12] This applies to the area of recreation and leisure as well. In a study of the relationship of family stress to caring for individuals with traumatic brain injury (6, 12, and 24 months postinjury), Hall et al.[13] reported that caregivers' most common complaints about their relatives were lack of involvement in leisure activities, fatigue, slowness, and forgetfulness. Therapeutic recreation specialists must include family members in each step of the rehabilitative process, including initial assessment, instruction sessions, community outings, home and community assessments, activity evaluations, resourcing, and discharge planning.

Family members may often be overwhelmed by the rehabilitation process and benefit from step-by-step guidance, practice, and continuing education. How-to information is helpful in providing structure, obtaining resource information, adapting recreation activity, ordering equipment, providing access to transportation, and ensuring safe participation in leisure pursuits. At the outpatient level, family members may appear to have a more peripheral role as they resume involvement in work and previous duties neglected during the acute phases of the injury. Every effort, including phone calls, home visits, flexible meeting times, and schedules, should be made to obtain and provide feedback. In addition to providing education and instruction, the therapeutic recreation specialist benefits from feedback by family members. Family members are often key to enabling community integration by providing needed assistance with planning, resourcing, and transportation, especially during the rehabilitation process and often following discharge.

□ TREATMENT INTERVENTION

As an individual who has sustained a traumatic brain injury begins to have periods of alertness, therapeutic recreation may be prescribed by the attending physiatrist (generally when the patient has reached Rancho level III or above). Patients who are functioning at Rancho levels III and IV may not be able to tolerate a full schedule of rehabilitation and generally have limited and inconsistent periods of alertness. The therapeutic recreation specialist evaluates the patient to determine the appropriateness of therapeutic recreation intervention. Appendix A at the end of this chapter lists sources of information for recreational skill evaluations. *Formal* involvement in recreation therapy may not be possible at this time because of agitation, confusion, and other factors.

□ ASSESSMENT

When appropriate, the therapeutic recreation specialist should conduct a formal therapeutic recreation assessment. The course of therapeutic recreation intervention is based on this assessment, including setting early identified short- and long-term goals and objectives, length of recommended treatment, and potential. The

therapeutic recreation specialist should focus the assessment on the following functional areas:

1. Premorbid lifestyle patterns
2. Leisure interests and specific skills
3. Capability for effective social communication and interaction
4. Capability for leisure activity planning and follow-through
5. Leisure satisfaction
6. Knowledge of necessary adaptations for involvement in leisure activity
7. Potential for active community reentry
8. Leisure resource awareness

The assessment information may be obtained through a combination of any of the following procedures:

1. Individual interviews with the patient and family members

Appropriate Rancho Level	Title and Source
I and up	Comprehensive Evaluation in Recreational Therapy–Physical Disabilities (CERT) Parker, Idyll-Arbor
II–V	The Fox, Based on Fox Activity Therapy Social Skills Assessment (Patterson), Idyll-Arbor
III and up	Recreation Participation Data Sheet Burlingame and Peterson, Idyll-Arbor
IV and up	Functional Assessment of Characteristics for Therapeutic Recreation (FACTR) Peterson, Dunn, Carruthers (1983), Idyll-Arbor
V and up	STILAP 1974 Navar and Peterson
V and up	STILAP 1990 (State Technical Institute's Leisure Assessment Process) Navar and Burlingame, Idyll-Arbor
V and up	Ohio Leisure Skills Scales on Normal Functioning (OLSSON) Olsson, Roy Jr., Associate Professor of Therapeutic Recreation, University of Toledo
V and up	The Bond-Howard Assessment on Neglect in Recreational Therapy (BANRT) Bond-Howard (1990), Ptarmigan West
V and up	Comprehensive Evaluation in Recreational Therapy Psych/Behavioral (CERT) Parker, Ellison, Kirby, Short, Idyll-Arbor
V and up	Maladaptive Social Functioning Scale (MASF) Idyll-Arbor
VI and up	Idyll-Arbor Leisure Battery (four assessments: Leisure Attitude Measurement, Leisure Interest Measurement, Leisure Motivation Scale, Leisure Satisfaction Measure) Idyll-Arbor (1990)
VI and up	Leisurescope Schenk, Leisure Dynamics
VI and up	Miranda Leisure Interest Finder, Miranda 1975 Leisure Counseling, Milwaukee Public Schools
VII and VIII	Leisure Diagnostic Battery (LDB) Witt and Ellis 1985, 1989, 1990, Venture Publishing
VIII	What Am I Doing? (WAID) Neulinger, The Leisure Institute

2. A review of available medical records and treatment team documentation

3. Clinical observation of both formal and informal socialization patterns

4. A home visit and community assessment as appropriate (pending cognitive level, length of stay)

5. Assessment of behavioral responses to various activities designed to assess cognitive, physical, and social skills

6. Administration of standardized tests

7. Administration of leisure questionnaires and worksheets (values, leisure education, time management, stress management, leisure resource inventory, telephone book use)

8. Administration of formal evaluation, as appropriate

The therapeutic recreation specialist should be familiar with a variety of assessment material; there is currently no specific standardized test designed for TBI pertaining to therapeutic recreation. The patient's cognitive level may also dictate which assessment tool is used. The therapist should be adept at obtaining information through observation and be aware of the patient's level of tolerance. Stumbo and Bloom[14] advise that "the assessment instrument or procedure must be valid, reliable and useable for this population." Table 32–1 provides a list of therapeutic recreation assessment tools, and Appendix B at the end of this chapter provides a list of assessment tool publishers.

The initial assessment should generally be completed within a specific time period designated by the hospital or program. After the therapeutic recreation specialist has completed the assessment, short- and long-term goals are identified. These are patient goals and must be individualized; measurable goals are set to evaluate improvement as a result of the treatment intervention.

The documented initial assessment for therapeutic recreation should contain assessment tools used and results of standardized tests, the patient's leisure interests, the impact of the injury as related to the patient's ability to pursue leisure activity interests, recommendations for therapeutic recreation intervention (including group treatment), long- and short-term goals, length of stay, and potential.

□ TREATMENT PROCEDURES

Treatment plans are based on the individual's goals and the assessment results. The therapeutic recreation specialist generally participates in an interdisciplinary team meeting to develop a comprehensive treatment plan for the patient. Recommendations for therapeutic recreation services may include individual treatment sessions, small and/or large group activity involvement, community reintegration outings, family instruction, and resource education. The patient and family, as well as the treatment team members, should be aware of and in agreement with the recommended treatment plan.

Following the initial assessment, the therapeutic recreation specialist should design a program to address the patient's current level of function (see Appendix C). Depending on the needs of the patient with TBI, the program should address social skills, behavior, mobility, cognitive skills (including memory, attention, and problem solving), communication, fine motor skills, visual-perceptual skills, and adjustment. The Therapeutic Recreation Services model designed by Gunn and Peterson[16] illustrates the phases of therapeutic recreation intervention.[8] The three phases of the model are (1) rehabilitation (focus on improving functional ability), (2) education (leisure education including introduction, instruction, training, and practice), and (3) recreation (acquired leisure skills participated in voluntarily). The needs of the patient determine the emphasis of treatment; it is not uncommon to combine aspects of all three phases into a therapeutic recreation treatment plan, depending on the patient's strengths and deficit areas. Sample goals that address the phases of the model include:

1. The patient will bowl three frames while ambulating with standby assistance on three of three trials (rehabilitation).

2. The patient will demonstrate ability to find the bowling alley listing in a phone book on three of three trials (education).

3. The patient will initiate participation in bowling at a neighborhood bowling alley during the weekend home visit (recreation).

In addition to setting goals, the model helps with designing treatment plans that incorporate improving function with teaching and active participation in recreation activity. Table 32–2 provides suggestions for activity intervention correlated to the cognitive levels of the Rancho Los Amigos Scale.[15]

□ GROUP TREATMENT

Group treatment can be a valuable component to the rehabilitation program for individuals with TBI. In addition to facilitating progress in specific task-related areas, group activity allows the therapist to observe the patient's response to so-

TABLE 32–2. Activity Suggestions

Rancho Cognitive Level	Goals/Emphasis	Therapeutic Recreation Intervention
II–III Localized response	▪ Increase arousal ▪ Increase awareness of environment	▪ Sensory stimulation including olfactory testing, tactile stimulation ▪ Music for brief intervals ▪ Large-screen visual films for brief intervals
IV Confused/agitated	▪ Provide maximum structure ▪ Improve orientation ▪ Increase tolerance for activity	▪ Multiple 1:1 short-term activities with breaks (in a quiet environment) including card games, matching activity, ball toss, recognition games ▪ Pictures, magazines, photo albums
V Confused inappropriate, nonagitated	▪ Increase attention ▪ Address social skills ▪ Improve orientation ▪ Provide structure ▪ Improve endurance	▪ Memory games ▪ Checkers, Connect Four ▪ Uno, War, Golf (cards) ▪ Simon ▪ 1:1 Horticulture, music, art activity ▪ Conversations about recreation ▪ Flash cards
VI Confused appropriate	▪ Increase orientation ▪ Increase recall ▪ Address social skills ▪ Provide structure ▪ Improve endurance ▪ Improve ability to choose activity ▪ Improve self-esteem	▪ Current events review ▪ Puzzles (simple) ▪ Checkers ▪ Memory games ▪ Basic sports (bowling, ball activity, pool) ▪ Drama ▪ Water activity ▪ Craft projects ▪ Letter writing ▪ Introduce group activity (games) ▪ Out-trips to low-stimulation settings
VII Automatic appropriate	▪ Improve recall and ability to plan for activity ▪ Improve awareness of safety issues ▪ Provide structure ▪ Improve sense of choice and control ▪ Improve community skills ▪ Improve physical and cognitive endurance	▪ Games (Mastermind, Skip-Bo, Rhyme or Reason, Jenga, Yahtzee, Scrabble) ▪ Logic puzzles ▪ Group activity, including leisure education, community skills, social skills, trivia games ▪ Activities to address planning ▪ Sports ▪ Arts/crafts ▪ Leisure counseling ▪ Leisure education ▪ Community-based treatment ▪ Computer activity ▪ Arcade games ▪ Cooking
VIII Purposeful appropriate	▪ Leisure skill refinement and exploration ▪ Improve ability to independently pursue leisure activity of choice	In addition to those of level VII, ▪ Advanced community-based treatment ▪ Set up for discharge at community locale ▪ Support groups ▪ Advanced games, logic puzzles ▪ Personal resourcing ▪ Involve in group leadership ▪ Fitness activity

Source: Adapted from Berger, J, and Regalski, A: Therapeutic recreation. In Rosenthal, M, et al (eds): Rehabilitation of the Adult and Child with Traumatic Brain Injury, ed 2. F A Davis, Philadelphia, 1990, with permission.

cial situations that incorporate increased stimulation, peer response, and elements of teamwork. The therapist should provide feedback about the patient's behavior in group situations to the patient, the treatment team, and family members. When planning to refer a patient to a particular group, the following factors should be considered:

1. The patient's current cognitive level and response to stimuli (most patients are not able to tolerate group activity unless they are at Rancho level VI or higher)
2. The type of group, including size, location (in-house or community based), and purpose
3. The patient's interest in group participation (currently and preinjury); group treatment is not a *must* for every patient
4. The patient's goals for group participation
5. The current mix of patients in the group

Each group designed for the patient with TBI should have specific protocols and purpose(s), as well as procedures for the group leader to follow. This will eliminate confusion when deciding whether a patient is appropriate for a particular group. Suggestions for therapeutic recreation groups include:

1. Leisure education topics, including adapted recreation (Table 32–3), management and planning, resourcing, and stress management, may be addressed in small groups facilitated by the therapeutic recreation specialist, possibly in conjunction with an occupational therapist.
2. Small group activities, including crafts, art, music, and games, may be facilitated by the therapeutic recreation specialist to address functional skill areas and the patient's ability to attend to an activity in a busy environment and work in cooperation with others. These small group activities also provide the patient with an opportunity to begin considering others and socialize in a structured setting.
3. Special events allow large group participation. Group activity planned in accordance with the calendar year, holidays, or seasons assists the patient with orientation to season and month. These activities allow the therapist to assess the patient's response to and tolerance for high stimulation.

Interdisciplinary groups should also be a component of the overall treatment program. Suggestions for interdisciplinary groups include:

1. Social skills
2. Support group
3. Fitness group (basic and advanced)
4. Community skills (basic and advanced)
5. Planning group

Therapeutic recreation specialists are highly trained in group leadership and should be involved conjointly with other disciplines to design specific groups according to patient needs. The groups may then be implemented or placed on hold, pending the current needs of the patients.

□ DISCHARGE PLANNING

The long-term goal established following the initial assessment should dictate the course of

---

TABLE 32–3. Examples of Adapted Recreation Activities

Virtually any activity can be modified or adapted to allow for participation.
- □ Board games with enlarged print for individuals with visual/perception deficits
- □ Bike riding on a tandem bike as a reintroduction to the activity for individuals with decreased safety/judgment or visual impairment
- □ Fishing with a rod holder for individuals with limited use of one or both upper extremities
- □ Golfing with adapted clubs (longer or shorter) for individuals in a wheelchair
- □ Swimming with a head float for individuals who hyperextend in the water
- □ "Reading" by listening to talking books for individuals with decreased or blurry vision and/or limited attention span
- □ Sewing/crocheting with a Velcro-attached aid for individuals who have limited hand movement and dexterity
- □ Skiing with a slant board, sit-ski, mono-ski, or bi-ski for individuals with paralyzed or amputated limbs, weakness, or excess tone
- □ Track (racing) with use of a specialized racing chair for individuals with paraplegia, quadriplegia, or cerebral palsy
- □ Hunting with use of a turret mount for individuals who use a wheelchair for mobility
- □ Card playing with an automatic card shuffler for individuals who have limited fine-motor skills in upper extremities
- □ Bowling in a wheelchair with use of a ball pusher or bowling ramp for individuals with mobility limitations

services provided, including possible needs at discharge. Although no one can predict at exactly what level of functioning a patient will be at discharge, most therapists should have a general plan in mind throughout the therapy program. Depending on the needs of the patient, the therapeutic recreation specialist should continually evaluate the program effectiveness, with the overall focus on the long-term goal and discharge from treatment. Discharge planning may necessitate just one session with a patient who is functioning for the most part independently, with emphasis on providing resources. For a more severely injured patient (requiring supervision), discharge planning may include developing home programs, providing daily schedules to structure free time, referral to a community-based agency, and resourcing for transportation, adapted equipment, and accessibility. If the patient is discharged from an inpatient unit to a day treatment program, the therapeutic recreation specialist should provide pertinent information to the therapists providing outpatient treatment. Each aspect of the therapeutic recreation program should contribute to the patient's ability to function and pursue leisure activities of choice. Individualized discharge plans are influenced by a number of factors, including severity of injury, family dynamics, patient motivation and participation in the treatment program, resource awareness, leisure history prior to injury, and adjustment to injury. The discharge plan may change during the course of treatment because of factors such as speed of recovery, behavioral issues, family issues, and medical concerns; the patient, family members, and treatment team should be aware of any changes made. The therapeutic recreation discharge plan should address the following concerns:

1. How much structure is required for the patient to initiate and pursue recreation activity?

2. What adaptations (if any) need to be made for the patient to pursue recreation activity?

3. Is transportation an issue? How will the patient get out to recreation?

4. Are there financial concerns that affect recreation activity pursuit?

5. Is the patient aware of recreation resources available (parks and recreation, community facilities, magazines, books, equipment, special services, continuing education)?

6. Has the patient's family been involved and instructed on recommendations for recreation activity pursuit?

7. What therapeutic activities should the patient continue to pursue to address deficit areas (computer activity, exercise, games, resourcing tasks, puzzles)?

8. Has the patient been provided with a home program that includes therapeutic activity suggestions, status, and recommendations?

9. Does the patient and/or family know how to contact the therapeutic recreation specialist if questions arise following discharge?

"Appropriate management of discretionary time enhances the client's expression, self-concept, social interaction skills and community involvement."[16] The discharge plan should adequately address each of these factors.

◻ COMMUNITY-BASED REHABILITATION

As hospital lengths of stay continue to decrease, outpatient and community rehabilitation services (including day treatment, cognitive retraining programs, and transitional living services) have risen to the forefront as a means to accomplish rehabilitation goals. Teaff and Van-Hyning[17] studied third-party reimbursement of therapeutic recreation specialists and found that specialists working on inpatient units often have difficulty completing the necessary interventions prior to discharge. Individuals who have sustained a mild brain injury often receive minimal, if any, inpatient rehabilitation but may require outpatient services to resume involvement in preinjury activities. Resources and assistance should be provided for successful return to the community.

Community integration is often a primary focus of the rehabilitation program at the outpatient level. The goal is to maximize functional skills that allow the patient to return to a variety of settings (work, school, home, community) with as much independence as possible.[18] Leisure and recreation programs provide a significant component to the community reintegration of individuals who have sustained TBI.[19]

At the onset of outpatient treatment, the therapeutic recreation specialist should obtain and review information regarding therapeutic recreation services that may have been provided on the inpatient rehabilitation unit. Every effort should be made to complete a thorough but concise evaluation and to avoid duplication of service. The family members should be included in the assessment process and throughout the outpatient treatment program.

Home assessments, community evaluations, and resourcing are primary components of the outpatient therapeutic recreation program. The patient should be observed and receive therapeutic intervention in a variety of community settings, including the patient's home and community locale (restaurants, shopping centers, libraries, fitness centers, museums, parks). It is impossible to provide community reintegration services without taking the patient out into the community. Community outings as an individual and as part of a group should produce a variety of information that will benefit the patient and the entire rehabilitation team. If the patient resides in a transitional living facility, the therapeutic recreation specialist should coordinate services and provide recommendations to the staff, preferably through meetings and observation held at the facility.

The therapeutic recreation specialist should be an expert at resourcing and community outreach. Values clarification sessions, in conjunction with community reentry outings, may contribute to the total rehabilitation of people with brain injuries.[20] Patients should receive not only resources but also leisure education regarding how to resource for themselves.

Active involvement in physical recreation is a necessary part of the outpatient therapeutic recreation program.[21] Specific evaluations are helpful in this setting (e.g., biking, swimming, skiing, weight lifting, rollerblading, and bowling) to assess function and provide a basis for therapeutic intervention. Participation in ongoing community-based clinics (snow skiing, adapted water sports, basketball) is beneficial during outpatient treatment as a means to link patient and community. If an individual plans to attend a parks and recreation program following discharge, it is often helpful to take the individual on an outing to meet with the facilitators prior to discharge. Providing access to community activity through a facilitator or community-based liaison can assist with discharge planning and bridge the gap between therapy and discharge.[22]

In describing a model therapeutic recreation program for the reintegration of people with disabilities into the community, Bullock and Howe note, "Since recently discharged rehabilitation patients usually have more time available for recreation/leisure, the need for a reintegration model that not only focuses on recreation but also on social integration within the community becomes clearer."[23] This is especially true for the patient with TBI. These individuals are often unable to work or drive because of restrictions following the injury, and excess leisure time is frequently an issue. This, combined with cognitive deficits that affect planning and organization, contributes to feelings of lack of control, apathy, and possible depression. As patients participate in therapeutic recreation services at the outpatient level, it is hoped that their sense of empowerment and control will increase as they gain the skills and independence to reintegrate into the community.

Community Assessment/Skills

The following client skill areas may be addressed individually or in a group setting:

- Task organization
- Problem solving
- Time management
- Memory
- Social interactions
- Participation
- Safety and judgment
- Mobility and endurance
- Money management
- Community resource awareness

Home Assessment

To be addressed in the client's home or transitional living facility:

- Availability of needed recreation tools and supplies at home
- General routine and leisure time management
- Home accessibility
- Identification of community facilities near the home
- Identification of the client's ability to navigate in the community
- Meeting with the family to address their concerns regarding leisure and recreation

Resourcing

The therapeutic recreation specialist should have a comprehensive resource file, including information on:

- Adaptive equipment
- Activities (rules for games, therapeutic activity suggestions)
- Associations
- Barriers information
- Books
- Camps
- Clinics (adapted golf, water skiing, sports)
- County information
- Laws (e.g., ADA)
- Local special event information
- Maps
- Out-trip site information and local facilities
- Parks and recreation information
- Periodicals

- Support groups
- Therapeutic activities (art, equestrian, music)
- Transportation
- Traumatic brain injury
- Travel

☐ CASE STUDIES

Case 1 ■ A 20-year-old woman sustained TBI in an automobile accident. Her initial Glasgow Coma Scale score was 6. She was noted to be in a post-traumatic amnesia for 10 days. She began inpatient rehabilitation at Rancho level IV. Prior to the injury, she was attending a community college for nursing and living in an apartment with a roommate. After a review of the available medical record, the therapeutic recreation specialist began the assessment. During the initial assessment, the therapeutic recreation specialist noted the patient to be alert and oriented to herself only. She appeared confused and distractible and was using a wheelchair on the unit because of limited insight and decreased safety. She stated that she was unable to complete a written assessment because of the inattention and cognitive deficits. The therapist used the CERT Scale for physical disabilities and the FACTR during the assessment. The first session lasted 30 minutes (including breaks).

The therapeutic recreation specialist met with the patient's mother to obtain further information to complete the assessment. Per the patient's mother, prior to the injury she participated in the following activities: Cooking, going out with friends, exercise, board games, and reading romance novels. Her mother characterized her as "independent and outgoing."

Upon completion of the initial assessment, the therapeutic recreation specialist noted the following deficits: disorientation, impaired short-term memory, impulsivity, decreased awareness of safety issues, decreased attention, decreased ability to tolerate activity and stimulation, and decreased self-awareness of leisure activity interests. As a result of these deficits, the patient required supervision, structure, and frequent breaks for leisure activity. She was unable to initiate involvement in leisure activity. Recommendations for therapeutic recreation included individual treatment sessions twice a week to address the deficit areas and increase the patient's ability to tolerate full activity sessions, gradual introduction to small group activity as tolerated, and family instruction for information on structuring and encouraging leisure activity during weekend visits home. The long-term goals were: "The patient will initiate involvement in a leisure activity of her choice when provided with structured activity choices as demonstrated by the ability to choose from a list of suggestions on nine out of ten occasions. The patient will consistently be able to independently identify leisure activity interests. The patient will tolerate involvement in small group activity as demonstrated by no episodes of agitation. The patient will participate in community outings of choice, a minimum of twice a week, with supervision." The short-term goal at the onset of treatment was: "The patient will participate in one-to-one, structured recreation activity for 15 minutes without a break." The estimated length of stay on the inpatient unit was 2 months.

After 1 month, the patient was functioning at Rancho level VII and had begun participation in small group treatment (a social skills group facilitated by therapeutic recreation and speech therapy). She responded well to feedback and increasingly recalled activity participation and plans. Her insight continued to be impaired. During community integration outings, she required supervision because of decreased judgment and limited ability to problem solve in unfamiliar situations. The patient began to assume increased responsibility for group activities, and her mother noted she was initiating routine activity involvement at home. At this time, the patient began to express frustration at the amount of supervision she needed and her inability to drive or return to her previous living situation in the apartment. She benefited from involvement in constructive therapeutic recreation activity to increase her feelings of control over her situation. She asked the therapist about working out at a health spa. Prior to the patient's discharge, the therapeutic recreation specialist contacted the outpatient therapist to provide feedback and recommendations for continued therapeutic recreation, including participation in an exercise program at a community-based health spa.

The patient was discharged home with her mother following a 7-week inpatient stay on the rehabilitation unit. At the time of discharge, she had reached Rancho level VII. The therapeutic recreation specialist, in addition to contacting the outpatient facility, provided the patient and her mother with a comprehensive packet of recreation resource information and a home activity program, including suggestions for continued therapeutic activity involvement. It was noted at discharge that the patient had met the long-term goal established at the onset of her inpatient rehabilitation program.

Case 2 ■ A 45-year-old man sustained a TBI in an automobile accident. According to the medical record, his initial Glasgow Coma Scale was 5. He also sustained four rib fractures, a right ulnar fracture, and a left proximal tibial fracture. He was in post-traumatic amnesia for approximately 4 weeks. He received inpatient rehabilitation for 6 weeks. During this time he progressed from Rancho level V to level VI. He was discharged to the care of his sister, who provided 24-hour supervision. He began outpatient therapy with a 5-day-a-week program. Prior to the injury, he worked full-time as a bus driver. He lived with his wife and their two young children.

The initial therapeutic recreation assessment included an interview with the patient, administration of the Leisure Interest Questionnaire, Leisure Interest Measurement, Leisure Satisfaction Measure, and Leisure Motivation Scale. The patient required verbal guidance to read directions for the assessments, as well as breaks throughout the session. He identified five leisure interests (when provided choices): exercise, fishing, gardening, watching football, and playing games with his children. He was unable to state whether he had done any of these things since his injury.

According to the patient's sister, he was generally sitting in his room and watching television, which she noted to be unlike his preinjury activities. She described him as "highly active" before the injury. She also stated that he was not initiating chores or socializing. The patient's sister agreed to participate in instructional sessions, with the emphasis on increasing the amount of structure provided for the patient.

In the initial assessment, the therapeutic recreation specialist noted impaired short-term memory and executive functioning skills, impaired attentional functions, decreased temporal orientation, and decreased mobility because his left leg could not bear weight. As a result of these deficits, the patient required supervision and structure to pursue leisure activity. He also required education for adapting physical activities. Recommendations for therapeutic recreation included individual sessions twice a week to address the deficit areas and provide leisure education, involvement in a community skills group two days a week, family instruction sessions, a home assessment, and referral to the community-based fitness group when full weight bearing was achieved. The long-term goals were: "The patient will consistently initiate and pursue recreation activities of his choice when provided structure, including use of a journal and daily check list. The patient and his family will be able to identify a minimum of five community-based recreational resources in their community. The patient will independently pursue an exercise and fitness program with distant supervision." The estimated length of stay for outpatient therapeutic recreation was 6 months.

During the course of treatment, the patient participated in a variety of leisure educational sessions, community integration outings (individual and in a group), leisure counseling sessions,

and active recreation pursuit. The therapeutic recreation specialist met with the patient's sister and wife at the outpatient facility to provide instruction, resource information, and obtain feedback. The therapeutic recreation specialist completed two home visits to assess the patient's level of involvement in activity at home and in his neighborhood and to provide education for the family. The patient participated in a fitness group (weight lifting, swimming and aquatic exercise, basketball, treadmill, and stationary bike) three days a week conducted by the therapeutic recreation specialist and physical therapist when he was able to bear weight on his left leg during the last 3 months of his outpatient treatment. He planted and tended a vegetable garden for 3 months at the outpatient clinic.

The patient eventually progressed to Rancho level VII. After 5 months of outpatient therapy, he was independently following a routine exercise and swimming program with distant supervision. Now living at home with his wife and children, he participates in household chores, supervises child care, and has started a garden. Family members assist with transportation for community-based activity. He expresses frustration at driving restrictions but is compliant. Social contact with friends has resumed. Before discharge from therapeutic recreation, the therapeutic recreation specialist assisted the patient with registering for a parks and recreation special services program in his community, which provided door-to-door transportation. It was noted that the patient met the long-term goal established at the onset of his outpatient rehabilitation program.

◻ CONCLUSION

This chapter has reviewed the roles of therapeutic recreation and the therapeutic recreation specialist in the rehabilitation of patients with TBI. Through involvement in prescribed functional activities, active recreation, leisure education, and community integration, the therapeutic recreation specialist provides patients with TBI opportunities to improve physical ability, build confidence, improve cognitive functioning, strengthen communication and interpersonal skills, manage stress, cope with the injury, and strive toward achieving their full potential. The therapeutic recreation specialist recognizes the need that all individuals have to choose and pursue meaningful recreation involvement; filling time does not mean *healthy leisure lifestyle*. Scientific literature continues to identify leisure as an area of concern of postinjury. As hospital lengths of stay shorten, the role of the therapeutic recreation specialist in community-based settings should expand, with emphasis on full reintegration into the community. By incorporating phases of therapeutic recreation services throughout the continuum of rehabilitation, including community reentry, the identified problems related to leisure functioning can be minimized.

Further research is warranted to assess outcomes specific to therapeutic recreation intervention for patients with TBI. Therapeutic recreation assessment instruments designed for individuals who have experienced a TBI would assist the therapeutic recreation specialist with accuracy and validation in planning the treatment program. Reimbursement issues will also need to be addressed, especially with the trend toward managed care.

Psychological well-being and feelings of self-worth are dramatically influenced by the amount of satisfaction an individual receives from leisure and recreation activities.[24] Therapeutic recreation intervention improves feelings of well-being by providing the tools, adaptations, education, participation, and resources necessary for the individual with TBI to maintain a satisfying leisure lifestyle and contribute to society.

REFERENCES

1. Schalèn, W, et al: Psychosocial outcome 5–8 years after severe brain lesions and the impact of rehabilitation services. Brain Inj 8:49–64, 1994.
2. Oddy, M, Humphrey, M, and Uttley, D: Subjective impairment and social recovery after closed head injury. J Neurol Neurosurg Psychiatry 41:611, 1978.
3. Ponsford, JL, Olver, HH, and Curran, C: A profile of outcome: 2 years after traumatic brain injury. Brain Inj 9:1–10, 1995.
4. McClean, A, Dikmen, SS, and Temkin, NR: Psychosocial recovery after head injury. Arch Phys Med Rehabil 74:1041–1046, 1993.
5. Dikmen, S, Machamer, J, and Temkin, N: Psychosocial outcome in patients with moderate to severe head injury: 2 year follow-up. Brain Inj 7:113–114, 1993.
6. Perry, J: Rehabilitation of the neurologically disabled patient: Principles, practice and scientific basis. J Neurosurg 58:799–816, 1983.
7. Coyle, CP, et al: Benefits of Therapeutic Recreation: A Consensus View. Idyll-Arbor, Ravensdale, Wash, 1991.
8. Gunn, S, and Peterson, C: Therapeutic recreation program design: Principles and procedures. Prentice Hall, Englewood Cliffs, NJ, 1978.
9. American Therapeutic Recreation Association/National Therapeutic Recreation Society: Therapeutic recreation: Responding to the challenges of health care reform (joint statement). September 1994.
10. Berryman, D, James, A, and Trader, B: The benefits of therapeutic recreation in physical medicine. In Coyle, CP, Kinney, WB, and Shank, JW: Benefits of therapeutic recreation: A consensus view. Idyll-Arbor, Ravensdale, Wash, 1991.
11. Burton, LA, and Volpe, B: Social adjustment scale assessments in traumatic brain injury. Journal of Rehabilitation Oct–Dec, 1993, pp 34–37.
12. Brooks, DN: The head-injured family. J Clin Exp Neuropsychol 13:155–158, 1991.
13. Hall, KM, et al: Family stressors in traumatic brain injury: A two year follow-up. Arch Phys Med Rehabil 75:876–884, 1994.
14. Stumbo, N, and Bloom, C: The implications of traumatic brain injury for therapeutic recreation services in rehabilitation settings. Therapeutic Recreation Journal 3:64–79, 1990.
15. Berger, J, and Regalski, A: Therapeutic recreation. In Rosenthal, M, et al (eds): Rehabilitation of the Adult and Child with Traumatic Brain Injury, ed 2, FA Davis, Philadelphia, 1990.
16. Paulson, R: A comprehensive therapeutic recreation service in rehabilitation. In Maynard, M, and Chadderon, L (eds): Leisure and Lifestyle. MS University Center for International Rehabilitation, 1984.
17. Teaff, J, and VanHyning, T: Third-party reimbursement of therapeutic recreation services within a national sample of United States hospital. Therapeutic Recreation Journal 22:31–37, 1988.
18. Evans, B, and Lauria, B: Day treatment programs: Maximizing the independence of brain injured persons who have returned to the community. Cognitive Rehabilitation January/February:20–24, 1988.
19. Fazio, S, and Fralish, K: A survey of leisure and recreation programs offered by agencies serving traumatic head injured adults. Therapeutic Recreation Journal 22:46–54, 1988.
20. Zoerink, D, and Lauener, K: Effects of a leisure education program on adults with traumatic brain injury. Therapeutic Recreation Journal 3:19–28, 1991.
21. Fines, L, and Nichols, D: An evaluation of twelve week recreational kayak program: Effects on self-concept, leisure satisfaction and leisure attitude of adults with traumatic brain injuries. Journal of Cognitive Rehabilitation, September/October:10–15, 1994.
22. Baker-Roth, S, et al: The impact of therapeutic recreation community liaison on successful re-integration of individuals with traumatic brain injury. Therapeutic Recreation Journal, 4:316–323, 1995.
23. Bullock, C, and Howe, C: A model therapeutic recreation program for the reintegration of persons with disabilities into the community. Therapeutic Recreation Journal, 1:7–17, 1991.
24. Riddick, C: Leisure satisfaction precursors. Journal of Leisure Research 18:256–259, 1986.

A p p e n d i x A— **Recreational Skill Evaluations**

Biking Assessment
Susan Popek-Boeve
DMC Rehab Center Novi
42005 W. 12 Mile
Novi, MI 48377-3113   (248) 305-7575

Bowling Assessment
Susan Popek-Boeve
DMC Rehab Center Novi
42005 W. 12 Mile
Novi, MI 48377-3113   (248) 305-7575

But Utilization Skills Assessment (BUS)
Burlingame and Peterson
Idyll-Arbor, Inc.
25119 S.E. 262 St.
Ravensdale, WA 98051-9763   (206) 432-3231

Cross Country Skiing Assessment
Peterson
Idyll-Arbor, Inc.
25119 S.E. 262 St.
Ravensdale, WA 98051-9763   (206) 432-3231

Leisure Questionnaire
Susan Popek-Boeve
DMC Rehab Center Novi

42005 W. 12 Mile
Novi, MI 48377-3113   (248) 305-7575

Roller Blading Assessment
Susan Popek-Boeve
DMC Rehab Center Novi
42005 W. 12 Mile
Novi, MI 48377-3113   (248) 305-7575

Roller Skating Assessment
Susan Popek-Boeve
DMC Rehab Center Novi
42005 W. 12 Mile
Novi, MI 48377-3113   (248) 305-7575

Swimming Assessment
Susan Popek-Boeve
DMC Rehab Center Novi
42005 W. 12 Mile
Novi, MI 48377-3113   (248) 305-7575

Therapeutic Recreation Discharge Session
Susan Popek-Boeve
DMC Rehab Center Novi
42005 W. 12 Mile
Novi, MI 48377-3113   (248) 305-7575

A p p e n d i x B— **Assessment Tool Publishers**

Idyll-Arbor, Inc.
25119 S.E. 262 Street
Ravensdale, WA 98051-9763   (206) 432-3231

Nancy Navar
132 Wittich Hall
University of Wisconsin–LaCrosse
LaCrosse, MI 54601   (608) 785-8207

Dept. of HPHP
Health Education Building
University of Toledo
2801 W. Bancroft
Toledo, OH 43606

Ptarmigan West
1061 Josh Wilson Road
Mt. Vernon, WA 98273-9619   (206) 428-9785

Leisure Dynamics
10106 Bear Paw Lane
Panama City, FL 32404   (904) 722-9270

Milwaukee Public Schools
Director of Municipal Recreation and Adult
   Education
P.O. Drawer 10-K
Milwaukee, WI 53201

Venture Publishing
1640 Oxford Circle
State College, PA 16803   (814) 234-4561

The Leisure Institute
R.D. #1, Hopson Road, Box 416
Dolgeville, NY 13329   (315) 429-9563

Appendix C— Suggested Resources for Therapeutic Recreation Treatment Programs

Life Management Skills I and II
(reproducible activity handouts)
Kork, Azok and Leutenberg
Wellness Reproductions, Inc.
23945 Mercantile Rd.
Beechwood, OH 44122-5924   (800) 669-9208

Therapeutic Fun for Head Injured Persons and
  Their Families
Group Activities for Head Injured Persons
  (Books I and II)
Community Skills Program
Counseling and Rehabilitation, Inc.
1616 Walnut #800
Philadelphia, PA 19103

Leisure Education: A Manual of Activities and
  Resources
N Stumbo and S Thompson (1986)

Venture Publishing, Inc.
1640 Oxford Circle
State College, PA 16803   (814) 234-4561

Sports and Recreation for the Disabled
M Paciorek and J Jones (1994)
Cooper Publishing Group, LLC
P.O. Box 562
Carmel, IN 46032

The Relaxation and Stress Program
Davis, Robbins-Eshelman, and McKay (1988)
Idyll-Arbor, Inc.
25119 S.E. 262 Street
Ravensdale, WA 98051-9763   (206) 432-3231

Learning to Survive (training packet)
Family Survival Project
1736 Divisadero Street
San Francisco, CA 94115

Case Management and Life Care Planning in Brain Injury Rehabilitation

JANE MATTSON, PHD, OTR

The sequelae of traumatic brain injury (TBI) include deficits in function in wide-ranging areas involving everyday skills that require differing degrees of mental alertness, information processing, planning, execution, and mental monitoring. Thus, TBI can affect so many areas and necessitate care by so many medical specialists that, at times, services overlap and care can become fragmented. Overlap of services can have serious financial repercussions; fragmentation of care can cause gaps in service, which leave injured individuals lost and languishing when they could be progressing. Case management and life care planning provide a cohesive structure for health care and rehabilitation service delivery following TBI. This structure allows any shortcomings in service delivery to be detected and corrected, thus assuring that the most effective treatments are available to—and accessed by—the brain injured individual at every level, from acute care to community reentry. During the past three decades, acute and postacute rehabilitation programs dedicated to the needs of people who have had TBI have increased in number. During that time, the discipline of case management emerged, followed shortly thereafter by life care planning. Since that time, these two disciplines have become inextricably linked in the rehabilitation and long-term support of individuals with acquired brain injury.

☐ DEFINITION OF CASE MANAGEMENT

The Case Management Society of America (CMSA), which is comprised of specialists in health care, law, education, administration, insurance, and management, defines *case management* as "a collaborative process which assesses, plans, implements, coordinates, monitors and evaluates options and services to meet an individual's health needs [and] to promote quality cost-effective outcomes."[1] This definition indicates the complexity of the case manager's responsibilities.

Above all, a case manager is an advocate for the individual who has sustained an injury. As such, the case manager must take into consideration the needs of the injured individual and the family, as well as the resources of the payer. As Smith[1] suggests, if we view the patient, the provider, and the payer as the points of a triangle, case managers would be properly placed right in the middle because they play a central role in facilitating the empowerment of the individual, as well as collaboration, communication, and problem solving between family and providers.

The philosophy of case management is that all individuals who suffer from catastrophic illness or injury should be afforded the services of a case manager. From the outset, the case manager facilitates communication so that the patient and the family are as knowledgeable as possible and so that the patient will ultimately go on to a brighter, more independent future. The following is an example of what can be accomplished with appropriate case management.

Case 1 ■ Tammy sustained a severe traumatic brain injury when she was 2 years old. Although she was making excellent progress, she was clearly going to have severe physical limitations, cognitive limitations, and, presumably, behavioral and social deficits. Just prior to her injury, she had learned to walk and climb. She was not adept at coloring or forming numbers. She had no ability to read. Her memory was only beginning to emerge. In a case such as this, it would be easy to leave Tammy in a classroom with children who had cerebral palsy and mental retardation. However, Tammy really required a customized education program to reach her potential.

Careful testing was completed with Tammy, and a program was developed within the school system. This required training the special education personnel, the teacher, and therapists to develop a sequential learning strategy for Tammy. She was given more occupational and physical therapy because she demonstrated the potential to learn. A private facilitator came into the school when Tammy was 3½ to further enhance her educational capability and to carry over her gains into the home setting.

By the time Tammy was 5½ and entering kindergarten, she had developed many social and behavioral skills, which allowed for significant mainstreaming. Cognitively, it was clear that she would function in the borderline range of intelligence, rather than in the severe range. Motorically, she was able to show dominance of one hand, and, with the use of a computer, she was able to achieve better communication.

During the next few years, Tammy developed even more skills and became a functional classroom ambulator. Although socially she was unable to maintain the level of her peers, she clearly was well above the children with whom she had started her education. Several new strategies were developed to help her adapt to her disability and to achieve higher goals. She was socially immature in some ways, but she worked well with animals, and therapists used small animals to help her develop social responsibility, which carried over into her home life.

The future is brighter for a child such as Tammy because of the careful coordination of the school district, school and private therapists, a facilitator, and funding from a private insurance company. Eventually, Tammy will use the system for assistance with achieving supported work or even gainful employment. Although she may never live on her own, Tammy will clearly be able to live in a supported living setting as a result of the carefully structured care plan that was developed and revised for her as time went on.

❑ OBJECTIVES

Case management functions to bring intentionality into the confusing medical culture. *Intentionality* is defined as "the centering and the setting of a focused purpose in every situation, with the purpose being the higher good and the most beneficial outcome for everyone involved."[2] A case manager who operates with the knowledge that, in brain injury, no two cases are ever the same can be very creative; each brain injured individual follows a unique path in terms of outcome and needs. Thus, in effect, each case requires the development of a unique paradigm. Within the framework of intentionality, case management has three main objectives. The first and foremost is to improve the person's functional capability and quality of life. For example, by means of ongoing evaluation, a knowledgeable case manager can recognize when a treatment is not working and effect a change. The second objective of case management is to ensure that available funding is spent wisely so that no one is paying for services that are not necessary or effective. The third objective is to educate the family about acquired brain injury and available services to foster independent decision making, which is necessary both for the short term and the long term. Often, a case manager is the only individual who remains consistently involved with the patient and the family over the course of treatment.

❑ WHO IS A CASE MANAGER?

Although, in the beginning, case management was practiced without clear rules and regulations, by the 1990s, case managers were required to maintain national certification and professional licensure. A case manager should have a baccalaureate degree from a program in health and human services. To be of service to the brain injured individual, the case manager should also have specific training in brain injury rehabilitation and a minimum of 24 months of experience in working with this population. As with all other professionals involved in traumatic brain injury rehabilitation, a case manager must pursue ongoing education, be able to conduct research and gather information to establish appropriate resources, and be able to critically analyze potential barriers to the patient's achievement of goals.[1]

In conjunction with this strong foundation and background, a case manager must possess a thorough knowledge of each patient's diagnosis, prognosis, and outcome goals and familiarity with available health and social services, as well as funding. The CMSA supports these standards; similar qualifications are recommended by the American Congress of Rehabilitation Medicine and its brain injury special interest group.

☐ CASE MANAGEMENT IN POSTACUTE PROGRAMS

Eventually, there is an end to formal rehabilitation services, and it is the case manager's role to bridge the gap.[3] A case manager can provide better preparation for discharge. In creating postacute treatment plans, many different services must be considered, including day programming, residential long-term care, and the use of group treatment versus individual treatment. For example, people who do not have stable family settings will not benefit from transitional living if they will always require formal supervision. A funder is more likely to provide creative reimbursement to maintain appropriate discharge into the community when there is case management.[4]

☐ FACILITATION FOR FAMILIES

The victims of severe brain injury are not a random cross-section of society; they tend to be economically active young adults. Consequently, with severe or even mild brain injury, families are faced with a very different person who may be tangibly altered by the physical disabilities, such as reduced mobility and speech difficulties, and emotionally and cognitively impaired with problems in executive function, mood, apathy, lack of inhibition, and poor judgment. An enormous family burden develops after brain injury. This burden is usually lifelong and affects the social functioning of the entire family.[5] Thus, the case manager must understand the psychological distress of the family. Some families are more vulnerable than others, and some are better able to cope

with the stresses. Some can provide care, and some cannot. Therefore, an individual analysis by a case manager can be critical in determining how lifelong needs will be met following brain injury. In the home or community setting, a case manger's role is to make certain that the shift takes place in the nuclear social system rather than in the individual, who is not capable of such adjustments.

In brain injury cases, family rights have to be examined along with the rights of the brain injured individual, and often a case manager acts both to separate these sometimes conflicting needs and to meld them by developing a life care plan that accomplishes the most favorable outcome for both the family and the individual. Once the injured individual's formal rehabilitation phase is concluded, the case manager's role is often extremely complicated because it often involves dealing not only with the needs of the individual but also with dysfunctional and disparate family members.

Although it is clear that, following even a mild brain injury, life may never be the same, a case manager can show the injured individual and the family what life has to offer. When appropriate steps are taken, a knowledgeable case manager can demonstrate that the words *no* and *never* do not belong in the lexicon because often what is considered impossible may simply take longer to achieve.

☐ THE GOALS OF CASE MANAGEMENT

Improved Outcomes

Following brain injury, deficits in function are likely in wide-ranging areas involving everyday skills that require differing degrees of mental alertness, information processing, planning, execution, and mental monitoring of daily actions. Diffuse brain injury disrupts the performance of real-life skills. Moreover, the inability of brain injured patients to integrate skills—that is, to select and use a group of skills collectively and sequentially to solve real-life problems—seems to be one of the most disabling consequences of TBI. The patient is unable to generate integrative actions that are appropriate to the context. Classical rehabilitation aims at physical restoration through functional skills retraining, with the expectation that the patient will use every restored skill as circumstances require. This approach assumes that the patient will integrate each restored skill within the context of the clusters of skills and routines needed for daily life. However, brain injury rehabilitation differs from this classic conception, and a rehabilitation program must focus not only on redeveloping individual skills but also on restoring the patient's ability to integrate these skills in problem-specific ways.

Case management can and should begin almost immediately following injury, during the period of acute care, if possible. It is always more difficult when a case manager becomes involved later because both time and money will have been irretrievably lost. It may also take time to break down preconceived biases that would not have been formed if the case manager had become involved earlier. Nonetheless, it is never too late to initiate case management. Even a case manager who becomes involved 6 months, a year, or several years following brain injury can still help shape outcome by providing a pathway for better function and greater life satisfaction.

Outcome has been extremely difficult to quantify in traumatic brain injury cases.[1] By doing a cost-benefit analysis that describes the disability, life-years gained, medical complications avoided, and marital disruptions avoided, the case manager can evaluate both the cost and the consequences of treatment. It can provide an estimate of the value of resources utilized in each program.

Because so many personnel are involved in any given traumatic brain injury case, it is important that the accountability for outcome and value rest with one professional, often the case manager.[6] A case manager who has the necessary training and experience to understand the short- and long-term financial, psychological, physical, social, and vocational consequences of brain injury can effect a number of outcomes. For example, as reported by Evans and Watke,[6] the impact of external case management on neurorehabilitation outcomes can be significant. A study was completed with 979 consecutive patients admitted to one neurorehabilitation program between 1989 and 1994. Of these, 137 were selected and provided with external case management. A single case manager was chosen to minimize differential case management practices. In both the control group and the study group, the primary funding was through traditional accident and health insurance, including workers' compensation. All of the patients in the study also had internal case management provided by the program. Outcomes were reported in three basic areas: (1) returning the injured person to the least restrictive environment (generally home), (2) assisting the person in achieving the highest level of function in terms of activities of daily living (ADLs), and (3) returning the person to a competitive workplace, school, or avocational setting.

Evans and Watke[6] reported that outcome superiority was demonstrated for externally case-managed patients. These patients were shown to improve and to maintain outcome during follow-up. Significant improvements in patient status were demonstrated across all outcome measures, especially in the return to work category. Referral practices were also favorably influenced by external case management; the externally case-managed patients in this study received postacute neurorehabilitation generally 5 months sooner than the strictly internally managed group.[7]

Cost Containment

Case management is often synonymous with cost management. A capable case manager understands public and private reimbursement issues, is aware of available providers, and correlates this information with the needs of the individual and the family to ensure that the best possible services are provided in the most appropriate settings, at reasonable costs. For example, in the 1980s and 1990s, marketers, whose primary motive was profit, would attempt to sway a family to use a particular rehabilitation center without regard for the family's or the injured individual's real needs. An independent professional case manager can counter such inappropriate recommendations.

Case management can affect the cost of care by improving communication and providing service delivery without waste. Often, transportation for the family, ordering of equipment, the redesigning of a home, and setting up of care can be implemented by one individual to save time and money. When treatment of a patient is diffused among many providers, as is often the case in brain injury rehabilitation, it is important to have a case manager who is responsible for controlling financial risk by arranging for the provision of the right treatment at the right time. By recommending against a suggested treatment or change of service, a case manager often is not negatively impacting outcome.

Case managers should have positive relationships with funding agencies. The case manager may be an employee or consultant of a particular funding source and should know the philosophy of the funder, understand policy language, and be able to influence the funder to live up to the contract as well as to spend extracontractually to expedite outcome. Case managers may educate funders about brain injury and its implications. The teaching process should be furthered through claims seminars and dissemination of teaching materials. In addition, the case manager must explain the value of case coordination in assuring the provision of appropriate, cost-effective services.

Comparisons between providers can be made available by requiring programs and providers to demonstrate outcome results. The case manager may demand effective goal setting and discharge planning prior to admission. When high-quality outcomes are not reached, the case manager should communicate displeasure to the provider and also recommend financial disincentives on the part of the funder in response to poor-quality of service delivery or failure to reach desired outcome in a timely manner.

Consumers generally develop trusting relationships with case managers. A case manager has a moral responsibility to perform well as a consumer advocate. Sometimes, effective teaching as well as careful listening must occur before trust develops. To create a positive link between funder and consumer, a case manager should demonstrate to the injured individual and family that spending large amounts of money does not ensure a positive outcome and that careful spending, which is often arrived at through creative case management, is more often tied to more beneficial solutions.

◻ COMPONENTS OF CASE MANAGEMENT

A case manager's interventions must be timely. In addition, because the effects of brain injury vary significantly, a case manager must be flexible to properly manage the care of each individual.[2] When a case manager coordinates the delivery of services, the entire care process is streamlined, outcome is maximized, and costs are kept appropriate. The following steps are basic to any case.

Evaluation

A case manager gathers all relevant data by reading available medical records and by speaking with family members and treatment providers.[8] A case manager then conducts a thorough, objective evaluation of the injured individual regarding the current status of (1) physical/medical needs, (2) psychosocial needs, (3) environmental needs, (4) financial needs, (5) vocational needs, (6) ability to provide self-care or need for a long-term care setting, (7) cognitive capability, and (8) potential for community reintegration.

Planning, Goal-Setting, and Facilitation

With the patient and the family, the case manager develops goals and a treatment plan that will enhance the patient's outcome and limit a payer's liability. The case manager must establish measurable goals to meet the individual's ability to utilize resources and to help the family plan a care process that will move the individual along a pathway toward stable health and adaptation. Contingency plans should be incorporated with each step to anticipate potential complications with service delivery or outcome.[1] The patient and the family will be the primary decision makers. Once a treatment plan has been developed, a case manager assists with its implementation by actively facilitating communication between all team members and the family. In this way, should the need arise, modifications in plans or goals can be made promptly.

Advocacy

The patient's and the family's unique needs and goals are always considered in the development of any treatment plan. When a thoughtfully prepared plan is implemented, the individual is supported and the family is empowered to become self-reliant. By advocating for early referral for any necessary treatment or services, the case manager ensures that progress remains steady. In addition, from the outset, by means of clear, thorough communication between the case manager and the family, family members are taught to act as advocates for the patient.

Reevaluation

As time goes on and the patient's status and needs change, the case manager makes timely reevaluations to see where the patient is in relation to the goals established in the planning stage. If progress is not being made, the case manager must define and advocate for any necessary adjustments.

Problem Solving

Case managers are in a unique position in that they not only discover and document problems but also come up with solutions; a case manager can bring a commonsense approach to an idea gone haywire. Once initial goals have been established, the case manager focuses on maintaining accountability regarding both maintenance of quality of care for the patient and the reporting of the efficacy of treatment to payers.[1] During all evaluations, a case manager looks for the following situations, which require correction:

- Overutilization of services
- Underutilization of services
- Overlapping services
- Premature discharge from an appropriate level of care
- Use of ineffective treatment
- Medical or psychological complications
- Lack of understanding of acquired brain injury on the part of patient and/or family
- Lack of family support
- Inadequate community reentry plan
- Lack of financial support
- Noncompliance with workable plan

□ LIFE CARE PLANNING

In keeping with the CMSA[1] definition of case management, *life care planning* can be defined as a road map or blueprint that directs the process aimed at meeting an individual's health needs and promoting high-quality, cost-effective outcomes. In developing a life care plan, a case manager creates a clear picture of the services, equipment, and financial resources that will be necessary to meet the brain injured individual's needs throughout his or her lifetime. Thus, a life care plan provides a case manager and the family with an outline of what is needed for the long term. Once a life care plan has been developed, a case manager assists the family with its implementation, which includes the procuring and financing of this care. In combination with the appropriate case management background and a carefully developed life care plan, a case manager can ensure that specialized assessment techniques are utilized when appropriate, that treatment approaches are carried out in optimum settings, and that the ethical and moral facts of every decision are considered.

History of Life Care Planning

In the early days of brain injury rehabilitation, lifelong living was not often part of the thought process. When long-term goals were not established at the outset, however, the care plan often did not contain a framework for the provision of all services necessary throughout the patient's lifetime. With a carefully developed life care plan, a case manager can empower an individual with a brain injury and the family to develop a lifelong living model, which goes well beyond rehabilitation. This approach does not necessarily reject the therapeutic model; rather, it incorporates therapeutic principles into it.[9–12]

Life care planners are traditionally case managers with backgrounds in nursing, occupational therapy, physical therapy, neuropsychology, or a medical speciality. Because the parameters of outcome are less defined in traumatic brain injury than in other disabilities, to develop a realistic life care plan, a life care planner must have an understanding of the etiology and the medical aspects of brain injury. Only then can a realistic, workable life care plan be developed, aimed at preventing medical complications.[3]

The idea of a life care plan as a case management tool was developed by Paul Deutsch and Fred Raffa in 1981.[13] In addition to being essential for effective case management, life care plans are used in litigation matters and in workers' compensation cases to set reserves and to control costs. This often results in unrealistic or inflated costs. However, every successful case manager knows that high costs are not synonymous with high-quality care and that each life care plan must be rationally developed to be unique and specific to the individual in question.

Because life care planning is often used for establishing appropriate reserves by anticipating costs of future medical and supportive care needs, growth trends must be considered. Because the growth of costs depends on the recent and long-term history of economic changes in each area, a life care planner should work with an economist. In addition, to fund future goals and services by investing today, the present value must be calculated. Once present value is determined, a figure can be established for the amount of money needed in today's dollars to provide a specific sum at a future date. There are numerous discount rates, which correspond to long-term Treasury rates. An economist should use the appropriate discount rate and calculate the present value for the costs over the duration of the life care plan.[14] Whether a life care plan is to be utilized by a risk management organization, an insurance company, or members of the individual's family, its content should be the same. A life care plan must be based on an impartial assessment of the individual's current condition and his or her current and long-term health care needs. These needs are separated into time periods, and quality of life issues are addressed at each life stage.

Although case management can and should begin almost immediately after an injury for the patient to achieve optimum, expeditious progress, a life care plan should be developed at a later time (usually within 2 years of injury), when realistic long-term goals can be established.[15]

The Elements of a Life Care Plan

The parts of a life care plan are interdependent; from the description of the injury to the determination of needs and the laying out of the financial strategy for meeting those needs, each segment depends on the accuracy and legitimacy of the others. Only when each section is as precise and objective as possible will the plan, in its entirety, be fully individualized and realistic, providing a comprehensive, unbiased picture of the client's current and future needs. In preparing a life care plan, a case manager typically analyzes and addresses the following areas.

CARE

Care includes nurses, facilitators, short- or long-term subacute and postacute programs, group homes, and supported living settings. Care may also include summer camps, residential schooling, and vocational retraining. The utilization of family members should be considered along with the needs of family members. It should also be considered that the individual's needs will change significantly with aging.

REHABILITATION

Rehabilitation may involve physical, occupational, speech, and recreational therapies in inpatient, outpatient, or home-based settings. Rehabilitation may include diagnostic testing and evaluations. It may also include the use of a psychologist or a neuropsychologist and interplay between therapists, teachers, and facilitators. It may include public and private education personnel and education engineering.

FUTURE MEDICAL CARE AND SURGICAL INTERVENTION

This category includes procedures and treatment that are anticipated or known to be required, as well as treatment of potential complications.

DURABLE EQUIPMENT

Durable equipment includes wheelchairs, computers, augmentative communications systems, and aids for independent living that are commonly used. Prosthetics and orthotics may also be included.

MEDICATIONS

For a brain injured individual, medication may be required for seizure prophylaxis, pain management, and treatment of infection. Medications may also be used to improve arousal and attention. Because a number of different medications may interfere with others, a sophisticated understanding of the medications is essential.

DISPOSABLE ITEMS

Disposable items may include diapers, catheters, bed pads, skin lotions, nasogastric tubes and supplies, and tracheostomy tubes and supplies.

TRANSPORTATION

The transportation category includes hand controls or a modified, wheelchair-accessible van, or it may be simply providing a transportation allowance for an individual who is unable to drive.

HOME MODIFICATION

If the brain injured individual requires a wheelchair, home modifications may be necessary, including the construction of a wheelchair-accessible bathroom with a roll-in shower, modification of kitchen counters and/or appliances to facilitate reaching, and installation of ramps at the entrances of the house.

COUNSELING

In brain injury, neuropsychological counseling is often recommended for work on adjustment and cognitive issues, as well as for support.

❑ DEVELOPING A LIFE CARE PLAN: THE PROCESS

The first step in the development of a life care plan (Fig. 33–1) is to thoroughly review all pertinent medical records, including discharge summaries and consultation reports. The second step is to interview the patient's family, preferably in the home setting, where an appreciation of the family dynamics can be obtained, along with a sense of the individual's premorbid health status, lifestyle, and interests. These elements are essential for any future planning and goal setting. In addition, during the inter-

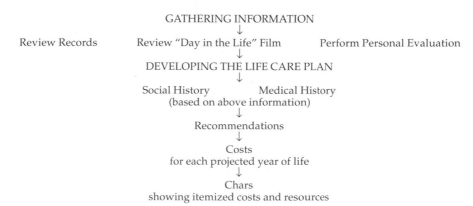

Figure 33–1. Steps in preparing a life care plan.

view in the home setting, the living space can be assessed for potential renovations. The third step is to identify long-term care issues by speaking with members of the treatment team.

Often, two care options are recommended for the same period. For example, a life care plan may provide for care in the home or community setting, as well as in a residential or institutional setting. The purpose of providing such alternatives is to enable the family to make educated decisions in their efforts to provide the best possible care for the brain injured individual.

☐ LIFE CARE PLANNING FOR CHILDREN: SPECIAL CONSIDERATIONS

Life care planning is especially challenging in pediatric cases because there is little information available as to how much improvement can be expected during the course of a child's development. Following brain injury, any individual may suddenly "take off" in terms of improvement, even several years after the injury. Alternatively, an individual can become more and more disabled and eventually handicapped by comorbidity problems or aging. Some individuals are simply not able to reach expected goals. Children with severe injuries may have moderate or even mild sequelae at outcome. Therefore, it is recommended that a full life care plan is not completed until at least 2 years after injury in pediatric cases. Even then, a life care plan should be completed in an algorithmic manner because outcome in adulthood may be much more positive (or negative).

Although with young adults, outcome is somewhat more predictable, it is still recommended that 18 months to 2 years elapse before the development of a life care plan. In addition, life care plans for children and young adults should have contingency plans for placement in a long-term residential setting when their parents are no longer able to cope because of their own aging.

☐ ETHICAL CONCERNS

Because of the impact of medical and technological advances in the care of persons after traumatic brain injury, survival has increased dramatically in the last 30 years. More than 600,000 traumatic brain injuries occur each year in the United States, with at least 50,000 cases requiring long-term, high-cost care. There has also been an escalation of litigation; some individuals have been awarded in excess of $10 million following traumatic brain injuries.[5] However, simply winning this kind of award does not ensure a favorable outcome.

The increasing prevalence of brain injured individuals in America is not only a sign of progress but also a symbol of personal tragedy. Although increased survival demonstrates the power of our medical delivery system to save and extend life, it also signifies personal devastation for more then 200,000 persons per year, most of whom are between 16 and 35 years old.[16] Survival at any cost creates substantial long-term care needs of indefinite duration. Often these individuals have severe injuries that can be devastating emotionally, cognitively, physically, and financially.

Once survival is assured, quality of life issues arise, including consideration of whether lifelong support should be used. In helping the family to make this determination, a case manager must be careful not to operate with a hedonistic view, which holds that human life is for the pursuit of pleasure. Thus, especially during the acute phase of treatment, decisions must be made on a case-by-case basis.

Perhaps the most difficult issue in bioethics is that of social justice in the allocation of resources. The sheer costs of providing for the needs that follow brain injury strain the boundaries that guide our thinking of what constitutes fair allocation of health and rehabilitation services. Although this problem is not unique to brain injury, proper allocation of resources is often much more difficult to define in a brain injury case. This difficulty is caused by the extraordinary resource needs of these individuals and the inability of many such individuals to express their own preferences and desires. There is never a single compelling solution in these cases. Each time such a situation arises, the case manager must choose the best possible solution from many potential plans.

☐ THE ECONOMIC RATIONALE FOR CASE MANAGEMENT

A case manager's negotiating, communication, and problem-solving skills are critically important in dealing with potential funders. In few other cases is the advocacy role so important. Because the case managers are independent of a brain injury program, they can represent the needs of both the injured individual and the funder. In this way, the case manager can often help to steer a course that a rehabilitation program cannot do from within.

As funding options narrow, case managers must see to it that precious resources are not wasted. In addition, a case manager can sometimes persuade a funder, a family, or a provider to go beyond the norm and come up with more creative solutions for financing long-term treatment of the brain injured individual.

It has been shown that, when case management expertise is introduced into the care of catastrophically injured patients, significant cost reductions can result.[17] As the pressure mounts to provide low-cost alternatives to rehabilitation hospitals, there has been a tremendous shift of treatment out of hospitals into postacute and subacute care.

With creative alternatives, spending less at strategic points can often enhance functional outcome. For example, by utilizing 3 part-time days for rehabilitation, thus stretching out total rehabilitation days, and by training caregivers to carry out rehabilitation strategies at home, individuals with TBI can begin to relearn skills in their own environment. Another example of reducing costs but maintaining quality would be a case manager's recognition that a particularly skilled but geographically distant therapist may make more of an impact than a local therapist. In this case, the individual would re-ceive therapy once or twice per month rather than weekly. This cost-effective solution organizes the best-quality care.

In the area of TBI, studies indicate that early intervention in the form of clinically expert rehabilitation facilitates a more rapid step-down to a lower-cost level of care.[18] Cope and Hall[20] demonstrated that early initiation of rehabilitation in a specialized acute brain injury program resulted in a 50 percent reduction in total acute and rehabilitation hospital days compared with a matched group of equally severely injured patients who were referred to the program after a delay. This finding has been replicated by Hall and Wright.[21] However, at times, a low-cost alternative may be truly inappropriate for a certain individual or in a particular situation.[19] A case manager must be alert to this possibility and, when the situation arises, advocate for what is appropriate. This can be seen in the following case history.

Case 2 ■ Three months after a mugging, Tommy was ready to be discharged from an acute rehabilitation setting, but he still had ongoing issues that required medical attention. He was not yet continent of bowel and bladder, but these skills were emerging. He had multiple fractures of both legs and his left upper extremity, which were healing but may have necessitated more surgery. Tommy was lacking in initiative as well as in judgment and safety awareness. He needed to be tied into a wheelchair because he would become forgetful and attempt to get up when no one was there to assist him.

Tommy's parents needed to work full-time to maintain their insurance and support their family. The home was located on a street where there was a significant amount of traffic. Rather than working toward returning Tommy to his home, the insurance company recommended placement in a nursing home that supposedly had a brain injury program. In truth, the nursing home had only part-time physical and occupational therapists and a physiatrist who came in twice per week. They did not have much experience with brain injury or community reentry. They were not well aware of all the other issues that would be important for Tommy over time. In addition, insurance was prepared to cover only 90 days of his stay in a nursing home; the insurance company assumed that Medicaid would then become the primary payer.

By utilizing a case manager, the hiring and training of a part-time facilitator was accomplished at two-thirds of the cost of the nursing home for the proposed 90 days. Tommy's parents were able to reintegrate him into his home setting. The case manager also helped the family to determine how the home could be made as barrier-free as possible.

Together, the case manager and the facilitator developed community resources so that Tommy was able to participate in day programming that was reimbursed by the Office of Vocational Rehabilitation. In addition, the family was able to develop a volunteer staff to work with Tommy when they could not be at home. With this approach, each day was properly structured for Tommy. At the end of 3 months, the insurance company accomplished its goal of cost containment. More important, Tommy was able to successfully reacclimate to the community, maintain the gains he had achieved in rehabilitation, and make further gains. The insurance company was willing to continue to pay for rehabilitation reevaluations and to allow an occupational therapist, a physical therapist, and a speech therapist to come into the home setting on a supervisory basis

Cost Effectiveness with Case Management

We live in a complex world, in which health care delivery has become a set of variables determined by the marketplace financiers. Managed care trends allow limited brain injury rehabilitation and support. A case manager can often help estimate reasonable capitation rates in managed care settings by facilitating agreement between the payer and the provider as to an appropriate length of stay and the best way of handling of possible complications. In this way, appropriate care is assured for the injured individual at the same time that cost containment is secured for the insurer. For example, a physician may believe that physical therapy in the hospital setting is imperative 5 days per week, but, in truth, a facilitator may be able to assist the individual in reaching the same goals in the home setting.

Today, because the costs of rehabilitation are high, to receive funding, a brain injury program must document its services and convince the payer of its contribution to a positive outcome. However, in the past two decades, services have been funded without verification of their effectiveness in brain injury rehabilitation.[19] The rehabilitation field has gone from an era when coma stimulation was considered ridiculous to an era when documentation of appropriate coma management and stimulation was used to provide a basis for obtaining funding for further treatment. Now, in a managed care environment, funding for coma stimulation is often denied. This circular scenario represents only the tip of the iceberg; in many other areas it is extremely difficult to prove that specific courses of action have led to desired outcomes. Without documented proof of efficacy, in a reimbursement environment that is governed by economic principles, many high-quality rehabilitation efforts are not considered cost-effective. Thus, quality of care is a double-edged sword. Often, a case manager can recognize when a program is not delivering care effectively, when the major difficulties in a case are not being resolved, or when the individual is not maximizing his or her outcome within the parameters of available resources. To do so, rehabilitation case managers must use more common sense and express themselves with greater focus and clarity than ever before.

It is essential that funders understand that services that are clearly appropriate for the injured individual will also be cost-effective in the long run. To that end, case managers are working to build a better understanding of brain injury and its sequelae by providing critical information to the insurance industry and the government on an ongoing basis.

Case Management in a Managed Care Environment

In managed care programs, as in other areas, case managers can make a true difference. The case manager is often in a unique position to challenge funders to providing the dollars that will enable a person to continue to receive appropriate services over the long term. Health maintenance organizations (HMOs) find that case management is beneficial to them.[8] Case managers provide utilization review, preadmission screening, concurrent review, discharge planning, and postdischarge services for patients whose care is funded through an HMO. Case managers are, in effect, good gatekeepers who facilitate efficient admissions into rehabilitation settings. HMO case managers often must communicate and negotiate early in the course of a patient's rehabilitation to obtain an appropriate amount of care. In working with an HMO, a case manager must be able to document the fact that creative blending of nontraditional services may result in a lower cost overall and measurably better health status.

Managed care programs are being incorporated more and more into Medicaid Model Waiver programs and into workers' compensation plans. At larger HMOs, there is often one department for ordering durable medical equipment and another for medications. All rehabilitation services are generally under contract with specific providers, and even home nursing care is often contracted out.

◻ TIMING FOR CASE MANAGEMENT

In the best-case scenario, a case manager becomes involved with an individual and the family directly after the injury. More often, a case manager becomes involved months or even years later, and much reeducation and counseling must be done. Ideally, only one case manager would be involved over the years on a diminishing basis. With brain injury, a minimum of several years of case management is recommended. However, this is often impossible because such factors as relocation of the injured individual or restriction of funding. Therefore, from the outset, the case manager will teach the family members to advocate for the injured individual. It is most important that the case manager avoid discontinuity and that information flow so that goals can be set and decision making can be achieved expeditiously. In this way, program performance will live up to expectations. To this end, case managers should not undertake a brain injury case if they will soon be leaving or for some other reason cannot devote at least 3 months (the permissible length of involvement of many managed care plans). If possible, the case manager should know the probable length of involvement so that expectations are known at the outset.

◻ THE FUTURE

Into the next millennium, the number of available brain injury programs will probably decrease as funding diminishes. Nevertheless, rehabilitation professionals must continue to effect functional adaptation and reintegration of skills in the brain injured population. To this end, funders need to understand that the standard allowance for exclusively facility-based physical, occupational, and speech therapies may not apply and that the use of facilitators in lieu of nursing services can be more beneficial for desired outcome. In addition, recent studies have shown not only that privately hired facilitators are more cost-effective than agency-based nurses but also that patients report greater life satisfaction and return of function when they, with the aid of their therapists, train their own caregivers. Increasingly, a case manager's role will be to introduce to the funder the concept of going "extracontractual"—that is, going outside a policy's language and constraints to obtain home-based modalities in lieu of traditional services such as registered nursing care or inpatient therapies.

At this time, case managers are being integrated into all forms of reimbursement in an effort to maximize outcome. In brain injury cases, where needs are lifelong, case management has been and will remain a strong component of the rehabilitation process. As a growing number of brain injured individuals are being supported by Medicaid, more and more states are using case managers to ensure continuity of care and cost containment. Thus, the case manager's role has a firm place in both the private and public sectors in a cooperative effort to provide appropriate long-term care and/or timely community reintegration for the brain injured individual. A case manager can add the cohesion that it takes to ensure that high-quality rehabilitation planning, fair spending, and excellent service delivery occur and that the brain injured individual achieves the maximum possible autonomy.

REFERENCES

1. Smith, DS: Standards of practice for case management: The importance of practice standards. The Journal of Case Management 1:6, 1995.
2. Killette, B: Intentionality: Case management revisioned. The Case Manager 5:51, 1994.
3. Jacobs, H, Blatnick, GS, and Sandhorst, J: What is lifelong living and how does it relate to quality of life? J Head Trauma Rehabil 5(1):1, 1990.
4. Mullahey, C: The case manager *is* the catalytic collaborator in managed care. The Journal of Case Management 1:7, 1995.
5. Livingston, M, and Brooks, D: The burden of families: A review. J Head Trauma Rehabil 3(4):6, 1988.
6. Evans, RW, and Watke, M: Catastrophic neurologic injury: Improving outcomes through case management. The Case Manger 6:83, 1995.
7. Frey, WR: Quality management: Protecting and enhancing quality in brain injury rehabilitation. J Head Trauma Rehabil 7(4):1, 1992.
8. Gerson, V: HMO case management. The Case Manager 6:79, 1995.
9. Jacobs, H: Los Angeles head injury survey procedures and preliminary findings. Arch Phys Med Rehabil 69:425, 1988.
10. Condelulci, A, Gretz, M, and Lasky, S: The societal role of valorization. J Head Trauma Rehabil 72(1):49, 1987.
11. DeJong, G, and Batavia, AI: Societal duty and resource allocation for persons with severe traumatic brain injury. J Head Trauma Rehabil 4(1):1, 1989.
12. Lehr, E: Community integration after traumatic brain injury: Infants and children. In Bacy-y-Rita, P (ed): Comprehensive Neurologic Brain Rehabilitation, vol 2. Demos, New York, 1989, p 223.
13. Weed, R, and Riddick, S: Life care plans as a case management tool. The Case Manager 3:36, 1992.
14. Deutsch P, et al: Life Care Plans for the Head Injured: A Step-by-Step Guide. P M Deutsch Press, Orlando, Fla, 1989.
15. Papastrat, L: Outcome and value following brain injury: A financial provider's perspective. J Head Trauma Rehabil 7(4):11, 1992.
16. DeJong, G, Batavia, A, and Williams J: Who is responsible for the lifelong well-being of a person with a head injury? J Head Trauma Rehabil 5(1):9, 1990.
17. Ashley, M, Persel, C, and Krych, D: Changes in reimbursement climate: Relationship among outcome, costs

and payor type in the postacute rehabilitation environment. J Head Trauma Rehabil 8(4):30, 1993.

18. Cope, DN, and O'Lear, J: A clinical and economic perspective on head injury rehabilitation. J Head Trauma Rehabil 8(4):1, 1993.

19. Frederickson, M, and Cannon, N: The role of the rehabilitation physician in the postacute continuum. Arch Phys Med Rehabil 76:5, 1995.

20. Cope, DN, and Hall, KM: Head injury rehabilitation: benefit of early intervention. APMR 63:433, 1982.

21. Hall, KM, and Wright, J: The benefit of early intervention in traumatic brain injury rehabilitation: a replication study. Unpublished manuscript, 1994.

(A page number followed by an "F" indicates a figure; a page number followed by a "T" indicates a table.)

ISBN 0-8036-0391-6